Neuroscience for Clinicians

EDUARDO E. BENARROCH

Professor of Neurology, Department of Neurology, Mayo Clinic, Rochester, MN, USA

Neuroscience for Clinicians

Basic Processes, Circuits, Disease Mechanisms, and Therapeutic Implications

OXFORD
UNIVERSITY PRESS

OXFORD
UNIVERSITY PRESS

Oxford University Press is a department of the University of Oxford. It furthers the University's objective of excellence in research, scholarship, and education by publishing worldwide. Oxford is a registered trade mark of Oxford University Press in the UK and certain other countries.

Published in the United States of America by Oxford University Press
198 Madison Avenue, New York, NY 10016, United States of America.

Library of Congress Cataloging-in-Publication Data
Names: Benarroch, Eduardo E., author.
Title: Neuroscience for clinicians : basic processes, circuits, disease mechanisms, and therapeutic implications / Benarroch, Eduardo E.
Description: New York, NY : Oxford University Press, 2021. |
Includes bibliographical references and index.
Identifiers: LCCN 2020036519 (print) | LCCN 2020036520 (ebook) |
ISBN 9780190948894 (hardback) | ISBN 9780190948917 (epub) |
ISBN 9780190948924 (online)
Subjects: MESH: Nervous System Physiological Phenomena | Nervous System Diseases—physiopathology | Nervous System Diseases—metabolism |
Molecular Structure | Cell Physiological Phenomena
Classification: LCC RC346 (print) | LCC RC346 (ebook) | NLM WL 102 |
DDC 616.8—dc23
LC record available at https://lccn.loc.gov/2020036519

DOI: 10.1093/med/9780190948894.001.0001

1 3 5 7 9 8 6 4 2

Printed by Sheridan Books, Inc., United States of America

CONTENTS

PREFACE

Over the past few years, and at an accelerating pace, several technological advances have provided new approaches to our understanding of the organization, function, and mechanisms of disease affecting the human nervous system. Examples include genomics, transcriptomics, epigenomics, proteomics (and other "omics"), the ability to record activity from neuronal ensembles in-vivo, brain mapping, and machine learning (colloquially "artificial intelligence"). Preceding, and now in parallel with these developments, elegant techniques both in-vitro and in experimental animals, primarily rodents and in some cases primates (replacing the cats used in classical experiments), have yielded an enormous amount of data and provocative insights into the function and dysfunction of the nervous system. These approaches range from optogenetics, calcium imaging, and multielectrode recordings to transgenic mouse models of disease. All these advances now allow in many cases to localize a "lesion" responsible for the manifestation of neurologic disease not only at one particular structure but also at a particular domain of a protein, an intracellular process, or at large-scale brain networks. Accordingly, the classification of neurological disorders have extended to introduce categories such as "tauopathies," "synucleinopathies" "channelopathies," "synaptopathies," and others.

Yet, the primary roles of the clinical neurologists have remained essentially unchanged: recognizing the manifestations of neurologic disease, trying to determine their pathological and (hopefully) pathophysiological substrate, deciding how to rationally and integrally treat patients, and conveying this information and experience to trainees. Whereas the foundations provided by the "fathers" of neuroscience and clinical neurology, from Sherrington and Cajal to Charcot, Broca, and Babinski, are still fundamental to the successful accomplishment of these tasks, clinicians now face new challenges and opportunities. One such challenge is to incorporate the tremendous amount of new information and insight provided by the major technological advances over the past two decades into the care of patients. The opportunities include the ability, from the bedside, to provide observations and ask fundamental questions about disease mechanisms and new rational therapies, to be addressed at the bench in research laboratories. Over the years, the increased specialization required to master individual approaches to neurologic disease have led to the formation of "tribes" of clinicians or researches, each with their individual dialects sometimes hardly understandable between groups. This has the potential risk of widening rather than closing the gap for translation. However, notable exceptions such as development of antisense oligonucleotides to treat spinal muscular atrophy and amyloidosis indicate that need not be the case. These and other examples emphasize the need for the clinician to understand some of the molecular and cellular processes underlying neural function, dysfunction, and interactions at synaptic, circuit, and system levels that underlie both normal behavior, from motor to social, and the manifestations of neurologic disease.

The main aim of this book is to help, from one clinician to another, to navigate this journey. The first section includes separate chapters reviewing basic cellular processes such as organization of cell membranes, mechanisms of signaling, DNA and RNA metabolism, proteostasis, vesicular trafficking, cytoskeletal organization, axonal transport, functions of axon and myelin, mitochondrial metabolism, and mechanisms of neural injury and repair. The second section includes chapters focused on mechanisms of communication and cells interactions, including function of ion channels, synaptic transmission, organization of the different neurotransmitter systems. The third section includes chapters on interactions among neurons, astrocytes, microglia, and their microenvironment. The fourth section includes chapters focused on the organization and interactions of circuits in the cortex, thalamus, brainstem, and spinal cord underlying the different behavioral states, sensory processing and motor control. The fifth section includes chapters on systems critical for survival including pain, autonomic, and hypothalamic functions. The last section includes chapters on cognitive neuroscience, including emotion, social behavior, memory, language, and executive functions.

Whereas the emphasis of this book is on concepts from basic neuroscience and mechanisms of neurologic disease in all chapters I provide brief clinical correlations, without entering into details that are best covered in available excellent clinical neurology books. There are also excellent books in basic neuroscience, many of them now classics. The aim of this book is not to provide a deep and authoritative discussion on basic neuroscience topics bur rather to attempt to bridge the gap from basic to clinical neuroscience from a clinician's standpoint.

I would like to acknowledge several of my colleagues in the Department of Neurology at the Mayo Clinic, Rochester MN, who provided me with invaluable feedback about the chapters of this book. J. Eric Ahlskog, M.D., Ph.D.; Farwa Ali, M.B.B.S.; Bradley W. Boeve, Hugo Botha, M.B., Ch.B.; Jeffrey W Britton, M.D.; Anhar Hassan, M.B., B.Ch.; Charles L. Howe., Ph.D.; David E. Jones, M.D., Ph.D., Keith A. Josephs, M.D.; Christopher J. Klein, M.D.; David S. Knopman, M.D.; Marc C. Patterson, M.D.; Margherita Milone, M.D., Ph.D.; Andrew McKeon, M.B., B.Ch., M.D.; Shirlene Sampson, M.D., M.S.; Paola Sandroni, M.D., Ph.D.; Gregory A. Worrell, M.D., Ph.D. are all experts that have made important contributions in their respective fields. I have incorporated many of their valuable comments, which have greatly improved the quality of the chapters of this book. I also thank Ms. Dhanalakshmi Narayanan and Ms. Jordan McAndrew from Oxford University Press for their editorial assistance.

Section I

Molecular and Cellular Mechanisms

1 Overview: Cellular Components of the Nervous System and Disease Mechanisms

OVERVIEW

Both normal and abnormal functions of the nervous system reflect the activity of networks organized at multiple hierarchical levels.[1] Their scale ranges from cell-specific gene and protein expression and intracellular processes (nanoscale and microscale) to synaptic interactions and microcircuit ensembles (mesoscale), to large circuits involving interactions among several brain areas (macroscale) (Figure 1.1). At each hierarchical level, networks can be decomposed into distinct units or "modules."[2] Neurons are primarily responsible for initiation, processing, and transmission of information, and their function is affected by their reciprocal interactions with glial cells and their environment (Figure 1.2). The aims of this introductory chapter are to briefly review (1) some of the current methods used to study the genetic and molecular signature of neural cells and assess the function of single neurons and neuronal ensembles; (2) the functions of neurons, glial cells, and their microenvironment; (3) the approaches to brain mapping; and (4) the basic molecular and cellular processes that provide disease pathways for neurologic disorders.

EXPERIMENTAL APPROACHES TO STUDY THE NERVOUS SYSTEM

Over the past few decades, a large number of new tools and techniques have been generated for neuroscience research, including but not limited to brain gene expression atlases, genetically encoded proteins to monitor and manipulate neuronal activity, and methods for imaging and mapping brain circuits.[3]

Genetic and Molecular Profiling

Genome-wide molecular profiling assesses the genome, epigenome, transcriptome, and proteome of single cells.[4–6] The transcriptomes of brain regions are organized into modules of coexpressed genes that reflect the cellular composition of the tissue.[7,8] High-throughput methods have been used to analyze morphological and biochemical signatures of different types of neurons and glial cells.[9] High-throughput DNA sequencing and bioinformatics approaches, such as next-generation sequencing have allowed for development of phenotype-specific gene panels to study neurologic disorders.[10] Single-cell RNA sequencing (RNA-seq) and cTag-crosslinking and immunoprecipitation (CLIP), together with candidate single-gene studies, have provided insight into mechanisms of normal mRNA metabolism and disease-associated perturbation of mRNA homeostasis. High-resolution proteomics analysis using multiepitope affinity purifications and mass spectroscopy has unraveled the architecture and molecular diversity of proteins such as voltage-gated ion channels and neurotransmitter receptors.[11] Metabolomics is the study of small molecule intermediates and products of metabolism and provides an instantaneous snapshot of the physiology of a cell.

Characterization of Cell Types

Several methods have allowed for single-cell classification using a combination of morphological, physiological, and molecular criteria. These include dye-filling of neurons characterized by their electrophysiology; patch-clamp recordings followed by extraction of the cellular content

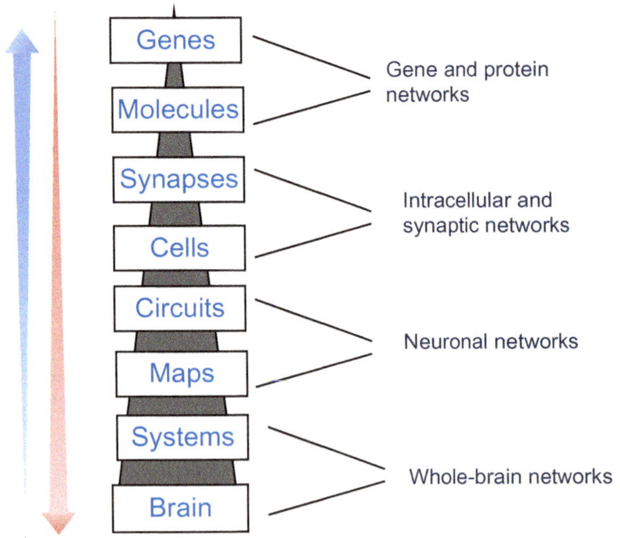

FIGURE 1.1 Hierarchical organization of neural networks. The nervous system is organized into different hierarchical levels each consisting of interconnected networks. The genetic level includes epigenetic control of DNA transcription and mechanisms of DNA repair. The molecular level includes mRNA metabolism and proteostasis. The cellular and synaptic levels include mechanisms of intracellular signaling and synaptic transmission and plasticity. Neurons are organized into networks and circuits that provide the basis functional maps that form the basis for motor, sensory, autonomic, emotional, and cognitive systems. These systems become integrated in large-scale networks to control behavior.

for single-cell RNA sequencing; and imaging neurons by light or electron microscopy following calcium imaging, among others.[9] Multiplexed fluorescence in situ hybridization (FISH) and in situ sequencing methods can be applied to brain sections to examine cell distribution patterns in specific areas, such as the hippocampus.[12] These studies show that no neuronal or glial cell type is homogeneous. The properties of these cells change during development, maturation, and environmental signals, reflecting both genetic or epigenetic mechanisms and responses to synaptic activity, neurotransmitters, hormones, and circadian influences.

Optogenetics and Chemogenetics

Optogenetics involves the genetic manipulation of selected cell types to express and activate light-gated ion channels or light-driven ion pumps to allow for optical control of cell activity.[13–15] This procedure requires the use of viral vectors to deliver the optogenetic construct and the insertion of a light probe. For example, channelorhodopsin 2 is a nonselective cation channel that is directly activated by blue light when bound by chromophores and allows the passage of cations into the cell, eliciting cell excitation. In contrast, the green-light-driven outward proton pump archaerhodopsin-3 mediates light-driven cell hyperpolarization and inhibition. Optogenetics has been extensively utilized as a tool to study neuron–neuron, neuron–glia, and glia–glia interactions with a high spatial and temporal resolution, both in vitro and in vivo. Chemogenetic technology involves the use of designer receptors exclusively activated by designer drugs (DREADDs).[16] These receptors are engineered receptors that can be activated by inert drug-like molecules that provide remote control of cellular signaling and thus neuronal activity.[17] DREADDs are typically expressed via virally mediated gene transduction in association with promoters that allow their selective expression in specific subtypes of neurons or glial cells or transgenic approaches.

Multiple Electrode Arrays and Optical Imaging

Multiple-electrode neurophysiology involves the implantation of up to 100 or more electrodes to study the activity of many neurons simultaneously, often in different brain regions. This tool maintains the spatial and temporal precision of single neuronal recordings and allows examining neurons in the global context of functioning of other neurons.[18] This approach has led to the identification of synchronized oscillatory activity in neuronal populations. Optical imaging allows simultaneous recording of activity from hundreds of neurons and/or glial cells in vivo at a single cell level using molecular indicators of voltage[19] or intracellular calcium levels.[20] For example, multi-photon calcium imaging in vivo allows collection of information from thousands of neurons simultaneously.[21,22]

CELLS OF THE NERVOUS SYSTEM AND THEIR FUNCTION

The normal function of the nervous system depends on reciprocal interactions among nervous, glial cells, blood vessels, and extracellular matrix (ECM) (Figure 1.2). Neurons and glial cells are the primary components of the central nervous system (CNS). There are an estimated 10^{11} neurons in the human brain; the glia:neuron ratio is in general ≤ 1:1.[23] In the neocortex, oligodendrocytes represent 45%–75% of glial cells; astrocytes 10%–49%; and microglia 10%;[24,25] NG2 glia (oligodendrocyte precursors) represent 5%–10% of glial cells in the human brain.[25] However, the ratio varies in different parts of the brain and with age and gender. The peripheral nervous system (PNS) consists of neurons, Schwann cells, and glial cells distributed in peripheral or enteric ganglia.

Neurons

Neurons are the electrically excitable cells in the nervous system; they can generate action potentials and process

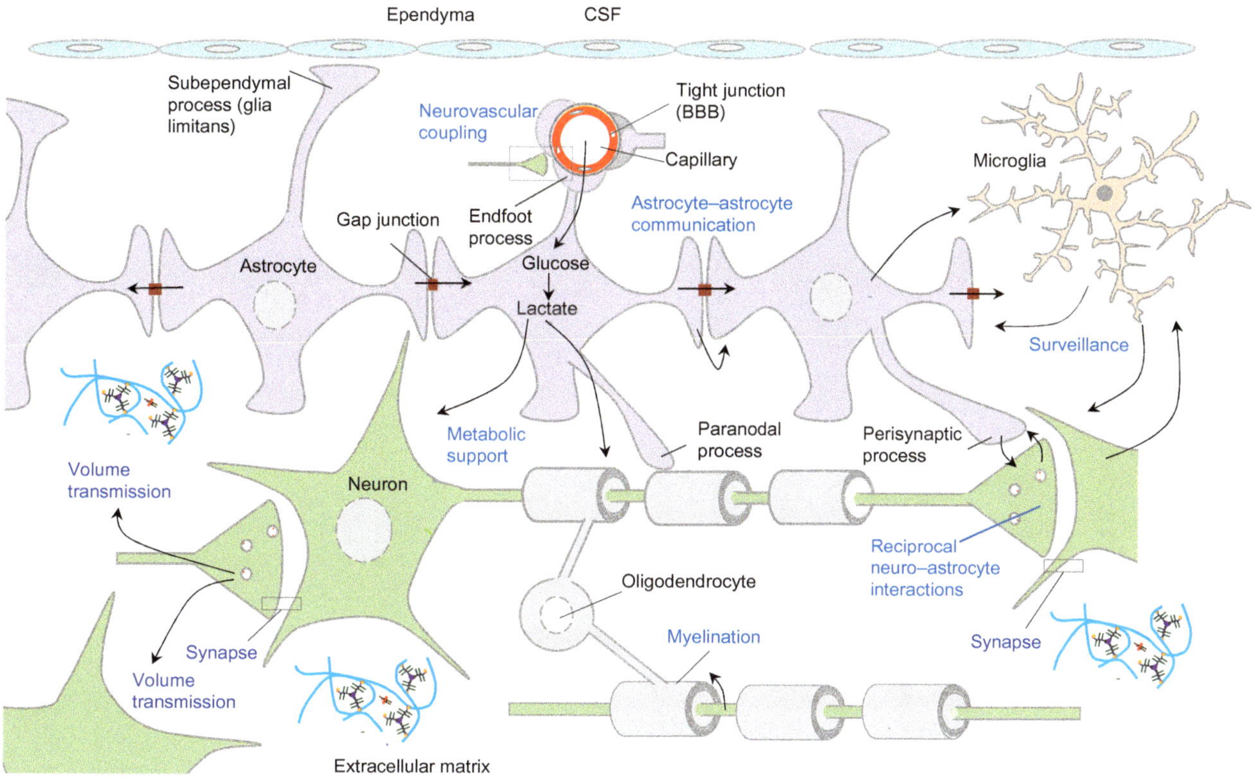

FIGURE 1.2 Components of the nervous system.

The nervous system consists of neurons, glial cells, blood vessels, and extracellular matrix that interact with each other. Neurons are connected primarily via chemical synapses but can also release neurotransmitters to the extracellular space to affect other cellular elements. Astrocytes are interconnected via gap junctions and paracrine mechanisms and contain perisynaptic processes that participate in reciprocal neuron–glia interactions and endfeet that cover the surface of cerebral blood vessels and are a critical component of the neurovascular unit, including the blood-brain barrier (BBB). Astrocytes have a major role in neurovascular coupling and metabolic support of active neurons and oligodendrocytes, in part via supply of lactate. Astrocytes also extend processes (glia limitans) that contact the ependyma in the wall of the ventricles containing the cerebrospinal fluid (CSF). Mature oligodendrocytes are responsible for formation and maintenance of myelin in the CNS. Microglial cells have a surveillance function and maintain cellular, synaptic, and myelin homeostasis.

and transmit information. They include many different subtypes that can be classified on the bases of their soma size, dendritic and axonal shapes and branching, resting membrane potential, firing patterns, and protein expression.[9] Neurons are extremely complex cells. Each neuronal compartment contains different functional domains with a unique distribution of membrane in channels, receptors, adhesion molecules, scaffold proteins, cytoskeletal proteins, and organelles. The typical example is that of pyramidal cells in the cerebral cortex (Figure 1.3). Typically, the dendrites and soma receive synaptic inputs. In many neurons, such as pyramidal cells of the cerebral cortex and Purkinje cells dendrites harbor dendritic spines that receive excitatory synapses, contain clustered receptors in postsynaptic densities, and provide the substrate for activity-dependent synaptic plasticity. The axons consist of the axon initial segment (AIS), which is the site of generation of the action potential, conductive axon, and presynaptic terminal. Myelinated axons consist of nodes of Ranvier, paranodes, juxtaparanodes, and internodes. The presynaptic terminal contains the synaptic vesicles clustered in presynaptic active zones via scaffold proteins, and proteins involved in calcium-triggered exocytosis.

Each cell compartment is the site of fundamental cellular processes that are of particular relevance in neurons given their phenotypic heterogeneity, presence of long axons, electrical and synaptic activity resulting in high metabolic demands, and need for both rapid and long-term responses to environmental signals (Figure 1.4). They include epigenetic control of mRNA transcription, mRNA metabolism, protein quality control in the endoplasmic reticulum (ER), and degradation by the ubiquitin/proteasome system and

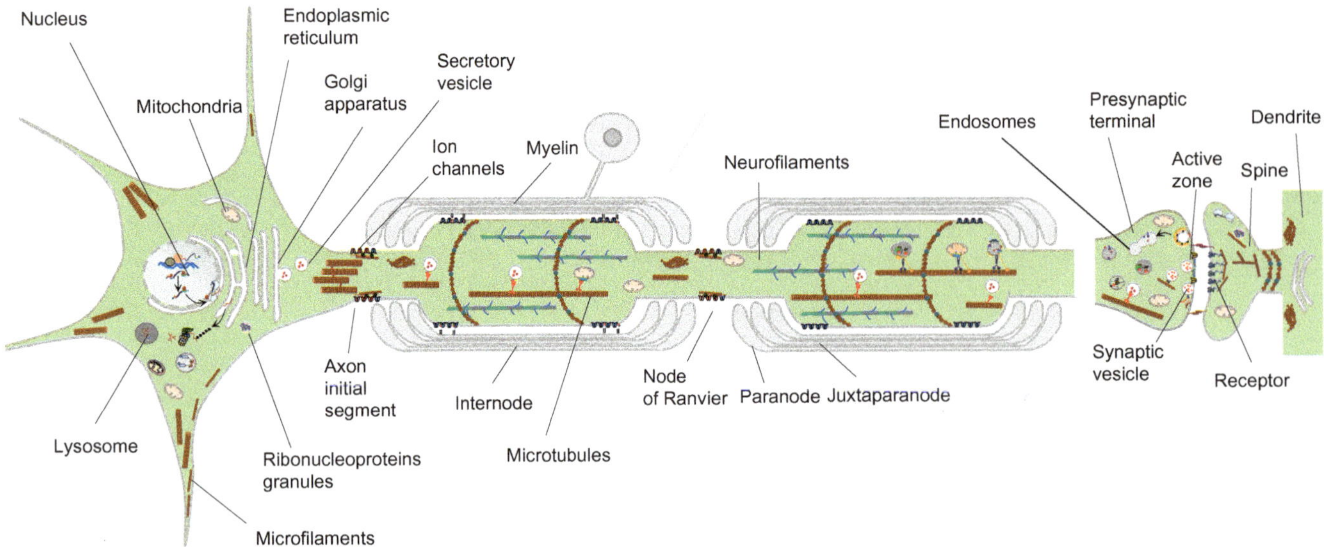

FIGURE 1.3 Functional compartments of neurons.
Neurons are extremely complex cells that consist of a cell body or soma, dendrites, and one axon. Each neuronal compartment contains a unique distribution of membrane in channels, receptors, adhesion molecules, scaffold proteins, cytoskeletal proteins, and organelles. Typically, the dendrites and soma receive synaptic inputs. In many neurons dendrites contain dendritic spines. The cell body contains the nucleus and the initial components of the secretory system, including the endoplasmic reticulum, Golgi apparatus, and secretory vesicles. The cell body contains most of the neuronal lysosomes that degrade material provided by endosomes and autophagic vesicles. The axons consist of the axon initial segment and a conduction portion that in myelinated axons includes the nodes of Ranvier, paranode, juxtaparanode, and internode. The presynaptic terminal contains the synaptic vesicles clustered in presynaptic active zones via scaffold proteins, and proteins involved in calcium-triggered exocytosis. The cytoskeleton, including actin microfilaments, microtubules, and neurofilaments, has a unique organization in different portions of the neurons.

the autophagy/lysosomal systems. The neuronal cytoskeleton includes actin microfilaments, microtubules, and neurofilaments. Vesicular trafficking in neurons includes exocytosis of synaptic vesicles, followed by endocytosis and formation and maturation of endosomes, which allow recycling of membrane components of their degradation via the lysosomes. Both the secretory and the endocytic pathways depend on normal axonal transport that involves motor proteins and is fueled by ATP. Neurons are highly dependent on mitochondrial metabolism for production of ATP, which is critical for maintenance of ion gradients, axonal transport, synaptic function, and protein quality control.

Astrocytes

Astrocytes are crucial for development, homeostasis, communication, and response to injury in the CNS. Their functions include structural and growth factor support during development and repair; formation and maintenance of the blood-brain barrier (BBB); activity-dependent regulation of local cerebral blood flow (CBF) and neuronal metabolism; maintenance of ion and water homeostasis in cells, myelin, and extracellular fluid; regulation of neurotransmitter levels at synapses; coordination of activity of neuronal networks; antioxidant protection; response to injury; and repair in the CNS[26,27] (Figure 1.5). Astrocytes are morphologically and functionally heterogeneous, consist of different functional compartments and are interconnected via gap junctions. Their perisynaptic processes participate in reciprocal interactions with presynaptic and postsynaptic terminals; their endfeet cover the surface of cerebral blood vessels and are a critical component of the neurovascular unit, participating in activity-dependent neurovascular coupling, metabolic support, and neurotransmitter and ion homeostasis at synapses. Astrocytes coordinate neuronal network activity via signal propagation throughout the astrocytic network. They also provide metabolic support and antioxidant protection to active neurons and oligodendrocytes.

Oligodendrocytes

Mature oligodendrocytes are responsible for formation and maintenance of myelin in the CNS (Figure 1.5). Oligodendrocyte precursor cells originate during development but are also present throughout the adult CNS and undergo activation, recruitment, and maturation required for

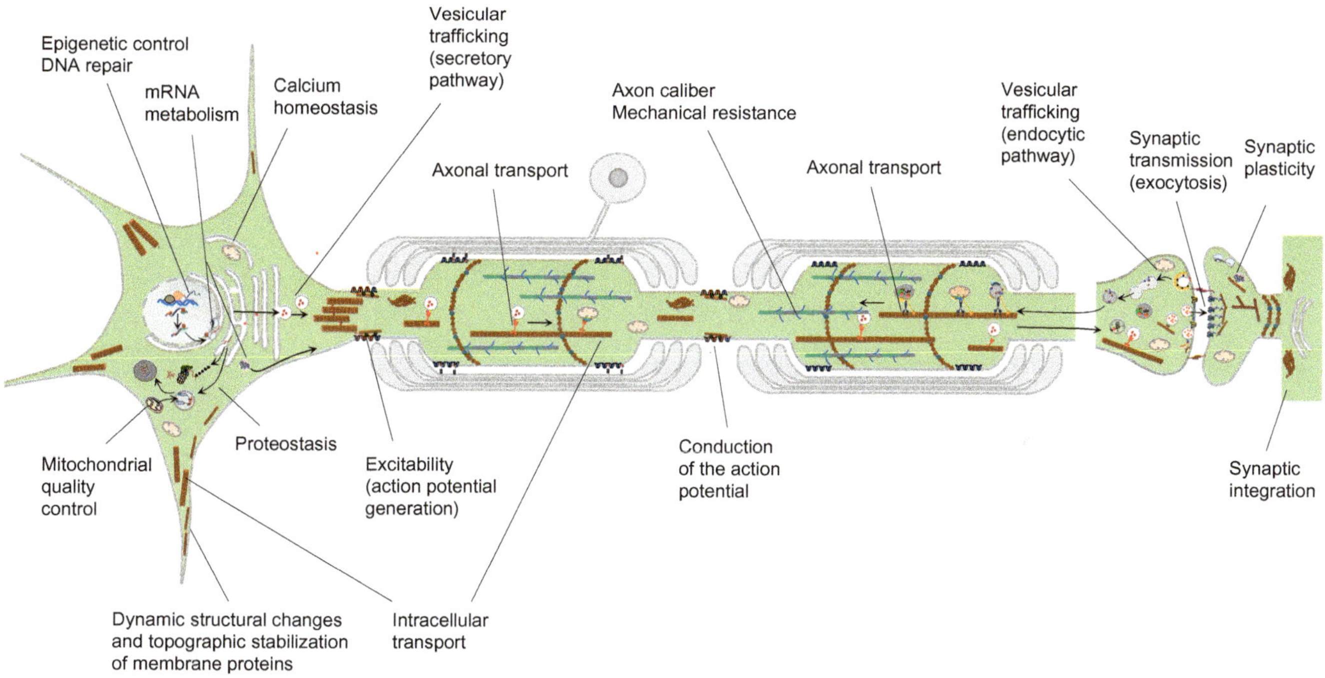

FIGURE 1.4 Main cellular processes in neurons.
Each cell compartment is the site of fundamental cellular processes. These include epigenetic control of mRNA transcription and DNA repair, and mRNA metabolism controlled by mRNA-binding proteins. The quality control of protein maturation in the endoplasmic reticulum (ER) and degradation by the ubiquitin/proteasome system and the autophagy/lysosomal system prevent accumulation of misfolded proteins. Vesicular trafficking occurs via the secretory pathway that involves the endoplasmic reticulum and Golgi complex. Exocytosis of synaptic vesicle is a fast, specialized form of secretion triggered by calcium influx. Endocytosis retrieves synaptic vesicles and other material from the extracellular space. Endosomes target endocytic material back to the Golgi complex or the plasma membrane or alternatively to the lysosome for degradation. Both the secretory and the endocytic pathway depend on normal axonal transport that involves motor proteins and is fueled by ATP.

remyelination after injury. Oligodendrocytes participate in reciprocal interactions with the axon. Signals from axons control activity-dependent oligodendrocyte proliferation and myelination; myelin supports several aspects of axonal function, structure, and maintenance. Oligodendrocytes provide metabolic support to the axon both directly and via interactions with astrocytes.

Microglia

Microglial cells are the immune cells of the CNS and represent approximately 10% of the total brain cell population. The primary role of microglia is to maintain cellular, synaptic, and myelin homeostasis both during development and normal function of the CNS and in response to CNS injury. Microglia are classified into "surveilling" microglia with a ramified morphology and present in the uninjured CNS, and "effector" (also referred to as "activated") microglia with an amoeboid morphology, and present at the sites of injury (Figure 1.5). Surveilling microglia actively extend thin, rapidly motile processes to actively survey their own parcel of brain parenchyma. Activated or effector microglia constitute a heterogeneous population that dynamically changes its phenotype, depending on the type of stimulus and microenvironment. Activated microglia are involved in programmed cell death and synaptic pruning during development and synaptic plasticity in the adult brain. In response to injury, activated microglia may exert not only proinflammatory and cytotoxic but also immunoregulatory and repair actions in response to different environmental cues.[28–30]

Schwann Cells

Schwann cells originate in the neural crest and have multiple functions in mature peripheral nerves. These include myelin formation, regeneration, and release of chemical signals that regulate neuromuscular organization. Myelinating Schwann cells are radially and longitudinally polarized cells. With myelination, Schwann cells organize into distinct membrane domains, each with a unique array of proteins, and a communicating set of cytoplasmic compartments. Schwann cell have a high degree of plasticity after injury.[31–34]

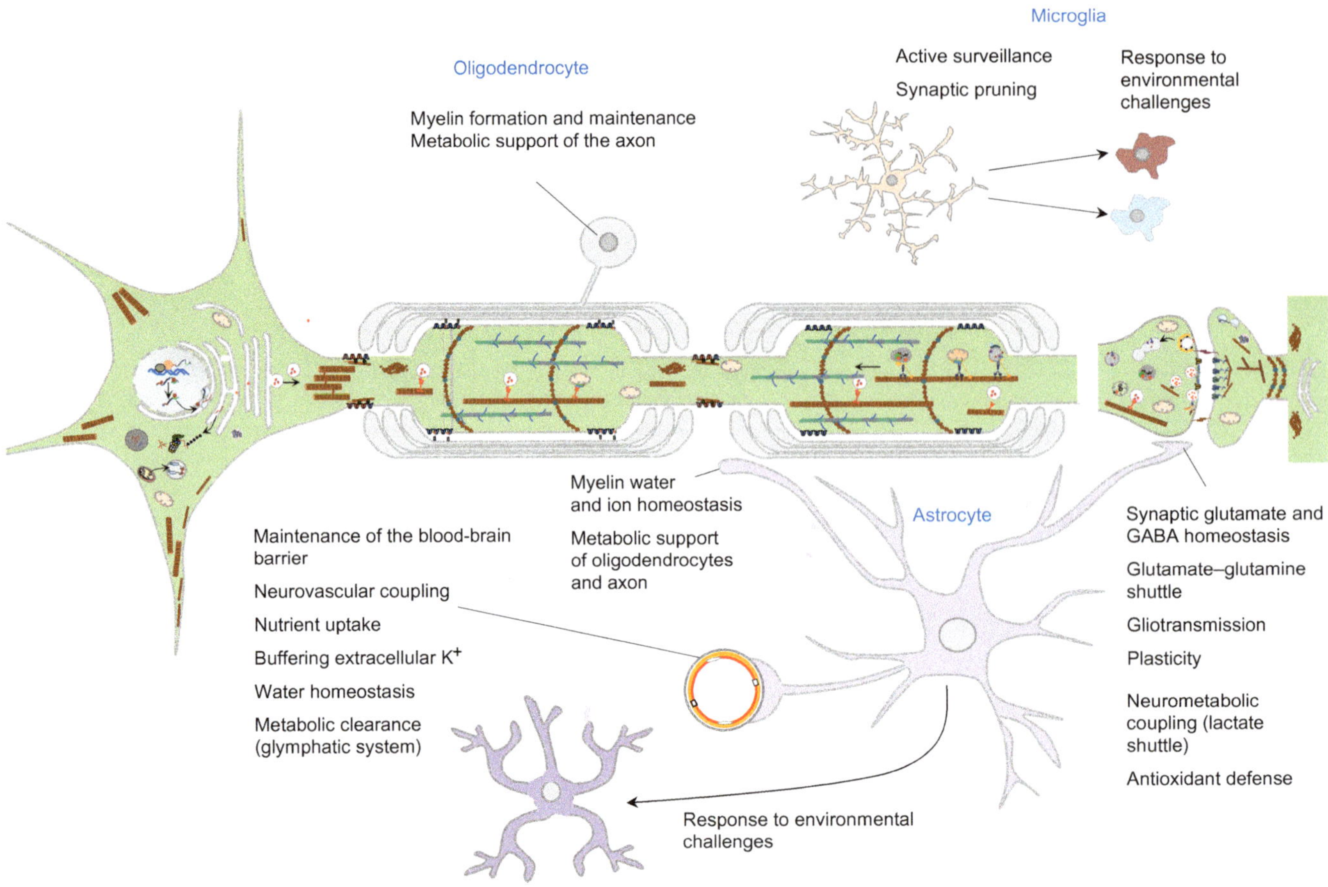

FIGURE 1.5 Functions of glial cells.
Astrocytes are involved in structural and growth factor support during development and repair; formation and maintenance of the blood-brain barrier; activity-dependent regulation of local cerebral blood flow and neuronal metabolism; maintenance of ion and water homeostasis in cells, myelin, and extracellular fluid; regulation of neurotransmitter levels at synapses; coordination of activity of neuronal networks; antioxidant protection; response to injury; and repair in the CNS. Oligodendrocytes are responsible for formation and maintenance of myelin in the CNS and participate in reciprocal interactions with the axon. Oligodendrocytes provide metabolic support to the axon both directly and via interactions with astrocytes. Microglia are classified into "surveilling" microglia and "effector" (also referred to as "activated") microglia.

NEURAL MICROENVIRONMENT

Neurovascular Unit, Blood-Brain Barrier, and Extracellular Fluid Dynamics

The structural and functional integrity of the CNS depend on the coupling between neural activity and CBF and the regulation of transport across the BBB. These two critical functions require the coordinated activity of a neurovascular unit that includes perivascular neurons, astrocytes, endothelial cells, pericytes, and vascular smooth muscle cells. All these cells participate in reciprocal interactions that are critical for local regulationof the CBF, BBB permeability, and homeostasis of the neuronal microenvironment, synaptic remodeling, neurogenesis, and angiogenesis.[35–38] Regulation of the CBF includes autoregulation in response to changes in blood pressure[39] and coupling of blood flow to local neuronal activity (functional hyperemia or neurovascular coupling), which reflects the effects of mediators released from active neurons[40,41] and surrounding astrocytes.[42] Capillary pericytes are a major player in control of CBF and BBB, and influence immune cell entry and angiogenesis.[43] The BBB is a key interface for molecular exchange between the blood and the brain interstitial fluid and depends on the presence of tight junctions and the polarized expression of ion channels, transporters, and receptors in endothelial cells.

The choroid plexus is primarily responsible for the production of cerebrospinal fluid (CSF).[44,45] The exchange of CSF and interstitial fluid promotes the clearance of interstitial solutes via the glymphatic and meningeal lymphatic systems.[46–48]

Extracellular Matrix

The ECM occupies the space between neurons and glial cells and accounts for 10%–20% of the total volume of the brain. During CNS development, the ECM provides a microenvironment that regulates cell migration, axonal guidance, and synaptogenesis during development. In the adult CNS it contributes to maintenance of synaptic stability and regulates repair following injury, in part by restricting aberrant remodeling. Molecules of the ECM may condense to create perineuronal nets, perisynaptic nets, or basement membranes that contribute to the BBB.[49,50]

SIGNALING AND LEVELS OF COMMUNICATION IN THE NERVOUS SYSTEM

Plasma Membrane, Ion Channels, and Intracellular Signaling

The cell membranes are lipid bilayers. Most membrane lipids are phospholipids; other components are sphingolipids and cholesterol. Sphingomyelin and gangliosides are stabilized via interactions with cholesterol at specific membrane microdomains known as lipid rafts. Membrane proteins undergo a continuous bidirectional trafficking between the membrane and the intracellular compartments. There are several fundamental transmembrane proteins critical for neuronal function and survival. The sodium-potassium ATPase is critical for maintenance of transmembrane ion gradients for neuronal excitability and drives secondary transporters required for nutrient, ion, and neurotransmitter homeostasis. Voltage-gated ion channels regulate the intrinsic electrophysiological properties of neurons. Neurotransmitter-gated ion channels (ionotropic receptors) mediate fast transmission of excitatory or inhibitory synaptic signals between neurons. The interactions among different subtypes of ion channels regulate neuronal excitability; shape, frequency, and pattern of firing of action potentials; propagation of the action potential along the axon; neurotransmitter release at synaptic terminals; dendritic integration of synaptic signals; and use-dependent plasticity.

Intracellular signaling involves different families of proteins and critically regulates membrane permeability, vesicular trafficking, cytoskeletal dynamics, synaptic events, gene transcription, and other functions. The mechanisms of intracellular signaling include the activity of G (guanosine nucleotide binding) proteins acting as molecular switches, activation of second messengers such as cyclic nucleotides and phospholipid metabolites, transient increases in intracellular Ca^{2+}, and regulation of protein phosphorylation mediated by balanced actions of protein kinases and protein phosphatases.

Synapses

Most interactions between neurons occur via chemical synapses, which are sites of bidirectional communication. The presynaptic terminal, synaptic cleft, and postsynaptic target membrane have a complex morphologic and molecular organization. Signaling molecules include amino acids, acetylcholine, monoamines, neuropeptides, lipid mediators, and nitric oxide. Glutamate is the primary excitatory neurotransmitter, and gamma-aminobutyric acid (GABA) is the most abundant inhibitory neurotransmitter. Presynaptic events include vesicular storage of neurotransmitter; trafficking, docking, and priming of the synaptic vesicles at the presynaptic active zone; Ca^{2+}-dependent neurotransmitter release by exocytosis; and endocytosis and recycling of synaptic vesicles. Neurotransmitter receptors undergo dynamic activity-dependent trafficking, which is a fundamental mechanism for synaptic plasticity. Neurochemical signals may diffuse via the extracellular space to act by a mechanism of volume transmission to affect neurons, glial cells and blood vessels located at a distance. Reciprocal interactions between neurons and astrocytes shape activity of individual synapses and neuronal ensembles.

Microcircuits, Local Circuits, and Neuronal Ensembles

Local patterns of synaptic connections and interactions involve small clusters of synapses termed microcircuits. They generally involve interactions between excitatory and inhibitory synapses forming subunits within the dendritic trees of individual neurons. Dendritic spines receive the majority of excitatory synapses in the CNS and are the fundamental sites for activity-dependent synaptic plasticity. Dendrites integrate excitatory and inhibitory inputs that eventually lead to generation of an axon potential in the AIS. The next level of complexity is the entire neuron, containing different dendritic subunits. Interactions between neurons constitute local circuits. These local circuits are then organized into columns, laminae, and topographic maps both within and between multiple brain regions.[51] Information processing in neuronal networks is critically dependent on the precise synchronization of ensembles of neurons both within local networks and across the relatively long distances between different brain regions. Whereas the average activity of individual neurons represents features of a stimulus, synchronization between neurons binds those features together and has a major role in whole-brain processing required for consciousness and cognition.[52] These synchronized neuronal oscillations are reflected by waves of electrical activity at different frequencies, which manifest as extracellular local field potentials that may be recorded with microelectrodes, electroencephalogram (EEG), and magnetoencephalogram (MEG).

COGNITIVE NEUROSCIENCE APPROACHES TO EXPLORATION OF BRAIN CONNECTIVITY AND FUNCTION

In parallel to the advances in genetic, molecular, and physiological techniques to characterize neurons, glial cells and cell ensembles, there have been important developments in neuroimaging and electrophysiological techniques to study human brain function and disorders.

In Vivo Neuroimaging

In vivo neuroimaging has provided further insight into structure and functional connectivity of the human CNS. This information is gathered from data provided by the Human Connectome Project. The combined use of different magnetic resonance imaging (MRI) modalities, including T1 and T2 weighted imaging to assess cortical thickness, myelin content, and cortical folding patterns,[53] diffusion tensor imaging to assess fiber tracts, and resting-state and task-functional MRI (fMRI) to assess functional connectivity,[54,55] has expanded the field of human connectomics.[56] For example, this approach has allowed the multimodal parcellation of the cerebral cortex.[55,57–61]

Resting-state fMRI is the most commonly used method to map whole-brain functional connectivity due to its high spatial resolution compared to the EEG or MEG.[62,63] This approach is based on synchronous fluctuations in low frequency blood-oxygen-level-dependent (BOLD) signal between different brain regions.[64] The BOLD signal is determined by changes in levels of deoxyhemoglobin and is a complex measure of blood flow, blood volume, and oxygen consumption that occurs as a consequence of change in energy demand due to neuronal activity, particularly ATP utilization to sustain excitatory synaptic interactions. However, the biological interpretation of this signal is still difficult.[64–66] In general, but not always, functional connectivity reflects structural connectivity. Whereas fMRI has substantially advanced the understanding of normal and pathological brain function, its utility in clinical settings has been limited, in part as a consequence of the low signal-to-noise ratio and reproducibility, especially at a single-subject level. The metabolic activity in different brain regions is primarily assessed using [^{18}F]glucose positron emission tomography (FDG-PET). The physiological interpretation of FDG-PET is based on the coupling between synaptic transmission and local glucose consumption.[67] As compared with BOLD fMRI, the FDG-PET measurements presumably indicate the steady state of neuronal activity and are less dependent on neurovascular coupling. Metabolic connectivity refers to the set of relationships between metabolic (usually FDG-PET) measurements in different brain regions, as determined statistically by the covariance or correlation between regions.[68]

Computational Network Approaches

System neuroscience uses multiple computational network approaches[69,70] to model the integration of brain activity, connectivity, and modulation into a particular cerebral module with a particular output. Numerous statistical methods have been used to capture BOLD or metabolic connectivity, including but not limited to voxel-wise interregional correlation analysis (seed correlation), independent component analysis (multivariate decomposition techniques), sparse inverse covariance estimation, and graph theory. Graph theory provides a mathematical framework to study the functional architecture of the brain.[71,72] In this framework, models represent the brain as a graph with a set of "nodes" that are connected by "edges" between nodes. The edges represent the strength of the correlation between the spontaneous neuronal activities between nodes derived from fMRI data, constrained by anatomical connectivity.[73] Nodes that are most tightly connected functionally with each other form a single "module." Nodes are subdivided into local nodes within modules and connector nodes with connections across modules. These connector nodes represent areas of the cerebral cortex that have access to information across multiple modules and coordinate connectivity within modules. Connector nodes include "connector hubs," which are densely interconnected forming a spatially distributed "rich club." Examples of rich club hub nodes include areas such as the posterior cingulate cortex, medial prefrontal cortex, and lateral parietal cortex.

Electrophysiological Approaches

Multielectrode intracortical recordings in patients undergoing preoperative evaluation have provided information about activity of neuronal ensembles in the cerebral cortex, basal ganglia circuit, thalamus, and other regions. These studies have provided the ability to detect responses of selected neuronal population during cognitive tasks and to identify abnormal firing patterns. Transcranial magnetic stimulation (TMS) allows the noninvasive stimulation of selected regions of the brains using different paradigms.[74] Stimulation is produced by generating a brief, high-intensity magnetic field by passing a brief electric current through a magnetic coil, which can excite or inhibit a small area of brain below the coil.[74]

PATHOPHYSIOLOGICAL CATEGORIES AND MECHANISMS OF NEUROLOGIC DISEASE

There are several common disease pathways shared in neurologic disorders (Figure 1.6).

Disorders of DNA Transcription and Repair

Mutations in genes directly linked to epigenetic regulation such as DNA methylation manifest with severe neurodevelopmental or neurodegenerative disorders. Epigenetic abnormalities may also have a major role in epilepsy and glioma. An estimated 10^5 DNA lesions occur daily in the mammalian genome as a consequence of spontaneous decay, replication errors, and cell metabolism, including reactive oxygen species produced by the mitochondria. There is an age-related accumulation of oxidative DNA damage in the brain, associated with a reduced capacity of DNA repair and neurodegeneration. One typical phenotype of defects

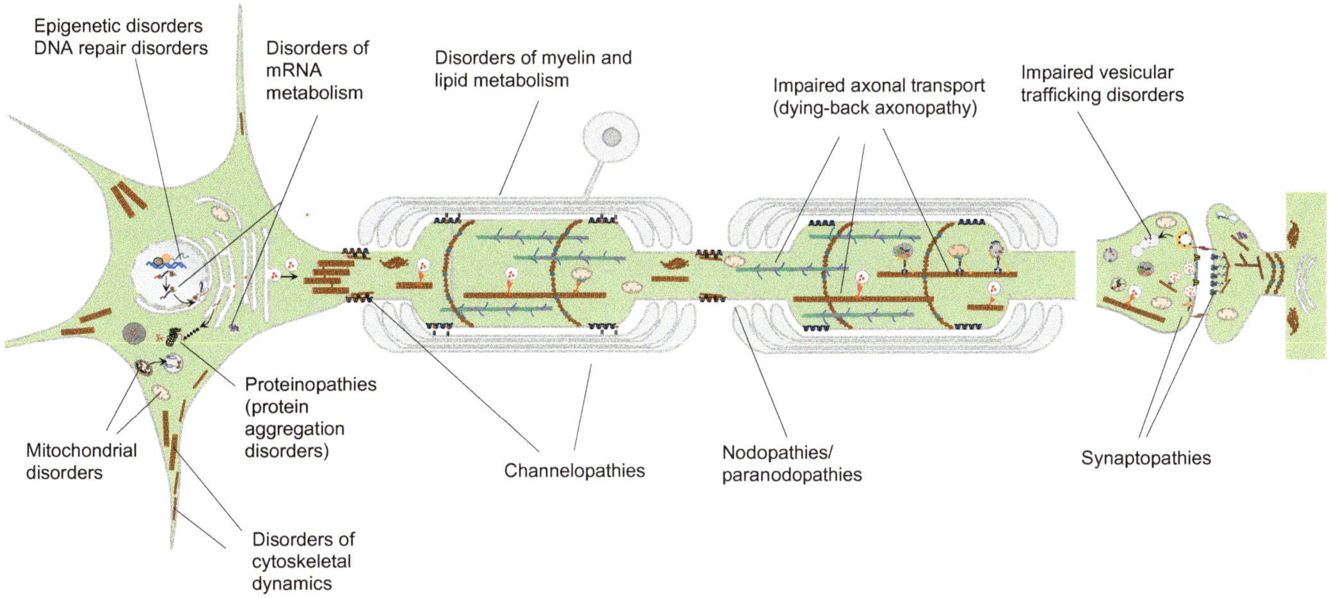

FIGURE 1.6 Disease mechanisms of neurological disorders.
Basic cellular processes can be affected by mutations or by environmental factors such as oxidative stress, impaired calcium metabolism, and inflammation. Whereas mutations affect individual proteins involved in this process, acquired disorders result from combinations of alterations in these hub pathways.

in DNA repair is that of some autosomal recessive cerebellar ataxias such as ataxia-telangiectasia.

Disorders of Messenger RNA Metabolism

Disorders affecting RNA-binding proteins affect transcription, splicing, and translation of mRNA. These disorders of ribostasis are typically associated with formation of nuclear or cytosolic aggregates of messenger ribonucleoprotein particles. For example, accumulation of cytoplasmic stress granules containing mRNA-binding proteins such as TAR-DNA binding protein of 43 kDA (TDP-43) is a hallmark of disorders such as amyotrophic lateral sclerosis (ALS) and frontotemporal dementia (FTD). Abnormal expansion of nucleotide repeats may produce toxicity through multiple pathogenic mechanisms. These include protein loss-of-function as in the case of Friedreich ataxia; RNA toxic gain-of-function as in the case of myotonic dystrophy; protein gain-of-function as in the case of diseases associated with polyglutamine(CAG) repeat expansions, such as Huntington disease and several autosomal dominant spinocerebellar ataxias; and repeat-associated non-AUG translation with formation of toxic polydipeptides, as in the case of CCGGG expansions in the chromosome 9 open reading frame 72 (*C9ORF72*) gene associated with familial ALS and FTD.

Disorders of Proteostasis

Impaired protein quality control, including protein maturation in the ER, heat shock protein function, or impaired activity of the ubiquitin-proteasome or the autophagy-lysosome system is major pathogenic hub in neurodegenerative disorders, also referred to as proteinopathies. In these disorders, proteins that normally have a major role in neuronal function, such as amyloid precursor protein, alpha-synuclein, or tau, accumulate in a misfolded conformation into fibrillary β-sheet-rich "amyloid" structures. This may lead to both a loss-of-function of the affected protein and a toxic gain-of-function of oligomers. This gain-of-function promotes the formation of aggregates that undergo cycles of nucleation and fragmentation and initiate a cascade of protein–protein interactions leading to neuronal dysfunction and death. These aggregates may also serve as templates or seed to elicit aggregation of their respective normal endogenous partners in neighboring cells, thereby having a "prion-like" behavior. Typical examples are synucleinopathies such as Parkinson disease (PD) or multiple system atrophy and primary or secondary tauopathies.

Disorders of Vesicular Trafficking, Cytoskeleton, and Axonal Transport

Impaired vesicular trafficking, cytoskeletal dynamics, and axonal transport are fundamental disease pathways in neurodegenerative disorders. These disorders typically affect selective populations of projection neurons with long axons and are associated with early loss of neuronal connectivity reflecting dying back neurodegeneration. Impaired axonal transport results in abnormal accumulation of cytoskeletal components such as neurofilament subunits, mitochondria, and or vesicular cargoes in the perikarya, proximal segment of the axons, or the distal portion of the axons. Impaired vesicular trafficking is a major disease mechanism in PD; impaired axonal transport is a hallmark in genetic or acquired disorders that manifest with hereditary spastic paraplegia, motor neuron disease, and motor neuronopathies, sometimes with overlapping phenotypes.

Mitochondria and Energy Metabolism

Mitochondrial disorders are subdivided into those directly related to defects in bioenergetics and metabolic functions; those reflecting impaired mitostasis; and adult-onset neurodegenerative disorders that affect axonal transport and autophagy. The major consequences of impaired mitochondrial oxidative phosphorylation (OXPHOS) are reduced ATP synthesis, oxidative stress, toxic accumulation of calcium in the cytosol and mitochondria, and increased mitochondrial membrane permeability leading to apoptosis. Mitochondrial disorders manifest with complex phenotypes, including encephalopathy, ataxia, progressive external ophthalmoplegia, basal ganglia dysfunction, peripheral neuropathy, myopathy, and optic neuropathy, which may occur in several combinations. Clinical features suggestive of mitochondrial disease include short stature, sensorineural deafness, diabetes mellitus, pigmentary retinopathy, and lactic acidosis.

Disorders of Complex Lipid Metabolism

Complex lipids including phospholipids, sphingolipids, and cholesterol have a crucial role in maintenance of membrane structure and dynamics as well as in intracellular signaling mechanisms. Disorders affecting metabolism or vesicular trafficking of complex lipids manifest with a wide range of phenotypes, including leukodistrophies, predominantly gray matter disorders and motor neuron disease. Leukoencephalopathies include primary disorders of myelin or oligodendrocyte (leukodystrophies), axonopathies, astrocytopathies, microgliopathies, and vasculopathies. A typical oligodendrocytopathy is Krabbe disease. Astrocytopathies include Alexander disease and microgliopathies include hereditary diffuse leukoencephalopathy with neuroaxonal spheroids and pigmented glia. Disorders affecting the gray matter include Niemann-Pick type C disease and GM2 gangliosidosis.

Inflammatory and Immune Disorders

Microglia and astrocytes are most commonly secondarily involved in mechanisms of CNS injury associated with inflammatory and immune responses.[75] Examples include traumatic injury, stroke, infections, demyelinating disease such as multiple sclerosis, and autoimmune encephalitis, where there is also disruption of the BBB. In these situations, microglia and astrocytes respond to mediators of innate or acquired immunity with proliferation, morphological changes, and upregulation of expression and release of cytokines, chemokines, and other products. The responses of microglia and astrocytes are not stereotyped, but rather include different phenotypes depending on the environmental setting. Whereas "pro-inflammatory" phenotypes promote cell and axonal injury, other phenotypes promote tissue repair. Inflammation is recognized as an important pathogenic mechanism in neurodegenerative disorders, chronic pain, and epilepsy. Autoreactive B cells can drive autoimmunity through production of antibody, immune complex formation; presentation of autoantigen to T cells, and production of cytokines. Autoimmune encephalitis may be due to antibodies directed either at cell surface antigens or at intracellular targets.

Channelopathies, Synaptopathies, and Nodopathies

Genetic, immune, or toxic disorders affecting ion channels, synaptic proteins, or structural proteins in the axonal nodes of Ranvier or paranodes, constitute an important group of neurologic disorders leading to neuronal dysfunction even in the absence of structural or metabolic changes. Genetic channelopathies affecting voltage-gated ion channels manifest with epilepsy, episodic ataxia, paroxysmal pain disorders, myotonia, or periodic paralysis. Autoimmune disorders affecting components of the voltage-gated potassium channels or ionotropic receptors manifest with limbic encephalitis with seizures, and in some cases excessive neuromuscular excitability. Synaptopathies resemble channelopathies as they can also manifest with paroxysmal movement disorders, seizures, ataxia, and hemiplegic migraine or, in some cases, congenital myasthenic syndrome. Nodopathies and paranodopathies are the consequence of antibodies affecting gangliosides or adhesion molecules critical for maintenance of the structural integrity and function of these components of the axon. They manifest with acute or chronic inflammatory polyradiculoneuropathies.

MECHANISMS OF CELL DEATH

Excitotoxicity, Calcium Overload, and Axonal Injury

In conditions such as hypoxia or ischemia, there is accumulation of glutamate in the synaptic and extrasynaptic spaces, leading to calcium-mediated cell toxicity, or excitotoxicity. One major consequence of calcium overload is impairment of mitochondrial function. Calcium also activates downstream damaging effectors such as the protease calpain, which proteolytically disrupts the cytoskeleton and other critical proteins. Excitotoxicity and disrupted calcium homeostasis not only affects neurons but also profoundly affects axons and oligodendrocytes.

Cell Death Pathways

Cell death is defined as either irreversible membrane permeabilization or cell complete fragmentation. "Accidental" cell death occurs in traumatic injury. In contrast, "regulated" cell death occurs in cells that experience unsolvable perturbation of homeostasis and can be triggered by intrinsic cell disturbances, such as DNA damage, accumulation of misfolded proteins in the ER, oxidative stress, or external activation of death receptors. There are two main morphologic manifestations of programmed cell death. Necrosis reflects membrane fragmentation and typically occurs in the setting of dissipation of mitochondrial potential, leading to impaired ATP production, disturbance in intracellular Ca^{2+} homeostasis, oxidative stress and membrane lipid peroxidation, or formation of pore complexes in the plasma membrane. Apoptosis is characterized by activation of caspases leading to fragmentation of nuclear DNA and is typically triggered by DNA damage and accumulation of misfolded proteins in the ER. Many forms of regulated cell death primarily or secondarily involve the mitochondria. They include intrinsic apoptosis, mitochondrial permeability transition-driven regulated necrosis, and parthanatos. Others, such as ferroptosis, are triggered by lipid peroxidation accelerated by intracellular iron.

CONTEMPORARY VIEW OF NEUROLOGIC DISORDERS

Multiple-Level Analysis of Neurologic Disease

Full understanding of neurologic disease requires the integration of neuronal and glial cell biology with neuronal networks and eventually with cognition and behavior. For example, epilepsy reflects enhanced excitability of cells, synapses, and networks. Several levels contribute to etiology and pathogenesis of this disorder, ranging from individual ion channels (e.g., genetic channelopathies), to individual cells and synapses (e.g., autoimmune synaptopathies) to networks (e.g., malformations of cortical development). Neurodegenerative disorders also reflect multiple interacting disturbances of intracellular processes, including ribostasis, proteostasis, impaired vesicular trafficking, and axonal transport, leading to accumulation of abnormal inclusions, mitochondrial dysfunction, oxidative stress, inflammation, and cell death. In these disorders, cellular disturbances lead to abnormalities at synaptic, network, and system levels. For example, in Alzheimer disease, impaired proteostasis leading to accumulation of Aβ oligomers and hyperphosphorylated tau produces dendritic loss, impairs axonal transport, affects synaptic plasticity, alters both local and large-scale network oscillations, and disrupts functional connectivity within episodic memory networks.

Machine Learning

The BRAIN (Brain Research through Advancing Innovative Neurotechnologies) initiative has promoted a new era in systems neuroscience, driven by technologies such as single-cell transcriptomics and proteomics, optogenetics, and large-scale multi-electrode arrays. The large datasets generated by these novel technologies require increasing computational power for analyses that provides the basis for machine learning. The same applies for databases derived from the Brain Connectome project. The traditional approach to localization of neurologic deficit by determining the most likely site of lesion to account for the patient's symptoms (classical lesion mapping) continues to be very helpful to localize lesions in the peripheral, spinal, and brainstem levels. However, movement disorders, and particularly disorders manifesting with high-order sensory, cognitive, or behavioral symptoms may not localize to a single region. Rather, they may result from functional alterations in several otherwise anatomically intact brain regions connected to the lesion site. A recent approach to this problem is lesion network mapping, where disparate lesions that result in the same symptoms are mapped on a normative resting-state connectivity database.[76] Multiscale modeling and artificial intelligence approaches may provide not only insight into disease pathophysiology but also the rationale to combine pharmacotherapy, genetic therapy, neuromodulation, and neurorehabilitation; personalize these therapies; and integrate diagnostic updates with reevaluation of therapy.

KEY POINTS

- Both normal and abnormal functions of the nervous system reflect the activity of networks with a scale ranging from cell-specific gene and protein expression to large circuits involving interactions among several brain areas.
- The function of neurons is affected by their reciprocal interactions with glial cells and their environment.
- Genome-wide molecular profiling shows that transcriptomes of brain regions are organized into modules of coexpressed genes.
- No neuronal or glial cell type is homogeneous, and their cell properties change during development and maturation and in response to environmental signals.
- Neurons are complex cells with different functional domains each with a unique distribution of membrane in channels, receptors, adhesion molecules, scaffold proteins, cytoskeletal proteins, and organelles.
- Neurons are highly dependent on mitochondrial metabolism for production of ATP, which is critical for maintenance of ion gradients, axonal transport, synaptic function, and protein quality control.
- Astrocytes have several crucial functions, including structural and growth factor support during development and repair, formation and maintenance of the blood-brain barrier, regulation of local cerebral blood flow, metabolic support to neurons and oligodendrocytes, maintenance of ion and water homeostasis, regulation of synaptic neurotransmitter levels, coordination of activity of neuronal networks, antioxidant protection, and response to injury.

- Oligodendrocytes participate in reciprocal interactions with the axon; axonal signals control oligodendrocyte proliferation and myelination; myelin supports several aspects of axonal function, structure, and maintenance.
- Microglia actively survey the brain parenchyma, participate in synaptic remodeling, and adopt different reactive phenotypes, depending on the type of stimulus and microenvironment.
- The structural and functional integrity of the central nervous system depends on the coupling between neural activity and cerebral blood flow via the neurovascular unit, regulation of transport across the blood-brain barrier, secretion and circulation of cerebrospinal fluid, and interstitial fluid dynamics in the brain.
- Plasma membrane transporters and ion channels are critical for control of neuronal survival and function, including excitability, conduction of the action potential, and neurotransmitter release.
- Intracellular signaling involving calcium dynamics and phosphorylation cascades regulates multiple cellular functions, including membrane permeability, vesicular trafficking, cytoskeletal dynamics, synaptic events, and gene transcription.
- Chemical synapses are sites of bidirectional communication.
- Dendritic spines receive the majority of excitatory synapses in the CNS and are the fundamental sites for activity-dependent synaptic plasticity.
- Information processing depends on the synchronization of ensembles of neurons both within local networks and across different brain regions.
- In most disorders, mechanisms of cell and axonal injury include excitotoxicity, intracellular calcium accumulation, or mitochondrial dysfunction, leading to cell death by mechanisms of necrosis or apoptosis. These common mechanisms provide multiple potential targets for neuroprotection.
- Multiscale modeling and machine learning approaches may provide insight into disease pathophysiology and help development of combined approaches to personalize therapy of neurologic disorders.

REFERENCES

1. Petersen SE, Sporns O. Brain networks and cognitive architectures. Neuron 2015;88:207–219.
2. Bertolero MA, Yeo BT, D'Esposito M. The modular and integrative functional architecture of the human brain. Proc Natl Acad Sci U S A 2015;112:E6798–6807.
3. Pollock JD, Wu DY, Satterlee JS. Molecular neuroanatomy: a generation of progress. Trends Neurosci 2014;37:106–123.
4. Shapiro E, Biezuner T, Linnarsson S. Single-cell sequencing-based technologies will revolutionize whole-organism science. Nat Rev Genet 2013;14:618–630.
5. Wagner A, Regev A, Yosef N. Revealing the vectors of cellular identity with single-cell genomics. Nat Biotechnol 2016;34:1145–1160.
6. Usoskin D, Furlan A, Islam S, et al. Unbiased classification of sensory neuron types by large-scale single-cell RNA sequencing. Nat Neurosci 2015;18:145–153.
7. Kelley KW, Oldham MC. Transcriptional architecture of the human brain. Nat Neurosci 2015;18:1699–1701.
8. Li M, Santpere G, Imamura Kawasawa Y, et al. Integrative functional genomic analysis of human brain development and neuropsychiatric risks. Science 2018;362.
9. Zeng H, Sanes JR. Neuronal cell-type classification: challenges, opportunities and the path forward. Nat Rev Neurosci 2017;18:530–546.
10. Silveira-Moriyama L, Paciorkowski AR. Genetic diagnostics for neurologists. Continuum (Minneap Minn) 2018;24:18–36.
11. Ponten F, Schwenk JM, Asplund A, Edqvist PH. The Human Protein Atlas as a proteomic resource for biomarker discovery. J Intern Med 2011;270:428–446.
12. Shah S, Lubeck E, Zhou W, Cai L. In situ transcription profiling of single cells reveals spatial organization of cells in the mouse hippocampus. Neuron 2016;92:342–357.
13. Boyden ES. A history of optogenetics: the development of tools for controlling brain circuits with light. F1000 Biol Rep 2011;3:11.
14. Boyden ES. Optogenetics and the future of neuroscience. Nat Neurosci 2015;18:1200–1201.
15. Deisseroth K. Optogenetics: 10 years of microbial opsins in neuroscience. Nat Neurosci 2015;18:1213–1225.
16. English JG, Roth BL. Chemogenetics: a transformational and translational platform. JAMA Neurol 2015;72:1361–1366.
17. Magnus CJ, Lee PH, Atasoy D, Su HH, Looger LL, Sternson SM. Chemical and genetic engineering of selective ion channel-ligand interactions. Science 2011;333:1292–1296.
18. Miller EK, Wilson MA. All my circuits: using multiple electrodes to understand functioning neural networks. Neuron 2008;60:483–488.
19. Antic SD, Empson RM, Knopfel T. Voltage imaging to understand connections and functions of neuronal circuits. J Neurophysiol 2016;116:135–152.
20. Chen TW, Wardill TJ, Sun Y, et al. Ultrasensitive fluorescent proteins for imaging neuronal activity. Nature 2013;499:295–300.
21. Peron S, Chen TW, Svoboda K. Comprehensive imaging of cortical networks. Curr Opin Neurobiol 2015;32:115–123.
22. Yang W, Yuste R. In vivo imaging of neural activity. Nat Methods 2017;14:349–359.
23. von Bartheld CS, Bahney J, Herculano-Houzel S. The search for true numbers of neurons and glial cells in the human brain: a review of 150 years of cell counting. J Comp Neurol 2016;524:3865–3895.
24. Pelvig DP, Pakkenberg H, Stark AK, Pakkenberg B. Neocortical glial cell numbers in human brains. Neurobiol Aging 2008;29:1754–1762.
25. Trotter J, Karram K, Nishiyama A. NG2 cells: properties, progeny and origin. Brain Res Rev 2010;63:72–82.
26. Khakh BS, Sofroniew MV. Diversity of astrocyte functions and phenotypes in neural circuits. Nat Neurosci 2015;18:942–952.
27. Verkhratsky A, Zorec R, Parpura V. Stratification of astrocytes in healthy and diseased brain. Brain Pathol 2017;27:629–644.

28. Paolicelli RC, Bolasco G, Pagani F, et al. Synaptic pruning by microglia is necessary for normal brain development. Science 2011;333:1456–1458.
29. Schafer DP, Lehrman EK, Kautzman AG, et al. Microglia sculpt postnatal neural circuits in an activity and complement-dependent manner. Neuron 2012;74:691–705.
30. Parkhurst CN, Yang G, Ninan I, et al. Microglia promote learning-dependent synapse formation through brain-derived neurotrophic factor. Cell 2013;155:1596–1609.
31. Boerboom A, Dion V, Chariot A, Franzen R. Molecular mechanisms involved in Schwann cell plasticity. Front Mol Neurosci 2017;10:38.
32. Ma KH, Svaren J. Epigenetic control of Schwann cells. Neuroscientist 2018;24:627–638.
33. Salzer JL. Schwann cell myelination. Cold Spring Harb Perspect Biol 2015;7:a020529.
34. Hyung S, Jung K, Cho SR, Jeon NL. The Schwann cell as an active synaptic partner. Chemphyschem 2018;19:1123–1127.
35. Abbott NJ, Friedman A. Overview and introduction: the blood-brain barrier in health and disease. Epilepsia 2012;53 Suppl 6:1–6.
36. Tajes M, Ramos-Fernandez E, Weng-Jiang X, et al. The blood-brain barrier: structure, function and therapeutic approaches to cross it. Mol Membr Biol 2014;31:152–167.
37. Liebner S, Dijkhuizen RM, Reiss Y, Plate KH, Agalliu D, Constantin G. Functional morphology of the blood-brain barrier in health and disease. Acta Neuropathol 2018;135:311–336.
38. Lecrux C, Hamel E. The neurovascular unit in brain function and disease. Acta Physiol (Oxf) 2011;203:47–59.
39. Strandgaard S, Paulson OB. Regulation of cerebral blood flow in health and disease. J Cardiovasc Pharmacol 1992;19 Suppl 6:S89–93.
40. Lecrux C, Bourourou M, Hamel E. How reliable is cerebral blood flow to map changes in neuronal activity? Auton Neurosci 2019;217:71–79.
41. Iadecola C. The neurovascular unit coming of age: a journey through neurovascular coupling in health and disease. Neuron 2017;96:17–42.
42. Cauli B, Hamel E. Brain perfusion and astrocytes. Trends Neurosci 2018;41:409–413.
43. Hirunpattarasilp C, Attwell D, Freitas F. The role of pericytes in brain disorders: from the periphery to the brain. J Neurochem 2019.
44. Spector R, Keep RF, Robert Snodgrass S, Smith QR, Johanson CE. A balanced view of choroid plexus structure and function: focus on adult humans. Exp Neurol 2015;267:78–86.
45. Lehtinen MK, Bjornsson CS, Dymecki SM, Gilbertson RJ, Holtzman DM, Monuki ES. The choroid plexus and cerebrospinal fluid: emerging roles in development, disease, and therapy. J Neurosci 2013;33:17553–17559.
46. Da Mesquita S, Fu Z, Kipnis J. The meningeal lymphatic system: a new player in neurophysiology. Neuron 2018;100:375–388.
47. Louveau A, Plog BA, Antila S, Alitalo K, Nedergaard M, Kipnis J. Understanding the functions and relationships of the glymphatic system and meningeal lymphatics. J Clin Invest 2017;127:3210–3219.
48. Engelhardt B, Carare RO, Bechmann I, Flugel A, Laman JD, Weller RO. Vascular, glial, and lymphatic immune gateways of the central nervous system. Acta Neuropathol 2016;132:317–338.
49. Testa D, Prochiantz A, Di Nardo AA. Perineuronal nets in brain physiology and disease. Semin Cell Dev Biol 2019;89:125–135.
50. Song I, Dityatev A. Crosstalk between glia, extracellular matrix and neurons. Brain Res Bull 2018;136:101–108.
51. Shepherd GM. Microcircuits in the nervous system. Sci Am 1978;238:93–103.
52. Singer W. Neuronal oscillations: unavoidable and useful? Eur J Neurosci 2018;48:2389–2398.
53. Destrieux C, Fischl B, Dale A, Halgren E. Automatic parcellation of human cortical gyri and sulci using standard anatomical nomenclature. Neuroimage 2010;53:1–15.
54. Arslan S, Ktena SI, Makropoulos A, Robinson EC, Rueckert D, Parisot S. Human brain mapping: a systematic comparison of parcellation methods for the human cerebral cortex. Neuroimage 2017.
55. Barch DM, Burgess GC, Harms MP, et al. Function in the human connectome: task-fMRI and individual differences in behavior. Neuroimage 2013;80:169–189.
56. Behrens TE, Sporns O. Human connectomics. Curr Opin Neurobiol 2012;22:144–153.
57. Glasser MF, Coalson TS, Robinson EC, et al. A multimodal parcellation of human cerebral cortex. Nature 2016;536:171–178.
58. Parisot S, Glocker B, Ktena SI, Arslan S, Schirmer MD, Rueckert D. A flexible graphical model for multi-modal parcellation of the cortex. Neuroimage 2017;162:226–248.
59. Ding SL, Royall JJ, Sunkin SM, et al. Comprehensive cellular-resolution atlas of the adult human brain. J Comp Neurol 2016;524:3127–3481.
60. Eickhoff SB, Constable RT, Yeo BTT. Topographic organization of the cerebral cortex and brain cartography. Neuroimage 2018;170:332–347.
61. Amunts K, Zilles K. Architectonic mapping of the human brain beyond Brodmann. Neuron 2015;88:1086–1107.
62. Damoiseaux JS, Rombouts SA, Barkhof F, et al. Consistent resting-state networks across healthy subjects. Proc Natl Acad Sci U S A 2006;103:13848–13853.
63. Power JD, Cohen AL, Nelson SM, et al. Functional network organization of the human brain. Neuron 2011;72:665–678.
64. Hall CN, Howarth C, Kurth-Nelson Z, Mishra A. Interpreting BOLD: towards a dialogue between cognitive and cellular neuroscience. Philos Trans R Soc Lond B Biol Sci 2016;371.
65. Logothetis NK, Wandell BA. Interpreting the BOLD signal. Annu Rev Physiol 2004;66:735–769.
66. Eickhoff SB, Thirion B, Varoquaux G, Bzdok D. Connectivity-based parcellation: critique and implications. Hum Brain Mapp 2015;36:4771–4792.
67. Magistretti PJ. Neuron-glia metabolic coupling and plasticity. J Exp Biol 2006;209:2304–2311.
68. Titov D, Diehl-Schmid J, Shi K, et al. Metabolic connectivity for differential diagnosis of dementing disorders. J Cereb Blood Flow Metab 2017;37:252–262.
69. Stephan KE, Iglesias S, Heinzle J, Diaconescu AO. Translational perspectives for computational neuroimaging. Neuron 2015;87:716–732.
70. Rigoux L, Daunizeau J. Dynamic causal modelling of brain-behaviour relationships. Neuroimage 2015;117:202–221.

71. Sporns O. Contributions and challenges for network models in cognitive neuroscience. Nat Neurosci 2014;17:652–660.
72. Veronese M, Moro L, Arcolin M, et al. Covariance statistics and network analysis of brain PET imaging studies. Sci Rep 2019;9:2496.
73. Hermundstad AM, Bassett DS, Brown KS, et al. Structural foundations of resting-state and task-based functional connectivity in the human brain. Proc Natl Acad Sci U S A 2013;110:6169–6174.
74. Hallett M. Transcranial magnetic stimulation: a primer. Neuron 2007;55:187–199.
75. Thurgur H, Pinteaux E. Microglia in the neurovascular unit: blood-brain barrier-microglia interactions after central nervous system disorders. Neuroscience 2019;405:55–67.
76. Boes AD, Prasad S, Liu H, et al. Network localization of neurological symptoms from focal brain lesions. Brain 2015;138:3061–3075.

2 Organization of Cell Membranes

OVERVIEW

The plasma membrane provides the interface between the cell and its environment; membranes in intracellular organelles including endoplasmic reticulum (ER), Golgi complex, vesicles, endosomes, lysosomes, and peroxisomes separate intraluminal from cytosolic compartments. Mitochondria contain an outer and an inner membrane that provide compartmentalization into an intramembranous space and a matrix. The plasma membrane is composed of lipids and proteins (Figure 2.1). The main membrane lipids are phospholipids, sphingolipids, and cholesterol. These lipids are asymmetrically distributed in the membrane bilayer and control the biophysical properties of the membrane, including fluidity and curvature for vesicle formation. Sphingomyelin and gangliosides interact with cholesterol at membrane microdomains known as lipid rafts. Phospholipids and sphingolipids provide metabolites that mediate intracellular or intercellular signaling. Glycolipids, particularly gangliosides, function in intercellular communication. Membrane proteins interact with the lipid bilayer and include integral and associated proteins. Integral membrane proteins traverse the lipid bilayer and include ion pumps, transporters, ion channels, receptors, and adhesion molecules. These proteins are localized into specific membrane domains by interactions with scaffolding and cytoskeletal proteins or with lipid drafts. Associated proteins are linked to the membrane via molecular anchors and also include receptors and adhesion molecules involved in cell–cell communication. Plasma membrane proteins undergo continuous recycling and can be inserted into or retrieved from the membrane. Myelin has a lipid-protein-lipid-protein-lipid structure formed by membrane expansion of Schwann cells in the peripheral nervous system and oligodendrocytes in the central nervous system. The aims of this chapter are to briefly review (1) the composition and dynamics of membrane lipids, (2) the function of some important membrane proteins, and (3) some representative examples of

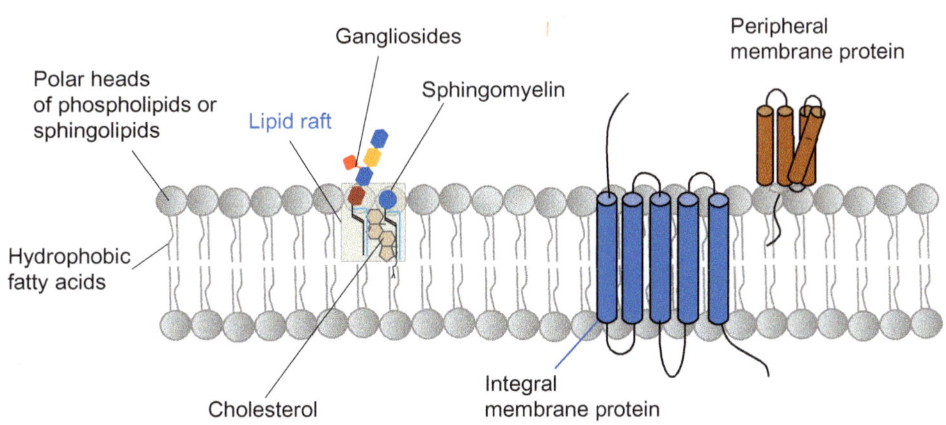

FIGURE 2.1 Organization of the plasma membrane.
Most membrane lipids are phospholipids, sphingolipids, and cholesterol. Sphingomyelin and gangliosides are stabilized via interactions with cholesterol at lipid rafts. Integral membrane proteins contain α-helices that traverse the lipid bilayer one or several times. Associated proteins are linked to the membrane via molecular anchors.

disorders affecting membrane lipids and transporter proteins. Disorders affecting membrane trafficking, ion channels, receptors, and myelin are discussed in other chapters of this book.

MEMBRANE LIPIDS

Lipids are amphipathic molecules with a small polar hydrophilic head and a large, hydrophobic tail consisting of fatty acids or isoprenoids. Most membrane lipids are phospholipids; other important components are sphingolipids and cholesterol. These lipids are asymmetrically distributed in the membrane bilayer; the different geometry and covalent interactions between their fatty acid chains determine their clustering into nano- or microdomains. Membrane lipids directly control the biophysical parameters of the membrane, including curvature, fluidity, and thickness. The saturation state of fatty acid affects the fluidity of the membrane, in concert with cholesterol. Membrane bending required for vesicle formation is regulated by local phospholipid metabolism or lipid exchange across the bilayer. The lipid composition varies in different cell membranes, driven by their dynamic interchange between compartments. Lipids are often synthesized in one intracellular compartment and must be transported to another compartment for membrane biogenesis. The intracellular transport of lipids from one membrane to another occurs via vesicular trafficking, direct transfer across membranes, and cytoplasmic transfer-exchange proteins.

Fatty Acids

Membrane lipids contain saturated and unsaturated fatty acids; an important example is arachidonic acid, which provides the substrate for production of signaling molecules such as prostaglandins and endocannabinoids. Some long polyunsaturated fatty acids cannot be synthesized de novo; they are provided from the diet and transported across the blood-brain barrier; some can also be synthesized in glial cells. The hydrophobic chains of fatty acids and isoprenoids are synthesized from acetyl coenzyme A (acetyl CoA). Coenzyme A is produced in the mitochondrial matrix by a complex reaction that includes phosphorylation of pantothenic acid by pantothenate kinase 2 (PANK2). Fatty acids are synthesized by elongation of 2-carbon units via cycles of condensation, reduction, dehydration, and hydrogenation reactions catalyzed by fatty acid synthase. Fatty acids are degraded in the mitochondria and peroxisomes. In the mitochondrial matrix, they undergo β-oxidation to their final product acetyl CoA, which then enters the Krebs cycle. Long-chain acyl CoA synthase activates long-chain fatty acids at the outer mitochondrial membrane; a carnitine transport system then mediates the import of activated fatty acids to the matrix via three sequential steps mediated by carnitine palmitoyl transferase I, carnitine: acyl carnitine translocase, and finally carnitine: palmitoyl transferase II. Saturated very long-chain fatty acids undergo β-oxidation in the peroxisome; this process requires their incorporation via the peroxisomal membrane protein adenosine triphosphate (ATP)-binding cassette, subunit D (encoded by the *ABCD1* gene).

Phospholipids

Phospholipid biosynthesis occurs primarily in the ER. Phospholipids have a polar head consisting of a glycerophosphoryl ester moiety, and a hydrocarbon tail composed of two fatty acids (Figure 2.2). Membrane phospholipids derive from phosphatidic acid and include phosphatidylcholine (lecithin), phosphatidylethanolamine, phosphatidylserine, and the phosphoinositides. Cardiolipin is a typical phospholipid in mitochondria. Phospholipids are asymmetrically distributed in the plasma membrane. Positively charged phospholipids such as phosphatidylcholine and phosphatidylethanolamine are predominantly present in the outer leaflet; negatively charged phospholipids such as phosphatidylserine and phosphoinositides predominate in the inner (cytoplasmic) leaflet. This asymmetric distribution depends on the ATP-dependent activity of proteins called "flippases." Conditions that increase intracellular calcium (Ca^{2+}), such as anoxia, can activate "scramblases" that catalyze the externalization of phosphatidylserine to the outer membrane surface. Whereas transient and localized phosphatidylserine scrambling may be a general signaling mechanism associated with membrane fusion and exocytosis, phosphatidylserine exposure to the outer membrane surface also constitutes a signal for apoptosis.

The formation of a curvature of the plasma membrane involves the interaction of phospholipids and sphingolipids with plasma membrane binding proteins, and depends on the shape of the individual lipid, which is determined both by the size of their head group and the length and saturation of the acyl chains.

Phosphoinositides derive from phosphatidylinositol and are quantitatively minor membrane phospholipids; however they have two fundamental physiological roles: shaping the membrane curvature for vesicular biogenesis and intracellular signal transduction. Phosphatidylinositol is phosphorylated by phosphatidylinositol 4'kinase to phosphatidylinositol 4-phosphate (PI4P), which is further phosphorylated to yield phosphatidylinositol 4,5-bisphosphate (PIP2). This phospholipid has a major role in signal transduction pathways triggered by a many neurotransmitters. Alternatively, phosphatidylinositol 3'kinase (PI3K) catalyzes the production phosphatidylinositol 3,4,5-triphosphate (PIP3), which is a critical mediator of cell survival pathways triggered by growth factors. Different phospholipases cleave specific sites of membrane phospholipids, creating new lipid species that have affect membrane curvature formation, signaling function, or both[1] (Figure 2.1). Phospholipase A2 (PLA2) hydrolyzes the second carbon group of phosphatidylcholine producing arachidonic acid, which serves as substrate for synthesis of prostaglandin E2. Phospholipase

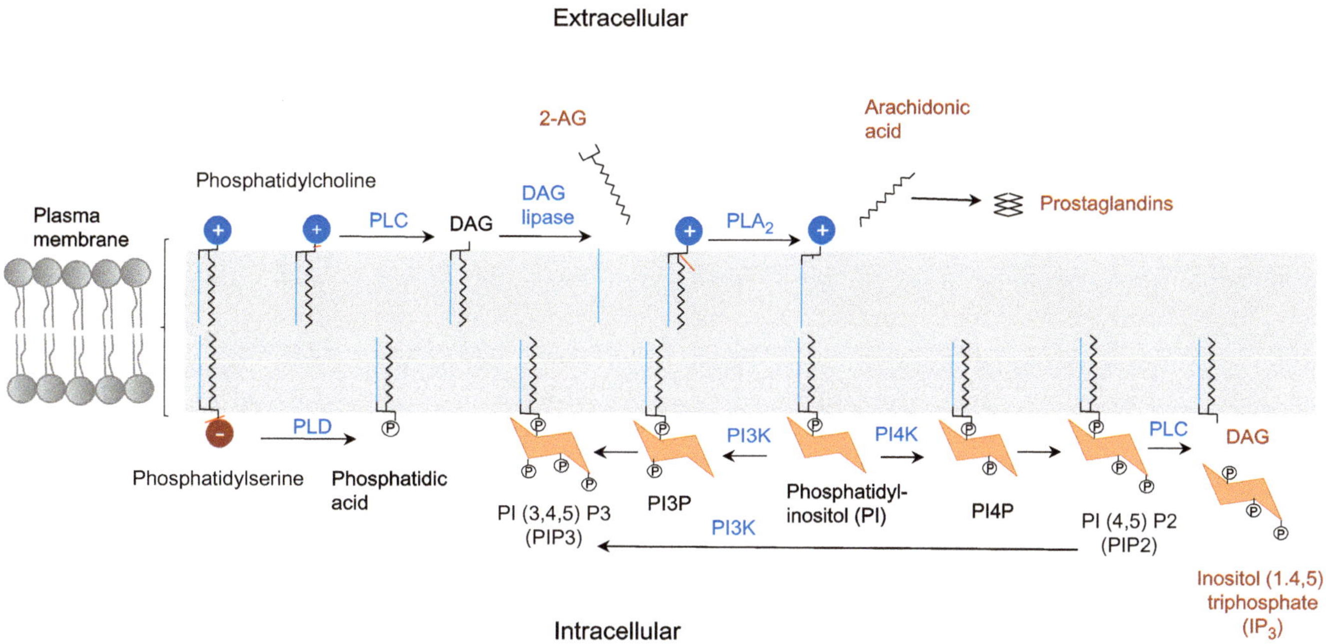

FIGURE 2.2 Organization and metabolism of membrane phospholipids.
Phosphatidylcholine and phosphatidylethanolamine are predominantly present in the outer leaflet of the membrane; phosphatidylserine and phosphoinositides predominate in the inner (cytoplasmic) leaflet. Phosphatidylinositol is phosphorylated by phosphatidylinositol 4'kinase (PI4K) to phosphatidylinositol 4 phosphate (PI4P), which is further phosphorylated to phosphatidylinositol 4,5 bisphosphate (PIP2). Alternatively, phosphatidylinositol 3'kinase (PI3K) catalyzes the production of 3-phosphoinositides, including phosphatidylinositol 3,4,5 triphosphate (PIP3). Phospholipase A2 (PLA2) produces lysolecithin and arachidonic acid; arachidonic acid serves as substrate for synthesis of prostanoids. Phospholipase D yields glycerol and phosphatidic acid. Phospholipase C (PLC) cleaves membrane PIP2 to yield diacylglycerol (DAG) and inositol triphosphate (IP_3), which are critical signaling molecules. Diacylglycerol is metabolized by a diacylglycerol lipase to the endocannabinoid 2-acylglycerol (2-AG).

D yields glycerol and phosphatidic acid, which functions as a signal molecule.[2] Phospholipase C cleaves membrane PIP2 to yield diacylglycerol (DAG) and inositol triphosphate, which are critical signaling molecules downstream of some neurotransmitter and growth factor receptors. Diacylglycerol is metabolized by a diacylglycerol lipase to the endocannabinoid 2-acylglycerol.

SPHINGOLIPIDS

Sphingolipids are more abundant in the outer than in the inner membrane leaflet. They contain a backbone consisting of the alcohol sphingosine combined with a long-chain fatty-acid-forming ceramide (Figure 2.3). Synthesis of ceramide occurs in the ER. Ceramide is transported to the Golgi apparatus, where it is converted to either sphingomyelin or glycosphingolipids. Ceramide combines with choline to produce sphingomyelin, which is the main sphingolipid in cell membranes, especially in the myelin sheath. Ceramide also combines with mono- or polysaccharides to form glycosphingolipids (also called glycolipids or cerebrosides) and gangliosides. The addition of neutral sugars and sialic acid molecules to ceramide occurs via actions of specific glycosyltransferases in the Golgi apparatus. These reactions are inhibited by miglustat. The most abundant cerebroside is galactosylceramide (galactocerebroside), which can be esterified by sulfate to produce sulfatides; both of them are enriched in CNS myelin.[3] Fatty acid hydroxylase 2 (FA2H) produces 2-hydroxylated fatty acids for ceramide species that are precursors for galactosylceramide and sulfatides. Alternatively, ceramide combines with glucose to produce glucosylceramide (glucocerebroside) or with a glucose-galactose-galactose trisaccharide to yield ceramide trihexoside (globoside).

Gangliosides

Gangliosides are glycosphingolipids that are particularly abundant in neurons and are expressed primarily at lipid rafts in the outer leaflet of the plasma membrane (Figure 2.3). They consist of a hydrophobic ceramide tail inserted in the membrane and a hydrophilic oligosaccharide moiety that is exposed extracellularly.[4] This carbohydrate portion consists of a variable backbone chain of neutral carbohydrates (galactose, glucose, and N-acetylgalactosamine) linked to one or more residues of negatively charged sialic

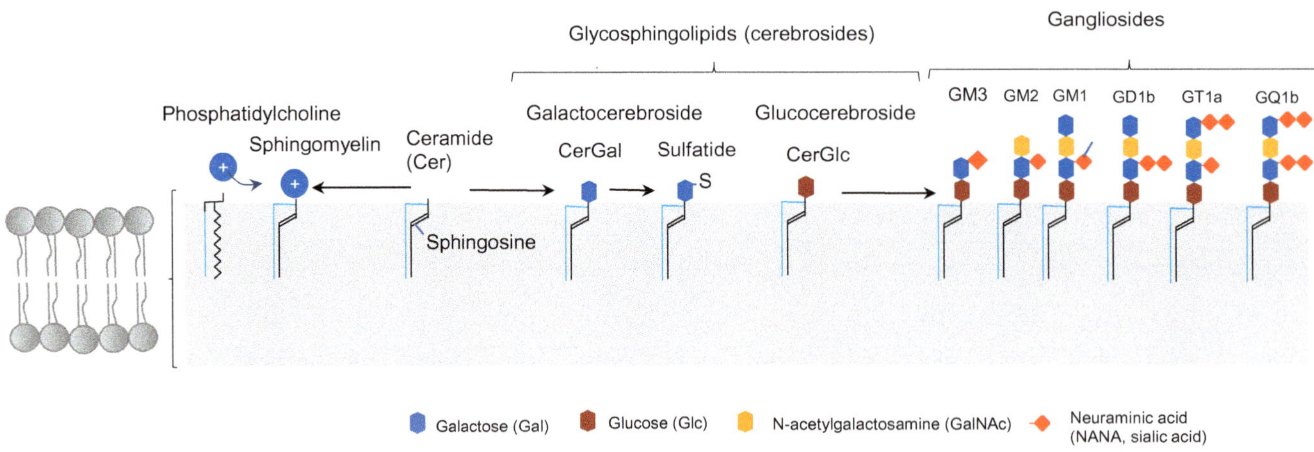

FIGURE 2.3 Organization of membrane sphingolipids.
Sphingolipids contain a backbone consisting of the alcohol sphingosine combined with a long chain 2-hydroxylated fatty acid forming ceramide. Ceramide combines with choline to produce sphingomyelin. Ceramide also combines with mono- or polysaccharides to form glycosphingolipids (also called glycolipids or cerebrosides) and gangliosides. The most abundant cerebroside is galactosylceramide (galactocerebroside), which can be esterified with sulfate to produce sulfatides. Ceramide combines with glucose to produce glucosylceramide. Gangliosides consist of a hydrophobic ceramide tail and a hydrophilic oligosaccharide moiety consisting of a variable backbone chain of neutral carbohydrates linked to one or more residues of negatively charged sialic acid (N-acetyl-neuraminic acid, NANA).

acid (N-acetyl-neuraminic acid). Gangliosides are named according to the nomenclature based on the number of sialic acid molecules, the length of the neutral sugar sequence, and the isomeric form. There is differential distribution of gangliosides in several regions of the nervous system and specific subcellular locations. For example GM1 is abundantly expressed in motor axons; GQ1b in oculomotor nerves; and GD1b in large dorsal root ganglion neurons. Gangliosides interact both laterally with transmembrane proteins located in the same membrane and with molecules in the opposing membrane. Gangliosides affect membrane proteins by influencing the fluidity of the plasma membrane and by the electrostatic effects of their negatively charged sialic acid residues. They have a major role in neuronal development and axonal growth, modulate function of ion channels and receptors, participate in Ca^{2+} channel homeostasis and signaling, and participate in cell–cell molecular interactions.

The constitutive degradation of sphingolipids and glycosphingolipids occurs via distinct acid hydrolases in the endosomes and lysosomes. Sphingomyelin is hydrolyzed back to ceramide by sphingomyelinase. Ceramide is hydrolyzed by ceramidase; sphingosine released from ceramide may become phosphorylated to sphingosine-1-phosphate. Glucosylceramide is degraded by β-glucocerebrosidase (β-glucosylceramidase), galactosylceramide by β galactocerebrosidase (β-galactosylceramidase), and sulfatides by arylsulphatase A. Alpha-galactosidase hydrolyzes the terminal α-galactose moieties from ceramide trihexoside.

Cholesterol

Cholesterol is a crucial component of mammalian membranes, as it stabilizes the lipid bilayers by intercalating at the interfaces between the head and tail regions of phospholipids. Sphingomyelin and gangliosides are stabilized via interactions with cholesterol at lipid rafts (Figure 2.1). The cholesterol content of the CNS is largely independent of dietary uptake or hepatic synthesis, as circulating cholesterol does not cross the blood-brain barrier. Cholesterol is formed from an isoprenoid backbone. The first steps of cholesterol synthesis are the formation of 3-hydroxy-3-methyglutaryl-CoA (HMG-CoA) in the cytoplasm followed by metabolism by the HMG-CoA reductase to mevalonate in the ER. Astrocytes are the main source of cholesterol for neurons. Astrocytes secrete cholesterol bound to apolipoprotein E (ApoE) via the ATP-binding cassette transporter protein family member A1 (ABCA1); neurons internalize ApoE-bound cholesterol via members of the low-density lipoprotein receptor (LDLR) family. Once in the cells, cholesterol passes through the late endosome system to the Golgi apparatus via a mechanism involving the late endosomal membrane protein Niemann-Pick type C (NPC) protein type 1 (NPC1) and its partner, the soluble lysosomal protein NPC2. In the CNS the main route of cholesterol elimination is its oxidation to form oxysterols, particularly 24-hydroxycholesterol, a process that is catalyzed primarily by members of the cytochrome P_{450} family. Oxysterols are major regulators of cholesterol homeostasis in the CNS; they act via liver X-activated receptors to prevent excessive intracellular accumulation of cholesterol.

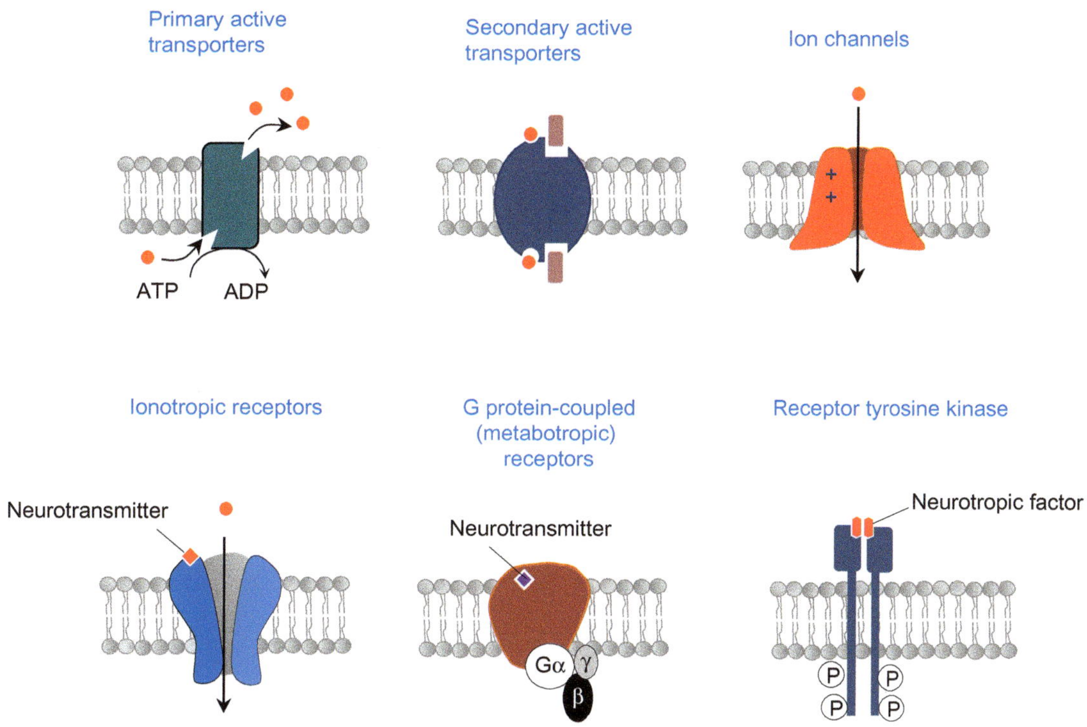

FIGURE 2.4 Examples of transmembrane proteins.
Most transmembrane proteins involved in cell signaling, homeostasis, and metabolism consist of several transmembrane helices that are usually closely packed. Examples include transporters, pumps, ion channels, neurotransmitter (NT) receptors and neurotrophin (NTF) tyrosine kinase receptors.

GENERAL FEATURES OF MEMBRANE PROTEINS

Membrane proteins are synthesized in polyribosomes attached to the ER. They include two types, integral and associated proteins. Integral membrane proteins consist of α-helices containing hydrophobic amino acids and traversing the lipid bilayer one or several times (Figure 2.1). These hydrophobic residues include stop-transfer sequences, which pause the translocation into the ER lumen and anchor the protein to the phospholipid bilayer. Some membrane-bound proteins are covalently linked to lipids, which promotes association of the protein to the lipid bilayer.

Structure and Localization of Membrane Proteins

Many transmembrane proteins, including transporters, pumps, neurotransmitter receptors, and ion channels have a critical role in cell signaling, homeostasis, and metabolism. (Figure 2.4). These proteins typically consist of a combination of different subunits. They include principal subunits that are primarily responsible for protein function, and auxiliary subunits that control membrane expression and function of the principal subunit. The function of transmembrane proteins is affected by their subunit composition, presence of auxiliary subunits, and posttranslational modifications, particularly phosphorylation. Transmembrane proteins are part of macromolecular complexes that include scaffold, adaptor, linker, and transducing proteins (Figure 2.5). Whereas the fluidity of the lipid bilayer permits their diffusion within the plane of the bilayer and dynamic interactions, membrane proteins are typically localized into specific domains, such as nodes of Ranvier or synaptic terminals in neurons or endfoot processes in astrocytes. This localization depends on networks of scaffolding, linker, and cytoskeletal proteins. Scaffold proteins are members of the large superfamily of membrane-associated guanylyl kinase homologs (MAGUKs), which contain different domains that allow their interaction with multiple partners, including membrane receptors, linker proteins, and signaling molecules.[5] A prototypical example of scaffold protein in the CNS is postsynaptic density protein-95 (PSD-95), which binds to ionotropic glutamate receptors at the postsynaptic densities in dendritic spines.[6] A typical example of a linker protein is ankyrin G, which, via interactions with spectrin, links voltage-gated sodium channels to the actin cytoskeleton at the axon initial segment and nodes of Ranvier.

Many proteins involved in signaling and cell–cell interactions are not transmembrane proteins but are associated proteins tethered to the outer leaflet of the plasma membrane. One important lipid modification of such proteins is

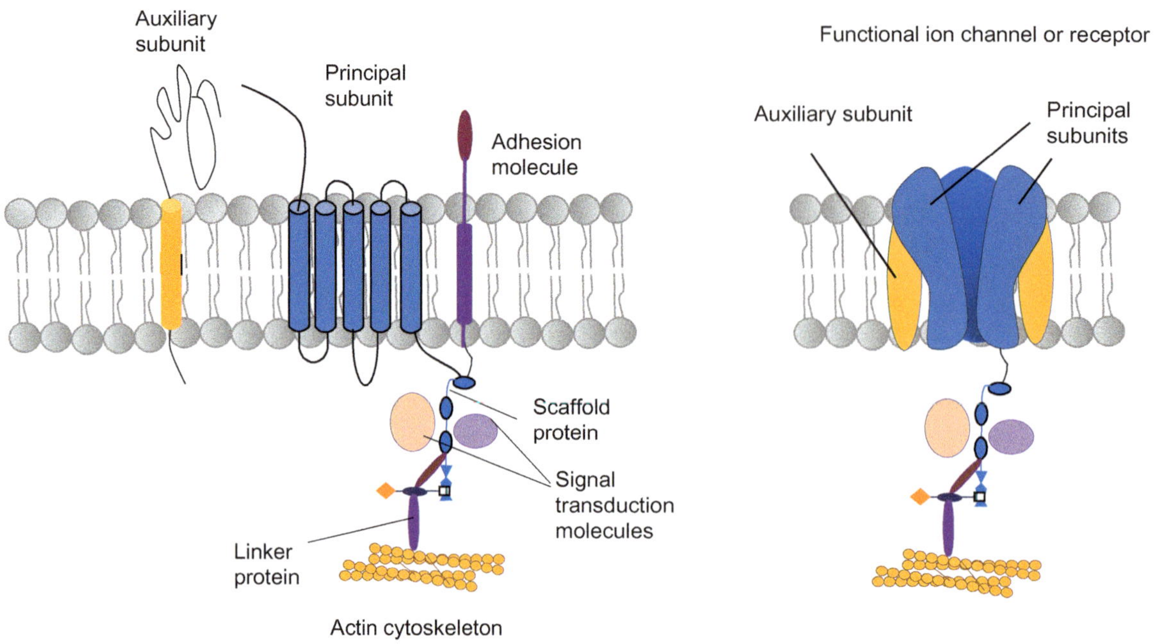

FIGURE 2.5 Organization of membrane protein complexes.
Membrane proteins involved in signaling include principal subunits primarily responsible for protein function and auxiliary subunits that control membrane expression and function of the principal subunit. Transmembrane proteins are part of macromolecular complexes that include scaffold, adaptor, linker, and transducing proteins. Scaffold proteins contain different domains that allow their interaction with multiple partners. Linker proteins interact with the actin cytoskeleton and anchor the multiprotein signaling complexes to specific functional domains of the membrane.

the formation of glycerophosphatidylinositol (GPI) anchors. These GPI anchors tether extracellular proteins such as prion proteins, receptors, adhesion molecules, and enzymes to the lipid rafts. The GPI anchor is synthesized and remodeled in a complex series of biochemical reactions that take place in the ER.[7] Lipid rafts also serve as platforms for localization and interaction of membrane proteins involved in vesicular transport and signaling, such as caveolins.

Dynamics of Membrane Proteins

Membrane proteins undergo a continuous bidirectional trafficking between the membrane and the intracellular compartments. Transmembrane proteins are synthesized, folded, and assembled in the ER and enter the secretory pathway, where they undergo posttranslational modifications in the Golgi apparatus. In the trans-Golgi network they are sorted into secretory vesicles targeted to the cell membrane; undergo anterograde transport via microtubules; and are inserted in the membrane via constitutive exocytosis. At the membrane, they undergo lateral diffusion within the plane of the membrane, and eventually become selectively localized in specific domains via interactions with scaffold and linker proteins, and ultimately the actin cytoskeleton. Membrane proteins, such as ligand-bound receptors, are recycled back to the cytoplasm via endocytosis. This process involves the formation of membrane invaginations via action of coating proteins such as clathrin, and incorporation into early endosomes that mature to late endosomes. Late endosomes may mature into vesicular structures that either allow membrane proteins to recycle back to the Golgi apparatus or plasma membrane or, alternatively, target them for lysosome degradation. In neurons, trafficking of membrane proteins, particularly receptors, is strongly affected by neuronal activity via mechanisms of phosphorylation or dephosphorylating of a variety of adaptor proteins. GPI-anchored proteins are synthesized in the cytoplasm, acquire their anchor during their transport to the ER, and are ultimately sorted to the outer leaflet of the membrane.

REPRESENTATIVE EXAMPLES OF MEMBRANE PROTEINS

Primary ATP-Dependent Transporters: Na^+/K^+ ATPase as the Prototype

Primary active transporters utilize energy from ATP hydrolysis to maintain transmembrane concentration gradients of sodium (Na^+), potassium (K^+), Ca^{2+}, and protons (H^+). These primary transporters include three main groups: P-type transporters such as the Na^+/K^+ ATPase, the membrane Ca^{2+} pumps, and the sarco/endoplasmic reticulum Ca^{2+} ATPase p (SERCA); the vesicular V0/V1 proton transporters; and the ATP-binding cassette (ABC) transporters. The Na^+/K^+ ATPase (sometimes referred to as sodium pump) is the most important example.[8] The Na^+/K^+ ATPase transports three Na^+ ions out of the cell in exchange for two K^+ ions with consumption of one ATP molecule. Activity of this transporter accounts for approximately 50% of total brain ATP consumption and is critical for maintenance of neuronal excitability via continuous restoration of transmembrane Na^+ and K^+ gradients, both at the steady state and following neuronal activity. The Na^+/K^+ ATPase also maintains the Na^+ gradient that drives secondary Na^+-coupled transporters such as the astrocytic excitatory amino acid transporters (EAATs). The functional Na^+/K^+ ATPase complex is composed of three subunits, α subunit, β subunit, and FXYD subunit. The α subunit is responsible for the catalytic activity and consists of 10 transmembrane helices containing the binding sites for Na^+ and K^+. This subunit undergoes phosphorylation and conformational transitions coupled to ATP hydrolysis and transport of ions. Of the four different isoforms of α subunit (α1–α4), three are expressed in the nervous system; the α1 subunit is expressed in neurons, glial cells, and throughout other tissues; the α2 subunit in astrocytes, oligodendrocytes, and skeletal muscle; and the α3 subunit in GABAergic neurons in the basal ganglia, cerebellum, and hippocampus and in photoreceptors.[8,9] The α1 subunit containing Na^+/K^+ ATPase has a major role in maintaining basal intracellular Na^+ level; the neuron specific α3-subunit-containing isoform participates in handling large transient increases in intracellular Na^+ during high neuronal activity. Neuronal activation also depolarizes the astrocyte membrane following the increase in extracellular K; the astrocyte-specific α2 subunit containing Na^+/K^+ ATPase clears extracellular K^+ to prevent further depolarization.[9]

The heavily glycosylated β subunit (including β1–β3 isoforms) targets the α subunit to the plasma membrane and functions as an intercellular adhesion protein. The Na^+/K^+ ATPase is often associated with a tissue-specific regulatory FXYD subunit that modulates the affinity of the enzyme for Na^+ and K^+ and is a target for phosphorylation. Intracellular Ca^{2+} inhibits enzyme activity by competing with Mg^{2+}, which is critical for ATP hydrolysis. The Na^+/K^+ ATPase is specifically inhibited by ouabain, digitalis, and several endogenous ouabain-like or digitalis-like steroids.

Another important example of P-family ATPases are those involved in maintenance of intracellular Ca^{2+} homeostasis. The ATP-dependent plasma membrane Ca^{2+} pump has high affinity for Ca^{2+} and is very sensitive to low Ca^{2+} concentrations; the smooth ER Ca^{2+} ATPase pumps Ca^{2+} from the cytosol to the ER for storage. Together with Na^+/Ca^{2+} antiporters these Ca^{2+} pumps act in concert to maintain a low concentration of cytosolic Ca^{2+} (~10^{-8} to 10^{-7} mol/l) in resting cells, which is critical to prevent cell toxicity.

The V0/V1 type primary transporters, termed vacuolar (V)-ATPases, pump protons (H^+) into the lumen of Golgi-derived organelles, including synaptic vesicles and lysosomes. In synaptic vesicles, the proton exchange drives storage of neurotransmitters; in endosomes and lysosomes V-ATPase activity is critical for acidification of intraluminal content. Finally, the ABC transporters participate in the transport of lipids and other amphiphilic molecules. Examples include ABC1, which is located in astrocytes and translocates cholesterol and phospholipids outward across the plasma membrane; and multidrug resistance proteins such as MDR1 or P-glycoprotein, which pumps drugs out of the cell and is highly expressed in the luminal membranes of brain endothelial and choroid plexus epithelial cells.

Solute Carrier Transporters

The solute carrier (SLC) group of membrane transport proteins include over 400 members organized into 65 families. These transporters contain several hydrophobic transmembrane domains and may function as either monomers or obligate homo- or hetero-oligomers. The *SLC* superfamily includes secondary active transporters that allow solutes to flow uphill against their electrochemical gradient by coupling to transport of a second solute such as Na^+ or H^+ downhill their concentration gradient driven by the ATP-dependent primary transporters, and facilitative transporters that allow solutes to flow downhill their electrochemical gradients.

One important example of secondary active transporters are the *SLC1* family, which includes EAATs that are expressed in astrocytes and neurons and are responsible for uptake of glutamate from the synaptic cleft. There is a tight functional coupling between these EAATs and the Na^+/K^+ ATPase, which generates the Na^+ gradient that drives the uptake of glutamate. Members of the *SLC6* subfamily of neurotransmitter transporters are Na^+/Cl^--dependent transporters that are involved in presynaptic reuptake of GABA, glycine, dopamine, norepinephrine, or serotonin. Transporters located in the membrane of synaptic vesicles are responsible for neurotransmitter storage and are driven by the proton gradient created by the vacuolar (V)-ATPases. Example include the vesicular glutamate transporters (SCL17 family) and vesicular monoamine transporters (SLC18 family).

A major example of facilitative transporters are members of the *SLC2* family that includes glucose transporters (GLUTs) involved in facilitated diffusion of glucose across the blood-brain barrier. GLUT1 is located in brain endothelial cells and the astrocytic endfeet covering the abluminal membranes of capillaries forming the blood-brain barrier and is critical for supply of glucose to the central nervous system. However, neurons can also take up glucose directly via GLUT3.

Several SLC transporters function as either antiporters or cotransporters. Antiporters exchange ions across the membrane according to their concentration gradients and independently of ATP. One important example of cation antiporter is the Na^+/Ca^{2+} exchanger (NCX, *SLC8* family), which has a major role in rapidly lowering high pulses of cytoplasmic Ca^{2+} by exchanging three Na^+ for one Ca^{2+} ion and is coupled with both the Na^+/K^+ ATPase and the Ca^{2+}

pumps. Other antiporters have a major role in regulation of pH and cerebrospinal fluid (CSF) production. For example the anion antiporter transports bicarbonate generated by CO_2 hydration by carbonic anhydrase both in astrocytes and in choroid plexus cells. Bicarbonate enters the cell in exchange with Cl^-. A decrease in intracellular pH triggers and efflux of protons in exchange for Na^+ via the Na^+/H^+ antiporter. An important example of cotransporters are the cation/chloride cotransporters, which have a major role in maintaining the transmembrane Cl^- gradient; this is critical both for volume regulation and for the synaptic effects of activation of $GABA_A$ and glycine receptors.[10] The K-Cl cotransporter 2 (KCC2) extrudes Cl^- from neurons maintaining a higher Cl^-concentration in the extracellular than in the intracellular space; the Na^+- K^+-2 Cl^- cotransporter 1 (NKCC1) mediates Cl^- influx and maintains a higher intracellular an extracellular Cl^- concentration.[11]

Aquaporins

Aquaporins (AQPs) are water channels consisting of homotetramers. AQP4 is expressed in the basolateral surface of ependymal cells (ventricular CSF-brain barrier); astrocyte subpial glial limitans (subarachnoid CSF-brain interface); perisynaptic astrocytic processes (neuronal-astrocyte interface); and particularly, at the astrocytic perivascular endfeet (blood-brain barrier). In the astrocyte endfeet, AQP4 is linked to the cytoskeleton in association with K^+ channels involved in coordinated regulation of cell volume and K^+ homeostasis. AQP1 is expressed in the apical surface epithelial cells of the choroid plexus; the Na^+/K^+ ATPase pumps Na^+ out of the apical surface of choroid epithelial cells and provides the osmotic gradient for extrusion of water through the AQP1 channel for CSF production.

Ion Channels and Neurotransmitter Receptors

Ion channels and receptors are members of different superfamilies and are critical to determine the electrophysiological properties and synaptic responses of neurons. These membrane proteins are described in more detail in other chapters of the book and only few examples will be briefly mentioned here. Voltage-gated Na^+, Ca^{2+}, and K^+ cation channels consist of a principal α subunit that forms the wall of the channel pore and auxiliary subunits. The elementary α subunit consists of six transmembrane segments (S1–S6) that have a modular structure: S1–S4 forms the selectivity filter and voltage sensor domain; the S5–S6 loop forms a pore domain. Ligand-gated ion channels, or ionotropic receptors, include three families. The cysteine residue family includes nicotinic acetylcholine receptor, 5-HT3 receptor, $GABA_A$ receptor, and glycine receptor. These receptors are pentamers consisting of several combinations of subunits, each with four transmembrane domains with the second domain forming the walls of the channel. The inotropic glutamate receptors are cation channels that contain three transmembrane domains and one reentrant cytoplasmic loop that forms the wall of the channel pore. Purinergic P2X receptors constitute the third family and are ATP-gated cation channels. G (guanosine nucleotide-binding) protein-coupled receptors are the largest family of receptors. They have seven transmembrane domains and contain both a ligand-binding site and G protein-interacting site. These receptors may occur as monomers or oligomers and are the most abundant receptors. Growth factor receptors bind neurotrophic factors, undergo dimerization and autophosphorylation, and triggers cell survival pathways.

Cell Adhesion Molecules

Cell adhesion molecules (CAMs) are cell surface proteins involved in cell-to-cell and cell-to-extracellular matrix (ECM) interactions and include several superfamilies. The immunoglobulin (Ig) superfamily comprises proteins that contain immunoglobulin-like domains with or without additional fibronectin III domains. Important examples are neural cell adhesion molecule (N-CAM) and L1, which have a critical role during development; myelin protein zero (MPZ, P0), involved in peripheral myelin compaction; and myelin associated glycoprotein (MAG), involved in myelin–axon interactions. In addition to serving as adhesion molecules, proteins of the Ig superfamily may initiate signal transduction cascades via their intracellular domains. The second major family are the cadherins that are stabilized by binding of Ca^{2+}, which is critical for their cell-to-cell adhesion function. Cadherins located on two opposing membranes bind to each other; and their full function requires their linkage to the actin cytoskeleton via catenins. The third family is that of integrins, which are major cell surface receptors responsible for cell adhesion to the ECM. Integrins are transmembrane heterodimers comprised of α- and β subunits with a large extracellular domain that recognizes ECM ligands such as laminin and fibronectin. Integrins form a link between the ECM and the actin cytoskeleton and are thus involved in mechanical stability and transduction in both the central and peripheral nervous system. Trans-synaptic CAMs organize synapse formation and control synapse morphology, receptor function, and synaptic elimination. One important example is transsynaptic synaptic adhesion interaction mediated by α- and β-neurexins, expressed in the presynaptic membrane and many postsynaptic partners, particularly neuroligins.[12]

DISORDERS OF MEMBRANE LIPID METABOLISM

Disorders of membrane lipid metabolism are an important disease pathway for neurologic disease. The prototype disorders reflect impaired endosome trafficking, lysosome hydrolase function, or mitochondrial metabolism.[13] They may affect primarily the gray or white matter and manifest with different phenotypes from infancy to adult life. This chapter and only a few points will be emphasized here

(Table 2.1). Mutations affecting enzymes involved in lipid metabolism are an important cause of upper and lower motor neuron disease.

Disorders of Sphingolipid Metabolism

Disorders affecting myelin glycosphingolipids may manifest with leukodystrophy.[14] Leukodistrophies manifest with an age-related phenotype, including regression of developmental skills spasticity, ataxia, optic atrophy, peripheral neuropathy, and behavioral changes. One typical example is metachromatic leukodystrophy due to mutations of *ARSA* gene encoding arylsulphatase A; deficit of this enzyme results in sulfatide accumulation reflected by sulfatiduria. Predominant involvement of the frontoparietal white matter and gallbladder are characteristic features. A second example is Krabbe disease due to *GALC* gene mutations producing β galactocerebrosidase deficiency; this leads to increased concentrations of galactosylceramide, which is toxic to oligodendrocytes. This disorder affects predominantly the periventricular and parietoocipital white matter. Other disorders of sphingolipid metabolism affect primarily the gray matter. Gaucher disease is due to homozygous mutations of the *GBA* (*GBA1*, *GCB*) gene encoding β glucocerebrosidase, leading to the buildup of glucosylceramide. Typical manifestations in infancy include irritability, opisthotonus, vertical gaze palsy. hepatomegaly, and conjunctival pingueculae. Heterozygous GBA/GCB mutations are a genetic risk factor for Parkinson disease.[15]

GM2 gangliosidoses are due to mutations of the *HEXA* gene encoding hexosaminidase A (Tay-Sachs disease) or the *HEXB* gene encoding hexosaminidase B (Sandhof disease), leading to inability to hydrolyze the N-acetylgalactosamine moiety of GM2 gangliosides and resulting in their accumulation predominantly in lysosomes of neurons. It is characterized by neurodegeneration preceded by activated microglia and astrocytes. GM2 gangliosidosis includes a severe early infantile, late infantile, juvenile and a rare late-onset form. The early infantile form is characterized by hypotonia. startle response, spasticity, blindness with a macular cherry red spot, seizures, and premature death. The late infantile and juvenile forms are characterized by psychomotor deterioration, spasticity, ataxia, seizures, and myoclonus. Adult-onset GM2 gangliosidosis may manifest with a proximal lower motor neuron disorder, cerebellar ataxia, or psychiatric disturbances, either alone or in various combinations.

Fabry disease is an X-linked disorder due to mutations of the *GALA* gene encoding α-galactosidase A, which hydrolyzes the terminal α-galactosyl moieties from glycolipids and glycoproteins.[16] This leads to accumulation of ceramide trihexoside, particularly in endothelial cells, heart, and kidneys. Fabry disease manifests with painful small fiber neuropathy, stroke, cardiac disease, renal disease, and cutaneous and eye findings. Enzyme replacement therapy with recombinant α-galactosidase A promotes a long-term slowdown of disease progression. Chaperone therapy (migalastat) is a currently approved therapy for Fabry disease and can only be used in patients with specific mutations.[16]

Niemann-Pick Type C Disease

Niemann-Pick type C (NPC) is an autosomal recessive lysosomal storage disorder caused by a failure in cholesterol trafficking, due to a due to mutations in the *NPC1* (95% of cases) or *NPC2* genes.[17–19] This disorder results in accumulation of unesterified cholesterol and sphingolipids in the late endosomes and lysosomes. Sphingosine accumulation may reflect impaired conversion of sphingosine to sphingosine-1 phosphate during endocytic processing. NPC has extreme clinical heterogeneity and its spectrum ranges from a rapidly fatal disorder in neonates to a neurodegenerative disorder in adults. Typical manifestations include vertical supranuclear palsy and hepatosplenomegaly. Delayed motor milestones, hypotonia, speech delay, cataplexy, and seizures occur in during childhood; psychiatric manifestations (such as atypical schizophrenia), dementia (mimicking frontotemporal dementia), dystonia, and ataxia occur in adolescence and adulthood. Neuropathological changes include accumulation of neurofibrillary tangles, neuronal degeneration, axonal dystrophy, and demyelination. Sphingosine appears to have a major role in inducing the NPC phenotype. Sphingosine accumulation may reflect impaired conversion of sphingosine to sphingosine-1 phosphate during endocytic processing. Whereas the definite diagnosis of NPC requires demonstration of *NPC1* or *NPC2* mutations, disease biomarkers include elevated levels of oxysterol species and the cholesterol metabolite 24-hydroxycholesterol. Sphingolipid quantification by mass spectrometry shows elevated levels of ceramide and monohexosylceramides. Miglustat reduces accumulation of downstream toxic glycosphingolipids by competitively inhibiting the first step of their biosynthesis.

Disorders of Lipoprotein Transport and Intermediate Lipid Metabolism

Genetic disorders affecting lipoprotein and cholesterol metabolism may indirectly affect the nervous system but produce prominent neurologic manifestations. Cerebrotendinous xanthomatosis (CTX) is caused by mutations in the *CYP27A1* gene encoding the mitochondrial cytochrome P-450 enzyme sterol 27-hydroxylase. This mutation interferes with the initial side-chain oxidation step of the sterol intermediates in the alternative bile acid pathway, resulting in reduced synthesis of 27-hydroxycholesterol and chenodeoxycholic acid and increased production of cholestenol, which accumulates in the brain and other tissues. Neurologic manifestations include ataxia, dementia, dystonia, epilepsy, spasticity peripheral neuropathy, and myopathy. Premature non-neurologic manifestations, such as tendon xanthomas, cataracts, diarrhea, atherosclerosis, osteoporosis, and pulmonary insufficiency distinguish CTX from other lipid-storage disorders. Magnetic

TABLE 2.1 *Disorders of Lipid Metabolism*

Disorder	Gene (protein)	Consequence	Therapeutic Approach
Disorders of sphingolipid metabolism			
Metachromatic dystrophy	*ARSA* (arylsulfatase A)	Sulfatide accumulation	HSCT
Krabbe disease	*GALC* (β galactocerebrosidase)	Galactosylceramide accumulation (toxic to oligodendrocytes)	HSCT
Gaucher disease	*GBA* (glucocerebrosidase)	Glucosylceramide accumulation and impaired lysosomal function	Enzyme replacement therapy (imiglucerase, velaglucerase, or taliglucerase) Miglustat or eliglustat
Fabry disease	*GALA* (α-galactosidase)	Ceramide trihexoside accumulation in endothelium, heart, and kidneys	ERT Migalastat
GM2 gangliosidosis (Tay-Sachs disease)	*HEXA* (hexosaminidase A)	GM2 ganglioside accumulation in neurons	Miglustat? HSCT?
Disorders of cholesterol or and lipoprotein trafficking			
Niemann-Pick type C	*NPC1*, *NPC2*	Uunesterified cholesterol and sphingolipids (sphingosine) accumulation Sphingosine toxicity Elevated oxysterols	Miglustat
Cerebrotendinous xanthomatosis	*CYP27A1* (mitochondrial cytochrome P-450 enzyme sterol 27-hydroxylase)	Cholestanol accumulation	Chenodeoxycolic acid
Ataxia with vitamin E deficiency	*TTPA* (α-tocopherol transfer protein)	Impaired passage of vitamin E into general circulation	Large-dose vitamin E supplementation
Abetalipoproteinemia	*MTTP* (microsomal triglyceride transfer protein)	Altered secretion of apolipoprotein B-containing lipoprotein hypocholesterolemia and malabsorption of lipid-soluble vitamins	Lipid-soluble vitamin supplementation
Tangier disease	*ABCA1* (ABCA1 transporter)	Deficiency of high-density lipoprotein deficiency Deposition of cholesteryl esters in the reticuloendothelial tissues and peripheral nerves	Cholesteryl ester transfer protein inhibitors (dalcetrapib, anacetrapib) and reconstituted HDL
Peroxisomal disorders			
X-linked adrenoleukodystrophy Adrenomyeloneuropathy	*ABCD1* (ATP-binding membrane protein)	Impaired transport of VLCF for β-oxidation leading to accumulation of VLCFA	HSCT
Refsum disease	*PHYH* (phytanoyl-CoA hydroxylase)	Impaired α-oxidation of phytanic acid, which accumulates and is toxic to mitochondria	Dietary restriction Plasma exchange

ERT, enzyme replacement therapy; HDL, high density lipoprotein; HSCT, hematopoietic stem cell transplantation; VLCFA, very long-chain fatty acids resonance imaging (MRI) shows bilateral lesions in the dentate nucleus and white matter. Elevated levels of cholestanol in serum and urine together with brain MRI and *CYP27A1* mutation confirm the diagnosis of CTX. Early diagnosis and long-term treatment with chenodeoxycholic acid improve neurological symptoms.[20]

Ataxia with vitamin E deficiency (AVED) is caused by mutations in the α-tocopherol transfer protein gene (*TTPA*) leading to impaired passage of vitamin E into general circulation. Abetalipoproteinemia is due to altered assembly and secretion of apolipoprotein B-containing lipoprotein particles due to mutations in the microsomal triglyceride transfer protein (*MTTP* gene), resulting in hypocholesterolemia and malabsorption of lipid-soluble vitamins. Both AVED and abetalipoproteinemia manifest with a phenotype that resembles Friederich ataxia. Tangier disease is an autosomal recessive disorder due to mutations in the *ABCA1* gene encoding the ABCA1 transporter leading to severe high-density lipoprotein deficiency. It is characterized by deposition of cholesteryl esters in the reticuloendothelial tissues and peripheral nerves and manifests with enlarged tonsils, splenomegaly, and different neuropathy types.[21]

Peroxisomal Disorders

Peroxisomes are key multifunctional, dynamic, membrane-bound metabolic organelles, which contribute to the β-oxidation of fatty acids and the synthesis of myelin sheath lipids, as well as cellular redox balance.[22] Peroxisomes interact with the ER, mitochondria, lysosomes, and lipid droplets. Peroxisomal disorders can be divided into peroxisome biogenesis disorders and single enzyme defects.[23] Two relevant peroxisomal enzyme defects are X-linked adrenoleukodystrophy (X-ALD) and Refsum disease. X-linked adrenoleukodystrophy (X-ALD) and is caused by mutations in the *ABCD1* gene encoding an ATP-binding membrane protein that is necessary for the transport of saturated very long-chain unbranched fatty acids (VLCFA) across the peroxisomal membrane for their β-oxidation. Impaired oxidation results in increased VLCFA levels in plasma and cells. The clinical presentation of patients with X-ALD may vary considerably even within families and may reflect the age of onset and organ affected. The most frequent presentations are the severe cerebral ALD form typically with onset in childhood and the milder adrenomyeloneuropathy with onset in or after the third decade. Allogenic hematopoietic stem cell transplantation in an early stage prevents progression of disease of the cerebral form. Refsum disease is caused by impaired α-oxidation of phytanic acid, due to *PHYH* gene mutations leading to deficiency in phytanoyl-CoA hydroxylase. The resulting accumulation of phytanic acid serves as a biomarker of this disorder and is thought to induce oxidative damage and mitochondrial dysfunction. Typical manifestations include peripheral neuropathy, retinitis pigmentosa, anosmia, deafness, and ichthyosis. Treatment includes dietary restriction of phytanic acid in combination with plasmapheresis.

Neurodegeneration with Brain Iron Accumulation

Neurodegeneration with brain iron accumulation (NBIA) is a group of disorders characterized by dystonia, parkinsonism, spasticity, and other manifestations.[24,25] The major feature is iron accumulation in the globus pallidus and the substantia nigra, which may be visualized with MRI using gradient echo sequences, susceptibility-weighted imaging, T2*-weighted sequences and R* mapping. These areas naturally contain high iron concentrations and also have a high metabolic requirement. Retinal cells also have a high metabolic rate and are often affected in NBIA patients. NBIA may be associated with axonal swellings, and α-synuclein or hyperphosphorylated tau accumulation. All proteins defective in NBIA are known or suspected to be involved in mitochondrial function (Table 2.2). Of the mutations so far linked to NBIA, two have a direct role in iron metabolism: *FTL* (ferritin light chain) mutations producing neuroferritinopathy and *CPL* (ceruloplasmin) mutations producing aceruloplasminemia. Several NBIA-linked mutations affect genes related to membrane lipid metabolism. They include *PANK2* (pantothenate kinase 2) associated with pantothenate kinase-associated neurodegeneration (PKAN, NBIA type 1); *COASY* (coenzyme A synthase) associated with coenzyme A synthase–associated neurodegeneration (CoPAN); *PLA2G6* (phospholipase A2 group 6) associated with phospholipase A2-associated neurodegeneration (PLAN); *FA2H* (fatty acid 2 hydroxylase) associated with fatty acid 2-hydroxylase-associated neurodegeneration (FAHN); and potentially *C19orf12* (C19orf12) associated with mitochondrial membrane protein-associated neurodegeneration (MPAN). Both PANK2 and COASY are expressed in the mitochondrial matrix and are involved in CoA synthesis. PLA2G6 hydrolyzes glycerophospholipids to produce lysophospholipids and free fatty acids. FA2H catalyzes the 2-hydroxylation of fatty acids as precursors for synthesis of ceramide. Normal lipid metabolism is also necessary for maintenance of membrane structures in mitochondria and lysosomes. For example, PLA2G6-mediated neurodegeneration may reflect inability to remodel oxidized and damaged phospholipids. Other mutations associated with NBIA affect proteins involved in lysosomal membrane function and dynamics. For example, *ATP13A2* loss-of-function mutations produce Kufor-Rakeb syndrome. These mutations impair activity of the lysosomal ATPase 13A2, which functions as divalent cation transporter, and lead to accumulation of divalent ions such as manganese and secondary mitochondrial damage. The protein involved in beta propeller-associated neurodegeneration (BPAN) may have a critical role in autophagy.

TABLE 2.2 *Neurodegeneration with Brain Iron Accumulation*

Disorder (gene)	Function	Clinical Features	MRI Features
PKAN (*PANK2*)	Pantothenate kinase (coenzyme A synthesis)	Dystonia, parkinsonism, spasticity, pigmentary retinopathy, acanthocytosis,	T2 hyperintense signal surrounded by hypointense signal in the globus pallidus ("eye of the tiger" sign)
CoPAN (*CoASY*)	Coenzyme A synthesis	Intellectual disability, dystonia, spasticity, behavioral difficulties	T2 hypointense signal in globus pallidus and substantia nigra
PLAN *(PLA2G6)*	Calcium-independent phospholipase A2	Psychomotor regression, autism, dystonia, ataxia, parkinsonism, optic atrophy	Affects globus pallidus and substantia nigra, cerebellar atrophy
FAHN (*FA2H*)	Fatty acid 2-hydroxylase	Spasticity, ataxia, dystonia, optic atrophy, dementia, seizures	T2 hypointense signal in globus pallidus; diffuse cerebral atrophy, white matter changes
MPAN (*C19orf12*)	Mitochondrial membrane protein	Spasticity, dystonia, dementia, peripheral neuropathy	Medial medullary lamina streak between the external and internal segment of the globus pallidus
BPAN (*WDR45*)	Beta-propeller protein involved in autophagosome formation	Intellectual disability, impaired language, autism, seizures types, juvenile parkinsonism	"Halo" in the substantia nigra and cerebellar peduncles on T1 sequences
Kufor-Rakeb syndrome (*ATPA13A2*)	Divalent cation-transporter	Juvenile parkinsonism dementia	T2 hypointense signal in striatum, with global atrophy
Aceruloplasminemia (*CPL*)	Ceruloplasmin	Adult-onset retinal degeneration, diabetes mellitus, chorea, dystonia, ataxia	T2 hypointense signal in basal ganglia, thalamus, and dentate, without cavitation
Neuroferritinopathy (*FTL*)	Ferritin light chain	Adult-onset chorea or dystonia with subtle cognitive deficits	Cavitary lesions and T2 hypointense signals in the basal ganglia, dentate, and thalamus

CoPAN, coenzyme A synthase-associated neurodegeneration (CoPAN); *FAHN* fatty acid 2-hydroxylase-associated neurodegeneration; MPAN, mitochondrial membrane protein-associated neurodegeneration; PKAN, pantothenate kinase-associated neurodegeneration PLAN, phospholipase A2-associated neurodegeneration

Disorders Affecting Synthesis of the GPI Anchor

Several genetic disorders, mostly autosomal recessive but some X-linked, result from mutations of genes encoding different classes of phosphatidylinositol glycan biosynthesis enzymes involved in the complex pathway of GPI anchor synthesis.[7] Clinical phenotypes are often variable, even within the same mutated gene. Mutations of phosphatidylinositol glycan biosynthesis class A protein (PIGA), which adds a N-acetylglucosamine residue to phosphatidylinositol in the ER membrane, has been linked to paroxysmal nocturnal hemoglobinuria. Mutations affecting GPI anchor biosynthesis also cause a clinically heterogeneous spectrum of disorders including early-onset epileptic encephalopathy with severe muscular hypotonia, dysmorphism, multiple congenital anomalies, and early death; neurodegenerative encephalopathy with systemic iron overload; and intellectual disability and seizures (including West syndrome) with or without dysmorphism. Other manifestations include structural brain abnormalities, macrocephaly, increased birth weight, joint contractures, coarse facial features, and cardiac and renal abnormalities.[26]

DISORDERS AFFECTING MEMBRANE TRANSPORTERS

Membrane proteins are a fundamental target in neurologic disorders. Disorders of ion channels and receptors are discussed in different chapters. Disorders affecting two fundamental membrane transporters will be discussed here.

Impaired Na^+/K^+ ATPase Activity in Acquired Neurologic Disease

Impaired activity of the Na^+/K^+ ATPase is a primary mechanism of acute injury of neurons and glial cells in the setting of trauma, hypoxia, ischemia, hypoglycemia, and other conditions associated with failure of oxidative mitochondrial metabolism and ATP production.[9] Reduced function of the Na^+/K^+ ATPase results in inability to maintain the resting membrane potential and to restore transmembrane K^+ and Na^+ gradients, leading to membrane depolarization, abnormal excitability, and influx of Ca^{2+} via voltage- and glutamate-activated channels. Failure to maintain the transcellular Na^+ gradient also leads to a secondary failure of secondary transporters, such as EAATs in astrocytes and transporters involved in maintenance of cell volume, leading to excitotoxic injury and cytotoxic edema. Impaired Na^+/K^+ ATPase function may also have a role in epilepsy. In axons, impaired Na^+/K^+ ATPase lead to increase in intra-axonal Na^+, which promotes reverse operation of the Na^+/Ca^{2+} exchanger and accumulation of intra-axonal Ca^{2+}, resulting in axonal injury.

Genetic Disorders Affecting the Na^+/K^+ ATPase

Mutations affecting the Na^+/K^+ ATPase are either de novo variants or have dominant inheritance.[8] These mutations can produce defects in ATPase activity, ion affinity, ion leakage, or biosynthesis.[27] Disease variants in *ATP1A1* are found in cases of Marie-Charcot-Tooth type disease.[28] Mutations in the *ATP1A2* gene encoding the α2 subunit expressed in astrocytes cause familial hemiplegic migraine (FHM) type 2.[8,9] The proposed mechanism in FHM2 is increased predisposition to cortical spreading depression due to the astrocyte's inability to clear K^+ and glutamate from the extracellular space. Diverse functional abnormalities has been associated with *ATP1A2* mutations.[29] Other FHM genes include *CACNA1A*, encoding the α1 subunit of P/Q type (Cav2.1) voltage-gated Ca^{2+} channel (FHM1); *SCN1A*, encoding the α subunit of a the Na_v1 voltage-gated Na^+ channel (FHM3); and *PRRT2*, encoding proline rich repeat transmembrane protein 2, which regulates exocytosis. All mutations associated with FHM may also be associated with epilepsy or other paroxysmal syndromes.

Variants in *ATP1A3* produce several overlapping phenotypes. The most severe have onset in infancy and include alternating hemiplegia of childhood and early infantile epileptic encephalopathy. Milder phenotypes have onset in children and adults and include rapid-onset dystonia-parkinsonism; rapid-onset cerebellar ataxia; cerebellar ataxia, areflexia, pes cavus, optic nerve atrophy, and sensorineural deafness; relapsing encephalopathy and cerebellar ataxia; and fever-induced paroxysmal muscle weakness and encephalopathy.[8,9,30–32] The majority of heterozygous mutations in the *ATP1A3* gene cause both sporadic and inherited forms of rapid-onset dystonia-parkinsonism and alternating hemiplegia of childhood. Neurons in the basal ganglia, cerebellum, and hippocampus express primarily the α3 subunit of the Na^+/K^+ ATPase, which may explain the phenotype.[9] Rapid-onset dystonia-parkinsonism (DYT12) most often affects adolescents and young adults and is characterized by an abrupt onset and rapid evolution (over a period of hours to weeks) of orofacial dystonia, dysarthria, dysphagia, dystonic spasms predominantly in the upper limbs, and variable bradykinesia and postural instability with or without rigidity. The clinical onset often occurs after triggering events such as minor head injuries, running, alcohol binges, overheating, emotional stress, infections, or childbirth. These patients are usually nonresponsive to levodopa but may show symptomatic relief with benzodiazepines. Alternating hemiplegia of childhood may respond to calcium channel blockers, topiramate, ketogenic diet, and benzodiazepines. This indicates that the main pathogenic mechanism of impaired functioning of mutant α3 Na^+/K^+ ATPase is neuronal hyperactivity, consistent with impaired GABAergic inhibition. Severe *ATP1A3* mutations may be associated with gain-of-function that is potentially toxic. The α3 subunit containing Na^+/K^+ ATPase may directly interact with abnormal α-synuclein, tau, and amyloid-β, and may contribute to their cell-to-cell propagation. These intermolecular interactions may result in the formation of deleterious clusters/aggregates of pathogenic proteins, often at the vicinity of the synapses and act as diffusion-trap for membrane Na^+/K^+ ATPase, reducing the capacity to rapidly extrude Na^+ following neuronal activity and contributing to the neurodegenerative process.[9]

Glucose Transporter Deficiency Syndrome

Mutation of the *SLC2A1* gene encoding glucose transporter type 1 (GLUT1), involved in transport of glucose across the blood-brain barrier, produce GLUT1 deficiency syndrome, which manifests with a widely variable phenotype.[33] The classic phenotype is characterized by infantile-onset seizures, delayed neurologic development, acquired microcephaly, and complex movement disorders. Seizures in classic early-onset disease begin before age six months and include generalized tonic or clonic, focal, myoclonic, atypical absence, atonic, and unclassified forms. In some infants, apneic episodes and abnormal episodic eye-head movements may precede the onset of seizures. Cognitive impairment, ranging from learning disabilities to severe intellectual disability, is typical. The complex movement disorder includes ataxia, dystonia, and chorea; they may occur in any combination and may be continuous, paroxysmal, or continuous with fluctuations in severity influenced by environmental factors such as fasting, infections, or stress.

In addition to this classical phenotype, GLUT1 deficiency syndrome may manifest with a continuum that includes paroxysmal exercise-induced dyskinesia and epilepsy; paroxysmal choreoathetosis with spasticity; atypical childhood absence epilepsy; myoclonic astatic epilepsy, and other paroxysmal syndromes such as intermittent ataxia, choreoathetosis, dystonia, and alternating hemiplegia. The diagnosis of GLUT1 deficiency syndrome is established in a patient with suggestive clinical findings; normal blood glucose concentration; CSF glucose concentration inappropriately, low typically <40 mg/dL; and identification of a pathogenic *SLC2A1* variant by molecular genetic testing. If no pathogenic variant is identified, 3-O-methyl-D-glucose uptake in erythrocytes can be performed; results between 35% and 74% of controls are diagnostic. The ketogenic diet is highly effective in controlling the seizures and improving gait disturbance and is generally well tolerated. However, ketogenic diet is effective early in life but becomes less so as children mature, reflecting the different brain's substrate preference. Patients on a ketogenic diet should receive L-carnitine supplementation and proper hydration; they should avoid carbonic anhydrase inhibitors, carbohydrate-containing foods, intravenous fluids, medications that interrupt the state of ketosis, and valproic acid because it increases the risk of a Reye-like illness.

KEY POINTS

- Membranes are composed by of lipids and proteins.
- Phosphoinositides have a major role in shaping the membrane curvature for vesicular biogenesis and in intracellular signal transduction.
- Sphingolipids derive from ceramide and include sphingomyelin, glycosphingolipids, and gangliosides.
- The most abundant cerebroside is galactosylceramide, which can be esterified with sulfate to produce sulfatides; both of them are enriched in CNS myelin.
- Gangliosides have a major role in neuronal development and axonal growth, modulate function of ion channels, and participate in cell–cell molecular interactions.
- The constitutive degradation of sphingolipids and glycosphingolipids occurs via distinct acid hydrolases in the endosomes and lysosomes.
- Cholesterol is a crucial component that stabilizes the lipid bilayers.
- Integral membrane proteins include ion pumps, transporters, ion channels, receptors, and adhesion molecules.
- Transmembrane transport and signaling proteins consist of a combination of different subunits and form macromolecular complexes with scaffold, adaptor, linker, and transducing proteins.
- Transmembrane proteins are typically localized into specific domains of cells.
- Membrane proteins undergo a continuous bidirectional trafficking between the membrane and the intracellular compartments; they are targeted to the cell membrane via the secretory pathway and are recycled back to the cytoplasm via endocytosis.
- The Na^+/K^+ ATPase accounts for approximately 50% of total brain ATP consumption and is critical for maintenance of neuronal excitability and Na^+ gradients to drive secondary Na^+-coupled transporters.
- The solute carrier (SLC) family includes the excitatory amino acid transporters (EAATs) responsible for uptake of glutamate from the synaptic cleft; and the glucose transporter-1 (GLUT1), critical for supply of glucose to the central nervous system.
- Cell adhesion molecules (CAMs) mediate cell-to-cell and cell-to-extracellular matrix (ECM) interaction critical for neural development, mechanic stability, and synaptic organization.
- Metachromatic leukodystrophy and Krabbe disease are disorders of metabolism of myelin glycosphingolipids producing leukodystrophy with age-dependent clinical manifestations; hematopoietic stem cell transplantation may slow progression at early stages.
- Fabry disease is an X-linked disorder that may manifest with a painful peripheral neuropathy or strokes in the young; migalastat may slow progression in individual cases.
- Homozygous mutations of the *GBA* (GBA1, GCB) gene encoding β glucocerebrosidase cause Gaucher disease; heterozygous GBA mutations are linked to Parkinson disease.
- Niemann-Pick type C (NPC) is caused by a failure in cholesterol trafficking; it is associated with increased levels of oxysterols, and is treatable with miglustat.
- Cerebrotendinous xanthomatosis (CTX) is associated with elevated plasma levels of cholestanol, and is treatable with chenodeoxycholic acid.
- X-linked adrenoleukodystrophy is a peroxisomal disorder affecting catabolism of very long-chain fatty acids, resulting in their increased levels in plasma and tissues; HSCT may slow disease progression at early stages in the childhood cerebral form.
- Refsum disease is a peroxisomal disorder resulting in accumulation of phytanic acid; treatments include avoidance of phytanic acid-containing foods and plasma exchange.
- Neurodegeneration with brain iron accumulation (NBIA) is frequently due to mutations of enzymes involved in lipid metabolism and affects myelinated axons and mitochondria.

- Mutations in the *ATP1A2* gene expressed in astrocytes cause familial hemiplegic migraine (FHM) type 2.
- Variants in *ATP1A3* produce alternating hemiplegia of childhood, early infantile epileptic encephalopathy, rapid-onset dystonia-parkinsonism, rapid-onset cerebellar ataxia;, and fever-induced paroxysmal muscle weakness.
- Mutations of the *SLC2A1* gene encoding glucose transporter type 1 (GLUT1) may manifest with atypical childhood absence epilepsy, variable cognitive impairment, paroxysmal exercise-induced dyskinesia and epilepsy, paroxysmal choreoathetosis with spasticity, and alternating hemiplegia; CSF glucose is typically <40 mg/dL and ketogenic diet is highly effective in controlling symptoms early in life.

REFERENCES

1. Lauwers E, Goodchild R, Verstreken P. Membrane lipids in presynaptic function and disease. Neuron 2016;90:11–25.
2. Yung YC, Stoddard NC, Mirendil H, Chun J. Lysophosphatidic acid signaling in the nervous system. Neuron 2015;85:669–682.
3. Aggarwal S, Yurlova L, Simons M. Central nervous system myelin: structure, synthesis and assembly. Trends Cell Biol 2011;21:585–593.
4. Schnaar RL. The biology of gangliosides. Adv Carbohydr Chem Biochem 2019;76:113–148.
5. Ye F, Zeng M, Zhang M. Mechanisms of MAGUK-mediated cellular junctional complex organization. Curr Opin Struct Biol 2018;48:6–15.
6. Zhu J, Shang Y, Zhang M. Mechanistic basis of MAGUK-organized complexes in synaptic development and signalling. Nat Rev Neurosci 2016;17:209–223.
7. Ng BG, Freeze HH. Human genetic disorders involving glycosylphosphatidylinositol (GPI) anchors and glycosphingolipids (GSL). J Inherit Metab Dis 2015;38:171–178.
8. Clausen MV, Hilbers F, Poulsen H. The structure and function of the Na,K-ATPase isoforms in health and disease. Front Physiol 2017;8:371.
9. Shrivastava AN, Triller A, Melki R. Cell biology and dynamics of neuronal Na(+)/K(+)-ATPase in health and diseases. Neuropharmacology 2018:107461.
10. Ben-Ari Y, Khalilov I, Kahle KT, Cherubini E. The GABA excitatory/inhibitory shift in brain maturation and neurological disorders. Neuroscientist 2012;18:467–486.
11. Watanabe M, Fukuda A. Development and regulation of chloride homeostasis in the central nervous system. Front Cell Neurosci 2015;9:371.
12. Jeong J, Paskus JD, Roche KW. Posttranslational modifications of neuroligins regulate neuronal and glial signaling. Curr Opin Neurobiol 2017;45:130–138.
13. Platt FM, d'Azzo A, Davidson BL, Neufeld EF, Tifft CJ. Lysosomal storage diseases. Nat Rev Dis Primers 2018;4:27.
14. Kohler W, Curiel J, Vanderver A. Adulthood leukodystrophies. Nat Rev Neurol 2018;14:94–105.
15. Paciotti S, Albi E, Parnetti L, Beccari T. Lysosomal ceramide metabolism disorders: implications in Parkinson's disease. J Clin Med 2020;9.
16. van der Veen SJ, Hollak CEM, van Kuilenburg ABP, Langeveld M. Developments in the treatment of Fabry disease. J Inherit Metab Dis 2020.
17. Patterson MC, Clayton P, Gissen P, et al. Recommendations for the detection and diagnosis of Niemann-Pick disease type C: an update. Neurol Clin Pract 2017;7:499–511.
18. Bonnot O, Gama CS, Mengel E, et al. Psychiatric and neurological symptoms in patients with Niemann-Pick disease type C (NP-C): findings from the international NPC registry. World J Biol Psychiatry 2017:1–10.
19. Sobrido MJ, Bauer P, de Koning T, et al. Recommendations for patient screening in ultra-rare inherited metabolic diseases: what have we learned from Niemann-Pick disease type C? Orphanet J Rare Dis 2019;14:20.
20. Nie S, Chen G, Cao X, Zhang Y. Cerebrotendinous xanthomatosis: a comprehensive review of pathogenesis, clinical manifestations, diagnosis, and management. Orphanet J Rare Dis 2014;9:179.
21. Mercan M, Yayla V, Altinay S, Seyhan S. Peripheral neuropathy in Tangier disease: A literature review and assessment. J Peripher Nerv Syst 2018;23:88–98.
22. Islinger M, Voelkl A, Fahimi HD, Schrader M. The peroxisome: an update on mysteries 2.0. Histochem Cell Biol 2018;150:443–471.
23. Waterham HR, Ferdinandusse S, Wanders RJ. Human disorders of peroxisome metabolism and biogenesis. Biochim Biophys Acta 2016;1863:922–933.
24. Arber CE, Li A, Houlden H, Wray S. Review: Insights into molecular mechanisms of disease in neurodegeneration with brain iron accumulation: unifying theories. Neuropathol Appl Neurobiol 2016;42:220–241.
25. Hayflick SJ, Kurian MA, Hogarth P. Neurodegeneration with brain iron accumulation. Handb Clin Neurol 2018;147:293–305.
26. Fauth C, Steindl K, Toutain A, et al. A recurrent germline mutation in the PIGA gene causes Simpson-Golabi-Behmel syndrome type 2. Am J Med Genet A 2016;170A:392–402.
27. Sweadner KJ, Arystarkhova E, Penniston JT, Swoboda KJ, Brashear A, Ozelius LJ. Genotype-structure-phenotype relationships diverge in paralogs ATP1A1, ATP1A2, and ATP1A3. Neurol Genet 2019;5:e303.
28. Lassuthova P, Rebelo AP, Ravenscroft G, et al. Mutations in ATP1A1 cause dominant Charcot-Marie-Tooth type 2. Am J Hum Genet 2018;102:505–514.
29. Friedrich T, Tavraz NN, Junghans C. ATP1A2 mutations in migraine: seeing through the facets of an ion pump onto the neurobiology of disease. Front Physiol 2016;7:239.
30. Prontera P, Sarchielli P, Caproni S, et al. Epilepsy in hemiplegic migraine: genetic mutations and clinical implications. Cephalalgia 2018;38:361–373.
31. Rosewich H, Ohlenbusch A, Huppke P, et al. The expanding clinical and genetic spectrum of ATP1A3-related disorders. Neurology 2014;82:945–955.
32. Heinzen EL, Arzimanoglou A, Brashear A, et al. Distinct neurological disorders with ATP1A3 mutations. Lancet Neurol 2014;13:503–514.
33. Pearson TS, Akman C, Hinton VJ, Engelstad K, De Vivo DC. Phenotypic spectrum of glucose transporter type 1 deficiency syndrome (Glut1 DS). Curr Neurol Neurosci Rep 2013;13:342–347.

3 Intracellular Signaling

OVERVIEW

Cells in the nervous system communicate via a wide range of chemical signals that may be released from neurons or glial cells and participate in bidirectional communication. These extracellular signals act via membrane receptors and affect multiple cellular functions through several intracellular transduction pathways that regulate the phosphorylation state of many target proteins, known as phosphoproteins. These downstream signaling cascades may be triggered by activation of G (guanosine nucleotide-binding) protein-coupled receptors (GPCRs), tyrosine kinase receptors, and other receptors or by directly transient increase in intracellular calcium (Ca^{2+}). Activation of GPCRs triggers second messengers such as cyclic nucleotides or products of hydrolysis of membrane phospholipids that promote Ca^{2+} release from stores in the endoplasmic reticulum (ER). The final effects of these cascades depend on activation of protein kinases or protein phosphatases that tightly control the phosphorylation state of fundamental membrane, cytosolic, cytoskeletal, and nuclear proteins. These intracellular mechanisms regulate neural development, growth and survival, electrophysiological behavior, synaptic transmission and plasticity, responses to injury, and repair. These signaling pathways are involved in most if not all neurodegenerative and neurodevelopmental disorders. The aims of this chapter are to review (1) the mechanisms of communication in the nervous system, (2) the G proteins as molecular switches, (3) the second messenger cascades triggered by activation of GPCRs, (4) the mechanisms that control intracellular Ca^{2+} transients, and (4) some examples of protein kinases and phosphatases of relevance in neurologic disorders. This chapter thus serves as an introduction to many processes that will be discussed in more detail in other chapters of this book.

BASIC FORMS OF INTERCELLULAR COMMUNICATION IN THE NERVOUS SYSTEM

Several chemical signals mediate cell–cell interactions in the nervous system. They include amino acids, acetylcholine, monoamines, neuropeptides, purines such as ATP and adenosine, lipid mediators; growth factors; cytokines; and adhesion molecules. These signals act via a wide range of receptors in their target cells.

Classical Neurotransmission

Classical neurotransmission refers to the rapid, precise transmission of excitatory or inhibitory signals between cells and is largely mediated by amino acids or acetylcholine acting via ionotropic receptors clustered at postsynaptic sites across the presynaptic active zone. Inotropic receptors are neurotransmitter-gated cation (Na^+, Ca^+) or Cl^- channels, which respectively trigger fast excitatory or inhibitory effects on postsynaptic targets, thereby strongly regulating their probability of triggering an action potential.

Neuromodulation

Neuromodulation refers to the mechanisms by which neurochemical signals influence the efficacy of synaptic transmission at presynaptic or postsynaptic levels. Presynaptic modulation affects the probability of neurotransmitter release from presynaptic terminals, which depends on availability of synaptic vesicles at release zones and the state of activity of presynaptic voltage-gated Ca^{2+} channels. Postsynaptic modulation determines the responsiveness of the postsynaptic target and depends on the opening probability of potassium (K^+) or Ca^{2+} channels that control cell excitability. Both presynaptic and postsynaptic modulation are mediated by GPCRs that may be activated by amino acids, acetylcholine, neuropeptides, purines, and lipids released not only from neurons but also from glial cells.

Plasticity and Trophic Signals

Signals from neurotransmitters, neurotrophic factors, cytokines, and adhesion molecules trigger complex downstream transduction cascades that eventually lead to changes in the phosphorylation state of a large number of cytosolic proteins, components of the cytoskeleton, and transcription factors. These signals are critical for neural development, differentiation, survival, connectivity, and use-dependent synaptic plasticity by affecting gene transcription, site-specific protein translation, receptor trafficking, cytoskeletal dynamics, protein quality control, macromolecule degradation by autophagy, and apoptosis.

PROTEIN PHOSPHORYLATION AS A FINAL COMMON SIGNALING EVENT

The control of protein phosphorylation is the major final mechanism for regulation of cell function. Under basal conditions, the phosphorylation level of a particular phosphoprotein is determined by the equilibrium between the activity of protein kinases and protein phosphatases (Figure 3.1).

General Concepts

Protein kinases are subdivided into two groups: serine/threonine kinase and tyrosine kinases. Over 85% of phosphoproteins are phosphorylated on serine residues; 12% on threonine residues; and less than 2% on tyrosine residues. Protein phosphorylation depends on ATP and requires the presence of a divalent cation. Phosphorylation typically induces conformational changes in the target protein affecting its activity, subcellular location, or association with other proteins. Most protein kinases are inactive at the basal state and require activation prior to substrate phosphorylation. Some kinases contain autoinhibitory phosphorylation sites, others are inactivated through interaction with an inhibitor subunit of another protein, and many are also be subject to allosteric modulation. Many kinases have interaction domains that confine the enzymes to specific subcellular locations. Many proteins can be phosphorylated at more than one site by several kinases; phosphorylation at distinct sites may result in distinct, similar, synergistic, competitive, or opposing effects. Phosphorylated proteins can be converted back to their unphosphorylated state by protein phosphatases.

Signal Mechanisms Regulating Protein Phosphorylation

There are two main signal mechanisms by which extracellular signals can affect the phosphorylation state of target proteins. Most neurotransmitters utilize an indirect mechanism that involves GPCRs that trigger second messenger cascades leading to activation of second messenger–dependent serine/threonine kinases, which propagate the intracellular signal (Table 3.1). In contrast, neurotrophic factors or cytokines may affect phosphorylation of target proteins through direct interaction with a membrane receptor with intrinsic tyrosine kinase activity. The signal from the receptor tyrosine kinases is then propagated downstream by phosphorylation cascades involving serine/threonine kinases, which are activated in the cytosol independently of second messengers (Table 3.2). Unlike protein kinases, phosphatases are generally active at a basal state but can also respond to intracellular signals. There are both serine-threonine and tyrosine protein phosphatases. Whereas the serine/threonine phosphatases participate in transduction signaling by opposing the effects of serine/threonine kinases, many protein tyrosine phosphatases function as membrane receptors for extracellular signals (Table 3.3). There is a complex crosstalk between the different protein kinases and phosphatase signaling cascades. Calcium serves a major role in signal transduction pathway as it can activate either protein kinase of protein phosphatases in response to different signals.

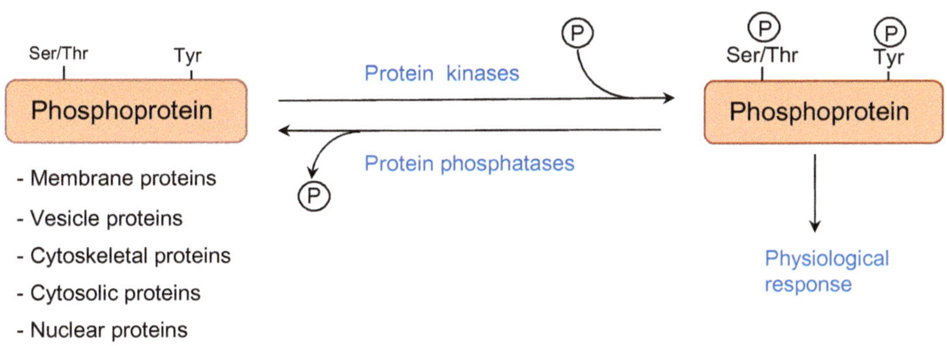

FIGURE 3.1 Control of protein phosphorylation.
The phosphorylation level of a particular phosphoprotein depends on the equilibrium between the activity of protein kinases and protein phosphatases that may target serine (Ser)/threonine (Thr) or tyrosine (Tyr) residues.

TABLE 3.1 *Second Messenger–Dependent Protein Kinases*

Kinase	Activating Messenger	Function (examples)
Protein kinase A	Cyclic AMP	Synaptic plasticity
Protein kinase C	Diacylglycerol and calcium (Ca^{2+})	Synaptic plasticity Growth factor signaling
Protein kinase G	Cyclic GMP	Nitric oxide signaling
Calmodulin (CaM) kinases	Ca^{2+}/Calmodulin	Synaptic plasticity
AKT (protein kinase B)	Phosphoinositide 3'kinase (PI3K)	Growth factor signaling
Ribosomal 6 kinase (RSK)	mTOR complex 1	Protein translation

G PROTEINS AS MOLECULAR SWITCHES

G proteins bind guanosine diphosphate (GDP) or guanosine triphosphate (GTP) moieties and function as molecular switches that undergo a regulatory cycle cycling between an inactive GDP-bound and an active GTP-bound state (Figure 3.2). This switch is turned on by signals that function as guanine nucleotide exchange factors (GEFs) and promote the interchange of GDP from GTP bound to the G protein, and antagonized by guanine nucleotide dissociation inhibitors. G proteins have an intrinsic GTPase that turns off their activity through hydrolysis to their bound GTP back to the GDP; this process is promoted by GTPase-activating proteins (GAPs). In the case of GPCRs, regulators of GPCR-signaling proteins stimulate this GTPase activity.

There are two main families of G proteins, monomeric Ras-like GTPase proteins and heteromeric G proteins coupled to GPCRs.

Small Ras-Like Proteins

Monomeric small G proteins are critical for intracellular events involving membrane and vesicle dynamics. In their inactive GDP-bound state they are localized to the cytoplasm, and in the GTP-active state they interact with cell membranes. Small Ras-GTPases have a major role in multiple cellular processes, including, but not restricted

TABLE 3.2 *Examples of Second Messenger–Independent Protein Kinases*

Kinase	Relevance
Extracellular signal-regulated kinase (ERK)	Final effector of the Ras-survival pathway Effector of synaptic plasticity pathways
Janus kinase (JAK)	Mediates effects of cytokines via signal transducer and activator of transcription (STAT)
c-JUN terminal kinase (JNK)	Stress response kinase activated by inflammation, oxidative stress, and other stimuli. Promotes apoptosis
p38 mitogen-activated kinase	Stress response kinase. Involved in synaptic plasticity and inflammatory responses
Cyclin-dependent kinase 5 (CDK5)	Shuttles between the cytosol and the nucleus during the cell cycle. Targets signal proteins, inhibitors of protein phosphatases, and receptors. Inhibits cell cycle progression
Glycogen synthase kinase 3 (GSK-3)	Unlike other kinases, active at resting state. Inhibits and is inhibited by other kinases. Typically inhibits signaling and structural proteins and transcription factors. Main tau phosphorylating kinase
PTEN-induced putative kinase 1 (PINK1)	Binding the mitochondrial membrane promotes recruitment of Parkin for mitophagy
Leucine repeat rich kinase 2 (LRRK2)	Regulates multiple function including lysosomal trafficking of α-synuclein

TABLE 3.3 *Serine/Threonine Phosphatases*

Phosphatase	Relevance
Calcineurin (protein phosphatase 2B, PP2B)	Activated by Ca^{2+}, mediates depression of glutamatergic synapses Activated by immunophilins (e.g., cyclosporine A) and regulates mitochondrial membrane permeability
Protein phosphatase 1 (PP-1)	Its inhibition by D1 receptor-mediated signaling via DARPP-32 promotes plasticity in the striatum
Phosphatase and Tensin homolog (PTEN)	Tumor suppressor protein that inhibits the PI3K-AKT pathway
Laforin	Regulates the mTORC1 pathway Inhibits glycogen synthesis in neurons

DARPP-32, dopamine and cAMP regulated phosphoprotein of 32 kDA; mTORC, mammalian (mechanistic) target of rapamycin complex; PI3K, phosphatidylinositol 3'kinase

to, vesicle targeting to the presynaptic terminal, cytoskeletal dynamics, nucleocytoplasmic transport, and growth factor signaling (Table 3.4). Mutations affecting these small Ras-GTPases have been associated with several neurologic disorders. For example, mutations of Rab7, which has a critical role in maturation of late endosomes, are an important cause of hereditary axonal peripheral neuropathy. These functions and disorders of small GTPases are described in other chapters of this book.

Heterotrimeric G Proteins and G Protein-Coupled Receptors

Heterotrimeric G proteins mediate the classical effects of GPCRs. These receptors constitute the largest family of receptors (Table 3.5). The genes that encode members of the GPCR superfamily in humans encompass about 4% of the entire genome. The GPCRs are integral membrane proteins that are typically targeted to the cholesterol- and sphingolipid-rich lipid rafts. GPCRs arrange into a tertiary structure resembling a barrel, with their seven

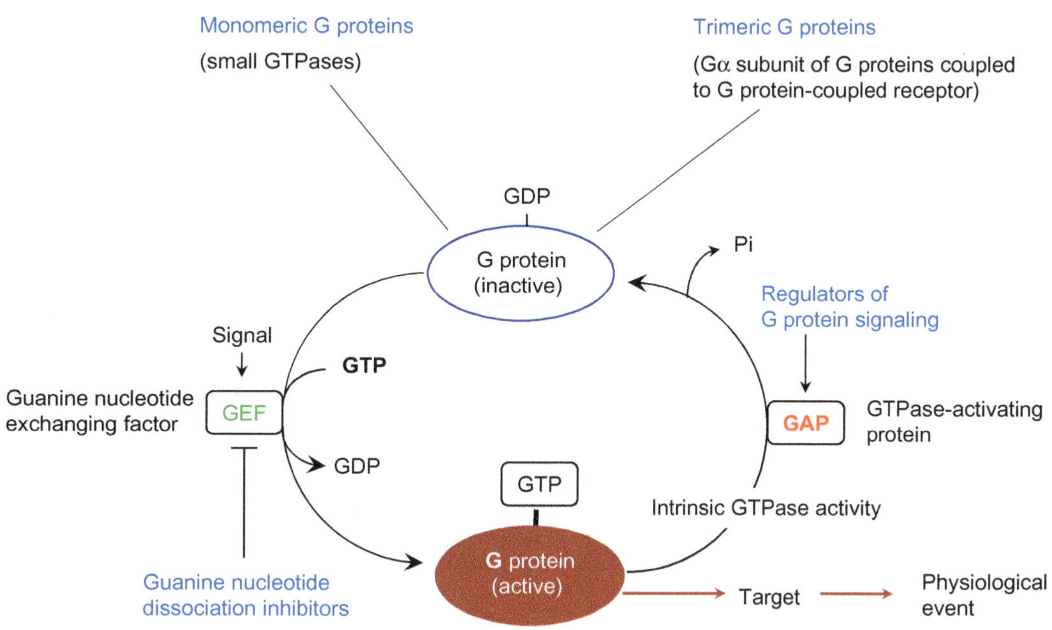

FIGURE 3.2 G proteins as molecular switches.
G proteins bind guanosine diphosphate (GDP) or guanosine triphosphate (GTP) moieties and undergo cycling between an inactive GDP-bound and an active GTP-bound state. This switch is turned on by guanine nucleotide exchange factors (GEFs) and antagonized by guanine nucleotide dissociation inhibitors. The intrinsic GTPase activity of the G protein turns off their activity through hydrolysis to their bound GTP back to the GDP.

TABLE 3.4 *Examples of Small Ras-Like GTPases*

Family Member	Function and Examples (function)
Ras	Growth factor signaling
Rab	Vesicular trafficking. Examples: Rab 3 (synaptic vesicles). Rab5 (early endosomes), Rab7 (late endosomes)
Rho	Dynamics of actin cytoskeleton
Rheb	Regulation of mechanistic target of rapamycin (mTOR) signaling
Ran	Nucleocytoplasmic transport

transmembrane helices forming a cavity within the plasma membrane that serves as a ligand-binding domain. Whereas GPCRs in general act as monomers, some are obligatory dimers; one of the monomers binds the neurotransmitter and the other couples to the G protein. Many types of GPCRs may form heterodimers with other receptors or form receptor mosaics where the different receptors interact both physically and functionally, so that one receptor modulates via allosteric mechanisms the features another receptor of the assembly.[1] In these complexes, the response of each GPCR to its ligand depends not only on its own conformation but also on its allosteric interactions with the other receptors of the macromolecular assembly.

Heteromeric G proteins consist of three distinct subunits, Gα, β, and γ; the Gα subunits confer functional specificity and provide the basis for classification of G proteins into distinct subfamilies.

Dynamics of GPCRs Signaling

In the absence of stimuli, heterotrimeric G proteins are in an inactive state where Gα subunits are bound to GDP forming a Gαβγ heterotrimeric complex (Figure 3.3).

Ligand binding at the extracellular side of a receptor leads to conformational changes in the cytoplasmic side of the receptor that initiates signal transduction. This involves the change from a GDP-bound to a GTP-bound Gα subunit, leading to the dissociation of the trimer into a Gα-GTP and a βγ complex. Gα-GTP acts on effector enzymes to initiate second messenger cascades, whereas the βγ complex directly interacts with membrane ion channels.

There are several mechanisms that turn off the GPCR signal. One such mechanism is dissociation of the ligand from the receptor and the GTPase activity of the Gα subunit, leading to reassociation of the Gαβγ heterotrimer; regulators of GPCR signaling (RGS) proteins act on Gα subunits

TABLE 3.5 *Examples of Heteromeric G Protein-Coupled Receptors*

Signal	Receptor (examples)
Classical neurotransmitters	Metabotropic glutamate receptors (mGluRs) $GABA_B$ receptor Muscarinic cholinergic M1 and M2 families Dopamine receptors D1 and D2 Adrenergic receptors (α1, α2, and β subfamilies) Serotonin receptors (5-HT1, 5-HT2, 5-HT6–7) Histamine receptors (H1, H2, and H3)
Purines	P2Y receptors for ATP Adenosine A1 and A2 receptors
Peptides	Neuropeptide receptors Hormone receptors
Lipids mediators	Endocannabinoid CB1 and CB2 receptors Prostaglandin receptors
Sensory transduction	Opsin receptors Melanopsin receptors Melatonin receptors Olfactory receptors Taste (sweet, umami)

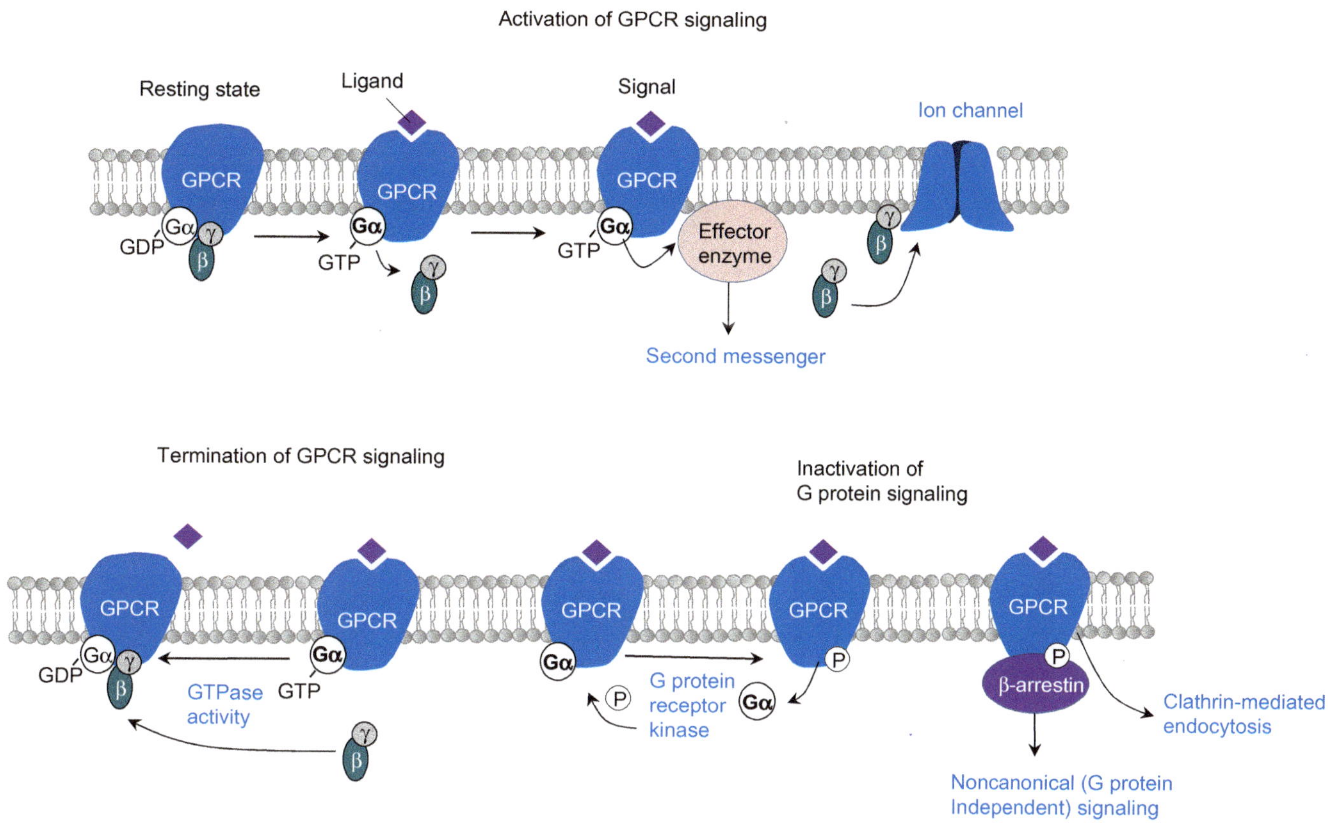

FIGURE 3.3 G protein-coupled receptors (GPCRs) and heteromeric G proteins.
In the absence of stimuli these G proteins are in an inactive state where Gα subunits are bound to GDP forming a Gαβγ heterotrimeric complex. Ligand binding triggers the change from a GDP-bound to a GTP-bound Gα subunit, leading to the dissociation of the trimer into a Gα-GTP and a βγ complex, both of which having signaling function. The signal is terminated when the ligand dissociates from the receptors and the Gα subunit hydrolyzes GTP to GDP. G protein receptor kinases phosphorylate the GPCR leading to its dissociation from the G protein. Phosphorylation of GPCRs also increases their affinity for β-arrestin, which promotes endocytosis of the ligand-bound GPCR or initiation of noncanonical GPCR signaling.

and stimulate their GTPase activity. GPCR phosphorylation by G protein receptor kinases leads to dissociation of the receptor from the G protein and terminates signaling. Phosphorylation of GPCRs also increases their affinity for the binding of scaffold proteins called β-arrestins. Beta arrestins prevent G-protein coupling and promote endocytosis of the ligand-bound GPCR. Beta arrestins may also recruit other proteins, leading to the creation of signaling complexes that initiate noncanonical GPCR signaling, independent of the G protein.[2]

As ligand-receptor binding promotes receptor internalization, it provides a mechanism regulating the number of GPCRs expressed on the membrane. Agonist deprivation or receptor blockade leads to upregulation of surface expression of the receptor; this may lead to an abnormal response to the agonist, as occurs, for example, in the case of D2 receptors after chronic antipsychotic treatment. In contrast, chronic exposure to the agonist results in receptor downregulation; in the case of opioids this predisposes to opioid withdrawal symptoms.

TRANSDUCTION CASCADES TRIGGERED BY GPCRS AND THEIR CLINICAL IMPLICATIONS

GPCRs are classified on the bases of their sequence homology and functional similarity into several classes.[3] According to the type of G proteins, activation of GPCRs triggers different downstream transduction cascades (Figure 3.4).

$G_{s/olf}$ Signaling

Proteins of the $G\alpha_s/G\alpha_{olf}$ family stimulate membrane-bound adenylyl cyclase, which catalyzes the formation of cyclic adenosine monophosphate (cAMP) from ATP. The major downstream signal of cAMP is protein kinase A (PKA), which phosphorylates several targets, including membrane receptors and ion channels, cytoskeletal proteins, phosphatase inhibitors, and transcription factors. Cyclic AMP also directly binds to and modulates cyclic nucleotide-gated channels. The cAMP signal is terminated

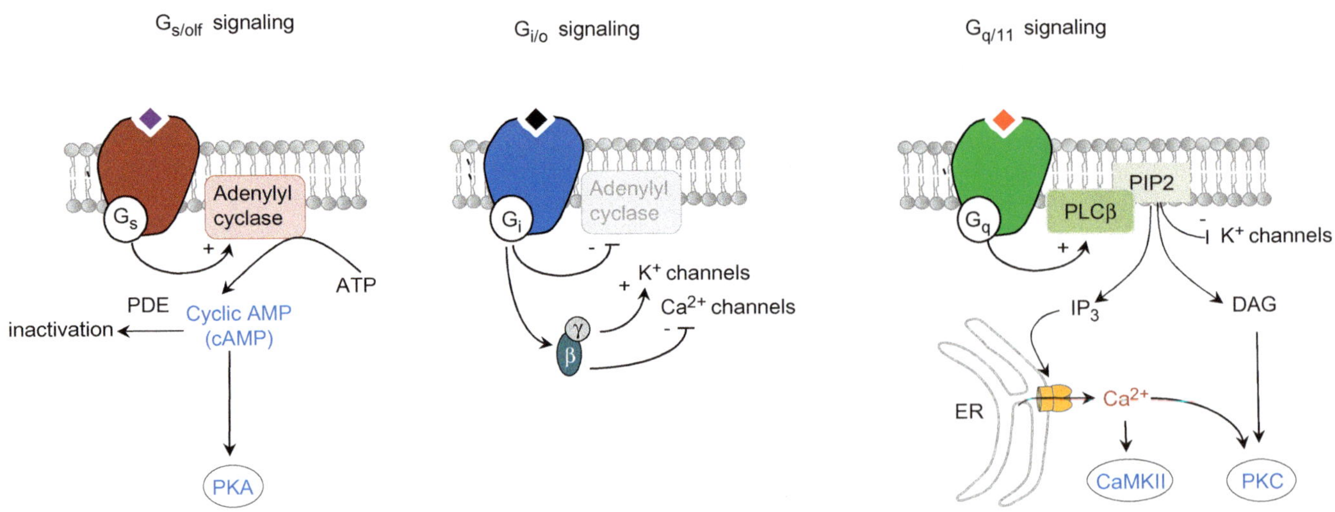

FIGURE 3.4 Classical signal transduction cascades of G protein-coupled receptors.
Proteins of the $G\alpha_s/G\alpha_{olf}$ family stimulate membrane-bound adenylyl cyclase, which catalyzes the formation of cyclic adenosine monophosphate (cAMP) from ATP. The major downstream signal of cAMP is protein kinase A (PKA), which phosphorylates several targets. The cAMP signal is terminated by its hydrolysis by cAMP phosphodiesterases (PDEs). Ligand binding to GPCRs coupled to $G_{i/o}$ signaling leads to inhibition of adenylyl cyclase via the $G\alpha_{i/o}$ subunit and dissociation of the βγ subunit complex; this complex directly activates K^+ channels and inhibits presynaptic voltage-gated Ca^{2+} channels. Activation of receptors coupled to G_q family proteins leads to activation of phospholipase C (PLC), which hydrolyzes membrane phosphatidylinositol 4,5 bisphosphate (PIP2), yielding diacylglycerol (DAG) and inositol triphosphate (IP_3). Since PIP2 is important for the function of K^+ channels, activation of this pathway typically results in reduced K^+ currents and increased cell excitability. Inositol triphosphate binds to IP_3 receptors (IP_3R, ITPR) in the endoplasmic reticulum (ER), leading to Ca^{2+} release; DAG together with Ca^{2+} activates protein kinase C (PKC).

by its hydrolysis by cAMP phosphodiesterases (PDEs). Several GPCRs utilize the G_s/G_{olf} signal transduction cascade.

One typical example is the dopamine D1 receptor in the striatum. These receptors are coupled to $G\alpha_{olf}$ and activate adenylyl cyclase 5 (encoded by the *ADCY5* gene), and this signal is terminated by cAMP hydrolysis by PDE10. Mutations leading to gain-of-function of *ADCY5* or loss-of-function of *PDE10* exaggerate D1 receptor signaling via this pathway and produce a variety of hyperkinetic movement disorders, including paroxysmal chorea, myoclonus, and dystonia.[4,5]

$G_{i/o}$ Signaling

Ligand binding to GPCRs coupled to $G_{i/o}$ signaling leads to inhibition of adenylyl cyclase via the $G\alpha_{i/o}$ subunit and dissociation of the βγ subunit complex, which directly interacts with membrane ion channels. The major effects are activation of K^+ channels leading to reduced neuronal excitability and inhibition of presynaptic voltage-gated Ca^{2+} channels resulting in inhibition of neurotransmitter release. Many receptors are coupled to this signal transduction pathway and involved in both presynaptic and postsynaptic inhibition. Some important examples are $GABA_B$, dopamine D2, norepinephrine α2, serotonin 5-HT1, opioid, and cannabinoid CB1 receptors. The crosstalk between these different receptors via a common $Gi_{/o}$ transduction pathway provides the rationale for the use of α2 receptor agonists both for potentiating opioid analgesia[6] and managing opioid withdrawal,[7] or the use of $GABA_B$ agonists (baclofen), alpha 2 agonists (such as tizanidine), and cannabinoids for management of pain and spasticity, and the beneficial effect of the alpha 2 agonist dexmedetomidine in baclofen withdrawal.[8] The *GNAO1* gene encodes the $G\alpha_o$ subunit of several inhibitory GPCRs. Loss-of-function *GNAO1* mutations produce severe early-onset epileptic encephalopathy; in contrast, gain-of-function *GNAO1* mutations produce chorea and other hyperkinetic movement disorders.[9]

G_q Signaling

Activation of receptors coupled to G_q family proteins leads to activation of phospholipase C (PLC), which hydrolyzes membrane phosphatidylinositol 4,5 bisphosphate (PIP2) yielding diacylglycerol (DAG) and inositol triphosphate (IP_3). Since PIP2 is important for function of K^+ channels, activation of this pathway typically results in reduced K^+ currents and increased cell excitability. Inositol triphosphate binds to IP_3 receptors (IP_3R, ITPR) in the ER, leading to Ca^{2+} release; DAG together with Ca^{2+} activates protein kinase C (PKC), which acts on several targets and has a major role in synaptic plasticity. Examples of GPCRs coupled to G_q include class 1 metabotropic glutamate receptors involved in synaptic plasticity; cholinergic muscarinic M1 receptors involved in attention, orexin (OX) receptors involved in maintenance of wakefulness, and neurokinin 1 (NK1) receptors for substance P mediating pain. However, one mediator of the G_q pathway is diacylglycerol, which is also substrate for synthesis of endocannabinoids. Endocannabinoids act as retrograde signals that inhibit neurotransmitter release via presynaptic CB1 receptors. Furthermore, PKC may phosphorylate glutamate receptor subunits, leading to receptor internalization, reduced membrane expression, and thus depression of excitatory synapses. The G_q–IP_3R–PKC pathway has a major role in plasticity of synapses on Purkinje cells in the cerebellum; mutations or affecting components of this pathway produce ataxia.[10–12]

Other Signal Transduction Pathways Involving GPCRs or Cyclic Nucleotides

Guanylyl cyclases catalyze the formation of cyclic guanosine monophosphate (cGMP) from GTP; cGMP directly regulates ion channels and also activates protein kinase G (PKG). Membrane-bound guanylyl cyclases bind directly to ligands such as natriuretic peptides. In contrast, nitric oxide directly diffuses across membranes and activates cytoplasmic guanylyl cyclase. In the retina, activation of the G protein rhodopsin by light closes cGMP-gated cation channels responsible for the dark current in photoreceptor cells, which is the first signal step of phototransduction. Cyclic GMP also mediates the vasodilator effects of nitric oxide and mediates some of its neuromodulator effects via PKG. The effects of cGMP signaling are terminated by action of cGMP phosphodiesterases such as PDE5, which is inhibited by drugs such as sildenafil. The common cGMP signaling pathway may contribute to retinal toxicity of sildenafil when used as a vasodilator.[13,14]

Arrestins and Non-G Protein–Mediated Effects of G Protein-Coupled Receptors

GPCRs may trigger signal transduction cascades independently of their interactions with G proteins. Upon phosphorylation by GPCR kinases, the GPCR dissociates from the G protein, which is referred to as homologous desensitization, and recruits scaffold proteins known as arrestins. Arrestins block the GPCR interactions with G proteins and in turn recruit signaling complexes to mediate non-G protein–mediated signaling.[15,16] There is increased beta 2 arrestin expression in Alzheimer disease, which may promote amyloid beta production and thus provide a potential therapeutic target for reducing amyloid pathology and GPCR dysfunction in this disorder.[17]

CALCIUM SIGNAL

Calcium is a fundament signal in the brain, both in physiological and in pathological conditions. In most cells, the free Ca^{2+} concentration in the cytosol is maintained in the nanomolar range (~ 100 nM), which is four orders of magnitude less than in the extracellular Ca^{2+} in blood and CSF. Cytosolic Ca^{2+} concentration and signaling function are determined by the interplay among several factors: (1) influx via different types of Ca^{2+} permeable channels; (2) release from intracellular stores, primarily the ER; (3) efflux through the membrane via transporters, pumps, and exchangers; (4) sequestration in intracellular stores, particularly the ER; and (5) intracellular binding proteins that function as Ca^{2+} buffers (Figure 3.5).

Sources of Calcium Influx into Cells

There are four major pathways for influx of Ca^{2+} into the cell. The most important is via voltage-gated Ca^{2+} channels that are activated by depolarization. An important second route is via Ca^{2+}-permeable ligand-gated channels (ionotropic receptors), such as glutamatergic N-methyl-aspartate receptors (NMDARs) in neurons and P2X receptors for ATP in glial cells. A third is via transient receptor potential (TRP) channels, such as those expressed in nociceptive and thermoreceptive afferents and in astrocytes.[18] Calcium influx may also occur via a store-operated Ca^{2+} entry via membrane channels activated upon emptying of the ER stores.[19]

Calcium Release from Intracellular Stores

Calcium is stored in the ER in association with binding proteins and may be released from ER stores in response to extracellular signals. There are two receptor mechanisms that trigger Ca^{2+} release from the ER. One is via activation of IP_3Rs (ITPRs) by IP_3 produced upon GPCR-triggered G_q-coupled signaling, discussed earlier.[20] The second is via Ca^{2+}-induced Ca^{2+} release mediated by ryanodine receptors (RYRs).[21] In astrocytes, release of Ca^{2+} from the ER can result in Ca^{2+} wave that moves through the entire cell following a gradient of $Ca^{2+}$from the source of release. In skeletal muscle, depolarization of T-tubule membranes, in response to motor neuron inputs via nicotinic cholinergic receptors and propagated sodium currents, leads to conformational changes in voltage-dependent Ca^{2+} channels resulting in activation RYRs and Ca^{2+} release from the sarcoplasmic reticulum; this is the fundamental machinery for excitation-contraction coupling, referred to as "couplon."[22] A similar mechanism mediates sympathetic beta adrenergic receptor–triggered excitation-contraction coupling in cardiac muscle. Mutations affecting this coupling mechanism lead to diseases of striated muscle, dubbed "couplonopathies," such as malignant hyperthermia and catecholaminergic polymorphic ventricular tachycardia.[22] An increase in store-operated calcium entry is also relevant in the pathogenesis of malignant hyperthermia.[22]

Mechanisms Preventing Excessive Intracellular Calcium Accumulation

There are two major Ca^{2+} efflux pathways in cells. One is mediated by the plasma membrane Ca^{2+} ATPase (PMCA) and responds to minimal increases in intracellular Ca^{2+}.

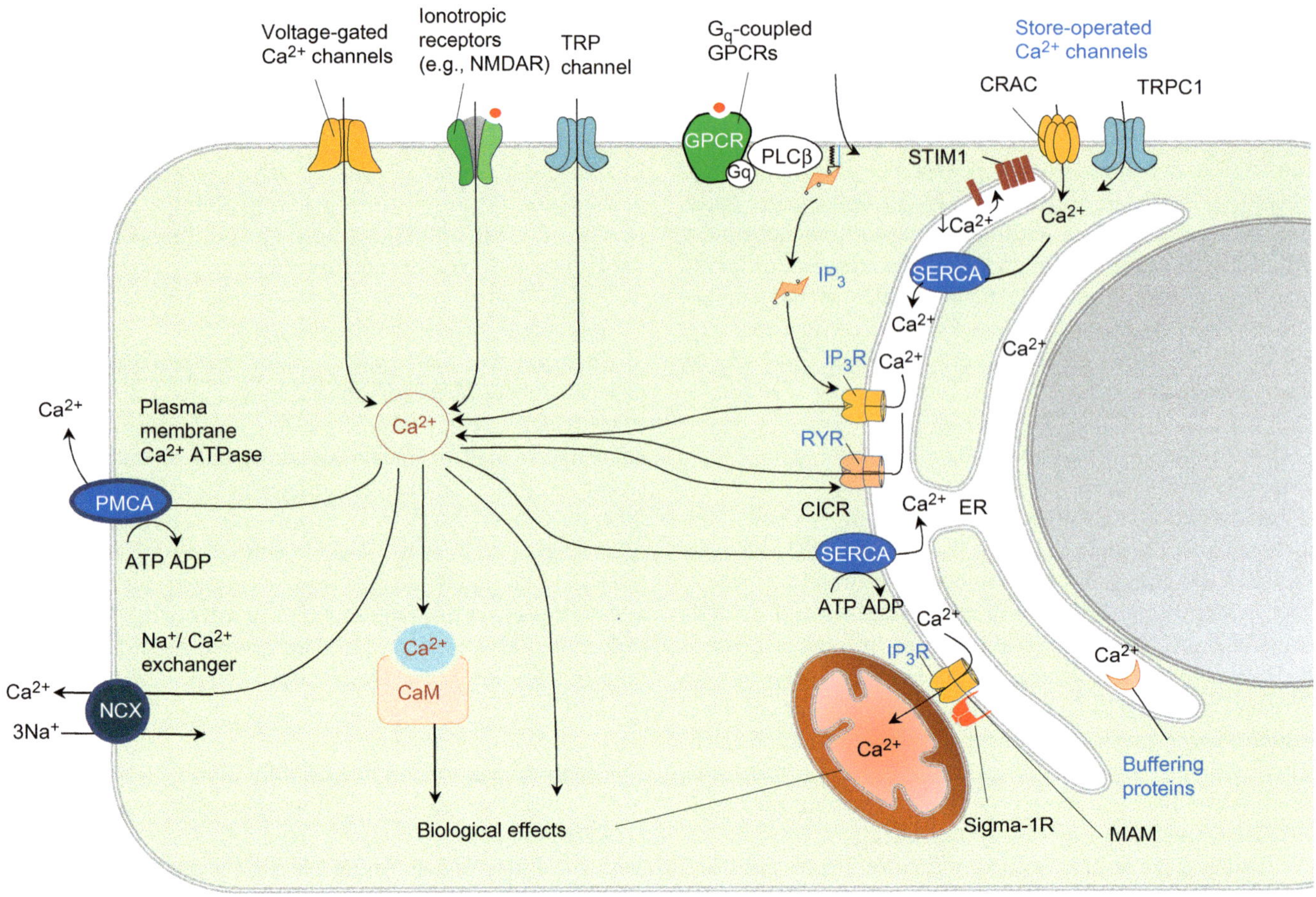

FIGURE 3.5 Calcium signaling.
The most important source of influx of Ca^{2+} into the cell is via voltage-gated Ca^{2+} channels. Others include Ca^{2+}-permeable ligand-gated channels such as N-methyl-aspartate receptors (NMDARs) or via transient receptor potential (TRP) channels. Release of Ca^{2+} from the ER occurs via inositol triphosphate (IP_3) receptors (IP_3Rs) upon activation of G_q-coupled G protein-coupled receptors (GPCRs) or via Ca^{2+}-induced Ca^{2+} release (CICR) mediated by ryanodine receptors (RYRs). Upon endoplasmic reticulum (ER) luminal Ca^{2+} depletion, Ca^{2+}-sensing stromal interaction molecule 1 (STIM1) allows clustering and trapping of membrane Orai1 subunits (not shown), which assemble into active Ca^{2+}-release-activated Ca^{2+} channels (CRACs). There, Ca^{2+} efflux is mediated by the plasma membrane Ca^{2+} ATPase (PMCA) and the Na^+/Ca^{2+} exchanger (NCX). Calcium is pumped back into the ER via sarcoendoplasmic reticular Ca^{2+}ATPases (SERCAs). The mitochondria and ER contact each other at specific ER domains called mitochondria-associated ER membrane enriched in sigma-1 receptors (Sig-1Rs), which function as molecular chaperones. Calcium is an important effector of several signaling pathways. Its effects frequently involve interactions with a large number of proteins; the typical example is calmodulin (CaM).

Whereas PMCA pumps are of minor importance to the bulk regulation of neuronal Ca^{2+}, they are important in Ca^{2+} regulation at specific subplasma membrane microdomains containing enzymes relevant to neuronal function.[23] Mutations of neuron-specific *PMCA 3* are linked to cerebellar ataxia; *PMA 2* mutations produce deafness.[23] The second and more powerful mechanism of Ca^{2+} extrusion is via the electronic Na^+/Ca^{2+} exchanger (NCX), which is bidirectional and voltage-sensitive. Under resting conditions the NCX exports one Ca^{2+} ion and imports three Na^+ ions. When the membrane is depolarized or when there is excessive accumulation of intracellular Na^+, the NCX functions in reverse; Na^+ is extruded while Ca^{2+} is imported into the cells. Reverse operation of the NCX has a major role in promoting intracellular Ca^{2+} accumulation, leading to excitotoxic cell injury in the setting of energy failure[24] and secondary axonal injury in the setting of demyelination.[25]

Maintenance of Endoplasmic Reticulum Calcium Stores

Calcium can leak from the ER into the cytoplasm and is pumped back into the ER via sarcoendoplasmic reticular Ca^{2+}ATPases (SERCAs), which sequester two Ca^{2+}

ions per molecule of ATP hydrolyzed and maintain a high Ca^{2+} content in ER.[26] Impaired SERCA-mediated $Ca2^{+}$ homeostasis may have a major role in neurodegeneration.[27] Within the ER, Ca^{2+} is buffered by multiple binding proteins, including calsequestrin and calreticulin. These proteins also function as molecular chaperones that promote folding and maturation of nascent proteins in the ER. If ER stores of Ca^{2+} are rapidly depleted through IP_3-mediated release, there is activation of a mechanism known as store-operated Ca^{2+} entry, which is essential to maintain an appropriate intracellular Ca^{2+} homeostasis and prevent cell damage.[19]

Endoplasmic Reticulum–Mitochondrial Interactions and Calcium Homeostasis

Mitochondria have a complex function in calcium dynamics. Mitochondria migrate toward domains of high Ca^{2+} flux near the plasma membrane and the ER, including the presynaptic membrane, where is there is high ATP requirement for vesicle recycling and Ca^{2+} extrusion by the plasma membrane Ca^{2+} ATPase. The mitochondria and ER contact each other at specific ER domains called mitochondria-associated ER membrane. These domains are enriched in ceramide and proteins such as the sigma-1 receptor (Sig-1R), which functions as a molecular chaperone that sustains the correct conformation of the IP_3R to ensure proper Ca^{2+} passage from the ER to the mitochondria.

Calcium Effector Mechanisms

Calcium is a critical regulator of many cellular functions. Its effects frequently involve interactions with a large number of proteins; the typical example is calmodulin (CaM), which activates several effectors pathways and also binds to and directly regulates voltage-gated ion channels. Mutations of ion channel subunits affecting their interaction with CaM are linked to epilepsy, cardiac arrhythmias, and other disorders.[28] Influx of Ca^{2+} activates CaM kinase II (CaMKII), which phosphorylates ion channels, receptors, transporters, pumps, signaling molecules, and cytoskeletal proteins and translocates to the nucleus, where it activates transcription.[29] The Ca^{2+}/CaM signal also activates the phosphatase calcineurin, resulting in protein dephosphorylation. Calcium thus provides for a crosstalk among intracellular signal transduction pathways. It activates some isoforms of adenylyl cyclase and PKC. In pathological conditions, excessive accumulation of intracellular Ca^{2+} triggers several potential cell-damaging cascades, including those mediated by nitric oxide synthase; the Ca^{2+}-activated protease calpain, and endonucleases, as discussed in chapter 12.

GROWTH FACTOR SIGNALING

Neurotrophic factors have a major role in development, growth, differentiation, survival, and plasticity in the nervous system. They activate downstream cascades that promote protein synthesis and inhibit cell death mechanisms of apoptosis and autophagy. There are several families of neurotrophic factors. Members of the neurotrophins family, such as nerve growth factor and brain-derived neurotrophic factor act via a canonical pathway that is initiated by tyrosine kinase receptors (Figure 3.6). Upon binding of growth factors, these receptors undergo dimerization and *trans*-autophosphorylation at their tyrosine residues, which leads to recruitment of signal proteins to the membrane.

Survival Signals Triggered by Growth Factors

Activation of tyrosine kinase receptors initiates three canonical survival pathways: the Ras-mitogen-activated protein kinase (MAPK), the phosphatidylinositol 3'kinase (PI3K)/AKT (protein kinase B) pathway; and the phospholipase Cγ (PLCγ) pathway. Upon binding of growth factors, tyrosine kinase receptors recruit, via an adaptor protein, a guanosine nucleotide–exchanging factor that activates the small G protein Ras by promoting the switch from inactive Ras-GDP to active Ras-GTP, which is recruited to the complex. Ras activates the MAPK pathway, which is a cytosolic signaling cascade that sequentially involves phosphorylation and activation of several serine/threonine protein kinases. The final effectors of this signaling cascade are the extracellular signal receptor kinases (ERKs), which target several downstream cytosolic and nuclear molecules, including membrane proteins, other protein kinases, and transcription factors. The second major survival pathway involves PI3K, leading to membrane recruitment, phosphorylation, and activation of AKT/protein kinase B. This serine/threonine kinase is a critical effector for cell survival by eliciting inhibitory phosphorylation of several targets that in basal conditions inhibit cell growth or promote cell death by apoptosis. The third survival pathway involves PLCγ, resulting in release of inositol phosphates and activation of PKC.

Mammalian (Mechanistic) Target of Rapamycin

The mechanistic (mammalian) target of rapamycin (mTOR) is a fundamental mediator of synaptic plasticity, cell growth, and survival pathways (Figure 3.5).[30,31] It is a ubiquitously expressed serine threonine protein kinase that forms two functionally distinct signaling complexes, mTOR complex 1 (mTORC1) and mTOR complex 2 (mTORC2). Activation of mTORC1 requires Rheb (Ras homologous enriched in brain), a small Ras-like GTPase that in its active GTP-bound form associates mTORC1 to the lysosomal membrane. In basal conditions, the functional complex formed by the tuberous sclerosis (TSC) proteins TSC1 (hamartin) and TSC2 (tuberin) inhibits mTORC1 signaling by stimulating the Rheb GTPase activity, thereby promoting the switch from an active GTP-Rheb to inactive GDP-Rheb. Growth factors, neurotransmitters, dietary amino acids, cell energy state, and cellular stress regulate

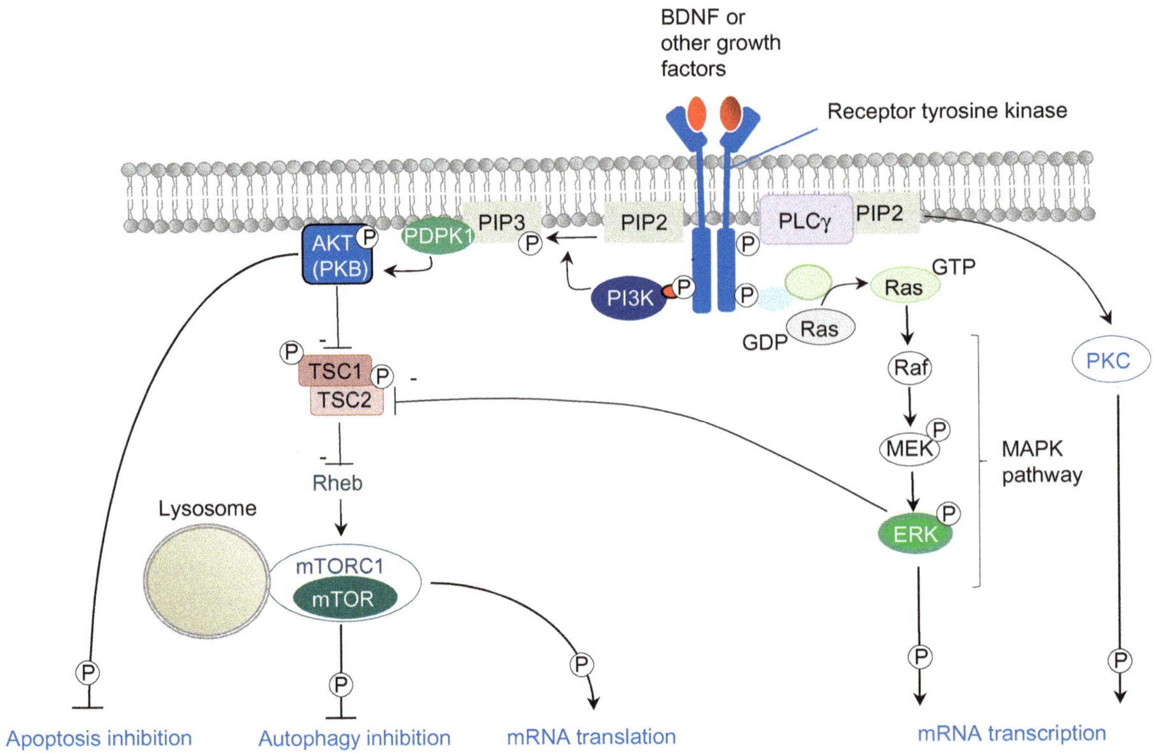

FIGURE 3.6 Growth factor signaling.
Members of the neurotrophins family, such as brain-derived neurotrophic factors (BDNFs), act via a canonical pathway that involves tyrosine kinase receptors. Upon binding of growth factors, these receptors undergo dimerization and autophosphorylation, allowing interaction with adaptor molecules and initiation of three major canonical survival pathways: the Ras–mitogen-activated protein kinase (MAPK) pathway, the phosphatidylinositol 3'kinase (PI3K)/AKT (protein kinase B) pathway; and the phospholipase C γ (PLCγ) pathway. Ras activates the MAPK pathway, which involves sequential phosphorylation and activation of the serine/threonine protein kinases including Raf, MAPK/extracellular signal receptor kinase (MEK), and extracellular signal receptor kinases (ERKs). The PI3K pathway involves phosphorylation of phosphatidylinositol 4,5 bisphosphate (PIP2) to produce phosphatidylinositol 3,4,5 triphosphate (PIP_3), which activates the phosphoinositide-dependent kinase 1 (PDPK1)(PDK-1), resulting in activation of AKT (also called protein kinase B, PKB). The phospholipase C (PLC)γ pathway results in activation of PKC. The mammalian (mechanistic) target of rapamycin (mTOR) acts as a critical effector of growth factor signaling by forming two functionally distinct multiprotein signaling complexes, mTOR complex 1 (mTORC1) and mTOR complex 2 (mTORC2) (not shown). Activation of mTORC1 requires Ras homologous enriched in brain (Rheb), which in its GTP-bound form associates mTOR to the lysosomal membrane and is critical for mTORC1 kinase activity. Growth factors and amino acids activate mTORC1 signaling via a final common indirect mechanism that involves inhibition of activity of a functional complex formed by the tuberous sclerosis (TSC) proteins TSC1 (hamartin) and TSC2 (tuberin).

mTORC1 activity via their effect on TSC-mediated inhibition. In particular, both growth factors and excitatory synaptic activity trigger phosphorylation cascades that inhibit TSC activity and thus activate mTORC1 signaling. The two major kinases eliciting inhibitory TSC phosphorylation and thus mTORC1 activation are PI3K/AKT and ERK. The mTORC1 kinase phosphorylates several downstream targets, leading to activation of mRNA translation, protein and lipid synthesis, and inhibition of autophagy. Whereas mTORC1 is a potent inhibitor of autophagy, adenosine monophosphate (AMP)-activated kinase (AMPK) promotes autophagy as one component of the response to cellular energy depletion.

OTHER SIGNALING PATHWAYS

Cytokine Signaling

Cytokines, including chemokines, interferons, interleukins, and tumor necrosis factor, are involved in immune signaling and also mediate reciprocal neuron-glia interactions. Inflammatory cytokines, reactive oxygen species, and other stress stimuli activate the c-Jun N-terminal kinase (JNK) and the p38 MAPK pathways. Both JNK and p38 MAPK phosphorylate numerous proteins in the nucleus, cytosol, and mitochondria, thereby regulating cell growth, differentiation, survival, and apoptosis. Many cytokines, such as interleukins and interferons, bind to cell-surface

TABLE 3.6 *Disorders Associated with Mutations Affecting Protein Kinases or Phosphatases (examples)*

Gene (protein)	Disorder
PINK1 (PTEN-induced kinase 1)	Early onset, juvenile parkinsonism
LRRK2 (Leucine repeat rich kinase 2)	Parkinson disease
TBK1 (TANK-binding kinase)	Amyotrophic lateral sclerosis
NEK1 (NIMA related kinase 1)	Amyotrophic lateral sclerosis
PTEN (Phosphatase and Tensin homolog)	PTEN deficiency hamartoma syndromes
EPM2A (Laforin glycogen protein phosphatase)	Lafora disease

receptors, leading to their dimerization and recruitment of receptor-associated Janus kinases (JAKs). JAKs are tyrosine kinases that phosphorylate and thus activate each other. The signal transducer and activator of transcription (STAT) proteins bind to the receptor and become tyrosine-phosphorylated by JAKs; this causes STATs to dissociate from the receptor. These activated STATs form hetero- or homodimers that translocate to the nucleus to induce transcription. JAK-STAT signaling interacts with other cell-signaling transduction pathways and is typically associated with inflammation and apoptosis; it is also involved in mechanisms of astrocyte differentiation and axonal repair.

Glycogen Synthase Kinase 3

Glycogen synthase kinase 3 (GSK3) is a multifunctional kinase that targets other kinases, cytoskeleton associated proteins such as tau, and transcription factors. GSK3 is involved in a number of central intracellular signaling pathways that regulate innate and adaptive immune responses, cellular proliferation, migration, glucose metabolism, and apoptosis. Two properties distinguish GSK3 from other kinases. GSK3 is active at basal state and is inhibited by phosphorylation by other kinases; phosphorylation by GSK3 usually inhibits the activity of its downstream targets, including other kinases.

ABNORMAL PHOSPHORYLATION AS A DISEASE MECHANISM

Essentially all neurologic disorders are associated directly or indirectly with disturbances in intracellular signaling, Ca^{2+} homeostasis, and protein phosphorylation, in various combinations. Whereas the signal transduction pathways described earlier are ubiquitous in both neural and non-neural cells, in some cases disturbances produce neurologic deficits that primarily affect a particular circuit or intracellular process. Only few examples will be mentioned here.

Disorders Due to Mutations Affecting Protein Kinases or Phosphatases

Protein kinases and phosphatases are involved in common pathogenic mechanisms of neurodegeneration, epilepsy, and developmental disorders, as discussed in other chapters of this book. Mutations affecting these proteins are also linked to different neurologic disorders (Table 3.6). For example, several kinases have been implicated in the pathogenesis of amyotrophic lateral sclerosis (ALS).[32] Examples include loss-of-function mutations of the *TBK1* gene encoding TANK-binding kinase, a serine/threonine kinase that phosphorylates p62/sequestosome (SQSTM), and optineurin (OPN), which function as autophagy receptors critical for proteostasis and mitostasis. Loss-of-function *SQSTM* or *OPTN* mutations have also been linked to familial ALS. Variants of the NEK1 (NIMA-related kinase 1) gene have also been identified in both familial and sporadic ALS. Overexpression of the nuclear isoform leads to abnormal chromatin condensation, DNA instability, and dispersal of the nuclear pore complex. NEK1 also interacts with multiple ALS-related gene products.

Abnormal Phosphorylation and Neurodegeneration

Abnormal protein phosphorylation is a fundamental disease pathway for neurodegeneration. The classical example is that of hyperphosphorylation of the microtubule-associated protein tau. Tau hyperphosphorylation is a hallmark of many neurodegenerative disorders, including Alzheimer disease (AD), tauopathies, and synucleinopathies. In general, increased tau phosphorylation reduces its affinity for microtubules and promotes its self-aggregation. Tau phosphorylation is tightly controlled by the balance between protein kinases and phosphatases.[33] Tau contains up to 85 residues that can be targeted by different kinases. They include serine/threonine kinases such as GSK3β, cyclin-dependent kinase 5 (CDK5), p38MAPK, casein-kinase 1, PKA, and CaMKII; and tyrosine kinases such as Fyn, among several others. Almost 40 putative phosphorylation sites may be target of GSK3β, which is a major contributor to tau hyperphosphorylation related to neurodegeneration, primarily due to impaired axonal transport. Tau phosphorylation at a tyrosine reside by Fyn kinase may also promote aggregation and mediated amyloid β (Aβ)-induced synaptic toxicity. Another major mechanism of neurodegeneration is abnormal phosphorylation of neurofilaments resulting in impairment of axonal transport. Many kinases can also impair axonal transport by phosphorylating subunits of motor proteins such as dynein and impairing their interactions with microtubules. Several such kinases have been implicated in ALS, including p38MAPK, JNK, GSK3β, and CDK5.[32] For example, the stress kinases p38MAPK and JNK are upregulated in mouse models of ALS; p38MAPK phosphorylates neurofilament medium- and heavy-chain proteins preventing their axonal transport, whereas JNK phosphorylates TAR-DNA-binding protein 43 (TDP-43) which is a major component of cytoplasmic inclusions in ALS and several forms of frontotemporal dementia. Increased activity of GSK3β may also impair axonal transport by phosphorylating dynein subunits or by disrupting ER–mitochondrial interactions. Upregulated CDK5 also impairs dynein-mediated transport whereas PTEN (phosphatase and tensin homolog)–induced kinase 1 (PINK1) may affect mitochondrial quality control and transport. Many kinases involved in ALS are also mediators or regulators of neuroinflammation. For example, TBK1 has a neuroprotective and anti-inflammatory effect by regulating the production of interferons α and β and modulating immune cell responses. Other kinases may contribute to ALS pathogenesis by affecting DNA/RNA metabolism or proteostasis.[32]

KEY POINTS

- Extracellular signals act via membrane receptors that trigger several intracellular transduction pathways affecting multiple cellular processes.
- Virtually all extracellular signals produce their physiological effects by regulating of the state of phosphorylation of their target proteins via protein kinases or phosphatases.
- Changes in the state of phosphorylation of membrane, cytosolic, cytoskeletal, and nuclear proteins regulate neural development, growth and survival, electrophysiological behavior, synaptic transmission and plasticity, responses to injury, and repair.
- G proteins function as molecular switches that undergo a regulatory cycle cycling between an inactive GDP-bound and an active GTP-bound state.
- Small Ras-GTPases are critically involved in growth factor signaling, endocytosis, mobilization of synaptic vesicles, actin cytoskeletal dynamics, and nucleocytoplasmic transport.
- G proteins consisting of Gα/β/γ subunits mediate the effects of GPCRs in response to a wide variety of neurotransmitters, hormones, and other signals.
- Upon ligand binding, the active Gα subunit regulates effector enzymes that trigger several second messenger–protein kinase cascades; the βγ complex directly modulates membrane ion channels.
- Many GPCR subtypes share common signal transduction pathways by activating the same type of G proteins.
- Control of cytosolic Ca^{2+} concentration in critical for both cell function and survival.
- Cytosolic Ca^{2+} concentration is determined by the interplay among influx through membrane channels, release from intracellular stores in the endoplasmic reticulum (ER) efflux through the plasma membrane, and sequestration in the ER.
- Calcium interacts with calmodulin (CaM) to regulate the phosphorylation of function of membrane, cytosolic, and nuclear proteins.
- Neurotrophic factors regulate development, growth, differentiation, survival, and plasticity via membrane tyrosine kinase receptors.
- The mechanistic (mammalian) target of rapamycin (mTOR) is a major downstream mediator of growth factor signaling and promotes cell growth and survival by promoting protein synthesis and suppressing autophagy.
- Essentially all neurologic disorders are associated, either directly or indirectly, with disturbances in intracellular signaling, Ca^{2+} homeostasis, and protein phosphorylation.

REFERENCES

1. Fuxe K, Borroto-Escuela D, Fisone G, Agnati LF, Tanganelli S. Understanding the role of heteroreceptor complexes in the central nervous system. Curr Protein Pept Sci 2014;15:647.
2. Guidolin D, Marcoli M, Tortorella C, Maura G, Agnati LF. G protein-coupled receptor-receptor interactions give integrative dynamics to intercellular communication. Rev Neurosci 2018;29:703–726.
3. Agnati LF, Guidolin D, Vilardaga JP, Ciruela F, Fuxe K. On the expanding terminology in the GPCR field: the meaning of receptor mosaics and receptor heteromers. J Recept Signal Transduct Res 2010;30:287–303.
4. Carecchio M, Mencacci NE. Emerging monogenic complex hyperkinetic disorders. Curr Neurol Neurosci Rep 2017;17:97.
5. Niccolini F, Mencacci NE, Yousaf T, et al. PDE10A and ADCY5 mutations linked to molecular and microstructural basal ganglia pathology. Mov Disord 2018;33:1961–1965.
6. Wampole CR, Smith KE. Beyond opioids for pain management in adult critically ill patients. J Pharm Pract 2019;32:256–270.
7. Kosten TR, Baxter LE. Review article: effective management of opioid withdrawal symptoms: a gateway to opioid dependence treatment. Am J Addict 2019;28:55–62.
8. Morr S, Heard CM, Li V, Reynolds RM. Dexmedetomidine for acute baclofen withdrawal. Neurocrit Care 2015;22:288–292.
9. Feng H, Sjogren B, Karaj B, Shaw V, Gezer A, Neubig RR. Movement disorder in GNAO1 encephalopathy associated with gain-of-function mutations. Neurology 2017;89:762–770.

10. Kerkhofs M, Seitaj B, Ivanova H, Monaco G, Bultynck G, Parys JB. Pathophysiological consequences of isoform-specific IP3 receptor mutations. Biochim Biophys Acta Mol Cell Res 2018;1865:1707–1717.
11. Shirafuji T, Shimazaki H, Miyagi T, et al. Spinocerebellar ataxia type 14 caused by a nonsense mutation in the PRKCG gene. Mol Cell Neurosci 2019;98:46–53.
12. Jarius S, Wildemann B. "Medusa-head ataxia": the expanding spectrum of Purkinje cell antibodies in autoimmune cerebellar ataxia. Part 1: Anti-mGluR1, anti-Homer-3, anti-Sj/ITPR1 and anti-CARP VIII. J Neuroinflammation 2015;12:166.
13. Martins J, Kolomiets B, Caplette R, et al. Sildenafil acutely decreases visual responses in ON and OFF retinal ganglion cells. Invest Ophthalmol Vis Sci 2015;56:2639–2648.
14. Yanoga F, Gentile RC, Chui TYP, et al. Sildenafil citrate induced retinal toxicity-electroretinogram, optical coherence tomography, and adaptive optics findings. Retin Cases Brief Rep 2018;12 Suppl 1:S33–S40.
15. Urs NM, Bido S, Peterson SM, et al. Targeting beta-arrestin2 in the treatment of L-DOPA-induced dyskinesia in Parkinson's disease. Proc Natl Acad Sci U S A 2015;112:E2517–2526.
16. Zhu J, Hu Z, Han X, et al. Dopamine D2 receptor restricts astrocytic NLRP3 inflammasome activation via enhancing the interaction of beta-arrestin2 and NLRP3. Cell Death Differ 2018;25:2037–2049.
17. Thathiah A, Horre K, Snellinx A, et al. Beta-arrestin 2 regulates Abeta generation and gamma-secretase activity in Alzheimer's disease. Nat Med 2013;19:43–49.
18. Moran MM. TRP channels as potential drug targets. Annu Rev Pharmacol Toxicol 2018;58:309–330.
19. Lopez JJ, Jardin I, Albarran L, et al. Molecular basis and regulation of store-operated calcium entry. Adv Exp Med Biol 2020;1131:445–469.
20. Hamada K, Mikoshiba K. IP3 receptor plasticity underlying diverse functions. Annu Rev Physiol 2020;82:151–176.
21. Abu-Omar N, Das J, Szeto V, Feng ZP. Neuronal ryanodine receptors in development and aging. Mol Neurobiol 2018;55:1183–1192.
22. Rios E, Figueroa L, Manno C, Kraeva N, Riazi S. The couplonopathies: a comparative approach to a class of diseases of skeletal and cardiac muscle. J Gen Physiol 2015;145:459–474.
23. Cali T, Brini M, Carafoli E. The PMCA pumps in genetically determined neuronal pathologies. Neurosci Lett 2018;663:2–11.
24. Bano D, Ankarcrona M. Beyond the critical point: an overview of excitotoxicity, calcium overload and the downstream consequences. Neurosci Lett 2018;663:79–85.
25. Spencer SA, Suarez-Pozos E, Escalante M, Myo YP, Fuss B. Sodium-calcium exchangers of the SLC8 family in oligodendrocytes: functional properties in health and disease. Neurochem Res 2020;45:1287–1297.
26. Britzolaki A, Saurine J, Klocke B, Pitychoutis PM. A role for SERCA pumps in the neurobiology of neuropsychiatric and neurodegenerative disorders. Adv Exp Med Biol 2020;1131:131–161.
27. Alvarez J, Alvarez-Illera P, Garcia-Casas P, Fonteriz RI, Montero M. The role of Ca(2+) Signaling in Aging and Neurodegeneration: insights from Caenorhabditis elegans models. Cells 2020;9:204–218.
28. Urrutia J, Aguado A, Muguruza-Montero A, et al. The crossroad of ion channels and calmodulin in disease. Int J Mol Sci 2019;20:400–414.
29. Takemoto-Kimura S, Suzuki K, Horigane SI, et al. Calmodulin kinases: essential regulators in health and disease. J Neurochem 2017;141:808–818.
30. Bockaert J, Marin P. mTOR in brain physiology and pathologies. Physiol Rev 2015;95:1157–1187.
31. Switon K, Kotulska K, Janusz-Kaminska A, Zmorzynska J, Jaworski J. Molecular neurobiology of mTOR. Neuroscience 2017;341:112–153.
32. Guo W, Vandoorne T, Steyaert J, Staats KA, Van Den Bosch L. The multifaceted role of kinases in amyotrophic lateral sclerosis: genetic, pathological and therapeutic implications. Brain 2020;143:1651–1673.
33. Wang Y, Mandelkow E. Tau in physiology and pathology. Nat Rev Neurosci 2016;17:22–35.

4 DNA: Epigenetic Control of Transcription and Repair Mechanisms

OVERVIEW

In cells, DNA is present in the nucleus and mitochondria. Nuclear DNA is organized into 46 chromosomes and consists of two long polynucleotide strands coiled into a double helix that contains the genetic code. Mitochondrial DNA encodes relatively few, but fundamental, mitochondrial proteins. DNA replication is a highly regulated process that involves different types of DNA polymerases, helicases, topoisomerases, and telomerases. In the nucleus, the DNA is packaged into chromatin together with histones and associated proteins. There are approximately 20,000 protein-coding genes in the human genome. Most (60%) of the genome is transcribed, and it has been estimated that roughly 12,000 genes are expressed in a given neuron. However, only about 1%–2% of the nuclear genome is transcribed into messenger RNA (mRNA) and encodes proteins; about 85%–90% is transcribed into noncoding RNAs (ncRNAs). Apart from DNA sequence, gene regulation is determined by epigenetic mechanisms, including DNA methylation, histone modifications such as acetylation and methylation that affect chromatin structure, and ncRNAs. These mechanisms may either promote or repress gene expression. Nuclear and mitochondrial DNA are exposed to damage by oxidative stress and other insults. Damaged DNA must be repaired to allow the proper reading of the genetic code. Whereas mature neurons are postmitotic cells, DNA replication and cell division also occurs in adult neurogenic niches. Progression through the cell cycle is driven by sequential activation of cyclin-dependent kinases. Abnormal epigenetic modulation, impaired DNA repair, and aberrant cell cycle entry are fundamental disease mechanisms in many neurologic disorders, including neurodegeneration and neoplasms. The aims of this chapter are to briefly review (1) the main epigenetic processes controlling DNA transcription; (2) the mechanisms of DNA damage and repair; (3) the checkpoint control of the cell cycle, and (4) examples of disorders affecting these processes.

STRUCTURE OF THE DNA AND CHROMATIN

The DNA is a polymer of nucleotides consisting of the purines adenine (A) and guanine (G) and the pyrimidines thymine (T) and cytosine (C), attached to a deoxyribose phosphate. The nuclear DNA consists of two long polynucleotide strands coiled into a double helix. The two DNA strands are complementary and are held together by hydrogen bonds between the A:T and G:C base pairs.

DNA Replication

DNA replication involves copying a complementary sequence of DNA using the opposite chain as a template. It occurs during the synthetic (S) phase of the cell cycle preceding cell division. DNA replication depends on different types of DNA polymerases (Pols). Pol α and -δ catalyze replication of nuclear DNA; Pol β is involved in nuclear DNA repair; and Pol γ (POLG) mediates DNA replication in the mitochondria. Before replication takes place, DNA helicases unwind the DNA molecule and open the double-stranded DNA into two single DNA strands. DNA polymerase moves along the template strand in a 3'–5' direction, and adds a nucleotide onto a preexisting 3'-hydroxyl (3'-OH) end of the newly forming strand. DNA ligases catalyze the formation of phosphodiester bonds between the 3'-OH ends of one nucleotide with the 5' phosphate (5'P) end of the next. Topoisomerases correct the overwinding or underwinding of DNA that occurs during DNA replication and transcription. Telomerase is a ribonucleoprotein that is recruited to single-strand 3' segments overhanging the telomeres at the ends of chromosomes; these segments cannot be replicated by DNA polymerase and thus grow shorter in every cell cycle. Telomerase functions as a reverse transcriptase, using RNA to elongate the ends of the chromosomal DNA and thus limit the shortening of the telomeres. The DNA molecule is cleaved by exonucleases and endonucleases.

Basic Structure of the Gene

The gene is composed of exons, introns, and a signal for polyadenylation. Exons are transcribed into coding mRNA that is translated into proteins; introns are interspersed between exons. A typical protein-coding gene contains multiple regulatory regions, including one or more enhancers and a promoter that drives transcriptional expression. The gene and its regulator elements are flanked by boundary elements or insulators. Intergenic regions that flank genes constitute 75% of DNA and consist largely of repetitive DNA sequences; these sequences appear multiple times and may be found in a series of adjacent clusters, called tandem repeats. Trinucleotide repeats may be present in either encoding or noncoding regions of genomic DNA. Once the length of the repetitive sequence passes a certain threshold, it tends to expand with increasing repeat size in successive generations. Some DNA sequences can self-replicate, and the additional copies might migrate to different portions within the genome as mobile elements, or transposons. Some sequences, called retrotransposons, may be inserted into DNA via reverse transcription of RNA.

Structure of Chromatin

The smallest unit of chromatin is the nucleosome. It consists of about 146 base pairs of DNA wrapped around a histone octamer, containing two each of the core histone proteins, H2A, H2B, H3, and H4) (Figure 4.1). Linker DNA folded around linker H1 histones connects nucleosomes together, forming a beads-on-a-string appearance that characterizes chromatin. Core histones contain basic residues that interact with the phosphate moieties of DNA, promoting its winding in the nucleosomes and thus restricting its access to the transcriptional machinery. There is a continuum of chromatin states from a condensed and transcriptionally inactive chromatin (heterochromatin) to open and transcriptionally active chromatin (chromatin) with the DNA template accessible to nuclear factors. Chromatin states critically modulate the execution of genomic programs, including activation of transcription, long-term gene silencing, genome imprinting, DNA replication and repair, and genome stability. Chromatin interacts with lamins and other proteins of the nuclear lamina that connect the nuclear lamina with the cytosolic cytoskeleton.

EPIGENETIC MECHANISMS

Epigenetic mechanisms regulate the function of single genes and gene networks and have a major role in brain development, adult neurogenesis, synaptic and network connectivity and plasticity, and inheritance of cognitive and behavioral traits.[1–3] The epigenome refers to several

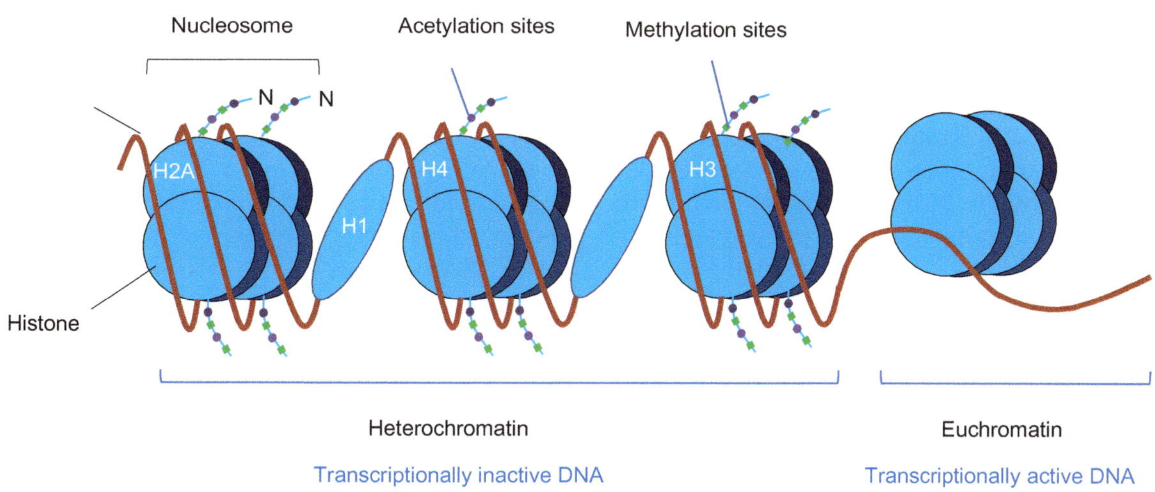

FIGURE 4.1 Structure of chromatin.
Chromatin is composed of DNA, histones, and associated proteins. The smallest unit of chromatin is the nucleosome, which consists of ~146 base pairs of DNA wrapped around a histone octamer containing two of each core histone proteins (i.e., H2A, H2B, H3, and H4). Linker DNA folded around linker H1 histones connects nucleosomes together forming chromatin. Chromatin states vary from a condensed and transcriptionally inactive chromatin (heterochromatin) to open and transcriptionally active chromatin (euchromatin).

TABLE 4.1 *Epigenetic Mechanisms*

Mechanism	Processes
Covalent modifications of DNA	DNA cytosine methylation (DNA methyltransferases, DMTs) Active cytosine demethylation (e.g., GADD45) Cytosine hydroxymethylation (Ten-Eleven-Translocation [TET] enzymes)
Histone posttranslational modifications	Lysine (K) acetylation (histone acetyl transferase, HAT) Lysine and arginine (R) mono-, di-, or trimethylation (histone methyl transferases, HMTs) Lysine and arginine demethylation Serine/threonine phosphorylation Monoubiquitination Poly (ADP) ribosylation
Noncoding RNAs	Short noncoding RNAs (e.g., microRNAs, small interfering RNAs (siRNAs) Long noncoding RNAs
Transcriptional repression	RE1-silencing transcription factor (REST)/Rest corepressor (coREST/syn3) system
Other mechanisms	ATP-dependent chromatin remodeling Histone subunit exchange Prion protein-based mechanisms

processes: DNA methylation and hydroxymethylation, histone posttranslational modifications, higher-order chromatin remodeling, DNA and RNA editing and regulation by ncRNAs (Table 4.1).

DNA Methylation and Hydroxymethylation

DNA methylation is the attachment of methyl groups to cytosine residues directly next to guanine residues (CpG sites) within the DNA molecule, yielding 5-methylcytosine (5-mC) (Figure 4.2). This process is mediated by DNA methyltransferases (DNMTs). There are three families of DNMTs; DNMT1 is primarily associated with maintaining DNA methylation patterns, whereas DNMT3a and DNMT3b are involved in adding new methylation marks. CpG dinucleotides constitute about 1% of the total human genome and 60%–80% are methylated; a small percentage of CpG dinucleotides are clustered within gene promoters and are referred to as CpG islands. DNA methylation at promoter regions typically represses the transcription of the associated gene. Methylated loci provide binding sites that are recognized by methyl-CpG binding domain proteins, including methyl-CpG binding protein 2 (MeCP2). These proteins regulate transcription and chromatin modifications and can repress gene expression by preventing the binding of transcription activators to DNA promoters. For example, MeCP2 functions as a dual transcriptional regulator of the *BDNF* gene encoding brain-derived neurotrophic factor (BDNF). Neuronal activity triggers calcium-dependent phosphorylation of MeCP2, thereby releasing MeCP2 from the promoter region and facilitating *BDNF* transcription. Methyl groups can be removed from DNA residues by several enzymes, including those activated by cell stress and involved in DNA repair, such as GADD45 (growth arrest and DNA damage-induced protein 45). The 5-methyl cytosine residues can be oxidized to 5-hydroxymethylcytosine by ten-eleven translocation (TET) enzymes. Unlike the case of 5-methylcytosine, the 5-hydroxymethylcytosine modification is typically associated with increased transcription.

Posttranslational Histone Modifications

Histone modifications constitute a fundamental mechanism of regulation of gene expression by affecting compaction and structure of chromatin, its interaction with transcription factors, and local and long-distance chromosomal reorganization (Figure 4.3). There is a broad range of histone-modifying and chromatin-remodeling enzymes that may serve as "writers" or "erasers" of epigenetic marks. Posttranslational modifications occur particularly at lysine (K) and arginine (R) residues of individual histone amino (N)-terminus tails and include acetylation, methylation, ubiquitination, and phosphorylation. Since core histones repress DNA transcription, their posttranslational modifications may either activate or inhibit gene expression, depending on the position of the residue that is covalently modified and its influence on chromatin structure. Histone acetylation, mediated by histone acetyl transferases (HATs), inhibits the interaction between histones and DNA, promoting the unwinding of the DNA and its exposure to the RNA

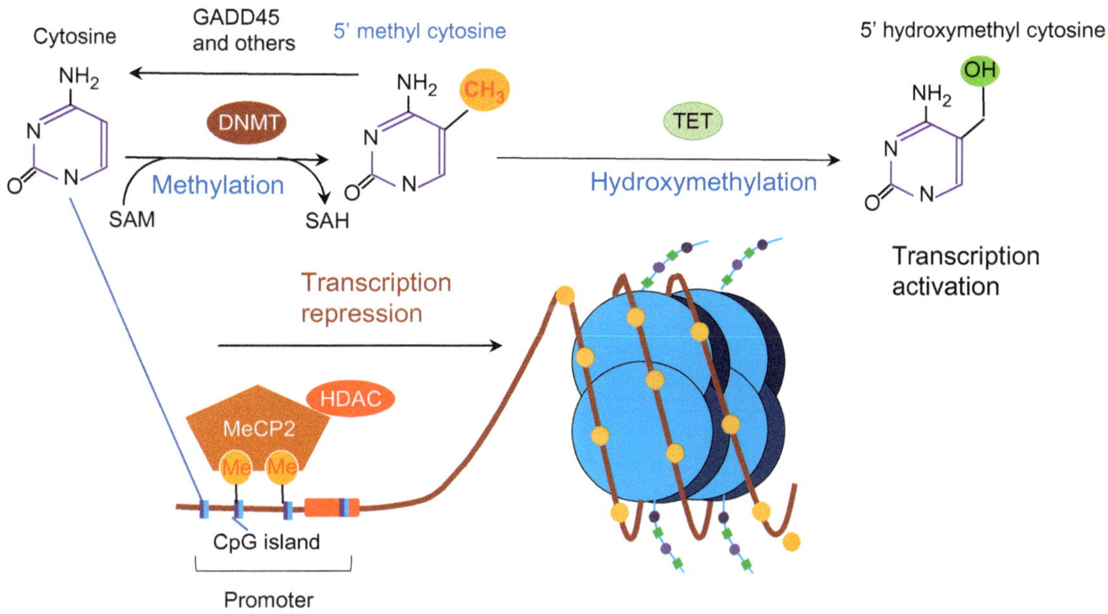

FIGURE 4.2 DNA methylation and hydroxymethylation.
DNA methylation is the attachment of methyl groups to cytosine residues directly next to guanine residues (CpG sites) within the DNA molecule, yielding 5-methyl cytosine (5-mC) This process is mediated by DNA methyltransferases (DNMTs) using S-adenoyslmethionine (SAM). Methylated loci provide binding sites that are recognized by methyl-CpG-binding domain proteins, including methyl-CpG-binding protein 2 (MeCP2), which recruits effector proteins such as histone acetyl transferases (HATs) that can repress gene expression. Proteins activated by cell stress and involved in DNA repair, such as GADD45 (growth arrest and DNA damage-induced protein 45) elicit DNA demethylation. The 5-mC residues can be oxidized to 5-hydroxymethylcytosine by Ten-Eleven Translocation (TET) enzymes. SAH, S-adenosylhomocyteine.

transcription machinery. In contrast, histone deacetylases (HDACs) provide a mechanism of transcriptional repression by removing the acetyl group and promoting histone interaction with DNA and its winding in the nucleosomes. Sirtuins are an important group of HDACs. Methylation of histones is controlled by histone methyltransferases (HMT) that catalyze the transfer of mono-, di-, or tri-methyl groups to lysine or arginine residues, and histone demethylases (HDMTs) that demethylate these residues. Histone methylation may have distinct effects depending on the residues targeted by these enzymes. For example, in the case of H3 histone, methylation of lysine 4 and lysine 36 residues (H3K4, H3K36) promotes an open chromatin structure and activation of gene expression, while methylation of lysine 9 and 27 residues (H3K9 HEK27) elicits silencing of transcription. Histone modifications work synergistically with DNA methylation to influence gene expression and chromatin structure.

The inhibitor of growth (ING) proteins serve as epigenetic readers of the H3K4Me3 histone mark of active gene transcription and target HAT or histone HDAC protein complexes, in order to alter local chromatin structure. These proteins are multidomain adaptor proteins that interact with numerous other proteins to facilitate their localization and regulate numerous biochemical pathways, acting as tumor suppressors.[4]

Noncoding RNAs

Noncoding RNAs (ncRNAs) are transcribed from both DNA strands and can be further processed to produce small and long species that interact in a sequence-specific manner with DNA, RNA, DNA:RNA complexes, and RNA-binding proteins. Noncoding RNAs mediate numerous epigenetic processes, including mRNA posttranscriptional processing. Short ncRNAs (< 200 nucleotides) include microRNAs (miRNAs), endogenous small interfering RNAs (siRNAs), and small nucleolar RNAs. MicroRNAs function primarily by mRNA silencing and posttranscriptional regulation of gene expression. Long ncRNAs (> 200 nucleotides) include intergenic ncRNAs, natural antisense transcripts, and ncRNA repeats. The mechanisms of long ncRNAs are more complex and heterogeneous than those of short ncRNAs. Some are transcribed from intergenic regions, whereas others have antisense function or overlapping interactions with protein-encoding genes. These long ncRNAs may regulate the transcription and posttranscriptional processing of the associated protein-coding gene; recruit transcriptional and epigenetic regulators at specific microdomains; modulate nucleocytoplasmic transport; and control local protein synthesis. Circular RNAs are a special type of ncRNAs that regulate the function of miRNAs and also control several other processes of mRNA metabolism, as discussed in the next chapter.

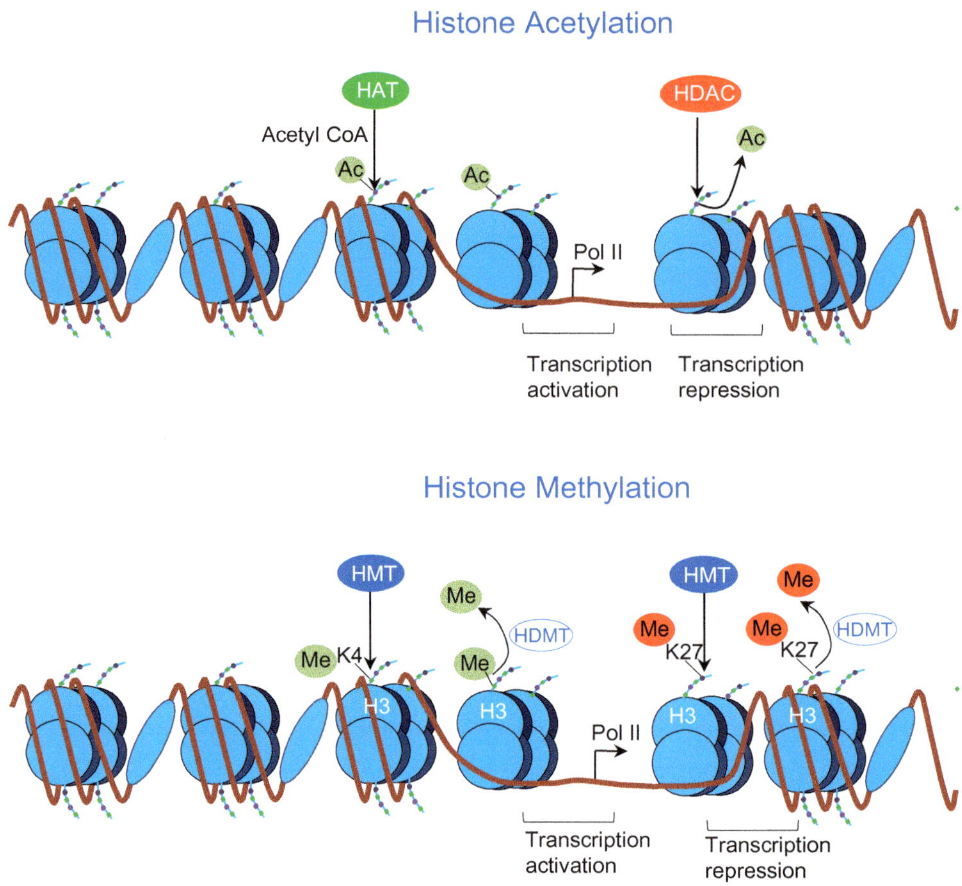

FIGURE 4.3 Posttranslational histone modifications.
Histone acetylation is mediated by histone acetyl transferases (HATs) using acetyl coenzyme A (acetyl CoA) as a donor; it inhibits histone interaction with DNA, promoting the unwinding of the DNA and allowing its exposure to the RNA transcription machinery. Histone deacetylases (HDACs) inhibit translation by promoting histone interaction with DNA. Methylation of histones is mediated by histone methyltransferases (HMTs) to lysine or arginine residues; histone demethylases (HDMTs) have an opposite role. Histone methylation may have distinct effects depending or the residues targeted by the enzyme. For example, H3 histone methylation of lysine 4 and lysine 36 (H3K4, H3K36) opens chromatin structure and activates while its methylation of lysine 9 and 27 (H3K9m HEK27) elicits transcription silencing.

Epigenetic Mechanisms for Metabolic Control of Gene Expression

There is a reciprocal regulation between intermediate metabolism and gene expression.[5,6] Several metabolites function as cofactors and regulators of various enzymes involved in epigenetic mechanisms. For example, methylation of DNA and histones is regulated by S-adenostylmethionine, which is synthesized from methionine and ATP by a reaction that requires vitamin B_{12} and folic acid derivatives as cofactors. As this reaction also produces S-adenosylhomocysteine, a potent inhibitor of all methyltransferases, the tightly regulated ratio between these two metabolites dynamically regulates DNA and histone methylation. The 5' methyl cytosine hydroxylase TET uses a reaction that requires α-ketoglutarate, ferrous iron, and molecular oxygen to upregulate gene expression. This reaction is inhibited by 2-hydroxyglutarate, an oncometabolite primarily produced by glioma cells bearing gain-of-function mutations of the isocitrate dehydrogenase (*ICDH*) genes. Histone acetylation is also sensitive to the availability of metabolites that serve as substrates or cofactors. Acetyl coenzyme A (acetyl CoA), a critical product of intermediate metabolism, provides the acetyl groups required for HATs to acetylate lysine residues of histones and promote transcription. This interaction coordinates responses of the transcription machinery to nutrient availability. In contrast, nuclear HDACs such as Sirtuins require oxidized nicotinamide adenine dinucleotide (NAD^+) for their activity; this allows regulation of transcription in the setting of starvation that leads to NAD^+ accumulation. Adenosine monophosphate (AMP)-activated protein kinase (AMPK), which is activated in conditions of energy deprivation and regulates metabolic pathways that promote ATP production, also elicits epigenetic regulation of chromatin dynamics by phosphorylating several histones and proteins involved in nucleosome remodeling.[6]

DNA DAMAGE AND REPAIR

In normal conditions, cells experience substantial DNA damage. It is estimated that about 10^5 DNA lesions occur daily as a consequence of spontaneous decay, replication errors, and cell metabolism, particularly reactive oxygen species (ROS) production by the mitochondria. Oxidative stress is the main cause of DNA damage in the nervous system. In addition to generating base modifications, ROS attack the DNA backbone and sugar moieties, leading to formation of DNA single-strand breaks that may block DNA replication and stall RNA polymerase progression during transcription. The DNA damage response consists of a series of processes that detect and repair the damaged DNA and coordinate repair with chromatin remodeling, transcription regulation, cell cycle progression, and apoptosis. There are several mechanisms of DNA repair[7–11] (Figure 4.4). Base excision-repair is the main pathway for removal

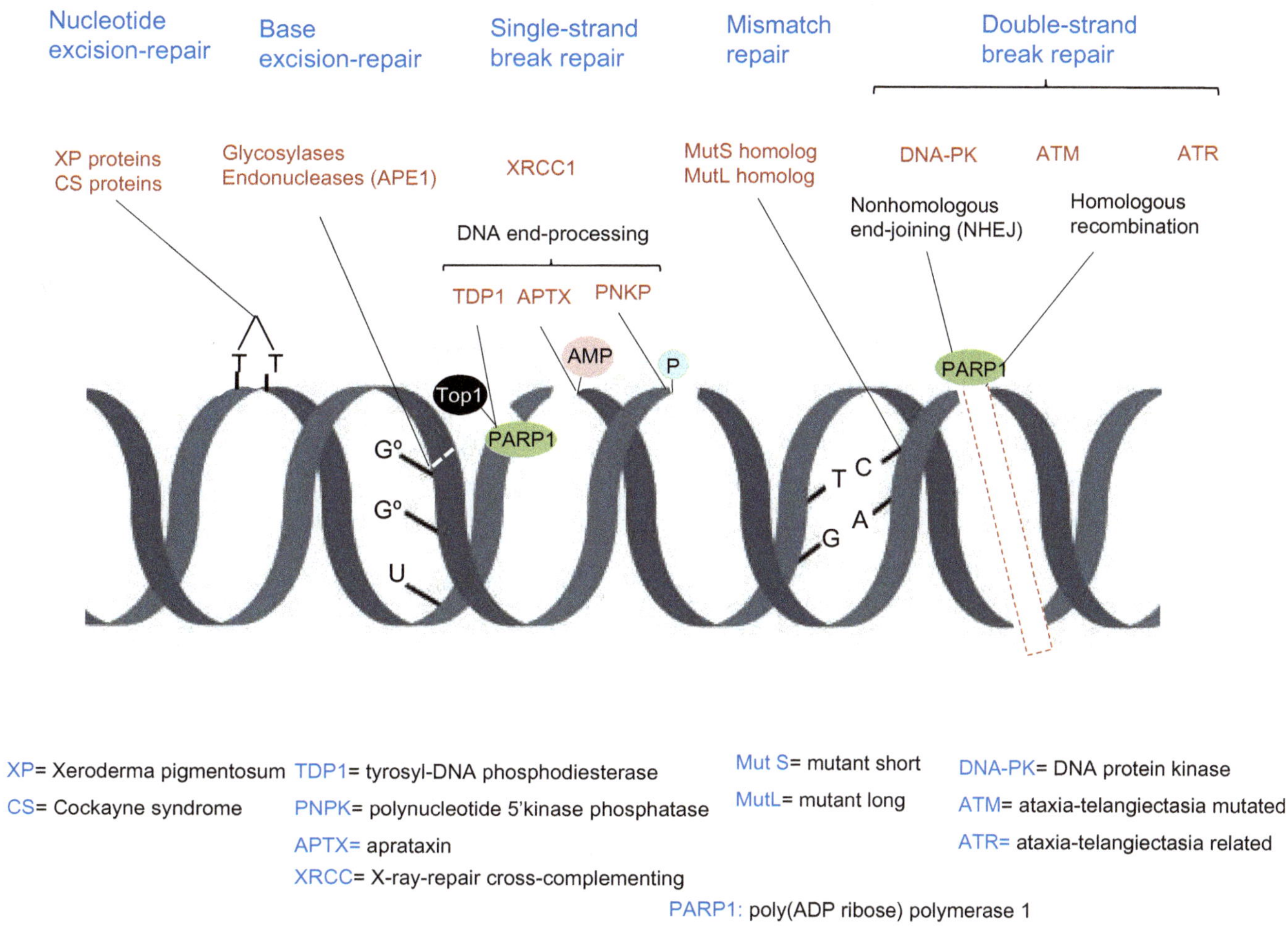

FIGURE 4.4 General mechanisms of DNA repair.
There are several mechanisms of DNA repair, including base excision-repair, nucleotide excision-repair; mismatch repair; single-strand break repair, and double-strand break repair. An early event in DNA repair is recruitment of poly(adenosine diphosphate [ADP] ribose) polymerase 1 (PARP1) to the site of DNA damage. A critical step is DNA end-processing via polynucleotide 3'kinase phosphatase (PNKP), which acts on the damaged 3'P terminus; tyrosyl-DNA phosphodiesterase 1 (TDP1), which hydrolyzes the phosphodiester bond between 3' ends and the catalytic tyrosyl residue of topoisomerase 1 (Top1); and aprataxin (APTX), which deadenylates the abnormal 5'AMP termini. X-ray-repair cross-complementing (XRCC) proteins provide a scaffold for several other DNA repair proteins, The nucleotide excision-repair system involves xeroderma pigmentosum (XP) proteins; transcription-coupled nucleotide excision-repair involves lesion recognition by Cockayne syndrome (CS) proteins. Mismatch repair involves a group of proteins homologous to the Mutator short (MutS) and Mutator long (MutL) proteins. Double-strand break repair is controlled by three master kinases: DNA-dependent kinase DMA-PK), ataxia-telangiectasia mutated (ATM), and ataxia-telangiectasia Rad3 (ATR) protein.

of bases affected by oxidative modifications in both nuclear and mitochondrial DNA. Single-strand break repair and double-strand break repair involve chromatin remodeling.

General Mechanisms

The response to DNA damage first involves DNA damage recognition; this is followed by resection of the affected site by exo- or endonucleases, DNA end-processing, filling the gap by action of DNA polymerases, and sealing of the nick by DNA ligases. One of the earliest events of DNA repair is recruitment of poly (adenosine diphosphate [ADP] ribose) polymerase 1 (PARP1).[12,13] This enzyme binds to sites of DNA breaks and subsequently modifies repair proteins, including protein kinases, nucleases, scaffold proteins, and histones, by adding of branches of poly (ADP) ribose residues derived from NAD^+; this process is called PARylation. A critical step in base excision-repair and single-strand break repair is DNA end-processing. The 3' and 5' termini of damaged DNA strands must be restored to conventional 3'-OH and 5'P moieties in order to fill the gap by action of DNA polymerases. There are three main DNA end-processing proteins. Polynucleotide 3'kinase phosphatase (PNKP) acts on the damaged 3'P terminus; tyrosyl-DNA phosphodiesterase 1 (TDP1) hydrolyzes the phosphodiester bond between 3' ends and the catalytic tyrosyl residue of topoisomerase 1 in topoisomerase 1 cleavage complexes; and aprataxin (APTX) deadenylates the abnormal 5'AMP termini resulting from abortive DNA ligase activity into normal 5'P ends. To complete DNA repair, gap filling may occur by insertion of either a single nucleotide (short-patch repair) or multiple nucleotides (long-patch repair). Many proteins serve as scaffolds to recruit other proteins involved in recognition, signal amplification, or execution of DNA repair. As an example, X-ray-repair cross-complementing (XRCC) proteins provide a scaffold for several DNA polymerases and ligases.

Specific Processes

The base excision-repair machinery is initiated by substrate-specific DNA glycosidases that detect and excise the damaged bases affected by oxidative modifications. This process is followed by activity of endonucleases that cleave the phosphoribosyl backbone, leaving a nick in the DNA. The nucleotide excision-repair system recognizes and corrects distortions in the helical structure of DNA, including pyrimidine dimers caused by ultraviolet radiation and DNA adducts in response to cis-platinum and other compounds. Nucleotide excision-repair occurs via two subpathways, global genomic repair and transcription-coupled repair; both processes involve several xeroderma pigmentosum (XP) proteins. Transcription-coupled nucleotide excision-repair also involves Cockayne syndrome (CS) proteins, which recognize the stalling of RNA polymerase at a lesion on the transcribed strand nucleotide.

Mismatch repair recognizes base-base mismatches that originate from errors or intermediates of DNA replication and is important to maintain genome stability. This repair process is important in regions containing short, repetitive DNA sequences, which are prone to DNA polymerase slippage errors that can lead to deleterious frameshift mutations. Single-strand breaks are one of the most common DNA lesions affecting the nervous system and most commonly result from oxidative attack by hydroxyl radicals; these breaks may also be due to abortive activity of DNA topoisomerase or erroneous incorporation of ribonucleotides into DNA. Double-strand break repair is tightly coordinated with chromatin remodeling and progression of the cell cycle. There are two major pathways for repair of double-strand DNA breaks, nonhomologous end-joining and homology-directed repair or homologous recombination. Nonhomologous end-joining is the direct religation of broken DNA without the use of a template. This is an error-prone mechanism that introduces mutations of genes and is essential to generate diversity of antigen receptors in immune cells. In contrast, homologous recombination requires the presence of a sister chromatid as a template and therefore only occurs during the S and G_2 phases of the cell cycle. Efficient homologous recombination requires a critical step of extensive DNA resection. This involves a complex consisting of MRE11 (meiotic recombination 11), RAD50 (DNA repair bridging protein 50), and NBS-1 (Nijmegen breakage syndrome-1), referred to as MRN complex. The resulting overhanging single DNA fragments undergo coating by a DNA repair bridging protein, forming a nucleoprotein filament that mediates strand invasion into the sister chromatid to search for the homolog template.

Ataxia-Telangiectasia Mutated Protein and Double-Strand Break Response

Ataxia-telangiectasia mutated (ATM) protein is a serine/threonine kinase that functions as the master regulator of the coordinated responses to DNA double-strand damage[14] (Figure 4.5). ATM is recruited at damaged sites via PARP1 and the MRN protein complex involved in DNA end-resection. At the level of DNA breaks, ATM phosphorylates and activates hundreds of substrate proteins, including other protein kinases, providing a mechanism for signal amplification. ATM also facilitates nonhomologous end-joining by activating DNA protein kinase. Furthermore, ATM promotes chromatin remodeling by phosphorylating the histone variant H2AX, triggering phosphorylation-ubiquitylation cascades affecting H1 histones. Importantly, ATM is also recruited and activated at the site of R-loops. These structures consist of DNA:RNA hybrids associated nontemplate single-stranded DNA and form at the site of DNA lesions that block transcription. ATM inhibits RNA transcription and further processing by the spliceosome at these sites. In contrast, the helicase senataxin (STX) prevents R-loop formation and promotes termination of transcription. Finally, ATM also regulates cell cycle and death pathways. One target for ATM phosphorylation is checkpoint kinase 2, which elicits cell cycle arrest. Another major

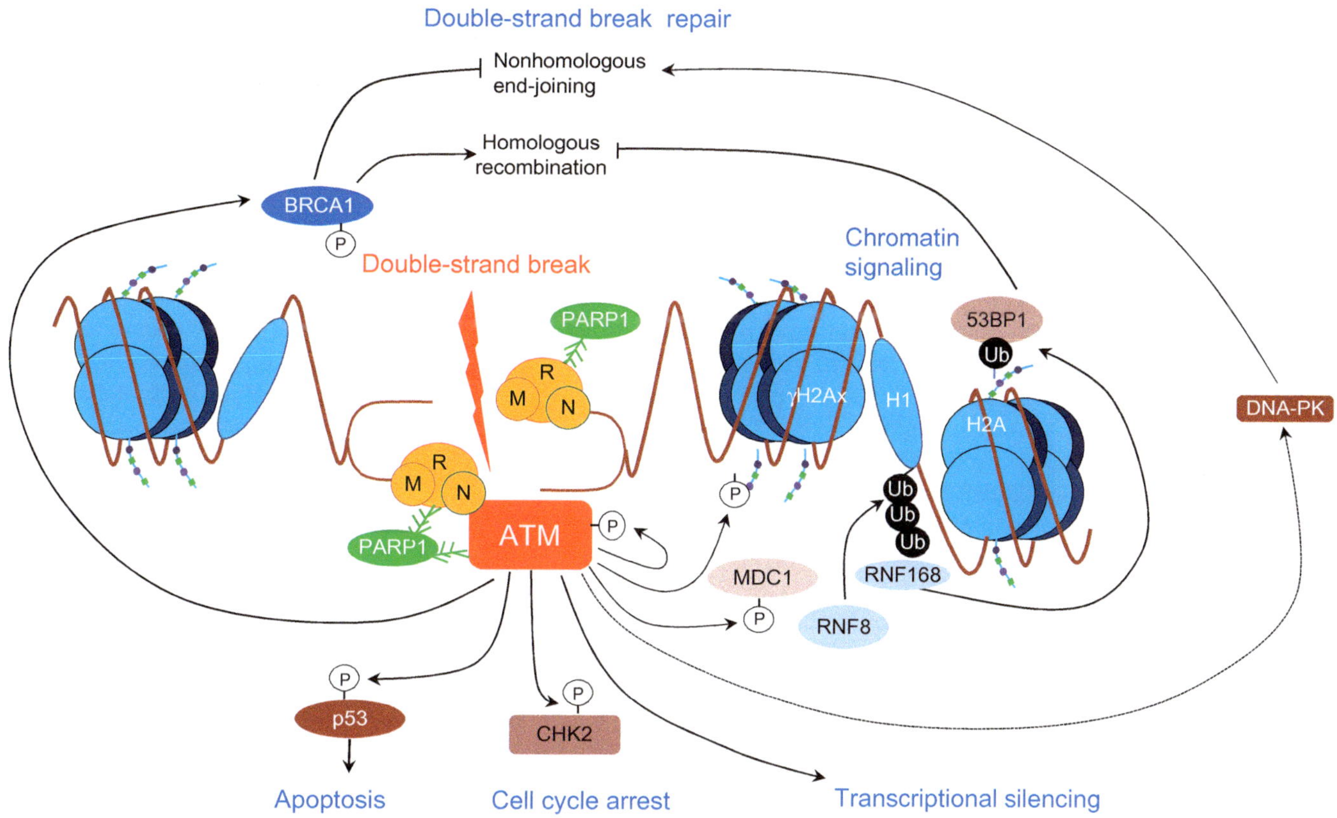

FIGURE 4.5 Ataxia-telangiectasia mutated (ATM) and DNA double-strand break response.
ATM is the master controller of responses to double-strand break. It binds to the site of DNA damage via interactions with poly adenosine diphosphate (ADP) ribose polymerase 1 (PARP11 and the MRN protein complex, consisting of MRE11 (meiotic recombination 11), RAD50 (DNA repair bridging protein 50), and NBS-1 (Nijmegen breakage syndrome -1), ATM phosphorylates and activates hundreds of substrate proteins. It stimulates DNA end-resection by phosphorylating C-terminal-binding protein–interacting protein (CtIP), a major activator of MRE11, and breast cancer 1 (BRCA)1 protein. ATM also promotes nonhomologous end-joining by activating DNA protein kinase (DNA-PK) and facilitating the accumulation of the p53-binding protein 1 (53BP1). ATM promotes chromatin remodeling by phosphorylating the histone variant H2AX yielding γH2AX; this recruits the mediator of DNA damage checkpoint 1 protein (MDC1) and triggers phosphorylation–ubiquitylation (Ub) cascades that are sequentially mediated by the ring finger 8 (RNF8) and RNF168 ubiquitin E3 targeting H1 linker histone and H2A histones, respectively. ATM activates the effector checkpoint kinase 2 (CHK2), which elicits cell cycle arrest, and p53, which triggers apoptosis. ATM is recruited and activated at the site of R-loops and elicits transcriptional silencing.

target is p53, the product of a tumor suppressor gene that promotes cell cycle arrest and triggers apoptosis.

CONTROL OF THE CELL CYCLE

Whereas neurons are largely postmitotic cells, they may aberrantly reenter the cell cycle in the setting of neurodegeneration. Adult neurogenesis still occurs in neurogenic niches such as the granule cell layer of the dentate gyrus of the hippocampus, which can make these cells particularly susceptible to the damaging effect of radiation therapy. The cell cycle is divided into four phases: G_1 (gap 1), S (synthesis), G_2 (gap 2), and M (mitosis). Appropriate transmission of genetic information depends on the accurate duplication of DNA during the S phase of the cell cycle and the segregation of the resultant sister chromatids during mitosis. In normal eukaryote cells, each event depends on the other, and replication of the genome and mitosis are alternative oscillating events.

Checkpoints and Cyclin-Dependent Kinases

Progression through the cell cycle is regulated at various checkpoints that monitor the efficacy and completion of events at each phase and stop the cycle if conditions are not perfect. The critical checkpoints are the G_1–S and the G_2–M transitions. Control at these checkpoints ensures that damaged DNA does not propagate, thereby preventing aberrant cell cycles that may result in translocations, amplification, and aneuploidy. Cell cycle progression at checkpoints is driven by the sequential activation of cyclin-dependent kinases (CDKs) that bind to partner proteins called cyclins. Each cyclin-CDK complex phosphorylates specific key proteins involved in the different phases of the cell cycle. The cyclin C/CDK3 complex marks the transition of cells into G1 in preparation for DNA synthesis. The passage through the G_1–S restriction point commits the cell to divide. The critical regulators are cyclin D and its catalytic partners, CDK4 and CDK6, which phosphorylate several proteins that control the G_1–S phase transition. A major target of phosphorylation the retinoblastoma protein (pRB). In its unphosphorylated state, pRB restricts cell growth by binding to the E2F1 transcription factor, thereby preventing its interaction with the cell transcription machinery and repressing expression of proteins required for DNA synthesis. Phosphorylation of pRB by the cyclin D/CDK4/CDK6 complex promotes dissociation of pRB from the E2F complex, thereby allowing progression to the S phase. DNA replication in the S phase is triggered by cyclin A/CDK2 and cyclin A/CDK1 complexes, and cell division in the M phase is regulated by the cyclin B/CDK1 complex. The integrity of the cell cycle is maintained by the timely degradation of cyclins by the ubiquitin-proteasome system and consequent inactivation of CDKs by cyclin dependent kinase inhibitors.

Signals Regulating Cell Cycle Checkpoints

Several signaling cascades regulate the cell cycle checkpoints. One important example is p53, which is activated by ATM in response to DNA damage. As a transcription factor, p53 regulates the S phase by activating expression of the CDK inhibitor p21, which halts the cell cycle. Growth factors promote degradation of p53 by the ubiquitin-proteasome system and thus facilitate the transition to the S phase. The cyclin-dependent kinase CDK5 has a major role in maintaining neurons in the postmitotic state. Unlike other cyclin-dependent kinases, CDK5 is a nucleocytoplasmic protein that is not activated by cyclins bur rather oscillates in and out of the nucleus during the cell cycle. During the S phase, CDK5 is exported from the nucleus to the cytoplasm, where it undergoes ubiquitin-proteasome mediated degradation. In postmitotic cells, CDK5 is imported to the nucleus where it inhibits cell cycle progression. In the cytoplasm, CDK5 phosphorylates a large number of substrates, including synaptic proteins and the microtubule-associated protein tau.

EPIGENETIC MECHANISMS OF NEUROLOGIC DISEASE

Epigenetic mechanisms are increasingly recognized as major disease pathways in genetic and acquired neurologic disorders.

Mutations Affecting Epigenetic Regulation

Mutations in genes directly linked to epigenetic regulation may manifest with either neurodevelopmental or adult-onset neurodegenerative disorders[3] (Table 4.2). A prototypical example is Rett syndrome, caused by mutations in the *MeCP2* gene on the X chromosome. Patients with Rett syndrome usually experience normal development until 6 to 18 months of age; they then develop a spectrum of symptoms including the loss of proper hand use, severe intellectual disability, loss of cognitive and motor skills, ataxia, and seizures. Mutations in *DNMT1* gene cause autosomal dominant hereditary sensory and autonomic neuropathy (HSAN) type 1E, a type of sensory neuropathy associated with dementia and hearing loss. *DNMT1* mutations have also been linked to autosomal dominant cerebellar ataxia with deafness and narcolepsy. Several intellectual disability syndromes are indirectly associated with epigenetic dysregulation and chromatin remodeling. The prototype is fragile X syndrome (FXS), an X-linked dominant disorder with variable penetrance that manifests with intellectual and emotional disabilities ranging from learning problems to mental retardation, mood instability, and autism spectrum disorders. The majority of FXS patients have large (> 200) expansions of CGG repeats in the 5'-untranslated region of the *FMR1* gene. This results in hypermethylation of the repeat region and reduction of expression of fragile X mental retardation protein, an RNA-binding protein that negatively regulates local translation of synaptic proteins in dendrites. Multiple genes associated with intellectual disability are regulated through imprinting. Imprinting refers to gene expression dependent on parent of origin as it is largely controlled by epigenetic mechanisms. An abnormal epigenetic mark that leads to improper gene expression from a specific paternal or maternal allele results in an imprinting disorder, which typically manifests with developmental delay and intellectual disabilities. Prototypical examples are Angelman syndrome and Prader-Willi syndrome. Angelman syndrome is caused by mutations in ubiquitin protein ligase E3A (*UBE3A*) gene, which is genomically imprinted so that only the maternally inherited copy is expressed in neurons. Topoisomerase I inhibitors such as topotecan could successfully reactivate the dormant paternal allele of *Ube3a* in neurons of a mouse model of this disorder and unsilence paternal *UBE3A* in induced pluripotent stem cell–derived neurons from these patients. Indotecan is a structural analogue Top1 inhibitor with greater biovailability and has a potential therapeutic role in this disease.

Epigenetic dysregulation may have an important contributory role in neurodegenerative disorders. For example, hexanucleotide (GGGGCC, G4C2) expansions in the intronic region of the *C9ORF72* gene are the most common cause of familial forms of amyotrophic lateral sclerosis associated or not with frontotemporal lobar degeneration. These expansions lead to hypermethylation of the CpG island located at the 5' end of the expansion and reduce *C9ORF72* mRNA transcript levels. Abnormal DNA methylation of presenilin 1 (*PSEN1*) and apolipoprotein E (*APOE*) gene may constitute genetic risks of Alzheimer's disease.

TABLE 4.2 *Neurologic Disorders Caused by Mutations in Epigenetic Regulator or Epigenetic Silencing of Genes*

Gene	Protein function	Disorder
DNMT1	DNA methylation	Hereditary Sensory and Autonomic Neuropathy type 1E Autosomal Dominant Cerebellar Ataxia with Deafness and Narcolepsy
MeCP2	Binds methylated CpG dinucleotides and promotes gene silencing	Rett syndrome
FMRP1	Fragile X mental retardation protein, RNA-binding protein that inhibits mRNA translation *FMRP* CGG expansion causes hypermethylation and reduced gene expression	Fragile X syndrome
CREBP	Transcriptional coactivator CREB-binding protein (CBP), which has HAT function	Rubinstein-Taybi syndrome (intellectual disability, growth deficiency, microcephaly, broad thumbs and halluces, and distinct facial features
RPS6KA3	Ribosomal protein S6 kinase, which modifies chromatin structure by interacting with CBP and phosphorylating histones	Coffin-Lowry syndrome (X-linked, manifested with intellectual disability, delayed development, and distinctive facial features)
ATRX	ATP-dependent chromatin-remodeler that interacts with histone methyltransferase and MeCP2	ATRX syndrome (X-linked mental retardation)
KDM5C	Histone demethylase	X-linked mental retardation
EHMT1	Histone methyltransferase	Kleefstra syndrome
NSD1	Histone methyltransferase	Sotos syndrome

Epigenetics and Epilepsy

Several epigenetic changes have been described in mouse models and in patients with epilepsy.[15] For example, DNA hypomethylation occurs shortly after induction of status epilepticus, whereas hypermethylation predominates upon development of epilepsy. Both DNMT1 and DNMT3 are upregulated in hippocampal issue in patients with temporal lobe epilepsy due to hippocampal sclerosis. This leads to global hypermethylation, including that of genes involved in neural development, remodeling, differentiation, and maturation. Following status epilepticus, there is decreased histone H4 acetylation in a gene encoding a glutamate receptor subunit, and increased acetylation of the *BDNF* promoter. Both miRNAs and long ncRNAs have also been found to be dysregulated in human temporal lobe epilepsy. For example, promoters of long ncRNAs targeting genes involved in pathways relevant to neural signaling and pharmacoresistance were found to be mostly hypermethylated in this condition. Status epilepticus is also associated with bidirectional changes in several long ncRNAs. Metabolic control of epigenetic mechanisms may also have a therapeutic role in epilepsy. For example, S-adenyosylmethione, the methyl donor for DNA and histone methylation, may have antiepileptic properties. Adenosine, which functions as an endogenous anticonvulsant via activation of inhibitory A1 receptors, may also prevent epileptogenesis by its effects on the S-adenosylmethionine:S-adenosylhomocysteine cycle, thereby reducing global DNA methylation.

Epigenetic Modulation of Metabolism in Glioblastoma

Reprogramming of cell metabolism has a pivotal role in initiation and progression of glioblastoma multiforme (GBM). Cell metabolism in GBM is characterized by increased Warburg effect (aerobic glycolysis), which is controlled by the glucose transporters GLUT1–4, and glycolytic enzymes regulated by several signaling pathways. A variety of epigenetic mechanisms contribute to regulation of cell metabolism in GBM and have therapeutic relevance.[6,16] For example, DNA methylation in the promoter region of the repair enzyme O-6-methylguanine-DNA methyltransferase (MGMT) is predictive of beneficial effect from alkylating agents such as temozolamide. Methylation on DNA sequences encoding glycolytic enzymes affect cell metabolism by silencing their expression. For example, pyruvate kinase isoform PKM2 regulates the final rate-limiting step of glycolysis and its expression is upregulated due to hypomethylation of the *PKM2* gene. Whereas other glycolytic enzymes such as glyceraldehyde 3-phosphate dehydrogenase and lactate dehydrogenase are also upregulated due to DNA hypomethylation in mesenchymal type GBM, they are downregulated due to DNA hypermethylation in *ICDH1* mutant GBM associated with more benign course. Histone acetylation, methylation, and demethylation can also affect cell metabolism and progression in GBM. For example, hyperacetylation of lysine 9 in histone H3 (H3K9) associated with promotor regions of glial cell-derived neurotrophic factor occurs in high grade but not low grade gliomas or normal astrocytes. The histone demethylase HDM1 decreases the inhibitory methylation of the lysine 4 residue of histone H3 (H3K4) and thereby activates the expression of oligodendrocyte lineage transcription factor 2 required for maintenance of GBM stem cells, while suppressing the p53 pathway, thus promoting GBM tumorigenesis and metastasis.

DEFECTS IN DNA REPAIR

Disruption of DNA repair may have distinct deleterious effects at different stages of neural development. Single-strand break repair and transcription-coupled nucleotide excision-repair in response to oxidative stress predominate at late stages of development and in the adult brain and their impairment is associated with aging and neurodegeneration.[17,18]

Aging and Neurodegeneration

There is an age-related accumulation of oxidative DNA damage in the brain. Some areas, such as the substantia nigra pars compacta, are particularly vulnerable to oxidative DNA modifications. With aging, there is reduction in the efficiency of base excision-repair due to decreased activity of DNA glycosylase and reduced ability for nonhomologous end-joining due to decreased activity of DNA protein kinase. There is also an age-dependent accumulation of mutations that can compromise the activity of DNA repair factors. DNA damage could progressively alter chromatin conformation and gene expression patterns via epigenetic mechanisms. One such mechanism is redistribution of Sirtuin 1, a NAD^+ dependent HDAC that accumulates at sites of double-strand breaks and stimulates activity of ATM. Oxidative damage and impaired repair in nuclear and mitochondrial DNA occurs in several neurodegenerative disorders. For example, there is accumulation of DNA strand breaks, reduction of double-strand break repair proteins and decreased base excision-repair ability in Alzheimer disease, and increased number of oxidative and single-strand breaks in neurons in amyotrophic lateral sclerosis. Studies in mouse models and cell lines show that mismatch repair, transcription-coupled nucleotide excision-repair, and base excision-repair can contribute to repeat instability and expansion in trinucleotide repeat disorders.[19] Repeat expansions trigger transient formation of unusual DNA structures, such as loop structures, which initiate DNA repair mechanisms. Mismatch repair mediators may promote expansion of CAG repeats, as in the case of the huntingtin (*HTT*) gene. Variants in mismatch repair proteins such as MutSβ (encoded by the *MSH3* gene) may influence the rate of somatic expansion in tissues that are vulnerable to repeat instability and neurodegeneration. MutSβ identifies DNA loop-outs in the CAG tracts and targets them for repair; incorrect repair could introduce short incremental CAG expansions in the *HTT* gene.

Autosomal Recessive Cerebellar Ataxias

Defects in DNA repair are a common disease pathway for several autosomal-recessive cerebellar ataxias (Table 4.3). These disorders are clinically and genetically heterogeneous and are characterized by cerebellar ataxia frequently associated with peripheral sensorimotor neuropathy. Defects in double-strand break repair not only affect the nervous system but also manifest with systemic effects, such as immunodeficiency and malignancy, due to genome instability. The prototype example is ataxia-telangiectasia, due to *ATM* gene mutations. It manifests with early-onset, progressive cerebellar ataxia with oculomotor apraxia and conjunctival telangiectasia, chorea, sensorimotor neuropathy, immunodeficiency with frequent sinopulmonary infections, and susceptibility to ionizing radiation and cancer. Ataxia with oculomotor apraxia (AOA) is a group of autosomal recessive disorders associated with impaired single-strand DNA break repair.[20] They are also characterized by cerebellar ataxia, oculomotor apraxia, chorea, myoclonus, and severe sensorimotor axonal neuropathy. In contrast to ataxia-telangiectasia, these disorders are not associated with immune deficiency or predisposition to cancer. Several genes linked to AOA encode proteins that are involved in DNA end-processing. AOA1 is due to mutations of the *APTX* gene encoding aprataxin and may be associated with hypoalbuminemia and hypercholesterolemia. AOA4 is due to the mutation of *PNPK* gene; *PNPK* mutations may also cause a severe neurodevelopmental disorder characterized by microcephaly, early-onset intractable seizures, and developmental delay. Mutations of the *XRCC1* gene encoding XRCC1, a molecular scaffold involved in DNA single-strand break repair, are associated with a phenotype resembling AOA4. Other forms of AOA reflect defects in control of DNA transcription. The typical example is AOA2, which is linked to mutations of the *STX* gene encoding senataxin, a DNA helicase critical to correct formation of R-loops comprising

TABLE 4.3 *Neurologic Disorders Due to Impaired DNA Repair*

DNA Repair Process	Protein (gene)	Disorder
Double-strand break	Ataxia-telangiectasia mutated (*ATM*) MRE11 (*MRE11*) AT and Rad3 (*ATR*) NBS ((Nijmegen breakage syndrome-1) (*NBS*) RAD 50	Ataxia-telangiectasia (A-T) AT-like syndrome ATR and Seckel syndrome Nijmegen breakage syndrome (NBS) NBS-like syndrome
Single-strand break	Aprataxin (*APTX*) Polynucleotide 5'kinase 3' phosphatase (*PNPK*) Tyrosyl DNA phosphodiesterase 1 (*TDP1*) *XRCC1*	Ataxia with oculomotor apraxia 1 (AOA1) Ataxia with oculomotor apraxia 4 (AOA4) Microcephaly with seizures Spinocerebellar ataxia with axonal neuropathy 1 (SCA1) Ataxia, oculomotor apraxia, and axonal neuropathy
Nucleotide excision-repair	Xeroderma pigmentosum (XP) proteins (*XPA-G, XPV*) Cockayne syndrome (CS) proteins (*CSA, CSB*)	Xeroderma pigmentosum Cockayne syndrome
R-loop correction	Senataxin (*STX*)	AOA2 ALS4

RNA/DNA hybrids. Senataxin mutations have also been linked to amyotrophic lateral sclerosis type 4 (ALS4). A phenotype resembling AOA2, and referred to as AOA3, has been linked to mutations in the *PI3KR5* gene encoding phosphatidylinositol 3'kinase regulatory subunit 5, which has a critical role in cerebellar development. Spinocerebellar ataxia with axonal neuropathy (SCAN1) is linked to mutations in the *TDP1* gene. SCAN1 is characterized by late-childhood-onset slowly progressive cerebellar ataxia, followed by progressive peripheral neuropathy. Abnormal repeat expansions of genes encoding proteins involved in DNA repair can also produce cerebellar ataxia. One example are AAGGG expansions in the *RFC1* gene encoding the large subunit of replication facilitation complex 1, which activates DNA polymerases δ and ε to promote the coordinated synthesis of both DNA strands during replication or after DNA damage. These mutations produce cerebellar ataxia, vestibular arreflexia, and sensory neuropathy syndrome (CANVAS). However, they have not been shown to affect DNA repair in-vitro.

Xeroderma pigmentosum (XP) and Cockayne syndrome (CS) are autosomal recessive disorders due to impaired transcription-coupled nucleotide excision-repair, which is a major mechanism of repair of DNA damage due to UV radiation.[21] Xeroderma pigmentosum is characterized by slow-healing sunburns after brief sun exposure and high risk of skin cancer. Approximately one-fourth of XP patients have neurological symptoms, including microcephaly, intellectual disability, hearing loss, ataxia, and neuropathy. Cockayne syndrome is a progeria syndrome characterized by photosensitivity, growth failure, intellectual disability, spasticity, ataxia, hearing loss and vision loss, joint contractures, and early mortality, but not cancer. Some patients have a combined XP-CS phenotype.

MECHANISMS OF NEURODEGENERATION IN DNA REPAIR DISORDERS

Defects of DNA repair elicit neuronal damage by several mechanisms, including p53-triggered apoptosis and excessive activity of recruitment of PARP1 (Figure 4.6).

Effects of p53 Signaling

The *TP53* tumor suppressor gene product, p53, has a critical role in the response to DNA damage and other forms of cell stress via both transcription-dependent and transcription-independent mechanisms.[22] As a transcription factor, p53 promotes the expression of p21, which promotes cell cycle arrest. In the presence of damaged DNA, p53 regulates different repair mechanisms, including homologous recombination, nucleotide excision-repair, base excision-repair, and mismatch repair through interactions with proteins critically involved in these processes. Within the mitochondria, p53 promotes apoptosis through displacement of antiapoptotic members of the BCL-2 family and direct activation of the proapoptotic factors.

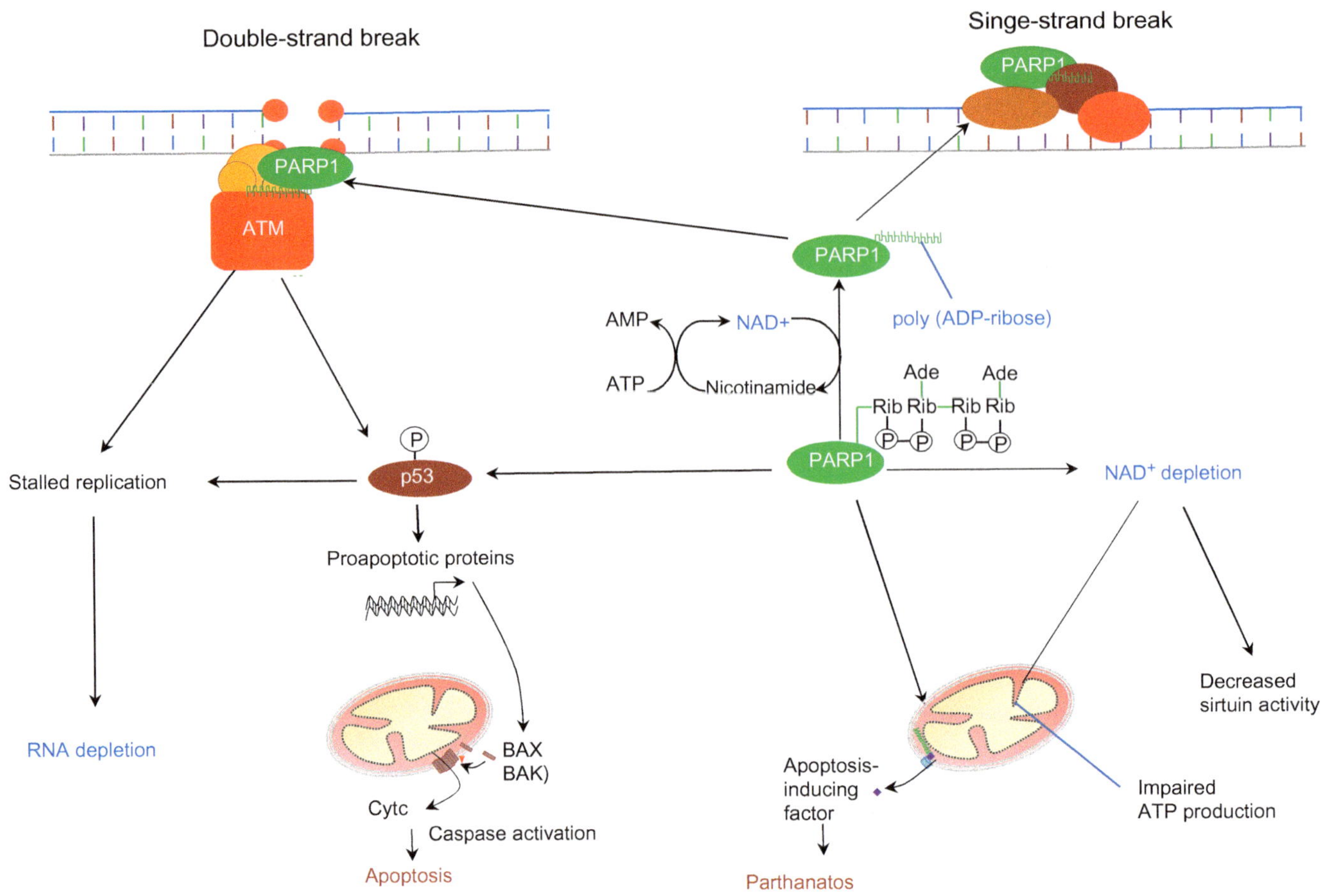

FIGURE 4.6 Consequences of DNA damage and DNA repair.
Defects of DNA repair elicit neuronal damage by several mechanisms, including p53-triggered apoptosis and excessive activity of poly(ADP ribose) polymerase 1 (PARP1) PARP1 is a fundamental component of the DNA damage-response machinery and utilizes nicotinamide adenine nucleotide (NAD+) and ATP to synthesize poly ADP-ribose (PAR) residues that can be added to a variety target proteins (PARrylation). Excessive PARP1 activation elicits cytotoxic effects by two main mechanisms. One mechanism is depletion of both NAD$^+$ and ATP utilized for PAR synthesis, with eventual bioenergetic and redox collapse. The second is accumulation of PAR polymers and PARylated proteins at the mitochondria, leading to dissipation the mitochondrial membrane potential. Hyperactivation of PARP1 also triggers a regulated form of programmed cell death known as parthanatos by binding of PAR polymers to a proapoptotic mitochondrial protein known as apoptosis-inducing factor (AIF), which translocates the nucleus and elicits large-scale DNA fragmentation and chromatin condensation.

Role of PARP1 in Cell Death Mechanisms

PARP1 is a fundamental component of the DNA damage response machinery and utilizes (NAD$^+$) and ATP to synthesize poly ADP-ribose residues.[12] Excessive PARP1 activation may produce cell injury through several mechanisms. One such mechanism is depletion of both NAD$^+$ and ATP utilized for PAR synthesis, with eventual bioenergetic and redox collapse. PARP-1 also competes with the histone deacetylase Sirtuin-1 for the same NAD+ pool, and thus increased PARP1 activation reduces activity of sirtuins. Hyperactivation of PARP1 also triggers a regulated form of programmed cell death known as parthanatos. This results from binding of PAR polymers to a proapoptotic mitochondrial protein known as apoptosis inducing factor (AIF), which translocates the nucleus and elicits large-scale DNA fragmentation and chromatin condensation. An emerging role of PARP1 is to participate, directly or indirectly, in the regulation of the intracellular trafficking of different transcriptional factors such as p53 and nuclear factor that activates kappa chain transcription in B lymphocytes (NFκB). PARP1 elicits PARylation and stabilization of p53 in mitochondria, making neurons prone to cell death; PARP1 regulates the nuclear import of NF-κB, which has an important role in neuroinflammation and also regulates neuronal survival and cell death through differential modulation of gene expression. PARP1 also activated the calcium-dependent protease calpain in conditions of excitotoxicity, which could be related to mitochondrial Ca^{2+} dysregulation caused by

PAR polymers. The potent nonselective PARP inhibitor PJ34 had neuroprotective effects in and experimental model of traumatic brain injury.[23]

Aberrant Cell Cycle Reentry in Neurodegenerative Disorders

In many pathological conditions there is a detrimental activation of the cell cycle machinery, which drives a cascade of DNA synthesis and consequent neuronal death.[24] There are several factors that may trigger abnormal cell cycle reentry in postmitotic cells such as neurons. For example, hypoxia activates hypoxia-induced factors that in turn cause upregulation of growth factors; this leads to downstream inhibition of p27 and thus increases activity of several cyclin/CDK complexes. During oxidative stress, reactive oxygen species increase cell cycle reentry by producing cumulative DNA damage leading to chromatin remodeling and activation of transcription factors such as E2F. During cell stress, CDK5 is translocated to the cytoplasm, thereby relieving its inhibitory effect on EF2-mediated cell cycle progression. Impaired activity of the ubiquitin-proteasome system results in accumulation of cyclins that are normally degraded by this system.

GENOME EDITING

Genome editing is the process of making precise and permanent changes in the genetic code.[25] Applications include disrupting gain-of-function mutations and replacing a target gene using excision-repair approaches. The first step is to program a DNA nuclease to bind to a precise DNA sequence and cut the DNA. The most commonly used nuclease platform is CRISPR (clustered regularly interspaced palindromic repeats) associated with Cas9 endonuclease. The Cas9 nuclease cleaves DNA after a conformational change produced by binding of a guide RNA to a complementary sequence in the target site. Nucleases create a site-specific double-stranded break in the DNA that activates repair through either nonhomologous end-joining or homology-directed repair. DNA repair at the site of the selected break can be utilized to either knock-out or introduce selected genes. One example is Duchenne muscle dystrophy, where genome editing aims to delete selective exons contained in pathological variants of the dystrophin gene to modify the phenotype from that of Duchenne to a Becker muscular dystrophy. Deletions of exons 43, 45, and 52 represent mutational "hotspot" regions in the dystrophin gene. Single guide RNAs can restore dystrophin expression by inducing exon skipping and reframing of the gene, restoring dystrophin expression. Another example is deletion of the CAG expansions of the *HTT* gene to treat Huntington disease In cell and animal models, CRISPR–Cas9 has been used to lower mutant HTT levels by blocking *HTT* transcription, excising CAG repeats, or selectively inactivating expanded CAG alleles.

Paradigms for gene editing includes ex-vivo and in-vivo gene editing. For ex-vivo editing, RNA- or protein-guided nucleases are used to alter or add DNA in cells that are extracted from the patient and purified, gene-edited, selected, expanded in cell culture, and given back to the patient by cell infusion or tissue injection. Patient-derived induced pluripotent stem cells can be subjected to ex-vivo gene editing and differentiated into neuronal or glial lineages for transplantation. These cells have been differentiated into sensory neurons for studying chemotherapy-induced peripheral neuropathy, oligodendrocyte precursor cells for study of demyelination in spinal cord injury repair,[25–27] and Schwann cells for peripheral and spinal cord injury therapeutics. Autologous bone marrow or adipose tissue-derived mesenchymal stems cells are emerging as a leading candidate cell platform for ex vivo therapies. In-vivo genome editing requires a gene-delivery vector such as adeno-associated virus (AAV), which does not integrate into the genome and can be delivered directly to cells in the CNS, PNS, or muscle to make changes in the genomic DNA within the tissue.

Materials such as biodegradable polymers such as lactic acid-to-glycolic acid (PLGA) can be used for drug delivery. DNA polymers can also be used as hydrogels for drug delivery;[28] they can also be incorporated to CRISPR systems and can be used as biosensors or as drug-delivery systems.[29]

KEY POINTS

- DNA is present in the nucleus and mitochondria.
- DNA replication involves different types of DNA polymerases, helicases, topoisomerases, and telomerases.
- Only about 1%–2% of the nuclear genome is transcribed into messenger RNA (mRNA) and encodes proteins; about 85%–90% is transcribed into noncoding RNAs.
- The gene is composed of exons transcribed into coding messenger mRNA, introns interspersed between exons, and a signal for polyadenylation.
- Chromatin is composed of DNA wrapped around histones.
- Epigenetic mechanisms include DNA methylation, histone modifications such as acetylation and methylation, and noncoding RNAs.
- DNA methylation, mediated by DNA methyltransferases, typically represses the transcription of the associated gene.
- Posttranslational histone modifications regulate DNA access to the transcriptional machinery: histone acetylation promotes and deacetylation inhibits transcription; changes in methylation may have distinct effects depending on the residues targeted.

- Noncoding RNAs mediate numerous epigenetic processes, including posttranscriptional processing of mRNA.
- Several metabolites function as cofactors and regulators of enzymes involved in epigenetic mechanisms.
- Oxidative stress is the main cause of DNA damage in the nervous system.
- One of the earliest events of DNA repair is recruitment of polyadenosyl diphosphate (ADP) ribose polymerase 1 (PARP1), which binds to sites of DNA breaks and subsequently modifies repair proteins
- A critical step in DNA repair pathways such as base excision-repair and single-strand break repair is DNA end-processing.
- Ataxia-telangiectasia mutated (ATM) protein is the master regulator of the coordinated responses to DNA double-strand damage.
- Cell cycle progression at checkpoints is driven by the sequential activation of cyclin-dependent kinases (CDKs) that bind to partner proteins called cyclins.
- Mutations in genes directly linked to epigenetic regulation may manifest with neurodevelopmental disorders such as Rett syndrome.
- *DNMT1* mutations cause autosomal dominant hereditary sensory and autonomic neuropathy type 1E, associated with dementia and hearing loss, *or* autosomal dominant cerebellar ataxia, associated with deafness and narcolepsy.
- Epigenetic dysregulation has an important contributory role in neurodegenerative disorders, epilepsy, and glioblastoma.
- There is an age-related accumulation of oxidative DNA damage in the brain, which is associated with reduced capacity for DNA repair.
- Defects in DNA repair are a common disease pathway for several autosomal-recessive cerebellar ataxias, such as ataxia-telangiectasia and ataxia with oculomotor apraxia.
- Defects of DNA repair elicit neuronal damage by p53-triggered apoptosis and excessive activity of recruitment of PARP1 leading both to depletion of substrates for energy metabolism and cell death by apoptosis (parthanatos).
- In many pathological conditions, there is a detrimental activation of the cell cycle machinery that drives a cascade of DNA synthesis.
- Genome editing is an emerging approach for treatment of neurologic disorders.

REFERENCES

1. Qureshi IA, Mehler MF. Epigenetics and therapeutic targets mediating neuroprotection. Brain Res 2015;1628:265–272.
2. Sweatt JD. The emerging field of neuroepigenetics. Neuron 2013;80:624–632.
3. Klein CJ, Benarroch EE. Epigenetic regulation: basic concepts and relevance to neurologic disease. Neurology 2014;82:1833–1840.
4. Dantas A, Al Shueili B, Yang Y, Nabbi A, Fink D, Riabowol K. Biological functions of the ING proteins. Cancers (Basel) 2019;11:1817–1843.
5. Li X, Egervari G, Wang Y, Berger SL, Lu Z. Regulation of chromatin and gene expression by metabolic enzymes and metabolites. Nat Rev Mol Cell Biol 2018;19:563–578.
6. Gongol B, Sari I, Bryant T, Rosete G, Marin T. AMPK: an epigenetic landscape modulator. Int J Mol Sci 2018;19:3238–3252.
7. Iyama T, Wilson DM, 3rd. DNA repair mechanisms in dividing and non-dividing cells. DNA Repair (Amst) 2013;12:620–636.
8. Sirbu BM, Cortez D. DNA damage response: three levels of DNA repair regulation. Cold Spring Harb Perspect Biol 2013;5:a012724.
9. Kowalczykowski SC. An overview of the molecular mechanisms of recombinational DNA repair. Cold Spring Harb Perspect Biol 2015;7:a016410.
10. Caldecott KW. DNA single-strand break repair. Exp Cell Res 2014;329:2–8.
11. Scharer OD. Nucleotide excision repair in eukaryotes. Cold Spring Harb Perspect Biol 2013;5:a012609.
12. Martire S, Mosca L, d'Erme M. PARP-1 involvement in neurodegeneration: a focus on Alzheimer's and Parkinson's diseases. Mech Ageing Dev 2015;146–148:53–64.
13. Ray Chaudhuri A, Nussenzweig A. The multifaceted roles of PARP1 in DNA repair and chromatin remodelling. Nat Rev Mol Cell Biol 2017.
14. Blackford AN, Jackson SP. ATM, ATR, and DNA-PK: the trinity at the heart of the DNA damage response. Mol Cell 2017;66:801–817.
15. Hauser RM, Henshall DC, Lubin FD. The epigenetics of epilepsy and its progression. Neuroscientist 2018;24:186–200.
16. Dong Z, Cui H. Epigenetic modulation of metabolism in glioblastoma. Semin Cancer Biol 2018;57:45–51.
17. Madabhushi R, Pan L, Tsai LH. DNA damage and its links to neurodegeneration. Neuron 2014;83:266–282.
18. Rulten SL, Caldecott KW. DNA strand break repair and neurodegeneration. DNA Repair (Amst) 2013;12:558–567.
19. Jones L, Houlden H, Tabrizi SJ. DNA repair in the trinucleotide repeat disorders. Lancet Neurol 2017;16:88–96.
20. Paucar M, Malmgren H, Taylor M, et al. Expanding the ataxia with oculomotor apraxia type 4 phenotype. Neurol Genet 2016;2:e49.
21. Natale V, Raquer H. Xeroderma pigmentosum-Cockayne syndrome complex. Orphanet J Rare Dis 2017;12:65.
22. Ho T, Tan BX, Lane D. How the other half lives: what p53 does when it is not being a transcription factor. Int J Mol Sci 2019;21:13–28.
23. Tao X, Chen X, Hou Z, Hao S, Liu B. Protective functions of PJ34, a Poly(ADP-ribose) polymerase inhibitor, are related to down-regulation of calpain and nuclear factor-kappaB in a mouse model of traumatic brain injury. World Neurosurg 2017;107:888–899.
24. Sharma R, Kumar D, Jha NK, Jha SK, Ambasta RK, Kumar P. Re-expression of cell cycle markers in aged neurons and muscles: whether cells should divide or die? Biochim Biophys Acta 2017;1863:324–336.
25. Porteus MH. A new class of medicines through DNA editing. N Engl J Med 2019;380:947–959.

26. Terzic D, Maxon JR, Krevitt L, et al. Directed differentiation of oligodendrocyte progenitor cells from mouse induced pluripotent stem cells. Cell Transplant 2016;25:411–424.
27. Parr AM, Walsh PJ, Truong V, Dutton JR. cGMP-compliant expansion of human iPSC cultures as adherent monolayers. Methods Mol Biol 2016;1357:221–229.
28. Wang D, Hu Y, Liu P, Luo D. Bioresponsive DNA hydrogels: beyond the conventional stimuli responsiveness. Acc Chem Res 2017;50:733–739.
29. Chen M, Luo D. A CRISPR path to cutting-edge materials. N Engl J Med 2020;382:85–88.

5 Messenger RNA Metabolism

OVERVIEW

Messenger mRNA (mRNA) conveys genetic information from DNA in the form of a sequence of nucleotides or codons (consisting of three base pairs each) that specifies the amino acid sequence for protein synthesis in the ribosome. The steps involved in this complex process are transcription, maturation, nucleocytoplasmic transport, translation, and decay (Figure 5.1). Overall, these processes are referred to as ribostasis. All steps of mRNA metabolism are coordinated and regulated by a large number of RNA-binding proteins (RBPs) that form complexes with mRNAs known as messenger ribonucleoprotein particles (mRNPs). RNA-binding proteins function as transcription factors, participate in mRNA maturation, promote nucleocytoplasmic transport, maintain mRNA in untranslated (silent) state during transport of mRNA granules to their final destination for local translation at specific sites of axon or dendrites, and control mRNA decay. Mutations affecting these RBPs are an important cause of neurodegenerative disorders including amyotrophic lateral sclerosis (ALS), frontotemporal lobar degeneration (FTLD) resulting in frontotemporal dementia (FTD), spinocerebellar ataxia, and others (Table 5.1). Most (85%–90%) transcribed DNA is transcribed into noncoding RNAs, which essentially control every step of mRNA metabolism. High-throughput sequencing methodologies, such as single-cell RNA sequencing (RNA-seq) and cTag-crosslinking and immunoprecipitation (CLIP), together with candidate single-gene studies, have provided increasing insight into mRNA metabolism. Perturbation of mRNA homeostasis is a fundamental mechanism in neurodegenerative disorders; many of them are associated with abnormal cytoplasmic accumulation of stress granules containing untranslated mRNAs and RNA-binding proteins. Nucleotide repeat expansions may cause impaired translation of the encoded protein; toxic mRNA gain-of-function leading to sequestration of splicing factors in the nucleus; toxic protein gain-of-function; and production of dipeptide repeats that prevent nucleocytoplasmic transport. The aims of this chapter are to briefly review: (1) the mechanisms of mRNA transcription and the role of inducible transcription factors and transcriptional repressors; (2) the basic aspects of maturation, transport, and translation of mRNA; (3) the role of mRNA-binding proteins in mRNA metabolism and formation of stress granules; (4) the function of microRNAs (miRNAs); and (5) some clinical correlations of impaired ribostasis, nucleotide repeat expansion disorders, and splicing disorders.

GENERAL MECHANISMS OF MESSENGER RNA TRANSCRIPTION

Each human gene is approximately 10,000 base pairs long; but only one-tenth of the gene actually codes for the amino acids that constitute the mature protein product. Within each gene, the DNA is fragmented into exons, which are the sequences that remain in the mature mRNA and code for the protein; introns that are removed from the primary transcripts during processing into mature mRNA, and a signal for polyadenylation that is transcribed into the mature mRNA. A typical protein-coding gene contains regulatory untranslated regions (UTRs) located upstream (5' UTR) and downstream (3' UTR) of the coding region, as well as multiple regulatory regions known as enhancers and promoters (Figure 5.2). Enhancer and promoter DNA

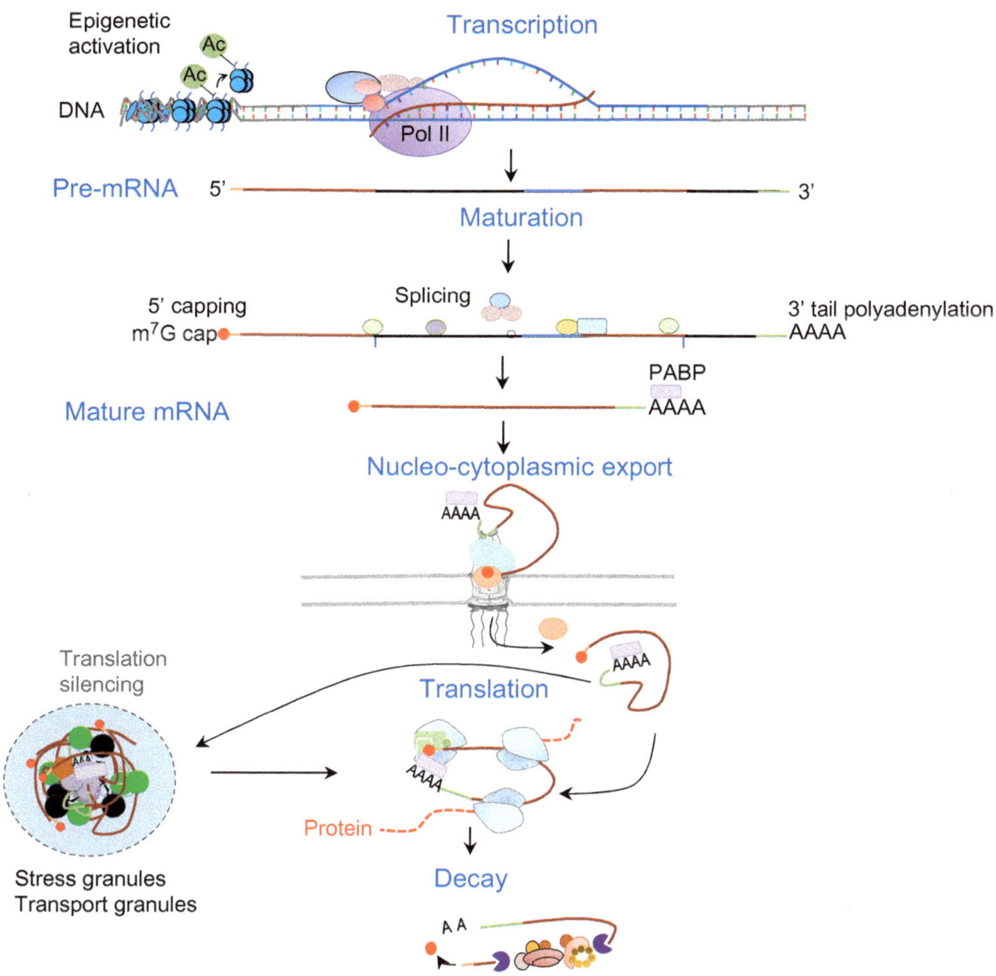

FIGURE 5.1 Overview of mRNA metabolism.

Metabolism of messenger RNA (mRNA) is critical for control of cell phenotype and includes several steps: transcription of DNA into a pre-mRNA, mRNA maturation, nucleocytoplasmic export and transport to specific cellular locations, translation into proteins, and decay. All these steps are seamlessly integrated and controlled by a large number of RNA-binding proteins, which interact with RNA forming messenger ribonucleoprotein particles. PABP, polyadenylate binding protein.

sequence motifs bind combinational arrays of transcription activators that recruit transcriptional co-activators.[1,2]

Basic Mechanisms: General Transcription Factors and Pre-Initiation Complex

In eukaryotes, mRNA transcription depends on RNA polymerase II (pol II), which is responsible for synthesis of both protein-coding mRNAs and various noncoding RNAs. Transcription starts at the core promoter region of DNA, and the key step is the formation of the pre-initiation complex. This complex consists of pol II, general transcription factors, and the Mediator co-activator complex. General transcription factors bind to various DNA sequences in the core promoter, including the TATA (thymine-adenine-thymine-adenine) box and other elements located upstream of the transcription start site. These sequences are the site of binding of the transcription factor TFIID, one of the general transcription factors that bind to the core promoter; these factors consist of several subunits, including TATA-binding protein (TBP) and TBP-associated factors (TAFs), including TAF15, which participate in basal transcription and function as co-activators. Components of this basal transcription complex are affected in neurodegenerative disorders. For example, trinucleotide repeat expansion of the *TBP* gene produces spinocerebellar ataxia 17 (SCA17), which is characterized by ataxia, cognitive decline, dystonia, parkinsonism, supranuclear gaze palsy, and autonomic dysfunction.[3] Mutations affecting TAF15 are linked to ALS.[4] The Mediator complex communicates signals from activating transcription factors to general transcription factors and to pol II. Enhancer sequences bind transcription factors, recruit chromatin modifying enzymes, and facilitate binding of pol II and general transcription factors to core promoters. Only one DNA strand, the antisense strand, serves as a template for transcription and is read by RNA pol II from the 3' end to the 5' end;

TABLE 5.1 *Examples of RNA-binding Proteins, Their Function, and Their Involvement in Disease*

Protein (gene)	Function (s)	Involvement in Disease
TDP-43 (*TABP*)	Regulation of mRNA transcription and splicing	Amyotrophic lateral sclerosis (ALS) Frontotemporal dementia (FTD) Hippocampal sclerosis
FUS/TLS (*FUS/TLS*)	Regulation of mRNA transcription and splicing DNA repair	FTD
TAF15 (*TAF15*)	Basal transcription and coactivation	ALS
Heterogeneous nuclear ribonucleoprotein (hnRNP) A1 and A2B1(*HNRP1*)	Inhibition of transcription Regulation of splicing	Multisystem proteinopathy
Fragile X mental retardation protein (*FMRP1*)	Silencing mRNA translation in transport granules mRNA editing, splicing, transport, and miRNA metabolism	Fragile X syndrome
Ataxin-2 (*ATXN2*)	Regulation of mRNA stability Translational repression in RNA granules Translation of select mRNA	Spinocerebellar ataxia type 2 Risk for juvenile ALS
Survival of motor neuron (*SMN1*)	Assembly of ribonucleoprotein complexes critical for splicing Axonal translation of mRNAs	Spinal muscular atrophy (SMA)
Muscleblind (*MBNL*)	Alternative splicing mRNA targeting	Myotonic dystrophy 1
Nova, Hu	Alternative splicing	Paraneoplastic neurologic syndromes

FUS/TLS, fuse in sarcoma/translocated in sarcoma; TAF15, TATA-binding protein-associated factor 15; TDP-43, TAR DNA finding protein-43

the complementary RNA is thus created in a 5' to 3' direction, matching the sequence of the non-template sense DNA strand.

Epigenetic Control of Transcription

As discussed in the previous chapter, the four major classes of epigenetic processes that regulate the function of single genes and gene networks are DNA methylation, changes in histone acetylation and methylation, chromatin remodeling, and regulation by noncoding RNAs.[5–7] Briefly, DNA methylation typically represses transcription via methyl-CpG-binding proteins that prevent binding of transcription activators to DNA promoters. In contrast, the 5-hydroxymethylcytosine mark is typically associated with increased transcription. Histone modifications regulate compaction and structure of chromatin, thus affecting DNA access to the transcription machinery. Histone acetylation promotes unwinding of the DNA and promotes transcription; in contrast, histone deacetylation represses transcription. Histone methylation may have either promoting or repressing transcriptional effects depending on the residues targeted.

Noncoding RNAs are transcribed from both DNA strands and are further processed to produce small and long regulatory RNA.[8] Short noncoding RNAs include miRNAs, endogenous small interfering RNAs (siRNAs), and small nucleolar RNAs. MicroRNAs have a major role in control of mRNA translation and decay. Long noncoding RNAs include intergenic noncoding RNAs, natural antisense transcripts, and noncoding RNA repeats. Long noncoding RNAs recruit transcriptional and epigenetic regulators at specific DNA loci, modulate nucleocytoplasmic transport, and control local protein synthesis. Circular RNAs are a special type of noncoding RNA that regulate the function of miRNAs and other processes.[9] RNA editing is a dynamic process that involves adenosine-to-inosine change mediated by adenosine deaminases or cytidine deaminases targeting the RNA or DNA. Editing selectively affects the properties of protein-coding genes regulating synaptic transmission and can modify miRNA biogenesis and alter the site of mRNA splicing, among other processes.

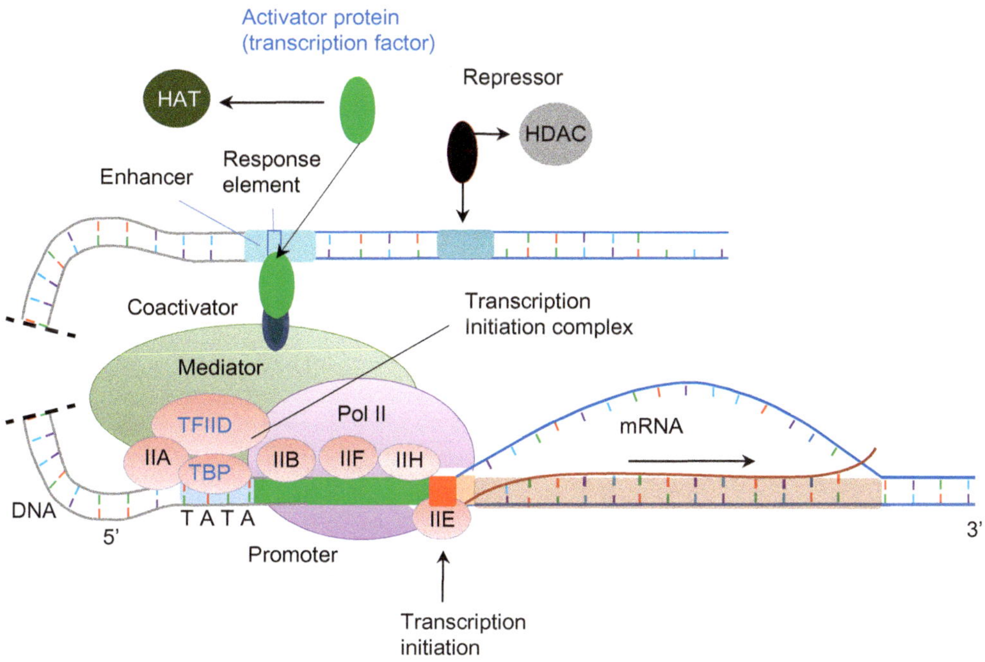

FIGURE 5.2 Basic machinery for transcription.

The key step of transcription is the formation of the pre-initiation complex at the core promoter region of DNA, which is the site of start of transcription. The pre-initiation complex is composed of RNA polymerase II (pol II), general transcription factors, and the mediator-coactivator complex. General transcription factors bind to various DNA sequences in the core promoter, including the TATA (thymine-adenine-thymine-adenine) box and other elements located upstream of the transcription start site. These sequences are the site of binding of the TATA-binding protein (TBP) subunit of the transcription factor IID (TFIID). Other components of the pre-initiation complex for mRNA transcription are the general transcription factors TFIIA, TFIIB, TFIIE, TFIIF, and TFIIH. Only one DNA strand, the antisense strand, serves as a template for transcription and is read by RNA pol II from the 3' end to the 5' end; the complementary RNA is thus created in a 5' to 3' direction. HAT, histone acetyltransferase; HDAC, histone deacetylase.

TRANSCRIPTIONAL REGULATION BY ENVIRONMENTAL SIGNALS

In addition to the basal transcription complex, other transcription factors, referred to as inducible transcription factors, mediate transcriptional control in response to a wide variety of extracellular signals. These inducible transcription factors that bind to enhancer regions of DNA adjacent to the regulated genes and have a major role in transcriptional regulation during development, growth, and maturation of the nervous system, use-dependent synaptic plasticity, response to injury, and survival.

Features of Inducible Transcription Factors

Inducible transcription factors contain a DNA-binding domain with a stretch of highly basic amino acids forming motifs that recognize specific DNA sequences called response elements within the regulatory regions of the target gene. Some transcription factors also contain an extracellular signal-sensing domain and transmit signals to the rest of the transcription complex. Transcription factors also regulate transcription through direct interactions with components of the DNA core promoter and with other transcription factors. Depending on the transcription factor and its interactions, gene transcription may be either up- or downregulated. Transcription factors regulate gene expression by several mechanisms, including stabilization of pol II binding to DNA, recruitment of co-activator or co-repressor proteins, and regulation of the acetylation or deacetylation of histones. Several extracellular signals, including neurotransmitters, hormones, growth factors, adhesion molecules, and cytokines, can trigger changes in gene expression via inducible transcription factors. A large number of inducible transcription factors mediate signaling cascades triggered by these environmental stimuli (Table 5.2). Many such transcription factors are activated by phosphorylation downstream of these signal transduction pathways. Others exist in an inactive form in the cytoplasm by binding to heat shock proteins or other inhibitory proteins; these "latent" transcription factors become activated by specific signals that elicit their relocation from the cytoplasm to the nucleus.

TABLE 5.2 *Examples of Inducible Transcription Factors*

Transcription Factor	Activators	Function
	Transcription Factors Activated by Extracellular Signals	
CREB	Activation of NMDAR, Ca^{2+} channels, and growth factor receptors via several protein kinases	Synaptic plasticity and cell survival via transcriptional activation after binding CBP
Fos-Jun (AP-1)	CREB	Immediate early gene products in response to synaptic activity
STAT	Jun activated kinases	Mediates effects of cytokines
	Latent Transcription Factors	
Steroid/thyroid hormone receptor superfamily of nuclear receptors	Cortisol Aldosterone Sex steroids Vitamin D Thyroxin Retinoid acid	Binding of hormone disinhibits the DNA-binding and transactivation domains allowing their translocation to the nucleus.
NFκB	Cytokines Growth factors Oxidative stress	Present in the cytosol in an inactive form bound to IκB protein; stimuli elicite IκB phosphorylation and allow translocation of NFκB to the nucleus, where it activates transcription of pro-inflammatory cytokines
Heat shock factor (HSF)	Accumulation of misfolded proteins	Molecular chaperone
Hypoxia-inducible factor (HIF)	Hypoxia-induced deoxygenation of proline residues and inactivation of VHL protein	Activation of genes encoding enzymes for glucose metabolism, VEGF, EPO, and others

AP-1, activating protein-1; CaM, calmodulin kinase; CBP, CREB-binding protein; CREB, cyclic adenosine monophosphate–response element-binding protein; EPO, erythropoietin; ERK, extracellular signal-regulated kinase; HAT, histone acetyltransferase; NFκB, nuclear factor that activates kappa chain transcription in B lymphocytes; NMDA, N-methyl-D aspartate; STAT, signal transduced and activation of transcription; VEGF, vascular endothelial growth factor; VHL, Von Hippel-Lindau protein

CREB as the Prototypical Inducible Transcription Factor

The prototypical example of signal-activated transcription factor is cyclic adenosine monophosphate (cAMP)– and calcium response element-binding protein (CREB) (Figure 5.3). CREB forms homo- or heterodimers that bind to the promoter sites of multiple target genes. CREB phosphorylation at its serine (Ser)[133] residue triggers transcriptional activation by allowing the recruitment of the transcriptional co-activator CREB-binding protein (CBP), which functions as a histone acetyl transferase and thus promotes transcription via epigenetic mechanisms. CREB mediates transcriptional activation in response to many extracellular signals, such excitatory synaptic activity via N-methyl-D-aspartate receptors (NMDARs) or activation of voltage-gated calcium channels, G protein-coupled receptor cascades, and tyrosine kinase receptor signals. All these signals activate downstream protein kinases that phosphorylate CREB and thereby promote transcription. CREB may also be activated by signaling complexes that form at active synaptic sites or at the site of injury and travel to the nucleus in association to adaptor proteins. Activation of CREB signaling is a fundamental mechanism of use-dependent synaptic plasticity and neuronal survival.[10] Phosphorylated CREB rapidly induces several hundred genes in response to excitatory synaptic activity. These include immediate-early genes encoding transcription factors such as c-Fos (which is a marker of synaptic activation), and genes encoding synaptic proteins, protein brain-derived neurotrophic factor (BDNF), and other plasticity and survival proteins. Mutations of the *CREBBP* gene encoding CREB or of the *CPB* gene encoding CBP are linked to the Rubinstein-Taybi syndrome; this disorder is characterized by growth and psychomotor delay, dysmorphic face and fingers, and mild to severe mental

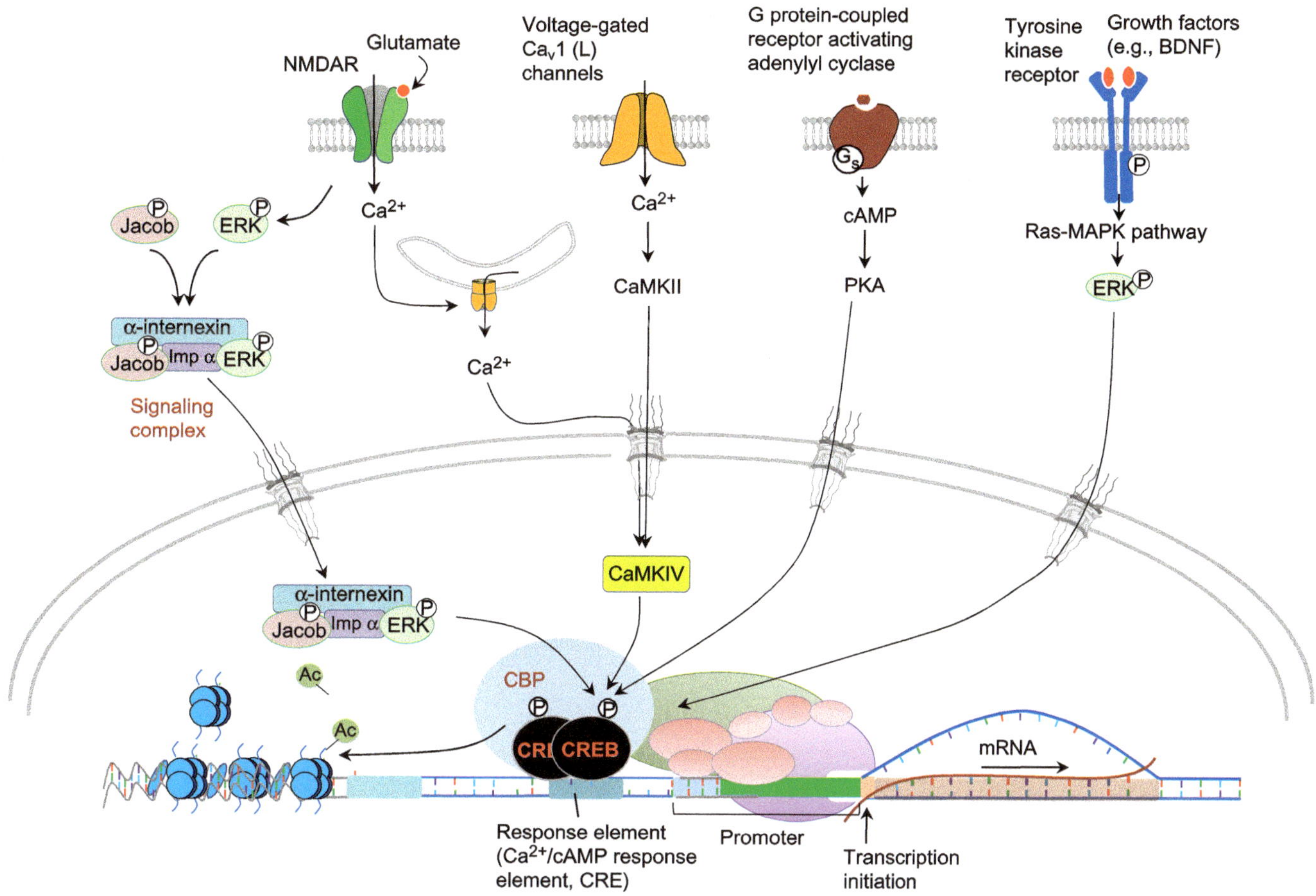

FIGURE 5.3 CREB as a prototype extracellular signal activated transcription factor.
Cyclic adenosine monophosphate (cAMP)–response element binding protein (CREB) is activated by several extracellular signals. They include activation of glutamatergic N-methyl-D aspartate receptors (NMDARs); calcium (Ca^{2+}) influx via voltage-gated $Ca_v1.1$ (L) channels; intercellular Ca^{2+} release by the endoplasmic reticulum; activation of G protein-coupled receptors positively coupled to G_s proteins; and activation of tyrosine kinase receptors for growth factors, such as brain-derived neurotrophic factor (BDNF). Several protein kinases activated by synaptic activity promote CREB phosphorylation at the serine 33 residue, leading to transcriptional activation; they include calmodulin (CaM) kinase IV, protein kinase A (PKA), and extracellular signal-regulated kinase (ERK). CREB may also be activated by signaling complexes including those containing Jacob, internexin, and phosphorylated ERK, which form at active synaptic sites or at the site of injury and travel to the nucleus in association to adaptor proteins such as importins. CREB phosphorylation allows the recruitment of the transcriptional coactivator CREB-binding protein (CBP), which functions as a histone acetyl transferase (HAT) and thus promotes transcription via epigenetic mechanisms.

retardation.[11] This reflects the importance of CREB-CBP signal in epigenetic activation of transcription.

Transcriptional Repression

Transcriptional repression has an important role in determining neural phenotype, both during development and in response to injury. The typical mediator is Repressor element-1 binding transcription factor (REST), also known as neuron-restrictive silencer factor[12] (Figure 5.4). REST acts via epigenetic remodeling to restrict the expression of neuronal genes by binding to a neuron-restrictive silencer element domain called Repressor element-1 binding site within target genes. REST then recruits coREST and other co-repressor proteins forming platforms that in turn recruit histone deacetylases and site-specific histone-methyltransferases and demethylases. REST also recruits chromatin remodeling and other proteins that promote gene transcription. Target genes for REST include those involved in axonal pathfinding, synaptogenesis, synaptic plasticity, and structural remodeling such as synaptic vesicle proteins, receptors, ion channels, transporters, and neuron-specific miRNAs. REST orchestrates the developmental switch of several key synaptic and extrasynaptic proteins, including NMDAR subunits and chloride transporters. These changes

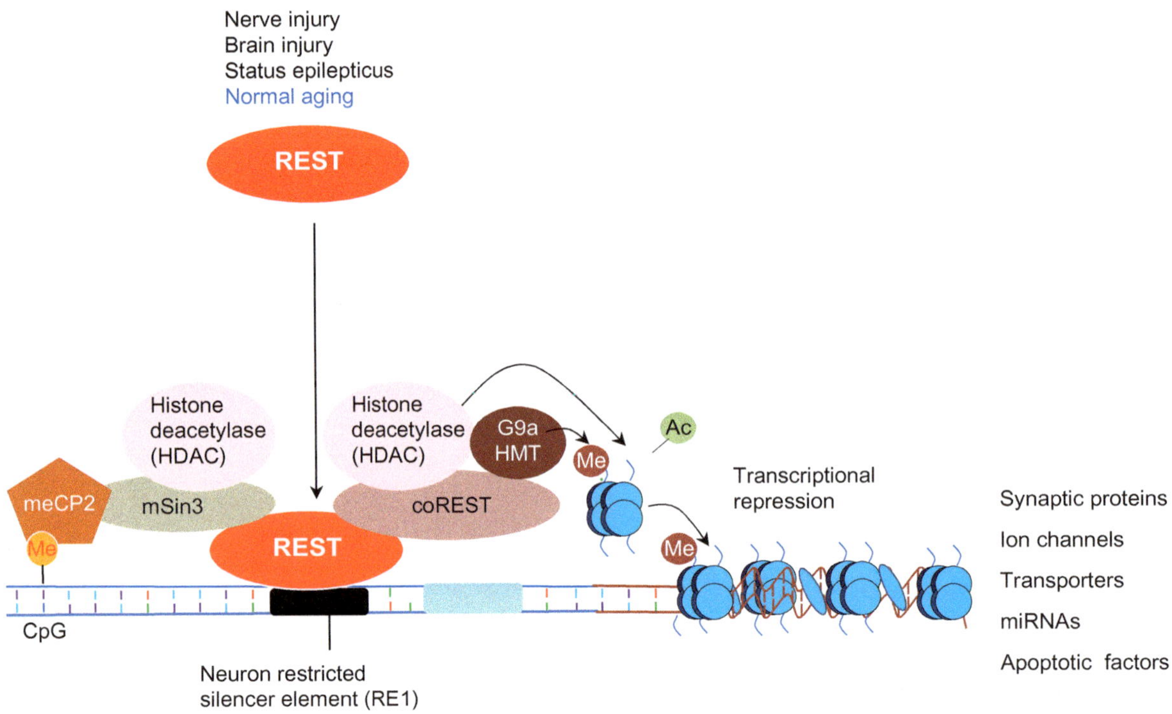

FIGURE 5.4 Transcriptional repression.
Repressor element-1 binding transcription factor (REST) binds the Repressor element-1 binding site within target genes and recruits coREST and other corepressor proteins forming platforms that in turn recruit histone deacetylases (HDAC), and site-specific histone-methyltransferases (HMT) and demethylases. REST also associates with methyl-CpG-binding protein 2 (MeCP2), which reads methylated DNA. REST not only silences but also recruits other proteins, which together activate REST target genes, including those encoding chromatin remodeling, promoting gene transcription. REST orchestrates the developmental switch of several key synaptic and extrasynaptic proteins. meCP2, methyl CpG binding protein 2.

are critical in regulating synaptic effects of excitatory and inhibitory neurotransmitters. Under physiological conditions, phosphorylation by several kinases typically reduces REST activity. The level of REST in neurons is also regulated by ubiquitin-dependent proteasomal degradation and autophagy/lysosomal pathways.

Loss of REST signaling is essential for acquisition of the neuronal phenotype during the final stages of neuronal differentiation. However, REST is also activated in differentiated neurons during periods when fine-tuning of genes is required for synaptic plasticity and neuroprotection, as occurs with normal aging. REST may also be upregulated in response to cytokines and epigenetic factors in ischemia, seizures, and other forms of injury. Activation of REST leading to reduced expression of potassium channels in axons is one of the several epigenetic alterations that occur in the setting of nerve injury or inflammation and contribute to neuropathic pain.[12]

MESSENGER RNA MATURATION

The transcribed region of DNA is first copied onto a primary transcript or pre-mRNA, which has to be further processed into a mature mRNA to be exported from the nucleus and initiate translation. During transcription, nascent mRNAs assemble with a set of RNA-binding proteins to form mRNPs that regulate both transcription and further steps of mRNA metabolism.[13–15]

Messenger RNA-Binding Proteins

There are approximately 1,000 RNA-binding proteins in a mammalian cell. These proteins regulate multiple steps of mRNA metabolism including transcription, splicing, transport, and degradation (Table 5.1).[15] Several mRNA-binding proteins affect several of these steps. Important examples include heterogeneous nuclear ribonucleoproteins (hnRNPs), TAR-DNA-binding protein 43 (TDP-43), and fused in sarcoma/translocated in liposarcoma (FUS). Mutations affecting these proteins are a fundamental disease mechanism in familial forms of ALS and FTLD.[16–18] TDP-43, encoded by the *TARDP* gene, is a primarily nuclear protein that shuttles between the nucleus and the cytoplasm, binds both DNA and RNA, and regulates the expression and splicing of multiple mRNA targets. It also has a major role in mRNA transport, transcriptional repression, miRNA biogenesis, stabilization of long noncoding RNA, and stress granule formation. FUS is also primarily a nuclear protein that functions in transcriptional regulation, pre-mRNA splicing, and other steps of mRNA processing and metabolism. FUS may also promote the DNA repair response by direct interaction with histone deacetylase 1. Both TDP-43 and FUS/TLS contain RNA recognition motifs, prion-like domains, and glycine-rich regions. Whereas TDP-43 specifically binds UG-rich sequences FUS/TLS lacks a linear consensus motif and its binding to target transcripts seems to be more position specific than sequence specific. However, these proteins may functionally interact with each other at several steps of mRNA metabolism. Whereas both TDP-43 and FUS are located primarily in the nucleus, they are also present in small amounts in the cytosol, where they bind to 3'UTRs of many mRNAs, regulating their stability, localization, translation, and dynamics. Several mRNA-binding proteins shuttle between the nucleus and the cytoplasm and are present in transport granules, where they primarily repress mRNA translation, as discussed later in this chapter. They include fragile X mental retardation protein 1 (FMRP1, *FMRP1* gene),[19] ataxin-2 (*ATXN2* gene) and others.[20]

Processing of Pre-mRNA

The processing of pre-mRNA occurs co-transcriptionally and includes addition of a 5' cap, 3' polyadenylation, and splicing (Figure 5.5). The 5' cap (also known as RNA 7-methylguanosine cap, or RNA m^7G cap) is a modified guanine nucleotide that is added to the 5' end of mRNA shortly after the start of transcription; this involves a cap-synthesizing complex recruited by pol II. The 5' cap is critical for mRNA recognition by the ribosome and protection from its degradation by RNAses. The covalent linkage of a polyadenylyl moiety to the 3' end of the mRNA, referred to as poly(A) tail also occurs during and/or immediately after transcription; this poly(A) tail is bound by polyadenylyl-binding protein 1 (PABP1), which is required for translation. Polyadenylation protects mRNA from degradation by exonucleases and is also important for transcription termination, export of the mRNA from the nucleus, and translation.

The final mature mRNA contains exon-coding sequences known as open reading frames (ORFs) that are translated into protein and untranslated regions (UTRs) at the 5′ and

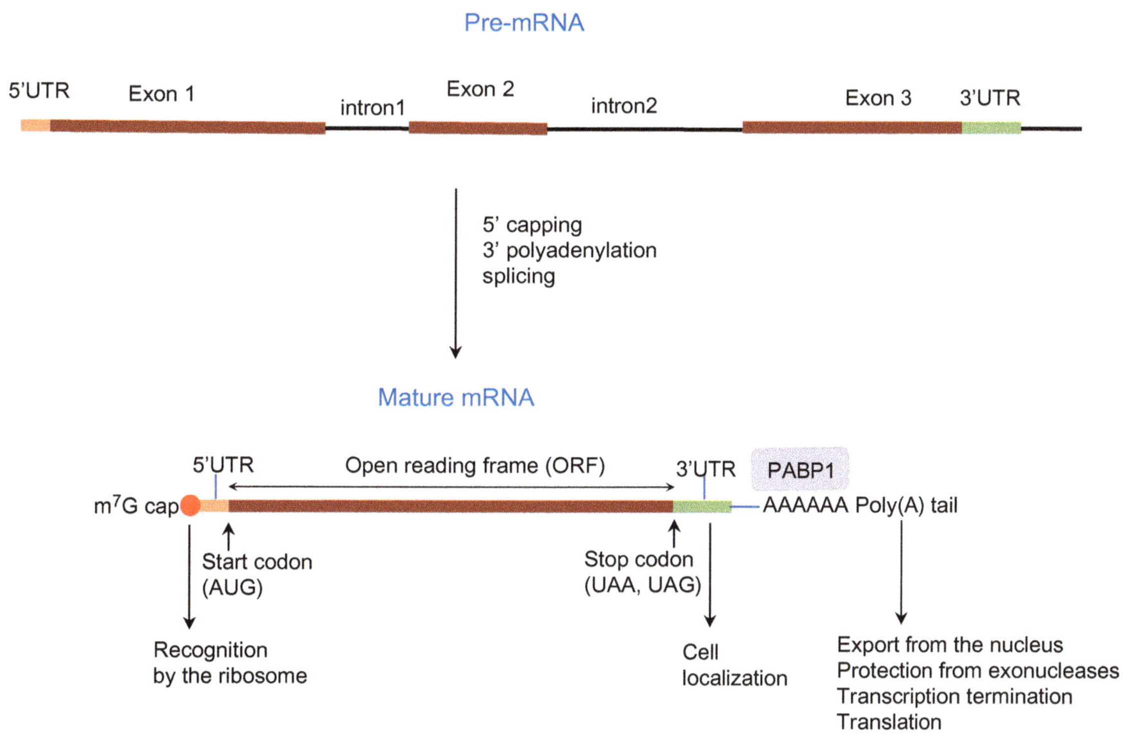

FIGURE 5.5 Processing on pre-mRNA.
The pre-mRNA undergoes maturation via addition of a 5' cap (also termed RNA cap, RNA 7-methylguanosine cap, or RNA m^7G cap), covalent linkage of a polyadenylyl moiety to the 3' end poly(A) tail and splicing. The poly(A) tail is bound by polyadenylyl binding protein 1 (PABP 1), which protects the mRNA from degradation by exonucleases. The final mature mRNA contains exon coding sequences known as open reading frame (ORF) that are translated into protein; and untranslated regions (UTRs) at the 5′ and 3′ ends of the molecule. Coding regions begin with the start codon (in general an AUG) and end with a stop codon (in general, UAA, UAG, or UGA) that signals termination of protein synthesis.

3′ ends of the molecule. Coding regions begin with the start codon (in general AUG) and end with a stop codon that signals termination of protein synthesis. The 5'UTR located before the start codon and the 3'UTR after the stop codon control stability, subcellular location, and translational efficiency of an individual mRNA. The 3'UTR also determines the cytoplasmic localization of mRNA and may contain sequences that allow the transcript to be localized to a particular cell region for translation.[21]

Control of Splicing

After completion of synthesis, the pre-mRNA undergoes splicing, which is the removal of the intron sequences and the joining together of the exon sequences to form mature mRNA. Splicing is often tightly coupled to transcription. During splicing, introns are excised and exons are ligated to each other in the 5′ → 3′ order in which they are encoded in the genome.[22] Splicing occurs in a large multiprotein complex called the spliceosome, which is composed of small nuclear ribonucleoproteins (snRNPs) that assemble during transcription of the pre-mRNA. The faithful assembly of spliceosome depends on survival of motor neuron (SMN) protein and associated proteins called gemins.[23] The splicing operation is critical, because any mistake of even a single nucleotide in the execution of the process would displace the triplet reading frame and interrupt the synthesis of the encoded protein. Loss-of-function mutations of *SMN1* gene encoding the SMN protein cause spinal muscular atrophy (SMA).[24,25] Alternative splicing generates different mRNAs by varying the exon composition of the same mRNA transcripts. This process thus generates functionally different proteins and contributes largely to phenotypic diversity in the nervous system. Alternative splicing is controlled by trans-acting proteins that bind to cis-acting sites on the pre-mRNA transcripts.[26] In addition to ubiquitously expressed splicing factors, there are specific RNA-binding proteins that regulate alternative splicing in neurons. Clinically relevant examples include neuro-oncological ventral antigen (Nova, also known as Ri)[27] and embryonic lethal abnormal visual (Elav, also known as Hu);[28] these splicing factors may be targeted by autoantibodies in the setting of paraneoplastic disease.[29] Another important splicing factor is Muscleblind-like protein (MBNL1).[30] Sequestration of MBNL1 into nuclear RNA inclusions in disorders such as myotonic dystrophy type 1 prevents appropriate splicing of target RNAs, which explains the complex phenotype of this disorder.[31–33] MBLN1 may modulate SMN localization and FUS toxicity by modulating stress granule dynamics.[34] Splicing mechanisms also generate circular RNAs, which are a special form of long coding RNAs that are enriched in the nervous system.[9] Circular RNAs are transported to dendrites and synaptic structures, are resistant to RNA exonuclease, and regulate several processes, including the effects of miRNAs.[31]

NUCLEOCYTOPLASMIC TRANSPORT

There is a bidirectional communication between the nucleus and the cytoplasm. This occurs through a highly regulated nucleocytoplasmic transport of RNAs, proteins, and ribonucleoproteins across the nuclear envelope via nuclear pore complexes.[35,36] The nuclear export of mRNAs is intrinsically linked to the co-transcriptional processing of nascent mRNA transcripts. Following nuclear export mRNA granules are targeted to different cellular destinations (Figure 5.6).

Nuclear Pore Complex and Cargo Transporters

The nuclear pore complex structures are large macromolecular complexes composed of highly conserved proteins called nucleoporins.[37] The nuclear pore consists of a symmetric core channel sandwiched between a ring attached to a nuclear basket and a ring attached to cytoplasmic filaments. Channel nucleoporins contain phenylalanine-glycine (FG) repeats that create a hydrogel meshwork within the nuclear pore that prevents the free passage of macromolecules. The transport of proteins and most RNAs across the nuclear pore requires their binding to cargo transport receptors (also known as karyopherins) that interact with these FG repeats. These cargo receptors include exportins that recognize nuclear export signals in cargoes that are transported from the nucleus to the cytoplasm, and importins that recognize nuclear localization signals and transport cargo from the cytoplasm to the nucleus. The directionality of transport is determined by small Ras-related nuclear protein (Ran)-GTPases. Cargoes containing a nuclear export signal and bound to exportins form a complex with Ran-GTP. Cytoplasmic cargoes to be imported to the nucleus form a complex with importins bound to Ran-GDP. Many RBPs contain nuclear localization signals that are recognized by importins; importin β2 (also called transportin-1) has a major role in import of mRNA-binding proteins back to the nucleus.[38] Some mRNA-binding proteins, such as TDP-43 and FUS are cargo substrates for both importins and exportins. Impaired nucleocytoplasmic transport of mRNA-binding proteins is a major disease mechanism in neurodegenerative disorders. Formation of abnormal large protein aggregates or assemblies may affect nucleocytoplasmic transport as a consequence of mislocalization of mRNA-binding proteins or through interactions with components of the nuclear pore complex. One important mechanism is via formation of toxic polydipeptides that interact with FG residues of nucleoporins and interfere with the transport of TDP-43 and other mRNA-binding proteins, as discussed later in this chapter.

Nucleocytoplasmic Export of Messenger Ribonucleoproteins

The passage of mRNPs from the nucleus to the cytoplasm utilizes an independent transport system.[39,40] Many mRNA-binding proteins that are recruited to the transcripts and regulate splicing also function as adaptors and regulators

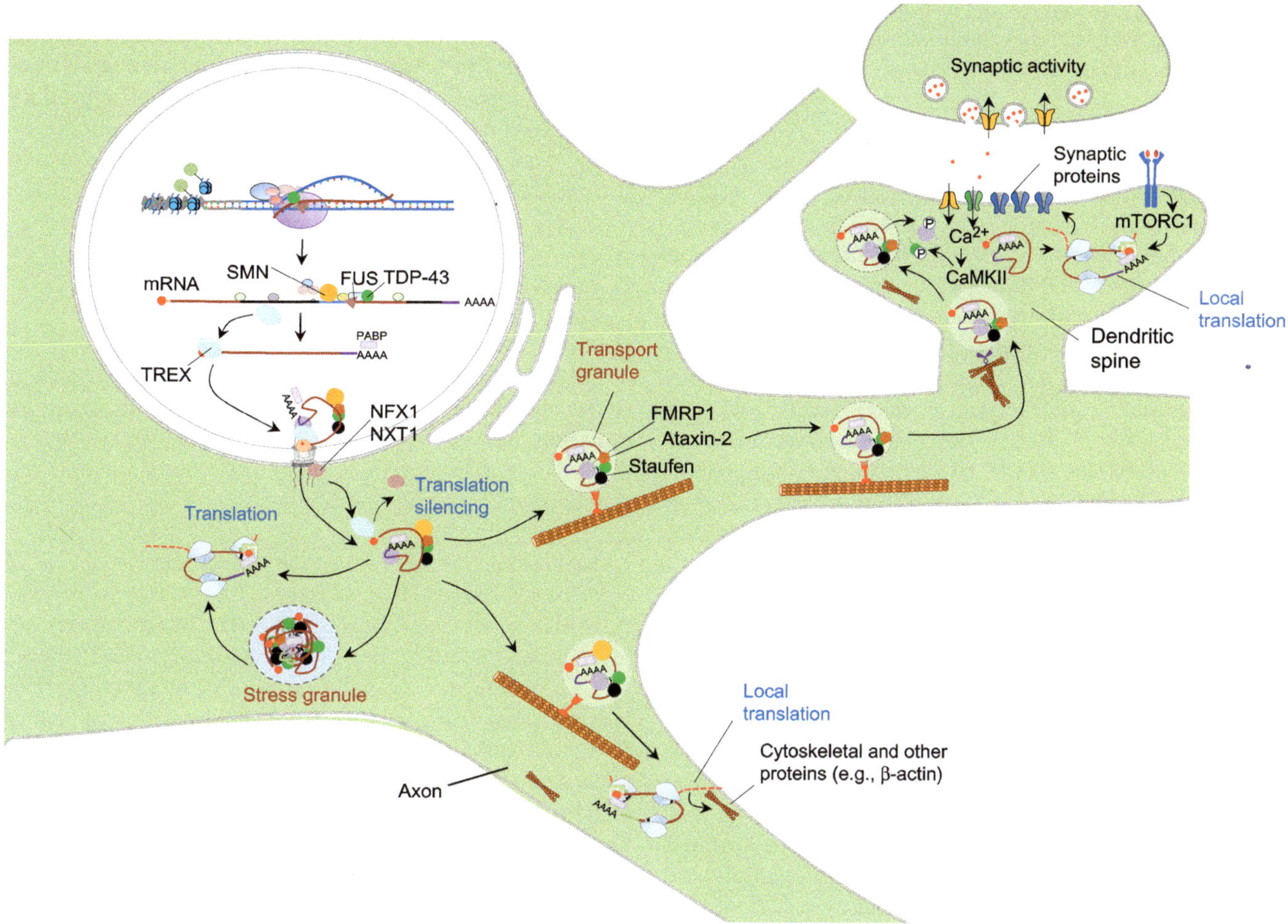

FIGURE 5.6 Nucleocytoplasmic and cytoplasmic transport of mRNA.
Nucleocytoplasmic transport of most mRNAs requires Transcription/Export (TREX) 1 complexes and transport factors such as Nuclear Export Factor 1 (NFX1) that interact with nucleoporins and thus allow transit of mRNAs through the nuclear pore. At the cytoplasmic face of the nuclear pore complex, NFX1 dimers encounter cytoplasmic filament nucleoporins and the protein GLE1, which activates the removal of the NFX1 dimers from the mRNA by action of DEAD-box helicases such as DDX19. In neurons, many ribonucleoprotein particles contain translationally silenced mRNAs that are transported in granules along microtubules from the nucleus to the axon or dendrites. Messenger RNAs are transported in a transcriptionally silent state via association with repressor proteins such as fragile X mental retardation protein 1 (FMR1), ataxin-2 (ATXN-2), and Staufen. For local translation to occur in dendrites, mRNAs have to be released from granules (unmasked) to be translated into synaptic proteins; this activity-dependent translation is promoted by mammalian (mechanistic) target of rapamycin (mTOR).

of mRNA export. The typical export receptor for mRNA is the transcription-coupled export (TREX) complex, which is recruited by the splicing machinery and binds to the capped 5' end of mRNA. Cargo mRNAs are then transferred from TREX to a conserved heterodimeric transport factor complex that mediates the bulk of mRNA export across the nuclear pore. The mRNPs that reach the cytoplasm undergo extensive remodeling to ensure that they do not reenter the nucleus. This remodeling is critical for maintaining the direction of mRNA export and preparing mRNAs for translation by the ribosome. Processing of mRNPs at the cytoplasmic face of the nuclear pore complex involves the cytoplasmic filament nucleoporins, including GLE1, which activate a helicase that removes the nuclear transport factor complex from the mRNP; this prevents reimport of mRNPs back from the cytosol to the nucleus.[39] Loss-of-function mutations in the *GLE1* gene produce autosomal recessive forms of motor neuron diseases.[41] *GLE1* mutations also cause a depletion of GLE1 at the nuclear pore in ALS patients.[42]

TRANSPORT OF MESSENGER RNA GRANULES FOR LOCAL TRANSLATION

There is compartmentalization of mRNAs in neurons. This depends on complex interactions among regulatory elements, or zipcode sequences in mRNAs and the effect of RNA-binding proteins that modulate mRNA trafficking to the dendrites and axon (Figure 5.6).

Zipcodes and mRNA-Silencing Proteins

A major determinant of local translation are zipcode sequences that are most commonly located in the 3' UTR of the mRNA. Alternative splicing and polyadenylation produce a large variety of zipcode regions or localization sequences in the 3'UTR of mRNAs, which specify the final destination of the splice isoform in axons and dendrites. The second major determinants of compartmentalization of mRNA transcripts in neurons are RNA-binding proteins that maintain the mRNA in an untranslated (silent) state during transport of mRNPs along microtubules until arrival to the site for local mRNA translation.[21,31,43] Important examples are FMRP1, ataxin-2 and Staufen. For translation to occur, mRNAs have to dissociate from these associated RNA-binding proteins; this typically involves phosphorylation of the RNA-binding proteins that silence the mRNA. However, these proteins also regulate other aspect of mRNA metabolism. For example, whereas ataxin-2 represses translation of select mRNAs, it also regulates mRNA stability by increasing mRNA polyadenylation thus promoting global translation. Ataxin-2 also prevents the deleterious accumulation of the RNA-DNA hybrid-harboring R-loop structures that prevent transcription.[20] Staufen is a double-stranded RNA-binding protein that is incorporated in RNA granules by both RNA-dependent and -independent interactions and participates in mechanisms of mRNA decay.

Local Translation in Axons and Dendrites

Transport of RNA granules allows locally regulated translation of mRNAs into proteins in dendritic and axonal subdomains.[44–47] Once assembled, mRNP granules interact with chaperone, adaptor, and motor proteins to undergo transport along microtubules to axons and dendrites. Mature axons contain the machinery for protein synthesis, including ribosomes and transfer RNAs, which are irregularly distributed and located close to the plasma membrane. Local translation is fundamental for axon growth during development, maintenance of axonal and synaptic function, response to injury, and communication of injury signals to the soma. Several RNA-binding proteins localized in the axon, including SMN, regulate the axonal location mRNA transcripts, for example, that encoding β-actin. The importance of SMN in this process explains the early involvement of the axons and neuromuscular junction in SMA.[48]

Synaptic activity triggers signaling cascades that unmask mRNAs for their local translation at active dendrites. For example, activity-dependent phosphorylation of FMRP1 elicits conformational changes in this transcriptional repressor triggering its dissociation from mRNAs, and allowing translation of synaptic proteins such as glutamate receptor subunits at the site of active dendrites. This is a fundamental mechanism of long-term potentiation of excitatory synaptic activity. FMRP1 interacts with postsynaptic proteins, modulating activity-dependent synaptic development, and balance between excitation and inhibition in neural circuits.[19] Mutations of *FMRP1* produce fragile X syndrome (FXS), which is the most common hereditary cognitive impairment that primarily reflects synaptic dysregulation.[48]

TRANSLATION OF MESSENGER RNA AND PROTEIN SYNTHESIS

Translation of mRNA into protein occurs in the ribosomes and involves four phases: initiation, elongation, termination, and recycling. A comprehensive description of this process is beyond the scope of this chapter and only few concepts will be emphasized here.

Formation of the Pre-Initiation Complex and mRNA Translation

Initiation of translation involves the interaction of key proteins called eukaryote initiation factors (eIFs) (Figure 5.7). The eukaryotic translation initiation factor (eIF) eIF2B is a key regulator of mRNA translation and is responsible for the activation of the G protein eIF2, which is required to allow translation initiation.[49] In the canonical translation initiation process, the first step requires the formation of a ternary complex consisting of GTP-bound eIF2, the initiator methionyl transfer RNA (Met-tRNA$_i^{Met}$) and the 40S ribosomal subunit.

This ternary complex interacts with other eIFs to form a pre-initiation complex that, once assembled, is recruited to the m^{7}G cap at the 5' end of the mRNA. This process requires the eIF4F complex, which consists of a cap-binding protein, a helicase, and a scaffolding protein that interacts with PABP1 bound to the 3' poly(A) tail of the mRNA. The pre-initiation complex scans the mRNA in 5' to 3' direction in search of the start codon, which is most often AUG. In addition to this canonical AUG codon translation, there is a mechanism of non-AUG translation that involves other codons (e.g., ACG or CUG) and alternative initial transfer mRNAs to form the pre-initiation complex.[50] Non-AUG translation occurs during development, in response to stressors, and in pathological conditions associated with nucleotide repeat expansions. After joining of the ribosomal 60S subunit to the 40S subunit forming a complete 80S ribosome, the second codon can be decoded in the aminoacyl site of the ribosome. During chain elongation, each additional amino acid is added to the nascent polypeptide chain. Elongation depends on eukaryotic elongation factors. Ribosomal pausing delays protein translation and aids the co-translational folding of the nascent polypeptide on the ribosome. Termination of elongation depends on the eukaryotic release factor 1, which recognizes the stop codons. Upon termination, the ribosome is disassembled and the completed polypeptide is released.

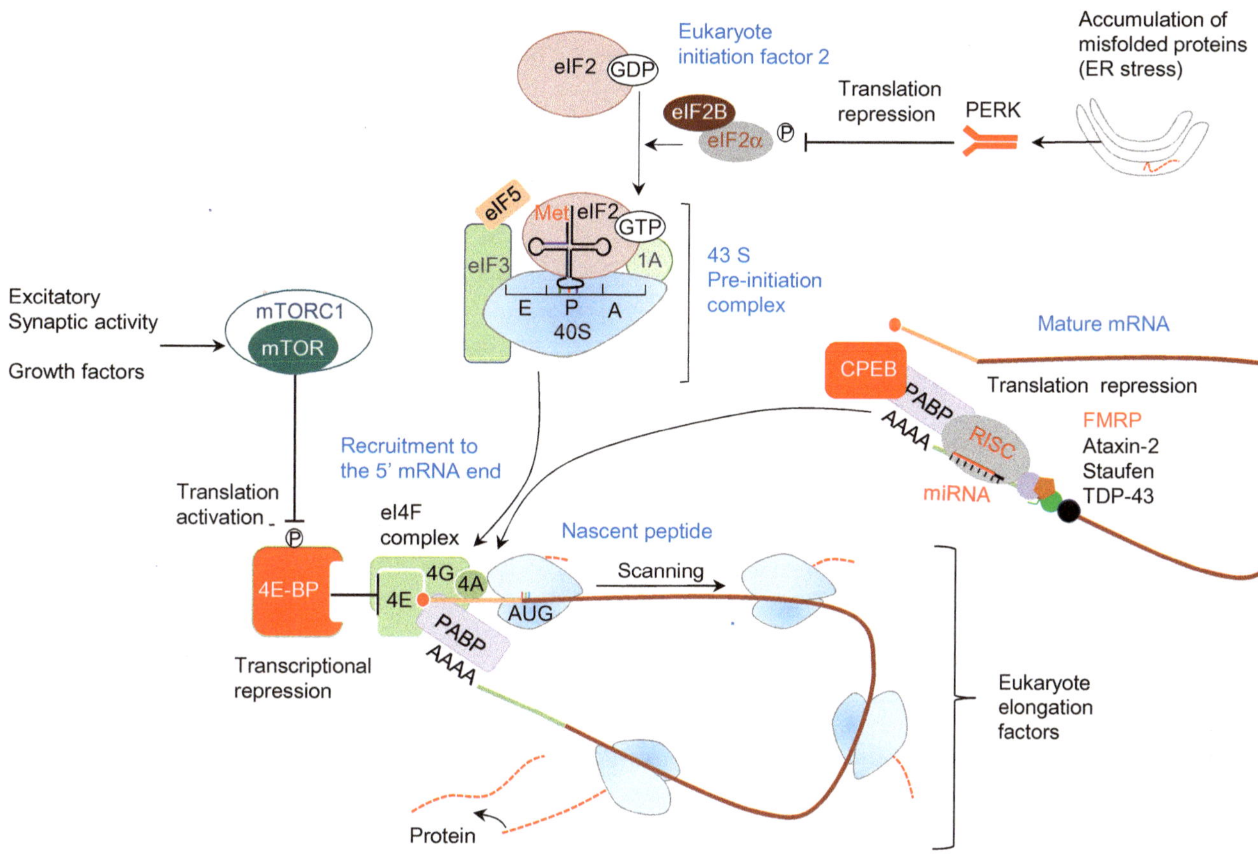

FIGURE 5.7 Overview of mRNA translation.

Translation of mRNA into protein occurs in the ribosomes and involves: initiation, elongation, termination, and recycling. Initiation involves key proteins called eukaryote initiation factors (eIFs). The first step is the formation of a ternary complex consisting of GTP-(guanosine triphosphate) bound eIF2, the initiator methionyl transfer RNA (Met-tRNA$_i^{Met}$) and the 40 S ribosomal subunit. This complex interacts with eIF1, eIF1A, eIF5, and eIF3 complex to form a 43 S pre-initiation complex. This complex is recruited to the m^{7}G cap at the 5'end of the mRNA by the eIF4F complex, consisting of the cap-binding protein eIF4E, the helicase eIF4A, and the scaffolding protein eIF4G, which binds PABP1 at the mRNA 3'end. The pre-initiation complex scans the mRNA in 5' to 3' direction in search of the start codon, which is most often AUG. After the eIF2-bound Met-tRNA$_i^{Met}$ anticodon base-pair with the peptidyl site of the ribosome, subsequent steps allow the joining of the ribosomal 60 S subunit, forming a complete 80 S ribosome. This allows the second codon to be decoded in the aminoacyl site. During chain elongation, each additional amino acid is added to the nascent polypeptide chain. Elongation depends on eukaryotic elongation factors. One important mechanism of regulation of mRNA translation is inhibition of the formation of the pre-initiation complex in the setting of cellular stress via protein kinase RNA-like endoplasmic reticulum kinase (PERK), which phosphorylates the α subunit of eIF2α. The EIF4 binding protein (4EBP) prevents the interaction of eIF4 with eIF4G, thus preventing cap-dependent initiation. Growth factors promote translation via activation of mammalian (mechanistic) target of rapamycin complex 1 (mTORC1), which phosphorylates 4EBP. Translation is also inhibited by several mRNA-binding proteins and microRNAs. CPEB, cytoplasmic polyadenylation element binding protein; PABP, polyadenylate binding protein; RISC, miRNA- induced silencing complex.

Regulation of mRNA Translation

There are several points of regulation of mRNA translation (Figure 5.7). One important mechanism is the inhibition of the formation of the pre-initiation complex in the setting of cellular stress. Several stressors, including reactive oxygen species, mitochondrial dysfunction, and endoplasmic reticulum (ER) stress due to accumulation of misfolded proteins activate stress-induced kinases, such as protein kinase RNA-like endoplasmic reticulum kinase (PERK).[51] PERK phosphorylates the eIF2α subunit of eIF2B, inhibiting formation of the ternary complex that is required by AUG-initiated translation. Therefore, as an initial response to cellular stress, there is a global suppression of translation allowing stress adaptation and recovery. Whereas PERK inhibits translation of most proteins, mRNAs encoding proteins that restore cellular homeostasis, such as endoplasmic reticulum chaperones are upregulated by PERK signaling and continue to be produced via non-AUG translation. The adaptor protein known as growth arrest and DNA damage-induced protein 34 (GADD34, which is activated downstream of PERK signaling, recruits protein phosphatase 1, which dephosphorylates of eIF2α, thus providing a feedback mechanism that allows reinitiation of normal translation. Mutations in *eIF2B* genes cause vanishing white matter disease, which is a fatal leukodystrophy that is triggered and exacerbated by different stressors, such as infections. Cells from patients with this disorder hypersuppress translation during ER stress, delaying stress-induced gene expression and interrupting the negative feedback loop that allows translational recovery from stress; small molecules targeting eIF2B or PERK rescue translation defects in these cells.[52]

Another major regulatory mechanism occurs at the level of cap-dependent translation initiation and is mediated by the eIF4-binding protein (4EBP), which prevents the formation of the eIF4F complex. Growth factors promote translation via activation of mammalian (mechanistic) target of rapamycin complex 1 (mTORC1), which phosphorylates 4EBP, permitting cap-dependent protein synthesis. As discussed earlier in this chapter, during mRNA transport in transport granules, translation is also inhibited by mRNA-binding proteins such as FMRP1,[19] ataxin-2,[20] and Staufen.[53] One important mechanism of inhibition of translation is by miRNAs.

MESSENGER RNA DEGRADATION

Degradation of mRNA is typically initiated by shortening of the 3' poly(A) tail, followed by removal of the 5' cap structure (decapping) and then digestion of the 5' to 3' ends. Messenger RNA riboprotein granules called processing (P) bodies contain mRNAs associated with translational repressors and components of the mRNA decay machinery. This machinery includes a decapping complex, an ATP-bound helicase, a 5',3' exoribonuclease, and components of mRNA nonsense-mediated decay. Nonsense-mediated decay recognizes and degrades aberrant mRNA transcripts harboring premature termination codons and alternatively spliced mRNAs encoding nonfunctional proteins. In the setting of cellular stress, nonsense-mediated decay may also recognize and degrade normally spliced mRNAs encoding normal transcripts, some mRNA-binding proteins, and miRNAs.[54] This mechanism is a fundamental effector of the unfolded protein response triggered by ER stress.

MicroRNA

MicroRNAs (miRNAs, miRs) are small, noncoding RNAs that function primarily by silencing mRNA translation and posttranscriptional regulation of gene expression. The human genome may encode up to 1,000 miRNAs. Whereas most miRNAs are found within cells, some are found in the extracellular fluid, blood, and CSF, and thus constitute potential disease biomarkers.[55,56]

Synthesis, Processing, and Formation of the miRNA-Silencing Complex

MicroRNAs are transcribed by pol II or pol III either from intergenic regions or introns of the hosting gene to yield a precursor termed primary miRNA (pri-miRNA) (Figure 5.8). The double-stranded RNA structure on the hairpin of pri-miRNA is recognized by the nuclear protein DiGeorge syndrome critical region 8 (DGCR 8) and cleaved by the RNA endonuclease Drosha to produce pre-miRNA. Pre-miRNAs are exported from the nucleus to the cytoplasm by exportin-5 using Ran-GTP. In the cytoplasm, the pre-miRNA hairpin is cleaved by the RNAse Dicer with the aid of TDP-43 to generate an approximately 22-nucleotide-long miRNA duplex consisting of a passenger strand, which is degraded, and a guided strand that is loaded and embedded into the Argonaut (AGO) protein to form the miRNA-induced silencing complex (miRISC). The miRISC binds to the complementary site in the 3'UTR of the target mRNA, inhibiting its translation. After the miRNA guides the miRISC to its target, AGO cleaves the target mRNAs if the matching is perfect; otherwise imperfect sequencing matching leads to loss of the 3' poly(A) tail and the 5' cap in the mRNA, leading to its destabilization and degradation by endo- or exonucleases. The miRNA can also prevent translation through inhibition of formation of the eIF4 complex. MicroRNAs can facilitate the formation of processing (P) bodies that sequester mRNAs from translation and destroy them.

Regulation, Functions, and Interactions with Circular RNAs

An individual miRNA can target up to thousands of mRNAs and inhibit protein translation. In addition, there are several noncanonical mechanisms of miRNA function. For example, some miRNAs may also bind to 5'UTR and other sites; some may sometimes activate translation; and some may relocate to the nucleus and target another miRNA primary transcripts and long noncoding RNAs. If the target miRNA is not available, the miRNA is detached from the miRISC complex and undergoes decay. There is crosstalk between miRNAs and epigenetics. Both DNA methylation and histone acetylation can regulate miRNA expression. Reciprocally, DNA methyltransferases and histone deacetylases may be regulated by miRNAs. Mitochondria are enriched in miRNAs and may regulate miRNA activity by miRNA storage, delivery to different cell compartments, or exchange within the mitochondrial network.

There is also a neuronal activity-dependent regulation of miRNAs in the CNS. Some miRNAs are particularly enriched in dendrites and synapses, and their expression may be up- or downregulated through different pathways.

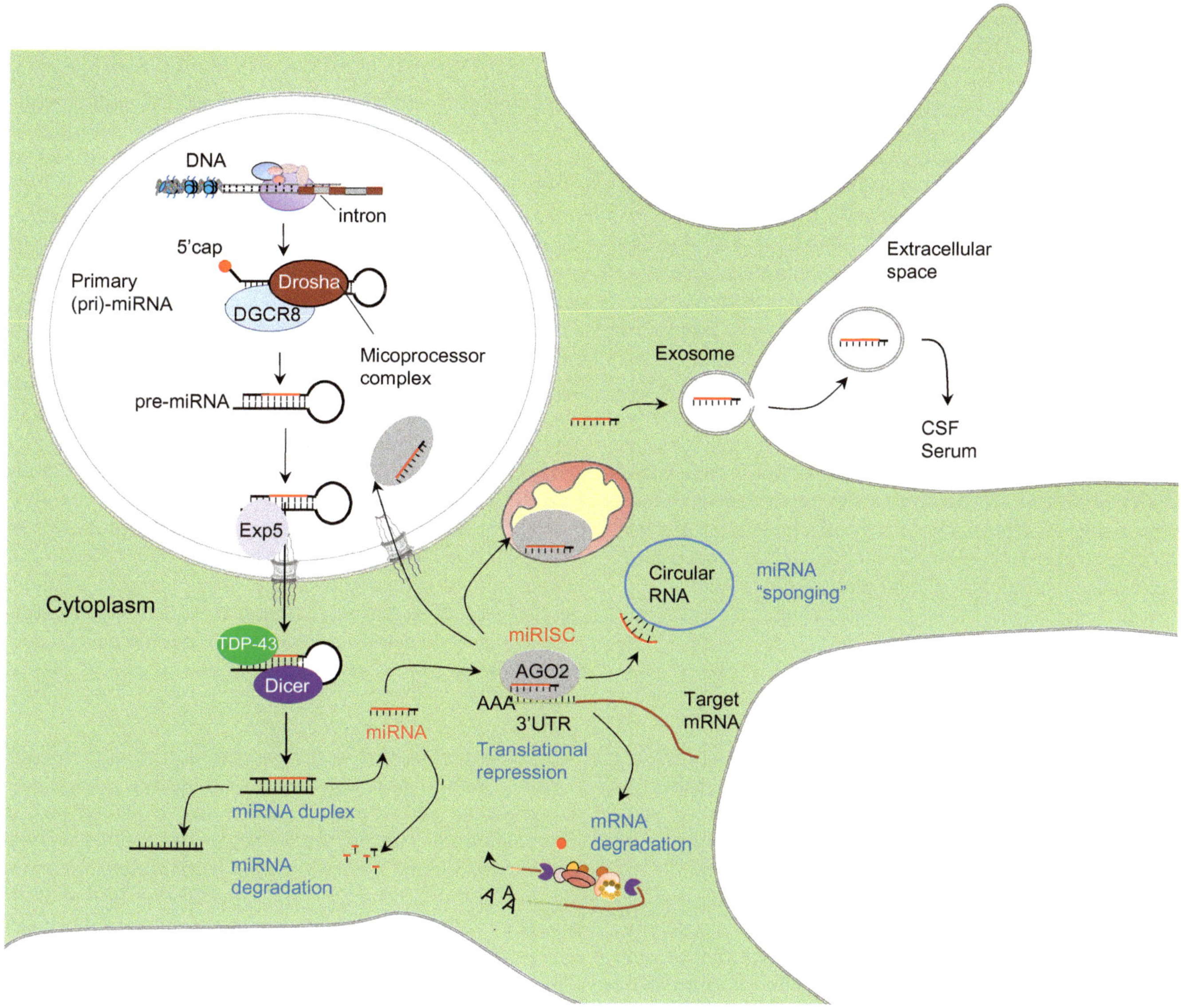

FIGURE 5.8 Biogenesis and functions of microRNAs.

MicroRNAs are transcribed by Pol II or Pol III to yield primary miRNA (pri-miRNA), which is recognized by the nuclear protein DiGeorge syndrome critical region 8 (DGCR 8) and cleaved by the RNA endonuclease Drosha to produce pre-miRNA. Pre-miRNAs are exported from the nucleus to the cytoplasm by exportin-5 in an energy-dependent process using Ran (**RA**s-related **N**uclear protein)-GTP. In the cytoplasm, the pre-miRNA hairpin is cleaved by Dicer with the aid of TAR DNA binding protein 43 (TDP-43) to generate a miRNA duplex. The passenger miRNA strand is degraded, whereas the guided strand is loaded embedded into the Argonaut (AGO) protein to form the miRNA-induced silencing complex (miRISC) that binds to the complementary site in the 3'UTR of the target mRNA. This leads to mRNAs cleavage by AGO, loss of the 3'pol (A) tail and the 5'cap, or mRNA destabilization and degradation by endo- or exonucleases. Some miRNAs may also relocate to the nucleus and target other miRNA primary transcripts or long no-coding RNAs. Some miRISCs can be recruited to mitochondria. Circular RNAs are able to "sponge" microRNAs and thereby relieve mRNA-coded messages from degradation and allow their translation. MicroRNAs can be secreted via exosomes, exert paracrine effects, and be detected in serum and CSF.

For example miR-132 is upregulated by synaptic activity. MicroRNAs such as miR-124 and miR-9 regulate several aspects of neural development, including proliferation and differentiation of neural stem cells, neuronal migration and circuit integration, dendritic complexity and spine biogenesis, axonal growth and guidance, and synaptic plasticity. Expression of some miRNAs is associated with CNS aging and brain response to injury. One example is miR-34a, which participates in tumor suppression and targets and silences multiple mitochondria-associated mRNAs.

Several transcription factors, including those activated during neuronal activity and oxidative stress, increase miR-34 expression. MicroRNAs regulate CNS inflammation in part via effects on microglia. For example, neuron-specific miR-124 and miR-9 are released from active neurons via exosomes and regulate the phenotype of microglia.

Circular RNAs are very stable in the cytoplasm and able to "sponge" miRNAs and thereby relieve mRNA-coded messages from degradation and allow their translation. For example, the antisense to the *cerebellar degeneration-related protein 1 transcript* (*CDR1as*) gene expresses a circular RNA (CDR1as) that binds to and inhibits miR-7 activity, thereby promoting translation of its target mRNAs. This is of potential clinical relevance, as miR-7 regulates an ubiquitin protein ligase that is essential for the clearance of βamyloid peptides and downregulates expression of α-synuclein.[37–57] Circular RNAs can stimulate the initiation and elongation of pol II-transcribed genes, contribute to downregulation of the expression of their cognate linear mRNA by negatively affecting linear splicing, and bind to proteins and impair the function of protein complexes related to translation and ribosome biogenesis.

ALTERED RIBOSTASIS AND NEURODEGENERATION

Disorders that directly or indirectly affect the functions of mRNA-binding proteins result in impaired transcription, splicing, and translation of mRNA. Many of these disorders are associated with abnormal formation or persistence of nuclear or cytosolic or mRNP aggregates.[15,58–60] Via protein–protein interactions, these aggregates may sequester other aggregation-prone mRNA-binding proteins, reduce the availability of other mRNAs for translation, and sequester other mRNA regulatory factors such as miRNAs and noncoding RNAs.

Formation and Dynamics of Stress Granules

When mRNA is not engaged in transcription, RNPs assemble into membraneless cytoplasmic structures, including stress granules and P bodies. Stress granules rapidly form in conditions that lead to impairment in translation initiation in the setting of cell stress (Figure 5.9). Stress granules, like transport granules or P bodies, are membraneless organelles formed by proteins containing disordered hydrophobic sequences that promote protein–protein interactions and liquid droplet formation. Formation of stress granules allows most mRNAs to be transiently placed on hold and shift translation toward synthesis of neuroprotective proteins, such as chaperones and repair enzymes. Stress granules contain untranslated mRNA transcripts, 40S ribosomal subunits, translation initiation factors, remodeling proteins, enzymes, and many other RNA-associated ribonucleoproteins, including TDP-43 and FUS. Nucleation of stress granules requires core RNA-binding proteins, including FMRP1.

Aggregation of the core nucleating proteins initiates a process that results in sequestration of mRNAs stalled in translation. The low complexity "prion-like" domains of mRNA-binding proteins such as TDP-43, FUS, and ataxin-2 mediate weak protein–protein interactions within the stress granules. These interactions produce conformational changes that may promote misfolding and β-sheet aggregation and result in the eventual transition into solid aggregates when these proteins accumulate, as in the setting of impaired translation or defective nucleocytoplasmic transport.[61] Stress granules consist of a stable core surrounded by a dynamic shell-like region and exchange components with each other and with P-bodies. In normal conditions, stress granules rapidly disperse in response to signal molecules, chaperones, or other proteins promoting their degradation. Assembly, disassembly, and transitions between the core and shell are driven by ATP and involve numerous proteins and RNA-remodeling complexes. The ATPases involved in dispersal and clearance of stress granules include RNA/DNA helicases, heat shock proteins (Hsp) 70 and 40; and valosin-containing protein (VCP). These proteins promote clearance of stress granule components via the ubiquitin-proteasome system and autophagy and also have a major role in proteostasis.

Accumulation of Stress Granules

Toxic accumulation of stress granules reflects the abnormal assembly of prion-domain-containing ribonucleoproteins into self-propagating amyloids.[61,62] Mutations of Hsp chaperones and impaired activity of proteins such as VCP may reduce clearance of misfolded proteins and stress granules by ubiquitination and autophagy. The crosstalk between mechanisms that maintain ribostasis and proteostasis may explain the clinical overlap of diseases primarily affecting each of these processes. Altered proteostasis may trigger the endoplasmic reticulum stress responses, which leads to mRNA translation inhibition and thus formation of stress granules. Abnormal accumulation of cytoplasmic stress granules is a pathological hallmark of many neurodegenerative disorders. The typical case is accumulation of TDP-43-containing stress granules, referred to as "TDP-43pathy." One important example is that of hexanucleotide (G_4C_2) repeat expansions of chromosome 9-open reading frame (*C9ORF72*) gene, which is the major cause of both sporadic and familial cases of ALS, FTLD, and ALS/FTLD.[63] Mutations in the gene encoding TDP-43 (*TARDBP*) have been identified in cases of both familial and sporadic ALS and in cases of FTLD. Accumulation of TDP-43 inclusions is also characteristic of FTLD associated with *GRN* (progranulin) mutations, multisystem proteinopathy associated with *VCP* mutations, and hippocampal sclerosis. These inclusions may also be associated with other disease-specific inclusions in Alzheimer disease (AD), Parkinson disease (PD), Huntington disease (HD), and tauopathies.

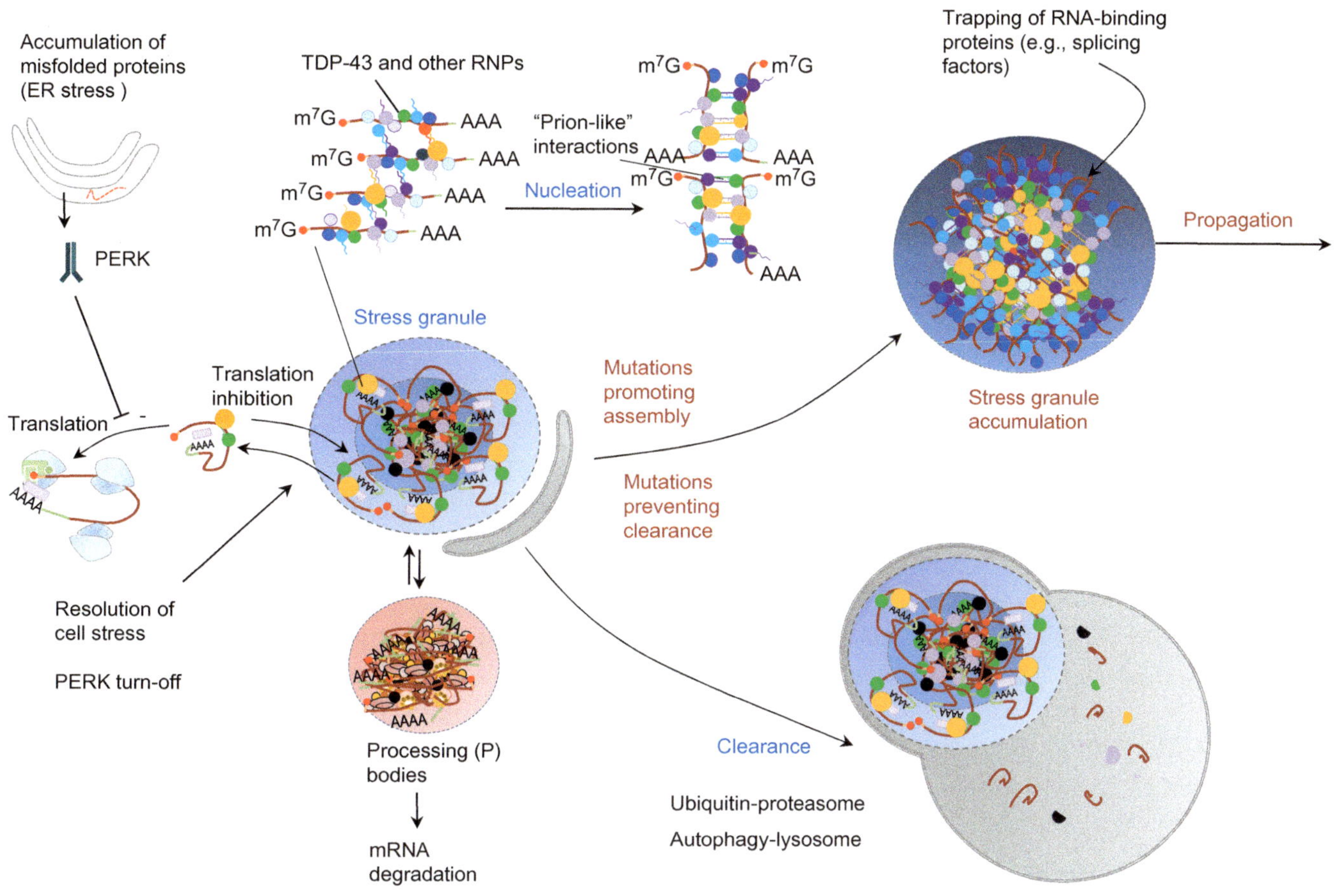

FIGURE 5.9 Formation and dynamics of stress granules.

Stalling of translation results in accumulation of stress granules. This results in part from activation of PERK in response to accumulation of misfolded proteins in the endoplasmic reticulum and other forms of cellular stress. RNA-binding proteins present in stress granules, such as TDP-43 and FUS/TLS, contain "prion-like" domains that allow protein–protein interactions responsible for nucleation of stress granules. Stress granules contain a stable core surrounded by a dynamic shell-like region, are transported via microtubules, and exchange components with each other and with processing (P) bodies. Stress granules readily disperse in response to signal molecules, chaperones, or other proteins promoting their degradation via ubiquitination and autophagy. These include several ATPases such as heat shock proteins (Hsps) and valosin-containing protein (VCP).

Impaired Nucleocytoplasmic Transport and Neurodegeneration

Impaired nucleocytoplasmic transport is increasingly recognized as a major disease mechanism in ALS, FTLD, HD, and AD.[64–66] This may occur as a consequence of formation of large protein aggregates or assemblies, mislocalization of mRNA-binding and transport proteins, or through interactions of toxic species with components of the nuclear pore complex. For example, TDP-43 aggregates in stress granules lead to mislocalization of importins and mRNA transport proteins, resulting in impaired nuclear import of TDP-43 from the cytoplasm. Impaired nuclear export may underlie the accumulation of aggregates of polyglutamine-expanded mutant huntingtin (HTT) in the nucleus in HD.[67–69] A major mechanism is interference of nuclear pore function via formation of toxic dipeptides formed by repeat-associated non-AUG (RAN) translation, as occurs downstream of hexanucleotide *C9ORF72* expansions.[70–73] Hyperphosphorylated tau (P-tau) can directly interact with components of the nuclear pore complex and components and disrupt nucleocytoplasmic transport.[74]

DISEASE MECHANISMS IN REPEAT EXPANSION DISORDERS

A large number of neurologic disorders are caused by expansion of nucleotide repeats (Table 5.3). The progressive expansion of the repeats over generations explains the phenomenon of anticipation, which is the tendency toward an early onset and more severe course in successive generations. The number of repeats correlates directly with severity of disease and earlier onset of disease. Expanded nucleotide repeats may produce toxicity through multiple pathogenic mechanisms.[31]

TABLE 5.3 *Repeat Expansion Disorders (Examples)*

Repeat (gene)	Disorder
GAA (*FXN*)	Friedreich ataxia
CGG (*FMRP*)	Fragile X mental retardation
CGG (*FMRP* premutation)	Fragile X tremor-ataxia syndrome (FXTAS)
CTG (*DMPK*)	Myotonic dystrophy 1
CTG (*ATXN8*)	Spinocerebellar ataxia (SCA) 8
CAG (*AR*)	Spinobulbar muscular atrophy (SBMA)
CAG (*HTT*)	Huntington disease
CAG (*ATXN1,2,3,7*)	(SCA1 (*ATXN1*), SCA2 (*ATXN2*), SCA3 (*ATXN3*), SCA7 (*ATXN7*)
CAG (*CACNA1A*)	SCA6
CAG CAG (T*BP*)	SCA17
CAG (*ATN*)	Dentorubropallidoluysian atrophy (DRPLA)
GCG (*PABPN1*)	Oculopharyngeal muscular dystrophy
GGC/*CGG* (*NOTCH2NLC*)	Neuronal intranuclear inclusion disease, leukoencephalopathy
CCTG (*CNBP/ZNF9*)	Myotonic dystrophy type 2
AAGGG (*RFC1*)	CANVAS (cerebellar ataxia, neuropathy, vestibular areflexia syndrome)
TTTCA (*SAMD12, RAPGEF2*)	Benign adult familial myoclonic epilepsies (BAFME) Familial cortical myoclonic tremor with epilepsy (FCMTE)
GGGGCC (*C9ORF72*)	Frontotemporal dementia, amyotrophic lateral sclerosis, chorea
CCCCGCCCCGCG (*CSTB*)	EPM1 myoclonic epilepsy (Unverricht-Lundborg disease)

AR, androgen receptor; ATN, atrophin; ATXN, ataxin; CACNA1A, α1A subunit of $Ca_v2.1$ (P/Q) channel; CNBP/ZFN9, cellular nucleic acid binding protein/zinc finger 9 protein); CSTB, cystatin B; DMPK, myotonic dystrophy protein kinase; FMRP1, fragile X mental retardation protein; FXN, frataxin; HTT, huntingtin; NOTCH2NLC, Notch homolog 2 N-terminal-like; PABPN1, polyadenylate-binding nuclear protein 1; RAPGEF2, Rap guanine nucleotide exchange factor; RFC1, replication facilitation complex 1, SAMD12, sterile alpha motif domain-containing 12

Protein Loss-of-Function

Loss-of-function may occur as a result of expansion in noncoding regions of DNA that may promote methylation and inactivation of the gene. One example is Friedreich ataxia, an autosomal recessive disease due to an expanded GAA repeat in the first intron of the *FXN* gene on chromosome 9q encoding for frataxin, a mitochondrial chaperone involved in formation of iron-sulfur clusters. Another example is fragile X syndrome caused by large (> 200 repeats) CGG repeat expansion in 5′UTR of the *FMR1* gene on chromosome Xq27.3 encoding FMRP1, resulting in DNA hypermethylation and transcriptional silencing with loss of gene function.

Toxic RNA Gain-of-Function

Disorders associated with GC-rich repeats residing in non-protein coding region of their respective disease genes may result from toxic RNA gain-of-function, due to abnormal nuclear accumulation of granules containing the abnormal mRNA associated with several ribonucleoproteins. These granules trap transcription and splicing factors required for normal mRNA metabolism. The typical example of this mechanism is myotonic dystrophy type 1, an autosomal dominant disorder caused by large unstable expansion of CTG repeats in the 3′UTR of the *DMPK* gene on chromosome 19, encoding for myotonin protein kinase. The normal *DMPK* gene 3'UTR contains 7 to 47 CTG repeats, which are stable on transmission. Normal subjects may have an allele with a low normal expansion (4–18) and another with a high normal expansion (19–37) but preferentially transmit to the offspring the allele with the larger expansion, a phenomenon called segregation distortion. Once the number exceeds 80 CTG repeats, there is a progressive increase in the likelihood of intergenerational expansion. The most severe form, congenital myotonic dystrophy, occurs in patients with large (> 500) CTG expansions, typically inherited from the mother. Proximal myotonic myopathy or myotonic dystrophy type 2 is linked to an expansion of CCTG repeats in intron 1 of the *CNBP/ZNF9* gene on chromosome 3q21 encoding a cellular nuclear acid binding protein/zinc finger protein 9. In both forms of myotonic dystrophy, the CTG expansion results in nuclear retention of CUG-containing mRNA species and accumulation of toxic granules in the nucleus. The CUG repeats bind to splicing factors such as MBLN1; this results in dysregulation of alternative mRNA splicing of multiple genes, which may explain the various disease manifestations. They include the *CLCN1* gene encoding the chloride muscle channel (myotonia), and genes encoding muscle bridging integratory protein 1 (weakness), insulin receptor (diabetes), cardiac sodium channel (arrhythmia), and cardiac troponin 1 (cardiomyopathy).

Another example of toxic RNA toxic-gain-of-function is that of *FMR1* gene premutations (55–200 CGG repeats). Some older carrier men develop fragile X tremor/ataxia syndrome (FXTAS), which manifests with ataxia, tremor, dementia, autonomic dysfunction, and white matter changes typically involving the middle cerebellar peduncle. Approximately 20% of carrier women manifest premature menopause. Nuclear accumulation of toxic mRNA products is also a pathogenic mechanism of spinocerebellar ataxia (SCA) type 8 (SCA8). This disorder is due to CTA/CTG expansions at the 3'UTR in a noncoding region of DNA, resulting in production of a natural RNA antisense of a gene called Kelch-like 1, which may be involved in cytoskeletal regulation. Neuronal intranuclear inclusion disease (NIID) is a severe adult-onset leukoencephalopathy due to GGC repeat expansion in the *NOTCH2NLC* gene. It manifests with dementia, cerebellar ataxia, peripheral neuropathy, autonomic dysfunction and in some cases tremor and encephalitis-like episodes. Skin biopsy shows intranuclear inclusions, which are also present in neurons and astrocytes. This disorder thus mimics FXTAS.

Toxic Protein Gain-of-Function

Toxic protein gain-of-function is a major mechanism of a large number of neurodegenerative disorders characterized by modest expansion (37 or more) of CAG repeats encoding polyglutamine (poly-Q) sequences. In general, these disorders affect specific components of the motor system, despite the fact that the mutated proteins carrying the CAG expansion are expressed in neural and non-neural tissues. Whereas these proteins have distinct functions, the main disease mechanism is not loss of function of the protein carrying the expanded polyglutamine but rather toxic gain of function leading to transcriptional dysregulation. Polyglutamine repeats are prone to formation of β-sheets promoting protein–protein interactions leading to accumulation of mRNA granules in the nucleus and trapping of proteins regulating mRNA metabolism. All CAG expansion disorders are autosomal dominant except spinobulbar muscular atrophy (SBMA), which is due to expansion in the androgen receptor gene on the X chromosome. The prototype CAG expansion disorder is HD, due to CAG repeat expansion in the first exon of the huntingtin (*HTT*) gene on chromosome 4p. Accumulation of mutant HTT exerts a toxic gain-of-function, such as impairment of clearance of abnormal protein aggregates by autophagy. Most normal subjects harbor 11 to 26 CAG repeats in the *HTT* gene; a repeat number of 27 to 35 confers no risk to the carrier but may expand between generations); a borderline number of CAG repeats (36–39) may or may not produce disease; more than 40 repeats confer a 100% lifetime risk of developing HD; and more than 60 repeats produce a juvenile form of disease.

Several forms of autosomal dominant cerebellar ataxia, including SCA1, SCA2, SCA3, SCA6, SCA7, SCA17, and dentorubropallydoluysian atrophy (DRPLA), are also due to CAG repeat expansions. SCA1 is due to expansion in the *ATXN1* gene encoding ataxin-1, a protein involved in transcriptional regulation. SCA2 is due to a long (>34) CAG expansion in the *ATXN2* gene; intermediate length repeats (27–33) are the most common genetic risk factor for ALS. SCA3 (Machado-Joseph disease) is due to a CAG expansion in the *ATXN3* gene encoding ataxin-3, which is a ubiquitin 3 ligase. SCA6 is due to a CAG expansion of the *CACNA1A* gene encoding the α1 subunit of the $Ca_v2.1$ (P/Q-type) voltage-gated calcium channel. SCA7 is due to CAG expansion of *ATXN7* gene encoding ataxin-7, a protein involved in transcriptional regulation in the CNS and retina, which explains the prominent visual loss that characterizes this disorder. SCA17 is linked to CAG/CAA repeat expansions in the *TBP* gene encoding for TATA-binding protein, a critical subunit of the transcriptional complex required for pol II function. Dentatorubropallidoluysian atrophy results from a CAG expansion of the *atrophin 1* (*ATN1*) gene and may reflect the combination of chronic blockade of the canonical autophagy pathway and upregulation of nucleophagy, resulting in marked nuclear pahtology.[75]

Repeat-Associated Non-AUG (RAN) Translation

Repeats may trigger toxicity through repeat-associated non-AUG (RAN) translation. The prototype is expansion of the (G_4C2) hexanucleotide in the first noncoding region of the *C9ORF72* gene.[71–73] Via RAN translation these *C9ORF72* hexanucleotide repeat expansions lead to the production of five different poly-dipeptide repeats: poly-glycyl-alanine (poly-GA) and poly-glycyl-arginine (poly-GR) from sense transcripts, poly-prolyl-alanine (poly-PA) and poly-prolyl-arginine (poly-PR) from antisense transcripts, and poly-glycyl-proline (poly-GP) from both sense and antisense transcripts. These toxic polydipeptide species bind many proteins, primarily those containing prion-like domains, including TDP-43, FUS, and FG-nucleoporins lining the nuclear pore.[76–78] Thus, repeat-containing transcripts of expanded *C9ORF72* not only form RNA foci that sequester and deplete RNA-binding proteins but also affect the nuclear pore meshwork interfering with nucleocytoplasmic transport.[76–78]

Another disease associated with RAN translation, oculopharyngeal muscular dystrophy, is a late-onset autosomal dominant disorder that manifests with ptosis and pharyngeal weakness. This disease is caused by small (8–13) CCG expansions in the first exon of the *PABP2* gene encoding PABP2, which binds the poly(A) tail of mRNA. These expansions trigger RAN translation leading to the formation of poly(A) oligomers that polymerize to form filamentous intranuclear inclusions in muscle cells. Other disorders in which RAN translation may have a pathogenic role include myotonic dystrophy type 1, SCA8, and FXTAs, all associated with CGG repeats.

DISORDERS DUE TO ABNORMAL MESSENGER RNA SPLICING

Approximately 15% to up to 50% of human genetic disorders are due to mutations affecting pre-mRNA splicing. These mutations may result in variation in the splice location and loss of function of that site by exposure of a premature stop codon, loss of an exon, or inclusion of an intron and disruption of the reading frame.[22,79]

One typical example of the importance of splicing in neurodegeneration is SMA, an autosomal recessive disease caused by loss-of-function mutations of the *SMN1* gene located in a telomere of chromosome 5q11.2-13 encoding the SMN protein.[24,25] The major feature of SMA is axonal dying back of spinal and bulbar motor neurons.[80] The severity of lower motor neuron weakness correlates with the amount of full-length SMN protein produced. The great heterogeneity in the age of onset and disease severity depends on several disease-modifying factors. Prominent among them is the expression of the *SMN2* gene located in the centromeric region of chromosome, which determines the degree to which SMN protein may be restored. However, *SMN2* cannot fully compensate for the loss of *SMN1* due to a C/T variation in exon 7 that causes a weakening of the 3' splice site and exon 7 skipping. This renders the *SMN2* gene transcriptionally inefficient and able to produce only 20% to 30% of full-length SMN protein, which is unstable and degraded. This has provided the bases for antisense nucleotide therapy, as discussed later. Another disorder associated with altered splicing is frontotemporal dementia and parkinsonism linked to chromosome 17 (FTDP-17), due to mutations of the *MAPT* gene encoding the microtubule associated protein tau.[81] Tau contains a microtubule assembly domain that comprises four-repeats (R1–R4) and flanking regions. There are six splice variants of tau that are distinguished by the presence or absence of the second repeat (R2), resulting in three repeat (3R) or four repeat (4R) isoforms. Because of the additional R2 repeat domain, 4R tau has higher affinity for microtubules and is more efficient in promoting microtubule assembly than 3R tau. Missense mutations that occur in or near the microtubule-binding domain reduce tau affinity for microtubules and increase its tendency to aggregate in the form of pathological hyperphosphorylated tau inclusions. Most of these splicing mutations occur within or near intron 10 encoding repeat R2 leading to an altered 4R to 3R tau ratio.[82,83]

ANTISENSE OLIGONUCLEOTIDES AND THERAPY OF NEUROLOGIC DISORDERS

Antisense oligonucleotides (ASOs) are 5–30 nucleotides long and are designed to be complementary to a sequence of mRNA or regulatory RNA. After parenteral administration the oligonucleotide enters the cell and binds the target RNA.

Mechanisms of Action

Depending on the targeted sequence, ASOs may trigger destruction of the mRNA by enzymatic cleavage, alter the splicing pattern of the pre-mRNA, or change of the function of a regulatory RNA.[84–87] Oligonucleotide-induced enzymatic cleavage or modification of the mRNA is potentially helpful when the targeted mRNA is mutated and encodes a pathogenic protein. Cleavage-inducing ASOs recruit enzymes such as RNAse H1 to the site of the mRNA where the ASO hybridizes, resulting in cleavage of the target mRNA. The second possible effect of ASOs is a change in the splicing pattern of the pre-mRNA, which is helpful when the default splicing produces a pathogenic product. Another mechanism is mRNA modification at the 5' cap or poly(A) site to prevent its translation. Finally, ASOs can also act through binding to miRNAs or other small RNA targets to inhibit their function. ASOs provide potentially valuable tools for treatment of repeat expansion disorders, as shown in two different mouse models of SCA2 due to *ATXN-2* mutations.[88] This approach has been explored in Huntington disease. Long noncoding RNAs are also targetable using antisense approaches. For example, silencing of a natural antisense RNA transcript of the *SCNA1* gene coding voltage-gated sodium channel Nav1.1 subunit resulted in upregulation of *SCNA1* expression and reduced seizures in a model of Dravet syndrome.

Applications in Neurologic Disease

Currently, oligonucleotides are FDA approved for treatment of Duchenne muscular dystrophy (DMD), infantile forms of SMA, and hereditary amyloid neuropathy associated with transthyretin (*TTR*) gene mutations. Duchenne muscular dystrophy is an X-linked caused by out-of-frame deletions of any of the 79 exons (most commonly exon 45) of the large *DMD* encoding dystrophin. These out-of-frame deletions result in production of an unstable and nonfunctional dystrophin that fails to connect the sarcolemma with the cytoskeleton; as a consequence muscle contractions elicit microtears in the sarcolemma and eventually muscle fiber cell loss. Antisense oligonucleotides can cause targeted exon skipping during pre-mRNA splicing and restore the frame of the primary DMD transcript. This results in production of dystrophin protein that is partially functional, thereby switching the phenotype from that of severe DMD to the less severe Becker muscular dystrophy. Eteplirsen hybridizes at site on exon 51, resulting in exon skipping; viltolarsen is designed to skip exon 53. Nusirensen is approved for treatment of infantile forms of SMA caused by loss of function *SMN1* mutations.[89] This ASO is directed to the intronic region 3' region to exon 7 of the *SMN2* gene, blocking the splicing signal that causes the exclusion of this exon from the transcript. As a consequence, the mRNA is processed to include the formerly missed exon 7 in the *SMN2* gene, which leads to the production of a functional SMN protein that rescues motor neurons. Another FDA-approved approaches for SMA include adeno-associated virus 9 (AAV) delivered *SM1* replacement (onasemnogene abeparvocec-xioi) and risdiplan, a small molecule that increases splicing efficiency at exon 7 in *SMN2* mRNA. Hereditary TTR amyloidosis is caused by several *TTR* gene mutations resulting in production of a mutant TTR protein that is prone to aggregation as amyloid deposits in peripheral nerves, heart, kidney, and other issues. Inotersen is an ASO and patisiran is a small interfering RNA that trigger cleavage of the mRNA encoding mutant TTR. Both drugs produce dose-dependent reduction of circulating TTR levels, limiting progression of the peripheral neuropathy.[90,91]

Therapy with ASO is being studied in Huntington disease and in ALS associated with superoxide dismutase 1 (SOD1) mutations.[92]

MicroRNAs as disease biomarkers and therapeutic targets

MicroRNAs have high specificity, are stable, and can be measured in many biological body fluids including plasma and CSF. However, their detection is challenging due to their small size, sequence similarity among various members, low level, and tissue- or developmental-stage-specific expression. One approach is to study the miRNA expression in serum exosomes, which are double lipid vesicles that are enriched in miRNAs and secreted by a variety of cells into peripheral body fluids. The membrane structure of exosomes protects miRNAs from degradation by RNA enzymes.

Dysregulation of miRNAs in Neurologic Disease

Several studies showed miRNA dysregulation in neurologic disease. However, the findings have been sometimes inconsistent and their clinical relevance is still to be determined. Only few examples will be briefly mentioned here. Several miRNAs increase in serum and CSF after stroke and remain elevated for several weeks to months beyond the acute recovery period. Some of the altered miRNAs, such as miR-34a, may participate in cardiovascular and endothelial function, angiogenesis, hypoxia, inflammatory/immune response, and cellular restoration. Individual miRNAs may have a beneficial or detrimental effect according to the cell of origin and their target. Many reports also showed miRNA changes in ALS; most of them show a global downregulation although some miRNAs are upregulated. Some miRNAs dysregulated in ALS are involved in neurodegeneration and apoptosis (e.g., miR-338, miR-142, miR-183), and others regulate biogenesis, degeneration, and reinnervation of striated muscle (e.g., miR-206, miR-133a, miR-133b, miR-27a). Results of miRNA analysis in muscle biopsies of ALS patients have been in general inconsistent and dependent on disease severity. MicroRNAs may also be potential epigenetic biomarkers for early detection of epilepsy and have therapeutic implications. For example, miR-324 is upregulated and inhibits expression of the potassium channel Kv4.2; inhibition of miR-324 decreased dendritic excitability and reduced susceptibility to status epilepticus in rodent models. Several miRNAs have also been found to be dysregulated in other neurologic diseases, such as AD and PD, as well neurodevelopmental disorders such as Rett syndrome and fragile X mental retardation and psychiatric disorders such as major depression.

MicroRNA-Based Therapies

MicroRNA-based therapies could be of potential value in management of selective groups of disorders. For example, studies in the superoxide dismutase 1 (SOD1) mouse model showed that intraventricular administration of adeno-associated virus 9, a single-stranded vector encoding an artificial miRNA against human SOD1, reduced mutant human SOD1 mRNA levels in motor neurons and exerted neuroprotective effects on spinal motor neurons. Anti-miRNA oligonucleotides provide an effective inhibition of miRNAs. Whereas the use of miRNAs as therapeutic targets is very promising, there are still limitations and challenges that require further validation in experimental models. For example, some miRNAs may have multiple targets and act differently at different disease stages and thus "off target" effects may cause unanticipated adverse results. Improved methods of drug delivery to the CNS may also be required to overcome the blood-brain barrier.

Key points

- The steps of mRNA metabolism include transcription of DNA into a pre-mRNA, maturation of mRNA, nucleocytoplasmic export, silencing and transport to specific cellular locations, local mRNA translation into proteins, and mRNA degradation.
- All these are regulated by mRNA-binding proteins and noncoding mRNAs.
- mRNA-binding proteins form complexes with mRNAs, forming messenger ribonucleoprotein particles (mRNPs).
- Noncoding RNAs include short noncoding RNAs such as microRNAs (miRNAs), long noncoding RNAs, and circular RNA.
- The basic mRNA transcription machinery includes RNA polymerase II (pol II), and a basic transcription initiation complex.

- Several extracellular signals trigger changes in gene expression via induction of transcription factors. CREB is the prototypical signal-activated transcription factor; it is activated by excitatory synaptic activity, growth factors, and other signals and promotes transcription of genes encoding synaptic and neuroprotective proteins.
- Transcriptional repression mediated by REST has an important role in determining neural phenotype, both during development and in response to injury.
- Concomitantly with transcription, mRNA undergoes a maturation process that includes addition of a 5' cap, polyadenylation, and splicing.
- Some mRNA-binding proteins, such as TDP-43 and FUS, affect multiple steps of mRNA metabolism.
- Splicing is a highly regulated process that occurs in the spliceosome, assembly of this multiprotein complex depends on survival of motor neuron (SMN) protein.
- Alternative splicing generates functionally different proteins from a single mRNA transcript; this process is regulated by proteins that may be a target of antibodies in paraneoplastic disorders.
- There is a bidirectional nucleocytoplasmic transport of RNAs and proteins across the nuclear envelope; this involves cargo proteins (importins or exportins) that interact with nuclear pore complex proteins called nucleoporins.
- mRNAs are targeted to specific compartments in axons or dendrites in transport mRNP granules together with mRNA-binding protein such as FMRP, ataxin-2 and Staufen, which prevent mRNA translation until its arrival to the destination for local translation.
- Local mRNA translation in axons is critical for axonal development and response to injury; local translation at dendrites is critical for synaptic plasticity.
- Initiation of mRNA translation requires the formation a pre-initiation complex that is recruited to the m^7G cap at the 5'end of the mRNA.
- In the setting of cellular stress, such as accumulation of misfolded proteins in the endoplasmic reticulum, there is inhibition of translation.
- Growth factors promote translation via activation of mammalian (mechanistic) target of rapamycin complex 1.
- MicroRNAs form a silencing complex that binds to the complementary site in the 3'UTR of the target mRNA; this leads to mRNA cleavage or degradation.
- MicroRNAs regulate multiple cellular functions and can be secreted via exosomes and detected in serum and CSF.
- Disorders affecting ribostasis are associated with accumulation of stress granules containing mRNA-binding proteins such as TDP-43, FUS, and ataxin-2.
- Impaired nucleocytoplasmic transport is as a major disease mechanism in neurodegenerative disorders.
- Expanded nucleotide repeats may produce toxicity through protein loss-of-function, RNA gain-of-function, protein gain-of-function, and repeat-associated non-AUG translation.
- Antisense oligonucleotides are FDA-approved for treatment of Duchenne muscular dystrophy, infantile forms of SMA, and hereditary amyloid neuropathy associated with transthyretin (*TTR*) gene mutations.

REFERENCES

1. Nogales E, Louder RK, He Y. Structural insights into the eukaryotic transcription initiation machinery. Annu Rev Biophys 2017;46:59–83.
2. Hantsche M, Cramer P. Conserved RNA polymerase II initiation complex structure. Curr Opin Struct Biol 2017;47:17–22.
3. Lin IS, Wu RM, Lee-Chen GJ, Shan DE, Gwinn-Hardy K. The SCA17 phenotype can include features of MSA-C, PSP and cognitive impairment. Parkinsonism Relat Disord 2007;13:246–249.
4. Kapeli K, Pratt GA, Vu AQ, et al. Distinct and shared functions of ALS-associated proteins TDP-43, FUS and TAF15 revealed by multisystem analyses. Nat Commun 2016;7:12143.
5. Day JJ, Sweatt JD. Epigenetic mechanisms in cognition. Neuron 2011;70:813–829.
6. Salta E, De Strooper B. Noncoding RNAs in neurodegeneration. Nat Rev Neurosci 2017;18:627–640.
7. Morris KV, Mattick JS. The rise of regulatory RNA. Nat Rev Genet 2014;15:423–437.
8. Briggs JA, Wolvetang EJ, Mattick JS, Rinn JL, Barry G. Mechanisms of long non-coding RNAs in mammalian nervous system development, plasticity, disease, and evolution. Neuron 2015;88:861–877.
9. Qu S, Yang X, Li X, et al. Circular RNA: a new star of non-coding RNAs. Cancer Lett 2015;365:141–148.
10. Greer PL, Greenberg ME. From synapse to nucleus: calcium-dependent gene transcription in the control of synapse development and function. Neuron 2008;59:846–860.
11. Korzus E. Rubinstein-Taybi syndrome and epigenetic alterations. Adv Exp Med Biol 2017;978:39–62.
12. Hwang JY, Zukin RS. REST, a master transcriptional regulator in neurodegenerative disease. Curr Opin Neurobiol 2018;48:193–200.
13. Achsel T, Bagni C. Cooperativity in RNA-protein interactions: the complex is more than the sum of its partners. Curr Opin Neurobiol 2016;39:146–151.
14. Harvey R, Dezi V, Pizzinga M, Willis AE. Post-transcriptional control of gene expression following stress: the role of RNA-binding proteins. Biochem Soc Trans 2017;45:1007–1014.
15. Lenzken SC, Achsel T, Carri MT, Barabino SM. Neuronal RNA-binding proteins in health and disease. Wiley Interdiscip Rev RNA 2014;5:565–576.
16. Purice MD, Taylor JP. Linking hnRNP function to ALS and FTD pathology. Front Neurosci 2018;12:326.

17. Hofmann JW, Seeley WW, Huang EJ. RNA binding proteins and the pathogenesis of frontotemporal lobar degeneration. Annu Rev Pathol 2019;14:469–495.
18. Butti Z, Patten SA. RNA dysregulation in amyotrophic lateral sclerosis. Front Genet 2018;9:712.
19. Davis JK, Broadie K. Multifarious functions of the fragile X mental retardation protein. Trends Genet 2017;33:703–714.
20. Ostrowski LA, Hall AC, Mekhail K. Ataxin-2: from RNA control to human health and disease. Genes (Basel) 2017;8:157–172.
21. Doyle M, Kiebler MA. Mechanisms of dendritic mRNA transport and its role in synaptic tagging. EMBO J 2011;30:3540–3552.
22. Cieply B, Carstens RP. Functional roles of alternative splicing factors in human disease. Wiley Interdiscip Rev RNA 2015;6:311–326.
23. Donlin-Asp PG, Fallini C, Campos J, et al. The survival of motor neuron protein acts as a molecular chaperone for mRNP assembly. Cell Rep 2017;18:1660–1673.
24. Ahmad S, Bhatia K, Kannan A, Gangwani L. Molecular mechanisms of neurodegeneration in spinal muscular atrophy. J Exp Neurosci 2016;10:39–49.
25. Beattie CE, Kolb SJ. Spinal muscular atrophy: selective motor neuron loss and global defect in the assembly of ribonucleoproteins. Brain Res 2018;1693:92–97.
26. Sebbag-Sznajder N, Raitskin O, Angenitzki M, Sato TA, Sperling J, Sperling R. Regulation of alternative splicing within the supraspliceosome. J Struct Biol 2012;177:152–159.
27. Saito Y, Yuan Y, Zucker-Scharff I, et al. Differential NOVA2-mediated splicing in excitatory and inhibitory neurons regulates cortical development and cerebellar function. Neuron 2019;101:707–720 e705.
28. Ogawa Y, Kakumoto K, Yoshida T, et al. Elavl3 is essential for the maintenance of Purkinje neuron axons. Sci Rep 2018;8:2722.
29. Darnell RB. RNA regulation in neurologic disease and cancer. Cancer Res Treat 2010;42:125–129.
30. Charizanis K, Lee KY, Batra R, et al. Muscleblind-like 2-mediated alternative splicing in the developing brain and dysregulation in myotonic dystrophy. Neuron 2012;75:437–450.
31. Wang ET, Taliaferro JM, Lee JA, et al. Dysregulation of mRNA localization and translation in genetic disease. J Neurosci 2016;36:11418–11426.
32. Hale MA, Johnson NE, Berglund JA. Repeat-associated RNA structure and aberrant splicing. Biochim Biophys Acta Gene Regul Mech 2019;1862:194405.
33. Lopez Castel A, Overby SJ, Artero R. MicroRNA-based therapeutic perspectives in myotonic dystrophy. Int J Mol Sci 2019;20.
34. Casci I, Krishnamurthy K, Kour S, et al. Muscleblind acts as a modifier of FUS toxicity by modulating stress granule dynamics and SMN localization. Nat Commun 2019;10:5583.
35. Raices M, D'Angelo MA. Nuclear pore complexes and regulation of gene expression. Curr Opin Cell Biol 2017;46:26–32.
36. Burns LT, Wente SR. From hypothesis to mechanism: uncovering nuclear pore complex links to gene expression. Mol Cell Biol 2014;34:2114–2120.
37. Wente SR, Rout MP. The nuclear pore complex and nuclear transport. Cold Spring Harb Perspect Biol 2010;2:a000562.
38. Twyffels L, Gueydan C, Kruys V. Transportin-1 and Transportin-2: protein nuclear import and beyond. FEBS Lett 2014;588:1857–1868.
39. Williams T, Ngo LH, Wickramasinghe VO. Nuclear export of RNA: Different sizes, shapes and functions. Semin Cell Dev Biol 2018;75:70–77.
40. Lin DH, Correia AR, Cai SW, Huber FM, Jette CA, Hoelz A. Structural and functional analysis of mRNA export regulation by the nuclear pore complex. Nat Commun 2018;9:2319.
41. Nousiainen HO, Kestila M, Pakkasjarvi N, et al. Mutations in mRNA export mediator GLE1 result in a fetal motoneuron disease. Nat Genet 2008;40:155–157.
42. Kaneb HM, Folkmann AW, Belzil VV, et al. Deleterious mutations in the essential mRNA metabolism factor, hGle1, in amyotrophic lateral sclerosis. Hum Mol Genet 2015;24:1363–1373.
43. Thomas MG, Pascual ML, Maschi D, Luchelli L, Boccaccio GL. Synaptic control of local translation: the plot thickens with new characters. Cell Mol Life Sci 2014;71:2219–2239.
44. Kar AN, Lee SJ, Twiss JL. Expanding axonal transcriptome brings new functions for axonally synthesized proteins in health and disease. Neuroscientist 2018;24:111–129.
45. Khalil B, Morderer D, Price PL, Liu F, Rossoll W. mRNP assembly, axonal transport, and local translation in neurodegenerative diseases. Brain Res 2018;1693:75–91.
46. Costa JC, Willis DE, DE Costa CJ, et al. To the end of the line: Axonal mRNA transport and local translation in health and neurodegenerative disease. Dev Neurobiol 2018 Mar;78:209–220.
47. Spaulding EL, Burgess RW. Accumulating evidence for axonal translation in neuronal homeostasis. Front Neurosci 2017;11:312.
48. Thelen MP, Kye MJ. The role of RNA binding proteins for local mRNA translation: implications in neurological disorders. Front Mol Biosci 2019;6:161.
49. Wortham NC, Proud CG. eIF2B: recent structural and functional insights into a key regulator of translation. Biochem Soc Trans 2015;43:1234–1240.
50. Kearse MG, Wilusz JE. Non-AUG translation: a new start for protein synthesis in eukaryotes. Genes Dev 2017;31:1717–1731.
51. Hughes D, Mallucci GR. The unfolded protein response in neurodegenerative disorders—therapeutic modulation of the PERK pathway. FEBS J 2019;286:342–355.
52. Moon SL, Parker R. EIF2B2 mutations in vanishing white matter disease hypersuppress translation and delay recovery during the integrated stress response. RNA 2018;24:841–852.
53. Heraud-Farlow JE, Sharangdhar T, Li X, et al. Staufen2 regulates neuronal target RNAs. Cell Rep 2013;5:1511–1518.
54. Goetz AE, Wilkinson M. Stress and the nonsense-mediated RNA decay pathway. Cell Mol Life Sci 2017;19:3509–3531.
55. Im HI, Kenny PJ. MicroRNAs in neuronal function and dysfunction. Trends Neurosci 2012;35:325–334.
56. McNeill E, Van Vactor D. MicroRNAs shape the neuronal landscape. Neuron 2012;75:363–379.
57. Akhter R. Circular RNA and Alzheimer's disease. Adv Exp Med Biol 2018;1087:239–243.
58. Ramaswami M, Taylor JP, Parker R. Altered ribostasis: RNA-protein granules in degenerative disorders. Cell 2013;154:727–736.

59. Maziuk B, Ballance HI, Wolozin B. Dysregulation of RNA binding protein aggregation in neurodegenerative disorders. Front Mol Neurosci 2017;10:89.
60. Nussbacher JK, Batra R, Lagier-Tourenne C, Yeo GW. RNA-binding proteins in neurodegeneration: Seq and you shall receive. Trends Neurosci 2015;38:226–236.
61. Harrison AF, Shorter J. RNA-binding proteins with prion-like domains in health and disease. Biochem J 2017;474:1417–1438.
62. Sheinberger J, Shav-Tal Y. mRNPs meet stress granules. FEBS Lett 2017;591:2534–2542.
63. Ling SC, Polymenidou M, Cleveland DW. Converging mechanisms in ALS and FTD: disrupted RNA and protein homeostasis. Neuron 2013;79:416–438.
64. Boehringer A, Bowser R. RNA nucleocytoplasmic transport defects in neurodegenerative diseases. Adv Neurobiol 2018;20:85–101.
65. Kim HJ, Taylor JP. Lost in transportation: nucleocytoplasmic transport defects in ALS and other neurodegenerative diseases. Neuron 2017;96:285–297.
66. Fahrenkrog B, Harel A. Perturbations in traffic: aberrant nucleocytoplasmic transport at the heart of neurodegeneration. Cells 2018;7:232–242.
67. Cornett J, Cao F, Wang CE, et al. Polyglutamine expansion of huntingtin impairs its nuclear export. Nat Genet 2005;37:198–204.
68. Gasset-Rosa F, Chillon-Marinas C, Goginashvili A, et al. Polyglutamine-expanded huntingtin exacerbates age-related disruption of nuclear integrity and nucleocytoplasmic transport. Neuron 2017;94:48–57 e44.
69. Grima JC, Daigle JG, Arbez N, et al. Mutant huntingtin disrupts the nuclear pore complex. Neuron 2017;94:93–107 e106.
70. Dormann D, Rodde R, Edbauer D, et al. ALS-associated fused in sarcoma (FUS) mutations disrupt transportin-mediated nuclear import. EMBO J 2010;29:2841–2857.
71. Jiang J, Zhu Q, Gendron TF, et al. Gain of toxicity from ALS/FTD-linked repeat expansions in C9ORF72 is alleviated by antisense oligonucleotides targeting GGGGCC-containing RNAs. Neuron 2016;90:535–550.
72. Freibaum BD, Taylor JP. The role of dipeptide repeats in C9ORF72-related ALS-FTD. Front Mol Neurosci 2017;10:35.
73. Cleary JD, Pattamatta A, Ranum LPW. Repeat-associated non-ATG (RAN) translation. J Biol Chem 2018;293:16127–16141.
74. Eftekharzadeh B, Daigle JG, Kapinos LE, et al. Tau protein disrupts nucleocytoplasmic transport in Alzheimer's disease. Neuron 2018;99:925–940 e927.
75. Baron O, Boudi A, Dias C, et al. Stall in canonical autophagy-lysosome pathways prompts nucleophagy-based nuclear breakdown in neurodegeneration. Curr Biol 2017;27:3626–3642 e3626.
76. Jovicic A, Mertens J, Boeynaems S, et al. Modifiers of C9orf72 dipeptide repeat toxicity connect nucleocytoplasmic transport defects to FTD/ALS. Nat Neurosci 2015;18:1226–1229.
77. Freibaum BD, Lu Y, Lopez-Gonzalez R, et al. GGGGCC repeat expansion in C9orf72 compromises nucleocytoplasmic transport. Nature 2015;525:129–133.
78. Shi KY, Mori E, Nizami ZF, et al. Toxic PRn poly-dipeptides encoded by the C9orf72 repeat expansion block nuclear import and export. Proc Natl Acad Sci U S A 2017;114:E1111–E1117.
79. Licatalosi DD, Darnell RB. Splicing regulation in neurologic disease. Neuron 2006;52:93–101.
80. Lanfranco M, Vassallo N, Cauchi RJ. Spinal muscular atrophy: from defective chaperoning of snRNP assembly to neuromuscular dysfunction. Front Mol Biosci 2017;4:41.
81. Mutreja Y, Combs B, Gamblin TC. FTDP-17 mutations alter the aggregation and microtubule stabilization propensity of tau in an isoform-specific fashion. Biochemistry 2019;58:742–754.
82. Lancaster E. Paraneoplastic disorders. Continuum (Minneap Minn) 2017;23:1653–1679.
83. Tobin WO, Pittock SJ. Autoimmune neurology of the central nervous system. Continuum (Minneap Minn) 2017;23:627–653.
84. Levin AA. Treating disease at the RNA level with oligonucleotides. N Engl J Med 2019;380:57–70.
85. Schoch KM, Miller TM. Antisense oligonucleotides: translation from mouse models to human neurodegenerative diseases. Neuron 2017;94:1056–1070.
86. Wurster CD, Ludolph AC. Antisense oligonucleotides in neurological disorders. Ther Adv Neurol Disord 2018;11:1756286418776932.
87. Scoles DR, Minikel EV, Pulst SM. Antisense oligonucleotides: A primer. Neurol Genet 2019;5:e323.
88. Scoles DR, Pulst SM. Oligonucleotide therapeutics in neurodegenerative diseases. RNA Biol 2018;15:707–714.
89. Neil EE, Bisaccia EK. Nusinersen: a novel antisense oligonucleotide for the treatment of spinal muscular atrophy. J Pediatr Pharmacol Ther 2019;24:194–203.
90. Benson MD, Dasgupta NR, Monia BP. Inotersen (transthyretin-specific antisense oligonucleotide) for treatment of transthyretin amyloidosis. Neurodegener Dis Manag 2019;9:25–30.
91. Hoy SM. Patisiran: first global approval. Drugs 2018;78:1625–1631.
92. Imbert M, Blandel F, Leumann C, Garcia L, Goyenvalle A. Lowering mutant huntingtin using tricyclo-DNA antisense oligonucleotides as a therapeutic approach for Huntington's disease. Nucleic Acid Ther 2019;29:256–265.

6 Proteostasis

OVERVIEW

The three-dimensional conformation of proteins is required for their proper function. Newly synthesized proteins undergo maturation in the endoplasmic reticulum (ER). Chaperones linked to protein synthesis in the ER stabilize and correctly fold newly formed proteins, whereas heat shock proteins (Hsps) in both the ER and cytoplasm recognize and bind immature or misfolded proteins until their maturation or refolding. If these protective mechanisms fail or become overwhelmed, the cell utilizes different interactive defense systems to prevent accumulation and aggregation of abnormal proteins. They include the ER-associated degradation (ERAD), the unfolded protein response (UPR), degradation via the ubiquitin-proteasome system (UPS), and the autophagy-lysosomal system. Overall, the control of protein maturation and clearance is referred to as proteostasis. As a consequence of mutations or environmental disturbances such as oxidative stress or posttranslational modifications, proteins undergo conformational changes that promote their misfolding. Impaired quality control and clearance by the UPS and the autophagy-lysosome system leads to accumulation of misfolded proteins and their incorporation into fibrillary β-sheet-rich structures referred to as "amyloids." Impaired proteostasis is a major disease mechanism in large group of neurodegenerative disorders, currently known as protein aggregation disorders. They include Alzheimer disease (AD), primary tauopathies, Parkinson disease (PD), and other synucleinopathies, Huntington disease (HD), amyotrophic lateral sclerosis (ALS), frontotemporal lobar degeneration (FTLD), prion disorders, and some forms of hereditary spastic paraplegia, Charcot-Marie-Tooth disease, motor neuronopathies, and myopathies. These disorders are associated with accumulation of characteristic fibrillary inclusions and autophagic vesicles. Toxic gain-of-function of the intermediate fibril monomers or oligomers promotes the formation of aggregates and initiates a cascade of protein–protein interactions resulting in neuronal dysfunction and death. These aggregates serve as templates or seeds to elicit aggregation of their respective normal endogenous partners in neighboring cells. Given the fundamental role of impaired proteostasis in neurodegeneration, there is intense basic and clinical research aimed to identify therapeutic approaches to improve proteostasis for neuroprotection. They include prevention of protein misfolding, upregulation of Hsps, increased autophagy, and modulation of the UPR, particularly PERK signaling. Many of these compounds are undergoing clinical trials. The aims of this chapter are to review: (1) the basic mechanisms of protein maturation in the ER, (2) the major mediators involved in the ERAD and UPR, (3) the heat shock response, (4) the ubiquitin proteasome systems, (5) mechanisms of autophagy, (6) the main pathophysiological consequences of protein misfolding in neurodegenerative disorders, and (7) representative examples of genetic disorders affecting protein quality control and clearance. Disorders of the autophagy and lysosome systems are discussed in the next chapter of this book.

PROTEIN MATURATION AND QUALITY CONTROL IN THE ENDOPLASMIC RETICULUM

Approximately one-third of all proteins are targeted to the secretory pathway, which includes the ER, Golgi apparatus, and secretory vesicles. The major role of the ER as the first compartment of this pathway is the synthesis and subsequent maturation of membrane and secreted proteins. Newly synthesized proteins entering the secretory pathway are first translocated across the ER membrane in an unfolded form. Protein folding in the ER begins cotranslationally and involves interactions with ER chaperones, N-glycosylation, and formation of disulfide bonds[1] (Figure 6.1). After maturation, proteins are transferred from the ER to the different components of the Golgi complex, where they are further

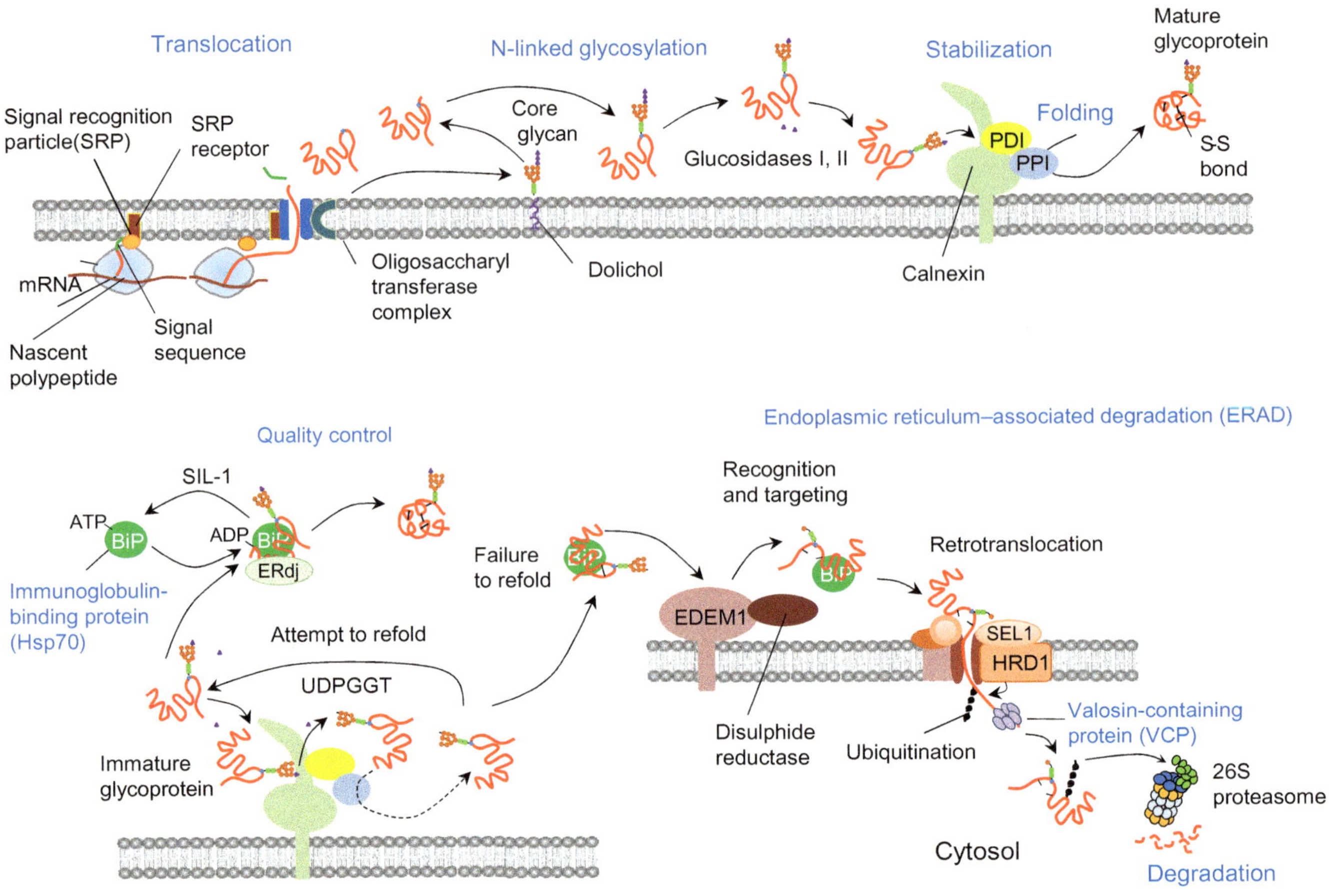

FIGURE 6.1 Protein maturation and quality control, and endoplasmic reticulum–associated degradation. Ribosomes containing mRNAs encoding secretory and integral membrane proteins are recruited to the ER via a signal sequence in the nascent polypeptide; this leads to recognition and binding by the signal recognition particle (SRP), and the complex is targeted to the ER, where it binds a SRP receptor and the signal sequence is then removed. Secretory proteins are modified by N-glycosylation. This process begins begins with a 14-sugar precursor containing two N-acetylglucosamide, nine mannose, and three glucose units assembled into the lipid carrier dolichol; the entire preassembled glycan is then transferred to the asparagine residue of nascent proteins by the oligosaccharyl transferase complexes. After removal of 2 glucose residues by glucosidases I and II, the glycopolypeptide chain binds to calnexin or calreticulin. Protein folding in the ER involves disulfide bonds protein via disulfide isomerases (PDIs) and proline isomerization via prolylpeptidyl *cis-trans* isomerases (PPIs). The ER chaperone immunoglobulin-binding protein (BiP), in its ADP-bound state binds the immature protein; the exchange of ADP for ATP releases the substrate; this involves the nucleotide exchange factor SIL1. The ER J-domain proteins (ERdjs) stimulate the ATPase activity of heat shock protein 70 (Hsp70). If the immature protein conformation persists the quality control sensor uridine diphosphate (UDP)-glucose: glycoprotein glucosyltransferase (UDPGGT) transfers glucose back to the unglucosylated protein to continue the attempts to fold properly. Glycoproteins that are unable to fold are diverted for endoplasmic reticulum–associated degradation (ERAD) by action of mannosidases, such as the ER degradation-enhancing α-mannosidase-like protein 1 (EDEM1), followed by activity of disulfide reductase. BiP then recruits the terminally misfolded proteins to the dislocation channel. Translocation to the cytoplasm is tightly coupled to that of substrate degradation and involves large sets of proteins organized around HRD1, a membrane-integrated ubiquitin E3 ligase that via its obligate partner sel-1 suppressor of lin-12-like (SIL-1), coordinates substrate recognition in the ER lumen with membrane dislocation and, via its ubiquitin ligase activity, recruits valosin-containing protein (VCP), which extracts ubiquilated proteins and targets them for degradation by the proteasome.

modified and then targeted to the different cell compartments, including the plasma membrane, synaptic vesicles, and lysosomes.[1]

Translocation and N-Glycosylation of Nascent Proteins

The canonical pathway for protein synthesis requires the docking of the mRNA:ribosome complex on the ER membrane during translation. Translation of secretory and integral membrane proteins starts in the cytosol; ribosomes are then recruited to the ER via a signal sequence of approximately the first 25 amino acids of the nascent polypeptide. The polypeptide is then recognized and bound by the signal recognition particle (SRP), which binds to a SRP receptor in the ER. Signal sequences help targeting and orienting the peptide during translocation across the lipid bilayer of the ER translocation pore, or translocon. The domain facing the ER lumen is recognized and cleaved by the signal peptidase complex that cleaves the short signal peptide, allowing the free protein to enter the ER. Proteins destined to be transmembrane (integral) proteins, such as ion channels and receptors, contain a stretch of hydrophobic residues, known as stop-transfer membrane anchor sequences, that pause the translocation and anchor the protein to the phospholipid bilayers. Proteins not destined to be integrated into the membrane enter the secretory pathway in the lumen of organelles.

Most proteins that traverse the secretory pathway, as well as intraluminal residues of transmembrane proteins, are modified by N-glycosylation.[2] N-glycans promote protein folding, stability, dimerization, trafficking, and localization. The formation of the core glycan is the product of a biosynthetic pathway that involves the sequential activity of different glycosyl transferases. These enzymes participate in the stepwise synthesis of a branched oligosaccharide containing two N-acetylglucosamine, nine mannose, and three glucose units assembled on the membrane lipid carrier dolichol. The entire preassembled glycan is then transferred from dolichol to the asparagine residue of nascent proteins by the multisubunit oligosaccharyl transferase, aided by associated complexes such as the translocon complex. Disorders affecting N-glycosylation manifest with a wide spectrum of neurologic manifestation, typically associated with abnormalities in multiple organ systems.[2]

Molecular Chaperones in the Endoplasmic Reticulum

Maturing nascent polypeptide chains are vulnerable to misfolding and aggregation, given their high concentration within the ER lumen. Molecular chaperones promote the efficient folding and prevent aggregation of immature proteins. There are two major chaperone systems in the ER, the classical chaperones and the carbohydrate-binding chaperone system. The classical chaperones are Hsps, which bind directly to the polypeptide chain, recognize exposed hydrophobic segments of immature or aberrant proteins, and are recruited to assist protein maturation. The master regulator of ER proteostasis is the Hsp70 chaperone immunoglobulin-binding protein (BiP), also known as glucose-regulated protein of 78 kDa (GRP78). As described below, Hsp70 chaperones are ATPases that in the ADP-bound state have high affinity for binding to the immature protein preventing them from premature folding; the exchange of ADP for ATP releases the substrate, which is then free to fold. The Hsp40 co-chaperone ER J-domain protein accelerates the ATPase activity of BiP, whereas the nucleotide exchange factor SIL1 assists the transition between the ADP-bound and ATP-bound state of BiP. Loss-of-function mutations of the *SIL1* gene encoding SIL1 are linked to Marinesco-Sjögren syndrome.[3] The second group of ER chaperones includes carbohydrate-binding lectin chaperones such as calnexin and calreticulin, which promote the efficient folding of glycoproteins by stabilizing folding events, preventing aggregation, and facilitating the formation of disulfide bonds.

Protein Folding in the Endoplasmic Reticulum

Secretory proteins have disulfide bonds and the majority also have proline residues close to these bonds in the primary sequence. Protein folding in the ER involves two processes, formation of disulfide bonds between cysteine residues and isomerization of proline residues. The first reaction involves protein disulfide isomerase (PDI) and endoplasmic reticulum protein 75 (ERp75).[4] Missense and intronic variants of PDI and ERp57 were associated with ALS.[5,6] The second protein-folding process involves prolylpeptidyl *cis-trans* isomerases (PPIs), including cyclophilins. These proteins may also have a role in neurodegeneration and neuroprotection.[7] Properly folded, proteins may stay in the ER and function locally or leave the ER to enter either the Golgi complex to be sorted to the plasma membrane, secretory vesicles, endosomes, or lysosomes or to the peroxisome.

Quality Control and Endoplasmic Reticulum–Associated Degradation

If the unfolded conformation of the protein persists after a single round of lectin chaperone binding, the quality control sensor uridine diphosphate (UDP)-glucose:glycoprotein glucosyltransferase transfers glucose back to the unglucosylated protein to reconstitute the glycan that can again associate to the lectin chaperone to continue the attempts to fold properly.[8] Glycoproteins that are unable to fold escape the otherwise futile calnexin/calreticulin cycle, are diverted for ERAD and ultimately degraded by the UPS[9,10] (Figure 6.1). The ERAD is a multistep process that includes substrate recognition and targeting, transfer or dislocation (retrotranslocation) of misfolded proteins across the lipid bilayer from the ER to the cytoplasm, addition of polyubiquitin adducts (ubiquitylation), and degradation by the proteasome. The substrates for the ERAD system include proteins that have not achieved a native mature structure because of mutation or translational dysfunction, or have failed to assemble into protein complexes. Misfolded glycoproteins are diverted for ERAD by action of mannosidases; this is followed by activity of a disulfide reductase that breaks the disulfide bonds of the immature protein. BiP then recruits the terminally misfolded nonglycosylated proteins to the dislocation channel. The process of substrate translocation from the ER to the cytoplasm (dislocation or retrotranslocation) is tightly coupled to that of substrate degradation. A large set of proteins is organized around a membrane-integrated ubiquitin E3 ligase, forming a hub that coordinates substrate recognition in the ER lumen with membrane dislocation and protein ubiquitylation.[11] This ubiquitin E3 ligase recruits valosin-containing protein (VCP) a cytoplasmic protein that is a member of the ATPase associated with multiple cellular activities (AAA-ATPase). VCP binds to ubiquitylated proteins, extracts them from across ER pores, and delivers them for degradation by 26S proteasomes in the cytoplasm. Of note, VCP couples ATP hydrolysis to segregation of polypeptides from other membranes, ribosomes, chromatin, and protein assemblies such as stress granules.[12,13] Mutations affecting VCP cause a large number of neurodegenerative disorders, including multisystem proteinopathy 1 and familial forms of ALS and FTLD, as discussed later in this chapter.[12] The ERAD system includes several membrane proteins relevant in neurodegenerative disorders, including erlin2; *ERLIN2* mutations are linked to hereditary spastic paraplegia (SPG18).[14] Membralin, a protein that interacts with erlin, interacts with gamma secretase and may protect against β-amyloid pathology.[13]

UNFOLDED PROTEIN RESPONSE (ENDOPLASMIC RETICULUM STRESS RESPONSE)

The UPR is a canonical protective mechanism to restore proteostasis in response to increased load of misfolded proteins in the ER or other forms of ER stress, such as those induced by hypoxia, disruption of Ca^{2+} homeostasis, and nutrient deprivation.[15–19] The UPR includes a translational and a transcriptional component (Figure 6.2). The translational component leads to the transient suppression of translation of most mRNAs into proteins. The transcriptional UPR consists of an initial neuroprotective phase involving activation of genes that promote protein folding and antioxidant responses; this may be followed by a secondary phase characterized by activation of genes that lead to apoptosis. The UPR is orchestrated by three transmembrane ER proteins: protein kinase RNA-like ER kinase (PERK), inositol-requiring protein 1α (IRE1α), and activating transcription factor 6 (ATF6). In normal conditions these proteins are maintained in an inactive state through their association with BiP; upon accumulation of misfolded proteins they dissociate from BIP, undergo activation via dimerization and autophosphorylation, and translocate to the cytoplasm.

Translational Unfolded Protein Response

Activated PERK inhibits translation of most proteins by phosphorylating the α subunit of eukaryote initiation factor 2 (eIF2α); this prevents the formation of the ternary complex required for initiation of cap-dependent AUG translation. By reducing global protein synthesis, PERK decreases the load of total proteins entering the ER, thus alleviating the protein burden to this organelle. PERK can also activate transcription of either neuroprotective or proapoptotic genes according to the cell context. For example, phosphorylated eIF2α activates the translation of mRNA-encoding activating transcription factor 4 (ATF4). This transcription factor upregulates expression of ER chaperones and proteins involved in redox control and amino acid metabolism. ATF4 also upregulates growth arrest and DNA damage-induced protein 34 (GADD34), which promotes dephosphorylation of eIF2α, thus providing a negative feedback on PERK signaling and allowing reinitiation of protein synthesis.

Transcriptional Unfolded Protein Response

The second component of the UPR is transcriptional activation, triggered by PERK (via ATF4), IRE1α, and ATF6. Whereas the initial effect of ATF4 is to promote transcription of neuroprotective genes, ATF4 upregulates transcription of propapoptotic genes if the ER stress is not resolved. One such effector is C/EBP homologous protein (CHOP), which initiates apoptotic signaling and promotes oxidative stress. IRE1α has both an RNAse and a kinase activity and can trigger neuroprotective or apoptotic pathways according to the cellular context. Upon activation, the RNAse domain of IRE1α cleaves the mRNA encoding X-box-binding protein 1 (XPB1), generating a spliced form that is a potent neuroprotective transcription factor. In addition, IRE1α targets a group of mRNAs and microRNAs for degradation via a process of regulated IRE1α-dependent decay; this alters expression of multiple proteins that participate in inflammation and apoptosis. The kinase activity of IRE1α allows its interaction with adaptor proteins that mediate crosstalk with other cellular stress pathways. The third effector of the UPR is ATF 6, which upon activation exits the ER and enters the Golgi apparatus, where it is undergoes sequential proteolysis to generate an active fragment that is translocated to the nucleus and induces expression of XPB1 and other neuroprotective genes involved in protein folding and ERAD. There is a functional crosstalk between the UPR and ERAD in response to accumulation of misfolded proteins.[9] These interactions have a major role in mechanisms of neurodegeneration.[19]

Sigma-1 Receptor and Endoplasmic Reticulum Stress Response

The sigma-1 receptor (Sig-1R) is an ER protein located at the interface between the ER and mitochondria and participates in the ER stress responses.[20] Sig-1R binds BiP, stabilizes IRE1α, and functions as a molecular chaperone that ensures proper Ca^{2+} transfer from the ER to the mitochondria, which is critical for normal mitochondrial function. Expression of the *SIGMAR1* gene is upregulated during ER stress. Activation of Sig-1R by reactive oxygen species derived from the mitochondria promotes the interaction between Sig-1R and IRE1α, which assures proper mitochondria-ER-nucleus signaling that promote neuroprotection. *SIGMAR1* mutations are linked to familial forms of ALS, with or without associated FTLD.[21]

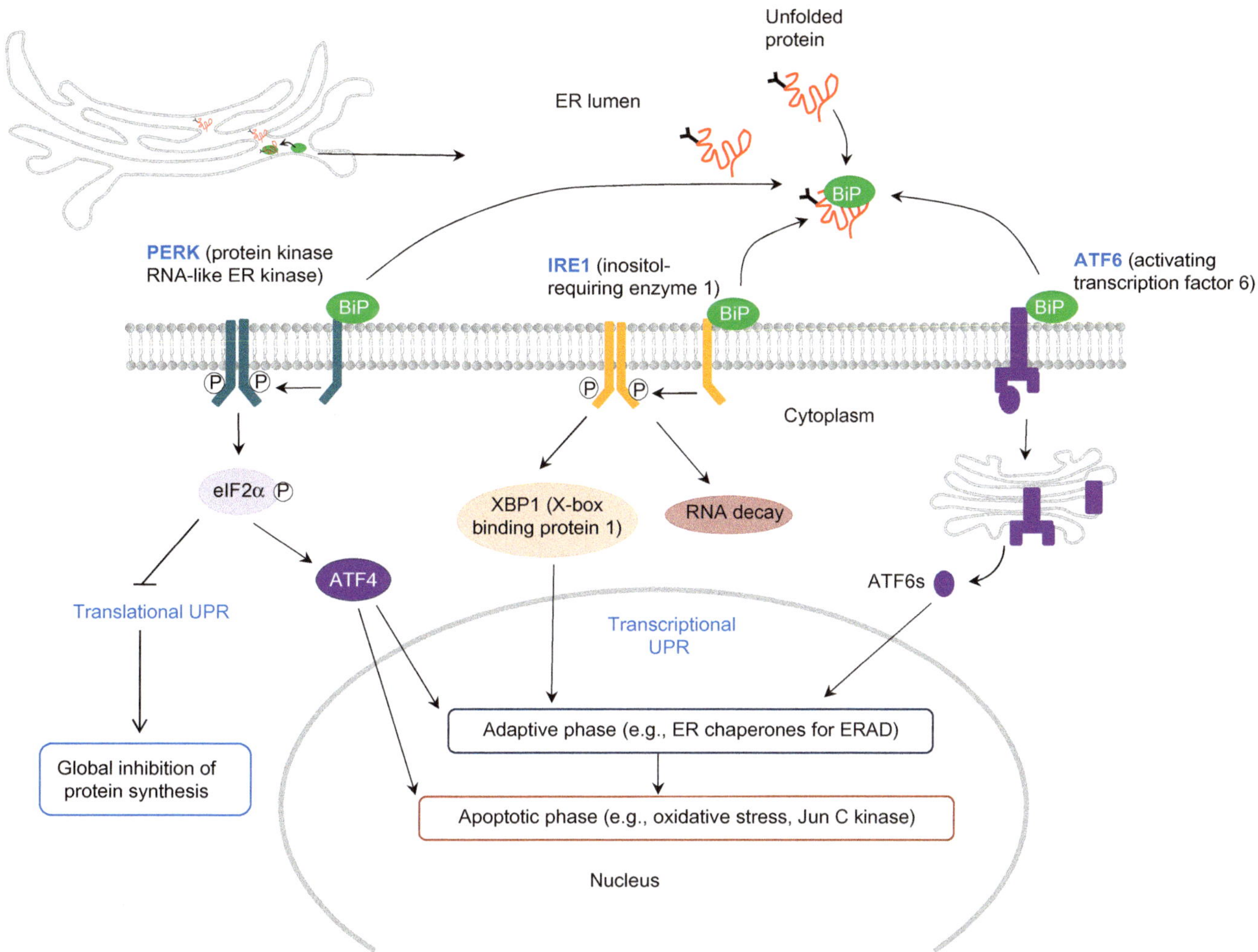

FIGURE 6.2 Unfolded protein response.

The unfolded protein response (UPR) includes a translational and a transcriptional component. The UPR is orchestrated by protein kinase RNA-like ER kinase (PERK), inositol-requiring protein 1α (IRE1α), and activating transcription factor 6 (ATF6), which in normal conditions are maintained inactive through their association with the immunoglobulin-binding protein (BiP) and dissociate from BiP upon accumulation of misfolded proteins. PERK inhibits translation by phosphorylating the α subunit of eukaryote initiation factor 2α (eIF2α). Phosphorylated eIF2α activates the translation of mRNA-encoding activating transcription factor 4 (ATF4). ATF4 upregulates the transcription of chaperones and other neuroprotective proteins, but if the ER stress is not resolved, ATF4 upregulates the pro-apoptotic transcription factors. The RNAse domain of IRE1α cleaves the mRNA encoding X-box-binding protein 1 (XPB1), generating a spliced form (XPB1s) that activates transcription of genes that promote ER biogenesis and endoplasmic reticulum–associated degradation (ERAD) responses. IRE1α also targets mRNAs and microRNAs for degradation via a process of regulated IRE1α-dependent decay. Upon activation ATF 6 exits the ER and enters the Golgi apparatus, where it is undergoes sequential proteolysis to generate an active fragment that is then translocated to the nucleus and exerts neuroprotective effects.

HEAT SHOCK PROTEINS

Heat shock proteins (Hsps) constitute a heterogeneous group of highly conserved molecular chaperones that are present in all cell compartments and provide the first line of defense against accumulation of misfolded, aggregation-prone proteins.[22,23] Heat shock proteins bind unfolded or misfolded proteins, interact with other mechanisms of proteostasis, and protect intracellular membranes, organelles, cytoskeleton, and nuclear proteins during stress conditions. Heat shock proteins are classified into several families based on their encoding genes and molecular weights. Important examples are Hsp90 (*HSPC* gene), Hsp70 (*HSPA* genes), Hsp60 (*HSPD* gene), Hsp40 (*DNAJ* genes), small Hsps such as Hsp22 and Hsp27 (*HSPB* genes), and Hsp11 (*HSPH* gene). Whereas some Hsps are constitutively expressed, most are rapidly induced in response to cellular stress resulting in the accumulation of denatured proteins. Accumulation of unfolded proteins triggers the heat shock response, which results in activation of *HSP* gene expression via the transcriptional activator heat shock factor-1 (HSF-1) (Figure 6.3). In the absence of cell stress, HSF-1 is constitutively expressed in the cytoplasm, where it is maintained in an inactive, monomeric state by association with Hsp90 and other Hsps. During cell stress, accumulated unfolded proteins compete with HSF-1 for binding to Hsps; ultimately HSF-1 is released, undergoes posttranslational modifications and trimerization, and translocates to the nucleus. In the nucleus, HSF-1 binds to heat-shock-element in the promoter region of several stress-inducible genes driving Hsp expression.

Chaperone Function of Heat Shock Proteins

Heat shock proteins can assist the refolding of misfolded proteins through three distinct ATP dependent actions: they can hold the clients in an unfolded state until they spontaneously achieve folding; unfold misfolded proteins and convert them into a native state; or function as "disaggregases" that forcefully unfold and solubilize preformed aggregates into natively refolded proteins. Hsp70 proteins are one of the most abundant chaperones; they are located in different cell compartments and participate in a broad range of activities. They include the Hsp70-homologous BiP, which is the major chaperone in the ER and cytosolic heat shock cognate 70 (Hsc70), which is involved in chaperone-mediated autophagy. Hsp70 proteins undergo an ATP-dependent

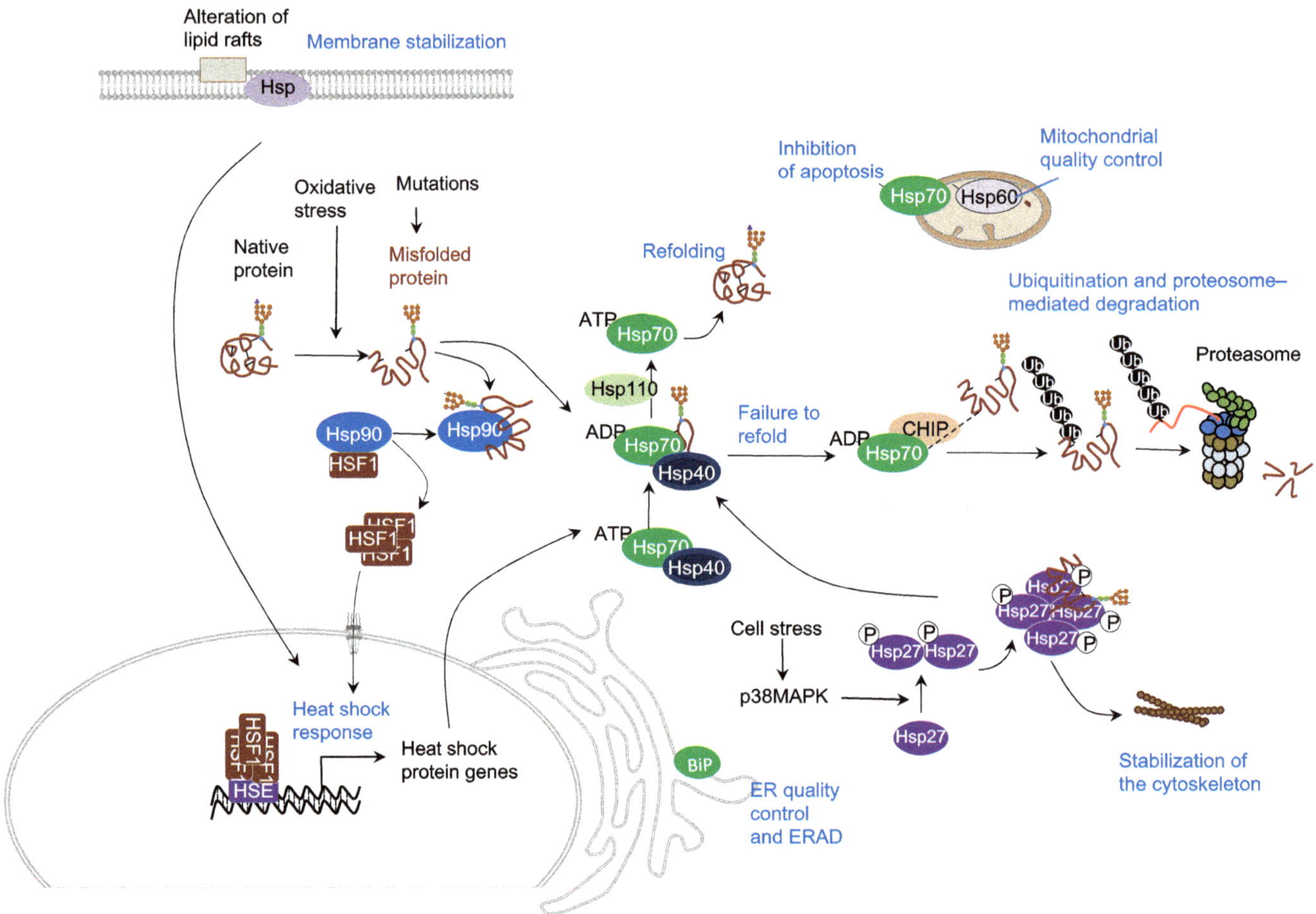

FIGURE 6.3 Heat shock response.

Accumulation of unfolded proteins during cellular stress promotes the dissociation of heat shock protein 90 (Hsp90) from heat shock factor-1 (HSF-1). HSF-1 then undergoes posttranslational modifications, trimerization, and translocation to the nucleus, where it activates expression of genes coding Hsps. Hsp70 proteins strongly bind to misfolded protein substrates and promote their refolding upon hydrolysis of ATP, which is promoted by cochaperones of the Hsp40 (*DNAJ*) family. Cochaperones such as Hsp110 act as nucleotide-exchanging factors removing ADP after ATP hydrolysis by HspA chaperones. The small Hsps (HspB) assemble into large, oligomeric structures resembling a hollow ball. They bind misfolded proteins, thereby preventing the formation of insoluble aggregates while keeping them available to other Hsp complexes.

transition between open and closed conformations of their substrate-binding domain. Once ATP hydrolysis is induced by cochaperones of the Hsp40 (*DNAJ*) family, the ADP-bound Hsp70 facilitates the refolding of their client proteins. In addition, Hsp70 can also unfold stable misfolded proteins and, together with Hsp40 and Hsp110, can have a disaggregase function and solubilize preformed protein aggregates. The Hsp110 co-chaperones are ATPases that, once guided to protein aggregates by Hsp70 and Hsp40, facilitate ADP release from Hsp70, retrieve proteins from aggregates, and thread them into nascent polypeptides. If protein misfolding is not repaired, the C-terminus of Hsc70-interacting protein (CHIP) binds to Hsp70 proteins, reducing their ATPase and chaperone activity, and then targets the misfolded proteins for degradation by the proteasome.

The mitochondrial chaperone Hsp60, like cytosolic Hsp70 can unfold stable misfolded proteins. Mutations of the *HSPD1* gene encoding Hsp60 cause a rare form of autosomal dominant hereditary spastic paraparesis (SPG13).[24]

The small Hsps of the *HSPB* gene superfamily share sequence homologies and assemble into large, oligomeric structures. Unlike other chaperones, these small Hsps are ATP-independent. Three relevant examples are αB crystallin (*HSPB5*); Hsp27 (*HSPPB1*), and Hsp22 (*HSPB8*). All small Hsps contain a conserved B-crystallin domain that mediates the formation of dimers, which form the building blocks for the formation of large dynamic oligomers. The activity of small Hsps is regulated by phosphorylation, primarily via p38 mitogen-activated kinases during cell stress. Small Hsps function as holding factors, binding unfolded or misfolded proteins and preventing their aggregation until the clients are delivered to other chaperones, such as the Hsp70/Hsp40 system. Mutations of genes encoding small Hsps have been linked to different neurologic disorders. Missense mutations in the *HSPB1* gene encoding Hsp27 and the *HSPB8* gene encoding HspP22 are associated with distal hereditary motor neuropathy (distal HMN type II) and Charcot-Marie-Tooth disease type 2.[25] Mutations affecting the Hsp40 protein B-crystallin produce adult-onset, desmin-related myofibrillar myopathy.[26]

The Hsp90 proteins are ATP-dependent chaperones that account for 1%–2% of cellular proteins and are present in various cellular compartments, including the cytosol, ER, mitochondria, and nucleus. Whereas Hsp90 proteins are constitutively expressed in normal conditions, their level increases during cell stress. These proteins bind a variety of clients such as protein kinases, nuclear receptors such as steroid receptors, transcription factors, and cell surface receptors. Since Hsp90 proteins stabilize unfolded proteins and inhibit their ubiquitylation, they can also favor the accumulation of toxic protein aggregates.

Other Neuroprotective Effects of Heat Shock Proteins

Several Hsps exert additional neuroprotective effects by acting as membrane stress sensors, promoting membrane stability, inhibiting apoptosis, and stabilizing the cytoskeleton. Stress-induced Hsp activation may occur in the absence of accumulation of misfolded proteins. One example is the Hsp response to changes in the physical properties of the membrane, such as membrane fluidity in cholesterol-rich domains (lipid drafts). Upon stress exposure, cholesteryl glycoside is rapidly formed in the membrane and induces HSF1 activation and Hsp70 production. Several Hsps also associate with the outer mitochondrial membrane and function as negative regulators of the mitochondrial pathway for apoptosis.[27] They may inhibit stress-induced signaling, reduce translocation of the proapoptotic proteins to the mitochondrial membrane, inhibit release and sequestering of cytochrome *c* in the cytosol, and arrest activation of caspases. Small Hsps may also regulate the dynamics of the structural elements of the cytoskeleton. For example, the interaction of Hsp27 with actin microfilaments prevents abnormal actin polymerization and thus disruption of the cytoskeleton upon exposure to cellular stress. Hsp90 promotes axonal regeneration by maintaining stability of signaling molecules such as protein kinases that drive axon degeneration, axon regeneration, and cell death. Hsp104 is a hexameric protein ATPase that functions as a disaggregase and has a role in the dissolution of stress granules.

UBIQUITIN-PROTEASOME SYSTEM

The UPS accounts for more than 80% of intracellular proteolysis. Ubiquitylation is a posttranslational modification that forms a bond between a lysine residue of the target protein and the carboxyl (C)-terminus of ubiquitin. Protein ubiquitylation is required both for degradation of short-lived proteins by the proteasome and for targeting substrates for autophagy. The ratio between these two degradative processes depends on amount of misfolded proteins and the physiological state of the cell.[28,29]

Ubiquitin System

The ubiquitin system includes four different classes of enzymes, E1–E4 (Figure 6.4). First, the ubiquitin-activating enzyme E1 (UBA1) hydrolyzes ATP, forming a thioester linkage with the cysteine residue of ubiquitin. The activated ubiquitin is then passed to the ubiquitin-conjugating enzyme E2; and finally E3 ubiquitin-protein ligases bind ubiquitin to the misfolded proteins. After the first ubiquitin has been attached, E3 ubiquitin ligases elongate the ubiquitin chain by creating ubiquitin–ubiquitin bonds leading to the formation of a polyubiquitylated misfolded peptide. There are hundreds of genes encoding ubiquitin E3 ligases, reflecting a high degree of specificity in target recognition. The E4 enzymes are E3-like enzymes that catalyze ubiquitin chain extension.

Several cytosolic or nuclear ubiquitin E3 ligases are involved in degradation of misfolded proteins or altered organelles in collaboration with molecule chaperones. One example

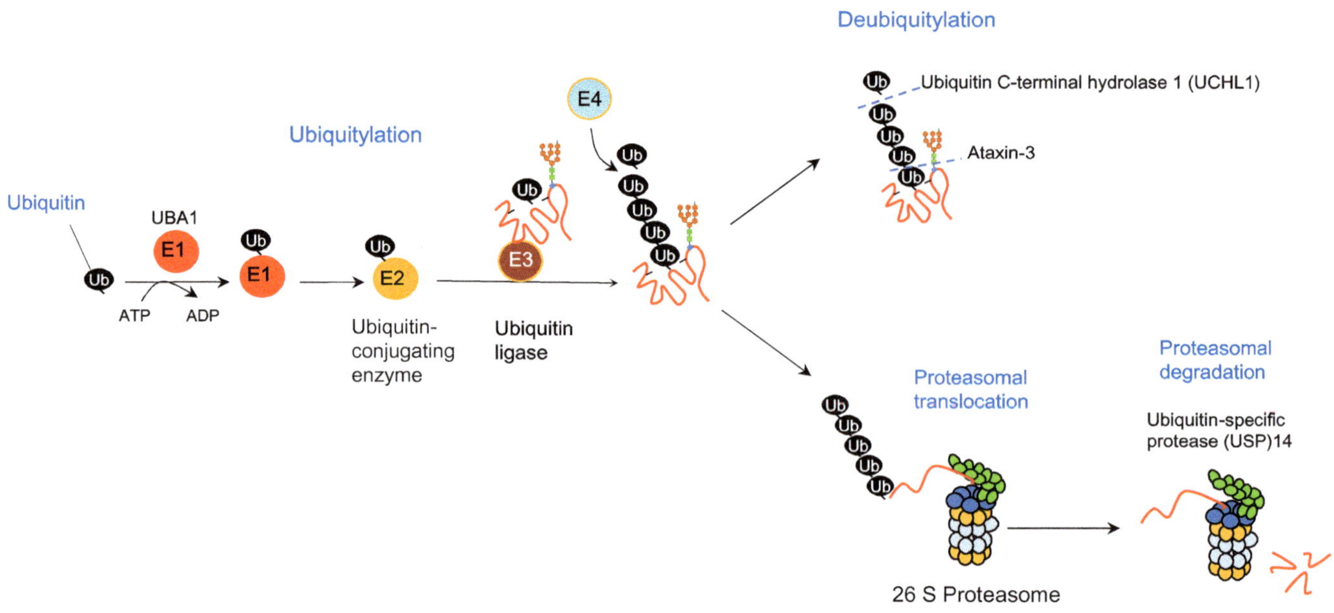

FIGURE 6.4 Ubiquitin–proteasome system.
The ubiquitylation system includes four different classes of enzymes, E1–E4. First, the ubiquitin-activating enzyme E1 (UBA1) hydrolyzes ATP, forming a linkage with ubiquitin. The activated ubiquitin is passed to the ubiquitin-conjugating enzyme E2; and E3 ubiquitin-protein ligases bind to the misfolded proteins and after the first ubiquitin has been attached elongate the ubiquitin, then creating ubiquitin–ubiquitin bonds leading to polyubiquitylated misfolded peptides that are targeted by degradation by the 26 S proteasome. Ubiquitin residues can be removed by deubiquitylating enzymes, including ataxin-3 and ubiquitin C-terminal hydrolases (UCHs).

is CHIP, which binds to Hsp70, reduces its chaperone activity and then functions as an E3 ubiquitin ligase that promotes proteasomal degradation of the misfolded protein. The substrates of CHIP include hyperphosphorylated tau and mutant superoxide dismutase 1 (SOD1). Ubiquitylation of damaged mitochondria is a fundamental mitochondrial quality-control mechanism that targets damaged mitochondria for autophagy (mitophagy). This process involves the ubiquitin E3 ligase parkin, which is recruited to the outer mitochondrial membrane by PTEN-induced putative kinase (PINK1). This process is further discussed in chapter 11. Monoubiquitylation modulates the activity, trafficking, and interaction of substrates in nondegradative processes. Substrates include H2A histones and various regulators of the endocytic pathway. Monoubiquitylation also promotes autophagic degradation of damaged peroxisomes.

Ubiquitin may undergo posttranslational modifications by phosphorylation, acetylation, and ribosylation. Ubiquitin modifications are highly dynamic and can be removed through the action of deubiquitylating enzymes, including ubiquitin-specific processing proteases and ubiquitin C-terminal hydrolases.[30] Deubiquitylating enzymes generally oppose the activity of E3 ligases by removing ubiquitin from target proteins. However, the effects of deubiquitylation are more complex, as in some cases deubiquitylation may regulate E3 ligase activity or promote degradation of E3 ligases. Examples of deubiquitylating enzymes are ubiquitin C-terminal hydrolase I (UCHL1) and ataxin-3. One target of deubiquitylation by ataxin-3 is the E3-ubiquitin ligase CHIP, which in turns ubiquitylates and increases activity of ataxin-3. Ataxin-3 also deubiquitylates and regulates the activity of parkin.

Several genetic disorders are due to mutations affecting components of the UPS. Mutations of the *UBA1* gene encoding E1 cause X-linked spinal muscular atrophy, associated with congenital contractures and fractures.[31] Several mutations affecting ubiquitylation or deubiquitylation have been linked to neurodegeneration. Mutations affecting the ubiquitin E3 ligase UBE3A are associated with Angelman syndrome.[32] *PARKIN* mutations leading to loss-of-function of parkin, are the most common causes of autosomal recessive juvenile onset PD, Mutations of the *UCHL1* gene encoding ubiquitin C-terminal hydrolase have also been linked to susceptibility to PD.[33] Trinucleotide (CAG) expansions of the *ATXN3* gene encoding ataxin-3 cause spinocerebellar ataxia (SCA) type 3, or Machado-Joseph disease, which is the most common SCA. Polyglutamine tract expansion in ataxin-3 leads to an inefficient deubiquitylation and increased clearance of proteins such as CHIP and parkin, thereby leading to accumulation of misfolded proteins and damaged mitochondria.[34]

Targets can also be conjugated to small ubiquitin-like modifier (SUMO) proteins. Sumoylation regulates several cellular processes including DNA damage response, transcriptional regulation, protein trafficking, and components of the UPS and autophagy.[35,36]

Targeting of Ubiquitylated Targets and Proteasomal Degradation

Ubiquitylation generates linkage-specific signals (degrons) on substrates destined for destruction (Figure 6.5). These ubiquitin-based degrons are recognized by specific adaptors that contain ubiquitin-binding domains; some adaptors deliver substrates to the central chamber of the 26 S proteasome, others deliver them to autophagic vacuoles, phagosomes, and lysosomes.[17] The polyubiquitin linkage at the lysine 48 residue is important for targeting proteins for proteasomal degradation. The proteasome is a large, multisubunit protease complex that includes a proteolytic 20 S core complex and a regulatory 19 S complex. The core complex is composed by four heptameric rings that confer its proteolytic activity; the 19S regulatory complex contains a hexameric ring of ATPase subunits. The 19S subunit receives the polyubiquitylated substrate, removes the ubiquitin, and unfolds the protein for translocation into the 20 S chamber.[17,37] Bortezomib, which is used for treatment of multiple myeloma inhibits approximately 30% of proteasome-mediated protein degradation. The primary dose-limiting toxicity of

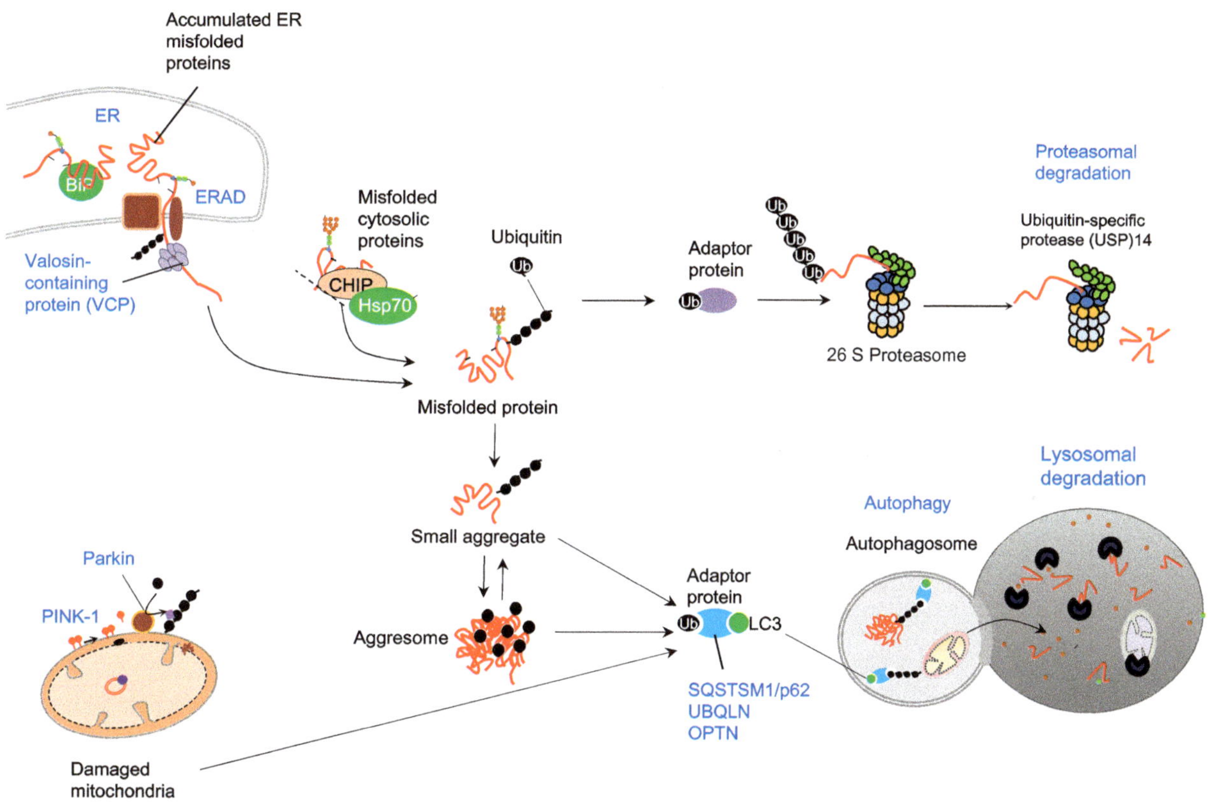

FIGURE 6.5 Targeting of ubiquitylated substrates for degradation.
The ubiquitin-based degrons are recognized by specific adaptors that contain ubiquitin-binding domains. Substrates for degradation include those originating from endoplasmic reticulum–associated degradation (ERAD) and extracted from the ER by valosin-containing protein (VCP). Misfolded cytosolic proteins bound to heat shock protein 70 (Hsp70) and remain misfolded are targeted for ubiquitin-proteasome degradation by the C-terminus of Hsc70 (Heat shock cognate)-interacting protein (CHIP). Adaptor proteins include sequestosome protein (SQSTM1, p62), ubiquilin (UBQL), and optineurin (OPN) and interact both with the ubiquitylated cargo and with microtubule-associated protein 1 light chain 3 (LC3) present in the autophagosome, leading to substrate degradation by autophagy. Ubiquitylation of damaged mitochondria is a fundamental mitochondrial quality-control mechanism that targets damaged mitochondria for autophagy (mitophagy). This process involves the ubiquitin E3 ligase Parkin, which is recruited to the outer mitochondrial membrane by PTEN (phosphatase and tensin homolog)-induced putative kinase (PINK1).

bortezomib is peripheral neuropathy, which typically affects sensory fibers.[38]

When terminally misfolded proteins escape from proteasomal degradation, the ubiquitin-tagged substrates tend to form aggregates. Histone deacetylase 6 (HDAC6) binds to the ubiquitin cargoes and temporally stores them in aggregates, whose content is eventually degraded by lysosomal hydrolases. In parallel with the HDAC6-dependent aggresome pathway, misfolded proteins and their aggregates are collected by specific adaptors that recognize ubiquitylated cargoes and target them for selective degradation by the autophagy-lysosomal system. These adaptor proteins include sequestosome protein (SQSTM1/p62), ubiquilin (UBQL), and optineurin (OPN).[39] Mutations of the *SQSTSM1* (SQSTM1/p62), *UBQLN2* (ubiquilin-2), or *OPTN* (optineurin) genes have been linked with ALS, FTLD, or both.[40] TANK-binding kinase 1 (TBK1) has a major role in autophagy and mitophagy, chiefly by phosphorylation of these autophagy adaptors.

AUTOPHAGY-LYSOSOMAL PATHWAYS

The autophagy-lysosome pathways digest ubiquitylated proteins, protein aggregates, stress RNA granules, and damaged cytoplasmic organelles such as mitochondria (mitophagy) or ER (ERphagy). Autophagic cargo also includes material incorporated via endocytosis and transported via endosomes and multivesicular bodies for lysosomal degradation. Autophagy includes three major types: microautophagy, chaperone-mediated autophagy, and macroautophagy (Figure 6.6). The lysosome is the final common organelle for all forms of autophagy. Under basal conditions, autophagy is inhibited by mammalian (mechanistic) target of rapamycin complex 1 (mTORC-1). The main autophagic processes involved in proteostasis and neurodegenerative disorders are chaperone-mediated autophagy and macroautophagy.

Chaperone-Mediated Autophagy

Chaperone-mediated autophagy accounts for a substantial proportion of the turnover of damaged or misfolded proteins, including huntingtin, α-synuclein, and tau. This process is highly selective and targets proteins bearing a lysosomal targeting pentapeptide motif KFERQ (lysine-phenylalanine-glutamate-arginine-glutamine) for delivery to lysosomes.[41–43] The KFERQ targeting motif is present in about 30% of cytosolic proteins and is exposed when there is a disruption of their tertiary structure due to unfolding, misfolding, or dissociation from a membrane. The Hsp70 member Hsc70 recognizes the KFERQ motif, and the chaperone-bound substrate binds to lysosomal-associated membrane protein (LAMP) 2. This protein is a protein translocation factor located in the cytosolic side of the lysosome. During chaperone-mediated autophagy, LAMP2A monomers are stabilized by the lysosomal chaperone Hsp90A1 and the substrates are translocated to the lumen of the lysosome. Since the targeted protein must be unfolded in order to be transported into the lysosome, chaperone-mediated autophagy can only degrade monomers; proteins organized in filaments or other aggregates are cleared via macroautophagy.

Macroautophagy

Macroautophagy is the most common form of autophagy, and is frequently referred to simply as autophagy. There are two main types of macroautophagy, basal (quality control) and starvation-induced macroautophagy.[44–47] Basal macroautophagy is an important quality-control mechanism that accepts and degrades polyubiquitylated proteins, protein aggregates, stress granules, and damaged mitochondria. Nutrient starvation-induced macroautophagy allows cells to mobilize energy from internal sources via degradation and recycling of cytoplasm constituents such as macromolecules. Macroautophagy involves three major steps, formation of a phagophore that engulfs cargo and then forms an autophagosome; transport of the autophagosome along microtubules; and fusion of the phagosome with endosomes and/or lysosomes (Figure 6.7). Formation of the autophagosomes requires membrane nucleation to form a phagophore, followed by elongation and finally closure of the phagophore. These processes involve highly regulated signaling events mediated by sequential activation of protein complexes encoded by autophagy (ATG) genes. The phagophore is a flat membrane cistern that elongates and curves into a double membrane that sequesters portions of the cytosol containing denatured proteins, RNA granules, lipids, carbohydrates, and old or damaged organelles. The initial step of phagophore formation is mediated by the unc-51-like kinase (ULK)1 complex and is inhibited by mTORC1. The next step is nucleation of the phagophore membrane and involves the phosphatidylinositol 3'kinase class III (PI3KIII) complex, also known as vacuolar sorting protein 34 (VPS34) complex, which includes the critical regulatory subunit Beclin-1. The VPS34 complex phosphorylates membrane phosphatidylinositol to phosphatidylinositol 3 phosphate; this step is required for elongation of the phagophore by recruitment of several adaptor proteins and lipid donors. Elongation of the phagophore involves two ubiquitin-like reactions that eventually lead to conjugation of microtubule-associated protein 1 light chain 3 (LC3) to phosphatidylethanolamine to yield LC3-II, which localizes to the membrane and facilitates the closure of the phagophore. LC3-II binds to adaptor proteins SQSTM1/p62, UBQL, and OPN that recognize ubiquitylated cargoes and target them for degradation.

Autophagosomes that are constitutively generated in distal axons undergo retrograde transport to the cell body via microtubules and eventually fuse with the lysosomes, forming autolysosomes. Autophagosomes may also initially fuse with late endosomes forming amphisomes that then fuse to the lysosome. Histone deacetylase 6 is an ubiquitin-binding deacetylase that targets protein aggregates, deacetylates tubulin, and promotes microtubule-mediated transport and fusion of autophagosomes with lysosomes. Huntingtin forms part of a multiprotein complex that interacts with

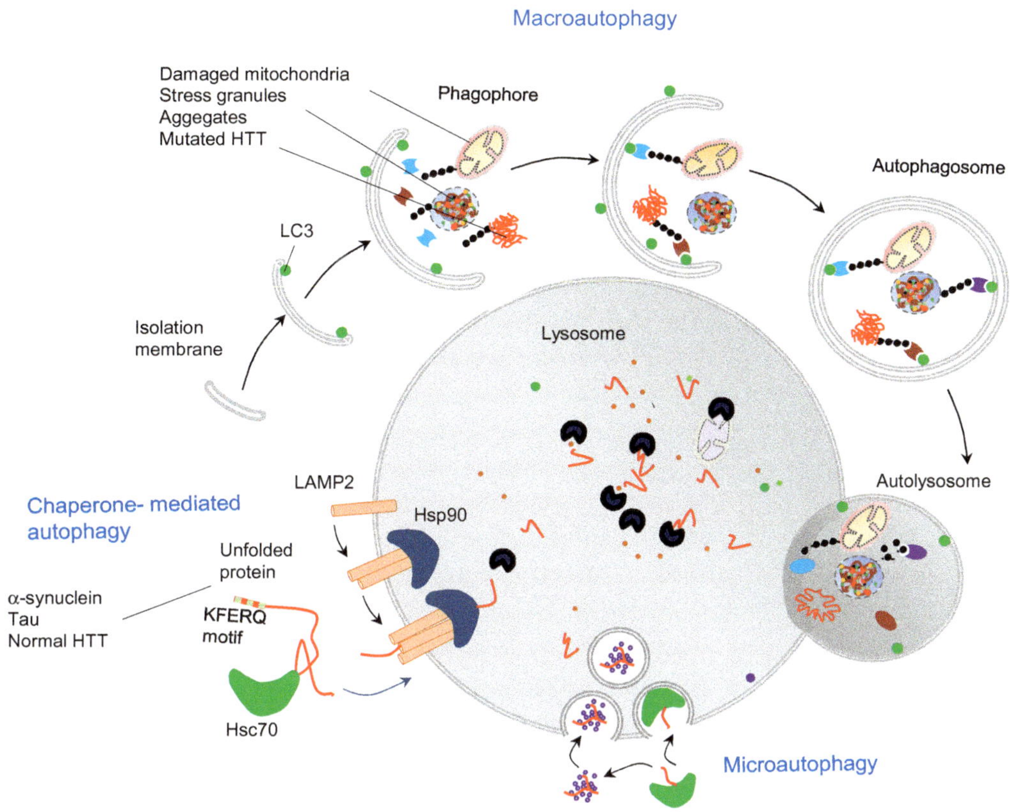

FIGURE 6.6 Mechanisms of autophagy.
Autophagy includes three major types: microautophagy, chaperone-mediated autophagy, and macroautophagy via formation of autophagosomes. Microautophagy involves pinocytosis of cytosolic regions surrounding lysosomes. Chaperone-mediated autophagy targets proteins bearing a lysine-phenylalanine-glutamate-arginine-glutamine (KFERQ) domain using the the heat-shock cognate protein 70 (Hsc70) as its Hsp70 chaperone and lysosomal LAMP2A as its receptor. Macroautophagy begins with the formation of an isolation membrane, or phagophore, that sequesters regions of the cytosol that include denatured proteins, lipids, carbohydrates, and old/damaged organelles. The phagophore eventually expands to become a mature autophagosome. The autophagosome is transported and then undergoes fusion either with the lysosome forming an autolysosome, or with the endosome forming an amphisome, then eventually fuses with the lysosome.

adaptors such as SQSTSM1/p62, with the ULK-1 complex, and with LC3, and thus participates in several steps of cargo loading to the autophagosome. Huntingtin also interacts with huntingtin-associated protein 1 to form a complex with motor proteins involved in axonal transport, thereby promoting the bidirectional microtubule-dependent transport of endosomes, autophagosomes, and lysosomes.

Crosstalk Between Autophagy and Apoptosis

Many stress pathways sequentially trigger autophagy and apoptosis within the same cell. There is a crosstalk between autophagy and apoptosis; in general, autophagy blocks the induction of apoptosis, and caspase activation during apoptosis inhibits autophagy. In most cases autophagy precedes and increases the threshold for apoptosis. Autophagy may reduce the levels of proapoptotic proteins, such as BAX proteins, in the cytosol. Reciprocally, the antiapoptotic protein Bcl2 interacts with Beclin-1 and prevents autophagy; Beclin-1 and other autophagic proteins are also targets of caspase-mediated cleavage. Caspase-mediated cleavage of these autophagic proteins also promotes the formation of products that localize to the mitochondria and sensitize cells to apoptosis. This crosstalk may facilitate the balanced cellular response to a given stress signal. For example, under basal conditions the tumor suppressor protein p53 is present in the cytosol and represses autophagy by interacting with a

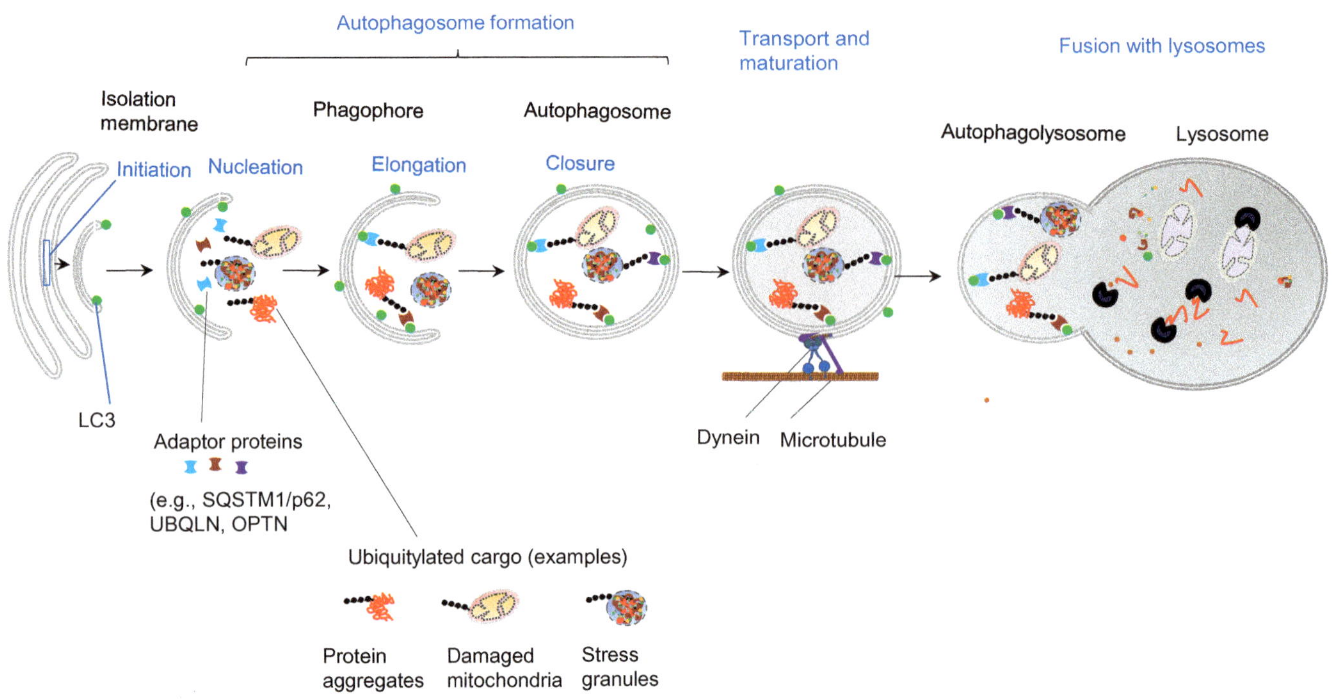

FIGURE 6.7 Steps involved in macroautophagy.
The first step of macroautophagy is phagophore formation resulting from nucleation of the phagophore membrane. This is followed by elongation of the phagophore membrane and then closure of the pagophore membrane, which involves s microtubule-associated protein 1 light chain 3 (LC3).

component of the ULK-1 complex required for phagophore formation. In response to cellular stress, p53 translocates to the nucleus and the mitochondrial matrix; this both facilitates the induction of autophagy and triggers apoptosis.

ALTERED PROTEOSTASIS IN NEURODEGENERATIVE DISORDERS

Altered proteostasis leads to accumulation of misfolded proteins in the form of toxic fibrillary oligomers and then aggregates and is a fundamental pathogenic hub in neurodegenerative disorders[15,19,23,46,48–53] (Table 6.1). In both genetic and acquired proteinopathies, there is accumulation of polyubiquitylated misfolded proteins forming inclusions that characterize the specific disorders (Table 6.2). The formation of these aggregates is the consequence of two interactive factors, the increased propensity of the protein to adopt a misfolded conformation, and the inability of the proteostatic systems to clear the abnormal protein. Several mechanisms may increase propensity of amyloid β (Aβ), tau, α-synuclein (α-SYN), huntingtin, PrP^c, or RNA-binding proteins such as TDP-43 to undergo conformational changes, misfolding, incorporation into fibrillary β-sheet-rich structures, and aggregation in the form of intracellular inclusions.[54] They include mutations affecting their primary structure, posttranslational modifications such as phosphorylation, oxidative stress, and protein–protein interactions with both normal and abnormal partners that serve as a "seed" via prion-like mechanisms (Figure 6.8). In some cases, there is interaction between two different types of proteins that promote their fibrillation. For example, hyperphosphorylated tau interacts with α-SYN in Lewy bodies; and α-SYN promotes tau phosphorylation. Typically almost all inclusions contain multiple proteins (for example, TDP-43 and tau); and inclusions with different morphology may have identical protein compositions. In addition to formation of aggregates, a fundamental neuropathological feature in proteinopathies is the accumulation of autophagic vacuoles, particularly autophagosomes, reflecting impaired trafficking and degradation of aggregates by lysosomes.

Mechanisms of Toxicity

In general, oligomers of misfolded proteins are more pathogenic than higher-order structures such as protofilaments and fibrils. Toxic gain-of-function of the intermediate fibril monomers promotes the formation of aggregates and initiates a cascade of protein–protein interactions. Neuronal dysfunction and death may occur due to loss-of-function of aggregated proteins, ER stress, mitochondrial dysfunction, synaptic toxicity, interference with axonal transport, and impaired function of the autophagy-lysosome system. Aggregates from different proteins may trigger converging pathways of toxicity. The precise mechanisms of

TABLE 6.1 *Proteins Involved in Neurodegenerative Disorders (Examples)*

Protein	Disorder
Amyloid β protein	Alzheimer disease
Tau	Alzheimer disease Familial FTLD/tau with parkinsonism Progressive supranuclear palsy Corticobasal degeneration Pick disease Chronic traumatic encephalopathy Argyrophilic grain disease Globular glial tauopathy Primary age-related tauopathy Aging-related tau astrogliopathy Subacute sclerosing panencephalitis
α-synuclein	Parkinson disease Dementia with Lewy bodies Multiple system atrophy Pure autonomic failure NBIA type I (PANK mutation)
TDP-43	Familial and sporadic ALS FTLD with motor neuron disease FTLD with *PGRN* mutations FTLD/ALS with *C9ORF72* expansion Multisystem proteinopathy (IBMPFD) due to *VCP* mutations Perry syndrome Hippocampal sclerosis
FUS	Familial ALS Atypical FTLD-U Neurofilament intermediate inclusion body disease Basophilic inclusion body disease
Prion protein (PrPc)	Sporadic Creutzfeld-Jakob disease (CJD) Familial CJD Fatal Familial and Sporadic Insomnia Gerstmann-Straussler-Scheinker disease Variant CJD Kuru
Proteins affected in trinucleotide repeat disorders (example)	Huntington disease (huntingtin, *HTT*) Spinocerebellar ataxias (ataxins 1, 2, 3, 6, 7,1 7, atrophin, others) Spinobulbar muscular atrophy (androgen receptor) Friedreich ataxia (frataxin, FTX) Fragile X syndrome and FXTAS (fragile X mental retardation protein)

ALS, amyotrophic lateral sclerosis; FTLD, frontotemporal lobar degeneration; FXTAS, fragile X tremor ataxia syndrome

cellular toxicity of aggregates are incompletely understood. Oligomeric forms of α-SYN may be more toxic than monomeric or fibrillary forms because of their ability to impair synaptic plasticity and form pores in the membrane that promote Ca^{2+} influx and cell toxicity. Impaired clearance by the autophagosome-lysosome system may result in the release of protein aggregates to the cell's surroundings via exosomes or other extracellular vesicles. These abnormal aggregates may then act in a prion-like mechanism by serving as a template that disrupts the conformation and promoting aggregation of normal proteins in the target cells, leading to disease propagation.

TABLE 6.2 *Cell Inclusions in Neurodegenerative Disorders*

Protein	Disorder	Inclusion
Amyloid β	Alzheimer disease	Neuritic plaque
Tau	Alzheimer disease Familial FTLD/tau with parkinsonism Progressive supranuclear palsy Corticobasal degeneration Pick disease	Neurofibrillary tangle Neurofibrillary tangle Tufted astrocytes Astrocytic plaques/ threads Pick bodies
α-synuclein	Parkinson disease (PD) /PDD/DLB Multiple system atrophy	Lewy body Glial cytoplasmic inclusions
TDP-43	Familial and sporadic ALS FTLD-TDP 43 Hippocampal sclerosis Multisystem proteinopathy	Cytoplasmic stress granules
FUS	Familial ALS Atypical FTLD Neurofilament intermediate inclusion body disease	Cytoplasmic stress granules NF (α-internexin) inclusion
Prion protein	Variant CJD	Kuru plaque
Nucleotide repeat disorders	Huntington disease Spinocerebellar ataxias	Intranuclear inclusions

ALS, amyotrophic lateral sclerosis; FTLD, frontotemporal lobar degeneration

Impaired ER Quality Control and Activation of the Unfolded Protein Response

Several ER quality-control mechanisms are affected in neurodegenerative disorders, leading to accumulation of misfolded proteins and ER stress. Accumulation of Aβ oligomers, or aggregates of α-SYN, phosphorylated tau, or mutant SOD1 in the ER lumen causes disruption of ER calcium homeostasis, suboptimal function of the calcium-binding chaperones calsequestrin and calreticulin, sequestration of the ER chaperone BiP, and impairment of the translocation step of the ERAD pathway. As a consequence, there is activation of the UPR in several neurodegenerative disorders.[9,18,19,55–58] There is upregulation of PERK and IRE1α signaling and their downstream effectors in neurons containing protein aggregations. The UPR is also a reaction to disrupted axonal integrity, and may be triggered by retrograde signals that are generated locally in the injured axon and propagate back to secondarily induce ER stress in the perikaryon. Endoplasmic reticulum stress and UPR activation also occur in disorders affecting the oligodendrocytes, such as multiple sclerosis, and in genetic white matter disorders such as Pelizaeus-Merzbacher disease and vanishing white matter disease. Studies on experimental models of demyelinating Charcot-Marie-Tooth disease showed that mutated peripheral myelin protein zero is retained in the ER and triggers the UPR in Schwann cells.

Upregulation of the Heat Shock Response

Studies in animal models and in brains obtained at autopsy show upregulation of the Hsp response in AD, PD, ALS, and HD. In these disorders, Hsps typically co-localize with abnormal protein aggregates. Whereas some Hsps are found in degenerating neurons, others are primarily expressed in astrocytes, microglia, and oligodendrocytes. Increased Hsp expression in neurodegenerative disorders may reflect an attempted compensatory mechanism. For example, studies in vitro showed that small Hsps bind α-SYN or Aβ fibrils and may transiently stabilize their structure and inhibit oligomerization. Overexpression of Hsp40/DNAJ family members prevents nuclear localization of mutant ataxin-1 and ataxin-3. The ability to induce Hsp response decreases with age. Both aging and neurodegenerative disorders are associated with altered membrane composition and membrane fluidity, which also trigger Hsp responses. For example, Aβ interacts with membrane lipids, proteoglycans, and membrane proteins, perturbing membrane structure and fluidity leading to activation of Hsp70.1. Peroxidation of membrane lipids leads to production of carbonylated form of Hsp70 that is cleaved and inactivated by calpain. The inability of Hsp70.1 to stabilize the inner lysosomal membrane results in increased lysosomal permeabilization and rupture, with the release of the proteases such as cathepsin, leading eventually to cell death.

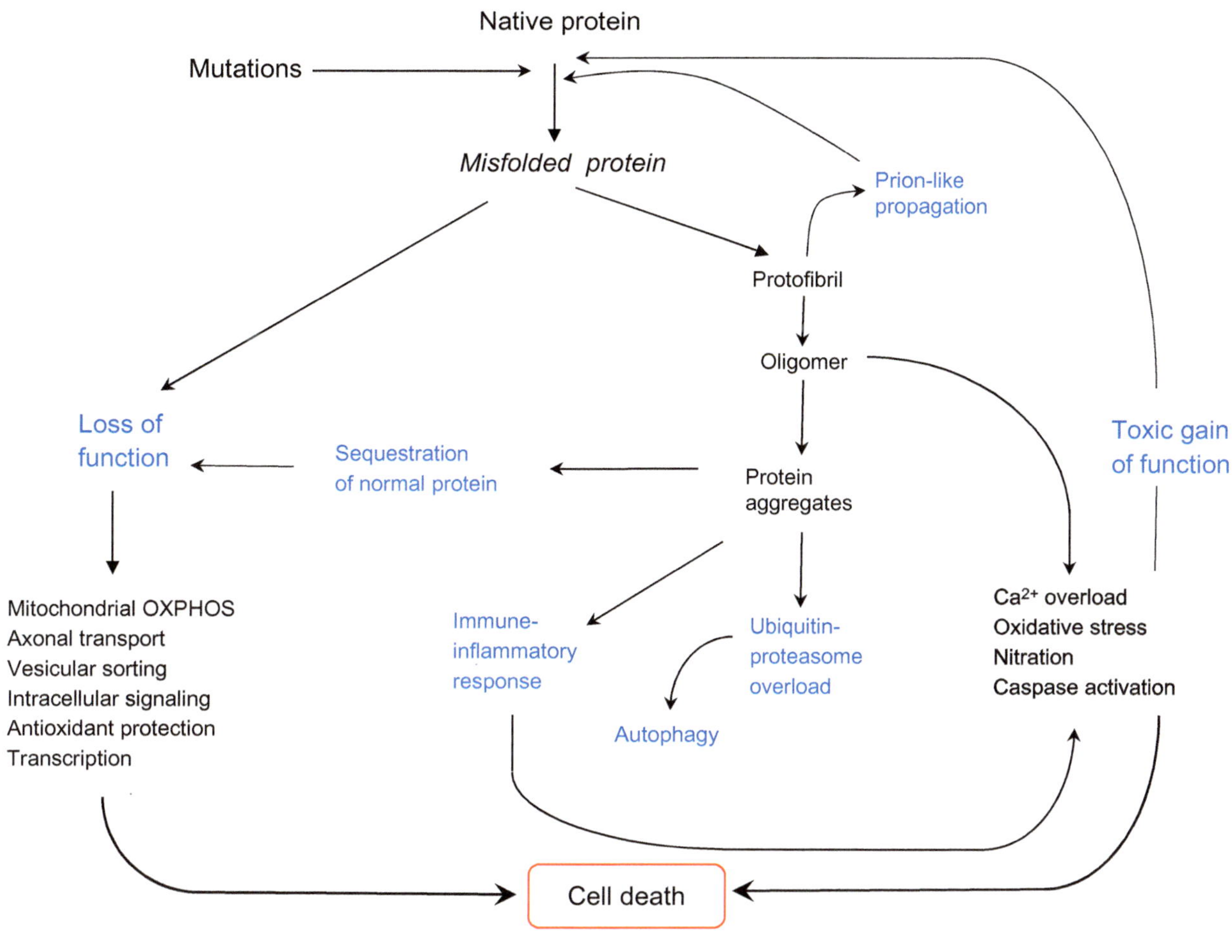

FIGURE 6.8 Mechanisms of cell injury in proteinopathies.
Altered proteostasis leads to accumulation of misfolded proteins in the form of toxic fibrillary oligomers and then aggregates, Mechanisms of proteoinopathies include mutations, posttranslational modifications, oxidative stress, and protein–protein interactions with both normal and abnormal partners that serve as a "seed" via prion-like propagation mechanisms.

Impaired Clearance by Autophagy

Disturbances of the autophagy-lysosomal system affect both quality-control mechanisms and cellular responses to stressors. Neurons are particularly vulnerable, as clearance of autophagosomes and fusion with lysosomes requires efficient intracellular transport over long distances. Inefficient clearance can result in backing up of cargo, further impairing axonal transport and effective autophagy. Impaired clearance by the autophagosome-lysosome system results in accumulation of dysfunctional mitochondria, leading to oxidative stress and apoptosis, which further impair the autophagy-lysosomal pathway. Impaired fusion of the autophagosome with the lysosome may result in the release of the autophagosome content, including protein aggregates, to the cell's surroundings via the unconventional protein secretion processes known as exophagy. Impaired autophagy may reflect mutations of proteins involved in vesicular trafficking and lysosomal function, as discussed in the next chapter, but is also a fundamental disease mechanism in late-onset neurodegenerative disorders (Table 6.3). For example, impaired chaperone-mediated autophagy is an important pathogenic mechanism in PD. As a consequence of mutations, posttranslational modifications, or interaction with oxidized dopamine, α-SYN can no longer be internalized and cleared by the lysosome. Instead, it becomes attached to the lysosome membrane and forms clusters that impair internalization and degradation of both itself and other substrates of chaperone-mediated autophagy. Hyperphosphorylated tau also interferes with autophagic flow.[50]

Prion-Like Propagation

Misfolded proteins incorporated into fibrillary β-sheet-rich amyloid structures undergo cycles of nucleation and fragmentation and may serve as templates or seeds to elicit aggregation of their respective normal endogenous partners, thus behaving like prions.[59,60] In the strict sense, prions are infectious proteinaceous agents that consist primarily of abnormal PrP protein (PrP^{sc}). Normal PrP^{c} is linked to the membrane via a glycerol phosphatidylinositol posttranslational modification and is involved in synaptic plasticity and

TABLE 6.3 *Examples of Mechanisms of Impaired Autophagy in Neurodegenerative Diseases*

Disorder	Process Affected	Mechanism
Alzheimer disease	Autophagosome induction	Early upregulation Reduced Beclin-1 expression
	Autophagosome-lysosome fusion	Cargo overload
	Chaperone-mediated autophagy (CMA)	Inefficient translocation of tau fragments across the lysosomal membrane
	Lysosomal acidification	*PSEN1* mutations impair V-ATPase function
Parkinson disease	CMA	Mutant α-SYN blocks autophagy receptors Mutant LRRK2 interferes with α-SYN clearance
	Substrate recognition	*PINK1* and *Parkin* mutations impair mitophagy
	Autophagosome maturation	Elevated TPPP/p25α impairs HDAC6 activity
	Lysosome digestion	*ATP13A2* mutations impair lysosomal acidification
Huntington disease	Phagophore formation	Aggregation of mTOR by mHTT
	Cargo recognition	Shielding p62/SQSTM1 binding sites by mHTT
	Autophagosome maturation	mHTT disrupts motility along microtubules
ALS, FTLD, or both	Cargo recognition	Mutations affecting cargo adaptors SQSTM1/p26, ubiquilin 2 (UBQLN2), and optineurin (OPTN) or TANK-binding kinase 1 (TBK1)
	Transfer of ubiquitylated substrates	*VCP* mutations decrease substrate delivery to the autophagosome (IBMPFD)
	Endosome-phagosome fusion	*CHM2B* mutation impair amphisome formation
	Autophagosome maturation	Dynactin (*DCTN1*) mutations impair autophagosome transport

ALS, amyotrophic lateral sclerosis; α-SYN, α-synuclein; CHMBP2, charged multivesicular protein 2B; FTLD, frontotemporal lobar degeneration; HDAC6, histone deacetylase 6; IBMPFD, inclusion body myositis-Paget disease-frontotemporal dementia; LRRK2, leucine-rich repeat kinase 2; mHTT, mutated huntingtin; mTOR, mammalian (mechanistic) target of rapamycin; PSEN, presenilin-1; SQSTM1, sequestosome 1; TPPP, tubulin polymerization-promoting protein; VCP, valosin-containing protein

myelin homeostasis via interactions with multiple partners. Abnormal PrP^{sc} multiplies by nucleation and fragmentation, forming highly ordered oligomers that incorporate endogenous PrP^{c}, thereby increasing in size. The different aggregates, or "strains," are transmitted between the same host species, resulting in different disease phenotypes. Sporadic Creutzfeld-Jakob disease (CJD) is the most common form of prion disease and has no yet identified cause. Acquired prion diseases induced by transmission of preexisting prions include iatrogenic CJD, variant CJD, and kuru. Genetic prion diseases due to mutations of the *PRNP* gene encoding PrP^{c} include familial CJD, Gerstmann-Straeussler-Scheinker syndrome, and fatal familial insomnia. Most *PRNP* mutations cause PrP^{c} misfolding and pathological aggregates. *PRNP* polymorphisms modulate susceptibility toward prion diseases in a strain-dependent manner. One important polymorphism occurs at codon 129, which can encode either a valine (V) or a methionine (M) and thus modify the disease phenotype. Most of a healthy population is heterozygous at this locus; homozygosity for either amino acid predisposes to sporadic CJD, to early onset of genetic CJD, and to variant CJD.

Accumulation of abnormal protein aggregates via a prion-like mechanism has been described in several neurologic disorders. One typical example is amyloid neuropathy, due either to accumulation of immunoglobulin light chain (AL amyloidosis) or to mutated transthyretin (hereditary TTR amyloidosis). Whereas misfolded proteins have a prion-like behavior, they have been referred to as "prionoids" because they have not yet been demonstrated to be transmissible between humans.[61,62] However, the most serious issue in domino liver transplantation using liver grafts from patients with TTR-related familial amyloid polyneuropathy is the development of iatrogenic transmitted TTR amyloidosis (de novo amyloidosis) in domino liver transplant recipients.[63] Drugs such as tafamidis or diflunisal stabilize mutant TTR reducing its aggregation. In PD patients who received embryonic neuronal transplants, grafts displayed α-SYN inclusions one or two decades after transplantation, indicating that α-SYN aggregates were able to spread from host to graft in a prion-like manner.[64] Brain homogenates from patients with multiple system atrophy (MSA) induced α-SYN phosphorylation, aggregation, and neuronal dysfunction in mice after serial inoculations; however, the development of these changes was dependent on the presence of a transgene encoding an aggregation-prone mutant of human α-SYN.[65] The MSA α-SYN prions are conformationally distinct from the misfolded α-SYN in PD patients.[66] One study showed that MSA prions robustly infected cells expressing wild-type α-SYN but were unable to replicate in cells expressing the mutant α-SYN.[67,68] In addition to fibrillary α-SYN, other abnormal proteins can also behave as prionoids. Tau aggregates may also spread in the brain in an orderly fashion which is characteristic of different tauopathies.[69] Hyperphosphorylation of tau not only promotes its precipitation as neurofibrillary tangles in AD but also promotes α-SYN neuropathology in PD.[70] Amyloid Aβ oligomers are able to self-propagate between neurons and generate aggregates in vitro. Furthermore, injection of human AD brain homogenates containing Aβ aggregates caused accumulation of amyloid plaques in mice overexpressing Aβ.

The seeding activity of prions and several nonprion protein aggegates is assessed using in-vitro amplification assays, including real-time quacking-induced conversion (RT-QuIC) and protein misfolding cyclic amplification (PMCA). For example, RT-QuIC in CSF is a reliable test for sporadic CJD; both RT-QuiC and PMCA has been more recently applied to detect α-SYN aggregation propensity both in CSF samples and skin biopsy of patients with synucleinopathies.

There are several potential mechanisms for prion-like transfer of abnormal fibrils between cells. These include diffusion through the cell membrane, ER-Golgi dependent exocytosis, nonclassical exocytosis, and secretion associated with exosomes or nanotubes.[71] An unconventional secretion pathway called misfolded-associated protein secretion involves recruitment of misfolded proteins to the ER for their deubiquitylation and their redirection to the endosomes for secretion. Some cleavage of amyloid precursor protein into Aβ occurs in endosomes, and some Aβ oligomers are released from cells via exosomes. Studies in transgenic mice expressing mutant human tau showed that tau-containing exosomes can transfer tau to cultured neurons and may promote seeding and propagation of abnormal tau in brains of normal mice. Studies in CSF of patients with AD show enrichment of exosomes containing hyperphosphorylated tau isoforms. Extracellular vesicles also have a role in prion-like intercellular spread of α-SYN aggregates. Release of α-SYN is Ca^{2+}-dependent and is increased by reduced lysosomal acidification. The direct interaction between α-SYN or Aβ oligomers and PrP^c may be important for their transfer between cells, as PrP^c may function as a conformation-specific sensor of disease-associated proteins.[72] Once the misfolded protein is released to the extracellular space, it is taken up by recipient cells. For example, uptake of α-SYN can occur via passive diffusion or via receptor-mediated endocytosis. Different cell surface proteins mediate the internalization of α-SYN interaction with its oligomeric or fibrillary forms. Propagation of TDP-43 aggregates contained in stress granules may also occur via exosomes.

GENETIC DISORDERS OF PROTEOSTASIS

Whereas impaired proteostasis is a major cell pathway for late-onset neurodegenerative disorders, it may also be the primary mechanism in genetic disorders due to mutations affecting key proteins involved in protein maturation, folding, quality control, and clearance (Table 6.4).

Disorders Affecting Protein Maturation and ER Quality Control

Congenital disorders of N-glycosylation of nascent proteins impair protein maturation and affect most organ systems. For example, mutations of the *PMM2* gene encoding phosphomannomutase 2, which generates the mannosylation donors for the formation of the core glycan complex, manifests with developmental delay, intellectual disabilities, hypotonia, seizures, neuropathy, and metabolic abnormalities in multiple organ systems.[2] Mutations of the *SIL1* gene encoding the nucleotide exchange factor required for the chaperone function of BiP are associated with Marinesco-Sjögren syndrome, an autosomal recessive disorder characterized by cerebellar ataxia, congenital cataracts, myopathy, developmental and mental retardation, hypogonadism, and skeletal deformities.[3] *SIL1* mutations have also been associated with myopathy, Dandy-Walker syndrome, spastic paraplegia, and motor neuronopathy. Mutations of the *ATF6* gene encoding an effector of the UPR cause autosomal recessive achromatopsia.[73] *SIGMAR1* mutations affecting the ER chaperone Sig-1R are linked to familial forms of ALS, with or without associated FTLD.[21] Overload of the ER may also occur with normally folded but polymerized proteins. This is the case in familial encephalopathy with neuroserpin inclusion bodies, which is characterized by dementia and epilepsy (including myoclonic epilepsy).[74] Neuroserpin is a member of the serine protease inhibitor family, and its mutations promote its polymerization within the ER without triggering the UPR. Neurotoxicity in this disorder reflects both toxic gain-of-function triggering a proinflammatory response and loss-of-function due to impaired neuroserpin secretion, leading to activation of proteolysis.[58,74]

Disorders Affecting Heat Shock Proteins

As mentioned earlier in this chapter, missense mutations in the *HSPB1* gene encoding Hsp27 and the *HSPB8* gene encoding HspP22 are associated with two distinct but overlapping phenotypes, distal hereditary motor neuropathy (distal HMN type II) and Charcot-Marie-Tooth disease type 2.[25] Mutations of the *HSPD1* gene encoding the mitochondrial chaperone Hsp60 cause a rare form of autosomal dominant hereditary spastic paraparesis (SPG13).[24] *HSPD1* polymorphisms may affect mitochondrial biogenesis and

TABLE 6.4 *Genetic Disorders Affecting Protein Maturation, Quality Control, and Degradation (Examples)*

Process	Gene (protein)		Phenotype
N-glycosylation	*PMM2*	Formation of N-glycan	Neurologic and multisystem disease
ER maturation	*SIL1*	Nucleotide exchange factor for BiP	Marinesco-Sjögren disease
ER-homeostasis	*SIGMAR1*	Chaperone at the ER-mitochondria interface	Familial ALS
Unfolded protein response (UPR)	ARF6	Effector of the UPR	Autosomal recessive achromatopsia
Heat shock protein	*HSPB1* (Hsp27) *HSPB8* (Hsp 22)	Chaperone and cytoskeletal protection	Distal hereditary motor neuropathy Charcot-Marie-Tooth 2 disease
	αB crystallin	Muscle chaperone	Myofibrillar myopathy
	HSPD1 (Hsp60)	Mitochondrial HSP	Hereditary spastic paraplegia
Ubiquitylation	*UBA1*	E1 ubiquitin-activating enzyme	X-linked spinal muscular atrophy with contractures
	UBA3	E3 ubiquitylating enzyme	Angelmann syndrome
	Parkin	E3 ubiquitylation for mitophagy	Early-onset PD
Deubiquitylation	*ATXN3* (ataxin-3)	Targets ubiquitylated Parkin and other substrates	Spinocerebellar ataxia 3
	UCHL1	Ubiquitin C-terminal hydrolase	Risk factor for familial PD

PMM2, phosphomannomutase 2

thus modify the severity of the most autosomal dominant hereditary spastic paraplegia associated with *spastin* mutations (SPG4) disrupting mitochondrial axonal transport.

Disorders Affecting the Ubiquitin System

As discussed earlier in this chapter, several mutations affecting ubiquitylation or deubiquitylation have been linked to neurodegeneration. Mutations of *UBA1* gene encoding the ubiquitin activating enzyme E1 cause X-linked spinal muscular atrophy associated with congenital contractures and fractures.[31] Ubiquitin E3 ligase UBE3A is implicated in in Angelman syndrome, which is characterized by intellectual disability, epilepsy, speech impairment, facial dysmorphism, and a characteristic behavioral phenotype of happy appearance and hyperactivity.[32] A missense variant in *CYLD*, which encodes a deubiquitinase has been recently identified in a large family with autosomal dominant FTD and ALS.[75] This variant resulted in increased deubiquitinase activity leading to impairment of autophagosome fusion to lysosomes.[75]

Disorders Due to Impaired Delivery of Ubiquitylated Proteins or Aggregates for Clearance

Mutations affecting proteins that target ubiquitylated proteins for degradation manifest with complex phenotypes affecting the CNS, neuromuscular system, and peripheral organs and is known as multisystem proteinopathy.[76] This is a heterogeneous, autosomal dominant adult-onset disorder that is characterized by a variable presentation, even within the same families. Multisystem proteinopathy typically manifests with inclusion body myopathy, Paget disease of bone, FTD, and ALS. These manifestations are associated with accumulation of cytoplasmic aggregates containing TDP-43 and other RNA-binding proteins. The first recognized genetic cause of multisystem proteinopathy are *VCP* mutations leading to loss-of-function of VCP. These mutations have also been associated with a spectrum of other diseases including hereditary spastic paraplegia, Charcot-Marie-Tooth type 2 disease, and different types of muscular dystrophy including distal myopathies or early onset PD. Mutations in the *HNRNPA2B1* and *HNRNPA1* genes promoting aggregation of heterogeneous nuclear ribonucleoproteins have also been linked to multisystem proteinopathy. In addition to *VCP* mutations, mutations affecting genes affecting autophagy adaptor proteins, including SQTSTM1/p62, OPTN, and TBK1, have also been linked to familial ALS/FTD.[77,78]

Disorders of the Autophagy-Lysosomal System

Impaired autophagy and lysosomal degradation are a fundamental pathogenic mechanism in some genetic neurodegenerative disorders. Many of these mutations have been linked to PD, as discussed in the next chapter. Briefly, mutations of both the *LRRK2* gene encoding leucine-rich repeat kinase 2 (LRRK2) and the *GBA* gene encoding lysosomal acid β-glucocerebrosidase (GCase), are the most common risk factors for PD. These mutations affect autophagic flux, impair degradation of α-SYN and other substrates by chaperone-mediated autophagy, and lead to α-SYN accumulation.[51,52] The endosome-lysosomal pathway is also affected in AD. Mutations of the *PS1* gene encoding presenilin-1 lead to impaired lysosomal acidification and thus proteolytic activity.

Several steps of autophagy are also affected in HD.[48] Whereas normal HTT is degraded both by the ubiquitin-proteasome system and lysosomes, mutated HTT is primarily degraded by autophagy. Mutated HTT impairs recognition of SQTSM/p62-bound cargoes by autophagosomes and their transport along microtubules for their fusion with the lysosomes.

KEY POINTS

- Normal cell function and survival depend on carefully regulated synthesis, folding, trafficking, and degradation of proteins, or proteostasis.
- Proteins undergo maturation and folding in the endoplasmic reticulum (ER) via N-glycosylation and formation of disulfide bonds.
- Tight quality-control mechanisms prevent the accumulation of misfolded proteins in the ER.
- The unfolded protein response, heat shock proteins, and degradation by the ubiquitin-proteasome and the autophagosome-lysosome system prevent the accumulation of misfolded proteins.
- The unfolded protein includes transient suppression of mRNA translation, transcriptional activation of neuroprotective genes, and, if ineffective, activation of genes that lead to apoptosis.
- Heat shock proteins bind to and promote repair of misfolded proteins and, if ineffective, target the misfolded proteins for degradation by the ubiquitin-proteasome system.
- Ubiquitylation targets proteins for degradation by the proteasome or autophagy-lysosome system.
- The autophagy-lysosome pathway digests ubiquitylated proteins, protein aggregates, stress RNA granules, and damaged cytoplasmic organelles.
- Impaired proteostasis with accumulation of protein aggregates is a fundamental disease mechanism in neurodegenerative disorders.
- Mutations or environmental disturbances such as oxidative stress may promote misfolding of normal cell proteins such as α-synuclein and render them prone to aggregation.
- Impaired quality control, degradation by the ubiquitin-proteasome system, or trafficking and degradation by the autophagosome-lysosome system have major roles in neurodegeneration.
- Misfolded proteins accumulate into fibrillary structures, forming inclusions that characterize the specific disorders.
- Degeneration results from toxic gain-of-function of the intermediate fibril monomers, promoting the formation of aggregates and initiating a cascade of protein–protein interactions and prion-like propagation.

REFERENCES

1. Braakman I, Hebert DN. Protein folding in the endoplasmic reticulum. Cold Spring Harb Perspect Biol 2013;5:a013201.
2. Freeze HH, Eklund EA, Ng BG, Patterson MC. Neurological aspects of human glycosylation disorders. Annu Rev Neurosci 2015;38:105–125.
3. Krieger M, Roos A, Stendel C, et al. SIL1 mutations and clinical spectrum in patients with Marinesco-Sjogren syndrome. Brain 2013;136:3634–3644.
4. Parakh S, Jagaraj CJ, Vidal M, et al. ERp57 is protective against mutant SOD1-induced cellular pathology in amyotrophic lateral sclerosis. Hum Mol Genet 2018;27:1311–1331.
5. Gonzalez-Perez P, Woehlbier U, Chian RJ, et al. Identification of rare protein disulfide isomerase gene variants in amyotrophic lateral sclerosis patients. Gene 2015;566:158–165.
6. Perri E, Parakh S, Atkin J. Protein disulphide isomerases: emerging roles of PDI and ERp57 in the nervous system and as therapeutic targets for ALS. Expert Opin Ther Targets 2017;21:37–49.
7. Gerard M, Deleersnijder A, Demeulemeester J, Debyser Z, Baekelandt V. Unraveling the role of peptidyl-prolyl isomerases in neurodegeneration. Mol Neurobiol 2011;44:13–27.
8. McCaffrey K, Braakman I. Protein quality control at the endoplasmic reticulum. Essays Biochem 2016;60:227–235.
9. Hwang J, Qi L. Quality control in the endoplasmic reticulum: crosstalk between ERAD and UPR pathways. Trends Biochem Sci 2018;43:593–605.
10. Mehrtash AB, Hochstrasser M. Ubiquitin-dependent protein degradation at the endoplasmic reticulum and nuclear envelope. Semin Cell Dev Biol 2018;93:111–124.
11. Preston GM, Brodsky JL. The evolving role of ubiquitin modification in endoplasmic reticulum-associated degradation. Biochem J 2017;474:445–469.
12. Ye Y, Tang WK, Zhang T, Xia D. A mighty "protein extractor" of the cell: structure and function of the p97/CDC48 ATPase. Front Mol Biosci 2017;4:39.
13. Zhu B, Jiang L, Huang T, et al. ER-associated degradation regulates Alzheimer's amyloid pathology and memory function by modulating gamma-secretase activity. Nat Commun 2017;8:1472.
14. Alazami AM, Adly N, Al Dhalaan H, Alkuraya FS. A nullimorphic ERLIN2 mutation defines a complicated hereditary spastic paraplegia locus (SPG18). Neurogenetics 2011;12:333–336.
15. Clayton BLL, Popko B. Endoplasmic reticulum stress and the unfolded protein response in disorders of myelinating glia. Brain Res 2016;1648:594–602.
16. Li S, Yang L, Selzer ME, Hu Y. Neuronal endoplasmic reticulum stress in axon injury and neurodegeneration. Ann Neurol 2013;74:768–777.

17. Rousseau A, Bertolotti A. Regulation of proteasome assembly and activity in health and disease. Nat Rev Mol Cell Biol 2018;19:697–712.
18. Smith HL, Mallucci GR. The unfolded protein response: mechanisms and therapy of neurodegeneration. Brain 2016;139:2113–2121.
19. Hetz C, Saxena S. ER stress and the unfolded protein response in neurodegeneration. Nat Rev Neurol 2017;13:477–491.
20. Delprat B, Crouzier L, Su TP, Maurice T. At the crossing of ER stress and MAMs: a key role of sigma-1 receptor? Adv Exp Med Biol 2020;1131:699–718.
21. Mancuso R, Navarro X. Sigma-1 receptor in motoneuron disease. Adv Exp Med Biol 2017;964:235–254.
22. Penke B, Bogar F, Crul T, Santha M, Toth ME, Vigh L. Heat shock proteins and autophagy pathways in neuroprotection: from molecular bases to pharmacological interventions. Int J Mol Sci 2018;19.
23. Ciechanover A, Kwon YT. Protein quality control by molecular chaperones in neurodegeneration. Front Neurosci 2017;11:185.
24. Bross P, Magnoni R, Bie AS. Molecular chaperone disorders: defective Hsp60 in neurodegeneration. Curr Top Med Chem 2012;12:2491–2503.
25. Echaniz-Laguna A, Geuens T, Petiot P, et al. Axonal neuropathies due to mutations in small heat shock proteins: clinical, genetic, and functional insights into novel mutations. Hum Mutat 2017;38:556–568.
26. Olive M, Goldfarb L, Moreno D, et al. Desmin-related myopathy: clinical, electrophysiological, radiological, neuropathological and genetic studies. J Neurol Sci 2004;219:125–137.
27. Kennedy D, Jager R, Mosser DD, Samali A. Regulation of apoptosis by heat shock proteins. IUBMB Life 2014;66:327–338.
28. Kwon YT, Ciechanover A. The ubiquitin code in the ubiquitin-proteasome system and autophagy. Trends Biochem Sci 2017;42:873–886.
29. Tai HC, Schuman EM. Ubiquitin, the proteasome and protein degradation in neuronal function and dysfunction. Nat Rev Neurosci 2008;9:826–838.
30. Todi SV, Paulson HL. Balancing act: deubiquitinating enzymes in the nervous system. Trends Neurosci 2011;34:370–382.
31. Jedrzejowska M, Jakubowska-Pietkiewicz E, Kostera-Pruszczyk A. X-linked spinal muscular atrophy (SMAX2) caused by de novo c.1731C>T substitution in the UBA1 gene. Neuromuscul Disord 2015;25:661–666.
32. Garcia Ramirez M, Csanyi B, Martinez Anton J, Delgado Marques M, Bauzano Poley E. [Genetic and clinical diagnosis of Angelman syndrome: Case Reviews]. An Pediatr (Barc) 2008;69:232–238.
33. Gorostidi A, Marti-Masso JF, Bergareche A, Rodriguez-Oroz MC, Lopez de Munain A, Ruiz-Martinez J. Genetic mutation analysis of Parkinson's disease patients using multigene next-generation sequencing panels. Mol Diagn Ther 2016;20:481–491.
34. Weishaupl D, Schneider J, Peixoto Pinheiro B, et al. Physiological and pathophysiological characteristics of ataxin-3 isoforms. J Biol Chem 2019;294:644–661.
35. Anderson DB, Zanella CA, Henley JM, Cimarosti H. Sumoylation: implications for neurodegenerative diseases. Adv Exp Med Biol 2017;963:261–281.
36. Vijayakumaran S, Pountney DL. SUMOylation, aging and autophagy in neurodegeneration. Neurotoxicology 2018;66:53–57.
37. Thibaudeau TA, Smith DM. A practical review of proteasome pharmacology. Pharmacol Rev 2019;71:170–197.
38. Staff NP, Podratz JL, Grassner L, et al. Bortezomib alters microtubule polymerization and axonal transport in rat dorsal root ganglion neurons. Neurotoxicology 2013;39:124–131.
39. Feleciano DR, Juenemann K, Iburg M, Bras IC, Holmberg CI, Kirstein J. Crosstalk between chaperone-mediated protein disaggregation and proteolytic pathways in aging and disease. Front Aging Neurosci 2019;11:9.
40. Majcher V, Goode A, James V, Layfield R. Autophagy receptor defects and ALS-FTLD. Mol Cell Neurosci 2015;66:43–52.
41. Catarino S, Pereira P, Girao H. Molecular control of chaperone-mediated autophagy. Essays Biochem 2017;61:663–674.
42. Kaushik S, Cuervo AM. The coming of age of chaperone-mediated autophagy. Nat Rev Mol Cell Biol 2018;19:365–381.
43. Alfaro IE, Albornoz A, Molina A, et al. Chaperone mediated autophagy in the crosstalk of neurodegenerative diseases and metabolic disorders. Front Endocrinol (Lausanne) 2018;9:778.
44. Damme M, Suntio T, Saftig P, Eskelinen EL. Autophagy in neuronal cells: general principles and physiological and pathological functions. Acta Neuropathol 2015;129:337–362.
45. Chu CT. Mechanisms of selective autophagy and mitophagy: implications for neurodegenerative diseases. Neurobiol Dis 2019;122:23–34.
46. Finkbeiner S. The autophagy lysosomal pathway and neurodegeneration. Cold Spring Harb Perspect Biol 2019;12(3):a033993.
47. Muller S, Brun S, Rene F, de Seze J, Loeffler JP, Jeltsch-David H. Autophagy in neuroinflammatory diseases. Autoimmun Rev 2017;16:856–874.
48. Koyuncu S, Fatima A, Gutierrez-Garcia R, Vilchez D. Proteostasis of Huntingtin in health and disease. Int J Mol Sci 2017;18.
49. Menzies FM, Fleming A, Caricasole A, et al. Autophagy and neurodegeneration: pathogenic mechanisms and therapeutic opportunities. Neuron 2017;93:1015–1034.
50. Caballero B, Wang Y, Diaz A, et al. Interplay of pathogenic forms of human tau with different autophagic pathways. Aging Cell 2018;17:(1):e12692.
51. Kinghorn KJ, Asghari AM, Castillo-Quan JI. The emerging role of autophagic-lysosomal dysfunction in Gaucher disease and Parkinson's disease. Neural Regen Res 2017;12:380–384.
52. Maiti P, Manna J, Dunbar GL. Current understanding of the molecular mechanisms in Parkinson's disease: targets for potential treatments. Transl Neurodegener 2017;6:28.
53. Martinez-Vicente M. Autophagy in neurodegenerative diseases: from pathogenic dysfunction to therapeutic modulation. Semin Cell Dev Biol 2015;40:115–126.
54. Douglas PM, Dillin A. Protein homeostasis and aging in neurodegeneration. J Cell Biol 2010 Sep 6;190(5):719–729.
55. Hetz C, Mollereau B. Disturbance of endoplasmic reticulum proteostasis in neurodegenerative diseases. Nat Rev Neurosci 2014;15:233–249.
56. Cabral-Miranda F, Hetz C. ER stress and neurodegenerative disease: a cause or effect relationship? Curr Top Microbiol Immunol 2018;414:131–157.
57. Medinas DB, Rozas P, Martinez Traub F, et al. Endoplasmic reticulum stress leads to accumulation of wild-type SOD1 aggregates associated with sporadic amyotrophic lateral sclerosis. Proc Natl Acad Sci U S A 2018;115:8209–8214.

58. Roussel BD, Kruppa AJ, Miranda E, Crowther DC, Lomas DA, Marciniak SJ. Endoplasmic reticulum dysfunction in neurological disease. Lancet Neurol 2013;12:105–118.
59. Scheckel C, Aguzzi A. Prions, prionoids and protein misfolding disorders. Nat Rev Genet 2018;19:405–418.
60. Kara E, Marks JD, Aguzzi A. Toxic protein spread in neurodegeneration: reality versus fantasy. Trends Mol Med 2018;24:1007–1020.
61. Duyckaerts C, Clavaguera F, Potier MC. The prion-like propagation hypothesis in Alzheimer's and Parkinson's disease. Curr Opin Neurol 2019;32:266–271.
62. Tamguney G, Korczyn AD. A critical review of the prion hypothesis of human synucleinopathies. Cell Tissue Res 2018;373:213–220.
63. Yoshinaga T, Yazaki M, Sekijima Y, et al. The pathological and biochemical identification of possible seed-lesions of transmitted transthyretin amyloidosis after domino liver transplantation. J Pathol Clin Res 2016;2:72–79.
64. Li JY, Englund E, Holton JL, et al. Lewy bodies in grafted neurons in subjects with Parkinson's disease suggest host-to-graft disease propagation. Nat Med 2008;14:501–503.
65. Prusiner SB, Woerman AL, Mordes DA, et al. Evidence for alpha-synuclein prions causing multiple system atrophy in humans with parkinsonism. Proc Natl Acad Sci U S A 2015;112:E5308–5317.
66. Peelaerts W, Bousset L, Baekelandt V, Melki R. a-Synuclein strains and seeding in Parkinson's disease, incidental Lewy body disease, dementia with Lewy bodies and multiple system atrophy: similarities and differences. Cell Tissue Res 2018;373:195–212.
67. Woerman AL, Kazmi SA, Patel S, et al. Familial Parkinson's point mutation abolishes multiple system atrophy prion replication. Proc Natl Acad Sci U S A 2018;115:409–414.
68. Steiner JA, Quansah E, Brundin P. The concept of alpha-synuclein as a prion-like protein: ten years after. Cell Tissue Res 2018;373:161–173.
69. Ayers JI, Giasson BI, Borchelt DR. Prion-like spreading in tauopathies. Biol Psychiatry 2018;83:337–346.
70. Zhang X, Gao F, Wang D, et al. Tau pathology in Parkinson's disease. Front Neurol 2018;9:809.
71. Liu S, Hossinger A, Gobbels S, Vorberg IM. Prions on the run: how extracellular vesicles serve as delivery vehicles for self-templating protein aggregates. Prion 2017;11:98–112.
72. Watts JC, Bourkas MEC, Arshad H. The function of the cellular prion protein in health and disease. Acta Neuropathol 2018;135:159–178.
73. Ansar M, Santos-Cortez RL, Saqib MA, et al. Mutation of ATF6 causes autosomal recessive achromatopsia. Hum Genet 2015;134:941–950.
74. Roussel BD, Lomas DA, Crowther DC. Progressive myoclonus epilepsy associated with neuroserpin inclusion bodies (neuroserpinosis). Epileptic Disord 2016;18:103–110.
75. Dobson-Stone C, Hallupp M, Shahheydari H, et al. CYLD is a causative gene for frontotemporal dementia—amyotrophic lateral sclerosis. Brain 2020;143:783–799.
76. Al-Obeidi E, Al-Tahan S, Surampalli A, et al. Genotype-phenotype study in patients with valosin-containing protein mutations associated with multisystem proteinopathy. Clin Genet 2018;93:119–125.
77. Brown RH, Jr., Al-Chalabi A. Amyotrophic lateral sclerosis. N Engl J Med 2017;377:1602.
78. Freischmidt A, Muller K, Ludolph AC, Weishaupt JH, Andersen PM. Association of mutations in TBK1 with sporadic and familial amyotrophic lateral sclerosis and frontotemporal dementia. JAMA Neurol 2017;74:110–113.

7 Vesicular Trafficking

OVERVIEW

The complex membrane organization of cells allows the compartmentalization of cellular processes within plasma membrane domains and specialized membrane-bound organelles. They include the endoplasmic reticulum (ER), Golgi complex, secretory vesicles, endosomes, autophagosomes, lysosomes, and intermediate organelles. These structures participate in three fundamental cellular pathways, the secretory pathway, endocytic pathway, and autophagy (Figure 7.1). The secretory pathway starts when proteins mature in the ER, is followed by cargo modification and then sorting in the Golgi complex, and ends with cargo targeting to either the cell membrane or specific organelles such as lysosomes. The secretory pathway also allows the release of neurochemical signals for intercellular communication. The endocytic pathway starts with the internalization of material via early endosomes, which mature to late endosomes. Endocytosed material may be recycled back to the different cell compartments via recycling endosomes, transported back to the cell body via retromer complexes, or delivered for degradation by the lysosome either directly or via the formation of multivesicular bodies (MVBs). Lysosomes are also the final site of degradation of material delivered by the autophagosome (autophagy). The contents from MVBs can be released to the extracellular space via exosomes. All these highly regulated processes involve complex interactions among many transmembrane, cytoskeletal, and adaptor proteins and membrane lipids. Impairment in vesicular biogenesis and dynamics is a prominent disease mechanism in many neurodegenerative disorders. The aims of this chapter are to review: (1) the mechanisms of vesicular trafficking in the secretory and endosome pathways; (2) the formation and maturation of autophagosomes; (3) the functions of the lysosomes; and (4) representative examples of disorders resulting from disturbances of vesicular trafficking.

GENERAL PROCESSES INVOLVED IN VESICULAR DYNAMICS

Vesicular trafficking involves tightly regulated processes, including vesicular biogenesis, transport along microtubules, and tethering and fusion of the vesicle membrane with the recipient compartment (Figure 7.2). During vesicular transport, lipid molecules are sorted into membrane vesicles that bud out of the donor membrane and travel to and then fuse with the recipient membrane.

Vesicular Biogenesis

Vesicular biogenesis involves molecular events that result in protein segregation in discrete membrane domains leading to focal membrane deformation (nucleation) followed by scission of a donor membrane forming a vesicle. Membrane nucleation requires coat proteins, such as coat complex (COP) proteins and clathrin. These coat proteins become linked to the cytoplasmic face of a donor membrane via adaptor proteins, and elicit focal changes in the shape of the membrane into curved structures. COPII-coated vesicles transport cargo from the ER to the Golgi apparatus, whereas COPI-coated vesicles mediate intra-Golgi transport and Golgi-to-ER retrograde transport. Clathrin-coated vesicles mediate endocytosis followed by transport from the endosomes to the Golgi apparatus as well as transport from the Golgi apparatus to endosomes.

Different membrane compartments have unique compositions of lipids, which are transported between compartments and have a major role in vesicular formation and dynamics. The formation of a curvature of the membrane around the coat involves the interaction of membrane-binding proteins with phospholipids and sphingolipids. The shape of the

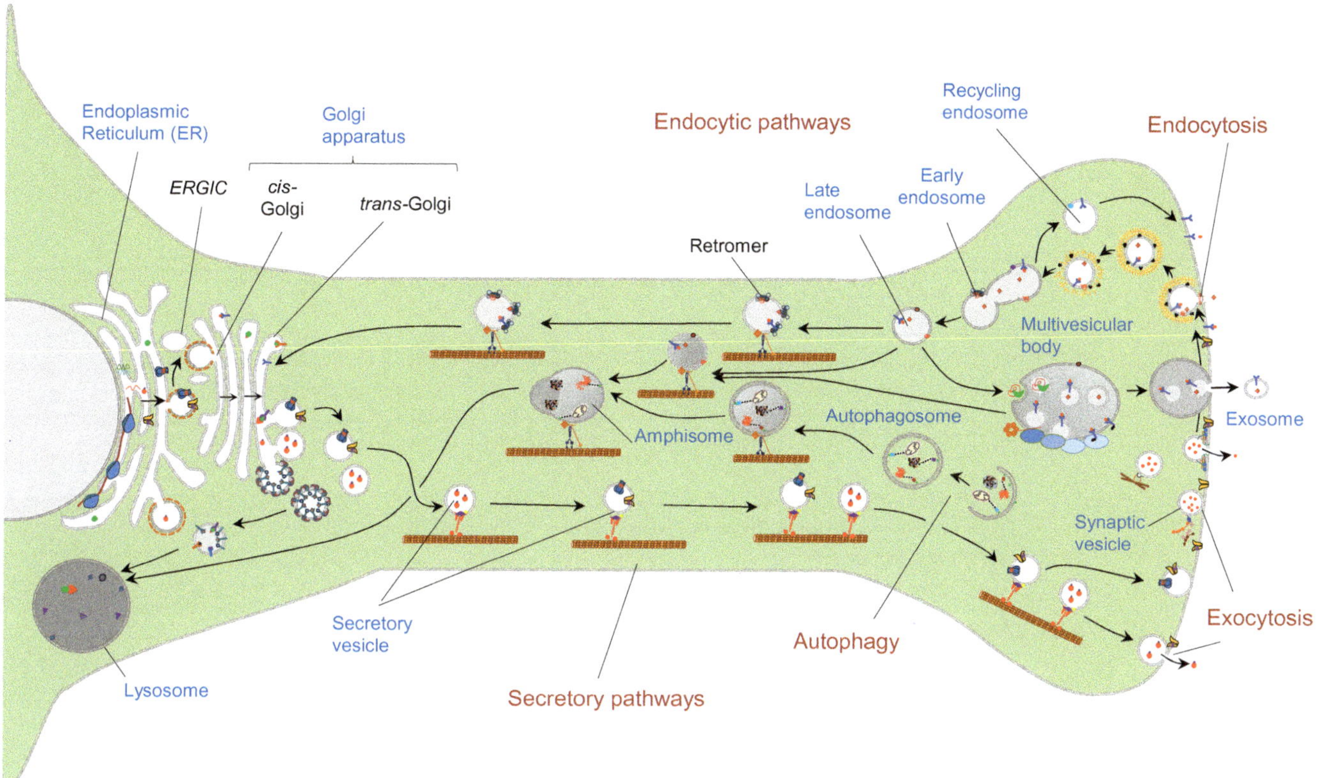

FIGURE 7.1 Overview of vesicular trafficking.
The membrane compartments involved in vesicular trafficking in cells include the endoplasmic reticulum (ER), the Golgi complex, secretory vesicles, endosomes, lysosomes, and intermediate organelles. The secretory pathway starts in the ER, is followed by cargo modification and sorting in the Golgi complex, and ends either in the cell membrane or in specific intracellular organelles. The endocytic pathway starts with the internalization of material via early endosomes that mature to late endosomes. Endocytosed material may also be recycled back to the different cell compartments via recycling endosomes. Content from late endosomes can be transported back to the cell body via retromer complexes; or delivered for degradation by the lysosome, either directly or via the formation of multivesicular bodies (MVBs). Lysosomes are also the final site of degradation of macromolecules, protein aggregates, and damaged organelles delivered by the autophagosome (autophagy). Autophagosomes may fuse with late endosomes to form amphysomes, that then fuse with the lysosome. The contents from MVBs can be released to the extracellular space via exosomes.

individual membrane lipid depends both on the size of the head group and the length and saturation of the acyl chains, and determines the direction of the membrane curvature, resulting either in invagination or evagination of the membrane. As the spherical bud begins to emerge, a tubular neck region begins to form in the membrane, aided by longitudinal force generated through interactions with the actin cytoskeleton. This is followed by vesicle pinch-off, or scission, which depends on dynamin, a guanosine triphosphatase (GTPase).

Once the vesicles are released from the donor membrane, heat shock protein (Hsp) chaperones and co-chaperones remove the clathrin coat.

Roles of Small GTPases and SNARE Proteins

Small GTPases function as molecular switches during vesicular transport and membrane trafficking, by cycling between an inactive GDP-bound form in the cytosol and an active GTP-bound form recruited to membranes. Different families of small GTPases are selectively distributed in the various vesicular compartments.[1,2] The main examples are Ras-analogous in brain (Rab)-GTPases, which participate at all stages of vesicle transport, from cargo selection to docking and fusion. Soluble N-ethylmaleimide-sensitive fusion protein attachment protein receptor (SNARE) proteins are critical for vesicular fusion events. SNARE proteins are divided into vesicle (v)-SNAREs and target (t)-SNAREs and contain an extended coiled-coil stretch of α-helices that mediate their mutual interactions, which allow membrane apposition and promote membrane fusion. The subtypes of SNARE proteins involved vary according to the specific process.

Roles of Cortical Actin and Microtubule-Dependent Transport

The actin cytoskeleton organizes into different structures at different cell compartments. In neurons and in other nonmuscle cells, actin filaments formed close to surface of

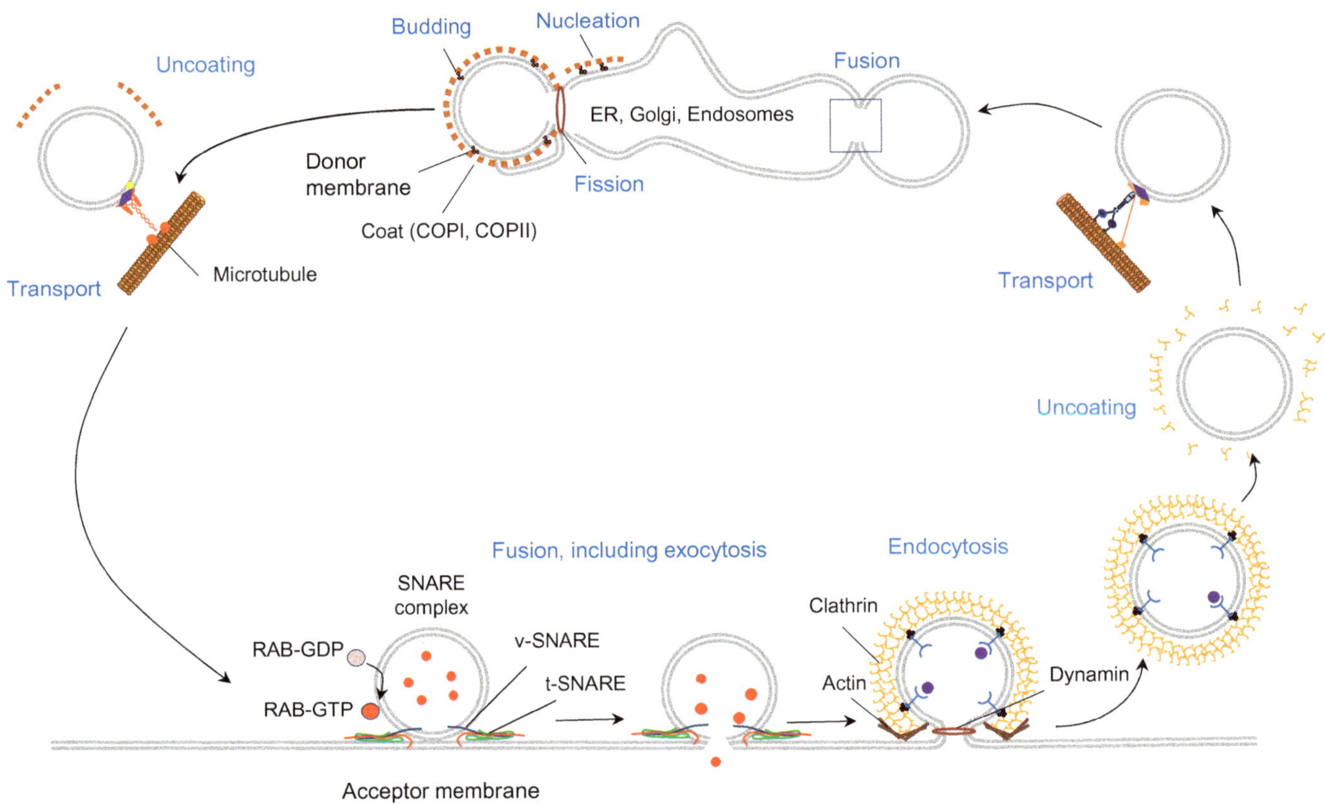

FIGURE 7.2 Processes involved in vesicular trafficking.
Vesicular biogenesis requires focal membrane deformation (nucleation) followed by scission of a donor membrane forming a vesicle. Membrane nucleation involves coat proteins. As the spherical bud begins to emerge, longitudinal forces generated through interactions with the actin cytoskeleton lead to the formation of a neck followed by vesicle pinch-off or scission, dependent on dynamin. Small RAB-GTPases function as molecular switches during vesicular transport and membrane trafficking. Soluble N-ethylmaleimide-sensitive fusion protein attachment protein receptor (SNARE) proteins are critical for vesicular fusion events. SNARE proteins are divided into vesicle (v)-SNAREs and target (t)-SNAREs. Intracellular transport of membrane cargo primarily occurs along microtubules.

membranes form a cortical actin network that controls both the functional topography of the plasma membrane and vesicular trafficking. Cortical actin modifies the physical properties of membrane such as tension, curvature, and diffusion of proteins and lipids; restricts secretory vesicle movement; interacts with their fusion and fission pores, and controls biogenesis of endosomes. The close proximity to the plasma membrane allows the interaction of the cortical actin network with the machinery for both exocytosis and endocytosis.[3] Intracellular transport of membrane cargo primarily occurs along microtubules. This requires the interaction of vesicular adaptor proteins with ATP-dependent molecular motors, including kinesins and the dynein/dynactin complex.

SECRETORY PATHWAY

Secretory proteins are synthesized on ER-bound ribosomes and translocated into the ER lumen, where they are folded, assembled, and glycosylated. Proteins are then sorted into budding vesicles that exit the ER and are transported forward to the Golgi complex, both directly and via the ER-Golgi complex intermediate compartment (ERGIC). After passing through the Golgi complex, where they are further modified, the different cargoes are sorted at the trans-Golgi network (TGN) via specialized vesicular carriers and then shipped out to the plasma membrane, lysosomes, or other destinations (Figure 7.1).

Endoplasmic Reticulum

The ER is a dynamic interconnected continuous membrane system that includes the nuclear envelope and the peripheral ER consisting of rough ER containing ribosomes, smooth ER, and the cortical ER. In neurons, the rough ER occupies the soma and proximal dendrites, particularly at branching points and close to synapses; the smooth ER predominates in more distal dendrites and forms a continuous tubular network along the axon. The ER maintains contact with other organelles such as mitochondria, plasma membrane, Golgi complex, and endosomes. The ER is the site for protein maturation, quality control, and response to misfolded proteins; participates in membrane sphingolipid biogenesis; and has a critical role in intracellular Ca^{2+} homeostasis.[4] The dendritic ER extends in dendrite spines, where it can adopt a conformation of stacked cisternae called the spine apparatus. The local production and supply of proteins at dendrites depends on localization of mRNAs at this level.

The morphology and dynamics of the ER depend on a large number of proteins that affect the curvature and remodeling the phospholipid bilayer and mediate ER interactions with the cytoskeleton (Figure 7.3). They include Reticulon proteins, related receptor-expression-enhancing proteins (REEPs) 1 and 2, atlastatin, and spastin. Reticulon proteins contribute to the bending of the membrane. Spastin severs microtubules and couples ER membrane remodeling with cytoskeletal dynamics. Atlastatin is a GTPase involved in formation of three-way junctions in the tubular ER. Mutations of these proteins are linked to autosomal dominant hereditary spastic paraplegia.[5–8] After properly folded, proteins and oligomers assembled in the ER and destined for the secretory pathway are selectively sorted and concentrated at specific domains of the membrane called ER exit sites. At these sites, the future secretory vesicles are coated with the COPII protein complex, bud off the ER, and then lose their coat. Vesicles then fuse with pre-Golgi intermediates in the ERGIC, which is a dynamic compartment that participates in bidirectional vesicular trafficking between the ER and the Golgi apparatus via interactions with microtubules.

Golgi Complex

The Golgi complex consists of flattened cisternae that are aligned in a parallel manner to form several stacks.[9] The Golgi complex includes the *cis*-Golgi network, which receives material from ER and contains glycosylation

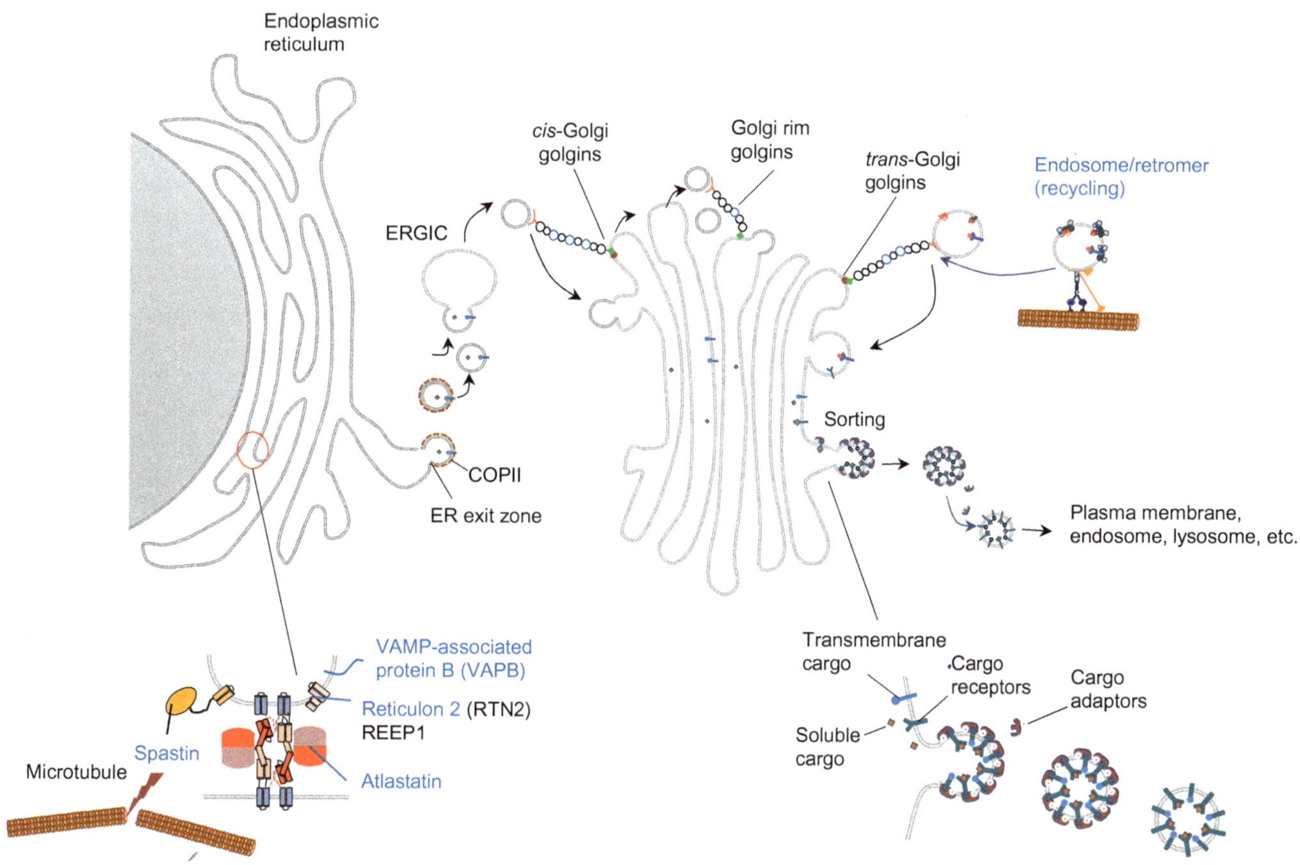

FIGURE 7.3 Biogenesis of the components of the secretory pathway.
Proteins involved in the formation and dynamics of the of the ER include Reticulon and related receptor-expression-enhancing proteins (REEPs), atlastatin-1, and spastin Golgins and are necessary for tethering events for membrane fusion, maintenance of Golgi cisternae, and interactions with the cytoskeleton. Vesicular sorting at the TGN (trans-Golgi network) involves recruitment of cytosolic cargo adaptors that recognize specific sorting signals within the cytosolic domains of transmembrane cargo molecules. Some proteins, in particular luminal proteins, are associated with cargo adaptors indirectly through transmembrane cargo receptors.

enzymes that process cargo proteins and lipids; and the TGN, which is the site of sorting of cargoes to their different post-Golgi compartments (Figure 7.3). The Golgi membranes also have a microtubule-organizing function in neurons. Posttranslational modifications of proteins at the Golgi complex include glycosylation, sulfation, phosphorylation, and proteolytic cleavage. Retrograde carriers recycle ER resident and misfolded proteins, signaling proteins, and proteins back to the ER while secretory cargo is moved onward through the Golgi stalks. In addition to sorting cargo for exit from the Golgi, the TGN also receives incoming material trafficked primarily via the endosome compartments. The Golgi apparatus is therefore a hub for membrane trafficking, given its central position in the secretory pathway and its interface with the endosomal system. The complexity of trafficking at the Golgi requires the highly specific recognition of transport vesicles at the various regions of this organelle. The structural integrity and interactions of the Golgi apparatus depend on proteins called golgins (Figure 7.3).[10] Golgins are necessary for tethering events for membrane fusion, maintenance of Golgi cisternae, and interactions with the cytoskeleton. Golgins are anchored to the Golgi membrane either directly or through binding to membrane-associated small GTPases, and may extend a considerable distance from the Golgi membrane. Golgins at the cis-Golgi capture vesicles bringing cargo from the ER, those at the cisternae rims tether intra-Golgi transport vesicles, and golgins at the TGN selectively capture endosome-derived vesicles. The Golgi apparatus depends on its interaction with microtubules to maintain its normal morphology. This interaction is requires a golgin called bicaudal D, which recruits the dynein/dynactin complex bound to microtubules. Mutation of the *BICD2* gene encoding Bicaudal 2 causes a dominant form of distal lower limb predominant spinal muscular atrophy (SMALED2).[11]

Cargo Sorting at the Trans-Golgi Network

At the TGN, proteins and lipids are sorted and packed into specific vesicles that utilize different trafficking routes for delivery of their cargoes to their final destinations.[12] Vesicular sorting involves recruitment of cytosolic cargo adaptors to the TGN membrane; these cargo adaptors recognize specific sorting signals within the cytosolic domains of transmembrane cargo molecules (Figure 7.3). Some proteins, in particular luminal proteins, associate with cargo adaptors indirectly through transmembrane cargo receptors, such as those that sort proteins to the lysosome. Many soluble enzymes are modified within the Golgi complex by the addition of mannose 6 phosphate and are then recognized by mannose 6 phosphate receptors (M6PRs) that mediate their sorting to the lysosome. The M6PR is localized not only at the TGN and endosomes but also at the plasma membrane and thus allows retrieval of extracellular proteins to be rerouted back to the endosomal and then the lysosomal compartment. This provides the basis for enzyme-replacement therapy for lysosomal disease.

TYPES OF SECRETORY PATHWAYS

Constitutive Versus Regulated Pathway

The constitutive pathway provides newly synthesized proteins and lipids to the membrane. Cargoes for this pathway include transmembrane proteins such as ion channels and receptors, which are packaged into common vesicles at the TGN and steadily delivered to the plasma membrane. The regulated pathway is responsible for the release of neuropeptides, trophic factors, and other signals for intercellular communication. In this pathway, after vesicles bud off from the TGN, they undergo a maturation process that creates secretion-competent dense core granules that are transported to nerve terminals, where the material is released to the extracellular space in response to a signal leading to influx of calcium (Ca^{2+}).

Synaptic Vesicle Exocytosis as a Special Form of Regulated Secretion

Release at classical neurotransmitters via exocytosis of synaptic vesicles at presynaptic active zones is a specialized and fast variant of secretory pathway (Figure 7.4). The presynaptic terminal harbors synaptic vesicles containing the chemical transmitters. In contrast to the regulated secretion of neuropeptides and growth factors, which are synthesized in the cell bodies, stored in secretory granules, and transported along the axons that reach the presynaptic terminals, exocytosis of synaptic vesicles is a fast process in which the neurotransmitters are synthesized and then stored in vesicles at the presynaptic terminals. These presynaptic terminals contain active zones that harbor clustered voltage-gated Ca^{2+}channels, which allows large Ca^{2+} influx in response to an action potential and fast release of neurotransmitter. The synchronous fusion of synaptic vesicles with the presynaptic membrane is mediated by a canonical SNARE mechanism involving the interaction of synaptic vesicle synaptobrevin (vesicle-associated membrane protein, VAMP) and the presynaptic plasma membrane syntaxin-1 and synaptosomal-associated protein-25 (SNAP-25). At presynaptic terminals, exocytosis depends on synaptotagmins, which are Ca^{2+}-sensing proteins located in the membrane of synaptic vesicles. Other important proteins involved in this process include Munc18 and complexin. SNAREs undergo a regulated assembly–disassembly cycle that involves the ATPase NSF (for N-ethylmaleimide-sensitive factor) acting via adaptor proteins called SNAPs (for soluble NSF-attachment proteins).

ENDOCYTIC PATHWAY

Endocytosis is the uptake of membrane surface and extracellular material by invagination or pinching off of the plasma membrane, resulting in the formation of an endosome. Endocytosis regulates several critical processes in neurons, including synaptic vesicle recycling, retrograde neurotrophic signaling, turnover and degradation of receptors and other

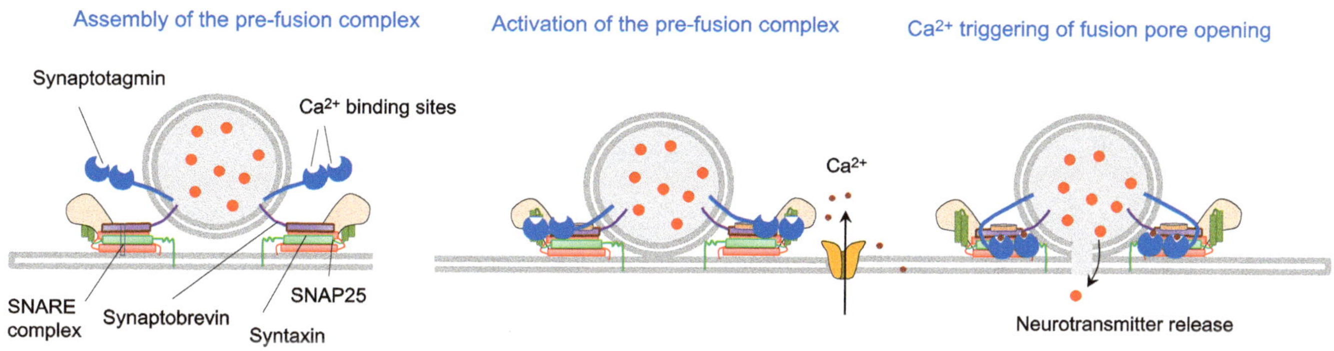

FIGURE 7.4 Exocytosis of synaptic vesicles.
Synchronous fusion of synaptic vesicles with the presynaptic membrane is mediated by the canonical SNARE mechanism involving the interaction of synaptic vesicle synaptobrevin 2 and the presynaptic plasma membrane syntaxin-1 and synaptosomal-associated protein-25 (SNAP-25). At presynaptic terminals, exocytosis depends on synaptotagmins, which are Ca^{2+}-sensing proteins located in the membrane of synaptic vesicles.

membrane proteins, synaptic plasticity, and axonal pathfinding during development.[13] Endocytosis is tightly coupled to exocytosis and retrieves the fused synaptic vesicle components from the neuronal surface, which is necessary to sustain a high rate of neurotransmission without depleting the recycling vesicle pools. Nerve growth factor and brain-derived neurotrophic factor are incorporated by endocytosis bound to their respective receptors in synaptic terminals, incorporated into endosomes, and transported back to the cell body. There are several forms of endocytosis. Clathrin-mediated endocytosis is the best-characterized endocytic pathway and the predominant route of vesicle retrieval. Bulk endocytosis internalizes a large area of plasma membrane, forming an endosome-like endocytic structure. The kiss-and-run mode of endocytosis represents the fast component of endocytosis, during which synaptic vesicles release their contents through a transient fusion pore and are retrieved rapidly without full collapse into the plasma membrane.

Clathrin-Mediated Endocytosis

Clathrin-mediated endocytosis involves four major steps: clathrin coat recruitment, vesicle budding, vesicle fission, and vesicle uncoating. These processes involve sequential recruitment of endocytic proteins[13,14] (Figure 7.5). The factors involved in initiation of endocytosis assemble at membrane sites enriched in phosphatidylinositol bisphosphate (PIP2) and generate a membrane template for clathrin assembly. Clathrin is composed by three large and three small polypeptide chains, which assemble to form a triskelion producing a basket-like lattice structure responsible for the formation of coated pits on the cytosolic phase of the membrane. Clathrin-mediated endocytosis is initiated at the presynaptic membrane by recruitment of the adaptor protein 2 (AP2) complex. The sequential steps involve the assembly and disassembly of protein scaffolds that bind acidic membrane phospholipids and stabilize or induce membrane curvature. These proteins are sequentially recruited and include epsin, endophilin, synaptojanin, and amphiphysin. Endophilin promotes membrane invagination by altering the composition of the donor membrane and recruits synaptojanin, a phosphatase that hydrolyzes PIP2 at the neck of the coated pits. The modular structure of some accessory proteins provides a scaffold for the assembly of other factors that synergistically stimulate nucleation of actin, which is necessary for elongation (tubulation) of the neck of the clathrin-coated vesicle. The last step of endocytosis is vesicular fission by action of dynamin. Amphiphysin recruits dynamin to tubular clathrin-coated pits, and promotes the GTPase activity of dynamin. Vesicular fission is followed by vesicle uncoating, which requires the actions of synaptojanin, the Hsp70 known as heat shock cognate protein 70 (Hsc70), and the Hsp40 co-chaperone auxilin (DNAJC6).

Altered endocytosis is an important mechanism in Parkinson disease (PD), as discussed later; for example, *SYNJ1* (synaptojanin) or *DNAJC6* (auxilin) mutations are linked with early-onset PD. The machinery for endocytosis is highly regulated and participates in other processes. For example, endophilin is functionally connected with the E3 ubiquitin ligase parkin and with leucine-rich repeat kinase 2 (LRRK2). LRKK2 phosphorylates the domain of endophilin that is critical for endocytosis and thus regulates the synaptic vesicle cycle.[15]

Role of Alpha-Synuclein in Synaptic Vesicle Cycling

Alpha-synuclein (α-SYN), encoded by the *SNCA1/PARK1* gene, is abundant at presynaptic terminals and interacts with synaptic vesicles to modulate membrane remodeling and vesicle recycling at nerve terminals.[16] It contains an N-terminal domain that interacts with membrane phospholipids, a hydrophobic domain, and a hydrophilic C-terminal domain with chaperone-like activity. Alpha-synuclein senses membrane curvatures and adopts an α-helix conformation upon interaction with negatively charged membrane lipids in the

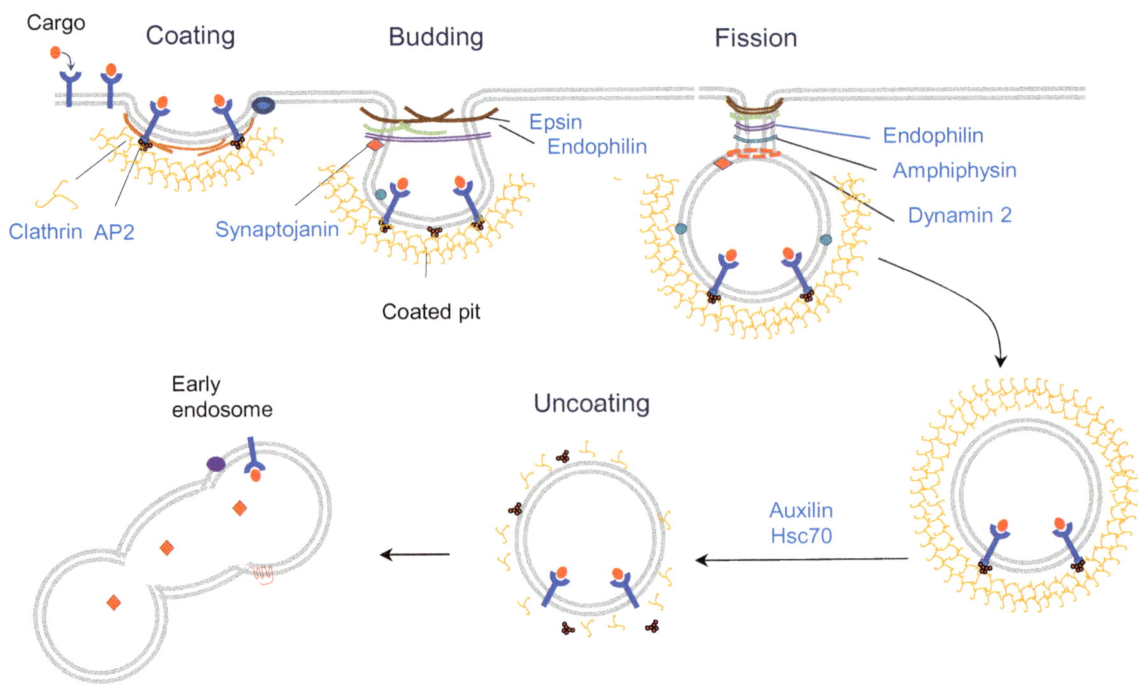

FIGURE 7.5 Clathrin-mediated endocytosis.
Clathrin-mediated endocytosis involves clathrin coat recruitment, vesicle budding, vesicle fission, and vesicle uncoating. The adaptor protein 2 (AP2) recruits clathrin; then clathrin-covered plasma membrane undergoes massive remodeling and invagination, resulting in the formation of clathrin-coated pits. Proteins involved in these processes include synaptojanin, endophilin, and amphiphysin. Membrane fission by dynamin is followed by disassembly of the clathrin coat. This involves the Hsp70 family member heat shock cognate protein 70 (Hsc70), aided by the Hsp40 chaperone auxilin (DNAJC6).

membrane of the synaptic vesicles. In the cytosol, α-SYN monomers may oligomerize stepwise and aggregate into β-sheet-rich amyloid fibrils.[17] Alpha-synuclein functions as a molecular chaperone that prevents the accumulation of unfolded or partly folded SNARE proteins, and thus has a critical role in the docking, priming, and fusion steps of exocytosis. For this chaperone function, α-SYN may cooperate with the co-chaperone cysteine string protein-α (CSPα, DNAJ5) to stabilize monomeric SNAP-25 and thus facilitate SNARE complex formation. The N-terminal α-helix is necessary for the regulatory role of α-SYN in receptor internalization and endocytosis. It also facilitates SNARE assembly by simultaneous binding to synaptobrevin and to membrane phospholipids, thereby functioning to bridge secretory vesicles and plasma membrane. Alpha-synuclein also promotes vesicle clustering and is involved in the vesicle priming stage and dilation of fusion pores during vesicle fusion. In contrast, both monomers and oligomers impair clathrin-mediated endocytosis; monomers impair clathrin uncoating, whereas dimeric α-SYN may impair vesicle fission.

Caveola-Mediated Endocytosis

Caveolae are small, flask-shaped invaginations of the plasma membrane that mediate endocytosis primarily at the cholesterol-rich lipid raft domains. Caveola-mediated endocytosis has an important role in neurotransmitter and calcium signaling, lipid regulation, and mechanosensation in muscle and other tissues. Caveolae are highly enriched of transmembrane scaffold proteins called caveolins, which recruit signaling proteins into the lipid rafts. Interactions among these proteins may either increase or dampen neurotransmitter signaling. For example, caveolin-receptor interactions may facilitate endocytosis and downregulation of G protein-coupled receptors following agonist binding. Caveolin-3 is the principal structural component of caveolae in skeletal muscle. Dominant mutations in the caveolin-3 *CAV3* gene cause a broad spectrum of clinical phenotypes, ranging from isolated hyperCKemia, to rippling muscle disease, to the most severe limb girdle muscular dystrophy and cardiomyopathy. These myopathies are associated with dramatic decrease of caveolae at the plasma membrane, resulting in abnormal response to mechanical stress.[18]

FORMATION AND MATURATION OF ENDOSOMES

The endocytic pathway is crucial for uptake of nutrients, cell surface receptor signaling, and several other key cellular processes.[19] Distinct compartments, such as early endosome, recycling endosome, late endosome, and lysosome, function in tandem to support protein recycling and degradation. Endocytic vesicles fuse with early endosomes, which function as a major sorting hub (Figure 7.6). The early endosomes allow receptor recycling back to the cell surface (rapid recycling pathway) or mature to late endosomes for receptor reuse and eventually degradation by the lysosome (degradation traffic or endolysosomal pathway).[20] Protein cargo may also be transported between the endosome and the TGN; many of the hydrolases present in the lysosome are

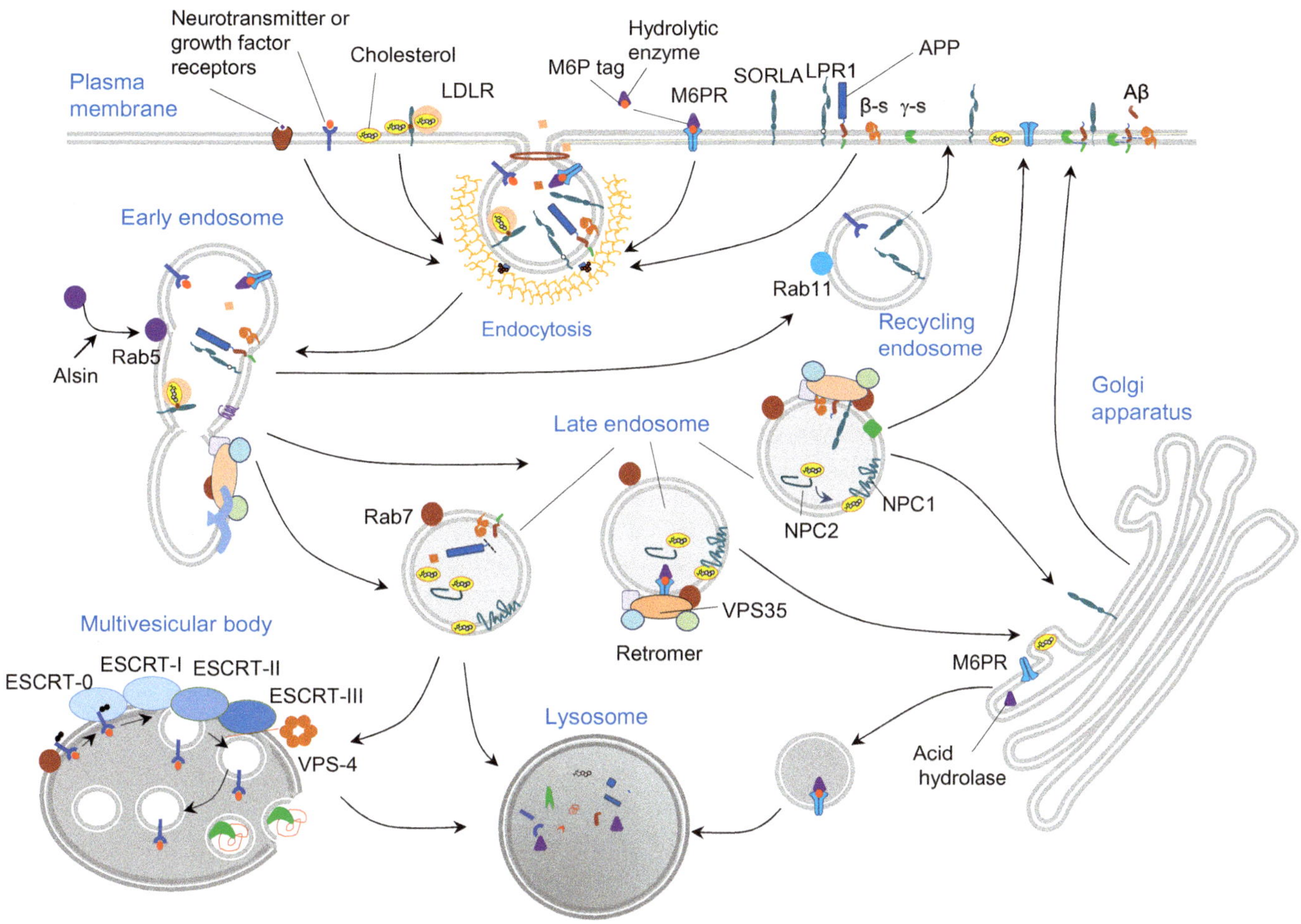

FIGURE 7.6 Formation and maturation of endosomes.

Endocytic vesicles fuse with early endosomes, which then mature to late endosomes, from which cargo proteins are sorted and delivered to several destinations. Cargo can be delivered to the lysosome either directly via formation of endolysosomes or indirectly via formation of multivesicular bodies (MVBs). Other cargoes pass through the TGN (trans-Golgi network) to be recycled to the plasma membrane or other organelles or rapidly traffic from early endosomes immediately back to the plasma membrane (rapid recycling pathway). The traffic of some cargoes from the endosome to the Golgi involves the formation of the retromer complex. Early endosomes express Rab5, which is activated by alsin, a protein mutated in familial amyotrophic lateral sclerosis (ALS). Following internalization into Rab5-containing early endosomes, cargo including receptors can rapidly recycled back to the plasma via recycling endosomes expressing Rab11, or can remain in endosomes that mature into late endosomes and MVBs via acquisition of Rab7. The retromer is recruited to endosomes and is required for shuttling of material from the endosome back to the TGN, including cation-independent mannose 6 phosphate receptors (M6PRs), amyloid precursor protein (APP), β-secretase-1, and sortilin-related receptor L with A repeats (SORLA, SORL1). The cargo recognition complex is composed of a heterotrimeric vacuolar protein-sorting (VPS) complex that includes VPS35. MVBs are formed in a process of inward invagination of endosomal membranes, via the successive recruitment of components of the endosomal sorting complex required for transport (ESCRT) complex. Neurons internalize cholesterol-containing ApoE particles bound to members of the low-density lipoproteins (LDL) receptor family. Once in the cell, cholesterol passes from the late endosome to the Golgi apparatus by action of the membrane-bound Niemann-Pick type C (NPC) protein 1 (NPC1) and its partner, the soluble protein NPC2.

recycled via this endosome–TGN transport system. Whereas newly synthesized hydrolases are trafficked via cargo receptors from the TGN to endosome for eventual transport to the lysosome, hydrolase receptors travel from endosome to TGN for reuse. This retrograde transport of cargo between endosome and TGN is mediated by a highly conserved retromer complex.[21,22]

The directionality and specificity of endosomal transport depend on several families of proteins, including Rab GTPases. The distinct endosomal compartments have distinct membrane phosphoinositide composition and expression of Rab proteins, some of them affected in neurologic disorders. Early endosomes express Rab5, a multifunctional protein that regulates early steps of endocytosis via interactions with numerous effectors, including huntingtin and huntingtin-associated protein. Rab5 is activated by the guanine-nucleotide-exchange factor alsin, encoded by the *ALS2* gene. Autosomal recessive *ALS2* mutations lead to a clinical spectrum of motor disorders including juvenile-onset amyotrophic lateral sclerosis (ALS2), primary lateral sclerosis, and hereditary spastic paraplegia.[23] Following internalization into Rab5-containing early endosomes, cargo including receptors can rapidly be recycled back to the plasma membrane via recycling endosomes expressing Rab11; or remain in endosomes that mature into late endosomes and MVBs via acquisition of Rab7. Rab7 has a critical role in vesicle recycling or targeting for degradation by the lysosome. Mutations of the *RAB7* gene produce Charcot-Marie-Tooth 2B (CMT2B), an autosomal dominant axonal primarily sensory neuropathy. These mutations enhance the cellular levels of activated Rab7 proteins, resulting in increased lysosomal activity and autophagy and impaired trafficking and signaling of neurotrophic factors; Rab7 mutations may also cause a loss of function.[24]

Retromer Complex

The retromer is a protein-trafficking complex recruited to endosomes and is required for shuttling of material from the endosome back to the TGN (Figure 7.6).[21,22] Molecules that are recycled via the retromer include cation-independent M6PR, which targets cathepsin D and other hydrolases to the lysosome; amyloid precursor protein (APP); β-secretase-1 (BACE1); sortilin-related receptor L (SORL1, SORLA), β2 adrenergic receptors, and the copper transporter ATP7A. The retromer consists of two subunits: a tubulation complex and a cargo recognition complex. The tubulation complex is responsible for remodeling of the endosomal membrane; this complex consists of several types of sorting nexins that interact with membrane phospholipids and bind to scaffold portions to induce curvature of the endosomal membrane. The cargo recognition complex is composed by a heterotrimeric vacuolar protein-sorting (VPS) complex that includes VPS35, which together with VP26 and VPS29 is responsible for recognition of and binding to cargo molecules and transport receptors. The retromer complex is recruited to the endosome via interactions of VPS35 containing heterotrimer with Rab7 present in the late endosome. Actin nucleation leads to the formation of a meshwork of actin filaments in the endosomes, which provides a driving force for retromer transport.[25]

Retromer dysfunction has recently been linked to several neurodegenerative diseases.[26] Mutations in the *VPS35* gene encoding vacuolar protein a core component of the retromer complex occurs in around 1% of late-onset, autosomal dominant familial PD.[22] Alpha-synuclein is normally degraded by lysosomal protease cathepsin, which is a cargo of the cation independent M6PR involved in retromer-mediated trafficking. A dysfunction in the retromer complex may cause improper or inefficient binding of this receptor to cathepsin D, thereby reducing the degradation of α-SYN in the lysosome. Retromer dysfunction has also been linked to amyloidogenesis in Alzheimer disease (AD). Amyloid precursor protein is normally transported to the Golgi and ultimately targeted to the plasma membrane via the secretory pathway. In the normal, non-amyloidogenic pathway, upon internalization by endocytosis, APP is cleaved sequentially by α-secretase and γ-secretase in the endosome, and then trafficked to the Golgi via the retromer and its binding partner, SORLA. In pathological amyloidogenic conditions, BACE1/β-secretase, a retromer cargo recycled between endosome and Golgi, cleaves APP at the endosome prior to γ-secretase cleavage. If there is retromer dysfunction, there is an improper recycling of both APP and BACE1, allowing residual APP to remain in the endosome and increasing APP processing via BACE1, yielding toxic amyloid-beta (Aβ) fragments.[27]

Multivesicular Bodies

Endocytic cargo can delivered to the lysosome either directly or indirectly via formation of multivesicular bodies (MVBs). Multivesicular bodies contain intraluminal vesicles that are formed in a process of inward invagination of endosomal membranes. This process is tightly controlled and depends on the successive recruitment of components of the endosomal sorting complex required for transport (ESCRT) complex[28,29] (Figure 7.6). The ESCRT complex consist of four different protein complexes. ESCRT-0 recruits the ESCRT machinery to endosomes; ESCRT-I binds ubiquitylated cargo and recruits ESCRT-II; ESCRT-II creates membrane invaginations containing ubiquitylated proteins; ESCRT-III pulls out these invaginations producing intraluminal vesicles and recruits the ATPase complex VPS4, which dissociates the ESCRT structure from the endosomal membrane. Multivesicular bodies can either be directed to lysosomes, where their content is degraded, or transported to the plasma membrane to release their content as exosomes. Like other components of the endocytic-lysosomal pathway, the ESCRT complex is involved in neurodegenerative disease. Mutations in *CHMP2B*, an ESCRT-III protein, have been identified in familial forms of frontotemporal dementia (FTD) and ALS.[30] Another ESCRT-III family protein, CHMP1B, interacts with the hereditary spastic paraplegia protein, spastin,[31] suggesting that defects in this association may compromise intracellular membrane trafficking events leading to motor neuron pathology.

Lipid Dynamics in the Endosome-Lysosome Pathway

Cholesterol and sphingolipids are synthesized and transported through the ER and Golgi systems to the plasma membrane, where they are concentrated at lipid rafts. Astrocytes secrete cholesterol bound to apolipoprotein E (ApoE) in the form of small high-density lipoprotein-like particles; neurons internalize cholesterol-containing ApoE particles by endocytosis via binding to members of the low-density lipoproteins (LDL) receptor family. Vesicles generated from the plasma membrane and formed during endocytosis are thus highly enriched with cholesterol and sphingolipids, which serve as both structural components and signaling modulators. Once in the cells cholesterol passes from the late endosome to the Golgi apparatus by action of the membrane-bound Niemann-Pick type C (NPC) protein 1 (NPC1) and its partner, the soluble lysosomal protein NPC2. From the Golgi apparatus, cholesterol is recycled back to the plasma membrane. Mutations affecting these proteins impair cholesterol trafficking and cause Niemann-Pick type C disease. Once taken into the cell, sphingolipids are either recycled back to the plasma membrane or transported through the endosomal system to the lysosome, where ceramide is degraded to produce free fatty acids and sphingosine. After egress from the lysosome, sphingosine is phosphorylated to sphingosine 1-phosphate and recruited to nascent endosomes to move to the ER, where it can be degraded by phosphatases to sphingosine and converted back to ceramide.

MACROAUTOPHAGY (AUTOPHAGY)

Macroautophagy (hereafter referred to as autophagy) is the mechanism by which macromolecules, protein aggregates, and damaged organelles such as mitochondria are targeted for degradation by the lysosomes.[32,33] Autophagy involves the formation of an autophagosome, which is transported via microtubules and fuses with lysosomes. As briefly discussed in the previous chapter, autophagosome formation involves several steps controlled by autophagy gene-encoded (ATG) proteins: membrane nucleation to form the phagophore, elongation of the phagophore, and closure of the phagophore to form the autophagosomes (Figure 7.7).

Phagophore Formation

The phagophore primarily originates from a specific ER membrane structure called the omegasome; other donors include the Golgi apparatus, endosomal membranes, plasma membrane, and ER–mitochondria contact sites. The initiation of phagophore formation requires the unc-51-like kinase (ULK) 1 complex. This step is inhibited by mechanistic (mammalian) target of rapamycin complex 1 (mTORC1) in the presence of nutrients or growth factors and activated by adenosine monophosphate-activated protein kinase (AMPK) during starvation. The next step is nucleation of the phagophore membrane, which involves the phosphatidylinositol 3'kinase class III (PI3KIII) complex, also known as vacuolar protein-sorting 34 (VPS34) complex. This complex includes components activated by ULK-1, the catalytic subunit VPS34, and the critical regulatory subunit Beclin-1. The PI3KIII/VPS34 complex relocates from the cytoskeleton to the phagophore and phosphorylates membrane phosphatidylinositol to generate phosphatidylinositol 3 phosphate. This produces cytosol-facing budding of the membrane and binds a tryptophan-aspartate (WD) repeat domain phosphoinositide interacting 1 protein (WIPI) that catalyzes the first of the next two steps that lead to elongation of the phagophore membrane.

Phagophore Elongation and Formation of the Autophagosome

Phagophore elongation involves two ubiquitin-like conjugation reactions mediated by several ATG proteins. The first reaction leads to the formation the ATG5-ATG12-ATG complex that has an ubiquitin E3 ligase-like activity. The second involves microtubule-associated protein 1 light chain 3 (LC3) and is initiated by conversion of pre-LC3 to LC3I, followed by its conjugation to phosphatidylethanolamine to yield LC3II with the help of the ATG5-ATG12-ATG6L complex. LC3II localizes to the membrane and facilitates the closure of the phagophore and formation of the autophagosome.

Maturation of the Autophagosome

Autophagy interacts with the endosome-lysosome system (Figure 7.1). In neurons, autophagosomes are mainly produced in the distal end of the axon and rapidly acquire late endosome markers such as Rab7, thereby gaining access to endosome-associated motor proteins required for their retrograde transport. Autophagosomes may merge with late endosomes to form amphisomes; axonal amphisomes and late endosomes undergo long-range retrograde transport while simultaneously maturing by acidifying their lumen and eventually fuse with mature lysosomes enriched in the cell body. Upon complete substrate degradation in the cell body, lysosomes undergo reformation to recycle membrane proteins and hydrolases for new rounds of lysosomal formation.

Single gene disorders of the autophagy may affect initiation and signaling, phagophore formation, phagophore maturation, autolysosome formation, or lysosome function.[34,35] As discussed later in this chapter, they affect various stages of central nervous system development, resulting in brain malformations, developmental delay, intellectual disability, epilepsy, movement disorders, and neurodegeneration.

LYSOSOMES

Lysosomes are the final organelles for degradation of material incorporated in vesicles via endocytosis or autophagy

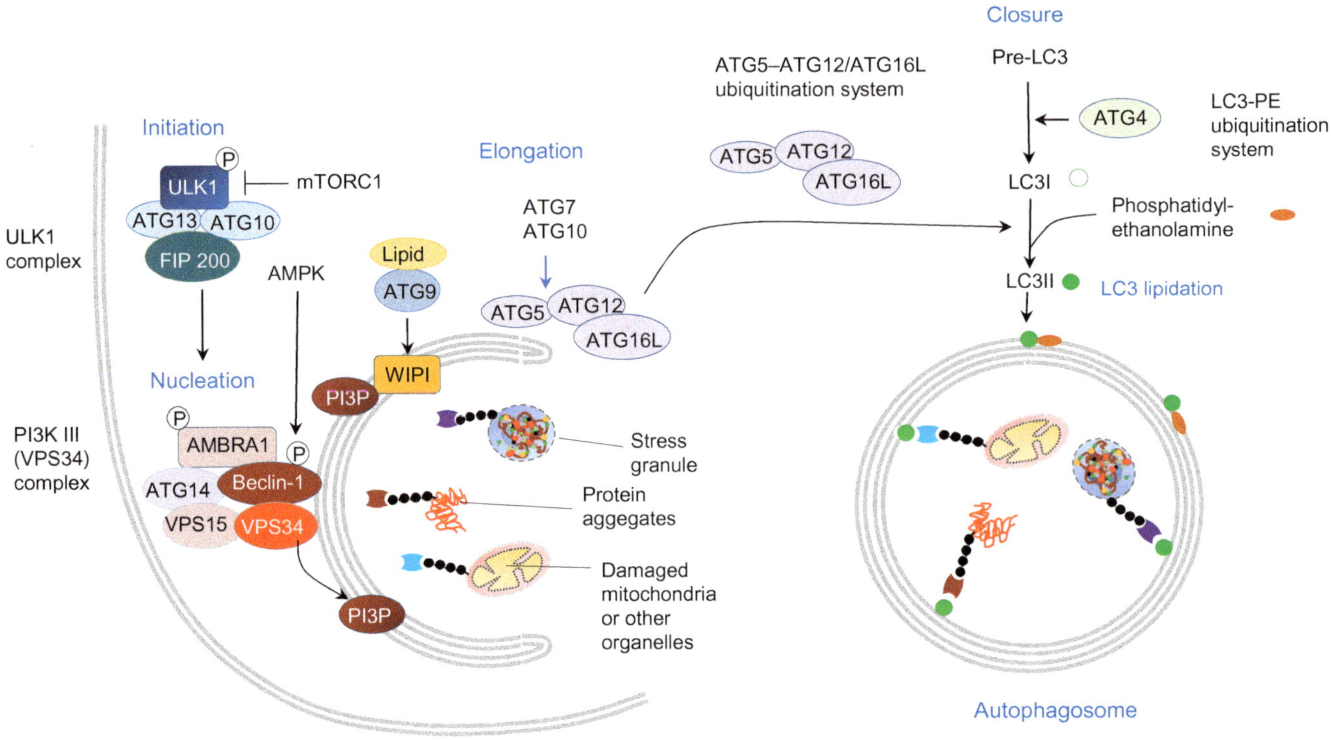

FIGURE 7.7 Formation of the autophagosome.

Formation of the autophagosomes involves several signaling events mediated by sequential activation of protein complexes encoded by autophagy (ATG) genes, including membrane nucleation to form the phagophore, elongation of the phagophore, and closure of the phagophore. The first step is the formation of the unc-51-like kinase 1(ULK1) complex, which includes ATG13, ATG101, and focal adhesion kinase (FAK) family kinase-interacting protein of 200 kD (FIP200). This first step is activated during starvation by adenosine monophosphate kinase (AMPK) and inhibited by mammalian target of rapamycin complex 1 (mTORC1). The next step is nucleation of the phagophore membrane, which involves the phosphatidylinositol 3'kinase class III (PI3KIII) also known as vacuolar protein-sorting 34 (VPS34) complex, which includes the catalytic subunit VPS34, the regulatory subunit Beclin-1, activating molecule in Beclin-1-regulated autophagy (AMBRA1), and VPS15. The PI3KII complex phosphorylates membrane phosphatidylinositol to phosphatidylinositol (3,4,5) triphosphate (PIP_3). PIP3 binds to WD (tryptophan-aspartate) repeat domain phosphoinositide-interacting 1 (WIPI) proteins and catalyzes the first of two steps that lead to elongation of the phagophore membrane. Elongation of the phagophore involves two ubiquitin-like reactions. The first is the conjugation of the ubiquitin-like molecule ATG12 to ATG5 with the help of the enzymes ATG7 and ATG10; the ATG5-ATG12 complex then combines with ATG16L1 to form the ATG5-ATG12-ATG complex, which has an E3 ligase-like activity. The second involves microtubule-associated protein 1 light chain 3 (LC3, ATG8). This is initiated by conversion of pre-LC3 to LC3I by the cysteine protease ATG4; LC3I is then conjugated to phosphatidylethanolamine to yield LC3II with the help of the ATG5-ATG12-ATG6L complex. LC3II localizes to the membrane and facilitates the closure of the phagophore.

(Figure 7.8). These spherical vesicles contain proteases, lipases, glycosidases, nucleases, and phosphatases that are optimally active at acidic pH (about 5.0). The endosomes and lysosomes maintain an acidic intravesicular pH by pumping protons (H^+ ions) from the cytosol across their membrane via the proton vacuolar ATPase (V-ATPase); this process is coupled with a countertransport of chloride (Cl^-) ions via the ClC-7 Cl^-/H^+ antiporter. Mucolipin 1 (transient receptor potential mucolipin, TRPML1) is a Ca^{2+}- and H^+-permeable cation channel that regulates the maturation of late endosomes to lysosomes. The lysosomal ATP13A2 ATPase regulates lysosomal function by functioning as a flippase transporting lipids or peptides from one membrane leaflet to the other, thereby controlling local lipid dynamics during vesicle formation and membrane fusion events.[36]

Biogenesis and Regulation by Nutritional State and Cellular Stress

Lysosome biogenesis is under the transcriptional control by transcription factor EB (TFEB).[37] TFEB is a master regulator of the lysosomal system; it coordinates the expression of lysosomal hydrolases and membrane proteins as well as autophagy proteins in response to pathways that sense nutritional conditions, lysosomal stress, and other stimuli (Figure 7.8). TFEB promotes transcription by binding to the "coordinated lysosomal expression and regulation" (CLEAR) motif

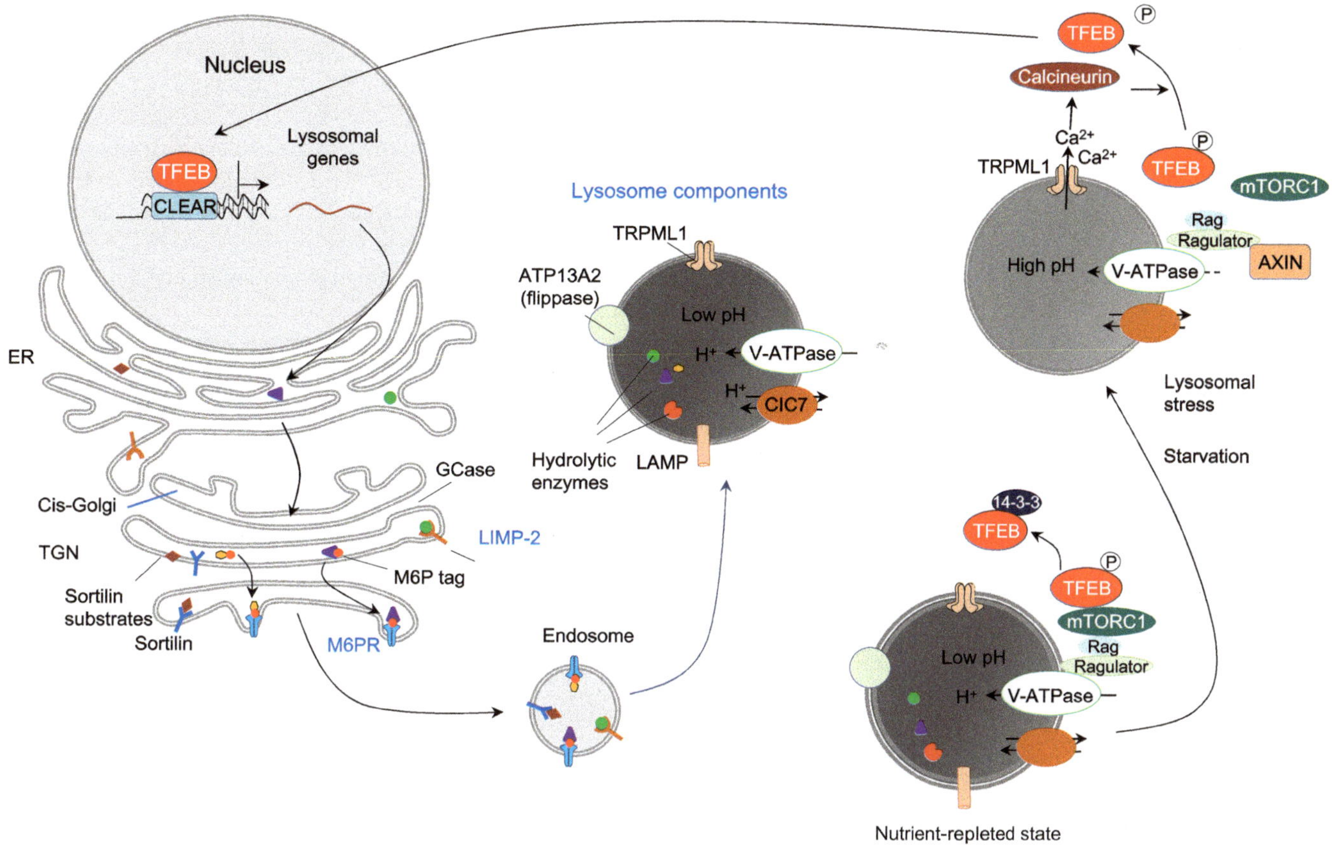

FIGURE 7.8 Lysosome biogenesis.

Lysosomes maintain an acidic intravesicular pH by pumping protons (H^+ ions) from the cytosol across their membrane via the proton vacuolar ATPase (V-ATPase); this process is coupled with a countertransport of chloride (Cl^-) ions via the ClC-7 Cl^-/H^+ antiporter. Mucolipin 1 (transient receptor potential mucolipin, TRPML1) is a Ca^{2+}- and H^+-permeable cation channel that regulates the maturation of late endosomes to lysosomes. The lysosomal ATP13A2 ATPase controls lipid dynamics during vesicle formation and membrane fusion events. Lysosome biogenesis is under the transcriptional control of transcription factor EB (TFEB), which binds to the "coordinated lysosomal expression and regulation" (CLEAR) motifs in the promoter regions of target genes. Soluble and membrane-bound proteins destined to the lysosome have sorting signals that are recognized by sorting receptors that allow proper delivery from the TGN to the endolysosomal system. These include the mannose 6 phospate receptors (M6PRs), sortilin 1, and lysosomal integral membrane protein type 2 (LIMP-2). LIMP-2 serves as a receptor for the transport of β-glucocerebrosidase (β-glucosylceramidase, GCase). Under conditions favorable for anabolism TFEB is sequestered in the cytoplasm due to its phosphorylation by mechanistic target of rapamycin complex 1 (mTORC1). The lysosome harbors a molecular complex that is able to sense multiple nutrients and consists of the V-ATPase, the amino acid transporter SLC38A9, Ragulator and Rag-GTP, which in turn recruits mechanistic mTORC1 to the lysosome. During starvation or lysosomal stress, there is formation of an alternative complex of Ragulator and V-ATPase with the scaffold protein AXIN, which causes mTORC dissociation from the lysosomal surface allowing TFEB translocation to the nucleus. Free Ca^{2+} stored in lysosomes coordinates adaptive cell responses upon release to the cytosol via mucolipin 1 (MCOLN1, TRPML1) channels, which results in activation of calcineurin and dephosphorylation TFEB, thus promoting its translocation to the nucleus.

in the promoter regions of target genes. Under conditions favorable for anabolism and cell growth, TFEB is sequestered in the cytoplasm as a consequence of its phosphorylation by active mTORC1. The lysosome harbors a molecular complex that is able to sense multiple nutrients, including amino acids, cholesterol, and glucose (Figure 7.8). In the nutritional repleted state, this complex recruits mTORC1 to the lysosome, where mTORC1 phosphorylates TFEB and prevents its translocation to the nucleus. In conditions of starvation or lysosomal stress, there is a switch to catabolic signaling and formation of an alternative complex that causes mTORC1 dissociation from the lysosomal surface. This results in dephosphorylation of TFEB, which translocates to the nucleus where it upregulates transcription of lysosomal and autophagy genes.

Free Ca^{2+} stored in lysosomes is an important signal that coordinates adaptive cell responses upon release to the cytosol via mucolipin 1 (TRPML1) channels. Several stress conditions, such as oxidative stress, which are associated with dysfunction of V-ATPase and increase in intralysosomal pH, trigger Ca^{2+} release via these channels. Focal increase in Ca^{2+} surrounding the lysosome activates calcineurin, which dephosphorylates TFEB, thus promoting its translocation to the nucleus. In addition, released lysosomal Ca^{2+} activates dynein-mediated retrograde transport of lysosomes to the perinuclear region, thereby facilitating autophagosome-lysosome fusion.

Lysosome Sorting Receptors and Membrane Proteins

As discussed earlier in this chapter, soluble and membrane-bound proteins destined to the lysosome have sorting signals recognized by sorting receptors that allow their proper delivery from the TGN to the endosomes and lysosomes.[38] They include cation-dependent and cation-independent M6PRs, lysosomal integral membrane protein type 2 (LIMP-2), sortilin, and SORLA/SORL1. Once the cargo is released in lysosomes, these receptors are recycled back to the TGN, in part via the retromer. The cation-independent M6PR is localized not only at the TGN and endosomes but also at the plasma membrane and thus allows retrieval of extracellular proteins to be rerouted back to the endosomal and then the lysosomal compartment. This provides the basis for enzyme-replacement therapy. Missing lysosomal enzymes provided exogenously can be modified with mannose 6 phosphate tags before administration, recognized by cation-independent MP6Rs in the plasma membrane, and taken from the extracellular compartment to be targeted to the lysosome. LIMP-2 serves as a receptor for the transport of β-glucocerebrosidase (GCase) from the ER to the lysosome. Sortilin allows the lysosomal sorting of the GM2 ganglioside activator prosaposin, acid sphingomyelinase, cathepsins, and progranulin. SORLA/SORL1 binds APP and is thus a central regulator of its processing by β-secretase (BACE) and γ-secretase.

The lysosome contains several lysosomal membrane proteins (LAMPs) that are involved in diverse functions, ranging from the acidification of the lysosomal lumen to the regulation of membrane fusion and fission events, import of sorting machineries, and recycling of lysosomal degradation products. For example, LAMP2A functions as a translocation factor for chaperone-mediated autophagy. Another clinically relevant example is transmembrane lysosomal protein 106B (TMEM106B), a glycoprotein that regulates lysosomal size, acidification, and transport. Increased TMEM106B expression promotes TFEB translocation to the nucleus (a marker of lysosomal stress), and reduces the number, maturation, and acidification of lysosomes.[39]

Progranulin and Lysosome Function

Progranulin, encoded by the *GRN* gene, is a highly conserved secreted protein that is expressed in the CNS and in peripheral tissues.[40] Both directly and via its conversion to granulins, progranulin regulates cell growth, survival, repair, and inflammation. Progranulin is incorporated into vesicles and follows the secretory pathway, undergoing regulated exocytosis in an activity-dependent manner. Once in the extracellular space, progranulin may either undergo cleavage to granulins by action of extracellular proteases or uptake into target cells via binding to SORLA/SORL1, which delivers progranulin via the endosome to the lysosome. Progranulin also has functional interactions with prosaposin, which functions as a molecular bridge between progranulin and M6PR, providing a direct route for progranulin to reach the lysosome. Progranulin may have several roles in formation and function of lysosomes. It binds TFEB; co-localizes with LAMP1; promotes lysosomal acidification by V-ATPases, and regulates levels of lysosomal proteins such as cathepsin D.

EXTRACELLULAR VESICLES

Extracellular vesicles are released from all cell types, including neurons and glial cells. Their composition and release vary with the state of the cell, including hypoxia and oxidative stress. There are three main types of extracellular vesicles: exosomes, microvesicles, and apoptotic bodies.[41]

Biogenesis

Exosomes originate from invagination of the endosomal-limiting membranes of intraluminal vesicles within MVBs and are released upon fusion of MVBs with the plasma membrane. The transport of MVBs to the plasma membrane depends on their interaction with actin and the microtubule cytoskeleton; fusion of MVBs with the plasma membrane for exosome release depends on SNAREs, tethering factors, and Rab GTPases. Microvesicles form by outward budding of the plasma membrane by a process that requires interactions between several membrane proteins. Apoptotic bodies are heterogeneous groups of cell fragments form during apoptosis and result from translocation of phosphatidylethanolamine from the inner to the outer leaflet of the plasma membrane. In addition to releasing apoptotic bodies and microvesicles, cells undergoing apoptosis also release exosomes that may trigger inflammatory responses.[42]

Cargo, Functions, and Potential Clinical Implication

Exosomes and microvesicles contain different proteins, lipids, and nucleic acids, and participate in intercellular communication, synaptic plasticity, maintenance of myelination, trophic support, and antigen presentation.[41,43] Extracellular vesicles provide material to target cells via receptor-ligand interactions at the surface of the membrane or internalization via endocytosis. This includes not only normal proteins but also abnormal protein aggregates. Thus extracellular vesicles may contribute to cell-to-cell propagation of abnormal fibrillary oligomers of synuclein, tau, and other proteins in neurodegenerative disease.[44] Exosomes also contain a large variety of nucleic acids, including microRNAs (miRNAs). Extracellular vesicles originating from neurons, glial cells, or endothelial cells may be present in the CSF and systemic circulation. Their transfer to the CSF increases in conditions associated with increased blood-brain barrier permeability. They can reach the systemic circulation through direct translocation into capillaries and draining venules, via the interstitial fluid into the CSF, or via meningeal lymphatics draining in the cervical lymph nodes. Extracellular vesicles have been extensively investigated as harboring potential biomarkers of neurodegeneration, including proteins and miRNAs, in disorders such as Alzheimer disease[45] and stroke.[46] Extracellular vesicles also have a role in neurodegenerative disorders in part by sequestering toxic oligomers and liberation of these oligomers from protein aggregates. As such, extracellular vesicles may also be a vehicle for prion-like propagation of misfolded proteins in neurodegenerative disorders. For example, misfolded α-SYN is secreted via exosomes in a calcium-dependent manner and by this mechanism propagates its cytotoxicity when taken up by neighboring cells. Rab11 participates in this process by recycling and secreting extracellular α-SYN via exocytosis.

IMPAIRED VESICULAR TRAFFICKING AS MAJOR MECHANISM OF NEUROLOGIC DISEASE

Disturbances of vesicular biogenesis and trafficking are increasingly recognized as a major disease mechanism in neurodegeneration. As discussed in the previous sections of this chapter, these alterations may be due to mutations affecting critical proteins involved in these processes. However, age-related processes such as oxidative stress can also affect vesicular dynamics. There are several comprehensive reviews on all these topics.[27,31–47] Disorders of vesicular biogenesis and dynamics manifest with overlapping phenotypes affecting motor neurons, including hereditary spastic paraplegia (Table 7.1), familial ALS, distal hereditary motor neuropathies (dHMN); spinal muscular atrophy (SMA) and axonal forms of Charcot-Marie-Tooth disease (CMT2) (Table 7.2). Impaired vesicular and maturation are also major disease mechanisms in PD, AD, frontotemporal lobar degeneration (FTLD) and Huntington disease (HD).

Hereditary Spastic Paraplegia

Several forms of hereditary spastic paraplegia (*SPG*–spastic gait genes) are associated with mutations linked to abnormalities in membrane trafficking and transport resulting in dying back axonopathy.[5–8,48] For example, autosomal dominant, uncomplicated hereditary spastic paraplegia has been linked to mutations of genes encoding proteins involved in ER shaping and modeling. The most common adult-onset form is SPG4, due to spastin mutations (*SPAST, SPG4*), which account for 40% of adult-onset cases. The most common early-onset form is SPG3, associated with atlastin-1 mutations. Other mutations associated with this phenotype include those of genes encoding Reticulon 2 (*RTN2, SPG12*), REEP1 (*SPG31*), and REEP2 (*SPG72*). Autosomal recessive, complex hereditary spastic paraplegia can be a manifestation of mutations affecting autophagosome formation and maturation. Two forms with onset in childhood or early adulthood are due to mutations affecting proteins involved in autophagosome-lysosome biogenesis. They include spatacsin (*SPG11*) and spastizin (*FYVE26, SPG15*) mutations.

TABLE 7.1 *Examples of Disorders of Vesicular Trafficking Associated with Hereditary Spastic Paraplegia (HSP)*

Protein (gene)	Function	Phenotype
Spastin (*SPAST*)	Microtubule severing Endoplasmic reticulum (ER) biogenesis	Autosomal dominant pure hereditary spastic paraplegia
Atlastatin-1 (*ATL-1*)	ER biogenesis	Early onset, AD, pure HSP HSAN
Reticulon 2 (*RTN2*)	ER biogenesis	Early onset, AD, pure HSP
REEP1 (receptor expression-enhancing protein-1 (*REEP1*)	ER biogenesis	Early onset, AD, pure HSP
Strumpelli 2	Endosomal biogenesis	Adult onset, AD, pure HSP
Spatacsin (*SPG11*)	Autophagosome maturation	Early onset, complex HSP with corpus callosum hypoplasia, optic atrophy, ataxia, intellectual disability, and peripheral neuropathy
Spastizin (*FYVE26*)	Lysosomal reformation	Early onset, complex spastic paraplegia with intellectual disability, pigmentary retinopathy, ataxia, amyotrophy, and thin corpus callosum

TABLE 7.2 *Examples of Disorders of Vesicular Trafficking Associated with Lower Motor Neuron Syndromes*

Protein (gene)	Function	Phenotype
Alsin (*Alsin*)	Guanine-nucleotide-exchange factor for Rab5	Autosomal recessive juvenile ALS (ALS2) Infantile-onset ascending hereditary spastic paraplegia
Vesicle-associated membrane protein-associated protein-B (*VAPB*)	Lipid transfer between the ER and Golgi complex	Late-onset spinal muscular atrophy (SMA) (ALS8)
Bicaudal-2 (*BICD2*)	Golgin that binds the dynein-dynactin complex	Autosomal dominant distal lower limb predominant SMA (SMALED2)
Seipin (*BSLC2*)	ER protein involved in lipid droplet metabolism	Upper limb distal hereditary motor neuronopathy (dHMN) V Autosomal dominant pure hereditary spastic paraplegia with amyotrophy (Silver syndrome)
Dynactin (*DNCT1*)	Retrograde transport motor	dHMN VII Perry syndrome
Dynein heavy chain (*DYNCH1*)	Retrograde transport motor	SMALED 1 dHMN Charcot-Marie-Tooth (CMT) 2
TUB4A	Tubulin α-4A isoform	ALS
Rab7 (*RAB7A*)	Component of late endosomes	CMT2B HSAN I
Family with sequence similarity 134, member B (*FAM134B*)	Receptor for ER autophagy	HSANIIB

HSAN, hereditary sensory and autonomic neuropathy

Spastizin participates in autophagosome maturation and interacts with spatacsin, forming a complex that maintains a pool of lysosomes competent to fuse with autophagosomes. SPG11 and SPG15 have a similar phenotype characterized by childhood- or adult-onset spastic paraplegia, intellectual disability, optic atrophy, cerebellar ataxia, polyneuropathy, pigmentary retinopathy, and thin corpus callosum; a typical finding in SPG11 is increased T2 signal in the forceps minor area of the corpus callosum resembling "ears of the lynx." Other forms of hereditary spastic paraplegia are due to mutations affecting mitochondrial chaperones, such as SPG7 due to mutations affecting paraplegin or SPG13 due to mutations of the *HSPD* gene encoding Hsp60. Another important mechanism of hereditary spastic paraplegia is impaired axonal transport, as occurs with mutations of the *KIF1A* gene encoding kinesin 1 (SPG30), or other kinesin genes, which are typically associated with a complex phenotype, including combination with ataxia, optic atrophy, or peripheral neuropathy.

Lower Motor Neuron Disorders and Peripheral Neuropathies

Some mutations affecting vesicular biogenesis and trafficking proteins manifest with lower motor neuron syndromes, either in isolation or with upper motor involvement.

ALS2 mutations produce autosomal recessive juvenile ALS and infantile-onset ascending hereditary spastic paraplegia; *VAPB* (vesicle-associated membrane protein-associated protein B) mutations produce an atypical form of familial ALS (ALS8) and late-onset spinal muscular atrophy; *BICD2* (Bicaudal 2) mutations cause a dominant form of distal lower limb predominant spinal muscular atrophy (SMALED2). Some genes linked to the dHMN phenotype are associated with ER dysfunction or impaired axonal transport. Mutations of the *BSCL2* gene encoding the ER protein seipin involved in lipid homeostasis have been linked to upper-limb-onset dHMN (dHMN type V), and to autosomal dominant hereditary spastic paraplegia with amyotrophy of hand and feet (Silver syndrome). Mutations of the *DNCT1* gene encoding dynactin, a critical component of dynein/dynactin complex required for retrograde axonal transport of vesicles and organelles, have been linked todHMN with vocal cord paralysis and facial weakness (dHMN type VII) and Perry syndrome.[49,50] Mutations of the *DYNCH1* gene encoding dynein, the dynactin partner for retrograde transport, have been be linked to autosomal dominant distal spinal muscular atrophy (SAMLED1), dHMN or CMT2 phenotypes. As mentioned earlier in this chapter, missense mutations of the *RAB7A* gene encoding for Rab7A produce CMT2B. HSAN has also linked to mutations of *ATLN*-1 encoding atlastatin-1, which is also associated with hereditary spastic paraplegia.

Parkinson Disease

Impaired vesicular trafficking, particularly affecting the endolysosomal pathway is a major pathogenic mechanism in PD[51–56] (Table 7.3). Impaired vesicle recycling may constitute a common pathogenic pathway shared by many PD risk genes, including *DNAJ6, SYNJ1, SYNT, LRRK2, VPS35,* and *TMEM230*.[57–59] Mutations of the *DNAJC6* gene encoding auxilin cause juvenile-onset PD, characterized by visual hallucinations, epilepsy, psychosis, and cognitive impairment. Mutations of the *SYNJ1* gene encoding synaptojanin produce early-onset PD with epilepsy. The *SYNT11* gene encoding synaptotagmin 11, which inhibits endocytosis in neurons, is associated with risk of PD. The most common *LRRK2* mutation (G210S) increases its kinase activity, which can impair vesicular trafficking and endolysosomal function. Loss-of-function *VPS35* mutations impair retromer function, resulting in accumulation of ceramide and impaired delivery of the cargo receptor required for cathepsin D targeting to lysosomes. Mutations of the *ATP13A2* gene encoding ATP13A2, a transmembrane lysosomal ATPase controlling lipid dynamics during vesicle formation, are linked to Kufor-Rakeb syndrome, a form of early-onset parkinsonism with dementia. Mutations of the *PL2AG6* encoding the calcium-independent phospholipase A2 β group VI causes slowly progressive dystonia-parkinsonism. In experimental models, loss of PL2AG6 affects the stability of VPS35 and causes retromer dysfunction, leading to impaired recycling of membrane sphingolipids, overload of lysosomes, and accumulation of ceramide. These findings suggest that impaired ceramide metabolism provides a mechanistic link between lysosomal storage disease and PD.[60] Increasing evidence indicates that Rab proteins have an important role in PD.[1] Loss-of-function mutations of the *RAB39B* gene cause an X-linked

TABLE 7.3 *Impaired Vesicular Trafficking as a Disease Mechanism in Parkinson Disease*

Gene (protein)	Function	Phenotype
SCNA (α-synuclein) triplication or mutation	Vesicular chaperone function for exocytosis and endocytosis	Autosomal dominant Parkinson disease (PD, PARK1, PARK4)
LRRK2 (Leucine-rich repeat kinase 2)	Regulates vesicular transport	Autosomal dominant PD (PARK8)
SYNJ1 (synaptojanin-1)	Clathrin vesicle tubulation and uncoating	Early-onset PD with epilepsy (PARK 20)
DNAJC6 (auxilin)	Hsp40 chaperone that aids clathrin vesicle uncoating	Juvenile PD with hallucinations, epilepsy, psychosis, and cognitive impairment
DNAJC13 (DNAJ homolog, subfamily C, member 13)	Hsp40 chaperone involved in endosome biogenesis	Autosomal dominant PD
VSP35 (vesicular protein-sorting 35)	Component of the retromer	Autosomal dominant PD
PLA2G6 (calcium-independent phospholipase A2-β Group VI)	Phospholipid remodeler, component of the retromer	Slowly progressive dystonia-parkinsonism (PARK 14)
ATP13A2 (ATPase 13A2)	Lysosome ATPase involved in endosomal and lysosomal maintenance	Autosomal recessive PD with dementia (Kufor-Rakeb syndrome, PARK9)
RAB39B (Rab GTPase 39B)	Vesicle recycling between the synaptic cell membrane, and endosomes	X-linked PD
RAB 32 (Rab GTPase)	Autophagy, mitochondrial dynamics, phagocytosis	Late-onset PD

recessive form of early-onset PD. Rab39 may function in the TGN, be expressed in different membrane compartments, and participate in α-synuclein homeostasis. Mutations in the *RAB32* gene cause late-onset familial PD. Rab32 participates in autophagy, mitochondrial dynamics, phagocytosis, and inflammation, and stabilizes normal α-SYN to the membranes of presynaptic vesicles. In its phosphorylated state, α-SYN strongly interacts with Rab8A, which may participate in the formation of α-SYN aggregates and the clearance of toxic oligomeric α-SYN species in the cell. Rab1A promotes formation of the autophagosome and may protect against α-SYN toxicity. In contrast, increased levels of α-SYN in dopaminergic cells may result in mislocalization of Rab1A from the ER and Golgi to the α-SYN aggregates, resulting in impaired autophagy and Golgi fragmentation. Alpha-synuclein aggregates also trap other Rab proteins, including Rab7 and Rab11, involved in recycling endosomes.

Impaired lysosomal function is also a major mechanism in PD. Duplication/triplication and point mutations in the *SNCA1* gene encoding α-SYN are associated with autosomal dominant familial PD. Upon α-SYN accumulation, the membrane-bound monomers undergo a conformational change to form β-sheet-rich intermediates (protofibrils), and then self-associate to form ring-like oligomers on the membrane. These oligomers can form transmembrane pores that disrupt the integrity of the membrane. Accumulated α-SYN also becomes attached to the lysosome membrane, forming clusters that impair degradation of other substrates and may also cause dysfunction in autophagy and endolysosomal and ER to Golgi trafficking. Impaired α-SYN degradation by cathepsin D in lysosomes may reflect impaired retromer assembly, as occurs with *VPS35* mutations. Mutations affecting genes encoding lysosomal enzymes are risk factors for development of PD. Whereas homozygous mutations of the *GBA* gene encoding lysosomal acid β-glucocerebrosidase (GCase) cause Gaucher disease, heterozygous mutations of the gene are among the most common risk factors for PD and dementia with Lewy bodies. The impaired sphingolipid metabolism due to reduced GCase activity is associated with impaired autophagic flux, accumulation of α-SYN oligomers, and mitochondrial dysfunction. In turn, α-SYN accumulation impairs trafficking of GCase.[61] Other genes encoding lysosomal enzymes are also risk factors for PD, including *SCARB2* (encoding LMP2, a GCase cargo receptor), *ASAH1* (acid ceramidase); *SMPD1* (acid sphingomyelinase 1); *CTSD* (cathepsin D); *CTSB* (cathepsin B,) and *ATPAVOA1* (vesicular proton ATPase).[60,61] The human transmembrane protein 175 (*TMEM175*) gene encoding a potassium channel located in late endosomes and lysosomes, is also a risk factor for PD.

Alzheimer Disease

As discussed earlier in this chapter, dysfunction of the retromer may promote amyloidogenic APP processing due to impaired recycling of APP and BACE1 from the endosome to the TGN. Accumulation of autophagosomes and autolysosomes in dystrophic neurites in both familial and sporadic AD in part reflects impaired lysosomal degradation. Accumulation of Aβ leads to Golgi fragmentation, which in turn accelerates Aβ production. Some *PS1* mutations affect lysosomal hydrolysis of APP by causing deficiency of a subunit of the V-ATPase necessary for lysosomal acidification. Genome-wide association studies showed that genes related to autophagy initiation and early autophagosome formation are risk factors for late-onset AD. These include the *PICALM* gene encoding the phosphatidylinositol-binding clathrin assembly protein, which has a key role in clathrin-mediated endocytosis. Altered PICALM protein levels in late-onset AD brains are associated with tau pathology and reduced levels of Beclin-1, a key component of complex required for autophagosome biogenesis.

Frontotemporal Lobar Degeneration

Frontotemporal lobar degeneration, either in isolation or in combination with ALS and associated with accumulation of TDP-43 inclusions (FTLD-TDP) has been linked to mutations of several genes encoding proteins involved in vesicular trafficking to the lysosome. Loss-of-function mutations of the *CHMP2B* gene encoding charged multivesicular body protein 2B, a component of the ESCRT-III complex, have been linked with familial FTLD. *CHMP2B*-associated FTLD is uniquely characterized by the presence of enlarged late endosomes and impaired endolysosomal fusion. Hexanucleotide repeat expansion of the *C9ORF72* gene reduces expression of the C9ORF72 protein, which functions as a guanine-nucleotide-exchanging factor for Rab8A and is a Rab1A effector that regulates Rab1A-dependent trafficking of the ULK-1 complex for the initiation of autophagy. C9ORF72 also binds inactive Rag GTPases, thereby affecting mTORC1 binding to lysosomes. Loss of C9ORF72 function results in enhanced nuclear translocation of TFEB, leading to altered lysosomal biogenesis and autophagy.[62] Mutations causing happloinsufficiency of the *GRN* gene encoding progranulin are a common cause of familial FTLD-TDP, which typically manifests with behavioral or language difficulties, and with asymmetric involvement of the frontal, temporal, and parietal lobes. However there is great phenotypic variability, including primary progressive aphasia, corticobasal syndrome, AD, or Lewy body disease. Single nucleotide polymorphisms of the *TMEM106B* gene may either increase or decrease the risk of developing FTLD-TDP. Studies in *Grn-/-* transgenic mice show that progranulin deficiency results in accumulation of TMEM106B as well as lysosomal abnormalities including lipofuscin accumulation during aging. These polymorphisms also modify the risk of FTLD-TDP associated with *C9ORF72* gene expansion, as well as that of AD and hippocampal sclerosis.

Huntington Disease

Several steps of autophagy are also affected in HD, a disorder due to expansion of CAG repeats encoding a polyglutamine tract in the *HTT* (huntingtin) gene. Normal huntingtin participates in many aspects of autophagy, including cargo recognition by the autophagosome for selective autophagy and autophagosome transport along microtubules for fusion with the lysosome. Mutant huntingtin interferes at different levels of the autophagic mechanisms, including cargo recognition and vesicular trafficking, thus impairing the access of endosomes and autophagosome to the lysosomes. Of note, *C9ORF72* mutations are not only the major cause of familial ALS/FTLD but also cause the most common HD phenocopy.

CHILDHOOD-ONSET DISORDERS OF VESICULAR TRAFFICKING AND LYSOSOMAL FUNCTION

Neurodegeneration Due to Impaired Autophagy

Lafora disease is a myoclonic epilepsy linked to autosomal recessive mutations of the *EPM2A* (epilepsy, progressive myoclonus 2A) gene encoding laforin, or the *EPM2B* gene encoding malin. Laforin is a dual specificity protein phosphatase and forms a complex with malin, which is a ubiquitin E3 ligase. The laforin-malin complex may increase autophagic flux by inhibiting mTORC1 and thus promoting formation of the phagophore. Lafora disease typically manifests in late childhood and adolescence occipital seizures, intractable tonic-clonic and other types of myoclonus, and rapid dementias. The disorder is characterized by the presence of glycogen-rich intracellular inclusions, called Lafora bodies and abnormally large lysosomes, indicating interruption of autophagic flux. Single-gene disorders of the autophagy may affect initiation and signaling, phagophore formation, phagophore maturation, autolysosome formation, or lysosome function.[34,35] These disorders prominently affect the central nervous system at various stages of development, leading to brain malformations, developmental delay, intellectual disability, epilepsy, movement disorders, and neurodegeneration. Two such disorders produce neurodegeneration with brain iron accumulation. Beta propeller protein-associated neurodegeneration (BPAN) is caused by X-linked dominant mutations of the *WDR45* gene encoding a member of the WIPI family of proteins that can bind to PI3P and regulates autophagosome formation and elongation. Mitochondrial member protein-associated neurodegeneration (MPAN) has been linked to mutation on chromosome 19 open reading frame 12 (*C19ORF12*), which encodes a protein that may be important for autophagosome formation.

Lysosome Storage Diseases

Lysosomal storage diseases are caused by genetic deficiencies of lysosomal proteins.[63] Many of these disorders are associated with increased lysosomal biogenesis, which is a compensatory mechanism to counteract lysosomal stress. For example, neuronal ceroid lipofucsinosis (NCL), or Batten disease, are primarily childhood neurodegenerative disorders associated with mutations in several genes (*CLN1 to CLN14*) encoding proteins with different cellular locations and functions and characterized by storage of autofluorescent material (ceroid lipopigment) in lysosomes. Many NCL proteins have been localized to lysosomes. For example, juvenile Batten disease is caused by mutations in the *CLN3* gene, which encodes a multipass lysosomal membrane protein involved in lysosome homeostasis. Homozygous *GRN* mutations cause NCL 11, which resembles other forms of NCL and manifests with progressive visual loss, cerebellar ataxia, and myoclonic seizures developing between 20 and 30 years of age. Mutations in the *SCARB2* gene encoding LIMP-2 cause a rare form of progressive myoclonus epilepsy often associated with action myoclonus-renal failure syndrome. Mutations in enzymes involved in M6PR-based trafficking of lysosomal enzymes result in mucolipidosis types II and III. Mutations of the *MLN1* gene encoding mucolipin 1 are linked to mucolipidosis type IV. Enzyme-replacement therapy is being used successfully for the treatment of some lysosomal storage disorders, including Fabry disease, Pompe disease, and CLN2 disease. Pharmacological activation of endogenous TFEB via oral administration of trehalose reduced neuropathology and improved phenotypes in mouse models of several lysosomal storage disorders, including a juvenile Batten disease, mucolipidoses, and multiple sulfatase deficiency, as well as models of AD and HD. Trehalose activates TFEB through the inhibition of the activity of AKT, a negative regulator of this key transcription factor for lysosome biogenesis.

KEY POINTS

- Normal cell function depends on highly regulated secretory, endocytic, and autophagy pathways.
- The secretory pathway involving the endoplasmic reticulum (ER) and Golgi complex is responsible for protein maturation, sorting, and delivery of transmembrane and secreted macromolecules.
- The ER is the site for protein maturation, quality control, and response to misfolded proteins; participates in membrane sphingolipid biogenesis; and has a critical role in intracellular Ca^{2+} homeostasis.
- The Golgi complex contains glycosylation and other enzymes that further process the proteins and lipids along the secretory pathway and is a critical hub for membrane trafficking.
- The different cargoes are sorted at the trans-Golgi network (TGN) via specialized vesicular carriers and then shipped out to the plasma membrane, lysosomes, or other destinations.
- The constitutive pathway delivers newly synthesized macromolecules to the membrane; the regulated pathway releases signals for intercellular communication.

- Exocytosis of synaptic vesicles at presynaptic active zones is a specialized and fast variant of secretory pathway.
- Alpha-synuclein interacts with synaptic vesicles to modulate membrane remodeling and vesicle recycling at nerve terminals.
- The endocytic pathway starts with the internalization of material primarily via clathrin-mediated endocytosis.
- Endosomal content can be transported back to the cell body via the retromer complex, recycled to cell compartments, or delivered to the lysosomes, either directly or via the formation of multivesicular bodies.
- Autophagy involves the formation of a phagophore, elongation and closure of the phagophore to form the autophagosomes, transport of the autophagosome via microtubules, and fusion of the phagosome with lysosomes.
- Lysosomes contain multiple enzymes that are optimally active at acidic pH.
- Lysosome biogenesis is tightly regulated in response to nutritional conditions, lysosomal stress, and other stimuli.
- Impaired vesicular trafficking is a major disease mechanism in hereditary motor disorders reflecting dying back axonopathy, including hereditary spastic paraplegia, familial ALS, distal hereditary motor neuropathies, and axonal forms of Charcot-Marie-Tooth disease.
- Impaired trafficking in the endolysosomal pathway is a major pathogenic mechanism in Parkinson disease.
- Impaired vesicular dynamics contributes to amyloidogenesis in Alzheimer disease and underlies some familiar forms of frontotemporal lobar degeneration.
- Mutations affecting the biogenesis of autophagosomes or lysosomes are an important cause of childhood neurodegenerative disorders, some of them amenable to enzyme-replacement therapy.

REFERENCES

1. Gao Y, Wilson GR, Stephenson SEM, Bozaoglu K, Farrer MJ, Lockhart PJ. The emerging role of Rab GTPases in the pathogenesis of Parkinson's disease. Mov Disord 2018;33:196–207.
2. Guadagno NA, Progida C. Rab GTPases: switching to human diseases. Cells 2019;8:909–916.
3. Papadopulos A. Membrane shaping by actin and myosin during regulated exocytosis. Mol Cell Neurosci 2017;84:93–99.
4. Schwarz DS, Blower MD. The endoplasmic reticulum: structure, function and response to cellular signaling. Cell Mol Life Sci 2016;73:79–94.
5. de Souza PVS, de Rezende Pinto WBV, de Rezende Batistella GN, Bortholin T, Oliveira ASB. Hereditary spastic paraplegia: clinical and genetic hallmarks. Cerebellum 2017;16:525–551.
6. Blackstone C. Hereditary spastic paraplegia. Handb Clin Neurol 2018;148:633–652.
7. Erfanian Omidvar M, Torkamandi S, Rezaei S, et al. Genotype-phenotype associations in hereditary spastic paraplegia: a systematic review and meta-analysis on 13,570 patients. J Neurol 2019.
8. Shribman S, Reid E, Crosby AH, Houlden H, Warner TT. Hereditary spastic paraplegia: from diagnosis to emerging therapeutic approaches. Lancet Neurol 2019;18:1136–1146.
9. Huang S, Wang Y. Golgi structure formation, function, and post-translational modifications in mammalian cells. F1000Res 2017;6:2050.
10. Witkos TM, Lowe M. Recognition and tethering of transport vesicles at the Golgi apparatus. Curr Opin Cell Biol 2017;47:16–23.
11. Koboldt DC, Waldrop MA, Wilson RK, Flanigan KM. The genotypic and phenotypic spectrum of BICD2 variants in spinal muscular atrophy. Ann Neurol 2020;87:487–496.
12. Guo Y, Sirkis DW, Schekman R. Protein sorting at the trans-Golgi network. Annu Rev Cell Dev Biol 2014;30:169–206.
13. Azarnia Tehran D, Kuijpers M, Haucke V. Presynaptic endocytic factors in autophagy and neurodegeneration. Curr Opin Neurobiol 2018;48:153–159.
14. Saheki Y, De Camilli P. Synaptic vesicle endocytosis. Cold Spring Harb Perspect Biol 2012;4:a005645.
15. Bae EJ, Kim DK, Kim C, et al. LRRK2 kinase regulates alpha-synuclein propagation via RAB35 phosphorylation. Nat Commun 2018;9:3465.
16. Huang M, Wang B, Li X, Fu C, Wang C, Kang X. Alpha-synuclein: a multifunctional player in exocytosis, endocytosis, and vesicle recycling. Front Neurosci 2019;13:28.
17. Snead D, Eliezer D. Intrinsically disordered proteins in synaptic vesicle trafficking and release. J Biol Chem 2019;294:3325–3342.
18. Dewulf M, Koster DV, Sinha B, et al. Dystrophy-associated caveolin-3 mutations reveal that caveolae couple IL6/STAT3 signaling with mechanosensing in human muscle cells. Nat Commun 2019;10:1974.
19. Scott CC, Vacca F, Gruenberg J. Endosome maturation, transport and functions. Semin Cell Dev Biol 2014;31:2–10.
20. Winckler B, Faundez V, Maday S, Cai Q, Guimas Almeida C, Zhang H. The endolysosomal system and proteostasis: from development to degeneration. J Neurosci 2018;38:9364–9374.
21. Trousdale C, Kim K. Retromer: structure, function, and roles in mammalian disease. Eur J Cell Biol 2015;94:513–521.
22. Williams ET, Chen X, Moore DJ. VPS35, the retromer complex and Parkinson's disease. J Parkinsons Dis 2017;7:219–233.
23. Chandran J, Ding J, Cai H. Alsin and the molecular pathways of amyotrophic lateral sclerosis. Mol Neurobiol 2007;36:224–231.
24. Liu H, Wu C. Charcot Marie Tooth 2B peripheral sensory neuropathy: how Rab7 mutations impact NGF signaling? Int J Mol Sci 2017;18:324–333.
25. Alekhina O, Burstein E, Billadeau DD. Cellular functions of WASP family proteins at a glance. J Cell Sci 2017;130:2235–2241.
26. Vagnozzi AN, Pratico D. Endosomal sorting and trafficking, the retromer complex and neurodegeneration. Mol Psychiatry 2019;24:857–868.
27. Klaips CL, Jayaraj GG, Hartl FU. Pathways of cellular proteostasis in aging and disease. J Cell Biol 2018;217:51–63.
28. Lefebvre C, Legouis R, Culetto E. ESCRT and autophagies: Endosomal functions and beyond. Semin Cell Dev Biol 2018;74:21–28.

29. Kaul Z, Chakrabarti O. Endosomal sorting complexes required for ESCRTing cells toward death during neurogenesis, neurodevelopment and neurodegeneration. Traffic 2018;19:485–495.
30. Parkinson N, Ince PG, Smith MO, et al. ALS phenotypes with mutations in CHMP2B (charged multivesicular body protein 2B). Neurology 2006;67:1074–1077.
31. Reid E, Connell J, Edwards TL, Duley S, Brown SE, Sanderson CM. The hereditary spastic paraplegia protein spastin interacts with the ESCRT-III complex-associated endosomal protein CHMP1B. Hum Mol Genet 2005;14:19–38.
32. Martini-Stoica H, Xu Y, Ballabio A, Zheng H. The autophagy-lysosomal pathway in neurodegeneration: a TFEB perspective. Trends Neurosci 2016;39:221–234.
33. Vijayan V, Verstreken P. Autophagy in the presynaptic compartment in health and disease. J Cell Biol 2017;216:1895–1906.
34. Ebrahimi-Fakhari D, Saffari A, Wahlster L, et al. Congenital disorders of autophagy: an emerging novel class of inborn errors of neuro-metabolism. Brain 2016;139:317–337.
35. Zhu Y, Runwal G, Obrocki P, Rubinsztein DC. Autophagy in childhood neurological disorders. Dev Med Child Neurol 2019;61:639–645.
36. Erro R, Picillo M, Manara R, Pellecchia MT, Barone P. From PARK9 to SPG78: the clinical spectrum of ATP13A2 mutations. Parkinsonism Relat Disord 2019;65:272–273.
37. Bajaj L, Lotfi P, Pal R, Ronza AD, Sharma J, Sardiello M. Lysosome biogenesis in health and disease. J Neurochem 2019;148:573–589.
38. Lie PPY, Nixon RA. Lysosome trafficking and signaling in health and neurodegenerative diseases. Neurobiol Dis 2019;122:94–105.
39. English AM, Hughes AL. Knowing when to let go: lysosomes regulate inter-mitochondrial tethering. Dev Cell 2019;50:259–260.
40. Kao AW, McKay A, Singh PP, Brunet A, Huang EJ. Progranulin, lysosomal regulation and neurodegenerative disease. Nat Rev Neurosci 2017;18:325–333.
41. Schneider A, Simons M. Exosomes: vesicular carriers for intercellular communication in neurodegenerative disorders. Cell Tissue Res 2013;352:33–47.
42. Kakarla R, Hur J, Kim YJ, Kim J, Chwae YJ. Apoptotic cell-derived exosomes: messages from dying cells. Exp Mol Med 2020;52:1–6.
43. Hessvik NP, Llorente A. Current knowledge on exosome biogenesis and release. Cell Mol Life Sci 2018;75:193–208.
44. Lee JG, Takahama S, Zhang G, Tomarev SI, Ye Y. Unconventional secretion of misfolded proteins promotes adaptation to proteasome dysfunction in mammalian cells. Nat Cell Biol 2016;18:765–776.
45. Cha DJ, Mengel D, Mustapic M, et al. miR-212 and miR-132 are downregulated in neurally derived plasma exosomes of Alzheimer's patients. Front Neurosci 2019;13:1208.
46. Jafarzadeh-Esfehani R, Soudyab M, Parizadeh SM, et al. Circulating exosomes and their role in stroke. Curr Drug Targets 2020;21:89–95.
47. Darios F, Stevanin G. Impairment of lysosome function and autophagy in rare neurodegenerative diseases. J Mol Biol 2020;432:2714–2734.
48. Hedera P. Hereditary myelopathies. Continuum (Minneap Minn) 2018;24:523–550.
49. Konno T, Ross OA, Teive HAG, Slawek J, Dickson DW, Wszolek ZK. DCTN1-related neurodegeneration: Perry syndrome and beyond. Parkinsonism Relat Disord 2017;41:14–24.
50. Hoang HT, Schlager MA, Carter AP, Bullock SL. DYNC1H1 mutations associated with neurological diseases compromise processivity of dynein-dynactin-cargo adaptor complexes. Proc Natl Acad Sci U S A 2017;114:E1597–E1606.
51. Vidyadhara DJ, Lee JE, Chandra SS. Role of the endolysosomal system in Parkinson's disease. J Neurochem 2019;150:487–506.
52. Rodriguez L, Marano MM, Tandon A. Import and export of misfolded alpha-synuclein. Front Neurosci 2018;12:344.
53. Robak LA, Jansen IE, van Rooij J, et al. Excessive burden of lysosomal storage disorder gene variants in Parkinson's disease. Brain 2017;140:3191–3203.
54. Rahman AA, Morrison BE. Contributions of VPS35 mutations to Parkinson's disease. Neuroscience 2019;401:1–10.
55. Abeliovich A, Gitler AD. Defects in trafficking bridge Parkinson's disease pathology and genetics. Nature 2016;539:207–216.
56. Pan PY, Zhu Y, Shen Y, Yue Z. Crosstalk between presynaptic trafficking and autophagy in Parkinson's disease. Neurobiol Dis 2019;122:64–71.
57. Weissbach A, Wittke C, Kasten M, Klein C. "Atypical" Parkinson's disease—genetic. Int Rev Neurobiol 2019;149:207–235.
58. Klein C, Hattori N, Marras C. MDSGene: closing data gaps in genotype-phenotype correlations of monogenic Parkinson's disease. J Parkinsons Dis 2018;8:S25–S30.
59. Trinh J, Zeldenrust FMJ, Huang J, et al. Genotype-phenotype relations for the Parkinson's disease genes SNCA, LRRK2, VPS35: MDSGene systematic review. Mov Disord 2018;33:1857–1870.
60. Lin G, Wang L, Marcogliese PC, Bellen HJ. Sphingolipids in the pathogenesis of Parkinson's disease and parkinsonism. Trends Endocrinol Metab 2019;30:106–117.
61. Taguchi YV, Liu J, Ruan J, et al. Glucosylsphingosine promotes alpha-synuclein pathology in mutant GBA-associated Parkinson's disease. J Neurosci 2017;37:9617–9631.
62. Wang M, Wang H, Tao Z, et al. C9orf72 associates with inactive Rag GTPases and regulates mTORC1-mediated autophagosomal and lysosomal biogenesis. Aging Cell 2020;19(4):e13126.
63. Parenti G, Andria G, Ballabio A. Lysosomal storage diseases: from pathophysiology to therapy. Annu Rev Med 2015;66:471–486.

8 Cytoskeleton

OVERVIEW

The neuronal cytoskeleton is primarily composed of microfilaments, intermediate filaments, and microtubules (Figure 8.1). All components of the cytoskeleton are dynamic structures that interact with each other to regulate dynamic changes in cell morphology and growth, functional compartmentalization, and intracellular transport. These functions are regulated by posttranslational modifications, particularly phosphorylation, and by a wide variety of interacting proteins. Actin microfilament dynamics is critical for axonal growth, activity-dependent changes in dendritic morphology, and topographic location of membrane proteins. Microtubules are polymers of tubulin, undergo cycles of polymerization and depolymerization, are stabilized by tau and other microtubule-associated proteins, and provide tracks for intracellular transport. Neuron-specific intermediate filaments consist of neurofilament light-(NfL), medium (NfM)-, and heavy-(NfH) chain proteins, as well as α-internexin or peripherin. They determine the axon caliber, provide mechanical resilience to the axon and serve as platforms for intracellular organelles. Glial fibrillary acid protein (GFAP) is the main intermediate filament of astrocytes. Nuclear lamins participate in regulation of the chromatin organization, import and export of transcription factors, and transduction of mechanical signals. Disorders affecting the composition and dynamics of the cytoskeleton thus strongly impair development, function, plasticity, and repair in the nervous system and constitute a major mechanism of neurodegeneration. The aims of this chapter are to review: (1) the structure and dynamics of microfilaments, microtubules, and neurofilaments; (2) the distribution and functions of these cytoskeletal elements in different compartments of neurons; (3) the function of GFAP, nuclear lamins, and septins; and (4) disorders resulting from mutations affecting cytoskeletal proteins.

MICROFILAMENTS

Microfilaments are composed of globular (G) actin subunits that polymerize to form filamentous (F) actin. Each microfilament consists of two helical, interlaced strands of subunits of approximately 6–7 nm in diameter and are assembled into bundles and networks. Actin polymerization, also called nucleation, starts with the self-association of three G-actin monomers to form a trimer that binds adenosine triphosphate (ATP). The ATP-bound actin binds the barbed end of the existing microfilament, and ATP is then hydrolyzed to ADP. Based on the turnover rate, actin filaments can be roughly divided into dynamic and stable pools.

Actin Structures

Actin filaments can be arranged in linear or in branched conformations, and together with stable microtubule arrays and neurofilaments, form the cytoskeleton in dendrites and axons (Figure 8.2). In neurons and in other nonmuscle cells, actin filaments underlying membrane surfaces form a cortical actin network. Cortical actin modifies the physical properties of the membrane and restricts the diffusion of proteins and phospholipids across the lipid bilayer, allowing the compartmentalization of the plasma membrane in different functional domains. The cortical actin network also interacts with the machinery for exocytosis and endocytosis. F-actin-based structures also include actin patches, longitudinal fibers, and rings. Actin patches are areas of enriched

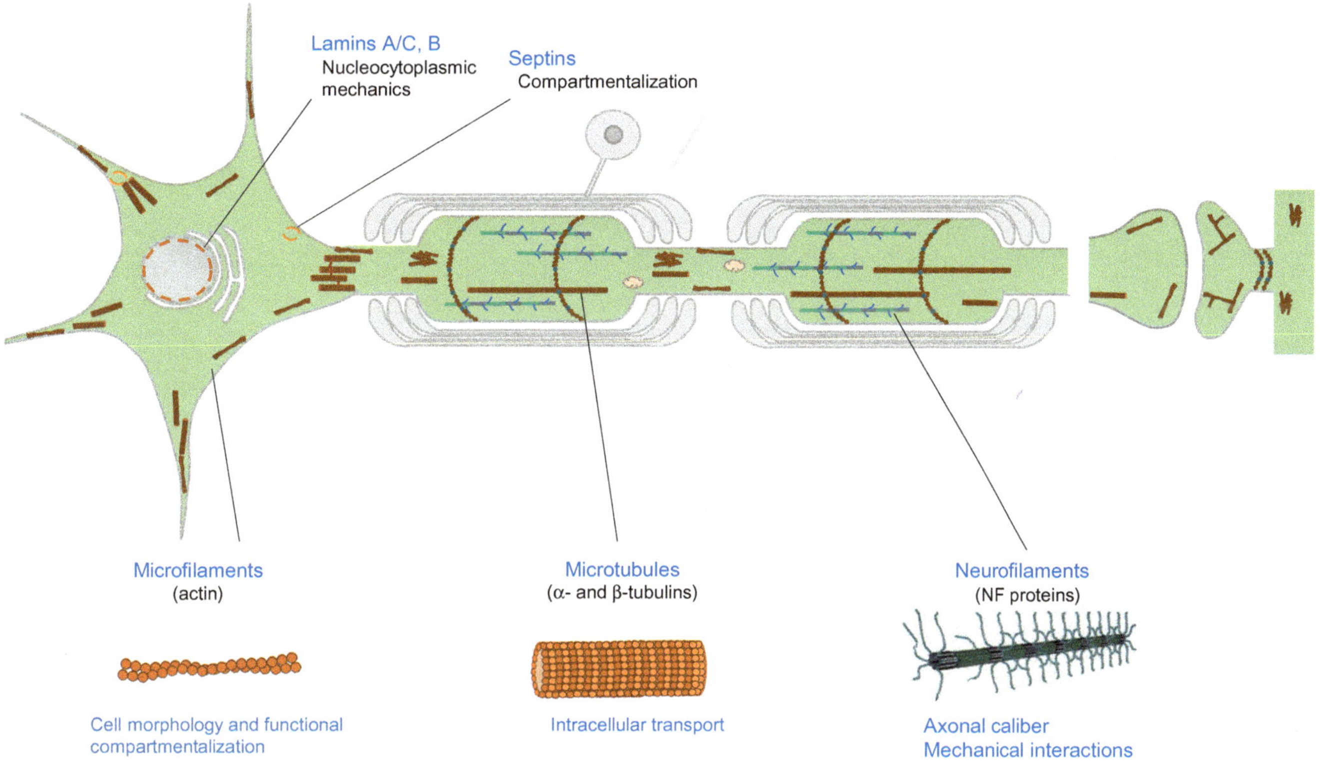

FIGURE 8.1 Components of the cytoskeleton in neurons.
The neuronal cytoskeleton is primarily composed of microfilaments, intermediate filaments, and microtubules. All components of the cytoskeleton are dynamic structures that interact with each other to regulate dynamic changes in cell morphology and growth, functional compartmentalization, and intercellular transport.

in branched F-actin; longitudinal actin are long bundles of F-actin that traverse along the lengths of dendrites; and actin rings are present in axons and in the necks of dendritic spines.

Actin-Binding Proteins

A large number of actin-binding proteins regulate the three-dimensional structure and dynamics of actin filament networks[1] (Table 8.1). Profilin binds monomeric actin and promotes the assembly of monomers. Elongation of F-actin, or actin nucleation, involves the action of formins and the actin-related protein 2/3 (Arp 2/3) complex, which also promotes the formation of a branched actin neurofilaments network. The F-actin-binding protein cortactin interacts with both the Arp2/3 complex and with scaffold proteins at the postsynaptic density in excitatory synapses. Formins nucleate unbranched actin filaments and are mainly involved in axon development and in the formation of a deep actin network within the axon.[2] Several actin filament-severing proteins have a major role in controlling actin turnover. The main example is cofilin, which regulates the G/F-actin pool by increasing the number of uncapped ends that may undergo polymerization. The activity of cofilin is tightly regulated via several mechanisms, including phosphorylation by calcium (Ca^{2+})-activated calmodulin kinase II (CaMKII) and dephosphorylation by calcineurin.[3] Gelsolin is a Ca^{2+}-dependent severing and capping protein that regulates filament length near the plasma membrane. Actin-binding proteins such cortactin, α-actinin, and drebrin stabilize the actin cytoskeleton by crosslinking F-actin in bundles or linking F-actin to membrane proteins. Drebrin also recruits microtubules to growth cones and dendritic spines. Myosin IIb binds actin and promotes contraction and remodeling of the actin network. Myosin Va is involved in transport of cargoes along the actin filaments and has an important role in coupling actin- and microtubule-based transport.

Extracellular Factors Controlling Actin Dynamics

Several extracellular signals, such as cell adhesion molecules and extracellular guidance cues, control actin dynamics during neuronal cell migration, axon pathfinding, axon–dendrite contact formation and dendritic spine plasticity. Integrins interact both with the actin cytoskeleton and with components of the extracellular matrix and initiate signals that affect actin dynamics and stability of dendrites and dendritic spines. A major factor for dendrite survival and

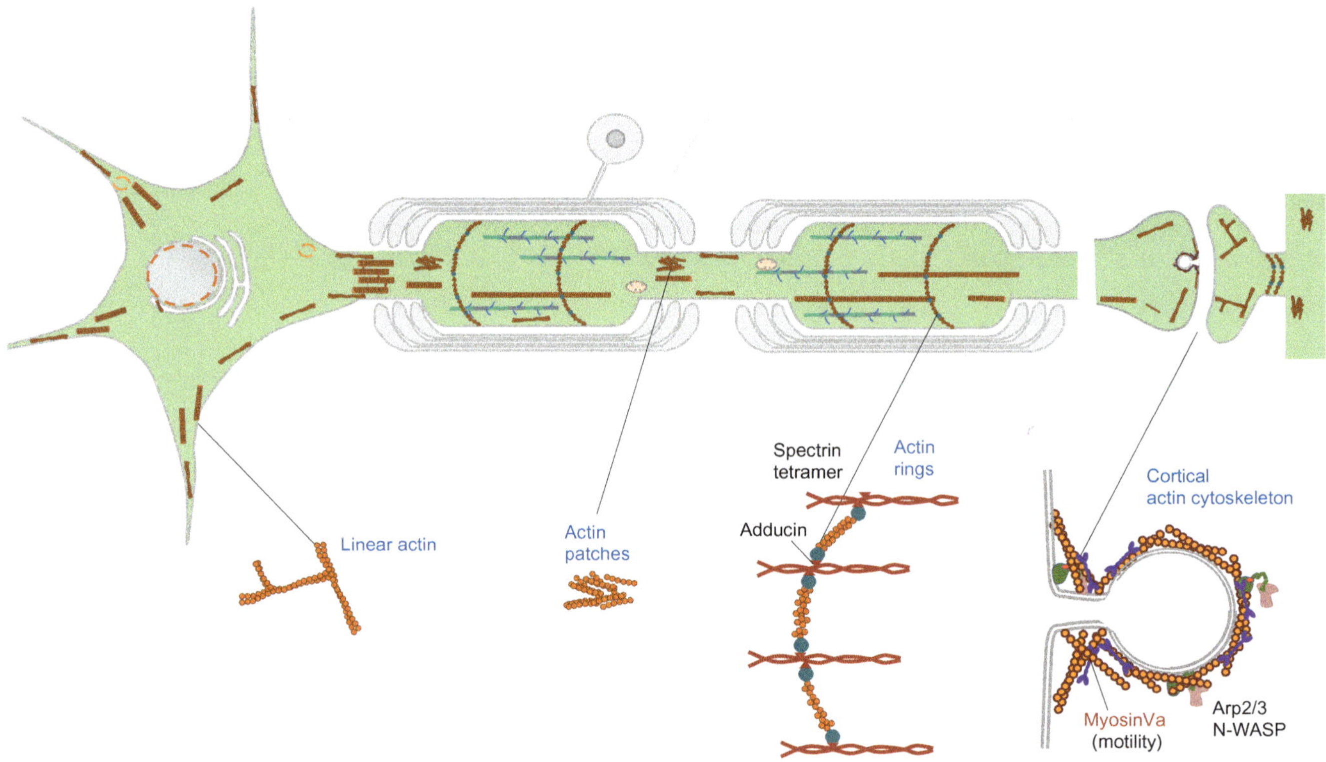

FIGURE 8.2 Actin structures.
Actin filaments can be arranged in linear or in branched conformations. The cortical actin network provides for functional compartmentalization of the plasma membrane and interacts with the machinery for exocytosis and endocytosis. Actin patches are enriched in branched F-actin. Longitudinal F-actin bundles traverse along the lengths of dendrites. Actin rings are present in axons and in the necks of dendritic spines; they are periodic cortical actin structures forming a lattice of actin filaments, capped by α-adducin, and crosslinked by α/β-spectrin.

stabilization is synaptic activity. Activation of glutamate N-methyl-D-aspartate receptors (NMDARs) and L-type Ca^{2+}-channels at excitatory synapses stabilizes dendritic branches and together with neurotrophic signaling via brain-derived neurotrophic factor (BDNF) modulates Ca^{2+} signaling and triggers multiple downstream pathways that affect actin dynamics and thus promote dendrite growth and stabilization. Cytoplasmic Ca^{2+} signaling is largely mediated by CaMKII, which regulates formation, growth, and branching of dendrites and stabilizes F-actin at synapses.

Control of Actin Dynamics via Rho-GTPases

Extrinsic signals regulate actin dynamics via small Rho (Ras-homologue) guanosine triphosphatases (GTPases), including Rac (Ras-related C3 botulinum toxin substrate1), Cdc42 (cell division cycle 42), and RhoA (Ras homologous member A) (Figure 8.3). The Rho, Rac1, and Cdc42 transduction pathways converge and diverge at different levels, and their downstream signals regulate actin filament polymerization and severing, contractility of actin-myosin complexes, and microtubule elongation. One important target of regulation by Rho GTPases is the actin-depolymerizing factor cofilin via its phosphorylation by LIMK (Lin-11, Isl-2, Mec-3 domain kinase) downstream of Rho GTPase signaling cascades. RhoA also controls elongation, branching, and severing of actin filaments via Rho kinase (ROCK), which stimulates assembly of contractile arrays of actin microfilaments and promotes their interaction with myosin IIb. Rac1 and Cdc42 inhibit cofilin via the p21-activated kinase (PAK) upstream of LIMK and promote assembly of branched actin filaments and thereby dendritic growth and elongation of the axonal growth cone. Rho GTPases are activated by growth factors, by adhesion molecules, and by guidance cue receptors such as slit, ephrins, netrins, and semaphorins (Figure 8.3). Activation of ionotropic glutamate receptors, BDNF, or chemoattractant molecules such as netrins leads to activation of CaMKII, which increases Rac1/Cdc42 and decreases RhoA activity, thereby promoting axonal and dendritic outgrowth. The actions of Rho GTPases depend on the developmental stage.[4] Several disorders affecting Rho-GTPase signaling have been associated with intellectual disability.[5] These disorders are typically associated with spine dysgenesis, with reduced density and immature shape of dendritic spines in cortical neurons.

TABLE 8.1 *Actin-Binding Proteins (Examples)*

Protein	Function in Neurons
Profilin	Actin nucleotide-exchanging factor
Arp2/3 complex	F-actin branching in growth cone and dendritic spine heads
Formins	Filament nucleation in filopodia, growth cone, and axons
Ena/VASP	Accelerates elongation and prevents capping
Adducin	Promotes F-actin and spectrin binding in actin rings
Tropomodulin	Stabilizes F-actin and decelerates actin
Spectrin	Couples F-actin cytoskeleton with the plasma membrane
α-actinin	Ca^{2+} sensitive, role in dendritic branching
ADF/cofilin	Binds and severs F-actin, enhances depolymerization
Gelsolin	Severs F-actin, directly activated by Ca^{2+}
Cortactin	Stabilizes F-actin, directly binds Arp2/3
Drebrin	Stabilizes actin and recruits microtubules into growth cones and dendritic spines
Microtubule-associated proteins (MAP) 1 and 2	Crosslink microtubules with F-actin, formation and stabilization of neurites
Formins	Simultaneous actin- and microtubule-binding protein
Cortactin-binding protein 2	Binds cortactin to microtubules
Myosin II	Network contraction, F-actin shearing, remodeling of actin network

Remodeling of Dendritic Spines and Synaptic Plasticity

Remodeling of the actin cytoskeleton in dendrites is a fundamental mechanism of activity-dependent long-term plastic changes in excitatory synapses.[6,7] Maintenance of long-term potentiation (LTP) of glutamatergic synapses relies on accumulation of F-actin in dendritic spines, leading to expansion of the spine head along with a shortening and widening of the spine neck. Excitatory synaptic activity results in release of L-glutamate and BDNF, which trigger downstream signals that activate Rac1 and Cdc42, promoting formation and maintenance of dendritic spines (Figure 8.3). During the early phase of induction of LTP there is a profound remodeling of the actin cytoskeleton through rapid periods of F-actin disassembly followed by periods of F-actin assembly. These changes reflect the rapid recruitment of actin, cofilin, and Arp2/3 and their synergistic actions in severing, capping, and branching of the actin filaments. Abnormalities in actin dynamics have a role in neurodegenerative disorders. Rods containing actin bound to cofilin may be the precursors of protein inclusions, eliciting dynamic actin remodeling disrupting cell function. For example, high extracellular levels of monomeric α-synuclein impair actin dynamics through the stabilization of microfilaments mediated by cofilin phosphorylation and loss of synaptic LTP.[8]

MICROTUBULES

Microtubules provide both the major tracks for intracellular transport and local cues for positioning of mitochondria and other organelles. Microtubules also interact with actin microfilaments to generate intracellular forces for both cell migration and dynamics of dendrites and axons, both during development and in response to synaptic activity.

Composition

Microtubules are dynamic polymers comprising tandem repeats of heterodimers of α- and β-tubulin[9] (Figure 8.4). Microtubule diversity reflects the expression of different α-tubulin (*TUBA*) or β-tubulin (*TUBB*) genes.[10] The α/β tubulin heterodimers assemble in a head-to- tail fashion to form a sheet or lattice of longitudinal protofilaments. Lateral interactions between neighboring protofilaments cause the sheet to close, forming fairly stiff hollow 25 nm tubes. Tubulins contain an amino (N)-terminal domain with residues that bind GTP; an intermediate domain that mediates interactions between protofilaments necessary for microtubule stability, and a carboxyl (C)-terminal that mediates microtubule interactions with motor and other microtubule-associated proteins. In neurons, microtubules typically organize at the Golgi apparatus or along existing microtubules. Microtubules are functionally polarized into a plus-end and a minus-end; the plus-end grows

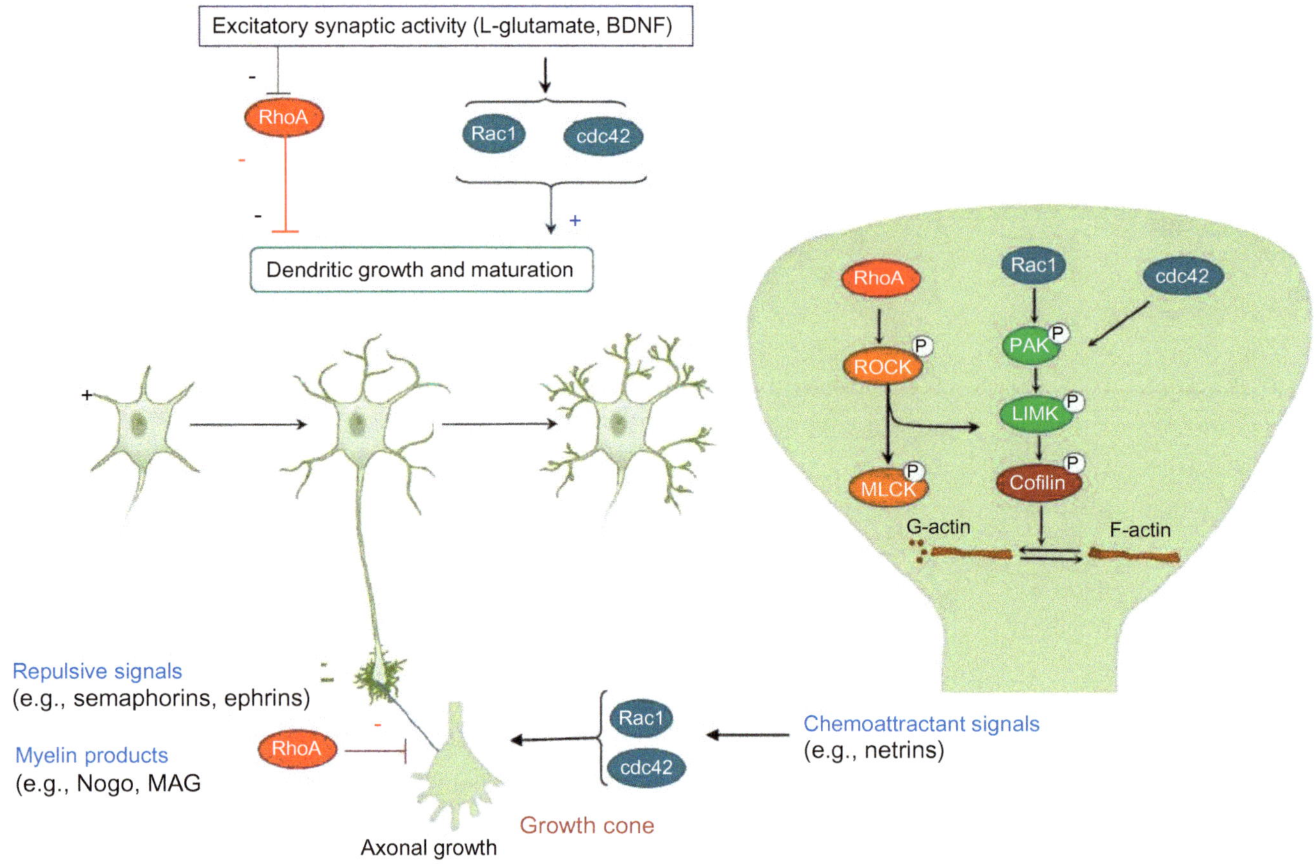

FIGURE 8.3 Rho proteins and regulation of actin dynamics.
Extrinsic signals regulate actin dynamics via small Rho (Ras-homologue) guanosine triphosphates (GTPases). They include Rac (Ras-related C3 botulinum toxin substrate1), Cdc42 (cell division cycle 42), and RhoA (Ras homologous member A). One important target of regulation is the actin depolarizing factor cofilin via its phosphorylation by LIM (Lin-11, Isl-2, Mec-3) domain kinase (LIMK). RhoA controls nucleation, elongation, branching, and severing of the actin filament network via the Rho kinase-LIM domain kinase (ROCK-LIMK). Rac1 and cdc42 inhibit cofilin via the p21-activated kinase (PAK)-LIMK pathway, Rho GTPases are activated by growth factors, adhesive ligands, and guidance cue receptors such as slit, ephrins, netrins, and semaphorins. Activation of ionotropic glutamate receptors, or effects of BDNF or chemoattractant increases Rac1/cdc42 and decreases RhoA activity to promote progression of axonal and dendritic outgrowth.

faster and undergoes more frequent depolymerization. At growing plus ends, GTP-bound α/β tubulin heterodimers are added to the exposed ends of linear protofilaments; this is followed by hydrolysis of the GTP bound to the β-tubulin subunit. The binding of GTP determines the structure and stability of tubulin heterodimers and the conformation of longitudinal protofilaments. Lateral interactions stabilize the interactions between protofilaments. Recent evidence indicates that GTP-tubulin islands can create points of microtubule rescue and regrowth and may be the mechanism underlying the high local microtubule dynamicity at presynaptic sites.

Dynamic Instability of Microtubules

Microtubules undergo periods of growth, shrinkage, and rest, depending on the continuous balance between assembly and disassembly.[11] The switch between phases of microtubule growth and disassembly is referred to as dynamic instability.[9] Hydrolysis of GTP bound by β-tubulin causes straight protofilaments to splay apart and curl outward, which produces microtubule depolymerization and shrinkage; this is called microtubule "catastrophe."

Tubulin undergoes several posttranslational modifications that regulate its stability, particularly acetylation, detyrosination, and polyglutamylation. Alpha-tubulin is acetylated by α-tubulin acetyltransferase and deacetylated by histone deacetylase 6 (HDAC6) and sirtuin 2. Acetylation increases microtubule resistance to mechanical breakage and might be especially important for increasing the longevity of microtubules in axons and may also have a role in specifying proper axonal pathfinding. The regulation of the α-tubulin tyrosination cycle is critical for proper neuronal differentiation and outgrowth, and influences axonal transport.

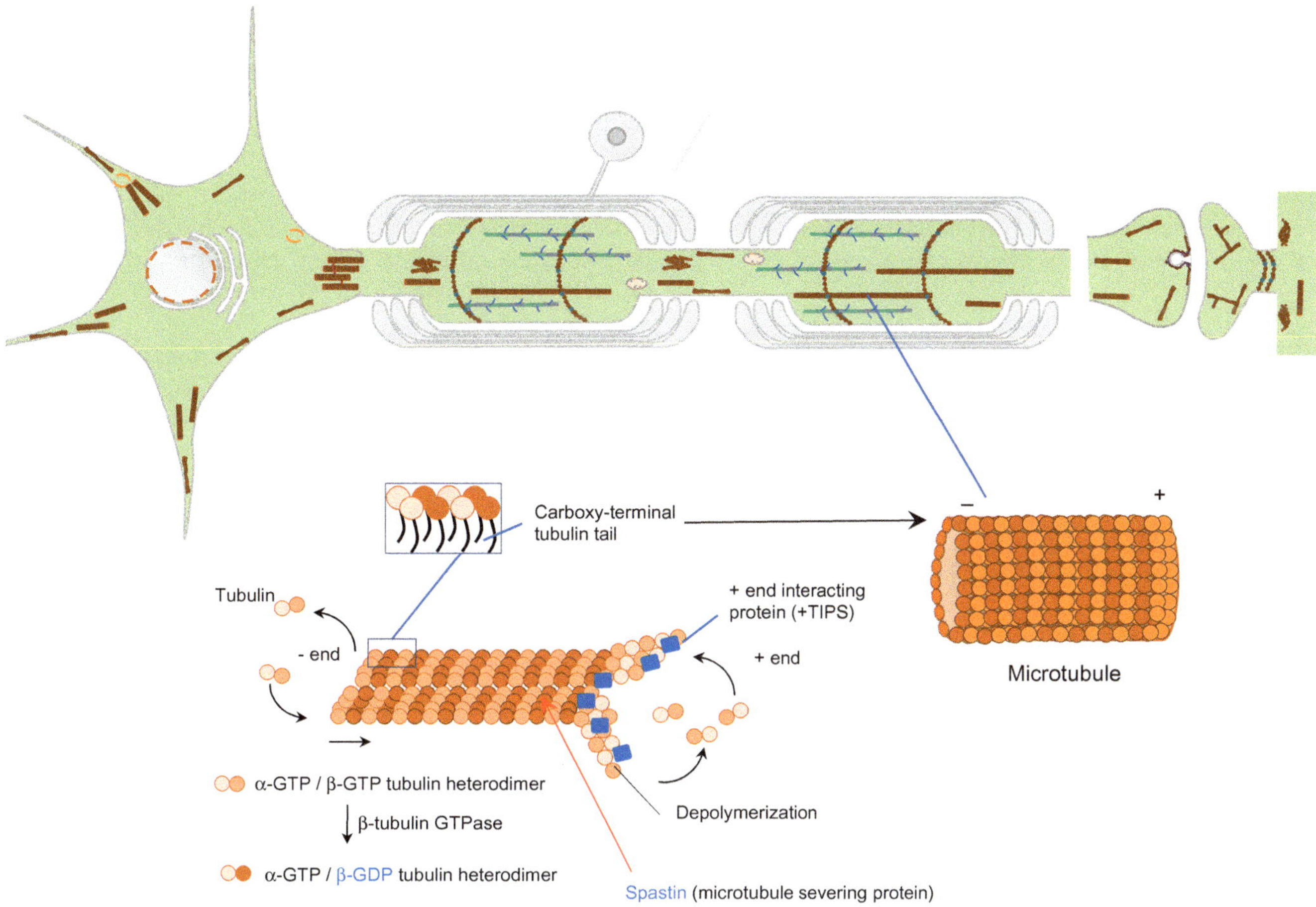

FIGURE 8.4 Composition and dynamic instability of microtubules.
Microtubules are dynamic polymers comprising tandem repeats of heterodimers of α- and β-tubulin. Microtubules are functionally polarized into a plus end and a minus end; at growing plus ends, GTP-bound α-/β-tubulin heterodimers are added to the exposed ends of linear protofilaments; this is followed by hydrolysis of the GTP bound to the β-tubulin subunit. Microtubules undergo periods of growth, shrinkage, and rest, depending on the continuous balance between assembly and disassembly. The switch between phases of microtubule growth and disassembly is referred to as dynamic instability. Hydrolysis of GTP bound by β-tubulin causes straight protofilaments to splay apart and curl outward, which produces microtubule depolymerization and shrinkage, this is called microtubule "catastrophe." Spastin and katanin are the main microtubule severing proteins in neurons.

Negatively charged glutamate residues can be sequentially added or removed from the C-terminal chain of α- and β-tubulin; the graded nature of this modification allows the fine control of several microtubule effectors, including spastin. Loss-of-function mutations in the deglutamylase CCP1 gene impair mitochondrial transport and cause infantile-onset neurodegeneration affecting the cerebellum, spinal motor neurons, and peripheral nerves.[12]

Proteins such as stathmin (STMN) promote microtubule instability by sequestering α/β-tubulin heterodimers or destabilizing the exposed microtubule protofilaments, which is necessary for normal axonal outgrowth and regeneration. Reduced STMN expression in motor neurons due to loss of TDP-43 function may contribute to the pathogenesis of amyotrophic lateral sclerosis (ALS) associated with *C9ORF72* mutations.[13] In contrast, compounds such as taxol or paclitaxel stabilize microtubules by counteracting the effects resulting from GTP hydrolysis. Spastin and katanin are the main microtubule-severing proteins in neurons; their action may release microtubule fragments that may be important for formation of axonal branches and dendritic development. However, the severing function of spastin in neurons is yet to be defined. Mutations of the *SPAST* gene encoding spastin are the most common cause of adult-onset, autosomal dominant pure hereditary spastic paraplegia.

Microtubule-Associated Proteins

Microtubule-associated proteins (MAPs) bind to the α- and β-tubulin monomers to regulate the stability, dynamics, and interactions of microtubules.[9] These MAPs bind directly to the tubulin dimers and in most cases stabilize microtubule structure, further encouraging polymerization. For example, plus-end tracking proteins (+TIPS) accumulate at the ends of the growing microtubules and prevent their depolymerization. Minus-end binding proteins, such as calmodulin-regulated spectrin-associated protein 2, stabilize microtubules and mediate actin–microtubule interactions. The numerous MAPs have been largely divided into two categories, type I includes the MAP1a and MAP1b found in the axons and dendrites, and type II includes MAP2 found mostly in dendrites and tau MAPT (tau) primarily present in axons.[14,15]

Tau: Structure, Functions, and Posttranslational Modifications

Microtubule-associated protein tau has a critical role in control of microtubule dynamics and axonal transport and is a primary target in many neurodegenerative disorders.[14,15]

Tau is encoded by the *MAPT* gene on chromosome 17q21 and is expressed primarily in neurons but also at low levels in oligodendrocytes and astrocytes.[14,15] Tau is a soluble protein that contains three domains. The N-terminal domain interacts both with membrane-associated proteins, allowing tau recruitment to lipid rafts, and with a subunit of dynactin, which is involved in retrograde transport. The central proline-rich domain harbors motifs that are targeted by protein kinases and regulates microtubule assembly, actin binding, and location. The C-terminal domain, the microtubule assembly domain, binds to microtubules; it includes a repeat domain with three of four repeat (R) regions (R1, R2, R3, R4), generated by alternative splicing out of R2. Four repeat (4R) tau has higher affinity for microtubules and is more efficient in promoting microtubule assembly than 3R tau.

Tau is primarily an axonal microtubule-binding protein. The axon initial segment (AIS) forms a retrograde barrier preventing tau movement toward the somatodendritic compartment. In axons normal tau binds to the interface between α/β heterodimers and promotes microtubule assembly, stabilizing microtubules either directly or by acting as a cross-bridge between microtubules and actin microfilaments. Tau can also inhibit HDAC6, thereby preventing microtubule depolymerization. Whereas tau may contribute to stabilization of microtubules, it primarily functions as a scaffold that targets protein kinases and phosphatases to microtubules, thus facilitating their interaction with motor proteins and other microtubule-associated protein substrates. A small amount of tau is present in dendrites, including dendritic spines, where it can regulate synaptic plasticity.[16]

Tau is subject to a wide range of posttranslational modifications, including phosphorylation, acetylation, and nitration. Many of these modifications strongly affect the probability for tau to form abnormal aggregates. Phosphorylation is the most common posttranslational modification and is tightly controlled by the balance between protein kinases and phosphatases. Important examples are glycogen synthase kinase 3β (GSK3β), cyclin-dependent kinase 5 (CDK5), protein kinase A, CaMKII, and tyrosine kinases such as Fyn, among several others. Tau is dephosphorylated primarily by protein phosphatase 2B. Tau hyperphosphorylation reduces its affinity for microtubules and promotes its self-aggregation.[17] Acetylation of tau at lysine residues in the microtubule-binding domain protects tau from increased phosphorylation and aggregation; however, acetylation at other lysine residues inhibits proteasome-mediated tau degradation.

Microtubules and Axonal Transport

Microtubules provide the tracks for intracellular transport, which is critical to deliver material to dendrites and axons.[18,19] Microtubule-based motors are essential for long-range transport of cargoes along the axon. The kinesin family of motor proteins mediate anterograde transport, which is directed toward the plus-end of microtubules and allows the delivery of membrane-bound organelles synthesized and packaged in the cell to the different compartments of dendrites, axons, and synaptic terminals. Cytoplasmic dynein forms a complex with dynactin and mediates retrograde transport, which is directed toward the minus-end of microtubules and allows both removal and degradation of materials via the endosome-lysosome systems and delivery of target-derived neurotrophic signals from the synaptic terminal or distal portions of the axon back to the cell body. Both anterograde and retrograde transport provide for the trafficking and turnover of cytoskeletal components.

CYTOSKELETAL REGULATION DURING DEVELOPMENT AND MAINTENANCE OF THE NERVOUS SYSTEM

The crosstalk between actin microfilaments and microtubules is crucial for development, maturation, and maintenance of the nervous system. During development, these cytoskeletal interactions produce the forces that are necessary for nuclear positioning, neuronal migration, and determining neuronal polarity. The first step in the architectural polarization of neurons is the sprouting of several short neurites from a spherical neuronal precursor; one of these neurites grows longer and becomes an axon, and the rest become dendrites. The tip of developing (or regenerating) axons consists of a growth cone that drives neuronal pathfinding during neurite outgrowth. Developing axons seek out synaptic partners by directed outgrowth mediated by the growth cone.

Dynamics of the Growth Cone

Neurite outgrowth is initiated both by polymerization of actin and by kinesin-mediated microtubule sliding.[20] Axon outgrowth exhibits three phases, protrusion, engorgement, and consolidation. Protrusion is the advancement of the leading edges of the growth cone, including a sheet-like structure called lamillopodium and finger-like extensions, or filopodia; this involves actin polymerization stimulated by dynamic microtubules that penetrate into the growth cone from the axonal shaft. Microtubule plus-end guidance into axonal branches is assisted by the actin cytoskeleton via interactions with septin 7, which is located at the base of filopodia, and drebrin, which is located along the proximal region of filopodia. Microtubules then stabilize the nascent neurites both by allowing the transport of vesicles and organelles into the developing protrusion and by promoting actin polymerization. In turn, actin promotes bundling of the microtubules to form a nascent neurite shaft. Actin-microtubule crosstalk engages different cytoskeletal regulators and involves various physical interactions, such as crosslinking, anchoring, and mechanical support. Large multidomain proteins or protein complexes bind both F-actin and microtubules and crosslink microtubules to act in bundles. Examples of such cross-linking proteins include tau, septins, and doublecortin.

Guidance Cues for Neuritic Growth

During development, guidance cues such as netrins, semaphorins, and ephrins provide directional information for the growing axons to reach their appropriate targets, in part by affecting the actin cytoskeleton via Rho GTPases. For example, netrins function as chemoattractant, eliciting growth cone extension by activating Rac and Cdc42. In contrast, semaphorins and ephrins elicit growth cone collapse and axon repulsion, both by activating Rho A and inhibiting Rac and Cdc42. The RhoA–Rho kinase pathway is also a key downstream intracellular effector of signals that prevent axonal regeneration following injury.

NEURONAL INTERMEDIATE FILAMENTS

Intermediate filaments constitute a family of related gene products that have been classified in five types (I–V) and are fundamental components of the cytoskeleton in neurons and astrocytes. Neurofilaments are the intermediate filaments in neurons; they have a major role in maintenance regulating axonal diameter and other mechanical functions and are involved in a variety neurodegenerative disorders.[21–23] Neurofilaments are very abundant in axons, particularly in myelinated axons, where they are highly organized into parallel arrays. Within these arrays individual neurofilaments are kept at a minimum distance from each other via side arms that project perpendicularly from a core. After axons establish synaptic contacts, signals from the myelinating glia elicit radial expansion of the axon.

Composition, Structure, and Dynamics

Neuron-specific intermediate filament subunits include the neurofilament triplet proteins, neurofilament light (NF-L, NfL), medium (NF-M, NfM), and heavy (NF-H, NfH) as well as α-internexin (in the central nervous system, CNS) and peripherin (in the peripheral nervous system, PNS).[24] All intermediate filaments have similar ultrastructure, forming 8–10 nm rope-like cytoskeletal filaments that may be several micrometers long. They all share a common structure characterized by three major domains: an N-terminal head domain, a central helical rod domain, and a C-terminal tail domain (Figure 8.5). The short head domain contains several sites for O-glycosylation and phosphorylation. The rod domain is shared with other members of the intermediate filament family and contains long stretches of hydrophobic repeats that mediate interactions between individual filament subunits, which coassemble to form dimers, protofilaments, and filaments. The C-terminal domain varies in the number of long glutamic and lysine-rich residues and determines the length of the different subunits. The backbone of the neurofilaments is mainly formed by NF-L (NfL), plus α-internexin or peripherin. NF-H (NfH) and NF-M (NfM) associate more peripherally and have long tail domains that are highly phosphorylated and project radially from the filament core to form side arms. These side arms maintain the minimal spacing between individual neurofilaments and between neurofilaments and microtubules. Although intermediate filaments are relatively stable cytoskeletal structures, they undergo degradation by calpains, the proteasome, and autophagy.

Intermediate filaments are regulated through their interactions with associated proteins, including 14-3-3 proteins, apoptosis-related proteins, kinases, and phosphatases.[24] Phosphorylation regulates intermediate filament solubility and binding to associated proteins. Neurofilament turnover via the ubiquitin-proteasome system involves a protein called gigaxonin. Gigaxonin functions as substrate adaptor for a E3 ubiquitin ligase complex that facilitates proteasome degradation of neurofilaments and other cytoskeletal proteins. Mutations of the *GAN* gene encoding gigaxonin produces giant axonal neuropathy, a rare neurodegenerative disorder of onset in infancy or early childhood and affecting both the PNS and CNS.

Axonal Transport of Neurofilament Proteins and Radial Growth of Axons

Neurofilament subunits undergo slow axonal transport along microtubules via ATP-dependent molecular motors at a rate of 0.2–1 mm/day. The slow transport of neurofilament and other cytoskeletal proteins by kinesin or dynein/dynactin motors may reflect short bursts of motility separated by long pauses. The rate of incorporation of transported neurofilament precursors into the stable neurofilament network is the major determinant of variation of neurofilament content along axons. The tight regulation of neurofilament content, particularly NF-L (NfL) and NF-M (NfM), and the phosphorylation state of the NF-M (NfM) and NF-H (NfH) tails are major determinants of the axon caliber and thus the cable properties of the axon. Myelination may signal changes in the phosphorylation state of the C-terminal domain of NF-M (NfM) to modulate axonal caliber. For example, myelin-associated glycoprotein regulates the radial expansion of axons by interacting with NF-M (NfM) and NF-H (NfH). Accumulation of hyperphosphorylated neurofilaments due to mutations and impairment of axonal transport is a hallmark of many peripheral and central neurodegenerative disorders.[21–23]

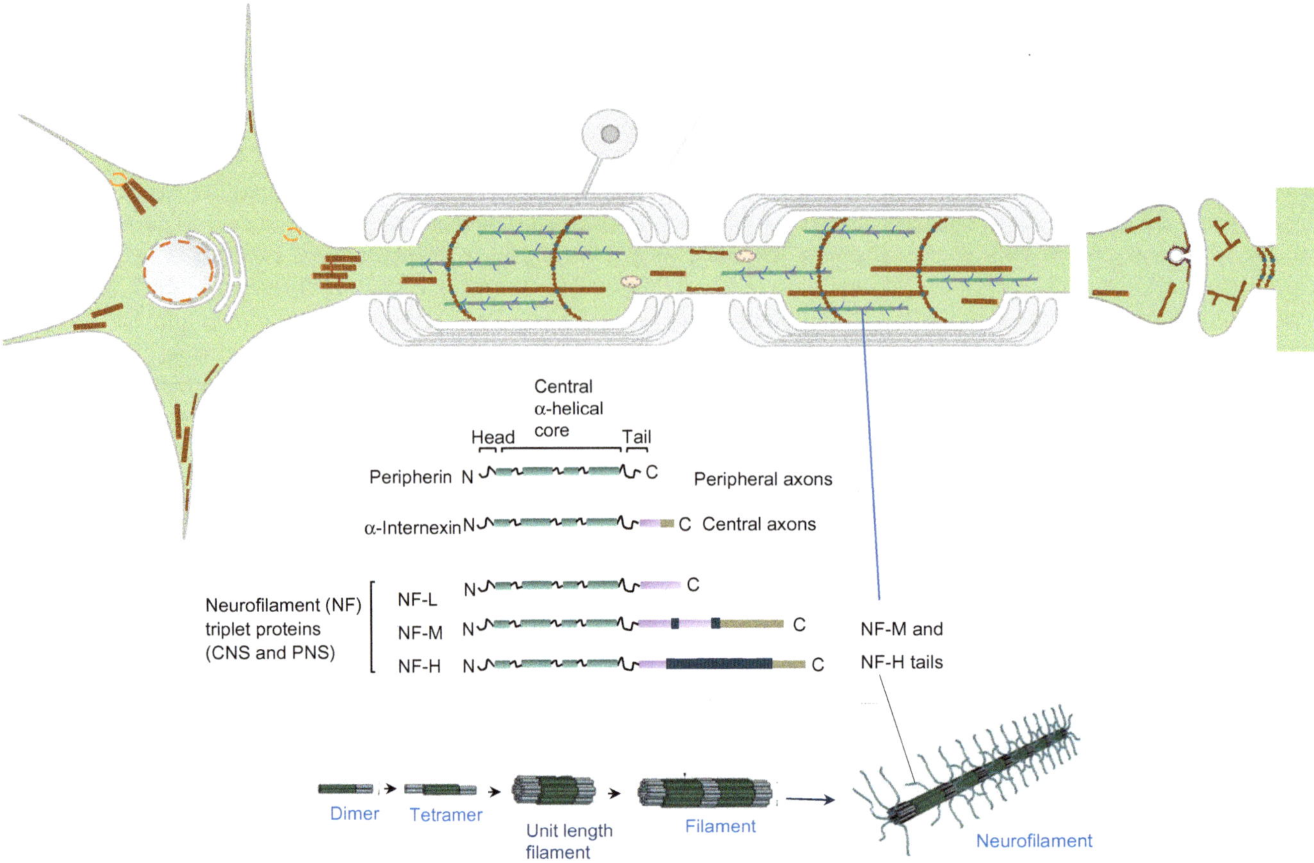

FIGURE 8.5 Structure and composition of neurofilaments.
Neuron-specific intermediate filament subunits include the neurofilament (NF) triplet proteins, neurofilament light (NF-L), medium (NF-M), and heavy (NF-H) as well as α-internexin (in the central nervous system) and peripherin (in the peripheral nervous system). All intermediate filaments share a common structure characterized by an N-terminal head domain, a central helical rod domain, and C-terminal tail domain. The rod domain mediates interactions between individual filament subunits, which coassemble with other subunits to form dimers, protofilaments, and filaments. The C-terminal domain varies in the number of long glutamic and lysine-rich residues and determines the length of the different NF subunits. The backbone of the neurofilaments is mainly formed by NF-L, plus α-internexin or peripherin. NF-H and NF-M have long tail domains that are highly phosphorylated and project radially from the filament core to form side arms and are critical determinants of axonal diameter.

Neurofilament Interactions with Other Organelles and Proteins

The neurofilament network interacts with many proteins, including actin, tubulin, spectrin, kinases, phosphatases, receptors, and molecular motors. Neurofilaments participate in active mechanical interactions with other cytoskeletal elements; they are linked to cortical actin via spectrins and to microtubules via tau and other microtubule-associated proteins. Neurofilaments form scaffolds for the endoplasmic reticulum (ER), endosomes, and synaptic vesicles. Myosin Va binds NF-L (NfL) and generates active ATP-dependent linkages with actin, promoting neurofilament motility and distribution of the ER and organelles in the axon. Neurofilaments interact with extracellular linker proteins, such as integrins and cadherin, which link these cytoskeletal structures with the extracellular matrix. This provides for mechanical interactions between the intracellular cytoskeleton and the extracellular environment that are critical for maintenance of axonal integrity in response to mechanical forces, which is particularly important in the PNS. Neurofilaments may also have important roles at synapses. Synaptic neurofilament assemblies are distinctive by their high proportion of α-internexin and low phosphorylation state of NF-M (NfM). This population of neurofilaments is particularly abundant in the postsynaptic regions of dendrites. Neurofilament subunits may be synthesized locally at the level of postsynaptic densities at dendritic spines of excitatory synapses, where they may regulate synaptic plasticity.

ORGANIZATION OF THE CYTOSKELETON IN AXONS AND DENDRITES

The different domains of neurons have distinct distribution and organization and dynamics of microfilaments, microtubules, and neurofilaments. This contributes to establish functional polarity and influences the structure and plasticity of axons and dendrites.

Axon Initial Segment

The different components of the axons have a unique cytoskeletal organization.[2] The proximal axon comprises a region that spans from the base of the soma to the end of the axon initial segment (AIS).[25] The AIS is characterized by small fascicles of microtubules and a dense subaxolemmal undercoat. Microtubules in the AIS are arranged as fascicles of three to six closely apposed microtubules connected by cross-bridges. The subaxolemmal undercoat consists of a complex of cytoskeletal proteins including actin, the scaffolding protein ankyrin G, and βIV-spectrin. Microtubules have a major role in organizing the AIS; they are connected to ankyrin G via plus-end binding proteins and stabilized via a microtubule cross-linking factor. The unique cytoskeletal organization of the AIS contributes to the intracellular barrier that prevents somatodendritic proteins to enter the axon. The area between the soma and the AIS constitutes the preaxonal exclusion zone, which is defined by its enrichment of both MAP2 and tripartite-containing motif protein 46 (TRIM46). At this region, somatodendritic cargoes are rerouted to the soma before entering the AIS. Some cargoes such as synaptic vesicles are trafficked to the axons, whereas lysosomes tend to be retained in the soma. The AIS also provides a barrier to the diffusion of tau and promotes its primary distribution in axons. Ankyrin G is the structural landmark of the AIS and links transmembrane proteins such as voltage-gated sodium and potassium channels to the actin and microtubule cytoskeleton.

Axon Shaft

The axon shaft contains two different actin cytoskeletal networks, a submembrane (cortical) and deep axonal networks (Figure 8.2). Cortical actin is organized in periodic actin ring structures consisting of a lattice of several short and stable actin filaments. These filaments are capped by α-adducin and cross-inked by α/βII and spectrin tetramers, forming a periodic actin-spectrin undercoat. These actin-spectrin ring complexes are immobile and stable; they provide both high resistance and flexibility to the axon, help organize the proteins in the membrane, and stabilize the underlying microtubules. In contrast, the deep axonal actin networks are highly dynamic and distributed along the axon in focal F-actin "hot spots," where actin is continuously polymerized and depolymerized, producing elongating actin polymers (actin trails) that extend in both anterograde and retrograde directions. These actin filaments may also contribute to short-range transport of vesicles in axons.

The axon shaft contains a succession of overlapping microtubules with their plus-end directed toward the axon terminal and minus-end directed toward the cell body. In the axon shaft, neurofilaments are organized in extensive parallel networks that fill the axoplasm and pack against one another in regular spaced arrays that slide easily in the axial direction along the axon. In peripheral axons, axoplasm regions encased in compact myelin are predominantly composed of neurofilaments with highly phosphorylated tails causing the neurofilaments to repel each other, thereby increasing the overall diameter of the myelinated segment, whereas at the nodes of Ranvier the lower degree of neurofilament phosphorylation reduces of axonal caliber and increases neurofilament density. Neurofilaments and microtubules also have a major role in maintaining trophic Schwann cell–axon and oligodendrocyte–axon interactions.

Dendrites

The organization of the cytoskeleton in dendrites has both similarities and differences with that in axons.[1,26] Glutamatergic synapses are frequently located on dendritic spines or can be found directly on the dendritic shaft. The most important parameter determining the degree of compartmentalization is the spine neck diameter, which depends on the organization of the actin cytoskeleton. Actin forms a ring at the base of the spines and dynamic patches within dendritic spines harboring excitatory synapses. In the dendritic shaft, F-actin forms actin patches and longitudinal fibers. Microtubules may invade dendrites and dendritic spines in response to increased neuronal activity. In dendrites, microtubules are organized in a complex, bipolar pattern and serve as roads for dynein- and to a lesser extent kinesin-driven cargo.

GLIAL FIBRILLARY ACID PROTEIN

Glial fibrillary acid protein (GFAP) is the main intermediate filament of astrocytes. It is also expressed in non-myelinating Schwann cells and enteric glial cells.

Structure and Processing

GFAP is encoded by a single gene on human chromosome 17q21, and its expression progressively increases with age. GFAP shares with other intermediate filaments a common structure characterized by an N-terminus head domain, a central helical rod domain, and a C-terminus tail domain. There are at least 10 GFAP isoforms resulting from alternative splicing. The GFAP-α isoform is the predominant form in the adult brain and spinal cord; GFAP-δ is preferentially expressed in neurogenic astrocytes in the subventricular zone; GFAP-β is highly expressed in non-myelinating

Schwann cells; and GFAP-γ in the corpus callosum. There are also four GFAP isoforms, referred to as GFAP+1, which are expressed in a subset of astrocytes throughout the brain, particularly in pathological conditions. GFAP is subject to numerous posttranslational modifications, including phosphorylation at the N-terminal head domain, which has a negative effect on GFAP filament assembly, as well as acetylation and citrullination producing epitopes that evoke autoimmune responses. Like neurofilaments, GFAP forms relatively stable cytoskeletal structures but undergoes turnover in part via degradation by the ubiquitin-proteasome system promoted by gigaxonin.[27]

Role of GFAP in Normal Astrocyte Function

GFAP interacts with microtubules, myosin, and actin microfilaments via several binding proteins and may have a role in astrocyte migration and mitosis. During mitosis, GFAP undergoes an increased phosphorylation of its head domain and movement to the site of daughter cell separation. GFAP expression may regulate astrocyte proliferation as well as Schwann cell proliferation in response to injury. GFAP may also regulate vesicle trafficking, including movement of vesicles releasing different gliotransmitters, vesicle recycling, and lysosome-mediated autophagy. GFAP may also contribute to astrocytic modulation of synaptic plasticity, organization of the astrocytic foot processes to induce blood-brain barrier properties in endothelial cells, and maintenance of normal CNS myelination. Mutations of the *GFAP* gene are linked to Alexander disease, a leukodystrophy with a variable, age-related phenotype.[28,29] The pathological hallmark is enlargement of the astrocytes, shortening of astrocytic processes, and accumulation of GFAP-containing aggregates (Rosenthal fibers) Many of the morphological and functional changes in astrocytes in Alexander disease mimic those of reactive astrocytes in a variety of neurologic disorders.

OTHER CYTOSKELETON-RELATED PROTEINS

Nuclear Lamins

Lamins are group IV intermediate filament proteins located in the nuclear lamina that underlies the inner nuclear membrane.[30,31] The nuclear lamina is an essential structural element of the nuclear envelope; it maintains the nuclear architecture and regulates DNA replication and chromatin organization. Nuclear lamins include lamin A, encoded by the *LMNA* gene, and lamin B, encoded by two separate genes, *LMNB1* and *LMNB2*. Lamin monomers associate in parallel homodimers that form head-to-tail polymers that interact with each other forming antiparallel protofilaments, which then associate to form 10 nm intermediate-like filaments. Posttranslational modifications, particularly phosphorylation, regulate lamin polymerization and insertion into the inner nuclear membrane. Lamins form the nuclear lamina scaffold adjacent to the inner nuclear membrane and interact with several inner nuclear membrane proteins that help anchor lamin filaments to the nuclear envelope. Lamin-binding proteins include emerin, nesprins, lamin B receptor, and lamin-associated polypeptides. Via these interactions, lamins participate in regulation of the chromatin organization, import and export of transcription factors across the nuclear envelope, and transduction of mechanical signals to the nucleus via interactions with the cytoskeleton. The mechanical roles of lamins and their effects on gene regulation suggest an interdependent regulation of these two functions. B-type lamins confer elasticity, while A-type lamins increase viscosity and stiffness to nucleus. Lamin A, emerin, nesprin, and the linker of the nucleoskeleton and cytoskeleton complex directly transmit forces from the extracellular matrix into the nucleus. These mechanical forces lead to changes in the molecular structure, modification, and assembly state of A-type lamins. This in turn activates a tension-induced "inside-out signaling" through which the nucleus feeds back to the cytoskeleton and the extracellular matrix to balance outside and inside forces. These functions regulate differentiation and may be impaired in lamin-linked diseases. Lamin-associated polypeptide 1 allows interaction of lamin A with cell cycle regulators. Lamin B receptor is a transmembrane protein that interacts with lamin B and chromatin via a protein that binds to methylated residues of histone, resulting in gene silencing. By this mechanism, lamin B participates in regulation of gene expression.

Septins

Septins are a family of proteins that are considered components of the cytoskeleton due to their filamentous appearance and association with cellular membranes, actin filaments and microtubules.[32,33] All septins are GTP-binding proteins that interact with each other to form heterohexamers or heterooctamers that assemble into filaments and rings. There are 13 septin (*SEPT*) genes in humans. Septins participate in a wide range of cellular processes by interacting with actin, microtubules, and membrane phospholipids. Septin assemblies function as scaffolds at the plasma membrane to regulate the distribution of membrane-bound proteins, regulate vesicle fusion events, couple membrane acquisition to autophagosome biogenesis, and facilitate the efficient fusion of autophagosomes to lysosomes. For example, septins can form arc-shaped or ring-like structures at the base of dendritic spines, which might contribute to establishment and stabilization of neuronal membrane curvature. Septin ring-like structures may also act as diffusion barriers that compartmentalize membrane proteins to specific cellular domains. Septins also participate in crosstalk between different cytoskeletal components, such as microtubule entry in dendritic spines, which depends on the presence of an F-actin mesh at the base of a target spine. Septin 9 has been linked to various intracellular functions, such as membrane trafficking and advancement of the axonal growth cone.

Mutations of the *SEPT9* gene encoding septin 9 are linked to hereditary neuralgic amyotrophy, an autosomal dominant disorder characterized by recurrent painful brachial plexus neuropathies.[34–36] Dysmorphic facial features are present in many but not all individuals. SEPT9 variants have also been identified in a kindred with Charcot-Marie-Tooth phenotype associated with cognitive deficits, including visual abilities and episodic memory.[37]

DEVELOPMENTAL DISORDERS ASSOCIATED WITH CYTOSKELETAL DYSFUNCTION

Disorders affecting actin or microtubule dynamics manifest with a variety of neurodevelopment disorders. Only some examples will be briefly discussed here.

Mutations Affecting Rho GTPase Signaling and Intellectual Disability

Intellectual disability (formerly referred to as mental retardation), is a common neurodevelopmental disorder characterized by a global impairment of cognition and adaptive behavior.[38] A pathologic hallmark in many of these disorders is spine dysgenesis, which is the presence of reduced density and immature shape of dendritic spines in cortical neurons. Some forms of these disorders are linked to mutations of genes encoding components or regulators of Rho GTPases, thereby affecting actin dynamics at dendritic spines. In these disorders the RhoA pathway is hyperactive while the Rac1 and Cdc42 pathways are consistently hypoactive.[5] Intellectual disability has been associated with mutations in more than 80 genes on the X-chromosome, some of which code for regulators or effectors of the small-GTPase family. They include oligophrenin 1 (*OPHN1*), *RAC1*, *PAK3*, Rac/Cdc42, guanine-nucleotide-exchange factor 6 (*aPIX*), *ARHGEF9*, *LIMK1*, and others.[5,38]

Tubulinopathies

Tubulinopathies encompass a group of disorders resulting in complex cortical malformations and due to mutations in genes encoding α-tubulin or β-tubulin isoforms such as *TUBA1A*, *TUBA8*, *TUBB2B*, *TUBB3*, *TUBB5*,and *TUBG1*.[39] This heterogeneous group of conditions has a wide spectrum of clinical severity reflecting abnormal neuronal migration and axonal growth and differentiation.[40–43] Many mutations impair the formation or stabilization of α/β tubulin heterodimers, the ability of microtubules to polymerize, or their dynamic properties, affecting axonal transport. Their clinical expression includes cortical malformation syndromes, various degrees of motor and intellectual disability, and seizures. Cortical malformations include microlissencephaly, lissencephaly, central pachygyria, polymicrogyria-like cortical dysplasia, and "simplified" gyral pattern with areas of focal polymicrogyria. Basal ganglia malformation, corpus callosum agenesis, and mild to severe cerebellar hypoplasia and dysplasia are frequent findings. *TUBA1* mutations may affect the interactions of α-tubulin with adaptor proteins involved in neural migration, such as doublecortin (encoded by the *DCX* gene) and lissencephaly 1 (encoded by the *PAFAH1B1* gene), thereby reproducing the phenotype resulting from mutations affecting these proteins. Similarly, some *TUBB3* mutations disrupt microtubule interactions with kinesin and produce phenotypes that resemble those associated with kinesin mutations, including sensorimotor peripheral neuropathy or congenital fibrosis of extraocular muscles.[41,42] Mutations of the *TUBB4A* gene have been linked to hereditary generalized dystonia with whispering dysphonia, hereditary spastic paraplegia, and leukodystrophy with hypomyelination and atrophy of the basal ganglia and cerebellum. These mutations interfere with motor protein binding to microtubules and impair mitochondrial transport.[44]

TAUOPATHIES

Neurodegenerative tauopathies constitute a heterogeneous group of disorders characterized by dementia and movement disorders (primarily atypical parkinsonism). They are characterized by abnormal accumulation of intracellular hyperphosphorylated tau filaments that form neurofibrillary tangles and other tau inclusions in neurons, glial cells, and frequently both[14,15,17,45] (Box 8.2). Tauopathies are subdivided according to the isoform and number of repeats of the abnormally accumulated tau inclusions. The four-repeat (4R) tauopathies include progressive supranuclear palsy (PSP), corticobasal degeneration (CBD), argyrophilic grain disease, primary age-related tauopathy, and globular glial tauopathy, whereas Pick disease is a 3-repeat (3R) tauopathy. Frontotemporal dementia and parkinsonism linked to chromosome 17 (FTDP-17, FTLD-tau) due to mutations of

BOX 8.2 TAUOPATHIES

Progressive supranuclear palsy
Corticobasal degeneration
Familial frontotemporal degeneration-tau
Pick disease
ALS-parkinsonism dementia complex of Guam
Postencephalitic parkinsonism
Argyrophilic grain disease
Primary age-related tauopathy
Chronic traumatic encephalopathy
Globular glial tauopathies
Aging-related tau astrogliopathy
Subacute sclerosing panencephalitis
Niemann-Pick type C disease
IgLON5 disease

the *MAPT* gene may be associated with accumulation of 3R tau, 4R tau, or both. These mutations typically cause abnormal *MAPT* splicing and produce several different clinical phenotypes, the majority of which include frontotemporal dementia. Other neurodegenerative disorders associated with tau pathology are referred to as secondary tauopathies; examples include Alzheimer disease (AD) and chronic traumatic encephalopathy. Neurofibrillary tangles in AD are paired helical and straight filaments, contain both 3R and 4R tau isoforms in a one-to-one ratio, similar to the isoform composition of tau in normal brain.

Mechanisms of Abnormal Tau Accumulation

The conversion of physiological forms of tau into pathological tau species may result from tau missplicing, aggregation, and posttranslational modifications. Tau contributes to the pathogenesis of tauopathies by undergoing misfolding and oligomerization into insoluble tau deposits. The aggregation propensity of tau depends on two hexapeptide motifs located in the second and third microtubule binding repeats. Further recruitment of tau monomers and dimers could lead to the formation of a nucleation center that after reaching a threshold size promotes tau oligomerization. Tau oligomers elongate into protomers, which adopt a cross-β-sheet structure typical of amyloid aggregates, and ultimately become the building blocks of neurofibrillary pathology. *MAPT* mutations affect the ratio of 3R and 4R tau isoforms and increase tau phosphorylation; 4R tau isoforms are more prone to aggregation. There is a co-occurrence of aggregated tau and α-synuclein in tauopathies and synucleinopathies. Tau and α-synuclein colocalize in the same neuronal compartments, particularly in axons. Moreover, tau fibrils are incorporated into Lewy bodies and colocalize with α-synuclein fibrils. Alpha synuclein promotes GSK3β-mediated tau phosphorylation by formation of a tripartite GSK3β/α-synuclein/tau complex. Proteolytic cleavage of tau could either generate fragments with a toxic gain of function triggering cell death cascade, or could induce and drive aggregation. Whereas soluble tau is preferentially degraded by the proteasome, pathological forms of phosphorylated tau are directed toward the autophagic-lysosomal system. Tau fragmentation by proteases such as caspases or hyperphosphorylation could lead to the formation of aggregates that exceed the capacity of the ubiquitin-proteasome system and promote tau degradation by the autophagy/lysosomal system.

Mechanisms of Tau Toxicity

The detrimental effects of pathological tau may be amplified by dysfunction of pathways involved in axonal transport, synaptic function, and protein quality control.[14] These pathological events could act synergistically and elicit cytotoxic effects, promote intercellular spreading of tau pathology, and affect both neurons and glia. Abnormal tau affects axonal transport by both compromising microtubule structure and disrupting the axonal transport machinery. Hyperphosphorylation, truncation, and acetylation of tau impair its interaction and its ability to stabilize microtubules. Tau also interferes with binding of the molecular motor proteins dynein and kinesin to microtubules. For example, tau sequesters the available kinesin and promotes release of cargo vesicles from kinesin by activating phosphorylation of kinesin by GSK3β.

Another typical feature of tauopathies is tau mislocalization in dendrites, leading to gain of toxicity. For example, in AD dendritic tau mediates Aβ toxicity by impairing normal excitatory synaptic transmission and activating the non-receptor-associated tyrosine kinase Fyn, which phosphorylates a subunit of the NMDAR and renders neurons susceptible to excitotoxicity. Whereas the presence of tau in axons protects microtubules from severing by spastin or katanin, dendritic tau recruits a tubulin tyrosine ligase that polyglutamylates the microtubules, increasing their susceptibility to cleavage. Accumulation of tau in dendrites also results in mislocalization of cargoes that are normally transported between the somatodendritic and axonal compartments and nerve terminals, such as mitochondria, vesicles, and neurofilaments. Mitochondrial dysfunction may also have a major role in tauopathy. Hyperphosphorylated tau interacts with the mitochondrial fission protein, dynamin-related protein 1 (Drp1), which results in increased fragmentation of mitochondria and mitochondrial deficiency in affected neurons. In AD, tau may interact with Aβ to affect mitochondrial integrity. Hyperphosphorylated tau may be recruited to stress granules in the nucleus; reduced normal activity of nuclear tau may disrupt chromatin dynamics and normal gene expression and predispose to oxidative stress-induced DNA damage.

Tau has prion-like properties. Pathological forms of tau can be transmitted transsynaptically and also taken up through cellular structures, suggesting additional trans-cellular propagation pathways. Tau secretion may be mediated through several different mechanisms, including unconventional secretion, exosomal release, and tunneling nanotubes. Neuronal activity enhances release of tau primarily via a nonvesicular, calcium-dependent mechanism. Secretion of tau is also mediated in part by exosomes, which display a propensity to seed aggregation of endogenous tau. Microglia-derived exosomes may be responsible for transmission of tau between neurons. Tunneling nanotubes have been identified as another mechanism by which tau aggregates may be transmitted through direct contact between neurons. Tau may be released by chaperone-dependent exocytosis via the presynaptic co-chaperone cysteine string protein-alpha (CSPα), which is involved in the release of several aggregated proteins through a noncanonical exocytosis pathway. Low-molecular-weight aggregates and short fibrils of recombinant tau can be internalized by endocytosis and by micropinocytosis by attaching to heparan sulfate proteoglycans in target cells, a mechanism shared with α-synuclein. Small tau oligomers may be the major tau species undergoing tau propagation. Tau propagation can be further accelerated through activation of inflammatory pathways involving microglia. Activated microglia may directly mediate tau propagation in part by tau release via exosomes.

Astrocyte Tauopathies

Astrocytic plaques, tufted astrocytes, ramified astrocytes, and globular astroglial inclusions are seen predominantly in primary tauopathies; thorn-shaped astrocytes and granular/fuzzy astrocytes occur in age-related tau astrogliopathy. Astrocytic tau pathology in this disorder may reflect a response to a repeated or prolonged pathogenic process such as blood-brain barrier dysfunction or local mechanical impact. Some of these findings overlap with the features of tau pathology seen in chronic traumatic encephalopathy (CTE). This condition is characterized by a distinct perivascular accumulation of hyperphosphorylated tau in neurons and astrocytes within cerebral sulci. Studies in mouse models show that traumatic brain injury induced neuronal production of the toxic compound *cis*-phospho tau, an abnormal and destructive isomer of the normal and benign *trans*-phospho tau leading to degeneration by via a process of "cistauosis."[46] In CTE, astroglial tau pathology is composed of 4R-immunoreactive thorn-shaped astrocytes similar to that found in aging-related tau astrogliopathy, whereas neurofibrillary tangles contain both 3R and 4R tau, with posttranslational modifications and conformations consistent with AD and primary age-related tauopathy.[47,48]

ROLE OF NEUROFILAMENTS IN NEUROLOGIC DISORDERS

Cellular stress induces transcription and translation of intermediate filaments. In this setting, intermediate filaments may have a protective role by providing mechanical support; serving as scaffold for binding of antiapoptotic proteins; regulating organelle positioning and function; and preventing excessive phosphorylation of propaptotic or other damaging proteins.[24] Many neurologic disorders are associated with axonal accumulation of neurofilaments in the form of axonal ovoids or torpedoes, reflecting impaired axonal transport (Figure 8.6).

Genetic Neurofilament-Associated Axonopathies

Mutations of NF proteins result in aggregation and impaired transport of neurofilaments, promoting their accumulation and leading to axonal dysfunction and degeneration.[49] Altered organization of the neurofilament network is followed by fragmentation of the Golgi complex, accumulation of mitochondria, decrease in neurite caliber, and later appearance of phosphorylated neurofilament subunits. Mutations in *NEFH*-encoding NF-H (NfH) have been associated with type 2C axonal form of Charcot-Marie-Tooth disease (CMT). Mutations in the *NEFL* gene encoding (NF-L (NfL) have been linked to several other less common forms of CMT including axonal CMT2E, demyelinating CMT1F, or intermediate forms.[50] Most *NEFL* mutations are missense mutations that disrupt the assembly and transport of neurofilament proteins with accumulations of neurofilament polymers.[23,51] Some other genetic diseases are characterized by prominent abnormal neurofilament accumulation in axons. Autosomal recessive spastic ataxia of Charlevoix-Saguenay (ARSACS) is caused by mutations of the *SACS* gene encoding sacsin, a protein with putative ubiquitin and chaperone function that may be involved in neurofilament turnover.[23] This disorder is the second most common worldwide cause of hereditary ataxia and is characterized by prominent peripheral neuropathy with accumulation and abnormal bundling of neurofilaments in affected neurons. Mutations of the *TRIM2* (tripartite motif containing 2) gene cause a rare early-onset, recessive form of CMT2R; TRIM2 is an E3 ubiquitin ligase that binds and ubiquitylates NF-L (NfL); this disorder is characterized by swollen axons with abnormal aggregation of neurofilaments in myelinated fibers. Giant axonal neuropathy is a rare fatal autosomal recessive neurodegenerative disorder of onset in infancy or early childhood affecting both the PNS and CNS. It is caused by mutations of the *GAN* gene encoding gigaxonin, which contains a Kelch-like E3 ubiquitin ligase domain and targets intermediate filaments for degradation. The neurofilament accumulation within "giant axons" is the most characteristic finding. However, there is also accumulation of GFAP in astrocytes and desmin in muscle.[23] Mutations of small heat shock proteins interacting with the cytoskeleton, such as HSPB1, HSPB3, and HSPB8 are linked to CMT disease and distal hereditary motor neuropathy (dHMN).[52] For example, mutations of the *HSPB1* gene encoding the small heat shock protein 27 (Hsp 27) produce CMT2F[53] whereas mutations of the *HSPB8* gene encoding Hsp22 produce CMT2L.

Neurofilament Accumulation in Neurodegenerative Disorders

Axonal accumulation of neurofilaments occurs in a wide range of neurologic disorders, including brain or peripheral nerve traumatic or ischemic injury, chronic inflammatory disorders such as multiple sclerosis, and neurodegenerative disorders such as ALS and PD. Neuronal intermediate filament inclusion disease (NIFID) is an early neurodegenerative disorder and heterogeneous clinical phenotype, dominated by frontotemporal dementia associated with pyramidal or extrapyramidal manifestations including poor levodopa responsive parkinsonism, and motor neuron disease.[55–58] This disorder is characterized by accumulation of large internexin-containing neurofilaments in swollen neurons, associated with neuronal loss and gliosis. Polymorphisms of the gene encoding NF-H (NfH) and certain mutations affecting the peripherin (*PRPH*) gene have been associated with susceptibly to ALS. Degenerating neurons in ALS show a 70% decrease in levels of NfL, α-internexin (INA), and peripherin mRNA post-mortem. TAR DNA-binding protein 43 (TDP-43), which forms cytoplasmic aggregates in ALS, binds and

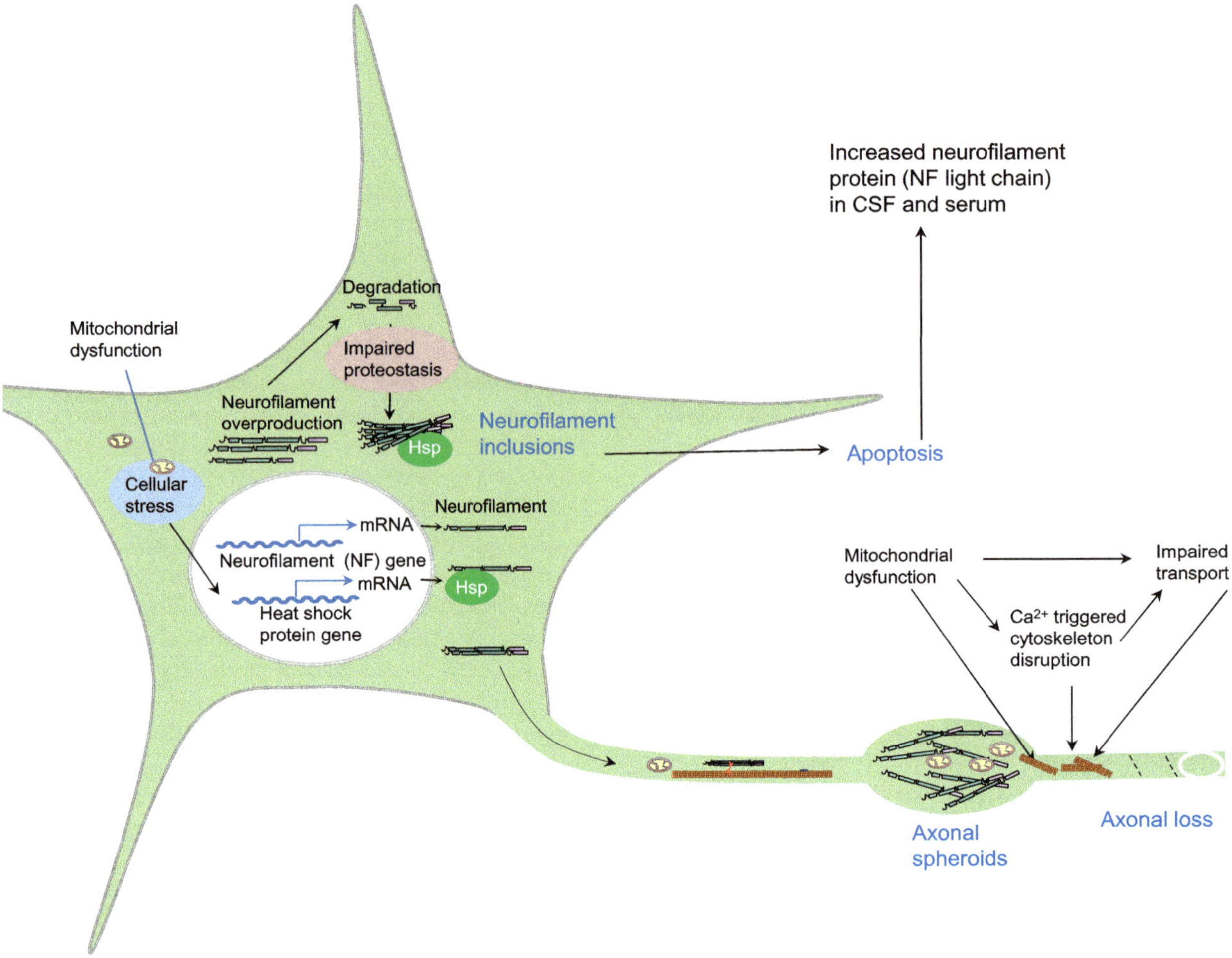

FIGURE 8.6 Neurofilament accumulation in neurodegenerative disease.
Cellular stress induces transcription and translation of intermediate filaments. Axonal accumulation of neurofilaments (NFs) in the form of axonal ovoids or torpedoes reflects impaired axonal transport due to several mechanisms. Disruption of the expanded axonal neurofilaments results in collapse and fasciculation of the filaments, forming ring-like structures surround organelles such as mitochondria in axonal segments showing atrophy, and whorls in swollen portions of the axon. Impaired axonal transport, disrupted calcium homeostasis, and mitochondrial dysfunction lead to dying back axonopathy, which, together with accumulation of intermediate filaments in the soma, eventually leads to cell death. Accumulation of intermediate filament subunits, including neurofilament light chain (NF-L) subunits in the cerebrospinal fluid and serum is a potential biomarker of cell and axonal injury and degeneration.

destabilizes or sequesters NEFL mRNA. Glutamate excitotoxicity and phosphorylation may alter neurofilament organization and axonal transport.

Neurofilament Proteins as Disease Biomarkers

There has been increased interest in the use of increased levels of neurofilament proteins in serum or CSF as a biomarker of the presence and progression neurodegenerative disorders.[23] For example, increased plasma NF-L (NfL) or NF-H (NfH) levels have been reported to serve as a measure of disease progression in ALS, brain injury, and multiple sclerosis. In these conditions, plasma levels reflect CSF levels. Increased CSF levels of GFAP are also detected in a wide variety of neurologic disorders, among the highest levels are found in astrocytopathies such Alexander disease and neuromyelitis optica spectrum disorders.[54]

LAMINOPATHIES

Lamin A Laminopathies

Mutations of *LMNA* and associated proteins are linked to Emery-Dreifuss muscular dystrophy (EDMD).[55] This disorder is characterized by early contractures of the elbow and Achilles tendons as well as posterior cervical muscles, leading to rigidity of the spine and the neck. Slowly progressive weakness and muscle wasting may occur in early childhood, initially with a predominant humeroperoneal distribution. Cardiomyopathy is clinically the most important aspect of the disease; conduction defects lead to a high risk of sudden cardiac death. *LMNA* (lamin A/C) mutations produce autosomal dominant or recessive EDMD (EDMD2) and mutations of the *emerin* gene cause X-linked EDMD (EDMD1). Mutations of *SYNE1* and *SYNE2* genes encoding nesprins have also been linked to EDMD. *SYNE1* mutations are also a common cause of autosomal recessive cerebellar ataxia (ARCA1) associated with spasticity, lower motor neuron involvement, myopathy, and cardiomyopathy. Missense mutations and splicing defects in *LMNA* have also been linked to autosomal dominant limb-girdle muscular dystrophy (LGMD1B), which may be accompanied by cardiac conduction defects in some patients.[56] An autosomal recessive *LMNA* mutation is linked to Charcot-Marie-Tooth disease type 2B1. Autosomal dominant *LMNA* mutations are a common cause of severe dilated cardiomyopathy.[57]

Lamin B Duplication

Duplication in *LMNB1*, encoding lamin B1, causes autosomal dominant leukodystrophy (ADLD).[58–60] This disorder has an insidious onset in the fourth or fifth decades of life with sympathetic autonomic failure followed by cerebellar and pyramidal signs and mild cognitive impairment. MRI shows diffuse, confluent, and symmetric increase in T2 signal in the frontoparietal and cerebellar white matter with sparing of the periventricular white matter and U-fibers; there can also be atrophy of the corpus callosum and increased T2 signal and atrophy of white matter of the spinal cord. The overexpression of lamin B1 causes premature arrest of oligodendrocyte differentiation without the autonomic manifestations. Allele-specific silencing may provide a potential therapeutic approach for this disorder.[61]

AUTOIMMUNE DISORDERS AFFECTING CYTOSKELETAL PROTEINS

Intermediate filaments in neurons and glial cells are targets of antibodies producing autoimmune encephalitis syndromes. For example, autoantibodies against MAP1B (microtubule-associated protein 1B) produce a paraneoplastic syndrome that may manifest with peripheral neuropathy, cerebellar ataxia, encephalopathy, and, when associated with other autoantibodies, also optic neuropathy, retinopathy, or movement disorders.[62] This autoantibody is a strong predictor of small-cell lung carcinoma. Autoantibodies against neuronal intermediate filaments can produce a paraneoplastic disorder (usually ataxia or encephalopathy) accompanying neuroendocrine lineage neoplasia.[63] Autoimmune GFAP astrocytopathy results from immunoglobulin G (IgG) autoantibodies directed against GFAP. The main clinical presentation includes meningitis (with prominent headache), encephalitis, and myelitis, either in isolation or in several combinations.[64]

KEY POINTS

- The cytoskeleton consists of microfilaments, microtubules, and intermediate filaments.
- Actin microfilaments have major role in growth, maintenance, and dynamic changes of growth cones and dendrites; location of proteins at specific membrane sites; and vesicle dynamics.
- Several extracellular signals control actin dynamics during neuronal cell migration, axon pathfinding, axon–dendrite contact formation, and dendritic spine plasticity.
- Remodeling of the actin cytoskeleton in dendrites is a fundamental mechanism of activity-dependent long-term plastic changes in excitatory synapses.
- Microtubules are dynamic polymers of α- and β-tubulin that undergo a continuous balance between assembly and disassembly.
- Microtubule-associated protein tau has a critical role in control of microtubule dynamics and axonal transport.
- Microtubules provide the tracks for intracellular transport, which depends on interactions with molecular motor proteins.
- The crosstalk between actin microfilaments and microtubules is crucial for development, maturation, and maintenance of the nervous system.
- Neurofilaments consist of neurofilament triplet proteins (NF-L (NfL), NF-M (NfL), and NF-H) (NfH) and associated proteins α-internexin or peripherin.
- Neurofilament subunit content and the state of the phosphorylation state of the NF-M (NfM) and NF-H (NfH) tails are major determinants of the axon caliber.
- Glial fibrillary acid protein is a primary component of intermediate filaments in astrocytes.
- Nuclear lamins participate in regulation of the chromatin organization, trafficking of transcription factors across the nuclear envelope, and transduction of mechanical signals from the cytoskeleton to nucleus.
- Septins interact with actin, microtubules, and membrane phospholipids; act as scaffolds at the plasma membrane; and participate in crosstalk between different cytoskeletal components.
- There are several neurodevelopmental disorders due to mutations affecting actin or microtubule dynamics, including those involving Rho GTPase signaling or tubulin subunits.
- Tauopathies constitute a heterogeneous groups of neurodegenerative disorders characterized by

accumulation of hyperphosphorylated tau aggregates in neurons and glia.

- Abnormal tau impairs microtubule-mediated transport, mislocalizes to dendrites promoting excitotoxicity, triggers mitochondrial dysfunction, interacts with another proteins involved in neurodegeneration, and propagates between cells.
- Neurofilament aggregations are both the cause and the consequence of axonal dysfunction and degeneration.
- Mutations of *LMNA* and associated proteins such as emerin are linked to Emery-Dreifuss muscular dystrophy; *LMNA* mutation also causes limb-girdle muscular dystrophy.
- *LMNB* duplication causes autosomal dominant leukodystrophy.
- *SEPT 9* mutations produce hereditary neuralgic amyotrophic neuropathy.
- Autoantibodies against MAP1B (microtubule associated protein 1B) produce paraneoplastic cerebellar ataxia, peripheral neuropathy, and encephalopathy and are strong predictors of small-cell lung carcinoma.

REFERENCES

1. Konietzny A, Bar J, Mikhaylova M. Dendritic actin cytoskeleton: structure, functions, and regulations. Front Cell Neurosci 2017;11:147.
2. Leterrier C, Potier J, Caillol G, Debarnot C, Rueda Boroni F, Dargent B. Nanoscale architecture of the axon initial segment reveals an organized and robust scaffold. Cell Rep 2015;13:2781–2793.
3. Kanellos G, Frame MC. Cellular functions of the ADF/cofilin family at a glance. J Cell Sci 2016;129:3211–3218.
4. Sit ST, Manser E. Rho GTPases and their role in organizing the actin cytoskeleton. J Cell Sci 2011;124:679–683.
5. Zamboni V, Jones R, Umbach A, et al. Rho GTPases in intellectual disability: from genetics to therapeutic opportunities. Int J Mol Sci 2018;19:1821–1838.
6. Hlushchenko I, Koskinen M, Hotulainen P. Dendritic spine actin dynamics in neuronal maturation and synaptic plasticity. Cytoskeleton (Hoboken) 2016;73:435–441.
7. Borovac J, Bosch M, Okamoto K. Regulation of actin dynamics during structural plasticity of dendritic spines: signaling messengers and actin-binding proteins. Mol Cell Neurosci 2018;91:122–130.
8. Bras IC, Lopes LV, Outeiro TF. Sensing alpha-synuclein from the outside via the prion protein: implications for neurodegeneration. Mov Disord 2018;33:1675–1684.
9. Kapitein LC, Hoogenraad CC. Building the neuronal microtubule cytoskeleton. Neuron 2015;87:492–506.
10. Breuss MW, Leca I, Gstrein T, Hansen AH, Keays DA. Tubulins and brain development—the origins of functional specification. Mol Cell Neurosci 2017;84:58–67.
11. Akhmanova A, Steinmetz MO. Control of microtubule organization and dynamics: two ends in the limelight. Nat Rev Mol Cell Biol 2015;16:711–726.
12. Shashi V, Magiera MM, Klein D, et al. Loss of tubulin deglutamylase CCP1 causes infantile-onset neurodegeneration. EMBO J 2018;37.
13. Klim JR, Williams LA, Limone F, et al. ALS-implicated protein TDP-43 sustains levels of STMN2, a mediator of motor neuron growth and repair. Nat Neurosci 2019;22:167–179.
14. Guo T, Noble W, Hanger DP. Roles of tau protein in health and disease. Acta Neuropathol 2017;133:665–704.
15. Wang Y, Mandelkow E. Tau in physiology and pathology. Nature reviews Neuroscience 2016;17:22–35.
16. Prezel E, Elie A, Delaroche J, et al. Tau can switch microtubule network organizations: from random networks to dynamic and stable bundles. Mol Biol Cell 2018;29:154–165.
17. Kneynsberg A, Combs B, Christensen K, Morfini G, Kanaan NM. Axonal degeneration in tauopathies: disease relevance and underlying mechanisms. Front Neurosci 2017;11:572.
18. Maday S, Twelvetrees AE, Moughamian AJ, Holzbaur EL. Axonal transport: cargo-specific mechanisms of motility and regulation. Neuron 2014;84:292–309.
19. Guedes-Dias P, Holzbaur ELF. Axonal transport: Driving synaptic function. Science 2019;366:642–687.
20. Dogterom M, Koenderink GH. Actin-microtubule crosstalk in cell biology. Nat Rev Mol Cell Biol 2019;20:38–54.
21. Kirkcaldie MTK, Dwyer ST. The third wave: intermediate filaments in the maturing nervous system. Mol Cell Neurosci 2017;84:68–76.
22. Yuan A, Rao MV, Veeranna, Nixon RA. Neurofilaments and neurofilament proteins in health and disease. Cold Spring Harb Perspect Biol 2017;9(4):a018309.
23. Gafson AR, Barthelemy NR, Bomont P, et al. Neurofilaments: neurobiological foundations for biomarker applications. Brain 2020;143:1975–1998.
24. Toivola DM, Strnad P, Habtezion A, Omary MB. Intermediate filaments take the heat as stress proteins. Trends Cell Biol 2010;20:79–91.
25. Leterrier C. The axon initial segment: an updated viewpoint. J Neurosci 2018;38:2135–2145.
26. Bucher M, Fanutza T, Mikhaylova M. Cytoskeletal makeup of the synapse: shaft versus spine. Cytoskeleton (Hoboken) 2019;77:55–64.
27. Lin NH, Huang YS, Opal P, Goldman RD, Messing A, Perng MD. The role of gigaxonin in the degradation of the glial-specific intermediate filament protein GFAP. Mol Biol Cell 2016;27:3980–3990.
28. Messing A. Alexander disease. Handb Clin Neurol 2018;148:693–700.
29. Olabarria M, Goldman JE. Disorders of astrocytes: Alexander disease as a model. Annu Rev Pathol 2017;12:131–152.
30. Osmanagic-Myers S, Dechat T, Foisner R. Lamins at the crossroads of mechanosignaling. Genes Dev 2015;29:225–237.
31. de Leeuw R, Gruenbaum Y, Medalia O. Nuclear lamins: thin filaments with major functions. Trends Cell Biol 2018;28:34–45.
32. Mostowy S, Cossart P. Septins: the fourth component of the cytoskeleton. Nat Rev Mol Cell Biol 2012;13:183–194.
33. Spiliotis ET. Spatial effects—site-specific regulation of actin and microtubule organization by septin GTPases. J Cell Sci 2018;131.
34. Ueda M, Kawamura N, Tateishi T, et al. Phenotypic spectrum of hereditary neuralgic amyotrophy caused by the SEPT9 R88W mutation. J Neurol Neurosurg Psychiatry 2010;81:94–96.

35. Klein CJ, Wu Y, Cunningham JM, et al. SEPT9 mutations and a conserved 17q25 sequence in sporadic and hereditary brachial plexus neuropathy. Arch Neurol 2009;66:238–243.
36. Serin HM, Yilmaz S, Kanmaz S, et al. A rare cause of brachial plexopathy: hereditary neuralgic amyotrophy. Turk Pediatri Ars 2019;54:189–191.
37. Grosse GM, Bauer C, Kopp B, Schrader C, Osmanovic A. Identification of a rare SEPT9 variant in a family with autosomal dominant Charcot-Marie-Tooth disease. BMC Med Genet 2020;21:45.
38. Ba W, van der Raadt J, Nadif Kasri N. Rho GTPase signaling at the synapse: implications for intellectual disability. Exp Cell Res 2013;319:2368–2374.
39. Bahi-Buisson N, Poirier K, Fourniol F, et al. The wide spectrum of tubulinopathies: what are the key features for the diagnosis? Brain 2014;137:1676–1700.
40. Tischfield MA, Cederquist GY, Gupta ML, Jr., Engle EC. Phenotypic spectrum of the tubulin-related disorders and functional implications of disease-causing mutations. Curr Opin Genet Dev 2011;21:286–294.
41. Romaniello R, Arrigoni F, Fry AE, et al. Tubulin genes and malformations of cortical development. Eur J Med Genet 2018;61:744–754.
42. Romaniello R, Zucca C, Arrigoni F, et al. Epilepsy in tubulinopathy: personal series and literature review. Cells 2019;8.
43. Poirier K, Lebrun N, Broix L, et al. Mutations in TUBG1, DYNC1H1, KIF5C and KIF2A cause malformations of cortical development and microcephaly. Nat Genet 2013;45:639–647.
44. Vulinovic F, Krajka V, Hausrat TJ, et al. Motor protein binding and mitochondrial transport are altered by pathogenic TUBB4A variants. Hum Mutat 2018;39:1901–1915.
45. Kovacs GG. Tauopathies. Handb Clin Neurol 2017;145:355–368.
46. Albayram O, Kondo A, Mannix R, et al. Cis P-tau is induced in clinical and preclinical brain injury and contributes to post-injury sequelae. Nat Commun 2017;8:1000.
47. Arena JD, Smith DH, Lee EB, et al. Tau immunophenotypes in chronic traumatic encephalopathy recapitulate those of ageing and Alzheimer's disease. Brain 2020;143:1572–1587.
48. Falcon B, Zivanov J, Zhang W, et al. Novel tau filament fold in chronic traumatic encephalopathy encloses hydrophobic molecules. Nature 2019;568:420–423.
49. Didonna A, Opal P. The role of neurofilament aggregation in neurodegeneration: lessons from rare inherited neurological disorders. Mol Neurodegener 2019;14:19.
50. Zhai J, Lin H, Julien JP, Schlaepfer WW. Disruption of neurofilament network with aggregation of light neurofilament protein: a common pathway leading to motor neuron degeneration due to Charcot-Marie-Tooth disease-linked mutations in NFL and HSPB1. Hum Mol Genet 2007;16:3103–3116.
51. Stone EJ, Uchida A, Brown A. Charcot-Marie-Tooth disease Type 2E/1F mutant neurofilament proteins assemble into neurofilaments. Cytoskeleton (Hoboken) 2019;76:423–439.
52. Vendredy L, Adriaenssens E, Timmerman V. Small heat shock proteins in neurodegenerative diseases. Cell Stress Chaperones 2020;(4):679–699.
53. Schwartz NU. Charcot-Marie-Tooth 2F (Hsp27 mutations): a review. Neurobiol Dis 2019;130:104505.
54. Lee Y, Lee BH, Yip W, Chou P, Yip BS. Neurofilament proteins as prognostic biomarkers in neurological disorders. Curr Pharm Des 2019;25:4560–4569.
55. Heller SA, Shih R, Kalra R, Kang PB. Emery-Dreifuss muscular dystrophy. Muscle Nerve 2019;61:436–448.
56. Gomez-Andres D, Dabaj I, Mompoint D, et al. Pediatric laminopathies: whole-body magnetic resonance imaging fingerprint and comparison with Sepn1 myopathy. Muscle Nerve 2016;54:192–202.
57. Guillin-Amarelle C, Sanchez-Iglesias S, Mera A, et al. Inflammatory myopathy in the context of an unusual overlapping laminopathy. Arch Endocrinol Metab 2018;62:376–382.
58. Alturkustani M, Sharma M, Hammond R, Ang LC. Adult-onset leukodystrophy: review of 3 clinicopathologic phenotypes and a proposed classification. J Neuropathol Exp Neurol 2013;72:1090–1103.
59. Finnsson J, Sundblom J, Dahl N, Melberg A, Raininko R. LMNB1-related autosomal-dominant leukodystrophy: clinical and radiological course. Ann Neurol 2015;78:412–425.
60. Mezaki N, Miura T, Ogaki K, et al. Duplication and deletion upstream of LMNB1 in autosomal dominant adult-onset leukodystrophy. Neurol Genet 2018;4:e292.
61. Giorgio E, Lorenzati M, Rivetti di Val Cervo P, et al. Allele-specific silencing as treatment for gene duplication disorders: proof-of-principle in autosomal dominant leukodystrophy. Brain 2019;142:1905–1920.
62. Gadoth A, Kryzer TJ, Fryer J, McKeon A, Lennon VA, Pittock SJ. Microtubule-associated protein 1B: Novel paraneoplastic biomarker. Ann Neurol 2017;81:266–277.
63. Basal E, Zalewski N, Kryzer TJ, et al. Paraneoplastic neuronal intermediate filament autoimmunity. Neurology 2018;91:e1677–e1689.
64. Flanagan EP, Hinson SR, Lennon VA, et al. Glial fibrillary acidic protein immunoglobulin Gas biomarker of autoimmune astrocytopathy: analysis of 102 patients. Ann Neurol 2017;81:298–309.

9 Axonal Transport

OVERVIEW

Neurons in the human central nervous system display highly complex axonal arbors that can branch thousands of times, reach hundreds of meters in total length, and contain hundreds of thousands of presynaptic sites. Since the main cellular machinery for synthesis and packaging of proteins and lipids is primarily located in the somatodendritic compartment, microtubule-based axonal transport is critical to deliver material to dendrites and axons.[1–4] Axonal transport supports synaptic function by delivering new synaptic vesicles and removing aged organelles from presynaptic sites. Anterograde axonal transport delivers membrane-bound organelles such as secretory vesicles, endosomes, and lysosomes to the different neuronal compartments. Retrograde transport allows removal and degradation of materials via the endosome-lysosome and autophagy pathways. It also delivers target-derived neurotrophic signals from the synaptic terminal or injury signals from the axon back to the cell body. Bidirectional transport provides for the trafficking and turnover of cytoskeletal components, mitochondria, and other organelles to generate and maintain the functional heterogeneity of dendritic and axonal subdomains. Axonal transport requires intact microtubules, motor proteins, and supply of ATP by mitochondria. The motor proteins for anterograde transport are members of the kinesin family. The motor protein for retrograde transport is cytoplasmic dynein in complex with dynactin (Figure 9.1). Axonal transport is regulated by posttranslational modification of the microtubules, microtubule-associated proteins, or both. The balance between kinesin and dynein/dynactin motors determines the direction of axonal transport. Fast axonal transport of membrane-bound organelles occurs at a rate of >0.5 mm/s, up to 400 mm/day; slow transport of cytoskeletal and cytoplasmic proteins is much slower at <0.1 mm/s, <8 mm/day[5] (Table 9.1). Impaired axonal transport is a fundamental disease mechanism in many neurodevelopmental and most neurodegenerative disorders. The main aims of this chapter are to review: (1) the general mechanisms of anterograde and retrograde axonal transport, (2) examples of axonal transport of different cargos, and (3) mechanisms of impaired axonal transport in representative neurologic disorders.

MOTOR PROTEINS FOR AXONAL TRANSPORT

Motor proteins are ATPases that bind directly to microtubules and indirectly to their respective cargoes via adaptor proteins. In the axon, microtubules are polarized into a minus-end in the cell body and a plus-end in the distal axons. Anterograde transport involves movement of cargo from the minus- to the plus-end of microtubules; retrograde transport occurs in an opposite direction.

Kinesins and Anterograde Transport

The kinesins drive anterograde transport by recognizing the plus-end of the microtubule. The kinesin (KIF) superfamily includes 15 families comprising more than 45 kinesins. Motors from the kinesin-1, kinesin-2, kinesin-3, and kinesin-4 families mediate anterograde transport in axons. Members of the kinesin 1 subfamily (*KIF5* gene) are rod-shaped heterotetramers composed of two heavy-chain (KHC) and two light-chain (KLC) subunits. The KHC consists of a terminal head motor region that binds microtubules and hydrolyzes ATP, a neck linker domain, a long stalk region, and a small globular tail that binds to cargo via adaptor proteins. There are at least six variants of kinesin-1. For example, kinesin-1A transports GABA receptors; kinesin-1B transports mitochondria; and kinesin-1C transports amyloid precursor protein (APP). Kinesin-2 motors can assemble into homo- or heterodimeric complexes and drive the anterograde transport of plasma membrane precursors, late endosomal vesicles, adhesion and signal molecules, and enzymes. Kinesin-3 motors (*KIF1A* gene) transport synaptic vesicle precursors. Upon binding to cargo, a conformation change unlocks the kinesin motor and allows it to bind to the microtubule; this occurs via

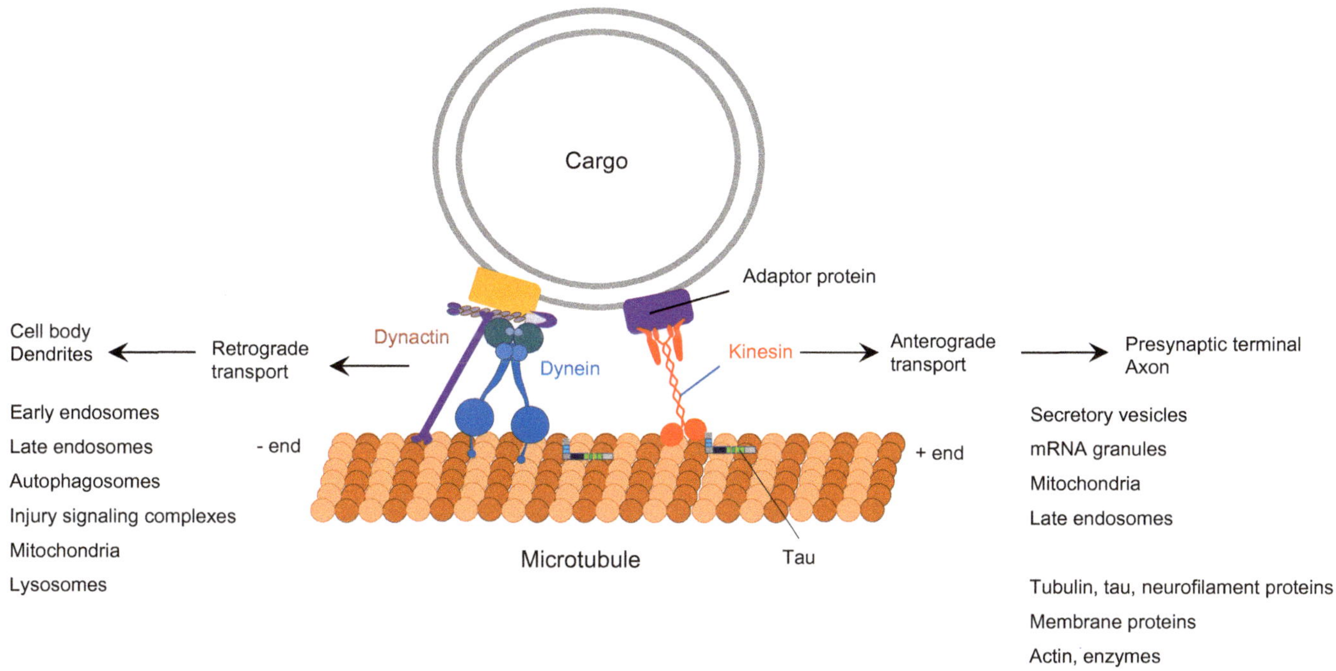

FIGURE 9.1 Overview of axonal transport.
Axonal transport requires intact microtubules, motor proteins, and supply of ATP by mitochondria. Anterograde axonal transport allows the delivery of membrane-bound organelles, such as secretory vesicles, endosomes, and lysosomes, to the different compartments of axons and to the synaptic terminals. Anterograde transport requires members of the kinesin family. Retrograde transport allows movement of endosomes, target-derived neurotrophic signals, and injury signals from the axon back to the cell body. The motor protein for retrograde transport is cytoplasmic dynein in complex with dynactin. Bidirectional transport provides for the trafficking and turnover of cytoskeletal components, mitochondria, and other organelles.

interaction between positive charges of kinesin and negative charges at the tubulin surface and is stabilized upon ADP/ATP nucleotide exchange in the kinesin motor domain. Posttranslational modifications of tubulin, accessory proteins, and microtubule-associated proteins may also modulate motor–microtubule interaction and transport initiation. For example, tubulin acetylation promotes the binding of kinesins to microtubules. After attachment of their motor domains to the microtubules and their tail regions to the cargo, kinesins "walk" along the microtubule; the kinesin front head remains bound to the microtubules and hydrolyzes ATP, which allows movement of the tail region toward the microtubule plus-end.

Dynein-Dynactin Complex and Retrograde Transport

Cytoplasmic dynein is the motor protein responsible for retrograde transport. Dynein is a large multisubunit complex composed of multiple polypeptide subunits. They include a core containing two catalytic dynein heavy-chain (DHC) subunits encoded by *DHCN* genes; two intermediate-chain subunits, four light-intermediate chain subunits; and several light-chain subunits. The DHC subunits have a globular motor domain with ATPase activity and bind to the microtubules; the dynein intermediate chain binds to a variety of membrane-bound organelle cargoes. The binding of the cargo to the intermediate and light chains of dynein involves interactions through the adaptor dynactin complex. The dynactin complex consists of a rod domain and a projecting arm with two microtubule binding sites. Dynactin includes the dynactin subunits 1 and 2 (encoded by *DCTN* genes), $p150^{glued}$, dynamitin, actin-related protein 1, and other subunits. There is a tight regulation of dynein activity in neurons. In the distal axon, microtubules are dynamic and enriched with plus-end binding proteins that recruit dynactin, leading to the initiation of retrograde transport by dynein. Several adaptor proteins, such as bicaudal 2 (BICD2) and lissencephaly-1 (Lis-1) bind directly to the dynein/dynactin complex and promote retrograde transport.

REGULATION OF AXONAL TRANSPORT

Several mechanisms regulate axonal transport of organelles and other cargoes. They include modification of the microtubule track through posttranslational tubulin modifications such as acetylation; influence of microtubule-associated proteins such as tau; biophysical properties of the

TABLE 9.1 *Direction and Rate of Axonal Transport for Different Cargoes*

Cargo	Main Direction	Rate
Synaptic vesicle precursors	Anterograde	200–400 mm/day
Secretory granules (neuropeptides or BDNF)	Anterograde	50–400 mm/day
Vesicles containing amyloid precursor protein	Anterograde	50–400 mm/day
Endosomal recycling vesicles	Retrograde	200 mm/day
Autophagosomes	Retrograde	40 mm/day
Lysosomes	Bidirectional	< 50 mm/day
Mitochondria	Bidirectional	< 50 mm/day
mRNA granules	Anterograde	20–200 mm/day
Membrane proteins	Anterograde	2–8 mm/day
Enzymes	Anterograde	2–8 mm/day
Actin	Anterograde	2–8 mm/day
Tubulin	Anterograde	0.2–1 mm/day
Tau	Anterograde	0.2–1, m/day
Neurofilaments	Anterograde	0.2–1 mm/day
Tetanus toxin	Retrograde	100–400 mm/day
Viruses	Retrograde	200 mm/day

motor proteins; localized activation or inactivation of kinesins or dynein; selective binding of these motor proteins to different cargoes via motor adaptors, and integration of opposing motors bound to the same cargo.

Interactions Between Kinesin and Dynein Motors

Most kinesins preferentially target cargo to the axon; only dynein transports cargo both along the axons and into dendrites. The organization of the cytoskeleton at the axon initial segment prevents the entry of dendritic cargo to the axon and the inappropriate transport of axon-targeted proteins into the soma and dendrites. Molecular motors interact competitively to determine the direction and speed of axonal transport. Many organelles and cytoskeletal proteins, including endosomes, autophagosomes, mitochondria, and intermediate filaments, bind simultaneously to both kinesin-1 and dynein, and are thus able to undergo bidirectional movement along microtubules in the axon. The net movement in one direction over long distances may be achieved via a stochastic "tug-of-war" between opposing kinesin and dynein motors. Due to the mixed polarity of the microtubule bundles in dendrites, a single motor type could mediate bidirectional transport of cargo transport. This antiparallel microtubule organization, together with the local organization of actin cytoskeleton in dendrites, provides the basis for the regulation of cargo trafficking and both functional and structural plasticity.

Phosphorylation-Dependent Regulation of Motor and Adaptor Proteins

One important determinant of the direction of transport is the state of phosphorylation of the kinesin and dynein motors, which strongly affects their respective affinity for their cargo and attachment of the microtubules. For example, phosphorylation of the kinesin light chain by glycogen synthase kinase 3β (GSK-3β) releases the transported vesicles from the kinesin-1 motor and thus inhibits anterograde transport. Other kinases may regulate axonal transport indirectly by regulating the activity of GSK-3β. For example activity of cyclin-dependent kinase 5 (CDK5) indirectly maintains GSK-3β in its inactive phosphorylated state thus promotes kinesin-based anterograde transport. In contrast, hyperphosphorylated tau, which accumulates in several neurodegenerative disorders, activates protein phosphatase 1, leading to dephosphorylation and activation of GSK-3β and thus inhibition of anterograde transport.[6] Some kinases such as neuronal c-Jun-N-terminal kinase (JNK3) phosphorylate the kinesin-1 head domain, thus inhibiting kinesin-1 movement along microtubules.[7] Phosphorylation may also affect axonal transport via its effects on adaptor proteins. For example, depending on its state of phosphorylation, the huntingtin-huntingtin adaptor protein 1 (HAP1) complex functions as a molecular switch between kinesin-1 and dynein motors, regulating transport of brain-derived neurotrophic factor (BDNF). Huntingtin phosphorylation in response to growth factor signals promotes recruitment of kinesin-1 and thus anterograde BDNF transport; huntingtin dephosphorization destabilizes kinesin-1 binding and promotes dynein-driven retrograde transport of BDNF.[8]

TRANSPORT OF SELECTIVE CARGOES AND FUNCTIONAL CORRELATIONS

Transport of Synaptic Vesicle Precursors and Dense Core Vesicles

Fast anterograde transport delivers membrane-bound organelles to synapses and axons (Figure 9.2). Synaptic vesicles are targeted to presynaptic terminals, whereas vesicles containing membrane-bound proteins such as voltage-gated channels and receptors are selectively targeted to distinct domains of the axons, such as the nodes of Ranvier or presynaptic membranes. The fast anterograde transport of synaptic organelles is primarily driven by members of the kinesin-3 family encoding KIF1A heavy chains. Coupling of kinesin-3 to synaptic vesicle precursors involves adaptor proteins such as α-liprin, which also interact with core components of the presynaptic terminal. Dense core vesicles packed with neuropeptides and trophic factors synthesized in the cell body are supplied to presynaptic release zones via fast anterograde transport also primarily via kinesin-3. In contrast, two important substrates of fast anterograde transport via kinesin-1 motors are BDNF and APP. Transport of BDNF-containing dense core vesicles is regulated by huntingtin, which functions as a scaffold for both kinesin-1 and dynein motors. Vesicles containing APP bind via the scaffolding protein JNK interacting protein 1 (JIP1) to both kinesin-1 and a subunit of dynactin. The relative affinity of JIP1 for kinesin-1 or dynactin is controlled by JNK-mediated phosphorylation; phosphorylated JIP1 promotes anterograde transport of APP; dephosphorylation promotes retrograde transport.

Transport of Signaling Endosomes

Retrograde axonal transport of signaling endosomes is critical for the neurotrophic effects of growth factors, such as nerve growth factor (NGF)[9] (Figure 9.3). Signaling endosomes formed during internalization of neurotrophins

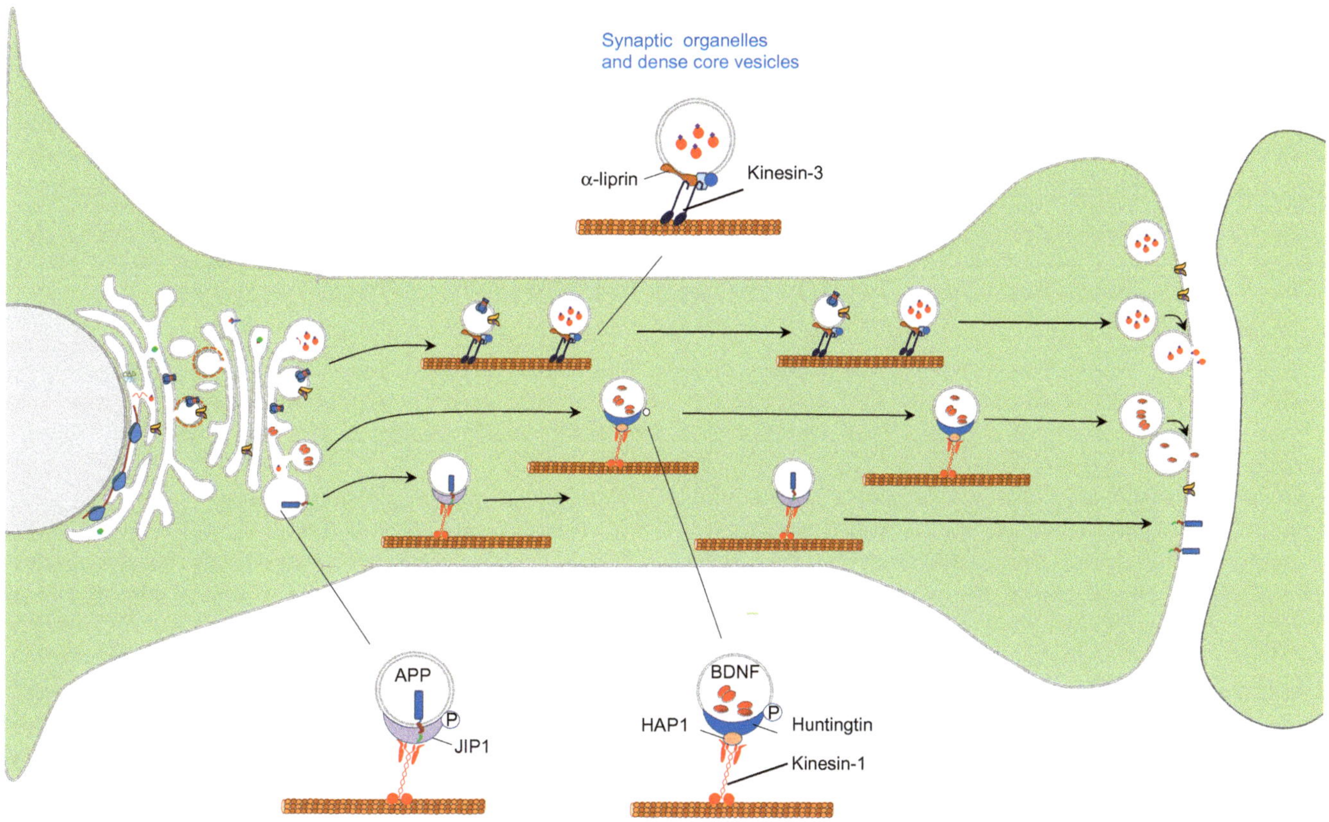

FIGURE 9.2 Transport of membrane-bound organelles to synapses and axons.
Anterograde transport of membrane-bound organelles is primarily driven by members of the kinesin-3 family. Coupling of kinesin-3 to synaptic vesicle precursors involves adaptor proteins such as α-liprin. Two important substrates of fast anterograde transport via kinesin 1 motors are brain-derived neurotrophic factor (BDNF) and amyloid precursor protein (APP). Transport of BDNF-containing dense core vesicles is regulated by huntingtin (HTT). The transport of APP requires binding to the scaffolding protein c-Jun N-terminal kinase (JNK) interacting protein 1 (JIP1).

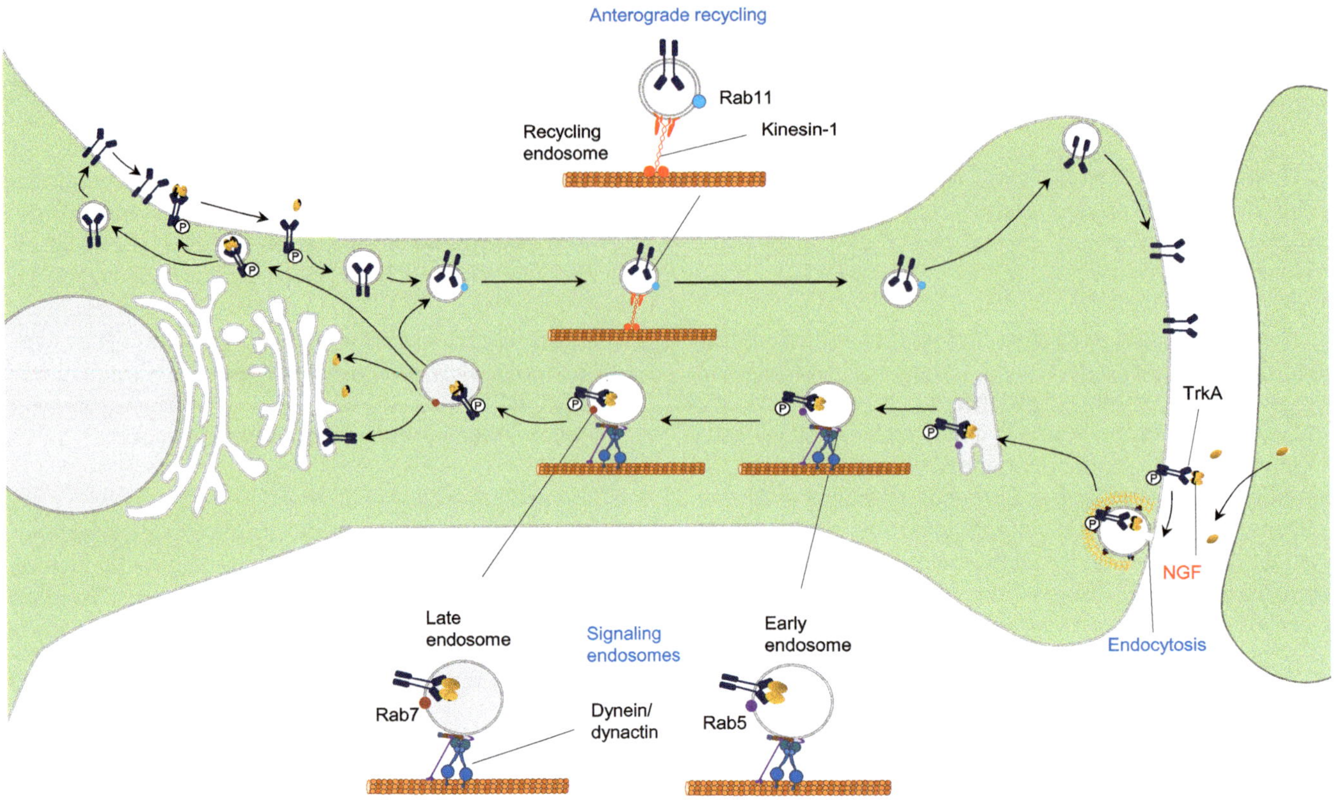

FIGURE 9.3 Transport of endosomes and neurotrophin signaling.
Axonal transport is critical for long-range neurotrophin signaling. For example, binding of nerve growth factor (NGF) to its tyrosine kinase A (TrkA) receptors receptor results in internalization of the NGF-TrkA complex, which is followed by retrograde transport via signaling endosomes, including early (Rab5-positive) and late (Rab7-positive) endosomes. Once these signaling endosomes reach the soma, NGF bound to TrkA can continue to signal for long periods due to local recycling (Rab11-positive) endosomes. Recycling endosomes can traffic Trk receptors anterogradely from the dendrites to the axon and to the synaptic terminal.

bound to their cognate tyrosine kinase (Trk) receptors.[10,11] For example, binding to NGF causes TrkA receptor dimerization and autophosphorylation, initiating canonical downstream growth and survival cascades. NGF-bound TrkA undergoes internalization via clathrin-dependent or caveolin-mediated endocytosis. Following internalization, the NGF-TrkA complex undergoes retrograde transport via signaling endosomes, including early (Rab5-positive) and late (Rab7-positive) endosomes.[11] The motility of signaling endosomes is regulated by the dynein adaptors such as Rab7-interacting lysosomal protein (RILP). Anchoring of Rab7 to the membrane of late endosomes and lysosomes by RILP is necessary for recruitment of both late endosomes and lysosomes to the dynein//dynactin motor complex. *RAB7* mutations are linked to Charcot-Marie-Tooth disease (CMT) 2B; this may reflect disruption of axonal transport of endosomes in sensory neurons.[12,13]

Once these signaling endosomes reach the soma, NGF bound to TrkA can continue to signal for long periods due to local recycling endosomes. In addition, TrkA receptors also undergo constitutive recycling at the soma in the absence of NGF binding, generating an endosomal receptor pool that can be recycled back to the axon or dendrites.[9,10]

Transport of mRNA Granules for Local Translation of Axonal Proteins

Transport of messenger RNA (mRNA) in transport granules consisting of ribonucleoprotein (RNP) complexes is an important mechanism of nonvesicular, long-distance transfer of signals between neuronal compartments[10,14–16] (Figure 9.4). This process allows local regulated translation of mRNAs into proteins in both dendritic and axonal subdomains. Mature axons contain the machinery for protein synthesis, including ribosomes and transfer RNAs, which are irregularly distributed and located close to the plasma membrane. Local translation in axons serves several functions. For example, it provides a mechanism for the cell to respond to environmental signals and thus locally express proteins involved in axon elongation and pathfinding in response to environmental signals during development. Local protein translation is also critical for maintenance and survival of mature axons and synaptic function in the adult nervous system. The

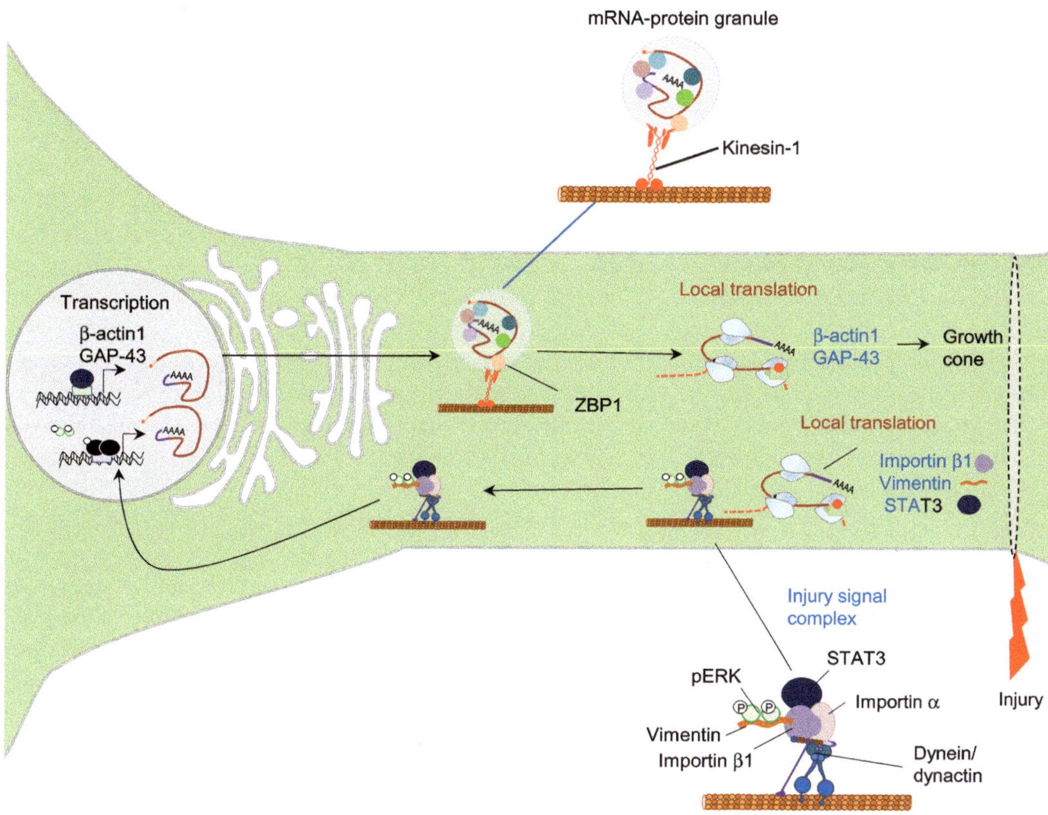

FIGURE 9.4 Retrograde transport of injury signals.
Axonal injury triggers local translation of mRNAs and retrograde transport of signals from the site of injury to the nucleus. Retrograde transport of transcription factors locally synthesized at the site of injury also occurs independently of endosomes via importin-dynein complexes to initiate axonal regeneration. One example is the local synthesis of signal transducer and activator of transcription (STAT) 3 and the nuclear import protein importin β1. Locally translated vimentin binds phosphorylated extracellular signal regulated kinase (pERK) and links it to dynein via importin β1. Several RNA binding proteins localized in the axon, including survival of motor neuron (SMN), and ZIP-binding protein 1 (ZBP1) regulate the axonal location mRNA transcripts, for example, that encoding β-actin.

axon transcriptomes contain mRNAs for multiple nuclear encoded mitochondrial proteins; local translation of these proteins in axons support mitochondrial function critical to maintain ATP production and protect against oxidative stress and injury. Finally, local mRNA translation in axons enables cells to respond to injury and communicate injury signals to the soma. This involves expression of nucleocytoplasmic transport factors and transcription factors that are assembled into signaling complexes that reach the nucleus by retrograde transport to promote transcription of genes required for axonal regeneration. Formation of ribonucleoprotein (RNP) granules protects mRNA from premature degradation, represses translation, and assures that mRNA transcripts arrive at the appropriate destinations. Once assembled, RNP granules interact with chaperone, adaptor, and motor proteins to undergo transport along microtubules to axons and dendrites. The kinesin motors are used for long-distance anterograde transport along microtubules, whereas myosin motors proteins are used for short-distance transport along actin microfilaments. Several RNA-binding proteins localized in the axon, including survival of motor neuron (SMN), regulate the axonal location mRNA transcripts, for example that encoding β-actin. Intracellular Ca^{2+} may impact the specificity for axonal mRNA translation.

Retrograde Transport of Axon Injury Signals

Axonal injury triggers local translation of mRNAs and retrograde transport of signals from the site of injury to the nucleus (Figure 9.4). Axonal mRNA translation and synthesis of dynein regulators affect dynein-mediated retrograde transport of membrane-bound vesicles. The dynein stimulators p150^{glued} (a component of the dynactin complex) and Lis-1 are synthesized locally in the distal axon and may provide an "on-demand" mechanism required for initiation of retrograde transport of signaling endosomes from the distal axon. Whereas many locally synthesized and retrogradely transported signals trigger neuroprotective responses, others may have a deleterious effect. Retrograde transport of transcription factors locally synthesized at the site of injury also occurs independently of endosomes via importin-dynein complexes to initiate axonal regeneration. One example is the local synthesis of signal transducer and activator of transcription (STAT) 3 and the nuclear import protein importin β1, followed by their transport to the nucleus in association with dynein. Local translation of other dynein cofactors and scaffolding proteins also generates non-endosomal signaling complexes that are retrogradely transported to the axon to reach the nucleus; these complexes enable phosphorylated signals to be transported over long distances while protecting them from dephosphorylation. For example, locally translated vimentin binds phosphorylated extracellular signal-regulated kinase (pERK) and links it to dynein via importin β1. This interaction shields pERK from dephosphorylation as the complex is transported from the site of injury to the nucleus.

Transport and maturation of Autophagosomes and Lysosomes

In many cell types, lysosomes and late endosomes are concentrated around the nucleus in relationship with the ER. Whereas there is no strong anterograde delivery of lysosomes from the cell body to the axon, there is a strong retrograde transport of lysosomes and late endocytic and autophagosomal organelles (Figure 9.5). The anterograde transport of late endosomes and lysosomes in axons is mainly mediated by kinesin-1 and kinesin-2. The retrograde motility of these organelles by dynein is regulated by JIP3 and RILP interacting with Rab7. Nutrient status modulates the recruitment of kinesin and dynein/dynactin motors to lysosomes, thereby regulating lysosomal position, signaling, and degrading functions. Starvation induces dynein/dynactin-dependent perinuclear clustering of lysosomes. This involves Ca^{2+} efflux from lysosomes and interaction of their membrane transient receptor potential channel mucolipin 1 with dynamitin, a component of the dynactin complex. Perinuclear location of lysosomes promotes their maturation and acidification, as well as their encounter with endosomes or autophagosomes. In contrast, nutrient repletion promotes the transfer of ER-associated kinesin to the lysosome and thus their anterograde transport. Late endosomes and lysosomes pause randomly along the axons; this provides for their even distribution, which may be optimal for their efficient fusion with autophagosomes. Endocytic substrates can be transported over long distances after transitioning from early endosomes to late endosomes. The Rab7 effector RILP interacts directly with the dynactin and promotes retrograde transport of late endosomes and lysosomes. Autophagosomes form constitutively in distal axons and initially show bidirectional oscillatory movement before engaging in retrograde transport; the accessory protein JIP1 inhibits kinesin-1 and allows unopposed dynein-based retrograde transport. Huntingtin and HAP1 also regulate autophagosome-bound motors.[17] Misregulation of autophagosome transport in Huntington disease (HD) results in inefficient autophagosome maturation and impaired autophagosome/lysosome fusion along the axon. The defective clearance of both polyglutamine tract-containing huntingtin aggregates and dysfunctional mitochondria by neuronal autophagosomes may contribute to neurodegeneration and cell death in HD. Ultimately, axonal autophagosomes and autophagolysosomes are conveyed to the soma for the final steps in the degradation of engulfed proteins and organelles and the recycling of their components.

Several presynaptic proteins regulate the endocytic and autophagic pathways and their concerted action modulates the pool size of synaptic vesicles by directing synaptic vesicles toward lysosomal degradation in the cell body. For example, endophilin A and synaptojanin 1, which are critically involved in endocytosis, promote autophagy. There is also a tight regulation of autophagosomal motility. For example, JIP1 binds to the autophagosome membrane protein LC3 blocking activation of kinesin-1 and thus leading to robust retrograde transport of the organelle. Late endosomes and phagosomes contain cholesterol-rich microdomains that provide a platform for recruitment of dynein motors. Recruitment of dynactin to these vesicles is a stepwise process that involves Rab7 and RILP and the activity of an oxysterol-binding protein that senses membrane cholesterol levels and regulates the attachment of dynactin on late endosomes.

Axonal autophagosomes commonly first fuse with the endosomes to yield amphisomes, which undergo long-range retrograde transport while simultaneously acidifying and maturing into lysosomes, and ultimately fuse with mature lysosomes in the cell body. The progressive decrease in intraluminal pH of endosomes, autophagosomes, and amphisomes as they are transported from the distal to the proximal axon indicates a coupling of retrograde transport with maturation of these lysosomal precursors. This acidification depends on vacuolar proton ATPase (V-ATPase). The robust transport of immature lysosomes from the distal axon to the cell body increases the probability for them to encounter anterogradely transported Golgi-derived vesicles delivering recently synthesized lysosomal enzymes. Upon complete substrate degradation in the cell body, the fully mature lysosomes likely undergo reformation and recycling of lysosomal enzymes and membrane proteins for new rounds of lysosomal formation. Lysosomes may also be directionally transported in dendrites. Proper lysosomal function is important for maintenance of plasticity at synapses. Lysosomal function maintains the homeostasis of synaptic proteins and regulates the structure and maintenance of dendritic spines. For example, back-propagated action potentials evoke lysosomal Ca^{2+} release that triggers lysosomal exocytosis leading to local release of cathepsin B; this lysosomal enzyme activates matrix metalloproteinase 9, which remodels the extracellular matrix to facilitate dendritic growth.

Mitochondrial Transport

Mitochondria include two populations, a large stable or stationary pool and motile mitochondria that constitute

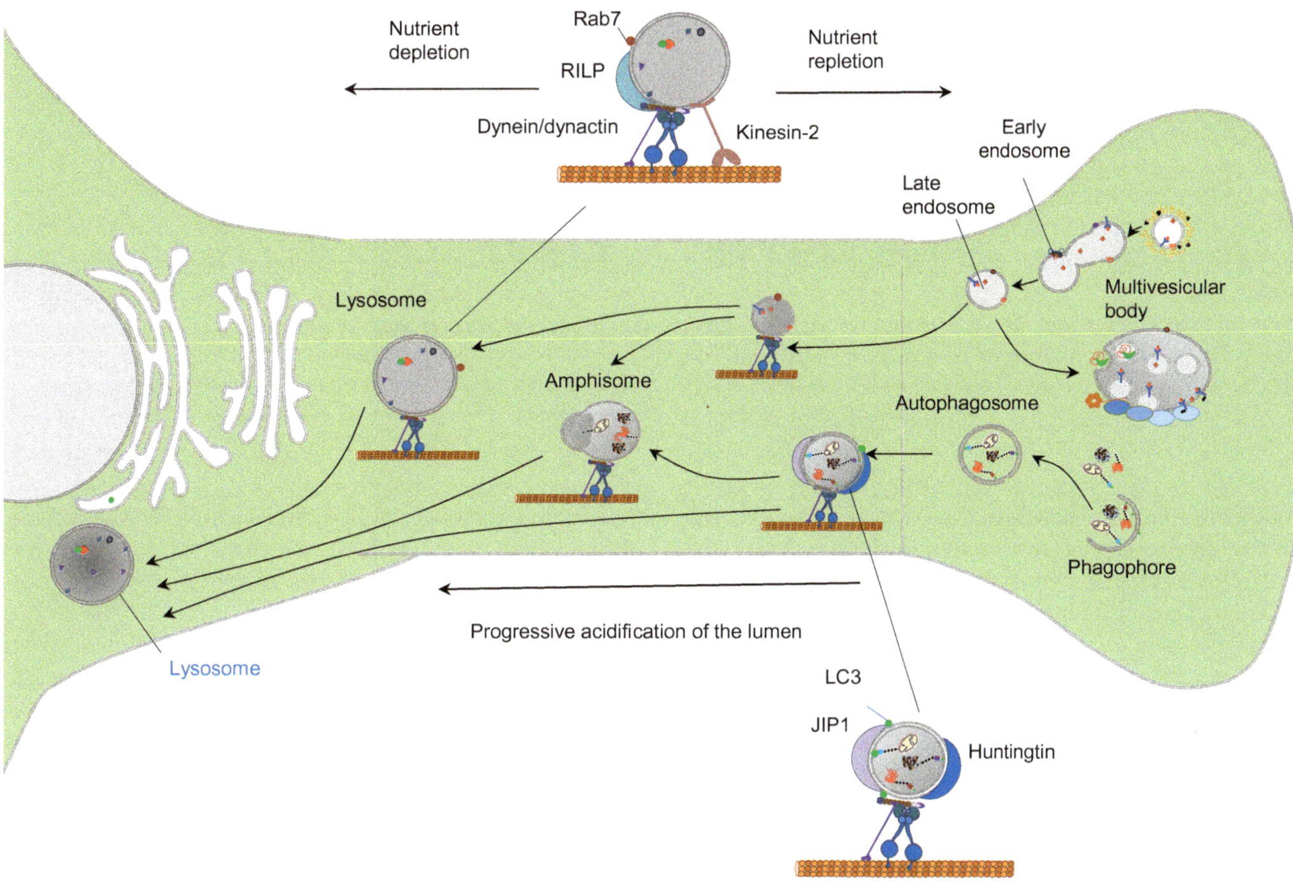

FIGURE 9.5 Transport and maturation of endosomes, autophagosomes, and lysosomes.
Perinuclear location of lysosomes promotes their maturation and acidification, as well as their encounter with endosomes or autophagosomes. Endocytic substrates can be transported over long distances after transitioning from early to late endosomes and then endolysosomes. Rab7 effector RILP (Rab7-interacting lysosomal protein), interacts directly with the dynactin and promotes retrograde transport of late endosomes and lysosomes. There is a progressive decrease in intraluminal pH of endosomes, autophagosomes, and amphisomes as they are transported from the distal to the proximal axon.

approximately 10%–15% of mitochondria. Mitochondria may undergo both anterograde (70%) and retrograde (30%) transport. Mitochondrial transport is a fundamental process required for their localization to sites of high energy demands, such as the synaptic terminals, nodes of Ranvier, and axonal growth cones.[18] It is unique in that it is characterized by frequent pauses and halting at sites of elevated in intracellular calcium (Ca^{2+}) in response to enhanced neuronal activity.[19–21] The mitochondrial transport machinery consists of a protein complex that includes the mitochondrial outer membrane protein mitochondrial Rho GTPase (MIRO) and the adaptor protein trafficking kinesin-binding protein (TRAK) 1 or 2. This machinery interacts with kinesin-1 (KIF5 heavy chain) or dynein motors for mitochondrial transport along microtubules. TRAK1 primarily localizes to axons, where it can bind either kinesin or dynactin/dynein; in dendrites, anterograde and retrograde transport mostly involves the MIRO/TRAK2 complex and is mediated primarily by dynein.[19–21]

Whereas some mitochondria need to be retained in the soma, others need to be transported and positioned along axons and dendrites to be concentrated in areas with high ATP consumption. Syntabulin is an adaptor protein that binds directly to KIF5 and attaches to the outer membrane of the mitochondria and may be required for anterograde transport to the presynaptic terminal. The huntingtin-binding protein HAP-1 associates with mitochondria and interacts with both kinesin and dynein/dynactin motors. Mitochondrial docking maintains the adequate number of stationary mitochondria in regions that require high ATP production and ability to buffer increased Ca^{2+}, such as dendritic spines and presynaptic terminals. Several signals converge on the MIRO/TRAK complex to immobilize mitochondria at such active sites. One important signal is increasing intracellular Ca^{2+}, resulting from influx via voltage-gated and neurotransmitter receptor channels. About half of mitochondria in the axon are stationed at presynaptic sites, where they are an important ATP source and regulate local Ca^{2+} levels. MIRO is a Ca^{2+}-binding protein that functions as sensor of local Ca^{2+} concentration. Increased Ca^{2+} arrests mitochondrial movement via binding to MIRO, producing a conformational change that reduces the number of kinesin molecules bound to the mitochondria or reduces microtubule interaction of MIRO-bound kinesin. Mitochondria also arrest their motility in response to increased extracellular glucose concentrations; this effect is mediated by posttranslational modifications of TRAK proteins.

Several protein tethers link the mitochondria to cytoskeletal filaments, thereby opposing motion. For example, syntaphilin is an axon-specific protein that is recruited and attached to the mitochondria outer membrane and binds to microtubules, thereby increasing the cytoskeletal forces that oppose motility. Calcium promotes binding of syntaphilin to both microtubules and kinesin-1 to act as a brake for mitochondria transport in the axon. Both axonal and dendritic mitochondria also dock along actin filaments, which are enriched at presynaptic terminals and dendritic spines. This may involve interactions with myosins that drive the short-range motion of mitochondria. Interactions with neurofilaments may also oppose mitochondrial motility in axons.

Transport of Cytoskeletal and Soluble Cytosolic Proteins

Slow axonal transport (0.2–10 mm/day) is subdivided into two categories: slow component a (SCa), which transports tubulin and neurofilament triplet (NF) proteins and other neurofilament subunits at rates of 0.2–1 mm/day; and slow component b (SCb), which transports cytosolic proteins at a rate of 1–10 mm/day. Except for the case of actin, slow axonal transport largely depends on microtubule-based transport and, in particular, kinesin-1 movement through the transient association of the soluble cargo with the motor. The different transport rates between fast and slow axonal transport reflect the different number of motor proteins and time engaged in active transport. One factor that curbs the axonal transport of cytoskeletal proteins is the density of the stationary cytoskeleton in the axon. The vast majority of neurofilament proteins are transported as assembled units or oligomers. In growing axons, transported neurofilaments establish a stationary network that elongates by end-to-end annealing of short neurofilaments to longer neurofilaments. Slow axonal transport also carries a large diverse pool of cytosolic proteins, including enzymes and adaptor proteins. These proteins may form spontaneously aggregated complexes that undergo dynamic recruitment to allow short bursts of anterograde transport by hitching a ride on passing vesicles. It is unknown to what extent neurons rely on slow axonal transport to supply soluble proteins to presynaptic sites. The sole reliance on this mechanism would severely limit the capacity of neurons with long axons or multiple harbors to rapidly adjust the supply upon sudden surges in local protein demand.

IMPAIRED AXONAL TRANSPORT AS A KEY MECHANISM IN NEURODEGENERATION

Impaired axonal transport due to disturbances in motor proteins, cargo adaptors, or cytoskeletal components is an important mechanism leading to both neurodevelopmental and neurodegenerative disorders.

Mutations Affecting Protein Motors or Their Adaptors

Mutations in microtubule-based motors or their cargo adaptors produce length-dependent axonopathies with overlapping phenotypes.[27] Advances in DNA-sequencing techniques have identified mutations in kinesin-1 and kinesin-3 as causative of a broad range of neurological disorders. De novo missense mutations in the *KIF1A* gene produce microcephaly, developmental delay, hypotonia, spastic paraparesis, cortical visual impairment, optic neuropathy, peripheral neuropathy, ataxia, epilepsy, and movement disorders.[25] Mutations in the KIF21A stalk region produce oculomotor nerve defects and congenital fibrosis of extraocular muscles. Mutations affecting kinesin and dynein motors or their adaptors produce a wide range of overlapping phenotypes, including hereditary spastic paraplegia, amyotrophic lateral sclerosis (ALS), and axonal Charcot-Marie-Tooth (CMT2) and other hereditary neuropathies. For example, loss-of-function mutations in kinesin family member 5A (*KIF5A*) affecting its cargo-binding tail domain have been associated with ALS.[24] In contrast, mutations affecting the motor domain of KIF5A cause hereditary spastic paraplegia (SPG10) and CMT2 phenotypes. Mutations in the *DYNC1H1* gene encoding the cytoplasmic dynein heavy chain, have been linked to CMT2 and spinal muscular atrophy–lower extremity predominant (SMALED). Missense mutations in the *DCTN1* gene encoding the $p150^{Glued}$ subunit of dynactin affect the initiation of retrograde transport and are directly implicated in Perry syndrome, which manifests with early-onset parkinsonism, depression, severe weight loss, and hypoventilation, with brain pathology characterized by TDP-43 immunostaining.[28] A distinct mutation within the same domain causes hereditary motor neuropathy with vocal cord paralysis (HMN7B) and distal and bulbar muscular atrophy.[29] Mutations in *BICD2*, which encodes an activating adaptor for dynein, lead to lower extremity prominent distal spinal muscular atrophy.[30,31] Mutations in scaffolding proteins can also lead to disease. As mentioned earlier in this chapter, *RAB7* mutations produce a predominantly sensory CMT2 phenotype due to disruption of endosome transport in sensory neurons.[32] Pathogenic expansion of the polyQ repeat region of huntingtin deleteriously affects the scaffolding functions of the protein, disrupting the axonal transport of multiple cargos, including BDNF, autophagosomes, and mitochondria[7,8,33]

Features of Impaired Axonal Transport in Neurodegenerative Disorders

Adult-onset neurodegenerative disorders, including Alzheimer disease (AD), tauopathies, Parkinson disease (PD) and other synucleinopathies, Huntington disease (HD), frontotemporal lobar degeneration (FTLD) and ALS, typically affect selective populations of projection neurons with long axons. The main cellular features of these disorders are accumulation of misfolded proteins and early loss of neuronal connectivity. These findings reflect dying back neurodegeneration due to impaired axonal transport.

In many neurodegenerative disorders distal axonopathy precedes cell death. There is abnormal accumulation of cytoskeletal components such as neurofilament (NF) subunits, mitochondria, and vesicular cargoes within the endolyosomal and autophagolysosomal compartments in the perikaryon, proximal segment of the axon, or in the distal portion of the axon. These accumulations reflect impaired axonal transport and may lead to neuritic pathology and local axonal swellings, including formation of spheroids or torpedoes.

Several potential mechanisms may lead to impaired axonal transport in these disorders. Posttranslational modifications of tubulin, motor proteins, or their adaptors may affect microtubule dynamics, cargo recognition, mitochondrial quality control, or vesicle trafficking. A major mechanism is dysregulation of phosphorylation of microtubule-associated and motor proteins.[34–36] In general, affected neurons have altered patterns of kinase activity and aberrant patterns of protein phosphorylation, as typically exemplified by tau and neurofilaments. This altered kinase activity also affects adaptor and motor proteins involved in axonal transport.

Consequences of Tau Hyperphosphorylation

Tau hyperphosphorylation is a prototypical mechanism of altered axonal transport in adult-onset neurodegenerative disorders.[6,22,23] Tau hyperphosphorylation reduces its affinity for microtubules and promotes tau self-aggregation, resulting in inhibition of axonal transport. This effect in part depends on a motif located in the extreme N-terminus of tau termed phosphatase-activating domain. This domain activates protein phosphatase 1, which in turn activates GSK-3β by dephosphorylation. Active GSK-3β not only phosphorylates tau but also kinesin light-chain subunits, promoting release of transported cargoes and inhibiting anterograde transport. There is increased activity of GSK-3β in both axons and synapses in AD and primary tauopathies. Increased tau phosphorylation not only occurs in AD and primary tauopathies but also has been shown in animal models of PD and ALS. There is a crosstalk among kinase pathways involved in neurodegeneration. For example, other kinases such as CDK5 phosphorylate tau and localize with neurofibrillary tangles in AD brains. Pathogenic Aβ oligomers activate casein kinase 2, which phosphorylates tau and inhibits axonal transport. Abnormal tau may also affect microtubule-based transport in astrocytes and oligodendrocytes.

Accumulation of Neurofilaments

Abnormal accumulation of neurofilaments is a pathological hallmark of several neurodegenerative diseases, including ALS, CMT2, giant axonal neuropathy, AD, PD, and intermediate filament inclusion disease. A major mechanism responsible for neurofilament accumulation is impaired axonal transport due to abnormal phosphorylation of neurofilament subunits. Hyperphosphorylation of neurofilament subunit tail domains impairs slow anterograde axonal transport. Studies on experimental models show that altered activity of motor proteins, such as absence of kinesin 1 (KIF5), mutations of dynein, or overexpression of dynamitin (a component of the dynactin complex) induce neurofilament accumulation in motor neurons. Another mechanism affecting neurofilament transport is abnormal stoichiometry of neurofilament subunits, including overexpression of neurofilament heavy chain (NF-H [NfH]) or peripherin and reduced levels of neurofilament light chain (NF-L [NfL]). As mentioned in the previous chapter, increased levels of NF-L (NfL) in the serum and CSF have been reported both in a variety of neurologic disorders, including AD, tauopathies, ALS, dementia with Lewy bodies, multiple system atrophy, vascular dementia, head trauma, stroke, and multiple sclerosis. Whereas NF-L (NfL) may be a general marker of neurodegeneration, it may have limited value for differential diagnosis between neurodegenerative disorders but may reflect disease severity and progression.

Impaired Retrograde Transport of Autophagosomes, Endosomes, and Lysosomes

Impaired vesicular trafficking and thus autophagosome-lysosomal function is an important mechanism in disorders such as PD, AD, HD, ALS, and FTLD.[37] In these disorders, there is accumulation of autophagic vesicles with incompletely degraded substrates in swollen dystrophic neurites, and focal accumulation of degradative organelles in axons. These abnormalities indicate impaired retrograde axonal transport and maturation of lysosomal precursors, including impaired acidification. For example, in AD intracellular Aβ peptides and oligomers bind the dynein intermediate-chain subunit and may competitively inhibit dynein recruitment to late endosomes and amphisomes, causing their accumulation in the distal axon. Retention of amphisomes and late endosomes may delay the lysosomal clearance of β-site APP-cleaving enzyme-1 (BACE1, β-secretase) increasing amyloidogenic APP processing and further production of Aβ. These events may create a vicious circle involving disruption of endolysosomal transport, Aβ production, and local extracellular release as seeds for plaque formation. Consistent with this pathogenic mechanism, APP gene duplication in a mouse model of Down's syndrome disrupted axonal transport of early endosomes containing NGF. This was associated with impaired maturation into enlargement of Rab5 containing early endosomes and impaired maturation into Rab7 containing late endosomes, preventing acidification of the lumen. High intraluminal pH may induce aberrant Ca^{2+} efflux from lysosomes, leading to hyperphosphorylation of the dynein intermediate-chain subunit. This may provide a common mechanism that links reduced lysosomal acidification and impaired retrograde transport of degradative organelles. This mechanism may be relevant not only to AD but also to other neurodegenerative disorders.

KEY POINTS

- Axonal transport is fundamental for neuronal survival and for maintenance of neuronal connectivity and synaptic function.
- Anterograde transport delivers membrane-bound organelles synthesized and packaged in the cell body to the axon and synaptic compartments, and allows traffic and turnover of cytoskeletal and metabolic components of dendrites and axons.
- Retrograde transport is necessary for removal and degradation of materials via the endosome-lysosome and the autophagy-lysosome systems and for delivery of target-derived neurotrophic signals or injury signals back to the cell body.
- Anterograde transport requires motor proteins of the kinesin family; retrograde transport involves cytoplasmic dynein in complex with dynactin.
- Axonal transport is regulated by posttranslational modification of the microtubules, microtubule-associated proteins, or both; properties of the motor proteins; and activation of motors by adaptors or other binding partners.
- Fast anterograde transport delivers membrane-bound organelles, synaptic vesicle precursors, and material dense core secretory granules to synapses and axons.
- Retrograde transport of signaling endosomes is critical to neurotrophic signaling.
- Transport of mRNA granules allows locally regulated translation of mRNAs into proteins in both dendritic and axonal subdomains.
- Axonal injury triggers local translation of mRNAs and retrograde transport of signals from the site of injury to the nucleus.
- The retrograde transport of lysosomes, late endosomes, and autophagosomes occurs as they mature, progressively decreasing their intraluminal pH.
- Mitochondria undergo either anterograde or retrograde transport and are immobilized at sites of high energy demand, such as the synaptic terminals and nodes of Ranvier, in response to local increase in intracellular calcium.
- Slow axonal transport allows movement of cytoskeletal components, such as tubulin and neurofilament subunits, as well as cytosolic proteins, to axons and synaptic terminals.
- Impaired axonal transport is an important mechanism of neurodevelopmental and neurodegenerative disorders.
- Adult neurodegenerative disorders are characterized by accumulation of misfolded proteins, early loss of neuronal connectivity, and neuritic pathology, reflecting dying back neurodegeneration (distal axonopathy) due to impaired axonal transport.
- Mutations in tubulin, kinesin, or dynein motors, or their adaptor proteins, cause a broad range of neurological disorders, including hereditary spastic paraplegia, ALS, and CMT2.
- Polyglutamine repeat expansion of huntingtin deleteriously disrupts axonal transport of brain-derived neurotrophic factor, mitochondria, and autophagosomes.
- Important features associated with impaired axonal transport in neurodegenerative disorders include tau hyperphosphorylation, axonal accumulation of phosphorylated neurofilaments, and impaired retrograde transport and maturation of autophagosomes, late endosomes, and lysosomes.

REFERENCES

1. Maday S, Twelvetrees AE, Moughamian AJ, Holzbaur EL. Axonal transport: cargo-specific mechanisms of motility and regulation. Neuron 2014;84:292–309.
2. Black MM. Axonal transport: the orderly motion of axonal structures. Methods Cell Biol 2016;131:1–19.
3. Notzel M, Rosso G, Mollmert S, et al. Axonal transport, phase-separated compartments, and neuron mechanics—a new approach to investigate neurodegenerative diseases. Front Cell Neurosci 2018;12:358.
4. Guedes-Dias P, Holzbaur ELF. Axonal transport: driving synaptic function. Science 2019;366:642–687.
5. Roy S. Seeing the unseen: the hidden world of slow axonal transport. Neuroscientist 2014;20:71–81.
6. Kneynsberg A, Combs B, Christensen K, Morfini G, Kanaan NM. Axonal degeneration in tauopathies: disease relevance and underlying mechanisms. Front Neurosci 2017;11:572.
7. Fu MM, Holzbaur EL. Integrated regulation of motor-driven organelle transport by scaffolding proteins. Trends Cell Biol 2014;24:564–574.
8. Saudou F, Humbert S. The biology of huntingtin. Neuron 2016;89:910–926.
9. Harrington AW, Ginty DD. Long-distance retrograde neurotrophic factor signalling in neurons. Nat Rev Neurosci 2013;14:177–187.

10. Spaulding EL, Burgess RW. Accumulating evidence for axonal translation in neuronal homeostasis. Front Neurosci 2017;11:312.
11. Villarroel-Campos D, Schiavo G, Lazo OM. The many disguises of the signalling endosome. FEBS Lett 2018;592:3615–3632.
12. Bucci C, De Luca M. Molecular basis of Charcot-Marie-Tooth type 2B disease. Biochem Soc Trans 2012;40:1368–1372.
13. Saveri P, De Luca M, Nisi V, et al. Charcot-Marie-Tooth type 2B: a new phenotype associated with a novel RAB7A mutation and inhibited EGFR degradation. Cells 2020;9:1028–1049.
14. Kar AN, Lee SJ, Twiss JL. Expanding axonal transcriptome brings new functions for axonally synthesized proteins in health and disease. Neuroscientist 2018;24:111–129.
15. Khalil B, Morderer D, Price PL, Liu F, Rossoll W. mRNP assembly, axonal transport, and local translation in neurodegenerative diseases. Brain Res 2018;1693:75–91.
16. Khalil B, Morderer D, Price PL, Liu F, Rossoll W. mRNP assembly, axonal transport, and local translation in neurodegenerative diseases. Brain Res 2018;1693:75–91.
17. Wong YC, Holzbaur EL. The regulation of autophagosome dynamics by huntingtin and HAP1 is disrupted by expression of mutant huntingtin, leading to defective cargo degradation. J Neurosci 2014;34:1293–1305.
18. Misgeld T, Schwarz TL. Mitostasis in neurons: maintaining mitochondria in an extended cellular architecture. Neuron 2017;96:651–666.
19. Barnhart EL. Mechanics of mitochondrial motility in neurons. Curr Opin Cell Biol 2016;38:90–99.
20. Panchal K, Tiwari AK. Mitochondrial dynamics, a key executioner in neurodegenerative diseases. Mitochondrion 2018;47:151–173.
21. Pareyson D, Saveri P, Sagnelli A, Piscosquito G. Mitochondrial dynamics and inherited peripheral nerve diseases. Neurosci Lett 2015;596:66–77.
22. Guo T, Noble W, Hanger DP. Roles of tau protein in health and disease. Acta Neuropathol 2017;133:665–704.
23. Wang Y, Mandelkow E. Tau in physiology and pathology. Nature reviews Neuroscience 2016;17:22–35.
24. Nicolas A, Kenna KP, Renton AE, et al. Genome-wide analyses identify KIF5A as a novel ALS gene. Neuron 2018;97:1268–1283 e1266.
25. Esmaeeli Nieh S, Madou MR, Sirajuddin M, et al. De novo mutations in KIF1A cause progressive encephalopathy and brain atrophy. Ann Clin Transl Neurol 2015;2:623–635.
26. Dafsari HS, Byrne S, Lin JP, et al. Goldberg-Shprintzen megacolon syndrome with associated sensory motor axonal neuropathy. Am J Med Genet A 2015;167:1300–1304.
27. Hines TJ, Gao X, Sahu S, et al. An essential postdevelopmental role for Lis1 in mice. eNeuro 2018;5.
28. Farrer MJ, Hulihan MM, Kachergus JM, et al. DCTN1 mutations in Perry syndrome. Nat Genet 2009;41:163–165.
29. Puls I, Oh SJ, Sumner CJ, et al. Distal spinal and bulbar muscular atrophy caused by dynactin mutation. Ann Neurol 2005;57:687–694.
30. Neveling K, Martinez-Carrera LA, Holker I, et al. Mutations in BICD2, which encodes a golgin and important motor adaptor, cause congenital autosomal-dominant spinal muscular atrophy. Am J Hum Genet 2013;92:946–954.
31. Rossor AM, Oates EC, Salter HK, et al. Phenotypic and molecular insights into spinal muscular atrophy due to mutations in BICD2. Brain 2015;138:293–310.
32. Cogli L, Piro F, Bucci C. Rab7 and the CMT2B disease. Biochem Soc Trans 2009;37:1027–1031.
33. Guedes-Dias P, Pinho BR, Soares TR, de Proenca J, Duchen MR, Oliveira JM. Mitochondrial dynamics and quality control in Huntington's disease. Neurobiol Dis 2016;90:51–57.
34. Millecamps S, Julien JP. Axonal transport deficits and neurodegenerative diseases. Nat Rev Neurosci 2013;14:161–176.
35. Brady ST, Morfini GA. Regulation of motor proteins, axonal transport deficits and adult-onset neurodegenerative diseases. Neurobiol Dis 2017;105:273–282.
36. Prior R, Van Helleputte L, Benoy V, Van Den Bosch L. Defective axonal transport: a common pathological mechanism in inherited and acquired peripheral neuropathies. Neurobiol Dis 2017;105:300–320.
37. Lie PPY, Nixon RA. Lysosome trafficking and signaling in health and neurodegenerative diseases. Neurobiol Dis 2018;122:94–105.

10 Axon and Myelin

OVERVIEW

The maintenance of the structure and composition of their axons is critical for neurons to transmit information. Axons differ in their diameter, degree of myelination, and functions (Table 10.1). There are several fundamental differences between peripheral and central axons (Table 10.2). In the peripheral nervous system (PNS), each Schwann cell myelinates a segment of the axon, is associated with a basal lamina, and promotes axonal regeneration after injury. In the central nervous system (CNS), oligodendrocytes each provide myelin to up to 40 axons, are not associated with a basal lamina, and their myelin products inhibit axonal regeneration. The myelin sheath is a multilayered stack of extended and uniformly thick plasma membrane that is wrapped in a spiral fashion around the axon. Myelinated axons consist of an axon initial segment (AIS), nodes of Ranvier, paranode, juxtaparanode and internode, and presynaptic terminal, each with a unique repertoire of ion channels, cytoskeletal organization, and function (Figure 10.1). The AIS contains clusters of voltage-gated sodium channels, is the site of generation of the action potential and provides a barrier for axonal transport between the somatodendritic and axonal compartments. The nodes of Ranvier resemble the structure of the AIS and support fast conduction of the action potential. The paranode functions as a barrier that prevents invasion of voltage -potassium channels from the juxtaparanode to the node. Voltage-gated potassium channels clustered in the juxtaparanode regulate axon excitability. The internode is surrounded by compact myelin that has both an insulator and a trophic function. Myelin has a unique lipid and protein composition, which differs in central and peripheral axons (Table 10.2). There are multiple reciprocal interactions between the axons and myelinating cells. Schwann cells and oligodendrocytes support axonal metabolism; active axons release signals that promote myelinating cell differentiation. Astrocytes participate in reciprocal interactions with both axons and oligodendrocytes to support axon and myelin homeostasis. Each domain of the axon has selective susceptibility to disease. Disorders of axons and myelin include hereditary and acquired peripheral neuropathies and leukoencephalopathies. The main aims of this chapter are to review: (1) the functional compartmentalization of myelinated axons; (2) the composition of myelin; (3) the trophic interactions between axons and glial cells; and (4) examples of disorders primarily affecting central or peripheral axons and myelin.

MOLECULAR DOMAINS IN MYELINATED AXONS

In myelinated axons, the AIS, nodes of Ranvier, paranode, juxtaparanode, and internode each have a unique molecular organization with differential expression of ion channels, adhesion molecules, cytoskeletal and structural proteins, extracellular matrix proteins, and signal transduction molecules[1–3] (Figure 10.2).

Axon Initial Segment

The AIS is located just after the axon hillock of the soma.[4] The AIS has a high density of clustered voltage-gated sodium channels (Na_v). $Na_v1.6$ channels are clustered at the distal portion of the AIS and are primarily responsible for the initiation of action potential in mature myelinated axons; Na_v 1.2 channels are present in the proximal portion of the AIS and mediate action potentials in unmyelinated axons; $Na_v1.1$channels are expressed in the AIS of some GABAergic neurons. The AIS also expresses several voltage-gated potassium channels (K_v), including $K_v1.1$, $K_v1.2$, and K_v7/KCNQ channels, which control the probability of action potential generation. The clustering of ion channels at the AIS depends on ankyrin G, which is the master regulator of the development and stability of the AIS. Ankyrin G is a linker protein that binds $Na_v1.6$ and K_v7 channels and links them to the underlying actin cytoskeleton through the scaffold protein β4 spectrin. The AIS expresses several cell adhesion molecules that belong to the L1 subfamily of immunoglobulins,

TABLE 10.1 *Types of Peripheral Axons*

Axon Type (diameter) Conduction Velocity	Type	Function
Large myelinated (12–20 μm) 70–120 m/s	Aα	Touch and Pacinian corpuscle afferent
	IA	Muscle spindle a primary ending afferents
	IB	Golgi tendon organ afferents
	α-efferent	α- motoneurons axons to extradural fibers
Medium myelinated (6–12 μm) 30–70 m/s	Aβ	Low-threshold (Ruffini) cutaneous afferents
	II	Muscle spindle afferents (secondary endings)
Small myelinated (2–6 μm) 4–30 m/s	Aς	Prickling pain and cold temperature Free nerve endings Visceral sensation (distension)
	III	Muscle pressure and pain afferents
	γ-efferent	γ-motoneurons axons to intramural (muscle spindle) fibers
	B	Preganglionic autonomic efferent
Unmyelinated (< 2 μm) 0.2–2	C	Burning pain and heat sensation Visceral pain afferents Low-threshold (affective touch) afferents
	IV	Muscle pain afferents

including neurofascin 186 (NF186) and neuronal cell adhesion molecule (NrCAM), which participates in the structural organization of the axon. The cytoskeletal organization of the AIS is characterized by small fascicles of microtubules connected by cross-bridges and a dense subaxolemmal undercoat containing a complex of ankyrin G, spectrin, and actin-binding proteins that link ankyrin G to the microtubule. These cytoskeletal structures form a selective molecular barrier that prevents the passage of dendritic and somatic proteins into the axon and that of axonal proteins to the somatodendritic component. The AIS is a plastic structure and its location may shift in an activity-dependent manner.

TABLE 10.2 *Differences Between Central and Peripheral Axons*

Axon Type	Peripheral	Central
Myelinating cell	Schwann cell	Oligodendrocyte
Relationship between myelinating cell and node of Ranvier	1:1	1: up to 60 axons
Regulation of Na^+ channel clustering	Schwann cell	Perinodal astrocyte
Predominant sphingolipid	Sphingomyelin	Galactocerebrosides and sulfatide
Typical myelin proteins	Myelin protein zero (Po) Peripheral myelin protein (PMP) 22 Periaxin	Proteolipid protein (PLP) Myelin oligodendrocyte glycoprotein (MOG) Oligodendrocyte specific protein
Basal lamina	Yes	No
Regeneration potential	High	Low (myelin inhibitors such as No-go and MOG)

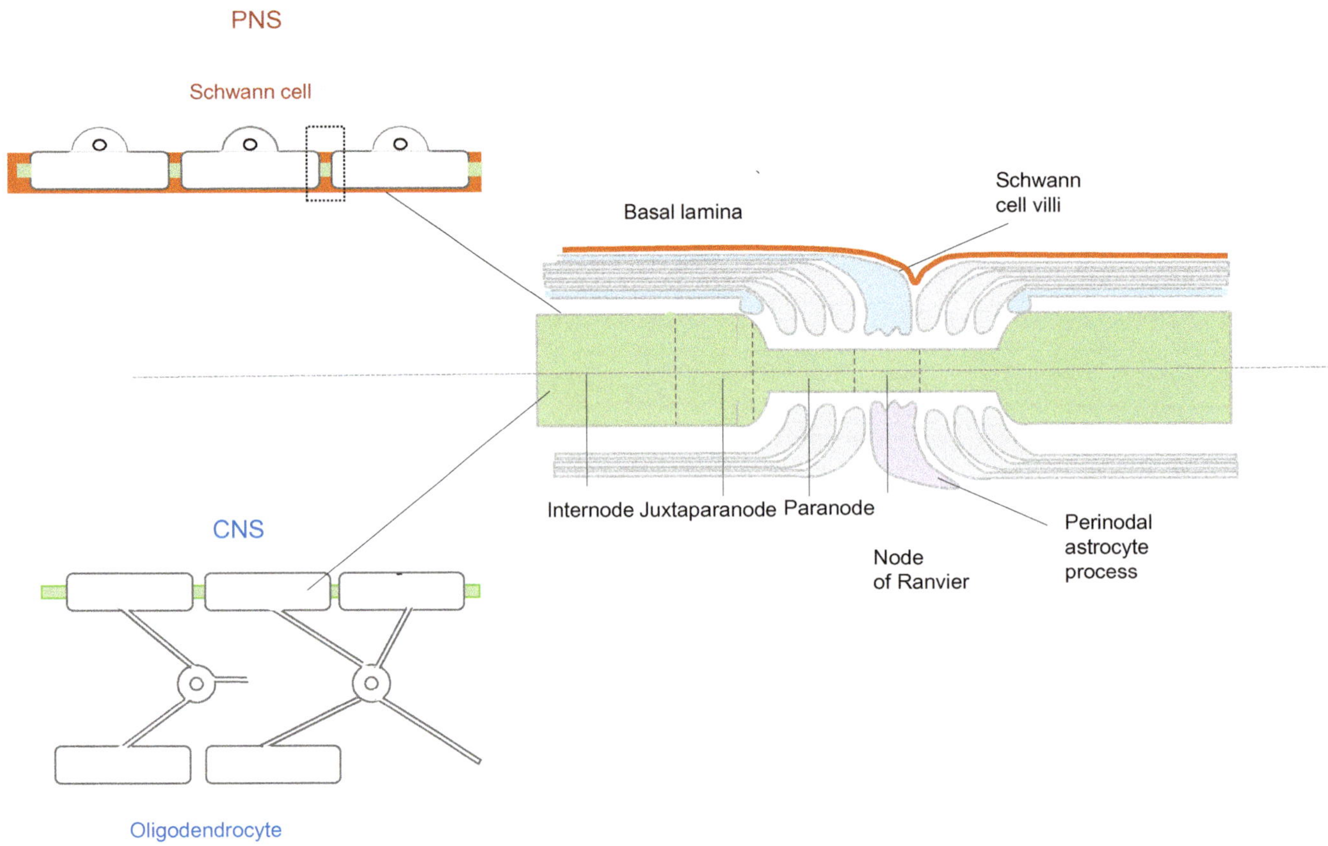

FIGURE 10.1 General organization of peripheral and central axons.
Myelination in the peripheral nervous system (PNS) involves Schwann cells; myelin in the CNS is produced by oligodendrocytes. An individual Schwann cell is responsible for myelination of a single internode; a single oligodendrocyte can contribute to myelin formation in up to 40 or more axons. Schwann cells are associated with a basal lamina, while central axons lack a basal lamina. In the PNS, the node is surrounded by Schwann cell microvilli. In the CNS, the nodes of Ranvier are often surrounded by perinodal processes of astrocytes, oligodendrocytes, or oligodendrocyte precursor cells.

Increased excitatory activity over a long period produces a shift of the AIS position to more distal portions of the axon, which may decrease probability of firing.

Node of Ranvier

The node of Ranvier is a ~1 μm long unmyelinated domain of the axon that enables saltatory conduction of the action potential.[1,2,5] The node of Ranvier is a hot spot containing clustered $Na_v1.6$ and $Na_v1.1$ channels, which are responsible for saltatory conduction of the action potential in myelinated axons. Nodal K_v3 and K_v7 channels dampen excitability and reduce the probability of reexcitation of the axon. Many of the adhesion molecules and cytoskeletal and scaffold proteins present in the AIS are also expressed at the nodes of Ranvier. Whereas development of the AIS primarily depends on the location of ankyrin G, the development of the node requires the influence of surrounding of myelinating glial cells. In peripheral axons, the node is surrounded by Schwann cell processes called microvilli (Figure10.2). These microvilli extend toward the nodal gap and produce the extracellular matrix protein gliomedin. Gliomedin is an adhesion molecule that binds microvilli to the axonal NF186-NrCAM complex and allows the recruitment and stabilization of other nodal components. Microvilli express transmembrane heparan sulfate proteoglycans that interact with extracellular matrix proteins, cytoskeletal proteins, and growth factors. The Schwann cell membrane opposing the basal lamina at the level of the node expresses dystroglycans, which interact with laminins. In the CNS, the nodes of Ranvier are often surrounded by perinodal processes of astrocytes, oligodendrocytes, or oligodendrocyte precursor cells, which may contribute to node maturation. Several adhesion molecules secreted by astrocytes, including heparan sulfate proteoglycans, and oligodendrocyte secreted proteins such as tenascin-R may participate in maturation of the node in CNS axons.

Paranode

As myelinating glia wrap around the axon, their cytoplasm is pushed to the edges, where it fills the loops of the

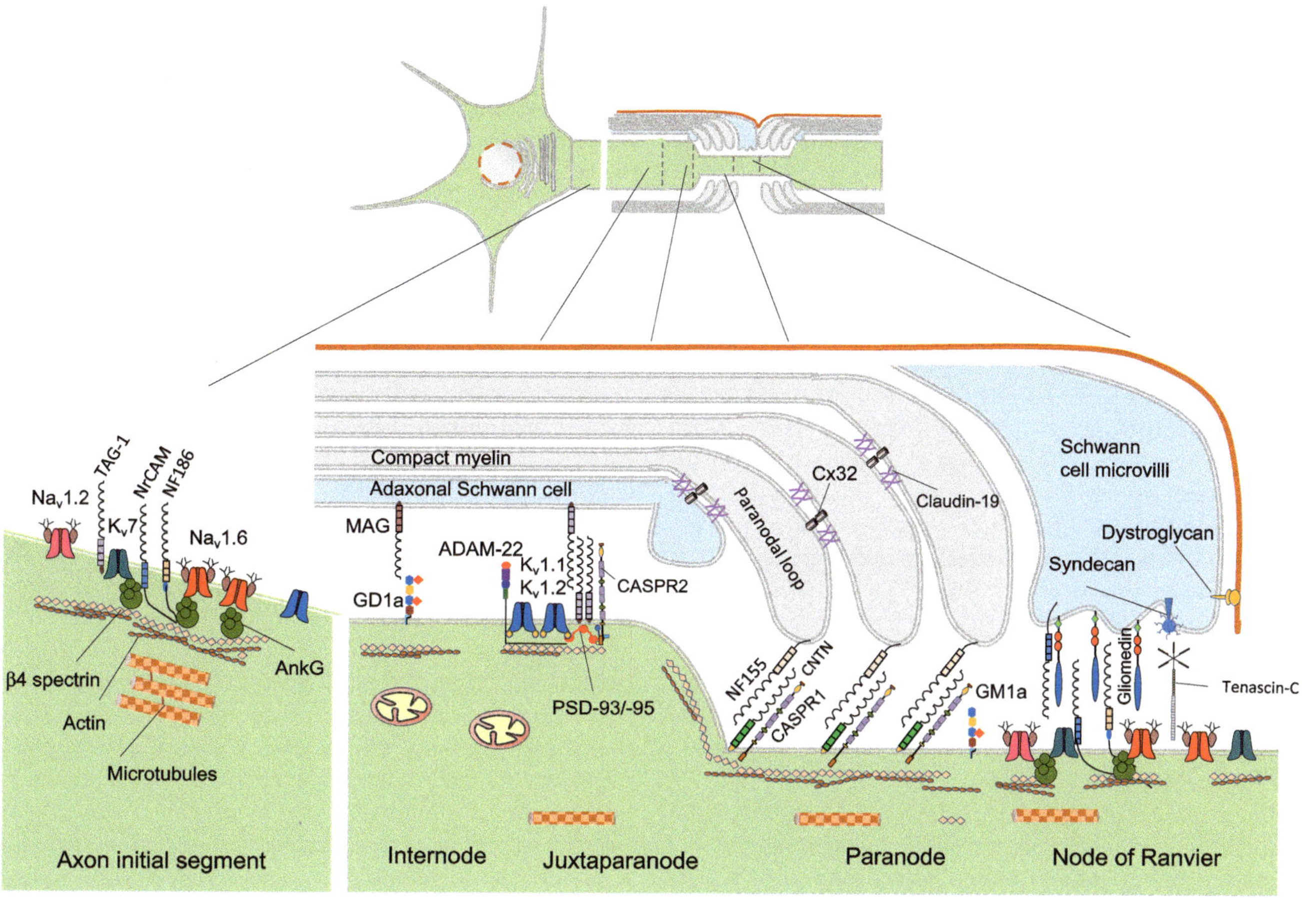

FIGURE 10.2 Molecular domains in myelinated axons.

The different compartments of the myelinating axons have a unique composition of ion channels, adhesion molecules, and adaptor proteins. The axon initial segment (AIS) has a high density of clustered Na$_v$1.6 voltage-gated sodium channels distally and Na$_v$ 1.2 channels proximally, as well as K$_v$1.1, K$_v$1.2, and K$_v$7 type voltage-gated potassium channels. The clustering of ion channels at the AIS depends on their interaction with ankyrin G. The AIS expresses several cell adhesion molecules, including neurofascin 186 (NF186), neuronal cell adhesion molecule (NrCAM), and transient axonal glycoprotein1 (TAG-1), and contactin-associated protein-2 (Caspr-2). The AIS is characterized by small fascicles of microtubules connected by cross-bridges and a dense undercoat of cytoskeletal proteins. Nodes of Ranvier contain clustered Na$_v$1.6 and Na$_v$1.1 as well K$_v$3.1 and K$_v$7.2/7.3. The node in peripheral axons is surrounded by Schwann cell microvilli, which produce gliomedin that binds the NF186-NrCAM complex. The paranodal loops attach to the axonemal through the formation of axon-glia septate junctions consisting of NF155, contactin (CNTN), and Caspr-1. The paranodal loops are interconnected by gap junctions consisting of connexin 32 (Cx32). The juxtaparanodes are enriched with K$_v$1.1 and K$_v$1.2 channels, which form a complex with CASPR2 and contactin/TAG-1. They also contain scaffolding proteins such as postsynaptic density protein (PSD)-93 and -95 and a disintegrin and metalloproteinase domain–containing protein-22 [ADAM-22]), which interacts with K$_v$1 and CASPR2. The compact myelin of the internode provides an insulating function. Myelin-associated glycoprotein (MAG) is present in the periaxonal membrane of the Schwan cell and mediates its interactions with the axon via gangliosides such as GD1a.

glial membranes that are attached to the axonal membrane. These loops, called paranodal loops, attach to the axonemal adjacent to the node through the formation of axon–glia septate junctions (Figure 10.2). These junctions comprise three major components: neurofascin 55 (NF155) present on the glial cell membrane, contactin anchored to the external surface of the axon, and contactin-associated protein-like 1 (CASPR1), which forms a complex with contactin and allows the interaction with the axoplasm and axonal cytoskeleton. These proteins are an important target of immune[6] or hereditary[7] nodo-paranodopathies. The link between the axon–glial septal junctions and the axonal cytoskeleton involves several scaffolding proteins, which contribute to the fence function of the paranode. A fundamental role of the paranode is to keep the K$_v$1 channels located in the juxtaparanodes segregated from the Na$_v$1.6 channels in the node. Paranodal complexes are also critical for maintenance of the axonal cytoskeleton. The paranodal loops are interconnected by gap junctions consisting of connexin (Cx) proteins, primarily Cx32 and Cx47. These gap junctions are involved in the passage of molecules between adjacent myelin membranes. Mutations affecting of the *GBJ1* gene encoding Cx32 are a major cause of X-linked Charcot-Marie-Tooth disease (CMTX).[8]

Although the paranodal loops are tightly attached to the axon via septate-like junctions, they form small triangular junctional clefts near the axon surface; this allows molecules to penetrate between the paranodal loops into the periaxonal spaces at the internodes. This extracellular pathway connects the extracellular space with the paranode and is important not only to deliver nutrients and metabolites but also to provide access to antibodies against paranodal antigens. The paranode is a particularly vulnerable region of the myelinated axon because it is an area of transition along the axonal microtubules; which can predispose of impaired axonal transport and axonal degeneration. The paranode is the main the site of formation of axonal swellings containing increased levels of phosphorylated neurofilaments, which reflects cytoskeletal disruption and is a hallmark of many disorders affecting the central or peripheral axons.

Juxtaparanode

The juxtaparanodes are enriched with K_v1.1 and K_v1.2 channels that control the probability of action potential generation and maintain the membrane in a slightly hyperpolarized state; that prevents back-propagation of the action and regulates burst firing. These channels form a complex with contactin and CASPR2, which allow their clustering in the juxtaparanode. The juxtaparanodes also contain scaffolding proteins such as postsynaptic density protein 95 (PSD-95) and a disintegrin and metalloproteinase domain–containing protein-22 (ADAM-22) which interacts with K_v1 channels and CASPR2. Antibodies against CASPR2 produce a wide spectrum of autoimmune disorders that include limbic encephalitis, movement disorders, sleep disturbance, hyponatremia, and typically peripheral nerve excitability manifested with neuromyotonia and neuropathic pain.[9]

Internode

The myelin sheath consists of a compact portion at the internode and juxtaparanode and a noncompacted portion forming the paranodal loops. The compact myelin of the internode provides an insulating function by increasing resistance and decreasing capacitance, which prevents loss of depolarizing current and promotes saltatory conduction of the action potential.[10] Under the electron microscopy, the compact portion has a periodic structure consisting of a dark layer (major dense line) that represents the fused proteins of the inner leaflets of the original cell membrane; a light line (intraperiod line) that represents tightly packed outer leaflets; and a still lighter line representing the lipid hydrocarbon chains at the outer membrane surface. When depicted in its unwrapped state, myelin is a large sheet of membrane with channel-like tubules at its borders. These cytoplasmic channels are integrated into an elaborate network of interconnected tunnels that allow distribution of molecules through the internode. In the CNS, the network can be further extended via gap junctions between oligodendrocytes with each other and with astrocytes.

Gangliosides and Regulation of Axonal Function

Gangliosides have a major role in the normal function of the axon.[11] Gangliosides are glycosphingolipids expressed primarily at lipid rafts in the outer leaflet of the plasma membrane. There is a differential distribution of gangliosides, both in several regions of the nervous system and in specific subcellular locations. For example GM1 is most abundantly expressed in motor nerves; GQ1b in oculomotor nerves; and GD1b in large dorsal root ganglion neurons. In peripheral myelinated axons, GM1 and GD1a are enriched at paranode regions; GM1 is also preferentially located at synaptic regions in some areas of the CNS. The motor nerve terminals at the neuromuscular junction are enriched with GM1, GD1a, GD1b, GQ1b, GQ1a, and GD3. Gangliosides interact laterally with transmembrane proteins located in the same membrane and with molecules located in the opposing membrane. Gangliosides influence membrane protein functions by affecting fluidity of the plasma membrane and by the electrostatic effects of their negatively charged sialic acid residues. They have a major role in neuronal development and axonal growth; modulate function of ion channels and receptors; participate in Ca^{2+} channel homeostasis and signaling; promote paranodal stability and synaptic transmission; and participate in cell–cell molecular interactions. Another important function of gangliosides, such as GM1 and GD1a, is to contribute to stability and maintenance of neuron–glia interactions at paranodes. Antiganglioside antibodies are associated with autoimmune peripheral neuropathies. In these disorders, immune attack targets glycan structures borne by glycolipids, particularly gangliosides concentrated in nerve myelin and axons.[12,13]

COMPOSITION OF THE MYELIN SHEATH

Myelin has a unique composition. The water content of myelin is 40%; the dry mass consists of 70–85 lipids and 15%–30% protein.

Myelin Lipids

The most abundant myelin lipid is cholesterol, which is concentrated in the outer leaflet of the membrane.[14,15] The most abundant phospholipid is phosphatidylethanolamine, which together with glycolipids is located in the cytoplasmic leaflet. Myelin is enriched with cerebrosides, primarily galactosylceramide and galactosylceramide sulfate (sulfatide). Peripheral myelin has considerably more sphingomyelin and less cerebroside and sulfatide than CNS myelin.

Intermolecular attractive forces between lipid molecules, particularly hydrogen bonds formed by galactosylceramide and sulfatides, lead to the formation of an organized and tightly packed myelin membrane. Mutations affecting these glycolipids are a major cause of leukodystrophy.[16,17] Mutations of the *ARSA* (arylsulfatase A) gene cause metachromatic leukodystrophy associated with excessive accumulation of sulfatides; mutations of the *GALC* (galactocerebrosidase) gene cause Krabbe disease. More than 50% of these glycolipids are hydroxylated in the endoplasmic reticulum (ER) by the fatty acid 2-hydroxylase (FA2H), which provides hydroxyl groups for the formation of hydrogen bonds. Loss-of-function *FA2H* mutations have been associated with various phenotypes including neurodegeneration with brain iron accumulation, hereditary spastic paraplegia (SPG35) and leukodystrophy with spasticity and dystonia spectrum; these mutations manifest white matter changes, hypointensity of the globus pallidus, ponto-cerebellar atrophy, and thin corpus callosum.[18]

Myelin Proteins

Myelin differs in protein composition in the CNS and PNS (Figure 10.3). The most abundant proteins are proteolipid protein (PLP) and myelin basic protein (MBP) as well as glycoproteins such as myelin protein zero (MPZ, P0), myelin oligodendrocyte glycoprotein (MOG), and myelin-associated glycoprotein (MAG). These proteins have fundamental functions in both compact and noncompact myelin and are affected in genetic or immune disorders (Table 10.3). Proteolipid protein contains four transmembrane domains, and has an important role in maintenance of compact myelin in central axons. It may have a role in oligodendrocyte migration and differentiation and in shuttling myelin proteins from the soma into the myelin sheaths. Myelin basic protein is located exclusively in the cytoplasmic surface and is the major protein in stabilizing the major dense line in the CNS. Myelin-oligodendrocyte glycoprotein is a transmembrane glycoprotein with an immunoglobulin domain that is located

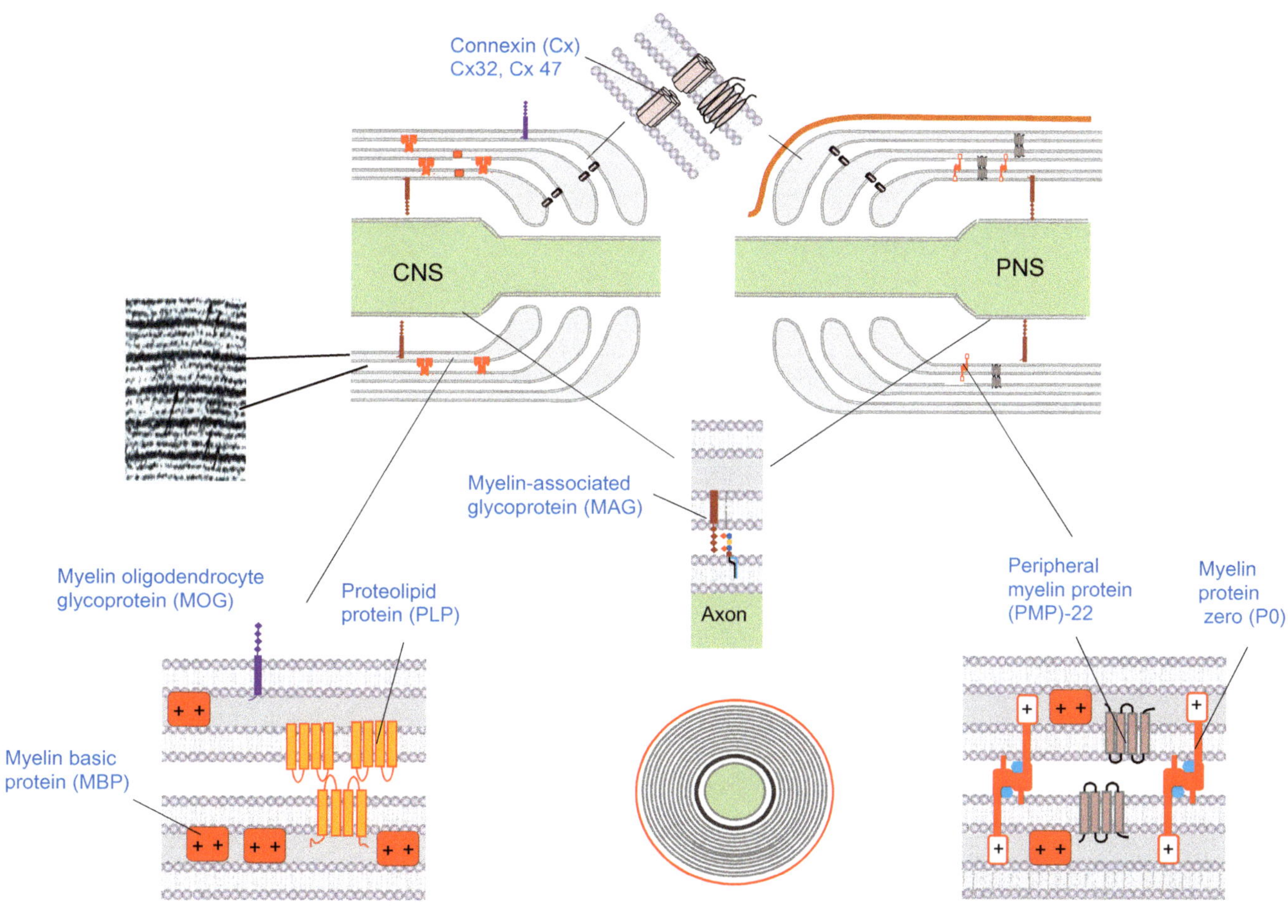

FIGURE 10.3 Myelin proteins in central and peripheral axons.

Myelin in central and peripheral axons differs in its protein composition. The most abundant proteins in central myelin are proteolipid protein (PLP) and myelin basic protein (MBP). The remaining are glycoproteins, including myelin protein zero (MPZ, P0), myelin oligodendrocyte glycoprotein (MOG), and myelin-associated glycoprotein (MAG). MPZ accounts for more than one-half of the proteins in peripheral myelin. Connexin-32 (Cx32) and Cx47 form gap junctions in the noncompact regions of myelin, including the paranodal loops.

TABLE 10.3 *Myelin Proteins*

Protein (gene)	Location	Function	Disease Association
Proteolipid protein *(PLP)*	CNS	Myelin compaction Oligodendrocyte differentiation	Pelizaeus-Merzbacher disease
Myelin basic protein (*MBP*)	CNS	Myelin compaction	Increased in CSF in demyelination
Myelin oligodendrocyte glycoprotein (MOG)	CNS	Located outside the myelin sheath Signal transmission to oligodendrocytes	Anti-MOG associated disorders: ADEM, optic neuritis, LETM, and others
Myelin protein zero (*MPZ*)	PNS	Myelin compaction	Several forms of CMT
Peripheral myelin protein-22 (PMP22)	PNS	Forms complex with MPZ Myelin assembly and maintenance	CMT1A (triplication) HNPP (deletion)
Myelin-associated glycoprotein (MAG)	PNS and CNS	Interactions with the axon Interaction between adjacent Schwann cell membranes	MAG antibodies associated with distal demyelinating neuropathy
Periaxin-2 (*PRX*)	PNS	Interaction with the ECM	CMT4F
Connexin 32 (*GBJ1*)	PNS CNS	Gap junction	CMTX Leukodystrophy

ADEM, acute disseminated encephalomyelitis; CMT, Charcot-Marie-Tooth disease; HNPP, hereditary neuropathy with predisposition to pressure palsies, LTEM, longitudinal extensive transverse myelopathy

in the outside surface of the myelin sheath and may function as a signal transduction molecule transmitting information from the extracellular matrix or adjacent myelin sheaths to oligodendrocytes. Myelin protein zero is a transmembrane glycoprotein with an extracellular immunoglobulin-like domain that mediates interactions between the outer surfaces of adjacent membranes and an intracellular portion that contributes to the stabilization of compact myelin in the PNS. Peripheral myelin protein-22 (PMP22) is an integral membrane protein present in compact myelin in peripheral axons. PMP22 may have a role in dynamic assembly and maintenance of peripheral myelin; it forms complexes with MPZ/P0, and the ratio between PMP22 and other myelin proteins is important for normal maintenance of myelinated axons. MAG is a relatively minor protein in both the CNS and PNS. MAG has a single transmembrane domain and is present in the periaxonal glial membrane of myelin sheaths, where it interacts with both glycoproteins and gangliosides in the axonal membrane, thereby participating in bidirectional signaling between the glia and the axon. In the PNS, MAG is also present in the Schmidt-Lanterman incisures, paranodal loops, and the outer mesaxon, reflecting its additional role in interactions between adjacent Schwann cell membranes. Connexin-32 (Cx32) and Cx47 form gap junctions in the noncompact regions of myelin, including the paranodal loops. These gap junctions are involved in the passage of molecules between adjacent myelin membranes. Other proteins expressed in oligodendrocytes include 2'3'-cyclic nucleotide phosphodiesterase, which promotes intracellular mRNA transport and cytoskeletal dynamics for outgrowth and differentiation of oligodendrocytes; and oligodendrocyte myelin glycoprotein, which is an important mediator of myelin-associated inhibition of axonal growth and myelination. There are many enzymes associated with myelin; they includes several protein kinases and phosphatases, enzymes involved in lipid and phosphoinositide metabolism, carbonic anhydrase, 5'nucleotidase, and Na^+/K^+ ATPase.

PERIPHERAL MYELINATION

Peripheral myelination depends on interactions among axons, Schwann cells, and basement membrane.

Development of Schwann Cells

Schwann cell precursors originate from neural crest progenitor cells that also give rise to sympathetic ganglia and sensory dorsal root ganglia neurons. There is a highly ordered developmental sequence that controls the progression of neural progenitor cells to become mature myelinating or nonmyelinating Schwann cells (Figure 10.4). Schwann cell precursors migrate with axons in the developing PNS

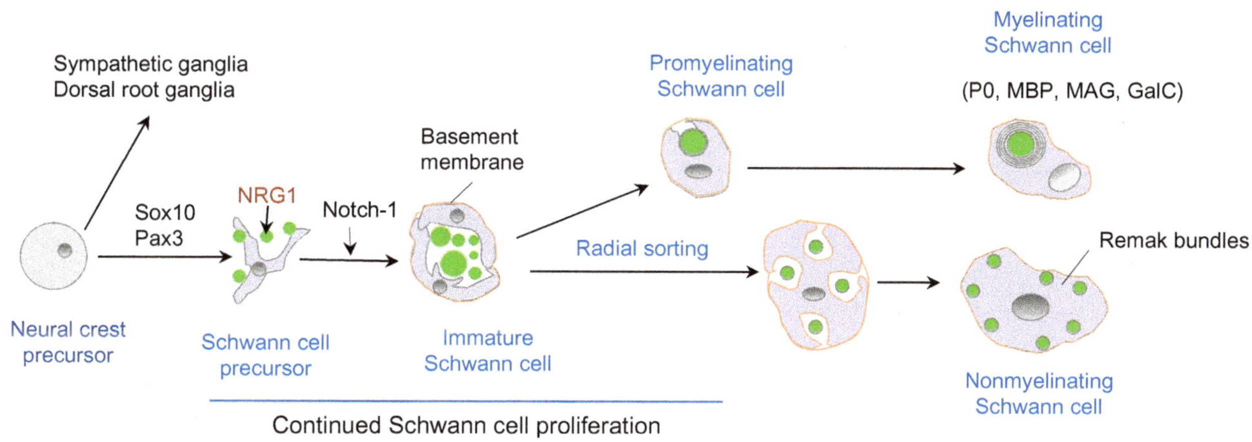

FIGURE 10.4 Development of Schwann cells.

Schwann cell precursors originate from neural crest progenitor cells. Some key transcription factors that govern the development of Schwann cell precursors from neural crest are Sox10 and Pax3. Axon-derived neuregulin-1 (NRG1) is the key regulator of Schwann cell precursors. Notch-1 signaling is important for this transition. Immature Schwann cells deposit a basal lamina. Promyelinating Schwann cells associate with a single axonal segment and differentiate into myelinating Schwann cells; nonmyelinating Schwann cells ensheath multiple small caliber axons forming Remak bundles.

and depend on axonal signals for survival. Axons provide trophic and mitogenic factors to Schwann cells, which in turn participate in normal development, long-term survival, and formation and the organization of nodes of Ranvier in the axon.[19–21] Axon-derived neuregulin 1 (NRG1) is the key regulator of Schwann cell precursor development and myelination. Schwann cell precursors become immature Schwann cells, which associate with many axons and continue proliferating but cease migrating. Immature Schwann cells deposit extracellular matrix (ECM) into an organized basal lamina that persists and matures through subsequent stages of Schwan cell development. Immature Schwann cells participate in a process called radial sorting, which separates axons destined to become myelinated from those that will remain nonmyelinated. During this process, immature Schwann cells interdigitate their cytoplasmic processes into the axon bundle and deposit ECM components into a basal lamina. Promyelinating Schwann cells become associated with a single axonal segment and differentiate into myelinating Schwann cells, Nonmyelinating Schwann cells ensheath multiple small caliber axons forming Remak bundles. In addition, Schwann cells sends signals such as vascular endothelial growth factor (VEGF) to mesenchymal cells to promote their differentiation into arteries, and other signals that promote their differentiation into perineurial and epineurial sheaths that surround mature nerves.

Signaling Mechanisms for Schwann Cell Differentiation, Radial Sorting, and Myelination

The development of Schwann cells and peripheral nerve myelination is controlled by a large number of signals from axons, ECM, and other sources.[19–22] Neuregulin 1 binds the tyrosine kinase ErbB2/3 receptors in Schwann cells and activates downstream canonical growth factor signal transduction cascades.[23] Signals from the ECM also trigger downstream cascades that promote myelination. One important example is cyclic adenosine monophosphate (cAMP) signaling cascades activated downstream of the G protein-coupled receptor GPR126. Critical regulators of PNS myelination include Notch1, which mediates axon–glial interaction and signaling, and the Wnt/β-catenin pathway, which controls radial sorting of axons.[22] During this process, both Schwann cells and axons also integrate influences from the ECM (laminin and collagen) which promote the remodeling of Schwann cell cytoskeletal components. An essential step in axo-glial signaling and radial sorting involves proteins called prohibitins.

CENTRAL MYELINATION

Oligodendrocyte development involves three stages: oligodendrocyte precursor cells (OPC), premyelinating oligodendrocytes, and mature oligodendrocytes[24–27] (Figure 10.5).

Oligodendrocyte Development

Oligodendrocyte precursor cells originate from neuroepithelial progenitor cells located in the ventricular zone in selected regions in the brain and spinal cord. Oligodendrocyte precursor cells express the neuron-glia 1 (NG2) chondroitin sulfate proteoglycan and platelet-derived growth factor (PDGF) receptor-α (PGDFR-α) and are specified in response to signaling by the secreted morphogen Sonic Hedgehog, derived from the floor plate. Oligodendrocyte precursor cells require substantial metabolic support to differentiate and critically depend on access to the vasculature

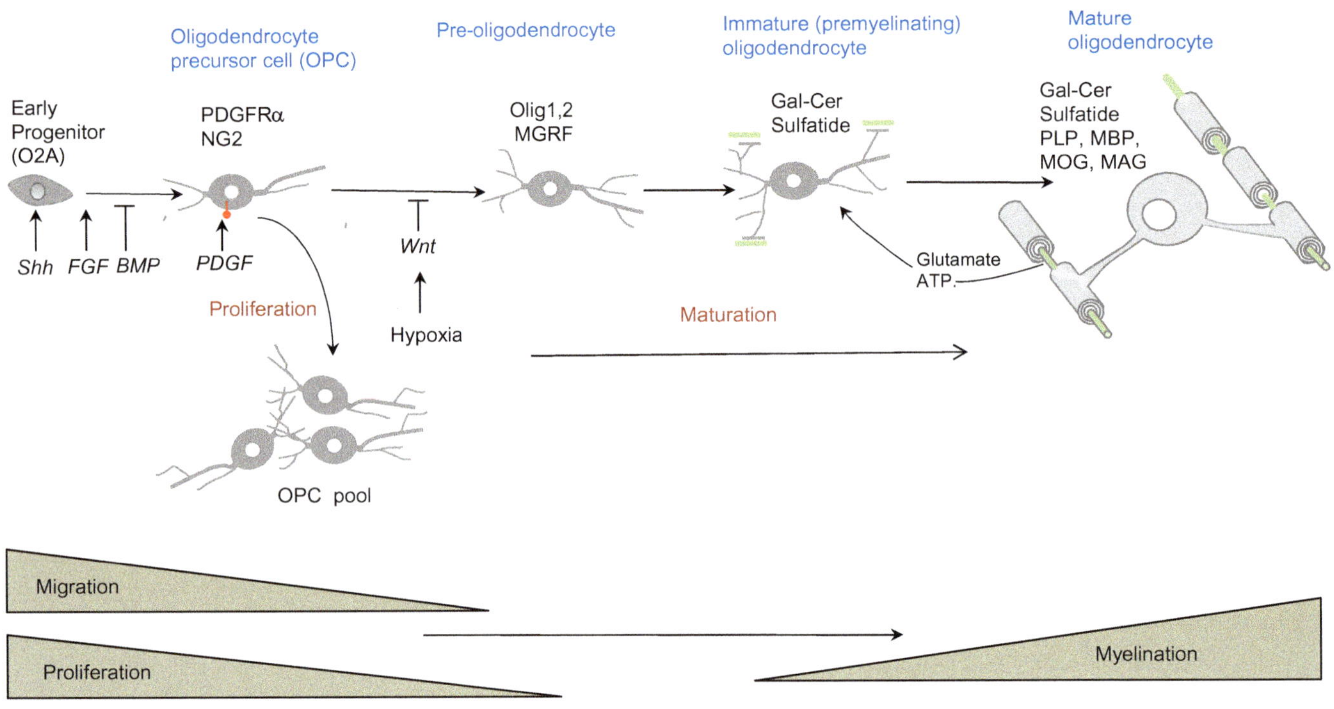

FIGURE 10.5 Oligodendrocyte differentiation.
Oligodendrocyte development involves three stages: oligodendrocyte precursor cells (OPCs), premyelinating oligodendrocytes, and mature oligodendrocytes. OPCs express the neuron-glia 2 (NG2) chondroitin sulfate proteoglycan and platelet-derived growth factor (PDGF) receptor-α (PGDFR-α) and are specified in response to signaling by the secreted morphogen Sonic hedgehog, derived from the floor plate. Sonic hedgehog (Shh), as well as Wnt. When premyelinating oligodendrocytes begin to branch to form multiple processes, they start producing galactosylceramide and sulfatide before synthesizing proteolipid protein (PLP) and myelin basic protein (MBP).

and oxygenation. In the setting of hypoxia, OPCs upregulate expression of hypoxia inducible factor, which via Wnt signaling inhibits their differentiation until proper metabolic support is available. Once the lineage of each oligodendrocyte is specified, tightly controlled feedback loops involving several transcription factors work to either maintain proliferating OPCs in their progenitor state and prevent their premature differentiation, or release them for differentiation into mature oligodendrocytes. Newly formed oligodendrocyte lineage cells express transcription factors such as NKX2.2 and oligodendrocyte transcription factor 2 (OLIG2), which together determine oligodendrocyte differentiation. OLIG2 directly induces the expression of SOX10, a transcription factor that is critical for oligodendrocyte maturation. SOX10 triggers several downstream cascades and directly activates several genes critical to the myelination process.[27] Nuclear receptors including the retinoid X receptors, vitamin D receptors, and thyroid hormone receptors also have a role in oligodendrocyte development and myelination. The expression of genes involved in fatty acid and cholesterol metabolism in oligodendrocytes is controlled by transcription factors of the sterol regulatory element binding proteins family and is activated by the mechanistic target of rapamycin (mTOR) pathway. Epigenetic regulation drives oligodendrocyte lineage progression and myelination. At the OPC stage, extracellular cues drive mainly inhibitory pathways that prevent differentiation and promote proliferation. At the onset of the differentiation process, histone deacetylase activity downregulates expression of the inhibitors that prevent differentiation. Some miRNAs and long noncoding RNAs also promote oligodendrocyte differentiation. During developmental myelination, the eukaryotic translation initiation factor 2B (eIF2B) has an oligodendrocyte cell–autonomous role in maintaining protein translation. Mutations of the *EIF2B* gene inhibit protein translation, delay recovery during the integrated cell stress response, and cause vanishing white matter disease.[28] The formation of CNS myelin starts when the OPCs become premyelinating oligodendrocytes, which begin to branch to form multiple processes to target axons and start producing galactosylceramide and sulfatide and then PLP and MBP. MBP translation requires anterograde mRNA transport followed by local mRNA translation at the cell processes in proximity to the developing myelin sheath. OPCs continue to divide throughout adulthood and form new myelinating oligodendrocytes producing progressively more and shorter internodes. Mechanical forces acting on the rigid cytoskeletal structures linked to nuclear components may interact with the epigenetic machinery to affect chromatin structure and induce transcriptional changes leading to differentiation.

Axon-Myelin Synapse and Activity-Dependent Control of Myelination in the CNS

A critical factor regulating myelination is neuronal activity (Figure 10.6). The normal formation of myelinated axons requires a precise matching between the number of oligodendrocytes generated from OPCs and the length of axons to be myelinated.[29] Oligodendrocytes receive functional axo-myelin synapses and express a variety of receptors for neurotransmitter released from electrically active axons, including glutamate, adenosine triphosphate (ATP), adenosine, brain-derived neurotrophic factor, and adhesion molecules such neuroligin 1.[30] All these transmitters influence all stages of oligodendrocyte development, primarily via Ca^{2+} dependent mechanisms.[30] Glutamate has a critical role in these axon–oligodendrocyte interactions, by activating Ca^{2+}-permeable α-amino-3-hydroxy-5-methyl-4-isoxazolepropionic acid receptors (AMPARs) expressed in the oligodendrocyte cell body and N-methyl-D-aspartate receptors (NMDARs) expressed in the processes forming the myelin sheath.[30] Whereas the intermodal axolemma expresses voltage-gated Ca^{2+} channels and may sense depolarization, it has limited access to extracellular Ca^{2+} due to the presence of the myelin sheath. Thus, the main source of Ca^{2+} in the axon is the ryanodine-sensitive intracellular Ca^{2+} stores in the ER, which are activated by Ca^{2+} influx via voltage-sensitive L-channels and Ca^{2+}-permeable AMPARs. Calcium influx may trigger vesicular release of glutamate from axons to activate NMDARs in myelin and thus Ca^{2+} influx in oligodendrocytes. These signals also influence, in

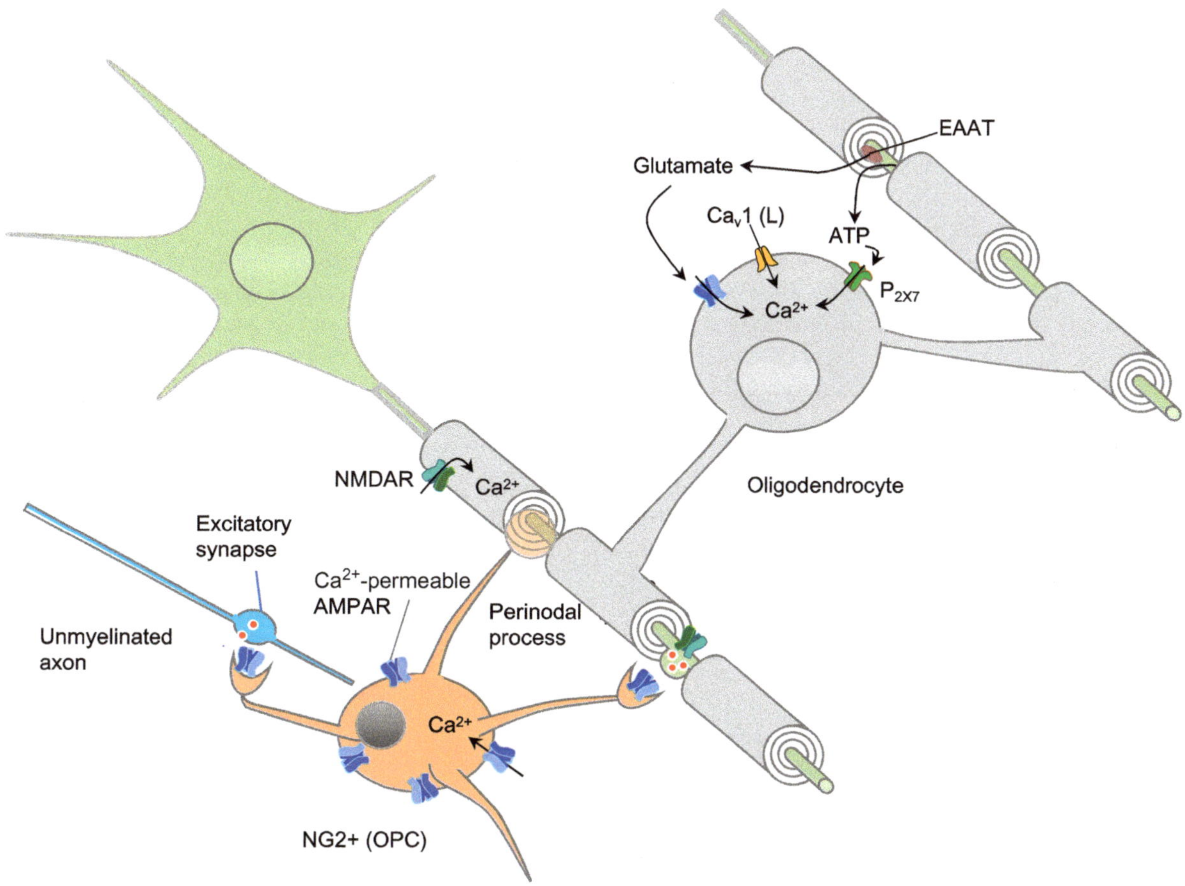

FIGURE 10.6 Activity-dependent control of myelination in the CNS.
A critical factor regulating myelination is neuronal activity. Oligodendrocyte precursor cells (OPCs) receive functional synapses from neurons. Neurotransmitters released by electrically active axons, including glutamate, adenosine triphosphate (ATP), and adenosine, can influence all stages of oligodendrocyte development, primarily via Ca^{2+} dependent mechanisms. Glutamate has a critical role in axon-oligodendrocyte interactions, by acting via α-amino-3-hydroxy-5-methyl-4-isoxazolepropionic acid receptors (AMPARs) predominantly expressed in the oligodendrocyte cell body and N-methyl-D-aspartate receptors (NMDARs) expressed in the processes forming the myelin sheath.

an activity-dependent manner, both short-term metabolic phenomena, such as increase in energy supply from the oligodendrocyte to an electrically active axon, and long-term changes in myelin nanostructure structure to modulate conduction of the action potential.[30] Activity-dependent myelin remodeling provides a mechanism for use-dependent synaptic plasticity and learning. However, excessive activity, as occurs in seizures, may foster abnormal proliferation of oligodendrocytes as occurs in glioma.

Environmental Signals Regulating Oligodendrocyte Differentiation

There are several extrinsic factors that regulate oligodendrocyte development and myelination. Astrocytes secrete several trophic factors that affect both oligodendrocyte development and remyelination after injury. Astrocytes are the main sources of growth factors such as PDGF-α and transforming growth factor (TGF)-β, which stimulate either OPC proliferation or differentiation into mature oligodendrocytes depending on their developmental stage. Ciliary neurotrophic factor, produced by both neurons and astrocytes, promotes OPC differentiation; insulin-like growth factor-1 also promotes oligodendrocyte development, differentiation, and survival. Remyelination following CNS injury requires activation, recruitment, and maturation of OPCs. Several extracellular cues, including growth factors, chemokines, cell–cell adhesion molecules, and ECM molecules regulate these processes. Up- or downregulation of expression of these molecules by signals produced during inflammation or other pathological conditions may strongly affect the probability of demyelination in disorders such as multiple sclerosis. Most extrinsic cues inhibit myelination. Reactive astrocytes secrete hyaluronan, chondroitin sulfate proteoglycans, tenascin C, end endothelin-1, which inhibit remyelination. Lesions also trigger expression of semaphorins, bone morphogenetic protein, and fibronectin, which inhibit OPC differentiation. Whereas surveilling ("resting") microglia secrete signals that sustain OPC production, reactive microglia may have different effects according to their phenotype.

RECIPROCAL TROPHIC INTERACTIONS BETWEEN AXONS AND GLIAL CELLS IN THE CNS

There are reciprocal trophic relationships between axons and oligodendrocytes. Active axons not only release signals that promote oligodendrocyte differentiation but also provide substrates for myelin formation. Reciprocally, myelin supports axon function and metabolism. Astrocytes also participate in reciprocal interactions with both axons and oligodendrocytes to support axon and myelin homeostasis (Figure 10.7).

Axonal Provision of Substrates for Myelin Synthesis

Active neurons provide substrates to the oligodendrocyte for synthesis of myelin lipids. Neurons synthesize N-acetylaspartate (NAA) in their mitochondria; NAA levels detected by magnetic resonance spectroscopy are a marker of axonal and neuronal integrity. NAA is transported out of the mitochondria and then released from neurons and transported to oligodendrocytes at the junction of the axon with the inner plasma membrane of the myelin sheath. In the oligodendrocyte, NAA is metabolized by aspartoacylase (ASPA), which removes acetate that is then converted to acetyl coenzyme A (CoA) by action of acetyl CoA synthetase I. As acetyl CoA is a precursor for lipid synthesis, the sequential activation of ASPA in axons and acetyl CoA synthetase I in oligodendrocytes is critical for the synthesis of myelin compounds, particularly galactocerebrosides, sulfatides, and cholesterol. Mutations producing *ASPA* loss of function result in Canavan disease, a cavitating leukodystrophy characterized by increased NAA levels in body fluids.

Myelin Support of Axonal Function

The classical function of myelin is as an electrical insulator facilitating conduction of the action potential, by reducing axolemma capacitance and thus the loss of electric charge across the axonal membrane. Another major role of myelin is to actively recruit ion channels and other axon membrane components into specific domains of the axon. Myelin also contributes to increased axonal diameter by inducing changes in the neurofilaments. Most of the volume of the axon is occupied by neurofilaments separated from each other by the side arms of neurofilament triplet (NF) subunits. The axon cytoskeleton is altered locally by contact with the glia. Myelin promotes phosphorylation of the tail domains neurofilament heavy (NF-H) and middle (NF-M) molecular weight proteins; this promotes the repulsion between their negative charges, thereby increasing axonal diameter.

Oligodendrocyte Support of Axonal Metabolism

Myelin also has a critical role in providing metabolic support to the axon. The axons require a constant supply of energy maintain the Na^+ gradient via the Na^+/K^+ ATPase, which is necessary to maintain excitability for action potential generation; to prevent excessive accumulation of Ca^{2+} in the axoplasm; and to support axonal transport.[31] The Na^+/K^+ ATPase is primarily located along the intermodal axon membrane. Local energy production is required to maintain axon function along its length. Since access of glucose to most axons is restricted by the hydrophobic barrier created by the presence of myelin, the supply of lactate from the oligodendrocyte to the axon is critical for metabolic support of the axon.[32] Lactate transport is mediated by monocarboxylic transporters (MCTs); oligodendrocytes primarily express MCT1; neurons express MCT2, and astrocytes express MCT4. According to the lactate shuttle hypothesis, heavily glycolytic cells, such as astrocytes, convert large amounts of pyruvate to lactate, which is transported to the extracellular fluids via MCT4; lactate is then transported by other MCTs into cells that are more dependent on oxidative metabolism.

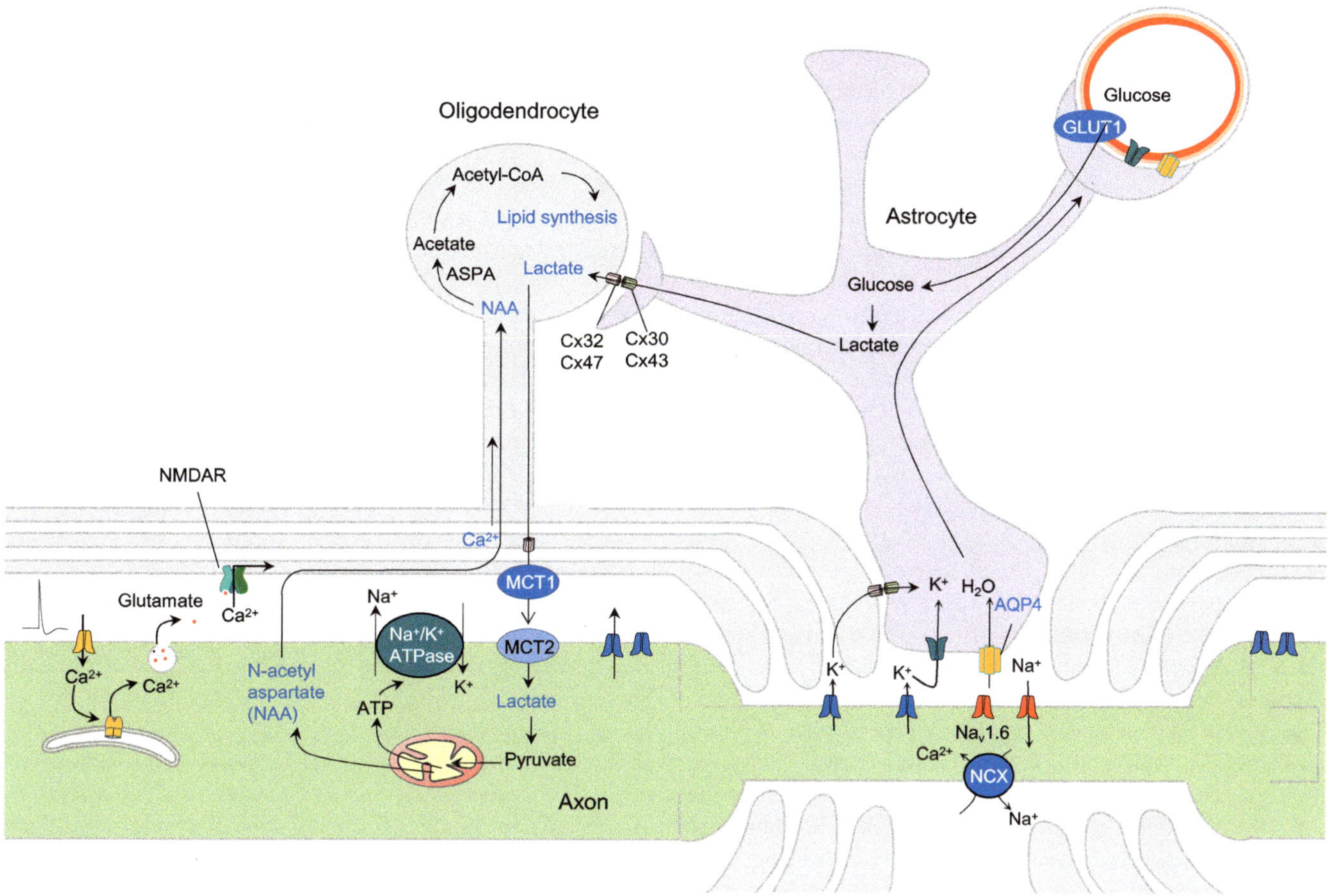

FIGURE 10.7 Reciprocal trophic interactions between axons and glial cells in the CNS.
Active neurons synthesize N-acetylaspartate (NAA), which is transported to oligodendrocytes and metabolized by aspartoacylase (ASPA), yielding acetyl coenzyme A (CoA) for lipid synthesis. The supply of lactate from the oligodendrocyte to the axon is critical for metabolic support of the axon. Lactate transport is mediated by monocarboxylic transporters (MCTs); oligodendrocytes primarily express MCT1, neurons express MCT2, and astrocytes MCT4. Astrocytes produce lactate, which is transported to oligodendrocytes, a process facilitated by gap junctions. Astrocytes express the water channel aquaporin 4 (AQP4) in their perivascular endfoot, subependymal, and subventricular, and perinodal processes. The functional coupling of AQP4 with the inward-rectifying $Ki_r4.1$ channels in the paranodal process is key for regulation of the ion and water environment in the axon.

These cells include neurons and oligodendrocytes where lactate is converted back to pyruvate and then used in the Krebs cycle for ATP production. Oligodendrocytes are critical intermediaries for the transport of lactate from astrocytes to the axon. The MCT1 is localized in myelin sheaths surrounding the axon and exports lactate from the oligodendrocyte to the axons, which incorporates lactate that can be used to support energy production. The main source of lactate for the oligodendrocyte is the astrocyte; these two types of glial cells make direct connections via heteromeric gap junction channels formed by Cx32 and Cx47 in oligodendrocyte and Cx30 and Cx43 in astrocytes. These gap junctions allow the passage of lactate from the astrocyte to the oligodendrocyte. Oligodendrocytes actively utilize lactate by oxidation and lipogenesis to synthesize myelin. Whereas oligodendrocytes may use lactate for their own energy needs, they primarily export lactate for metabolic support of the axon. Astrocytes can also deliver lactate directly to the axon at the nodes of Ranvier.[31]

Astrocyte Support of Oligodendrocyte Function

Oligodendrocytes are highly metabolically active cells as they have to support the production of membranes up to 100 times the weight of their cell body, Both during development and regeneration after CNS lesions fibrous astrocytes regulate the activity and function of oligodendrocytes.[33,34] Fibrous astrocytes provide extensively overlapping processes, supporting metabolic homeostasis in the white matter. Astrocytes have several important roles critical for oligodendrocyte survival and function. These include protection against glutamate-mediated excitotoxicity and oxidative stress; metabolic support, supply of iron; and regulation of myelin water and ion homeostasis. Astrocytes in the white matter express high levels of excitatory amino acid transporters and have a critical role in glutamate clearance. The high metabolic rate of oligodendrocytes leads to the production of toxic products, including reactive oxygen species. However oligodendrocytes have only a low concentration of antioxidant molecules such as glutathione and are therefore more vulnerable to ischemia or hypoxia than neurons. Oligodendrocytes thus depend on astrocyte uptake of glutamate and glutathione production for antioxidant protection and survival. Astrocytes are also critical to provide metabolic support to oligodendrocytes. In basal conditions both astrocytes and oligodendrocytes take in glucose directly from the blood via the glucose transporter-1 (GLUT1) However, during periods of increased neuronal activity or hypoglycemia, lactate produced by astrocytes serve as a major substrate to support energy metabolism both in oligodendrocytes and neurons.

Oligodendrocytes have a high demand for iron to sustain their basic metabolic needs and myelination; they have the highest concentration of ferritin-bound iron in the CNS. However, they must obtain iron from their environment. Astrocytes are the key regulators of iron availability in the CNS, given their extensive coverage of the surface of brain capillaries by their endfoot processes and thus their high ability to take up iron from the bloodstream. Iron enters the cytosol via its binding to transferrin, which is incorporated via endocytosis and released in the form of ferrous iron (Fe^{2+}) into the cytoplasm. Fe^{2+} is oxidized to Fe^{3+} by ceruloplasmin located on plasma membrane of astrocytes and then binds to transferrin to be transported to the brain extracellular fluid and other cells in the CNS. Transferrin is mainly synthesized and secreted by oligodendrocytes and choroid plexus cells.

Astrocytes express the water channel aquaporin 4 (AQP4) in their perinodal processes. The functional coupling of AQP4 with the efflux of K^+ via Kir4.1 channels in the paranodal process is key for regulation of ion and water environment in the axon and is also required for development and survival of oligodendrocytes. Contacts via gap junction between astrocytes and oligodendrocytes form a syncytium that supports the unidirectional flow of cytosolic content from the astrocyte to the oligodendrocytes. This coupling also provides for potential spatial K^+ buffering to dissipate high K^+ concentration on the oligodendrocyte and is critical for volume regulation in the myelin sheath.

PERIPHERAL NEUROPATHY

Peripheral neuropathies can be classified according to their distribution, temporal profile, type of fiber involved, pathophysiologic features, and cause. A comprehensive discussion of these disorders is beyond the scope of this chapter, and only some salient concepts will be emphasized here. The involvement of peripheral nerves may be focal, multifocal, or generalized; symmetric or asymmetric; and acute, subacute, fluctuating, or chronic progressive. The abnormality may be predominantly demyelinating or axonal; and the cause may be hereditary, immune-inflammatory, metabolic, or toxic. Nerve conduction velocities and needle EMG are important tools to identify whether the primary abnormality is demyelinating or axonal, but this may require confirmation with nerve biopsy.

Segmental demyelinating neuropathies are usually acquired and commonly affect sites of nerve compression early and produce asymmetric nerve involvement. Conduction slowing is more common in chronic disorders and conduction block in rapidly developing disorders. Axonal neuropathies result from either diffuse axonal degeneration or from dying back of the distal portion of the axon (distal axonopathy). These neuropathies show denervation changes on EMG, including fibrillation potentials, fasciculation potentials, and reduced recruitment, particularly in distal muscles.

Autoimmune Neuropathies

Immune peripheral neuropathies can be subdivided into (1) acute or subacute nodo-paranodopathies due to IgG antiganglioside antibodies and producing variants of Guillain Barré syndrome (GBS); (2) nodo-paranodopathies due to IgG4 autoantibodies targeting adhesion or adaptor molecules and producing a chronic inflammatory demyelinating (CIDP) phenotype; and (3) autoimmune neuropathies due to IgM antibodies producing specific syndromes (Table 10.4).[35–37] There are several forms of acute/subacute nodo-paranodopathies due to IgG1 and IgG3 antibodies targeting gangliosides and fixing complement. For example, GM1 antibodies produce acute motor axonal neuropathy (AMAN) in general in the context of *Campylobacter jejuni* infection; GDa1 antibodies produce AMAN with cranial nerve involvement; GQ1b antibodies are typically associated with Miller-Fischer syndrome, Bickerstaff's brainstem encephalitis acute bulbar palsy and extraocular motor weakness; GT1a antibodies with pharyngeal-cervical-brachial variant of GBS; and GD1b antibodies with sensory GBS with bulbar weakness. Of note, COVID-19 may present with a cranial neuropathy manifested with oculomotor paralysis and associated with GD1b antibodies in the setting of acute SARS-CoV2 infection.[38]

Nodo-paranodopathies associated with IgG4 antibodies targeting adhesion and adaptor molecules produce severe CIDP-like syndromes that do not respond to IVIG and require use with rituximab. Neurofascin-155 antibodies produce a CIDP syndrome with severe proprioceptive symptoms, distal weakness, cerebellar ataxia, cranial nerve involvement, and low-frequency tremor. Contactin-1 IgG4 produces CIDP with old age of onset and severe motor involvement and denervation; these autoantibodies may also produce an acute GBS-like disorder. Other CIDP-like nodo-paranodopathies are produced by autoantibodies targeting CASPSR1 (CIDP or GBS-like picture) and NF 168 (CIDP with glomerulosclerosis). Multifocal motor neuropathy (MMN) is a demyelinating neuropathy due to IgM antibodies against

TABLE 10.4 *Autoimmune Neuropathies*

Acute or subacute nodo-paranodopathies due to IgG or IgM antiganglioside antibodies	
GM1 (IgG)	Acute motor axonal neuropathy (AMAN)
GD1a (IgG)	AMAN. Guillain Barré syndrome (GBS) with cranial nerve involvement
GQ1b (IgG)	Miller-Fischer syndrome Bickerstaff's brainstem encephalitis; acute bulbar palsy; extraocular motor (EOM) weakness
GT1a (IgG)	Pharyngeal-cervical-brachial variant of GBS
GM2 (IgG or IgM)	GBS, may have limited cranial nerve palsies
GD1b	Sensory GBS with bulbar weakness COVID-19 associated cranial motor neuropathy
GalNAc—GD1A	Pure motor GBS
Nodo-paranodopathies) producing a CIDP-like picture due to IgG	
Neurofascin-155 (IgG4)*	CIDP with severe proprioceptive symptoms, distal weakness, cerebellar ataxia, cranial nerve involvement, and tremor.
Contactin-1 (IgG4)*	CIDP with old age of onset and severe motor involvement and denervation. May present as an acute GBS-like disorder
CASPR1 1 (IgG3, IgG4)	CIDP or GBS-like picture. Neuropathic pain
Neurofascin 168	CIDP with glomerulosclerosis
Sialogalactosyl ceramide (IgG)	CIDP with sensory ataxia
Other chronic neuropathies with typical manifestations	
Myelin-associated glycoprotein (MAG) (IgM)	Slowly progressive, predominantly sensory-ataxic, distal with demyelinating features on EMG Associated with MGUS
GM1 ganglioside (IgM)	Multifocal motor neuropathy(nodopathy)
Disialosyl gangliosides (GD1a, GD3, GQ1b)	Chronic ataxia neuropathy with opthalmoplegia, bulbar involvement, cold agglutinins, and disialosyl antibodies (CANOMAD) Associated with MGUS

CASPR1, contactin-associated protein 1; CIDP, chronic inflammatory demyelinating polyradiculoneuropathy; MGUS, monoclonal gammopathy of undetermined significance

the GM1 ganglioside producing motor conduction block at the node of Ranvier and thus should be considered a nodopathy rather than a CIDP variant. It manifests with asymmetric distal upper extremity weakness, cramps and fasciculations resembling motor neuron disease; increased weakness with cold (cold paresis); and partial motor conduction block at noncompressible sites.

Monoclonal gammopathies are an important cause of peripheral neuropathy and include IgM-associated disorders, non-IgM associated disorders, and light chain associated disorders. These disorders may manifest as a monoclonal gammopathy of undetermined significance (MGUS) or be the first manifestation of a hematological malignancy such as Waldentröm macroglobulinemia or multiple myeloma. IgM-associated peripheral neuropathy most commonly manifests with marked gait ataxia due to proprioceptive sensory loss in the feet and occasionally associated with tremor; this is known as distal acquired demyelinating symmetric (DADS) neuropathy. It is characterized by prolonged distal latencies on nerve conduction studies and by the presence of anti-MAG antibodies in 50% of cases. Other IgM-associated disorder is chronic ataxic neuropathy, ophthalmoplegia, IgM protein, cold agglutinins, and disialosyl antibodies (CANOMAD), which resembles Miller Fischer syndrome but is chronic rather than acute. There are two important examples of non-IgM associated neuropathies that may be occasionally mistaken for CIDP but have very different diagnostic and therapeutic implications. POEMS (polyneuropathy, organomegaly, endocrinopathy, plasma cell disorder and skin changes) syndrome is a length-dependent severe demyelinating polyneuropathy or polyradiculopathy associated with lambda light-chain restricted IgG or IgA and is characterized by high plasma vascular endothelial growth factor (VEGF) levels. POEMS is associated with osteosclerotic myeloma in 95% of cases. Immunoglobulin light chain (AL) amyloidosis is a systemic disorder that in about two-thirds of cases manifests with generalized autonomic failure and painful length-dependent sensory and motor axonal neuropathy that also affects small fibers.

Hereditary Peripheral Neuropathies

Hereditary neuropathies are a group of genetically heterogeneous disorders with a phenotype spectrum spanning from mildly symptomatic to severe disability. They account for as many as 50% of neuropathies, and many have been characterized by their genetic and molecular bases.[39,46] Next-generation sequencing (NGS) has greatly improved genetic diagnosis of hereditary neuropathies.[42,43] However standard NGS testing cannot identify nucleotide repeat expansion mutations. Because of overlapping phenotypes and inheritance patterns, gene names are being included in the nomenclature of inherited disorders including inherited neuropathies. A specific genetic diagnosis is important given the advancements in gene-specific therapy including small molecule chaperones, antisense oligonucleotides, RNA-interference, and viral gene delivery therapies. The most common form of Mendelian inherited neuropathy is Charcot-Marie-Tooth disease (CMT), also called hereditary motor and sensory neuropathy (HMSN). However CMT accounts for only a minority of the gene abnormalities among inherited neuropathies. Non-CMT hereditary neuropathies include motor only forms (hereditary motor neuropathy, HMN); sensory predominant forms (hereditary sensory and autonomic neuropathy, HSAN); episodic attack forms (hereditary neuropathy with pressure palsies, HNPP; hereditary brachial plexus neuropathy, HBPN); spastic forms (hereditary spastic paraplegia with neuropathy, complicated-HSP); spinocerebellar forms with neuropathy (spinocerebellar ataxias, SCAs); 5) inherited metabolic neuropathies; and mitochondrial neuropathy. There is a considerable phenotypic and genetic overlap among these categories.[43] Some inherited myopathies such as myofibrillary myopathy) and certain motor neuron disorders such as progressive muscular atrophy (SMA)[44] can present with symmetric lower motor neuron distal weaknesses, mimicking neuropathy. The preservation of ankle reflexes and absence of sensory loss suggest disorders other than hereditary neuropathies. Based on electrophysiological features (particularly motor nerve conduction velocities-NCV in the ulnar nerve) and pattern of inheritance, CMT (HSMN) disease has been classified into several subgroups: (1) CMT1 (HSMN1), an autosomal dominant demyelinating form with uniformly slowed motor NCV (< 38 m/s) and nerve hypertrophy from diffuse myelin and fibroblast lamellae (onion bulbs) on nerve biopsy; (2) CMT2 (HMSN2), an autosomal dominant axonal predominant neuropathy showing normal to borderline slow motor NCV (> 48 m/sec) with axonal atrophy; (3) CMT intermediate forms (motor NCV (35–45 m/s) with both axonal and demyelinating features and variable inheritance; (4) CMT4, an autosomal recessive, demyelinating form of CMT (AR-CMT1); and (5) X-linked CMT disease (CMTX). CMT3, or Déjérine-Sottas neuropathy with markedly reduction in motor NCV (<15 m/s) is not a separate category but a severe, infantile form of dominant or recessive mutations of some genes associated with demyelinating neuropathy. However, this classification is an oversimplification.[45] This has led to a new method of classification that uses three modules for each disease category[46]: a generic term (e.g., CMT, HSAN, etc.); phenotype (axonal, demyelination, or intermediate); inheritance (autosomal dominant, autosomal recessive, X-linked), and lastly, the causal gene name.[46]

Autosomal dominant demyelinating neuropathy (commonly referred as CMT1) causes distal weakness and atrophy, reduced distal sensation, decreased deep tendon reflexes, and variable foot and hand deformity. There are so far seven CMT1 subtypes and five causal genes identified. These genes encode proteins critical for myelin organization and maintenance. CMT1A is the most common form (more than 50% of all CMT and approximately 70% of CMT1 cases). It is caused by mutations (most often duplication) in the PMP22 (*PMP22)* gene. As discussed earlier in this chapter, PMP22 is a membrane glycoprotein of the compact myelin sheet; the amount of PMP22 is critical in formation and maintenance of compact myelin, but the exact molecular disease pathway of PMP22 overexpression remains unclear. CMT1B is caused by mutations of the MPZ/P0 (*MPZ)* gene; this protein is critical for stabilization of compact myelin. Rarely, *MPZ* mutations also cause late-onset axonal neuropathy (CMT2J) associated with pupillary defects (Adie's pupil).

Autosomal dominant axonal neuropathy (CMT2) accounts for ~30% of all genetically confirmed CMT cases. Over 30 subtypes and 33 causal genes have been identified in CMT2, and 10 genes are linked to intermediate types (motor NCV in an intermediate range). CMT2A is the most common form (accounting for approximately 15%–20% CMT) and is caused by mutations in mitochondrial fusion protein mitofusin 2 (*MFN2*), resulting in reduced mitochondrial mobility and leads to insufficient axonal transport of mitochondria.[47] Additional clinical features in CMT2A may include optic atrophy, hearing loss, vocal cord paralysis, and diaphragmatic weakness. It is extremely challenging to determine the subtype of CMT2 based on clinical presentations alone, as the disease mechanisms are diverse and in many cases incompletely defined. Some specific manifestations are associated with specific genes. For example CMT2B due to Rab7 (*RAB7*) mutations affecting axonal transport of late endosomes and lysosomes in sensory axons is characterized by severe sensory loss with foot ulceration and mutilation; CMT2C associated *TRPV4* (transient receptor potential vanilloid type 4) mutations is associated with vocal cord paralysis; and CMT2D associated with *GARS* (glycyl-transfer RNA-tRNA, synthetase) causes prominent distal upper-extremity weakness.

Several forms of CMT have been linked to mutations affecting cytoskeletal or axon transport proteins. These mutations can produce a variable phenotype. For example, dominant mutations of *NEFL* (neurofilament light chain) produce axonal (CMT2) neuropathy, whereas recessive *NEFL* mutations produce demyelinating (CMT1) neuropathy. NEFL-related disorders are frequently of early onset and may be associated with postural tremor and sensory or cerebellar ataxia. *DYNC1H1* mutations affecting cytoplasmic dynein heavy-chain dynactin cause a form of CMT2 characterized by congenital or early onset, of variable severity. These mutations have also been linked to dHMN and SMA, sometimes with associated pyramidal signs.

Autosomal recessive CMT is rare (less than 10% of cases) and can be demyelinating, axonal, or intermediate. CMT4 is a rare autosomal recessive demyelinating neuropathy that usually shows an early onset and severe, progressive course leading to loss of ambulation. These neuropathies also tend to be phenotypically complex with more bulbar weakness and respiratory involvement. Demyelinating CMT4 often presents with severe secondary axonal loss. So far, 12 causal genes have been identified linked to the CMT4 phenotype. These genes encode many kinds of proteins, including mitochondrial proteins, phosphatases in the endosomal pathway, endocytic recycling proteins, and trafficking proteins. They are expressed in Schwann cells and are necessary for the development and maintenance of peripheral axons. Molecular diagnosis in these disorders is challenging due to the low mutation frequency and high genetic heterogeneity. One of the most common forms is CMT4A due to mutations of the *GDAP1* (ganglioside-induced differentiation-associated protein) gene encoding a mitochondrial membrane protein that regulates mitochondrial fission and fusion. Patients with recessive *GDAP1* mutations have reduced mitochondrial fission, whereas patients with dominant *GDAP1* mutations have impaired mitochondrial fusion. The most severe CMT4 phenotypes (CMT4B1, CNT4B2) are related to mutations affecting myotubularin (*MTMR1* and *SBF2*), a lipid phosphatase that dephosphorylates 3-phosphoinositides that are critical for membrane dynamics; these neuropathies are characterized by folded myelin sheaths.

X-linked CMT due to mutations of *GJB1* gene encoding the gap junction protein connexin32 (CMTX1) is the second most common form of hereditary motor and sensory neuropathy, accounting for ~10%–15% all CMT cases. CMTX1 is X-linked dominant, and thus may also affect females although males are much more severely affected. As mentioned earlier in this chapter, connexin forms gap junctions in noncompact myelin at the paranodal region in Schwann cells and oligodendrocytes, having an important role in the homeostasis of both peripheral and central myelinated axons. This explains the development of white matter abnormalities associated with GJB1 mutations.

Hereditary sensory and autonomic neuropathy (HSAN) predominantly affects the sensory and autonomic nervous systems. Autosomal dominant HSAN1, the most common form, is linked to mutations of the *SPTLC* (serine palmitoyl transferase long chain base subunit 1) gene encoding the initial enzyme in sphingolipid biosynthesis and produces severe loss a Aα, Aδ, and C fibers. Patients with HSAN1 typically have lancinating leg pains and early-onset insensate foot ulcers leading to amputation. Mutations of the ATL1 gene, encoding atlastatin, which is linked to hereditary spastic paraplegia, also produce HSAN1D. Mutations of *DNMT1* encoding DNA methyltransferase, which is critical for epigenetic silencing of DNA transcription, cause HSAN1E; other phenotypes include cerebellar ataxia, deafness, and narcolepsy. HSAN 2–6 and 8 are autosomal recessive and manifest in infancy. HSAN2 is associated with distal sensory loss and arreflexia but no prominent autonomic manifestations; some forms are due to loss-of-function mutations of the *SCNA9* gene encoding the $Na_v1.7$ channel causing congenital insensitivity (HSAN2D); in contrast, *SCN9A* gain-of-function mutations cause paroxysmal pain syndromes. HSAN3 (familial dysautonomia, Riley-Day syndrome) are due to mutations of the *ELP1* (*IKBKAP*) gene encoding a component of the elongator complex for RNA polymerase II; it is characterized by insensitivity to pain, autonomic lability, loss of tears and lacrimation, and other features. HSAN4 and HSAN5 produces congenital insensitivity to pain and anhidrosis due to impaired nerve growth factor (NGF)-tyrosine kinase A (NTR1) signaling that is critical for development of nociceptive dorsal root ganglia and sympathetic neurons.

Distal hereditary motor neuropathy (dHMN) is characterized by slowly progressive, symmetrical, distal lower-motor-neuron weakness with reduced or absent reflexes. Many forms of dHMN also present with upper-motor-neuron features. A total of 19 causative genes have been described in dHMN or distal SMA, which have very similar phenotypes; there is also phenotypic overlap between dHMN and CMT2. An important cause is mutation of genes encoding small heat shock proteins (Hsps), *HSPB1* encoding Hsp27 (dHMN2A) and *HSPB8* encoding Hsp22 (dHMN2B); if sensory involvement is present, the disorders are classified as CMT2 subtypes. Similarly, dHMN5 linked to *GARS* mutations is characterized by upper-limb onset, if there is sensory involvement it is termed CMT2D.

Familial amyloid polyneuropathies (FAPs) are a group of autosomal dominant, multisystem disorders causing tissue accumulation of fibril aggregates of mutated precursor proteins of amyloid, most commonly transthyretin (TTR), but occasionally apolipoprotein A-1 (APOA1), and gelsolin. Patients with hereditary amyloid neuropathy from TTR mutations typically have a length-dependent small-fiber sensorimotor polyneuropathy with loss of temperature and pain sensations, autonomic dysfunction, cardiomyopathy, and sometimes nephrotic syndrome. The clinical course, penetrance, and age at onset vary significantly, even among persons with the same mutation. The first identified TTR mutation (Val30Met) is still the most common, but there are more than 100 amyloidogenic point mutations. Oral administration of tafamidis-meglumine prevents misfolding and deposition of mutated TTR. Two small oligonucleotide-based gene therapies, one using a small interfering RNA (patisiran) and one using antisense (inotersen) are FDA approved for treatment.

Axonal sensory neuropathy can be a prominent presenting feature in common varieties of SCA. Large-fiber sensory ataxia is typical of Friedreich ataxia and late-onset cerebellar ataxia, neuropathy, vestibular areflexia syndrome (CANVAS). These two disorders and many other hereditary ataxias with neuropathy are caused by repeat nucleotide expansions that generally cannot be identified by standard NGS platforms. Sensorimotor axonal peripheral neuropathy is an important feature of several forms of apraxia with oculomotor apraxia.

LEUKODYSTROPHIES

Leukodystrophies are genetic disorders that primarily affect the white matter in the CNS. Onset may be at any age; many are neurodegenerative, but others only affect white matter function. Based on the primary component of the white matter affected, leukodystrophies have been classified into: (1) primary disorders of myelin or oligodendrocytes, including disorders associated with hypomyelination, demyelination, or myelin vacuolation; (2) astrocytopathies; (3) leuko-axonopathies: (4) microgliopathies; (5) leukovasculopathies; and (6) other disorders[48–50] (Box 10.1). Leukodystrophies may reflect different underlying pathogenic mechanisms, including impaired lysosomal or peroxisomal enzyme-dependent degradation; mitochondrial respiratory chain dysfunction; altered amino acid and organic acid metabolism or messenger RNA translation; disturbed ion and water homeostasis; primary disorders of myelin proteins; altered microcirculation; impaired DNA repair; and many others.[48–50] A comprehensive discussion of this large topic is beyond the scope of this chapter. Some examples are also mentioned in another chapters of this book.

Primary Disorders of Oligodendrocytes and Myelin

Hypomyelinating disorders include Pelizaeus-Merzbacher disease associated with mutations of the *PLP1* gene on the X chromosome encoding proteolipid protein. This disorder is characterized by nystagmus within the first six months of life, hypotonia, feeding difficulties, cerebellar ataxia, and spasticity by six years of age. Deletions cause X-linked hereditary spastic paraplegia. MRI shows diffuse hypomyelination. Lack of myelin is thought to reflect oligodendrocyte death due to toxic gain-of-function of PLP1 causing ER stress and impaired PLP1 trafficking to myelin via vesicular transport. Autosomal recessive mutations of the *GJC2* gene encoding connexin 47 produce Pelizaeus Merzbacher-like syndrome.[49] Myelin disorders with demyelination are characterized by T1 hypointensity and confluent T2 hyperintensity on MRI. Demyelinating leukodystrophies include autosomal recessive metachromatic leukodystrophy (MLD), Krabbe disease, and X-linked adrenoleukodystrophy (X-ALD). Early recognition of these disorders is important as hematopoietic stem cell transplantation may alter disease progression in asymptomatic early-onset forms. Metachromatic leukodystrophy is due to mutations of the *ARSA* gene encoding lysosomal arylsulfatase A, leading to accumulation of sulfatides in the CNS, PNS, and non-neural tissues such as the gallbladder. Krabbe disease is due to mutations of the *GALC* gene encoding lysosomal alpha galactosidase, which is essential for degradation of lipids during myelin turnover. X-linked adrenoleukodystrophy is caused by mutations in the *ABCD1* gene encoding peroxisomal ATP-binding membrane protein, which is necessary for β-oxidation of saturated unbranched fatty acids, leading to accumulation of very long-chain fatty acids (VLCFAs).

Myelin disorders associated with myelin vacuolation include Canavan disease, due to mutation of the *ASPA* gene encoding aspartyl acylase. Infants with Canavan disease appear normal at birth but then show signs of slow development and hypotonia followed by macrocephaly, optic atrophy, spasticity, and seizures. High NAA levels may be neurotoxic and predispose to seizures or induce osmotic dysregulation resulting in demyelination and subcortical vacuolation. Other disorders associated with myelin vacuolation include X-linked CMT (CMTX) due to mutations of the *GJB1* encoding connexin-32; amino acid disorders such as homocysteine methylation defects; mitochondrial disorders; and mutations of the *CIC2* gene encoding a chloride channel.

Astrocytopathies

The prototype astrocytopathy associated with leukoencephalopathy is Alexander disease, an autosomal dominant disorder associated with mutations of the *GFAP* gene encoding glial fibrillary acid protein. Vanishing white matter disease is an autosomal recessive disorder due to mutations of the *EIF2B1* gene encoding eukaryote initiation factor 2B. This disorder may present at any age, mostly between 2 and 6 years, and is always fatal. The disorder is also known as childhood ataxia with central nervous system hypomyelination. The disease progresses slowly with superimposed episodes of deterioration following stress, infection, or minor head trauma. MRI is characterized by progressive rarefaction with cystic degeneration of the white matter and radial stripes extending between the ventricular wall to the subcortical regions. Megalencephalic leukoencephalopathy with subcortical cysts (MLC) is due to mutations of the *MLC1* or *MLC2* genes encoding an astroglial cell adhesion molecule.

Leuko-Axonopathies

Leuko-axonopathies affect both the white and the gray matter. They include GM1 gangliosidosis, associated with mutations of the *GLB1* gene encoding beta galactosidase,

BOX 10.1 CLASSIFICATION AND EXAMPLES OF LEUKODYSTROPHIES

Primary disorders of oligodendrocyte and myelin

Hypomyelinating disorders (gene and protein product)

- Pelizaeus-Merzbacher (*PLP1*, proteolipid protein1)
- Pelizaeus-Merzbacher-like (*GBJ2*, connexin-47)

Demyelinating disorders

- Metachromatic leukodystrophy (*ARSA*, aryl sulfatase A)
- Krabbe disease (*GALC*, galactocerebrosidase)
- X-linked adrenoleukodystropy (*ABCD1*, peroxisomal ATP-binding membrane protein)
- Multiple sulfatase deficiency (*SUMF1*, sulfatase modifying factor 1

Vacuolar disorders

- Canavan disease (*ASPA*, N-acetyl aspartate acylase)
- X-linked Charcot-Marie-Tooth-1 (*GBJ1*, connexin-32)
- Amino acid metabolism disorders
- Mitochondrial disorders

Astrocytopathies

- Alexander disease (*GFAP*, glial fibrillary acid protein)
- Vanishing white matter disease (*EIF2B*, eukaryote initiator factor for mRNA translation)
- CIC2 related disease (*CIC2*, chloride transporter)
- Giant axonal neuropathy (*GXN*, gigaxonin, and ubiquitin E3 ligase for intermediate figments)
- Aicardi-Goutières syndrome

Leuko-axonopathies

- GM1 gangliosidosis (*GALB*, beta-galactosidase)
- GM2 gangliosidosis (*HEXA*, hexosaminidase A)
- Infantile neuronal ceroid lipofuscinosis (CLN1) (*PPT*, palmitotyl protein thioesterase-1)
- Leukoencephalopathy with brainstem and spinal atrophy and high lactate (*ARS*, aspartate tRNA aminoacyl transferase).
- Leukoencephalopathy with basal ganglia and cerebellar involvement (*TUB4A*, tubulin beta 4A).
- AGC1-related disease

Microgliopathies

- Hereditary diffuse leukoencephalopathy with pigmented glia and neuroaxonal spheroids (*CSF-1*, colony stimulating factor 1)
- Nasu-Ahoka disease (*TREM2*, *TYRPBP*, signal transduction for microglia)

Leuko-vasculopathies

- Familial cerebral amyloid angiopathy (*APP*, amyloid precursor protein)
- Cerebral autosomal dominant arteriopathy with subcortical infarcts and leukoencephalopathy (CADASIL) (*NOTCH3*, Notch 3)
- Cerebral autosomal recessive arteriopathy with subcortical infarcts and leukoencephalopathy (CARASIL) (*HTRAS*, serine protease 1)
- Leukoencephalopathy with calcifications and cysts (*SNORD118*, ribosomal biogenesis)
- Cathepsin A-related arteriopathy with strokes and leukoencephalopathy (*CTAS*, cathepsin A)
- Cerebroretinal vasculopathies (*TREX1*, 3,5' hexonuclease)

Other disorders

- Cerebrotendinous xanthomatosis (*CYP27A*, cytochrome P45 27A)
- Adult polyglucosan storage disease (*GBE*, glycogen branching enzyme)
- Autosomal demining leukodystrophy with Lamin B mutations (*LMNB*, nuclear membrane protein)

and GM2 gangliosidosis due to mutations of the *HEXA* gene encoding hexosaminidase A. Other example is infantile neuronal lipofucsinosis (CLN)1 due to mutations of the *PPT* gene encoding lysosomal palmitotyl 1 protein thioesterase-1. Leukoencephalopathy with brainstem and spinal cord involvement and high lactate is due to mutations of the *DARS* gene encoding aspartate tRNA aminoacyl transferase. Hypomyelination with atrophy of the basal ganglia and cerebellum (HABC) is due to mutations of the *TUB4A* encoding tubulin beta 4A.

Microgliopathies

Primary microglial disorders result from loss-of-function mutations affecting the TREM2 (triggering receptor expressed in myeloid cells 2)/DAP12 (DNAX activating protein of 12 kD) or the colony stimulating factor 1 (CSF1)/CSF1 receptor (CSF1R) signaling pathways involved in microglial development. Mutations of the *TREM2* or *DAP2* genes produce polycystic lipomembranous dysplasia with sclerosing leukoencephalopathy (Nasu-Hakola disease). This is an autosomal recessive disorder that manifests with multiple bone cysts (due to impairment of osteoclasts) and early-onset progressive dementia associated with white matter lesions presumably related to abnormal microglial activation. Mutations of the *CSF1R* gene cause hereditary diffuse leukoencephalopathy with neuroaxonal spheroids and pigmented glia (ALSP).[51] This autosomal dominant disorder manifests primarily with relatively rapidly progressive frontal lobe dementia with prominent psychiatric symptoms, spasticity, parkinsonism associated with T2 hyperintensities in the anterior white matter, small cysts, thinning of the corpus callosum and small symmetric calcifications. Similar findings have been described in leukoencephalopathy associated with mutations of the *AARS2* gene encoding alanyl-transfer RNA synthetase 2.

Leuko-Vasculopathies

Small vessel disease in the CNS manifests with prominent involvement of the white matter.[52,53] Few cases are due to hereditary small vessel disease.[54] These disorders are discussed in chapter 23. The prototypical example of genetic leuko-vasculopathy is cerebral autosomal dominant arteriopathy with subcortical infarcts and leukoencephalopathy (CADASIL) associated with *NOTCH3* mutations.[55,56] CARASIL (cerebral autosomal recessive arteriopathy with subcortical infarcts and leukoencephalopathy) is associated with mutations of the *HTRAS* gene encoding a serine protease that regulates transforming growth factor- α signaling. Cathepsin A -related arteriopathy with strokes and leukoencephalopathy (CARASAL) is due to mutations of the *CTSAS* gene encoding cathepsin A. Cathepsin-A degrades endotheliun-1, a potent vasoconstrictor; there is increased endothelin-1 immunoreactivity in astrocytes, similar to other leuko-vasculopathies, which may contribute to long-standing vasoconstriction and hypoxia and inhibition of OPC maturation.[57] Other examples of leuko-vasculopathies are cerebral amyloid angiopathy and leukoencephalopathy with calcifications and cysts associated with mutations in in the *SNORD118* (snoRNA U8) involved in ribosomal biogenesis and function.

Other Disorders

Other hereditary disorders may primarily affect the white matter. They include cerebrotendinous xanthomatosis (CTX) due to mutation of the *CYP27A* gene encoding cytochrome P45 27A involved in bile acid metabolism; this disorder is associated with elevation of plasma cholestenol.[58] Polyglucosan body disease is due to mutations of the *GBE* gene encoding glycogen branching enzyme.[59] It manifests as a leukoencephalopathy with upper- and lower-motor-neuron dysfunction, neurogenic bladder, spastic gait, peripheral neuropathy, sensory loss, and dementia, with onset at 40–60 years or later. Some patients presented an asymmetric motor syndrome mimicking ALS. Polyglucosan bodies can be observed both in central axons in gray and white matter, peripheral nerves, skeletal muscle, and occasionally in myoepithelial cells of the axillary apocrine sweat glands. Autosomal dominant leukoencephalopathy is due to mutations of the *LMNB1* gene encoding nuclear lamin B and may associated with sympathetic failure.

The white matter in the central nervous system is a major target of immune attack in disorders such as multiple sclerosis, aquaporin 4 (AQP4) associated neuromyelitis optica spectrum disorder (NMOSD) and myelin oligodendrocyte glycoprotein (MOG) autoimmune encephalitis. These disorders may manifest with transverse myelitis, optic neuritis and signs and symptoms that allow there distinction on the basis of clinical and MRI findings. A discussion of these disorders is beyond the scope of this chapter.

KEY POINTS

- There are several fundamental differences between peripheral and central axons.
- Schwann cells provide myelin to peripheral axons, are associated with a basal lamina, and promote axonal regeneration after injury.
- Oligodendrocytes myelinate central nervous system axons, and their myelin products inhibit axonal regeneration.
- The AIS has a high density of clustered voltage-gated sodium channels responsible for the initiation of action potential in mature axons.
- The clustering of ion channels at the AIS depends on their interaction with ankyrin G.
- The AIS cytoskeleton provides a molecular barrier preventing the passage of both dendritic and somatic proteins into the axon.
- The AIS is a plastic structure and its location may shift in an activity-dependent manner.
- The node of Ranvier enables saltatory conduction of the action potential.
- The paranodal loops form axon–glia septate junctions consisting of proteins that are targets for autoimmune neuropathy.
- The paranode is a particularly vulnerable region of the myelinated axon.
- The juxtaparanodes contain $K_v1.1$ and $K_v1.2$ clustered by interaction with CASPR2, which is a target of autoimmune disease.

- Gangliosides influence plasma membrane fluidity, function of ion channels and receptors, paranodal stability and synaptic transmission.
- Myelin is enriched with cholesterol, phosphatidylethanolamine, galactosylceramide, and galactosylceramide sulfate (sulfatide).
- The main myelin proteins are proteolipid protein (PLP), myelin basic protein (MBP), myelin oligodendrocyte glycoprotein (MOG), myelin protein zero (MPZ), myelin-associated glycoprotein (MAG), peripheral myelin protein22 (PMP22), and connexin.
- Schwann cell precursors originate from the neural crest and eventually become mature myelinating or nonmyelinating Schwann cells.
- Immature Schwann cells deposit extracellular matrix that promotes a radial sorting of axons.
- Oligodendrocyte development involves three stages: oligodendrocyte precursor cells (OPCs), premyelinating oligodendrocytes, and mature oligodendrocytes.
- Relief from inhibitory neuronal signals is a major mechanism that modulates oligodendrocyte biogenesis.
- Neuronal activity is a major factor regulating myelination.
- There are reciprocal trophic interactions between axons and oligodendrocytes; axons provide N-acetyl aspartate to oligodendrocyte as a substrate for lipid synthesis; oligodendrocytes provide lactate from the astrocyte to the axons for metabolic support.
- Astrocytes have a major role in oligodendrocytes and myelin support via supply of lactate, glutamate uptake, production of glutathione, and regulation of ion and water homeostasis.
- Acute or subacute nodo-paranodopathies due to IgG targeting different gangliosides antibodies produce several variants of Guillain Barré syndrome
- Nodo-paranodopathies due to IgG4 autoantibodies produce severe forms of chronic inflammatory demyelinating neuropathy.
- IgM antibodies against myelin-associated glycoprotein (MAG) produce distal ataxic neuropathy; GM1 IgM antibodies produce multifocal motor neuropathy.
- Hereditary neuropathies account for as many as 50% of neuropathies, and many have been characterized using next-generation sequencing (NGS).
- The molecular pathways underlying inherited neuropathy are extremely diverse.
- *PMP22*duplications account for approximately 70% of demyelinating Charcot-Marie-Tooth (CMT) neuropathy.
- Mutations of *MFN2* encoding mitofusin-2 are the most common cause for axonal CMT.
- CMTX1-*GJB1* mutations affecting connexin-32 produce the second most common form of CMT neuropathy.
- Leukodystrophies have been classified into primary disorders of myelin or oligodendrocytes, astrocytopathies, leuko-axonopathies, microgliopathies, and leuko-vasculopathies.
- Pathogenic mechanisms in leukodystrophies include impaired lysosomal or peroxisomal degradation; mitochondrial respiratory chain dysfunction; altered amino acid and organic acid metabolism or messenger RNA translation; disturbed ion and water homeostasis; altered microcirculation; and many others.

REFERENCES

1. Debanne D, Campanac E, Bialowas A, Carlier E, Alcaraz G. Axon physiology. Physiol Rev 2011;91:555–602.
2. Chang KJ, Rasband MN. Excitable domains of myelinated nerves: axon initial segments and nodes of Ranvier. Curr Top Membr 2013;72:159–192.
3. Yermakov LM, Hong LA, Drouet DE, Griggs RB, Susuki K. Functional domains in myelinated axons. Adv Exp Med Biol 2019;1190:65–83.
4. Bender KJ, Trussell LO. The physiology of the axon initial segment. Annu Rev Neurosci 2012;35:249–265.
5. Rasband MN, Peles E. The nodes of Ranvier: molecular assembly and maintenance. Cold Spring Harb Perspect Biol 2015;8:a020495.
6. Uncini A, Vallat JM. Autoimmune nodo-paranodopathies of peripheral nerve: the concept is gaining ground. J Neurol Neurosurg Psychiatry 2018;89:627–635.
7. Karakaya M, Wirth B. Hereditary nodo-paranodopathies: genomic variants, not just autoantibodies, hit the protein. Brain 2019;142:2895–2897.
8. Wang Y, Yin F. A review of X-linked Charcot-Marie-Tooth disease. J Child Neurol 2016;31:761–772.
9. Binks SNM, Klein CJ, Waters P, Pittock SJ, Irani SR. LGI1, CASPR2 and related antibodies: a molecular evolution of the phenotypes. J Neurol Neurosurg Psychiatry 2018;89:526–534.
10. Franssen H. Physiology of myelinated nerve conduction and pathophysiology of demyelination. Adv Exp Med Biol 2019;1190:85–106.
11. Lopez PHH, Baez BB. Gangliosides in axon stability and regeneration. Prog Mol Biol Transl Sci 2018;156:383–412.
12. Goodfellow JA, Willison HJ. Guillain-Barre syndrome: a century of progress. Nat Rev Neurol 2016;12:723–731.
13. Willison HJ. Anti-ganglioside antibodies in peripheral nerve pathology. Methods Mol Biol 2018;1804:173–188.
14. Schmitt S, Castelvetri LC, Simons M. Metabolism and functions of lipids in myelin. Biochim Biophys Acta 2015;1851:999–1005.
15. Li ZH, Lu FF, Shao Q, Zhu M, Cao L. [Progress in metabolism and function of myelin lipids]. Sheng Li Xue Bao 2017;69:817–829.
16. Raymond GV. Leukodystrophy: basic and clinical. Adv Neurobiol 2017;15:365–382.

17. Lynch DS, Wade C, Paiva ARB, et al. Practical approach to the diagnosis of adult-onset leukodystrophies: an updated guide in the genomic era. J Neurol Neurosurg Psychiatry 2019;90:543–554.
18. Rattay TW, Lindig T, Baets J, et al. FAHN/SPG35: a narrow phenotypic spectrum across disease classifications. Brain 2019;142:1561–1572.
19. Taveggia C. Schwann cells-axon interaction in myelination. Curr Opin Neurobiol 2016;39:24–29.
20. Monk KR, Feltri ML, Taveggia C. New insights on Schwann cell development. Glia 2015;63:1376–1393.
21. Salzer JL. Schwann cell myelination. Cold Spring Harb Perspect Biol 2015;7:a020529.
22. Feltri ML, Poitelon Y, Previtali SC. How Schwann cells sort axons: new concepts. Neuroscientist 2016;22:252–265.
23. Pereira JA, Lebrun-Julien F, Suter U. Molecular mechanisms regulating myelination in the peripheral nervous system. Trends Neurosci 2012;35:123–134.
24. Bercury KK, Macklin WB. Dynamics and mechanisms of CNS myelination. Dev Cell 2015;32:447–458.
25. Simons M, Nave KA. Oligodendrocytes: myelination and axonal support. Cold Spring Harb Perspect Biol 2015;8:a020479.
26. Mayoral SR, Chan JR. The environment rules: spatiotemporal regulation of oligodendrocyte differentiation. Curr Opin Neurobiol 2016;39:47–52.
27. Elbaz B, Popko B. Molecular control of oligodendrocyte development. Trends Neurosci 2019;42:263–277.
28. Moon SL, Parker R. EIF2B2 mutations in vanishing white matter disease hypersuppress translation and delay recovery during the integrated stress response. RNA 2018;24:841–852.
29. Mount CW, Monje M. Wrapped to adapt: experience-dependent myelination. Neuron 2017;95:743–756.
30. Micu I, Plemel JR, Caprariello AV, Nave KA, Stys PK. Axo-myelinic neurotransmission: a novel mode of cell signalling in the central nervous system. Nat Rev Neurosci 2018;19:49–58.
31. Morrison BM, Lee Y, Rothstein JD. Oligodendroglia: metabolic supporters of axons. Trends Cell Biol 2013;23:644–651.
32. Saab AS, Tzvetanova ID, Nave KA. The role of myelin and oligodendrocytes in axonal energy metabolism. Curr Opin Neurobiol 2013;23:1065–1072.
33. Domingues HS, Portugal CC, Socodato R, Relvas JB. Oligodendrocyte, astrocyte, and microglia crosstalk in myelin development, damage, and repair. Front Cell Dev Biol 2016;4:71.
34. Li J, Zhang L, Chu Y, et al. Astrocytes in oligodendrocyte lineage development and white matter pathology. Front Cell Neurosci 2016;10:119.
35. Stathopoulos P, Alexopoulos H, Dalakas MC. Autoimmune antigenic targets at the node of Ranvier in demyelinating disorders. Nat Rev Neurol 2015;11:143–156.
36. Uncini A, Kuwabara S. Nodopathies of the peripheral nerve: an emerging concept. J Neurol Neurosurg Psychiatry 2015;86:1186–1195.
37. Rajabally YA, Stettner M, Kieseier BC, Hartung HP, Malik RA. CIDP and other inflammatory neuropathies in diabetes—diagnosis and management. Nat Rev Neurol 2017;13:599–611.
38. Dinkin M, Gao V, Kahan J, et al. COVID-19 presenting with ophthalmoparesis from cranial nerve palsy. Neurology 2020;95:221–223.
39. Ramchandren S. Charcot-Marie-Tooth disease and other genetic polyneuropathies. Continuum (Minneap Minn) 2017;23:1360–1377.
40. Kamil K, Yazid MD, Idrus RBH, Das S, Kumar J. Peripheral demyelinating diseases: from biology to translational medicine. Front Neurol 2019;10:87.
41. Murakami T, Sunada Y. Schwann cell and the pathogenesis of Charcot-Marie-Tooth disease. Adv Exp Med Biol 2019;1190:301–321.
42. Klein CJ, Foroud TM. Neurology individualized medicine: when to use next-generation sequencing panels. Mayo Clin Proc 2017;92:292–305.
43. Klein CJ. Charcot-Marie-Tooth disease and other hereditary neuropathies. Continuum 2020;26:1224–1256.
44. Liewluck T, Saperstein DS. Progressive muscular atrophy. Neurol Clin 2015;33:761–773.
45. Mathis S, Goizet C, Tazir M, et al. Charcot-Marie-Tooth diseases: an update and some new proposals for the classification. J Med Genet 2015;52:681–690.
46. Magy L, Mathis S, Le Masson G, Goizet C, Tazir M, Vallat JM. Updating the classification of inherited neuropathies: results of an international survey. Neurology 2018;90:e870–e876.
47. Santel A, Fuller MT. Control of mitochondrial morphology by a human mitofusin. J Cell Sci 2001;114:867–874.
48. van der Knaap MS, Bugiani M. Leukodystrophies: a proposed classification system based on pathological changes and pathogenetic mechanisms. Acta Neuropathol 2017;134:351–382.
49. Abrams CK, Scherer SS. Gap junctions in inherited human disorders of the central nervous system. Biochim Biophys Acta 2012;1818:2030–2047.
50. Van der Knaap MS, Schiffmann R, Mochel F, Wolf NI. Diagnosis, prognosis, and treatment of leukodistrophies. Lancet Neurol 2019;18:962–972.
51. Konno T, Kasanuki K, Ikeuchi T, Dickson DW, Wszolek ZK. CSF1R-related leukoencephalopathy: a major player in primary microgliopathies. Neurology 2018;91:1092–1104.
52. Vinters HV, Zarow C, Borys E, et al. Review: Vascular dementia: clinicopathologic and genetic considerations. Neuropathol Appl Neurobiol 2018;44:247–266.
53. Cannistraro RJ, Badi M, Eidelman BH, Dickson DW, Middlebrooks EH, Meschia JF. CNS small vessel disease: a clinical review. Neurology 2019;92:1146–1156.
54. Mancuso M, Arnold M, Bersano A, et al. Monogenic cerebral small-vessel diseases: diagnosis and therapy: consensus recommendations of the European Academy of Neurology. Eur J Neurol 2020;27:909–927.
55. Wang MM. Cadasil. Handb Clin Neurol 2018;148:733–743.
56. Wardlaw JM, Benveniste H, Nedergaard M, et al. Perivascular spaces in the brain: anatomy, physiology and pathology. Nat Rev Neurol 2020;16:137–153.
57. Bugiani M, Kevelam SH, Bakels HS, et al. Cathepsin A-related arteriopathy with strokes and leukoencephalopathy (CARASAL). Neurology 2016;87:1777–1786.
58. Salen G, Steiner RD. Epidemiology, diagnosis, and treatment of cerebrotendinous xanthomatosis (CTX). J Inherit Metab Dis 2017;40:771–781.
59. Cenacchi G, Papa V, Costa R, et al. Update on polyglucosan storage diseases. Virchows Arch 2019;475:671–686.

11 Mitochondria and Energy Metabolism

OVERVIEW

The function and survival of neurons critically depends on adenosine triphosphate (ATP) generated by mitochondrial oxidative phosphorylation (OXPHOS), which accounts for 20% of the body's oxygen consumption. The OXPHOS system includes the respiratory complexes I, II, III, and IV and the F_1-F_0 ATP synthase (complex V). In neurons, ATP is primarily consumed in maintaining resting membrane potentials and supporting presynaptic and postsynaptic events. In addition to ATP production, mitochondria have a critical role in reactive oxygen species (ROS) production and signaling; redox homeostasis; synthesis of iron-sulfur (Fe-S) clusters; protein import and processing; maintenance of intracellular calcium (Ca^{2+}) homeostasis; and metabolism of lipids, amino acids, nucleotides, and heme (Figure 11.1). The size, activity, and longevity of neurons requires the appropriate coordination of mitochondrial location with energy demands. The maintenance of mitochondria quality and distribution, referred to as mitostasis, depends on the interplay among finely balanced and dynamically regulated processes. They include mitochondrial biogenesis, protein quality control, fusion and fission, motility and docking, and clearance by mitophagy. Mitochondria respond to cell stress and may also be released from damaged cells as a "help me" signal. Mitochondria are also central to various mechanisms of regulated cell death. Neurologic disorders due to mitochondrial dysfunction include classical mitochondrial disorders directly related to defects in bioenergetics and metabolic functions; disorders directly affecting mitostasis; and adult-onset neurodegenerative disorders that indirectly affect mitostasis through defects in axonal transport and autophagy. The aims of this chapter are to review (1) the main functions of mitochondria; (2) the mechanisms of mitostasis, and (3) representative examples of mitochondrial disorders.

BIOGENESIS OF MITOCHONDRIA

Mitochondria are organelles composed of an outer mitochondrial membrane and an inner mitochondrial membrane, which delineate two aqueous compartments; the intermembrane space between the outer and the inner membrane and the mitochondrial matrix surrounded by the inner membrane (Figure 11.1).[1] The outer mitochondrial membrane is highly permeable to ions and small uncharged metabolites due to the presence of large channels called porins. In contrast, the inner mitochondrial membrane forms a tight diffusion barrier to ions and metabolites, which require transport via mitochondrial carrier proteins. The inner mitochondrial membrane forms invaginations or cristae that harbor the proteins of the respiratory chain. Salient features of mitochondria are that they contain their own DNA (mitochondrial DNA, mtDNA) inherited from the mother, and their negative membrane potential that drives several processes including transport and ATP production. The half-life of mitochondria in the brain is about 30 days. Single cells may contain different types of mitochondria with different sizes and morphologies and different copy numbers of mtDNA. This is referred to as heteroplasmy and reflects the constant out-of-phase fusion and fission of mitochondria resulting in a heterogeneous population. Heteroplasmy and copy numbers of mtDNA contribute to the variability of symptoms in mitochondrial disorders, particularly in maternally inherited disorders resulting in mutation of mtDNA. Disease manifestations and severity depends on the ratio between healthy and affected or mutated mitochondria, which may vary between cells and tissues.

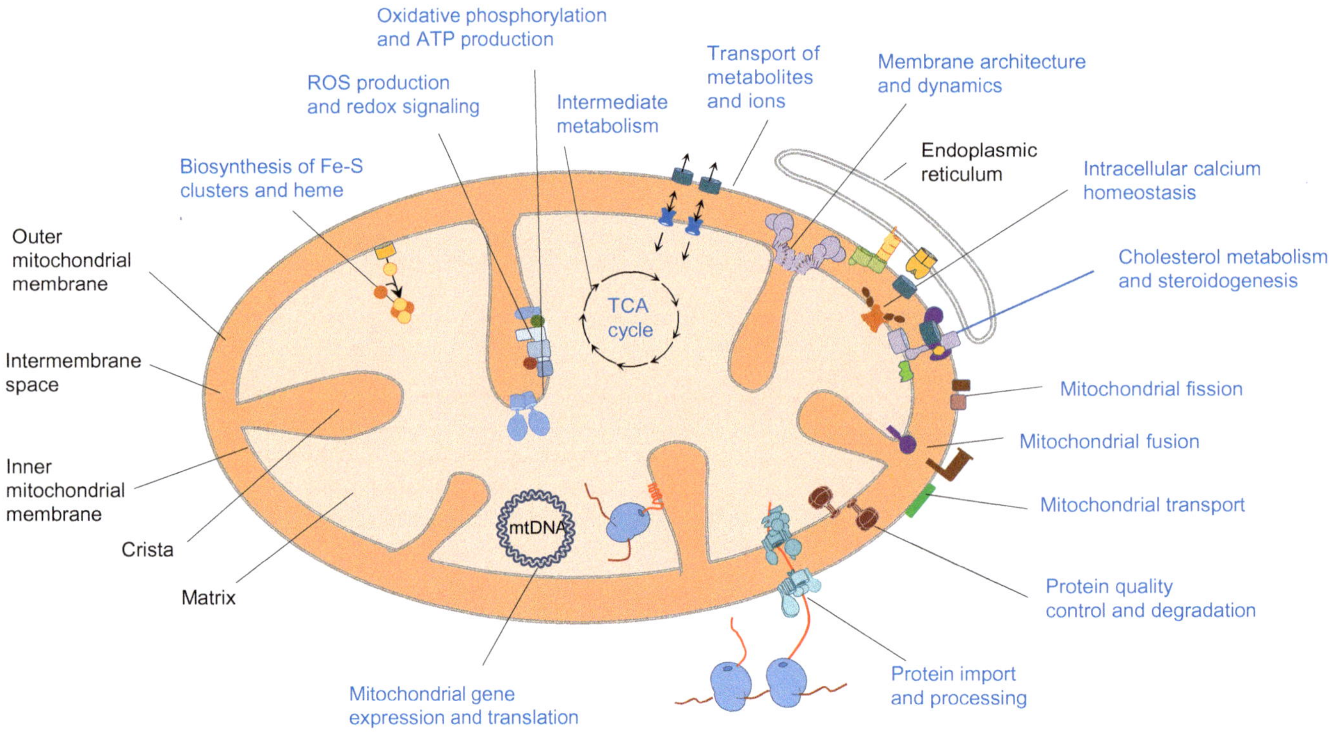

FIGURE 11.1 General structure and function of mitochondria.
Mitochondria are composed by an outer and an inner membrane, which delineate two aqueous compartments; the intermembrane and the mitochondrial matrix. The mitochondria are critical for intermediate metabolism via the tricarboxylic acid (TCA) cycle and ATP synthesis via oxidative phosphorylation (OXPHOS). They also have a critical role in reactive oxygen species (ROS) production and signaling; redox homeostasis; synthesis of iron-sulfur (Fe-S) clusters; protein import and processing; maintenance of intracellular calcium (Ca^{2+}) homeostasis; and metabolism of lipids, amino acids, nucleotides, and heme. The maintenance of mitochondria quality and distribution, referred to as mitostasis, depends on the interplay among finely balanced and dynamically regulated processes including fusion, fission, transport, quality control, and mitophagy.

Mitochondrial DNA

Mitochondria DNA is a small circular DNA that contains only 37 genes, has no introns, and encodes about 1% of all mitochondria proteins. They include 13 of the subunits of complexes I, III, IV, and V of the respiratory chain, 22 transfer RNAs and two ribosomal RNAs. Complex II components are encoded only by nuclear DNA. Most genes involved in maintenance of mitochondrial function are also located in nuclear DNA. The machinery required for maintenance of the mitochondrial genome is entirely encoded in the nucleus. It includes mtDNA polymerase γ (POLG), the helicase Twinkle (which allows mtDNA replication), and mitochondrial single-stranded DNA–binding protein (Figure 11.2). Other proteins that contribute to the organization of mtDNA include mitochondrial transcription factor A, which has a histone-like function and contributes to mtDNA organization, and mitochondrial DNA topoisomerase I. In addition, mtDNA replication requires a supply of nucleotides; the mitochondrial nucleotide pools are closely linked to cytosolic nucleotide metabolism. More than 1,300 genes encoded in nuclear DNA produce proteins that are targeted from the cytosol to the mitochondria. These include those involved the maintenance and expression of mitochondrial DNA and most components of the OXPHOS complex. Complex II and most subunits of complexes I, III, IV, and V are encoded by nuclear DNA.

Mitochondrial Biogenesis and Its Coupling to Energy Requirements

Mitochondrial biogenesis is the growth and division of preexisting mitochondria. In peripheral tissues, such as muscle, mitochondrial biogenesis is influenced by environmental stress such as exercise, caloric restriction, oxidative stress, and cell renewal and differentiation. The major regulator of mitochondrial biogenesis is peroxisome proliferator-activated receptor gamma coactivator 1-α (PGC-1α), which is a co-transcriptional regulation factor. PGC-1α activates several nuclear respiratory factors that drive transcription and replication of mtDNA and promote expression of several mitochondrial enzymes. A major regulator of mitochondrial biogenesis during acute energy crises is adenosine monophosphate-activated protein kinase (AMPK), which is activated in response to a reduction in ATP/AMP ratio and activates PGC-1α and nuclear respiratory factors.

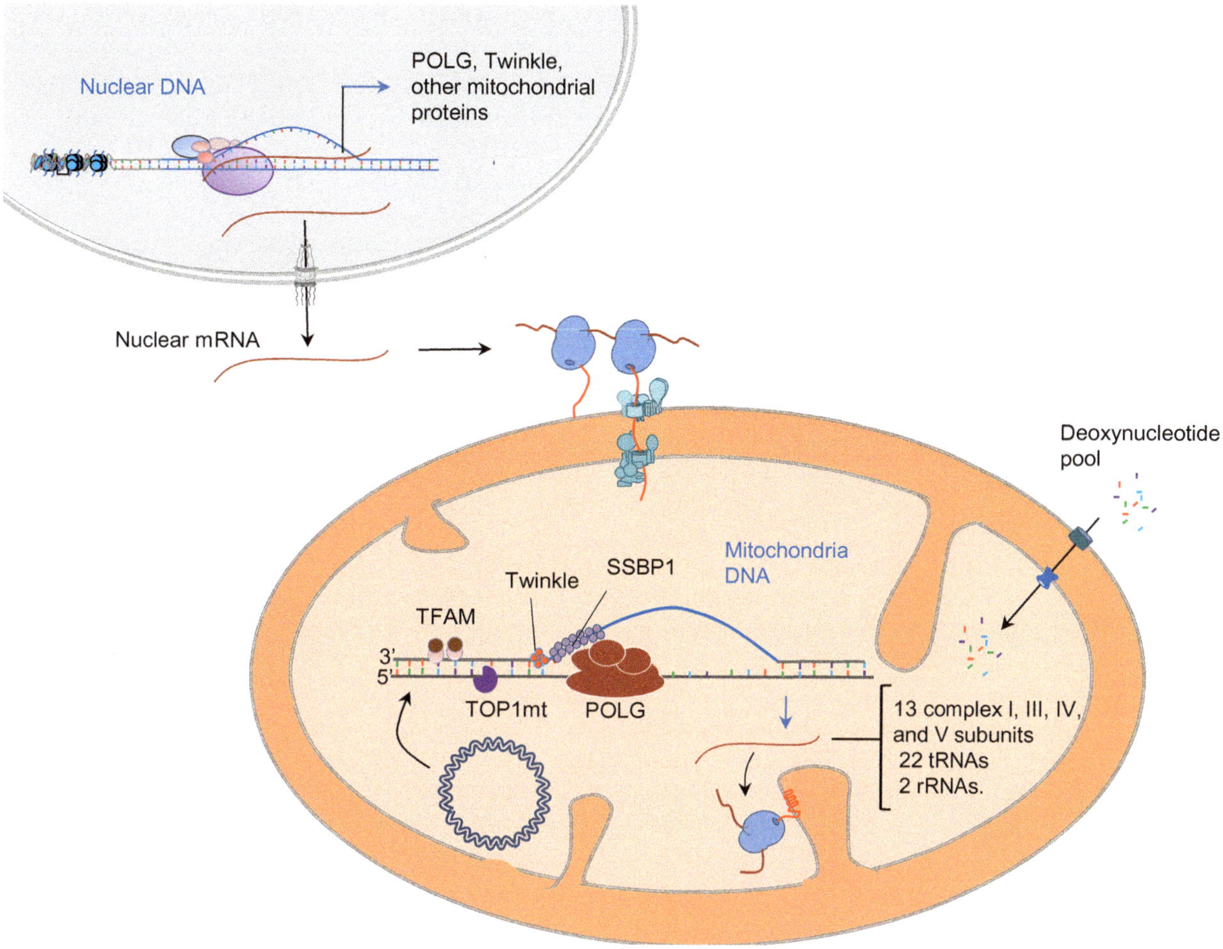

FIGURE 11.2 Synthesis of mitochondrial DNA.
The machinery for maintenance of the mitochondrial genome includes mtDNA polymerase γ (POLG), the helicase Twinkle that allows mtDNA replication, and mitochondrial single-stranded DNA–binding protein 1 (SSBP1). Other proteins that contribute to the organization of mtDNA include mitochondrial transcription factor A (TFAM) and mitochondrial DNA topoisomerase I (TOPmt). In addition, mtDNA replication requires a supply of nucleotides; the mitochondrial nucleotide pools are closely linked to cytosolic nucleotide metabolism.

Sirtuins (SIRTs) are nicotinamide adenine dinucleotide–(NAD) dependent acetylases that are also activated in the setting of energy depletion and differ in their subcellular location and function. SIRT1 is located in the nucleus and targets histones and transcription factors such as PGC-1α; SIRT 3 is present in the mitochondria, where it regulates several processes, including glucose utilization, fatty acid oxidation, and ROS levels. The estrogen-related receptor α (ERRα) regulates both nuclear genes devoted to mitochondrial functions and numerous mitochondrial DNA genes. Nearly half of the proteins encoded by the mitochondrial genome are regulated by ERRα. ERRα controls mitochondrial processes such as OXPHOS through a network of protein kinases, and regulates expression of sirtuins such as SIRT 3.This receptor also regulates mitochondrial biogenesis in association with PGC-1-related co-activator and via cross-talk with mitogen-activated protein kinase kinases and survival signaling kinases.

Mitochondrial Protein Synthesis

Proteome analysis shows that human mitochondria contain at least 1,500 different proteins. Only up to 15% of mitochondrial proteins are directly involved in energy metabolism; 20%–25% of these proteins maintain the mitochondria genome. Mitochondria contain their own protein synthetic machinery. Protein translation occurs in ribosomes (mitoribosomes) that incorporate transfer RNAs (tRNAs). Translation initiation in mitochondria (as in bacteria) requires formylated methionine tRNA, which distinguishes the initiator methionine from that used for peptide elongation. Mitochondria contain a unique set of 17 aminoacyl tRNA synthases. Respiratory chain subunits synthesized in the mitochondria are inserted in the inner membrane by coupling translational ribosomes to a protein called the oxidase assembly insertase. In addition to synthesis of components of the OXPHOS system, the mitochondria participates in biosynthesis of Fe-S complexes. Proteins that are involved in biogenesis and protein import machinery are essential housekeeping systems for normal mitochondrial function.[2]

Protein Import to the Mitochondria

As the majority of mitochondrial proteins are encoded by nuclear DNA and synthesized in the cytosol, they have to be imported into the mitochondria. The majority of these proteins targeted to the mitochondria contain an amino-terminal mitochondrial target sequence (called presequence). This allows their recognition by the translocase of the outer membrane (TOM) complex, which is the main gate for protein entry into the mitochondria. The TOM complex interacts with other protein complexes forming different supercomplexes that mediate protein sorting to different mitochondria compartments. Import of proteins into the mitochondrial matrix involves their passage through the TOM channel and translocation via translocase of the inner membrane 23 (TIM23); this process requires a proton gradient generated by the respiratory chain, ATP, and the mitochondrial heat shock protein 70 (mtHsp70). Precursors that become incorporated into the inner mitochondrial membrane can either become arrested in the TIM23 complex and released into the inner membrane or are first transported to the matrix and then inserted in the inner membrane by the oxidase assembly insertase. Proteins are translocated and inserted at the outer mitochondrial membrane by different mechanisms; some precursors are first translocated by the TOM complex to the intermembrane space and then inserted into the outer membrane by the sorting and assembly machinery complex.

Mitochondrial Protein Quality Control

Proteins synthesized or imported in the mitochondria are subject to a tight quality control. A key mechanism required for the turnover of these proteins involves a large inner membrane ATPase-dependent protease system. These proteases belong to the family of ATPases associated with multiple cellular activities (AAA family) and include inner membrane and matrix-exposed AAA proteases.[3–5] These proteases cleave or degrade different inner membrane proteins and are also involved in quality control and turnover of some matrix, intermembrane space, and outer membrane proteins. The matrix AAA complex is an inner membrane-anchored hexamer that is composed of homo- or heterooligomers of the peptidase subunit known as AFG3-like matrix AAA peptidase subunit-2 (AFG3L2) and paraplegin. These proteins degrade misfolded proteins. Absence of the chaperone function of AFG3L2 activates a metalloproteinase that cleaves the inner membrane-anchored protein optic atrophy 1 (OPA1), leading to remodeling of the mitochondrial membrane and mitochondrial fragmentation.

MITOCHONDRIAL MEMBRANE ARCHITECTURE AND MEMBRANE CONTACT SITES

Mitochondria form synapses both between each other and with organelles such as the endoplasmic reticulum (ER), Golgi complex, and nucleus. Mitochondrion–mitochondrion junctions are analogous to tight junctions with apposition between outer mitochondrial membranes from adjacent mitochondria. The cristae of two mitochondria bound by intermitochondrial junctions become coordinated in space and may participate in rapid signaling events.

Mitochondria-Associated Membrane (MAM)

The contact sites between the outer mitochondrial membrane and the ER are referred to as mitochondrial-associated membrane (MAM) and participate in mitochondrial membrane architecture and dynamics, metabolite and ion transport, protein and lipid biogenesis, mitochondrial Ca^{2+} homeostasis, lipid transfer, and mitochondrial fission and fusion events.[6]

The MAM is enriched with several proteins, including the inositol triphosphate receptor type 3 (ITPR3, IP_3R3), a Ca^{2+} release channel present in the ER, and the sigma 1 receptor (Sig-1R), an ER chaperone that ensures proper Ca^{2+} transfer from the ER to the mitochondria. The MAM also contains long-chain fatty acyl coenzyme A (CoA) synthetase that mediates the ligation of fatty acids with CoA and other cholesterol metabolites and has an important role in steroidogenesis.

Mitochondria Contact Sites and Crista Organizing System (MICOS)

The mitochondrial contact site and cristae organizing system (MICOS) of the inner mitochondrial membrane is crucial for maintenance of the architecture of the cristae.

The MICOS is enriched at the crista junctions and has an important role in formation of outer-inner membrane contact sites, thereby helping position the downstream translocation machineries close to the import channel TOM and the protein sorting and assembly machinery.[2] In the inner membrane, the core component of MICOS and a partner protein are in dynamic contact with the dimeric ATP synthase that mediates the last step of OXPHOS. Assembly of the major subcomplex of MICOS in relationship to the respiratory chain involves the mitochondrial-specific inner membrane dimeric phospholipid cardiolipin. MICOS is also connected to the machinery of mitochondrial fusion, including the inner membrane protein OPA1. The MICOS also interacts with the sorting and assembly protein complex in the outer membrane and thus indirectly with the TOM complex and the ER membrane.

MITOCHONDRIAL FUNCTIONS

Intermediate Metabolism

The metabolic pathways that provide substrate for the respiratory chain occur in the mitochondrial matrix and include the tricarboxylic acid cycle (Krebs cycle) and β-oxidation of fatty acids (Figure 11.3). In the adult brain, glycogen is predominantly present in astrocytes. Glycogenolysis and glycolysis are essential for astrocytic responses to increasing energy demand. The utilization of glucose by neurons and astrocytes differ in several important features. Neurons have a functional block of the phosphofructokinase, the rate-limiting enzyme for glycolysis, and cannot use this pathway as a source of ATP. Instead, neurons metabolize glucose via the pentose phosphate pathway, yielding nicotinamide adenine dinucleotide phosphate (NADPH), which protects against oxidative stress. Neurons have an active pyruvate dehydrogenase (PDH), which is the gatekeeper of mitochondria and allows them to utilize pyruvate efficiently to produce acetyl CoA as a substrate for the Krebs cycle. In contrast, astrocytes are highly capable for using glycolysis as a source of ATP and pyruvate whereas their PDH activity is tonically inhibited, which shunts pyruvate toward lactate production. Astrocyte-derived lactate is then shuttled to neurons and oligodendrocytes to serve as a fuel for metabolism. The oxidative metabolism of glucose in the Krebs cycle requires a critical thiamine-dependent step mediated by the PDH complex that metabolizes pyruvate into acetyl CoA. The second major source of acetyl CoA is oxidation of fatty acids. Long chain acyl CoA synthase activates long-chain fatty acids at the outer mitochondrial membrane; a carnitine transport system then mediates the import of activated fatty acids into the matrix via three sequential steps. These steps are mediated by the carnitine

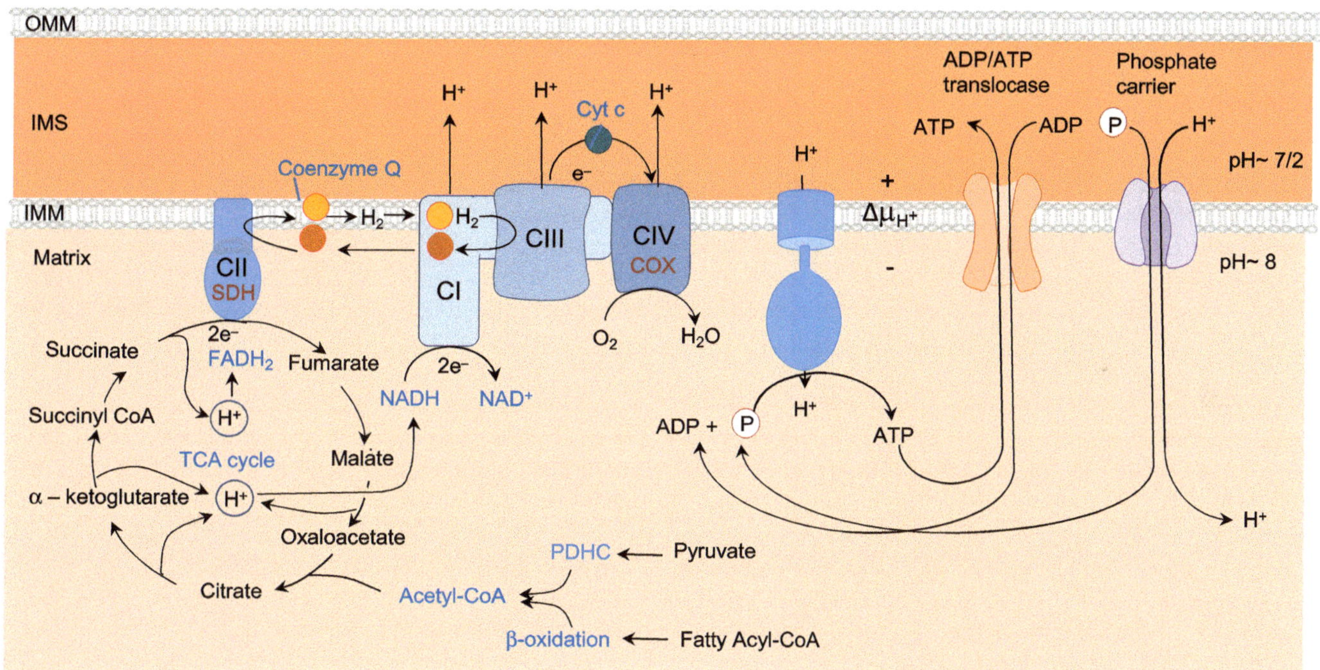

FIGURE 11.3 Krebs cycle and oxidative phosphorylation.

The metabolic pathways that provide substrate for the respiratory chain include the tricarboxylic acid cycle (TCA, Krebs cycle) and β-oxidation of fatty acids. Glucose is metabolized to pyruvate, which by action of pyruvate dehydrogenase (PDH) is converted to acetyl coenzyme A (acetyl CoA). Fatty acid β-oxidation is catalyzed by distinct enzyme complexes to yield acetyl CoA. The oxidative steps of the tricarboxylic acid cycle break down substrates to reduce nicotinamide adenine dinucleotide (NAD) to NADH and flavin adenine dinucleotide (FAD) to $FADH_2$. The oxidative phosphorylation (OXPHOS) system includes five multi-enzyme complexes (complex I–V) and two electron carriers, coenzyme Q and cytochrome c (cyt c). The electrons transferred from one respiratory chain complex to another drive the pumping of protons (H+) to the intermembrane space and generate an electrochemical gradient across the inner mitochondrial membrane. This proton gradient creates a motive force that is used by the F_1-F_0 ATP synthase (complex V) to phosphorylate ADP to produce ATP. ATP is transported out of the mitochondria by ATP-ADP translocase 1. A phosphate carrier allows the import of inorganic phosphate to the matrix.

palmitoyl transferase-I (CPT-I) in the outer mitochondrial membrane; the carnitine: acylcarnitine translocase that translocates the acylcarnitines to the mitochondrial matrix; and finally the carnitine: palmitoyl transferase II (CPT-II) in the inner mitochondrial membrane, which converts acylcarnitine back into acyl CoAs. Fatty acid β-oxidation in the matrix is catalyzed by distinct enzyme with specificity for short-, medium-, and long-chain fatty acids in the form of acyl CoAs that yield acetyl CoA. The oxidative steps of the tricarboxylic acid cycle break down substrates to reduce NAD to NADH and flavin adenine dinucleotide (FAD) to $FADH_2$ (Figure 11.3).

Oxidative Phosphorylation

Metabolism of a single molecule of glucose via aerobic glycolysis and OXPHOS yields 36 molecules of ATP, whereas anaerobic glycolysis yields only two ATP molecules. The OXPHOS system includes five multi-enzyme complexes (complex I–V) and two electron carriers, coenzyme Q and cytochrome c (Figure 11.3). Complex I, III, and IV form a supercomplex called respirasome, which serves as a hub for other protein complexes coupling energy metabolism with transport and other functions. NADH donates electrons to complex I and $FADH_2$ donates electrons to complex II; via these complexes electrons are transferred to coenzyme Q, or ubiquinone. Complex I (NAD: ubiquinone oxidoreductase), complex II (succinate: ubiquinone oxidoreductase), and complex III (ubiquinol: cytochrome c oxidoreductase) contain associated Fe-S centers; complex IV is also known as cytochrome c oxidase. The electrons are transferred from one respiratory chain complex to another by a series of reduction-oxidation (redox) reactions that drive the pumping of protons (H^+) to the intermembrane space via complexes I, III, and IV. This generates an electrochemical gradient across the mitochondrial membrane. Complex IV donates the electrons to oxygen, yielding water. The proton gradient across the inner mitochondrial membrane creates a motive force (called chemiosmotic potential) that is used by the F_1-F_0 ATP synthase (complex V) to phosphorylate ADP to produce ATP. ATP is transported out of the mitochondria by ATP/ADP translocase 1 or adenine nucleotide translocator (ANT), an antiporter located in the located in inner mitochondrial membrane. A phosphate carrier allows the import of inorganic phosphate to the matrix for the reaction with ADP.

Maintenance of the Mitochondrial Transmembrane Potential

A salient feature of normal mitochondria is their very negative membrane potential (-160 to -180 mV) across the inner mitochondrial membrane created by the H^+ pumping to the intermembranous space. This mitochondrial membrane potential not only drives ATP production but also is required for synthesis of Fe-S clusters, mitochondrial import of many nuclear-encoded proteins, and import of Ca^{2+} from the cytosol and the ER. Potassium (K^+) ions have an integral role in mitochondrial maintenance and function. The major K^+ channels in mitochondria are the large conductance Ca^{2+}-activated K^+ channel, the ATP-regulated K^+ channel and voltage-dependent K^+ channel $K_v1.3$; these channels are sensitive to changes in mitochondrial membrane potential. In response to K^+ influx driven by the high mitochondrial membrane potential across the inner membrane, the K^+/H^+ antiporter exchanges one matrix K^+ for one inner mitochondrial membrane H^+, thus maintaining mitochondrial volume and preventing matrix swelling. Uncoupling proteins are inner mitochondrial membrane proteins that function as facilitated transporters of H^+, dispersing the proton gradient generated by the respiratory chain across the inner mitochondrial membrane.

Reactive Oxygen Species (ROS) Production

Reactive oxygen species (ROS) are important signaling molecules released from mitochondria. Whereas ROS regulate several cellular functions, when produced in large quantities they elicit oxidative damage to membranes and DNA, particularly mtDNA, given its proximity to the electron transfer chain. The respiratory chain generates ROS via the reduction of molecular oxygen to superoxide ion (O_2^-), which occurs primarily via complex I and complex III. There are other sources of O_2^- production in the mitochondria, including the activity of the α-ketoglutarate dehydrogenase, pyruvate dehydrogenase, glyceraldehyde 3 phosphate dehydrogenase, and the electron-transfer flavoprotein (ETF) ubiquinone oxidoreductase (ETF-QO), which is an electron carrier involved in fatty acid β-oxidation and delivery of electrons to the ubiquinone pool in the mitochondrial respiratory chain. At the mitochondrial matrix, O_2^- is transformed to hydrogen peroxide (H_2O_2) by the manganese superoxide dismutase 2 (SOD2). Some O_2^- that escapes into the intermembranous space is dismutated by the copper-zinc SOD 1 (SOD1). Hydrogen peroxide is the only ROS species that can cross mitochondrial membranes and may affect cell behavior independently of its oxidative effects. Hydrogen peroxide is mostly metabolized in the cytosol by action of peroxiredoxins and glutathione peroxidases, which require NADPH as a cofactor.

Mitohormesis

Whereas high ROS levels have damaging effects, ROS may also trigger a neuroprotective mechanism known as mitochondrial hormesis or mitohormesis. This mechanism has been implicated in the neuroprotective effect of glucose deprivation, ketogenic diet, and physical exercise. Mitohormesis is both a bioenergetics and an antioxidant adaptation that primarily depends on increased expression and nuclear location of peroxisome proliferator-activated receptor γ coactivator 1α (PPR1α). Ketones, such as β-hydroxybutyric acid, increase retrograde electron transfer by increasing the $FADH_2$/ NADH ratio, leading to $FADH_2$-mediated reduction of the coenzyme Q pool via complex II. Beta hydroxbutyrate interacts with, and inhibits histone deacetylases, leading to increased transcription of antioxidant-promoting factors.

Calcium Homeostasis

Calcium microdomains and membrane contacts between the mitochondria and ER are crucial for cellular Ca^{2+} homeostasis (Figure 11.4). Intracellular Ca^{2+} is primarily sequestered within the ER and mitochondria via a strictly controlled bidirectional flow that occurs at the site of contact between the ER and the mitochondria. The Sig-1R functions as a ER chaperone that ensures proper Ca^{2+} transfer from the ER to the mitochondria via interactions with the ITPR3 (IP_3R3). When activated by inositol triphosphate, this receptor allows efflux of Ca^{2+} from the ER to the mitochondria. The voltage-dependent anion channel (VDAC) localized in the outer mitochondrial membrane, together with the cytosolic glucose-regulated chaperone Grp75, forms a complex with the ITPR3 at the level of the MAM, facilitating Ca^{2+} efflux from the ER to the mitochondria. The ER-mitochondrial junctions are also sites of localized H_2O_2 nanodomains, where H_2O_2 may potentiate Ca^{2+} release by regulating IP3R. The mitochondrial Ca^{2+} uniporter (MCU), is a transmembrane protein in the inner mitochondrial membrane that mediates Ca^{2+} entry to the mitochondria by forming a highly selective channel that is activated by interactions with mitochondria Ca^{2+} uptake proteins 1 (MICU1) and MICU2. These MICU proteins function as a Ca^{2+} sensor; their role is to regulate the threshold of cytosolic Ca^{2+} that allows efficient Ca^{2+} entry in the mitochondria. This prevents or reduces Ca^{2+} entry in the mitochondria at low cytosolic Ca^{2+} levels and thus also prevents futile Ca^{2+} cycles and energy cost required to maintain low

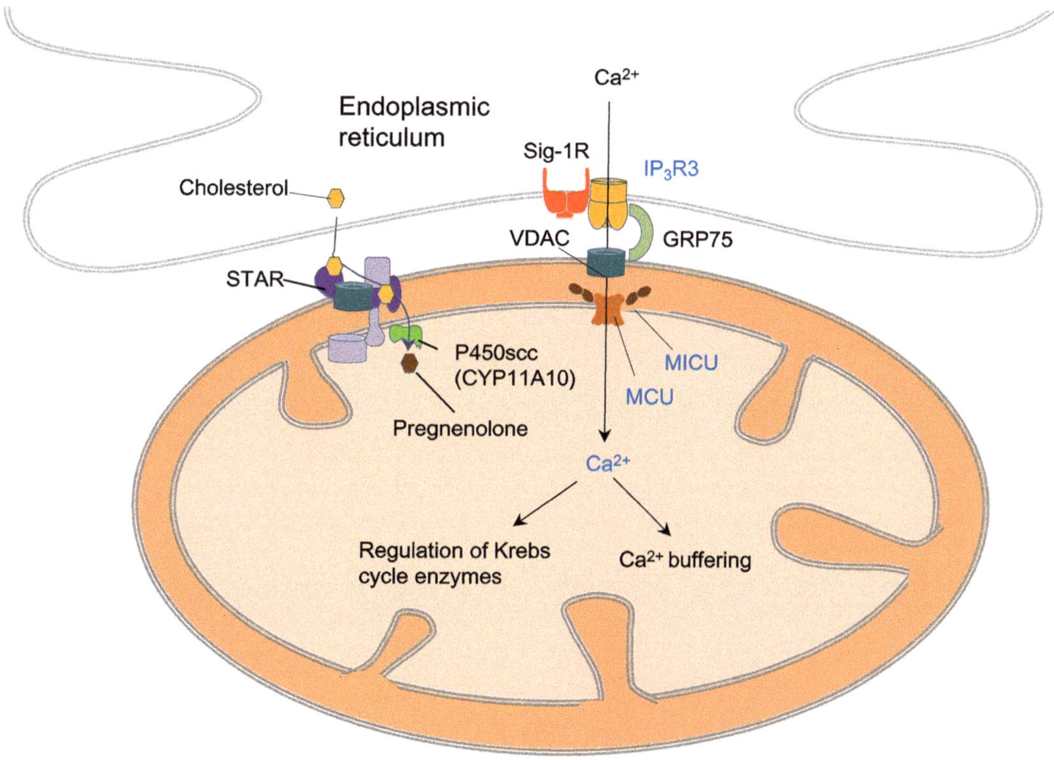

FIGURE 11.4 Role of mitochondria in calcium homeostasis and cholesterol metabolism.
The membrane contacts between the mitochondria and endoplasmic reticulum (ER) are crucial for cellular Ca^{2+} homeostasis. Calcium transfer from the ER to the mitochondria via interactions with the inositol 3 phosphate receptors ITPR3 (IP_3R3). The sigma 1 receptor Sig-1R functions as a chaperone that facilitates this process. The voltage-dependent ion channel (VDAC), together with the cytosolic glucose-regulated chaperone Grp75, forms a complex with the ITPR3 at the level of MAM, facilitating Ca^{2+} efflux from the ER to the mitochondria. The mitochondrial Ca^{2+} uniporter (MCU) mediates Ca^{2+} entry to the mitochondria by forming a highly selective channel that is activated by interactions with mitochondria Ca^{2+} uptake proteins 1 (MICU1) and MICU2. Cholesterol is transported from the outer to the inner mitochondrial membrane, where it becomes the substrate for the first enzyme of steroidogenesis cytochrome P450 side chain cleavage enzyme (P450SCC, CYP11A10). An outer mitochondrial membrane protein complex termed the transduceosome initiates cholesterol transfer by anchoring of the steroidogenesis acute regulatory protein (STAR) to an outer mitochondrial translocator protein.

mitochondrial Ca^{2+} concentrations. Loss-of-function mutations of *MICU1* gene are linked to early-onset proximal myopathy, progressive movement disorder, and intellectual disability.[7] Muscle biopsy shows focal loss of mitochondria and fragmentation of the mitochondrial network, but not classical features of mitochondrial myopathy.

Calcium exerts multiple physiological effects in mitochondria regulating the Krebs cycle and ATP production. For example, PDH, α-ketoglutaric dehydrogenase, and isocitrate dehydrogenase are all Ca^{2+}-regulated mitochondrial enzymes. Intramitochondrial Ca^{2+} also modulates soluble adenylyl cyclase and thus production of cyclic adenosine monophosphate (cAMP), which elicits phosphorylation and regulation of respiratory chain proteins. Thus mitochondrial Ca^{2+} signaling has a major role in coupling neuronal activity with metabolism. Mitochondrial Ca^{2+} transferring at junctional complexes also regulates mitochondrial fission and opening of the mitochondrial permeability transition pore that may be associated with tissue damage. Mitochondria are also tethered to the plasma membrane, where they can communicate with voltage-gated Ca^{2+} channels and regulate Ca^{2+} pumps, including the plasma membrane Ca^{2+} pump that extrudes Ca^{2+} from the cell. Mitochondria located just subjacent to the membrane may also regulate store-operated Ca^{2+} entry at ER--plasma membrane junctions; this mechanism is vital for Ca^{2+} reloading of the ER for maintenance of Ca^{2+} signaling. This is a redox-sensitive process that can be regulated by ROS generated in mitochondria.

Cholesterol Metabolism and Steroidogenesis

Mitochondria participate in several crucial steps of lipid metabolism, including long-chain fatty acid β-oxidation and steroidogenesis. The ER–mitochondrial contact sites are the center for intermembrane transport of cholesterol, phospholipids, and ceramide.[8] Phosphatidylserine and phosphatidylcholine are imported from the ER to the mitochondria. Cholesterol is synthesized in the ER and is then transported into the mitochondria, where it is transformed into steroids (Figure 11.4). Cholesterol is transported from the outer to the inner mitochondrial membrane, where it becomes the substrate for the first enzyme of steroidogenesis cytochrome P450 side chain cleavage enzyme (P450SCC, CYP11A10), located in the matrix side of the inner mitochondrial membrane. The transfer of cholesterol from the ER to the inner mitochondrial membrane involves a multimeric protein complex spanning the outer-inner mitochondrial membrane unit.[9] An outer mitochondrial membrane protein complex termed the transduceosome initiates cholesterol transfer, which involves the steroidogenesis acute regulatory protein (StAR) and the outer mitochondrial translocator protein (previously referred to as peripheral benzodiazepine receptor). Intracellular Ca^{2+} stimulates both cholesterol transfer and expression of StAR in the outer mitochondrial membrane.

Coenzyme Q (ubiquinone or CoQ) is an essential lipid that plays a role in mitochondrial respiratory electron transport and serves as an important antioxidant. CoQ synthesis derives from aromatic ring precursors and the isoprene biosynthetic pathway.[10] The synthesis of coenzyme Q involves multiple proteins, including a high-molecular mass multisubunit protein and lipid complex called the CoQ synthome (Coq3–Coq9 and Coq11) associated with the matrix site of the inner mitochondrial membrane, and Coq1, Coq2, and Coq10, which do not associate with the complex. Mutations of different *COQ* genes encoding several enzymes involved in this process produce COQ10 deficiency.[10]

Iron Metabolism

Iron is a key player in many cellular processes, including respiration, energy metabolism, myelin formation, and DNA synthesis. Iron is capable of accepting or donating electrons and has flexible redox activity; it is often incorporated as a prosthetic group of enzymes and structural proteins. However, iron can also participate in potentially harmful reactions such as ROS production. Therefore, cells have carefully regulated mechanisms that control acquisition, usage, and detoxification of iron to meet iron metabolic needs and prevent its toxic effects. Mitochondria are a key component of these regulatory mechanisms.[11] Depending on the cell type, they may contain up to 20%–50% of cellular iron. Cytosolic iron first crosses the outer mitochondrial membrane and is then imported through the inner membrane to the mitochondrial matrix by carrier proteins called mitoferrins that form a complex with the ATP binding cassette protein ABC10. Mitochondrial iron is primarily used for three metabolic pathways: heme synthesis, Fe-S cluster biogenesis, and iron storage. Heme is a complex of ferrous iron and protoporphyrin IX and is an important prosthetic group of several vital proteins, including hemoglobin, myoglobin, cytochromes, catalases, and peroxidases, where it is involved in oxygen transport and storage, electron transfer for redox reactions, signal transduction, and control of gene expression. The first step in the heme synthesis pathway occurs in the matrix and is the production of δ-aminolevulinic acid (ALA), which is transported to the cytosol to form porphobilinogen. Subsequent steps in the cytosol eventually lead to the formation to coproporphyrinogen III, which is then transported back to the mitochondria, where it undergoes oxidative decarboxylation to protoporphyrin IX. In the mitochondrial matrix, ferrous iron is inserted into protoporphyrin IX to form heme by action of ferrochelatase. Mitochondrial iron is also used for synthesis of Fe-S clusters, which are important prosthetic groups of several proteins, including NADH: ubiquinone oxidoreductase (complex I), electron transfer flavoproteins, and other proteins involved in metabolic pathways linked to energy metabolism.[12] The assembly of Fe-S clusters is a multistep process that requires a multimeric core complex that includes frataxin (FTXN);

FTXN regulates iron entry during Fe-S assembly and enhances the rate of sulfur transfer to a scaffold protein that forms the structural backbone for cluster assembly. Once formed into the scaffold, nascent Fe-S clusters are released and transferred to recipient proteins. Excessive iron can be stored in mitochondrial ferritin.

Metabolic Signaling to the Nucleus and Epigenetic Control

Mitochondria are positioned morphologically and functionally in close proximity to the nucleus and participate in mechanisms of chromatin remodeling and epigenetic control of gene expression by releasing several metabolic signals.[13] They include ROS and reactive metabolic intermediaries such as acetyl CoA, succinyl CoA, α-ketoglutarate; NAD^+, FAD, and S-adenosyl methionine. These metabolites are substrates for enzymes involved in epigenetic control of transcription, including DNA methyltransferases and histone acetylates. Other mitochondrial signals responding to cell energy levels, such as AMPK and PGC-1α, also translocate to the nucleus and regulate gene expression.

MITOSTASIS

Mitostasis encompasses the mechanisms by which the neurons preserve a healthy, functional pool of mitochondria by regulating the heir number and quality at each cell compartment. In many cell types, mitochondria form a highly interconnected and dynamic reticulum with ongoing divisions and reconnections. Mitochondria numbers and quality control are governed by several processes, including fusion fission, transport and docking, biogenesis, and mitophagy, biogenesis, and mytophagy.[14]

Mitochondrial Fusion and Fission

Mitochondrial fusion and fission control the length, shape, size, and number of mitochondria and maintain the overall morphology and functional properties of the mitochondrial population. Mitochondrial fusion enables the exchange of contents between mitochondria, allowing defective mitochondria to regain essential elements for their normal function, including components of the respiratory chain and mitochondrial DNA, in the setting of cell stress. Mitochondrial fusion depends on two members of the mitofusin (MFN) family, MFN1 and MF2, which are present in the outer mitochondrial membrane and form homo-oligomeric and hetero-oligomeric complexes with each other between apposing mitochondria (Figure 11.5). Fusion of the outer mitochondrial membrane is followed by fusion of the inner mitochondrial membrane mediated by the optic atrophy 1 (OPA1) protein, located within narrow junctional regions that insulate the cristae from the rest of the intermembrane space. OPA1 is imported into the mitochondrial intermembrane space and is first processed by matrix metalloproteinases followed by processing by other proteases such as paraplegin. Processing of OPA1 by presenilin-associated rhomboid-like (PARL) protease serves as a sensor of membrane potential across the mitochondrial inner membrane. In addition to their primary role in mitochondrial fusion, MFN2 and OPA1 also participate in regulation of the coupling of the mitochondrial respiratory chain and oxidative phosphorylation. Proteolytic activation of OPA1 is regulated by the output of oxidative phosphorylation; this provides for a match between mitochondrial morphology and the metabolic demands of the cell. MFN2 is enriched at the interface between the mitochondria and the ER (MAM); the areas of contact between these two organelles mark future sites of mitochondrial fission.[15]

Whereas interconnected mitochondria are present in the neuronal cell body, in order to enter the axon a mitochondrion must undergo fission, and then proper transport in the axon. Mitochondrial fission also facilitates apoptosis by regulating the release of intermembrane-space proteins into the cytosol, and facilitates the removal of dysfunctional mitochondria. Mitochondrial fission requires the recruitment of dynamin-like/related protein 1 (DLP1/Drp1), from the cytosol. Drp1 is a GTPase that assembles into punctate spots on the mitochondria and forms rings and spirals that encircle and constrict the mitochondrial tubule. The recruitment of Drp1 to the fission sites involves the adaptor proteins Fission 1 and a mitochondrial fission factor, which form different complexes anchored to the outer mitochondrial membrane. Ganglioside-induced differentiation-associated protein 1 belongs to the family of the glutathione-S-transferases and is anchored to the outer mitochondrial membrane, where it regulates mitochondrial fission. Mitochondrial elongation factor 1 is a protein anchored to the outer mitochondrial membrane that recruits Drp1 independently of Fission-1, negatively regulates mitochondrial fission, and promotes fusion.

Mitochondrial Transport and Docking

Mitochondria include a large stable or stationary pool and motile pool. Motile mitochondria may temporarily pause but tend to continue onward and only infrequently change direction. Mitochondrial motility patterns reflect the interplay among microtubules, motor proteins, adaptor complexes, and anchor mechanisms that oppose transport.[16–18] (Figure 11.6). Mitochondrial anterograde axonal transport requires the motor protein kinesin-1/KIF5); retrograde transport toward the minus-end requires the dynein/dynactin complex motor. Complex mitochondrial motility patterns, such as saltatory motion and direction changes, indicate that the relative number of active kinesin or dynein motors attached to the mitochondrion at a given time, as well as their mutually opposing forces, determines the net direction of movement. In dendrites, microtubule

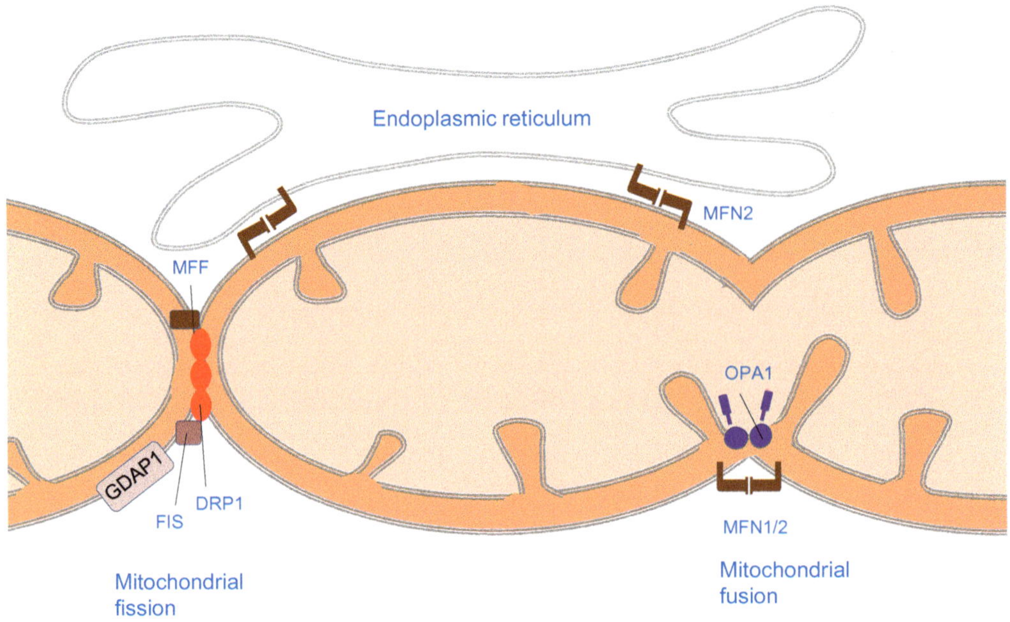

FIGURE 11.5 Mitochondrial fusion and fission.
Mitochondrial fusion depends mitofusin (MFN) 1 and MFN2, MFN1, which are present in the outer mitochondrial membrane and form homo-oligomeric and hetero-oligomeric complexes with each other between apposing mitochondria. Fusion of the outer mitochondrial membrane is followed by fusion of the inner mitochondrial membrane mediated by the optic atrophy 1 (OPA1) protein. Mitochondrial fission requires the recruitment of dynamin-related protein 1 (DRP1) from the cytosol. The recruitment of DRP1 to the fission sites involves the adaptor proteins Fission 1 (FIS) and a mitochondrial fission factor (MFF), which forms different complexes anchored to the outer mitochondrial membrane. GDAP1 (ganglioside-induced differentiation-associated protein 1 (GDAP1) regulates the fission process.

organization is heterogeneous and mixed, and in general dynein is primarily responsible for mitochondrial movement. Some mitochondria need to be retained in the soma, while others need to be transported and positioned along axons and dendrites to be concentrated in areas with high ATP consumption, such as presynaptic terminals and near the nodes of Ranvier. By this mechanism, mitochondria are immobilized in areas of high synaptic activity where demands for ATP and Ca^{2+} buffering are high. The distribution of mitochondria at synapses also affects synaptic transmission and strength; stable positioning of mitochondria at presynaptic boutons maintains a steady release of synaptic vesicles. The mitochondrial transport machinery consists of a protein complex that includes the mitochondrial outer membrane protein mitochondrial Rho GTPase (MIRO), which binds to kinesin-1 (KIF5 heavy chain) or dynein motors via the adaptor protein trafficking kinesin binding protein (TRAK). TRAK1 primarily localizes to axons where it can bind either kinesin or dynactin/dynein; in dendrites, anterograde and retrograde transport mostly involves the MIRO/TRAK2 complex. Syntabulin is an adaptor protein that binds directly to KIF5, attaches to the outer membrane to the mitochondria, and may be required for anterograde transport to the presynaptic terminal.

Mitochondrial docking maintains the adequate number of stationary mitochondria in regions that require high ATP production and ability to buffer increased Ca^{2+}, such as dendritic spines and presynaptic terminals. Several signals converge on the MIRO/TRAK complex to immobilize mitochondria at such active sites. One important signal is increasing intracellular Ca^{2+}resulting from influx via voltage-gated and neurotransmitter receptor channels. MIRO is a Ca^{2+}-binding protein that functions as a sensor of local Ca^{2+} concentration. Increased Ca^{2+} arrests mitochondrial movement by producing a conformational change in MIRO that reduces the microtubule interaction of MIRO-bound kinesin. Increased extracellular glucose concentrations may also arrest mitochondrial motility; this effect is mediated by posttranslational modifications of TRAK proteins by the enzyme O-glucose-N-acyl transferase. Syntaphilin is an axon-specific protein that is recruited and attached to the mitochondria outer membrane and binds to microtubules, thereby increasing the cytoskeletal forces that oppose motility. Both axonal and dendritic mitochondria also dock along actin filaments enriched at presynaptic terminals and dendritic spines and interact with neurofilaments that oppose mitochondrial motility in axons. The close membrane contacts between mitochondria and

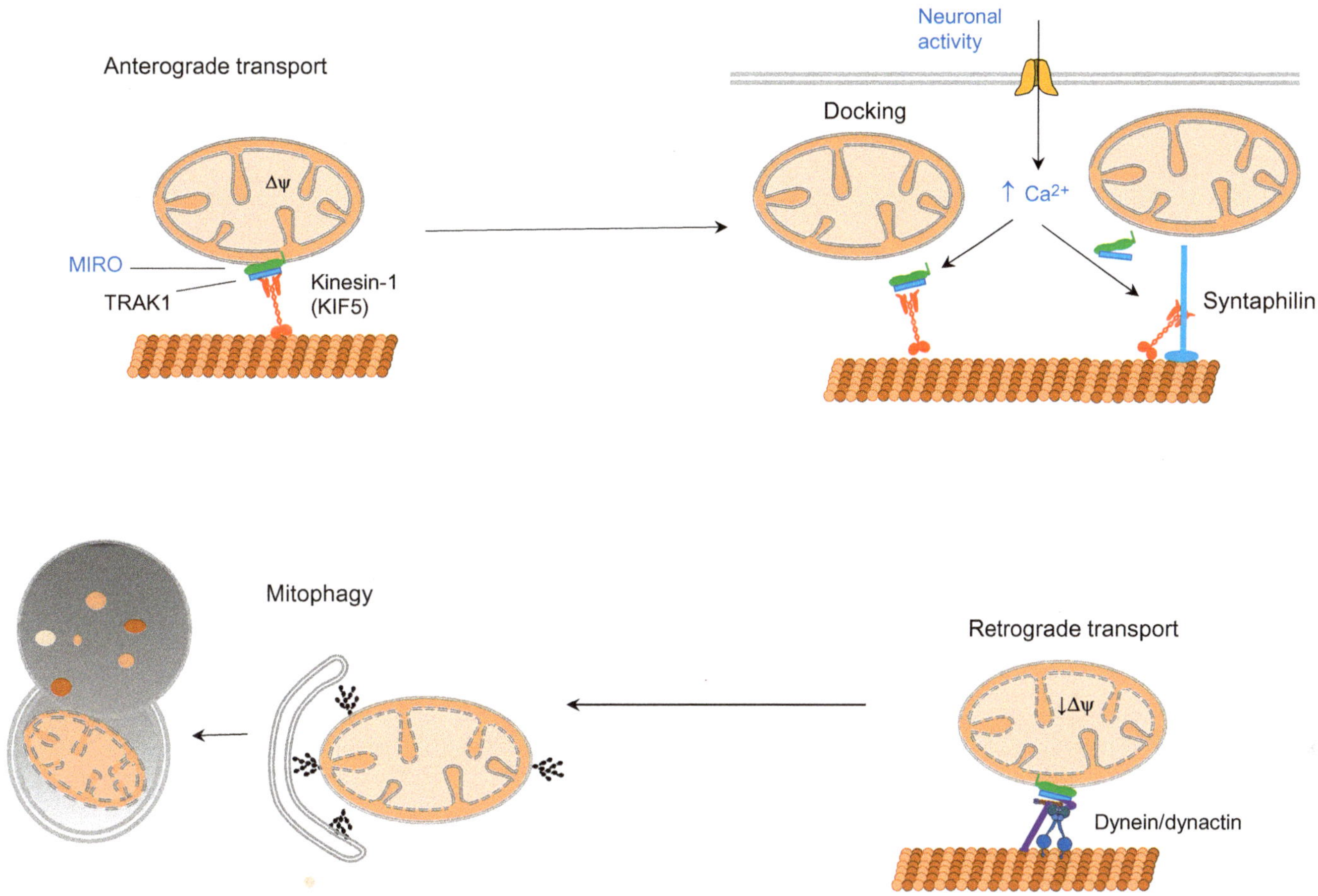

FIGURE 11.6 Mitochondrial transport and docking.
Mitochondrial anterograde axonal transport requires the motor protein kinesin-1/KIF5); retrograde transport toward the minus-end requires the dynein/dynactin complex motor. The mitochondrial transport requires the mitochondrial outer membrane protein Mitochondrial Rho GTPase (MIRO) that binds to kinesin-1 (KIF5 heavy chain) or dynein motors via the adaptor protein trafficking kinesin-binding protein (TRAK). Mitochondrial docking maintains the adequate number of stationary mitochondria in regions that require high ATP. Increased Ca^{2+} arrests mitochondrial movement via binding to MIRO, producing a conformational change that reduces the number of kinesin molecules bound to the mitochondria or reduce microtubule interaction of MIRO-bound kinesin. Syntaphilin is is recruited to the mitochondria and binds to microtubules, thereby increasing the cytoskeletal forces that oppose motility.

ER may also oppose mitochondrial movement as MIRO localizes at this high Ca^{2+} sites. Some evidence shows that mitochondria with high membrane potential preferentially migrate in the anterograde direction to synaptic regions with high metabolic demand whereas mitochondria with low membrane potential mostly move in the retrograde direction for destruction by the lysosomes, which are abundant in the cell body. However, mitochondria do not necessarily need to return to the soma for clearance.

Mitochondrial Quality Control and Clearance

Mitochondrial proteins are at high risk of damage and undergo misfolding, denaturation, oxidation, and glycation because of their proximity to the electron transport chain and other metabolic processes producing ROS. Neurons employ several quality control mechanisms that maintain mitochondrial health. They include protein degradation by proteases, mitochondria-derived vesicles, and mitophagy. The most relevant class proteases involved in removal of misfolded and denatured proteins are the mitochondrial AAA+ proteases such as paraplegin as discussed earlier. These proteases recognize hydrophobic domains that are exposed by oxidized or misfolded proteins and then unfold and degrade them. Mitochondrial-derived vesicles may remove large assemblies of proteins and lipids; this mechanism may be particularly important when a local stressor leads to accumulation of damaged proteins. Mitochondria-derived vesicles bud-off from the mitochondrion and can be targeted to multivesicular bodies for exocytosis, to lysosomes, or to peroxisomes.

Mitophagy targets entire or fragmented mitochondria for destruction by the lysosome (Figure 11.7). Mitophagy is

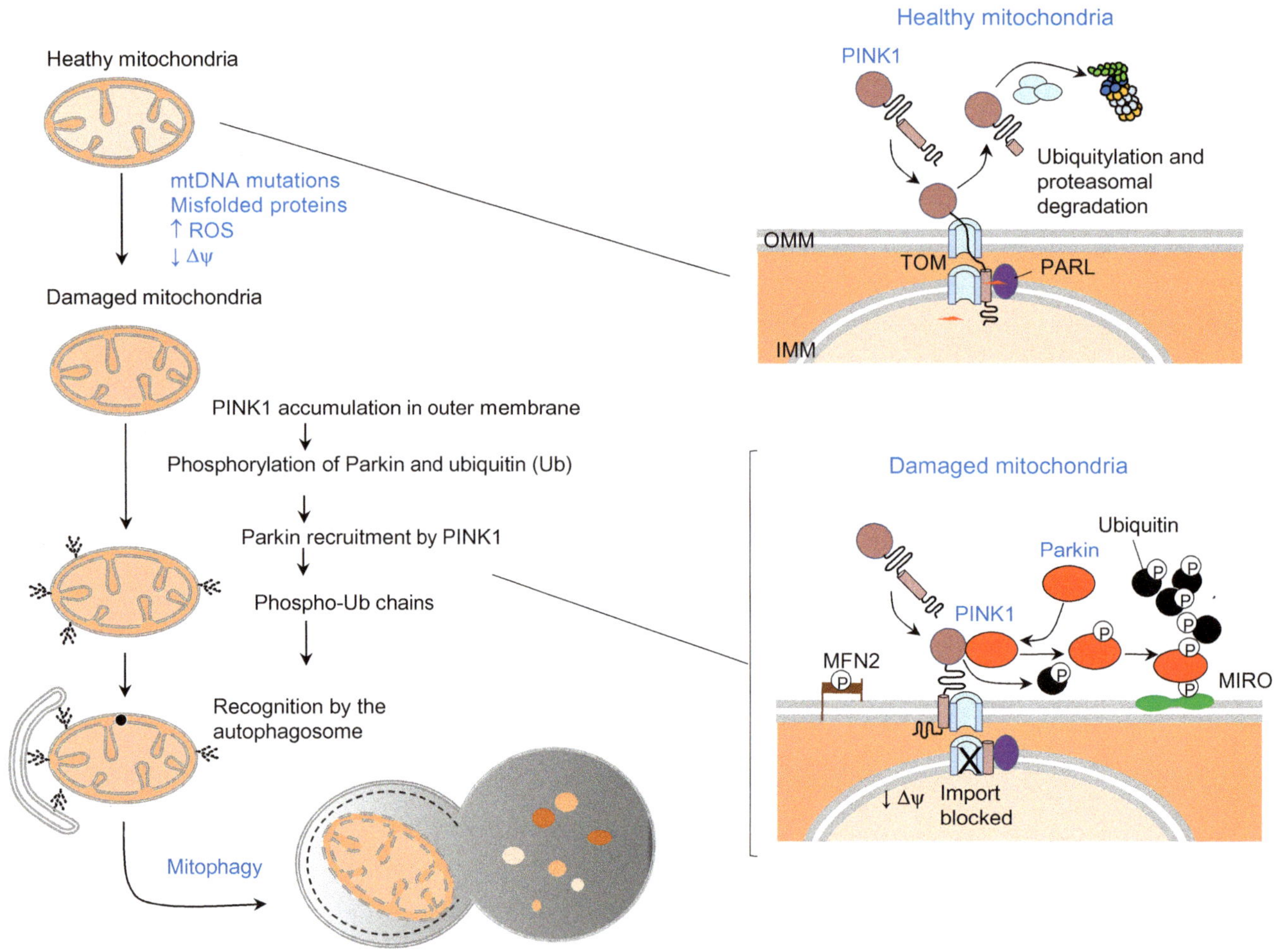

FIGURE 11.7 Mitophagy.

One key pathway for mitophagy involves PINK1 (phosphatase-tensin homolog-induced putative kinase 1) and the ubiquitin E3 ligase Parkin. PINK1 undergoes continuous synthesis and import to the inner mitochondrial membrane, where it undergoes proteolysis by mitochondrial enzymes such Presenilin-associated rhomboid-like (PARLI). If the mitochondrion loses its membrane potential or accumulates misfolded proteins PINK1is not degraded and stabilizes at the outer mitochondria surface, where it triggers mitophagy by phosphorylation of MFN2 and MIRO, as well as phosphorylation and activation of Parkin.

TOM, translocase of the outer membrane complex

a specialized form of autophagy that involves three stages: recognition of the mitochondrion to be targeted, formation of the autophagy membrane around the organelle, and fusion of the resulting mitoautophagosome to the lysosome. Mitophagy requires a specialized mechanism that recognizes a mitochondrion that requires clearance and thus recruitment to the autophagosome membrane. One key pathway involves mitochondrial serine/threonine kinase PINK1 (phosphatase-tensin homolog-induced putative kinase 1) and the ubiquitin E3 ligase Parkin.[19] PINK1 functions as a sensor of mitochondrial quality. It undergoes continuous synthesis and import to the inner mitochondrial membrane, where it undergoes proteolysis by mitochondrial enzymes such PARL1; this process is driven by the mitochondrial membrane potential. If the mitochondrion loses its membrane potential or accumulates misfolded proteins PINK1 is not degraded but instead becomes stabilized at the outer surface of the mitochondria. Stabilized PINK1 triggers mitophagy by phosphorylation of MFN2 and MIRO, as well as phosphorylation and activation of Parkin. Parkin binds to both phospho-MIRO and phospho-ubiquitin and is thereby recruited to the outer mitochondrial surface; this results in a positive feedback loop leading to addition of phospho-ubiquitin to the mitochondrial surface. Phospho-ubiquitin then binds to one of several mitophagy adaptors that recruit that recruit the membrane of the autophagosome. Parkin also initiates proteasomal degradation of several proteins in the outer mitochondrial surface, including MFNs and MIRO1. In addition, both PINK1 and Parkin can also mediate the formation of mitochondrial derived vesicles as an alternative to mitophagy; mitochondria can also be swept up along with other cytoplasmic component during macroautophagy. Mitochondrial derived vesicles could potentially be generated anywhere in the neuron and may be transported to the lysosomes. Mitophagy and macroautophagy of mitochondria may occur by lysosomes and autophagolysosomes in the axon as they move toward the cell body. In addition, axonal mitochondria may be shed and engulfed by glial cells. There is also local clearance of mitochondria via mitochondrial proteases. Mitochondrial proteases, such as paraplegin, may have an important role in continuously preserving mitochondrial quality in distal axons.

MITOCHONDRIA STRESS RESPONSE

The induction of mitochondrial stress response and activation of quality control pathways initiate retrograde signals from the mitochondria, which then activate transcription of genes that promote maintenance and enhanced quality control of the organelle.[20] Triggers of the mitochondria stress response include mtDNA defects, perturbations in mitochondrial translation and protein synthesis, impairment of the protein import machinery, and altered mitochondrial proteostasis. These perturbations induce imbalance between mitochondrial and nuclear-encoded OXPHOS complex subunits, leading to accumulation of components that cannot be assembled into complexes.

Mitochondrial Unfolded Protein Response

The mitochondrial unfolded protein response is a transcriptional response that is activated by several types of mitochondrial dysfunction, including impaired protein import, accumulation of misfolded proteins within the mitochondrial matrix, and perturbation of OXPHOS system. This stress response involves mitochondrial-to-nuclear communication via activating transcription factors (ATFs) that promote transcription of genes encoding mitochondrial chaperones and proteases involved in repair and recovery of the mitochondria network. These mitochondrial ATFs, such as ATF4 and ATF5, have both mitochondrial targeting and nuclear location sequences. In normal conditions they are imported into mitochondria and then degraded by a matrix-located protease; when mitochondria are damaged, they are targeted to the nucleus to regulate transcription. The mitochondrial unfolded protein response also involves chromatin remodeling. Mitochondrial stress induces nuclear translocation of cytosolic lysine methyltransferases that promote chromatin compaction and global gene silencing; some transcription factors interact with histone regions harboring mitochondrial stress response genes to maintain transcription required for the mitochondrial unfolded protein response.

Integrated Mitochondrial Stress Response

Defects in mtDNA maintenance and translation also trigger an integrated mitochondrial stress response that combines the transcriptional component of the mitochondrial unfolded protein response with metabolite and redox signaling. This response involves the early induction of the mitochondrial folate cycle. The folate cycle is an integral part of one-carbon metabolism and provides formylmethionine for mitochondrial RNA translation initiation. The redox-regulated methylene tetrahydrofolate reductase 2 is the regulatory enzyme for the mitochondrial folate cycle and mediates this mitochondrial stress response. Activation of the folate cycle provides the cell with nucleotides for DNA maintenance, glutathione as an antioxidant, and phospholipids and NADPH for membrane synthesis. Impairment of the folate cycle leads to imbalance of deoxyribonucleotide pools and causes mtDNA depletion. The integrated mitochondrial stress response in peripheral issues, including muscle, also causes mitochondrial release of mediators such as fibroblast growth factor 21, a metabolic cytokine, that elicits systemic effects. Increased levels of these mediators may be a marker of mitochondrial dysfunction in myopathies, but are not very specific.[20]

Extracellular Mitochondria as Signals of Cell Injury

Mitochondria may help regulate neuronal responses to oxidative stress. Whereas disruptions in the electron transport chain can lead to electron leak and the generation of ROS in mitochondria, these organelles are also enriched with antioxidant systems including manganese SOD, glutathione, thioredoxin, and thioredoxin reductase. Mitochondrial regulation of ROS and reactive nitric oxide species represents a major mechanism for protecting against oxidative injury in the CNS.[21] In some conditions, mitochondria can be released and transferred between cells.[22] For example, retinal neurons may transfer mitochondria to astrocytes for disposal and recycling.[23] Some mitochondrial components may contain damage-associated molecular pattern motifs and thus act as "danger signals."[24] For example, astrocytes may sense stress and transfer mitochondria into adjacent neurons at risk as a "help me" signal.[22] This may in part involve calcium-dependent release; tunneling nanotubes can also allow mitochondria to move between cells.[22]

GENERAL FEATURES OF MITOCHONDRIAL DISORDERS

Mitochondrial disorders can be broadly categorized into those primarily affecting OXPHOS and cell metabolism (classical mitochondrial disorders); those primarily affecting mitostasis; and neurodegenerative disorders affecting axonal transport or autophagy. Genetic mutations that disrupt nuclear DNA, mtDNA replication, its transcription into mRNA, or its translation are the most common cause of mitochondrial disease. These disorders lead to impaired OXPHOS due to failure in the assembly of respiratory chain. Primary disorders of mitostasis are caused by mutations of proteins involved in mitochondrial fusion, fission, protein quality control, and mitophagy. Adult neurodegenerative disorders associated with impaired mitochondrial transport and autophagy include tauopathies, Parkinson disease (PD), motor neuron disease, and peripheral neuropathy. Mitochondrial diseases are a group of genetic disorders that are characterized by dysfunctional mitochondria. There are several comprehensive reviews on mitochondrial disorders,[25–35] and only selected aspects will be emphasized in this chapter.

Disease Mechanisms in Classical Mitochondrial Disorders

The pathophysiology of mitochondrial diseases is complex, as they may result from mutations in mtDNA or nuclear DNA. Mitochondrial diseases can therefore have may any pattern of inheritance, including maternal inheritance for mtDNA mutations and autosomal and X-linked inheritance for nuclear DNA mutations; there are also reported sporadic cases due to de novo mutations. Mitochondrial DNA may be prone to point mutations due to its proximity to the respiratory chain predisposing to base damage by ROS, but has robust base excision-repair mechanisms. Most mtDNA single deletions occur in regions flanked by small repeat sequences and can occur during the repair process. Pathogenic mutations have been reported in all mitochondrial DNA genes. The largest group of primary OXPHOS defect genes encode structural subunits of one of the five respiratory chain complexes, factors required for their assembly, or biogenesis of the electron carriers CoQ (ubiquinone) and cytochrome c. Mitochondrial disorders are clinically and genetically heterogeneous, can present at any age, and manifest with a wide range of symptoms. They most often affect tissues that are highly dependent on aerobic metabolism, such as the brain, skeletal muscle, eyes, heart, and liver. In patients with mtDNA mutations the clinical presentation is further complicated by the presence of multiple mtDNA genomes in an individual cell, which can often lead to a mixture of mutated and wild-type genomes (heteroplasmy). The level of heteroplasmy is crucial in determining the extent of cellular dysfunction.

Mutations of mtDNA can be classified into mtDNA rearrangements (for example, sporadic, single, large-scale mtDNA deletions), mutations in genes involved in protein synthesis (for example, mutations in mitochondrial tRNA or mRNA), or mutations in genes encoding structural proteins such as respiratory chain subunits. Mendelian mitochondrial disorders due to nuclear DNA mutations include defects in mtDNA maintenance, mtDNA translation and mitochondrial homeostasis. Defects in mtDNA maintenance include mutations affecting mtDNA replication, deoxynucleotide triphosphate synthesis and/or salvage, mtDNA translation, mitochondrial tRNA-modifying proteins, mitochondrial mRNA-processing enzymes, mitochondrial aminoacyl-tRNA synthetases, or mitoribosomal proteins.

Consequences of Mitochondrial Dysfunction

The two major consequences of mitochondrial dysfunction are OXPHOS defects leading to impaired ATP synthesis and reduction of the mitochondrial membrane potential. Inadequate ATP synthesis results in inability to sustain the high energy demands of neurons, astrocytes, skeletal muscle cells, cardiomyocytes, and other tissues. Inadequate ATP synthesis can also increase the AMP/ATP ratio, leading to activation of AMPK and its multiple downstream signaling cascades. The decrease in the mitochondrial membrane potential, which is due to restriction of electron transfer and proton pumping, impairs not only ATP production but also synthesis of Fe-S clusters, mitochondrial import of many nuclear-encoded proteins, and import of Ca^{2+} from the cytosol and the ER. Inability of the mitochondria to sequester Ca^{2+} and prevent aberrant Ca^{2+} accumulation promote induction of cell death by opening of the mitochondrial permeability transition pore. Mitochondria with decreased membrane potential are also prone to cleavage of OPA1, triggering mitochondrial fission; and to stabilization and accumulation of PINK1 in the outer mitochondrial membrane, which triggers mitophagy. OXPHOS complexes I and III are the major sites of mitochondrial ROS generation. Whereas modest increase in ROS levels can trigger protective antioxidant responses, excessive production results in oxidation of proteins, lipids, and nucleic acid and triggers cell stress responses or cell death. Excessive ROS production may result from mutations affecting complexes I, III, and V or proteins that are key to ROS homeostasis. Defects in complex I inhibit NADH oxidation, leading to a decrease in NAD/NADH ratio, as reflected by an increase in plasma hydroxyacylcarnitine to acylcarnitine ratio. Decreased NAD^+ levels also inhibit SIRT1-PGC1α signaling and may potentially downregulate mitochondrial biogenesis. Mitochondrial disorders may also affect Krebs cycle intermediates and folate cycle, and lead to accumulation of toxic substances. For example, increased 2-ketoglutarate rate levels results in increased production of the 2-hydroxglutarate, which can inhibit enzymes such as hypoxia-inducible factor prolyl hydroxylases, leading to activation of hypoxic signaling and epigenetic changes. Increased levels of succinate lead to protein succinylation and transcriptional changes predisposing to tumors such as paragangliomas, pheochromocytomas, gliomas, and myomas.

PRIMARY DISORDERS OF MITOCHONDRIAL DNA

Classical Syndromes

The classical syndromes due to mtDNA mutations in adults include Leber hereditary optic neuropathy (LHON); Kearns-Sayre syndrome (KSS); mitochondrial encephalomyopathy, lactic acidosis, and stroke-like episodes (MELAS); myoclonic epilepsy with ragged red fibers (MERRF); and neuropathy, ataxia, and retinitis pigmentosa

(NARP). LHON is characterized by subacute, sequential, painless visual loss; whereas it typically occurs in isolation, it may be associated with multiple-sclerosis-like features (Harding syndrome). LHON is associated with mtDNA mutations affecting subunits of complex I, such as 11778 G>A (*MT-ND4* gene) 14448 T>C (*MT-ND6*) and 3460 G>A (*MT-ND1*). The axons of the optic nerve are unmyelinated before crossing the lamina cribosa and highly myelinated thereafter; the prelaminar axons are highly dependent OXPHOS and this explains the selective vulnerability of retinal ganglion cells in LHON. The various manifestations of KSS, MELAS, and MERRF exemplify the clinical complexity of mitochondrial disorders. In addition to their classical manifestations, clinical features suggestive of mitochondrial disease include short stature, sensorineural deafness, diabetes mellitus, pigmentary retinopathy, and lactic acidosis. KSS is associated with single large-scale mtDNA deletions and is usually sporadic. It is characterized by progressive external ophthalmoplegia, pigmentary retinopathy (due to degeneration of rod photoreceptors), elevated CSF protein (> 1 g/dl, due to involvement of the choroid plexus), cerebellar ataxia, cardiac conduction defects, myopathy, bulbar weakness, and dementia. MELAS is characterized by stroke-like episodes and can also include cerebellar ataxia, encephalopathy, seizures, cardiomyopathy, myopathy, and lactic acidosis. MERRF is characterized by progressive myoclonic epilepsy, ataxia, weakness, cardiomyopathy, myopathy, cardiac conduction detects and lactic acidosis. MELAS and MERFF are due to several mtDNA mutations or variants affecting transfer RNAs (*MT-T* genes) that globally affect mitochondrial protein synthesis. MELAS is associated with mutations of the *MT-TL1* gene encoding leucine tRNA; the most common mutation (3243A>G) leads to synthesis of unstable proteins that are inserted into the inner membranes, and recognized by chaperones for their extraction and degradation by proteases. MERRF is typically caused by mutations of the *MT-TK* gene encoding lysine tRNA; the most common mutation (8344A>G) results in stalling of the ribosome during translation elongation. NARP is due to m8993T>C mtDNA mutations of the *MT-ATP6* gene encoding mitochondrial ATPase 6. It is characterized by early childhood or adult-onset onset sensorimotor neuropathy, ataxia, and pigmentary retinopathy that can remain quiescent or stable into adulthood or can include seizures, learning disability, basal ganglia abnormalities, cardiac conduction defects, and other manifestations that form a clinical continuum with Leigh syndrome.

DISORDERS OF NUCLEAR DNA

Mutations Affecting Mitochondrial DNA Maintenance, Replication, and/or Repair

Disorders of mtDNA maintenance can cause mitochondrial DNA depletion or multiple deletions. Chronic progressive external ophthalmoplegia (CPEO) is an important clinical feature of mitochondrial disorders, and can be associated with several mutations affecting nuclear DNA. These disorders may originate from mutations affecting the core mtDNA replication machinery including POLG and Twinkle or from defects in nucleotide synthesis that lead to imbalance in the nucleotide pools. Mutations of the *POLG1* and *POLG2* genes encoding different subunits of mtDNA polymerase γ are the most common nuclear cause of mitochondrial disease. Autosomal recessive *POLG* mutations can cause a range of syndromes that differ in age of onset, severity, and combination of neurologic symptoms with muscle, liver, gut, or renal involvement. Infantile-onset forms include Alpers syndrome with mitochondrial DNA depletion. Some childhood onset disorders associated with mutations of the *POLG* gene are characterized by prominent ataxia and sensory axonal neuropathy. Examples include mitochondrial recessive ataxia syndrome and sensory ataxia neuropathy, dysarthria, and ophthalmoplegia (SANDO). Autosomal dominant *POLG* mutations can cause CPEO associated with ataxia, sensory peripheral neuropathy, parkinsonism, epilepsy, and premature ovarian failure. The spectrum of phenotypes associated with *POLG* mutations has led to the term POLG-related disorder. There is only a weak correlation between the specific *POLG* mutation and the phenotype. Autosomal dominant mutations of the *TWNK* gene encoding the mtDNA helicase Twinkle can cause isolated CPEO with or without proximal myopathy, exercise intolerance, sensorineural hearing loss, or parkinsonism, while recessive mutations cause a mtDNA depletion syndrome manifesting with early onset hepatic encephalopathy or with Perrault syndrome (deafness and gonadal dysgenesis).

Defects Affecting the Deoxynucleotide Triphosphate Pool (mtDNA Depletion Syndromes)

An adequate and balanced pool of deoxynucleotide triphosphates is necessary to provide precursors for mtDNA replication. A prototype disorder due to deficits of enzymes that control this balance is mitochondrial neurogastrointestinal encephalopathy (MNGIE) caused by mutations of the *TYMP* gene encoding thymidine phosphorylase. This disorder manifests with gastrointestinal dysmotility, CPEO, cachexia, demyelinating peripheral neuropathy and leukoencephalopathy due to depleted thymidine monophosphate activity. Other examples are mutations of the *TK* gene encoding thymidine kinase 2 producing ptosis, proximal myopathy, dysphagia, and respiratory insufficiency, and mutations of the *DGUOK* gene encoding deoxyguanosine kinase and producing limb girdle weakness, exercise intolerance, and muscle cramps.

Mutations Primarily Affecting OXPHOS Biogenesis

Pathogenic mutations have been reported in all mitochondrial OXPHOS genes. The largest group affects structural subunits of one of the five OXPHOS complexes, factors required for their assembly, or electron carriers such as coenzyme Q (CoQ or ubiquinone) and cytochrome c. Direct hit mutations affect nuclear DNA; they may affect any of all five complexes but most frequently involve the large complex I. The classical phenotype is Leigh syndrome, which is genetically very heterogeneous and can also be caused by mtDNA mutations. This disorder is characterized by acute episodes of neurodevelopmental regression followed by partial recovery, hypotonia, dystonia, hypopnea, dysphagia, encephalopathy, epilepsy, blindness, failure to thrive, and bilateral symmetric lesions throughout the CNS, particularly the basal ganglia, thalamus, brainstem, and cerebellar fastigial nuclei.

The respiratory chain subunits encoded by nuclear DNA must be correctly translated, transported, and directed to the mitochondrial inner membrane; assemble with other subunits; acquire prosthetic groups; and further assemble into supercomplexes. Mutations in genes involved in these pathways are referred to as "indirect" hits that affect OXPHOS function. For example, mutations of *SURF1* encoding an assembly factor for COX produces a phenotype that partially overlaps with that of Leigh syndrome and more often manifests with leukodystrophy and cardiomyopathy. Primary CoQ10 (ubiquinone) deficiency is included in the differential diagnosis of juvenile ataxias and infantile encephalomyopathies but may also produce steroid-responsive nephrotic syndrome and may show benefit from CoQ_{10} supplementation. Although primary CoQ10 deficiency often manifests with multisystem involvement, it can also lead to isolated myopathy.

Mutations Affecting Biogenesis of Fe-S Clusters

As mentioned earlier in this chapter, Fe-S clusters are found in OXPHOS complexes I–III and in other mitochondrial and cellular enzymes involved in steps of the Krebs cycle, fatty acid oxidation, and amino acid synthesis.[12] The most common neurologic disorder associated with impaired of Fe-S cluster biogenesis is Friedreich ataxia. This disorder is due to homozygous GAA (guanine-adenine-adenine) trinucleotide repeat expansion in the first intron of the frataxin (*FXN*) (*FTN*) gene on the long arm of chromosome 9 or less commonly by point mutations. Loss of frataxin function affects mitochondrial iron metabolism resulting in deficits of respiratory chain complexes, and metabolic enzymes such as aconitase, intracellular iron accumulation, and oxidative damage. Friedreich ataxia affects metabolically active cells such as large dorsal root ganglion and corticospinal neurons and manifests with cerebellar ataxia, oculomotor findings (square-wave jerks), severe proprioceptive sensory loss, areflexia, and Babinski sign. Associated findings include pas cavus, scoliosis, hypertrophic cardiomyopathy, and diabetes. Other disorders due to impaired Fe-S cluster biogenesis include X-linked sideroblastic anemia and ataxia due to mutations of the *ABCB7* gene encoding the ATP-binding cassette, subfamily B member 7 transporter present in the inner mitochondrial membrane; myopathies associated with *ISCU* mutations affecting the iron-sulfur complex scaffold protein and *FDX2* mutations affecting ferredoxin.[12] Mutations of the *BCS1L* encoding a protein involved in the assembly of Complex III produce GRACILE syndrome (growth retardation, aminoaciduria, cholestasis, iron overload, lactic acidosis, and early death) but may also manifest in adults with aminoaciduria, seizures, bilateral sensorineural deafness, and learning difficulties.[36]

Other Disorders Affecting Mitochondrial Biogenesis

In addition to genetic disorders affecting assembly of Fe-S clusters, other genes affect general mitochondrial biogenesis or homeostasis, including protein import, mitochondrial lipid or membrane composition, cristae organization, or quality control. One important example of impaired mitochondrial quality control is autosomal recessive complex hereditary spastic paraplegia due to mutations of the paraplegin (*SPG7*) gene, which is a component of the mAAA protease system involved in protein quality control. Clinical manifestations include spastic paraplegia, ataxia, optic atrophy, myopathy, and cerebellar atrophy. Mutations of the *AFG3L2* gene encoding AFG3L2 matrix AAA peptidase subunit-2, which is part of this protease complex, produce a similar phenotype known as autosomal dominant spinocerebellar ataxia type 28 (SCA28). Mutations of the *TAZ* gene encoding tafazzin, which catalyzes a transacylation step for remodeling of cardiolipin in the mitochondria inner membrane produce Barth syndrome, an X-linked disorder associated with myopathy, cardiomyopathy, neutropenia, exercise intolerance, and growth delay; this disorder may be amenable to enzyme restitution therapy using adenoviral vectors.[37] Mutations in the *ATAD3A* gene encoding the ATPase family AAA domain-containing protein 3 (ATAD3) that is crucial for normal mitochondrial-ER interactions results in cerebellar ataxia and dystonia.

DISORDERS OF MITOSTASIS

Disorders of fusion

Mutations of the *MFN2* gene encoding the outer mitochondrial membrane fusion protein MFN2 are a frequent cause of axonal Charcot-Marie-Tooth disease (CMT) type 2A. The age of onset varies from early childhood to adult life. The neuropathy ranges from a pure motor to sensorimotor phenotype, sometimes resulting in profound loss of proprioception. Up to 10%–20% of the affected subjects with early onset severe disease have optic atrophy. Cerebral white matter involvement with T2 hyperintensities can accompany the peripheral neuropathy. Loss-of-function mutations of the *OPA1* gene producing OPA1 haploinsufficency are responsible for the majority of cases of autosomal dominant optic atrophy (ADOA), which is the most common inherited optic nerve disease and is characterized by insidious-onset symmetrical visual loss typically starting in childhood. The age of onset, clinical course, and autosomal dominant inheritance distinguish *OPA1*-related ADOA from LHON. In addition to isolated optic neuropathy, *OPA1* mutations can produce a multisystem neurological disease that manifests with a variable combination of optic atrophy, sensorineural deafness, peripheral neuropathy, ataxia, myopathy, CPEO, spastic paraparesis of adult onset, and multiple sclerosis-like phenotype.

Disorders of Fission

A mutation in *DLP1* gene encoding Drp1 causes a lethal neurological disorder characterized by microcephaly, abnormal brain development, optic atrophy, truncal hypotonia, dysmorphism, lactic acidosis and elevated very long-chain fatty acid concentration. Recent evidence indicates that mitochondrial fission also has a major role in the pathogenesis neurodegenerative disorders, such as Huntington disease.[38] Mutant, but not normal huntingtin interacts with Drp1 and promotes mitochondrial fragmentation and loss of bidirectional mitochondrial transport. Mitochondrial fragmentation and redistribution may also have a pivotal role in mitochondria dysfunction and neuron apoptosis associated with abnormal prion protein accumulation.[39] Mutations of the *GDAP1* gene encoding ganglioside-induced differentiation-associated protein 1, which is anchored to the outer mitochondrial membrane and regulates fission, are responsible for CMT4A. This autosomal recessive sensorimotor neuropathy can be either predominantly axonal or demyelinating, and manifests in the neonatal period or early infancy with distal muscle weakness and atrophy, followed by development of vocal cord paresis.

Disorders of Mitophagy

Parkin (*PARK2*) and PINK1 (*PARK3*) mutations are associated with autosomal recessive early-onset Parkinson disease (PD). *PARK2* is the leading gene and accounts for almost 50% of familial and 18% of sporadic cases. However, *PARK2* mutations have also been detected in patients with adult-onset parkinsonism, clinically indistinguishable from idiopathic PD. Early-onset PD due to *PINK1* mutation, unlike *PARK2*-related early onset PD, is associated with Lewy body pathology.

SECONDARY INVOLVEMENT OF MITOCHONDRIA IN NEURODEGENERATION

Mitochondria are involved in essentially all neurodegenerative disorders.[40] They have a major role in mechanisms of cell death by apoptosis, production of damaging ROS, and impairment of axonal transport and other vital neuronal functions. Mitochondria are also a target of proteinopathies or other mechanisms of neurodegeneration. For example, accumulation of hyperphosphorylated tau may affect mitochondrial function by impairing mitochondrial transport, morphology, and bioenergetics.[41] Pathological tau impairs anterograde transport while promoting retrograde mitochondrial transport. Overexpression of tau enhances mitochondrial fusion producing perinuclear distribution of mitochondria, in part due to impaired ubiquitination and degradation of MFN2. Hyperphosphorylated tau also affects mitochondrial fission in part by interacting with Drp1 and may also alter mitochondrial membrane potential, promoting membrane permeability transition and apoptosis. Mitochondrial dysfunction also has a major role in amyotrophic lateral sclerosis (ALS), some forms of hereditary spastic paraplegia, cerebellar ataxia, and hereditary peripheral neuropathy. For example, RNA/DNA-binding proteins involved in ALS, such as TAR DNA binding protein (TDP)-43 and fused in sarcoma (FUS) are strongly linked to mitochondrial dysfunction.[42] Studies in animal models show changes in mitochondrial structure, plasticity, replication/copy number, mitochondrial DNA instability, and altered membrane potential in several subsets of motor neuron disorders. These mitochondrial abnormalities begin prior to the clinical and pathological onset of the disease. For example, there are defects in DNA break-ligation mediated by DNA ligase 3 (LIG3) which is necessary for both mitochondrial DNA replication and repair in FUS-associated ALS.[42]

KEY POINTS

- Mitochondria have a critical role in intermediate metabolism, oxidative phosphorylation (OXPHOS); reactive oxygen species (ROS) production; synthesis of iron-sulfur (Fe-S) clusters; maintenance of intracellular calcium (Ca^{2+}) homeostasis; and metabolism of lipids, amino acids, nucleotides, and heme.
- Mitostasis depends on the interplay among mitochondrial biogenesis, protein quality control, fusion and fission, motility and docking, and clearance by mitophagy.
- Mitochondria DNA (mtDNA) encodes about 1% of all mitochondria proteins; most genes involved in maintenance of mitochondrial function are encoded by nuclear DNA.
- Synthesis mtDNA depends on DNA polymerase gamma (POLG) and associated factors.
- Mitochondrial proteins are subject to a tight quality control by ATP-dependent proteases such as paraplegin, which degrade misfolded proteins.
- The contacts sites between the outer mitochondrial membrane and the endoplasmic reticulum (ER) have a major role in mitochondrial Ca^{2+} homeostasis, lipid transfer, and mitochondrial fission and fusion events.
- Complex I, III, and IV contain several subunits encoded both by nuclear and mitochondrial DNA, complex II subunits are encoded only by nuclear DNA.

- The mitochondrial respiratory chain is a major source of ROS, which are important signaling and potentially toxic molecules and may trigger mitohormesis.
- The mitochondrial Ca^{2+} uniporter mediates Ca^{2+} entry to the mitochondria and interacts with mitochondria Ca^{2+} uptake proteins.
- Calcium exerts multiple physiological effects in mitochondria regulating the Krebs cycle and ATP production.
- Mitochondria participate in long-chain fatty acid β-oxidation, steroidogenesis, and synthesis of coenzyme Q.
- In mitochondria, iron is primarily used for heme synthesis, Fe-S cluster biogenesis, and iron storage.
- Synthesis of Fe-S clusters requires a multimeric core complex that includes frataxin.
- Mitochondrial fusion depends on both mitofusin 2 (MFN2) and optic atrophy 1 protein (OPA1).
- Mitochondrial fission depends on dynamin-like/related protein 1 (DLP1/Drp1).
- Mitochondrial transport requires the mitochondrial Rho GTPase (MIRO) that binds to kinesin-1 or dynein motors via the trafficking kinesin binding protein (TRAK).
- Mitochondrial docking maintains at regions that require high ATP production and Ca^{2+} buffering, and is primarily triggered by increase in intracellular Ca^{2+}.
- Mitophagy targets mitochondria for destruction by the lysosome; it involves PINK1 (phosphatase-tensin homolog-induced putative kinase 1) and Parkin.
- Mitochondrial disorders include those primarily affecting OXPHOS; those affecting mitostasis; and neurodegenerative disorders affecting axonal transport or autophagy.
- The clinical presentation of mtDNA mutations is complicated due to heteroplasmy.
- The classical syndromes due to mtDNA mutations in adults include Leber hereditary optic neuropathy (LHON); Kearns-Sayre syndrome (KSS); mitochondrial encephalomyopathy, lactic acidosis, and stroke-like episodes (MELAS); myoclonic epilepsy with ragged red fibers (MERRF); and neuropathy, ataxia, and retinitis pigmentosa (NARP).
- *POLG* mutations are the most common nuclear cause of mitochondrial disease and can cause a range of syndromes including ataxia and sensory neuropathy, CPEO, parkinsonism, and epilepsy.
- Friedreich ataxia is due to impaired Fe-S cluster biogenesis.
- *SPG7* mutations affecting paraplegin impair mitochondrial protein quality control and produce autosomal recessive complex hereditary spastic paraplegia.
- *MFN2* mutations are the most frequent cause of axonal Charcot-Marie-Tooth disease (CMT) type 2A.
- *OPA1* mutations are responsible for the majority of cases of autosomal dominant optic atrophy.
- Abnormal mitochondrial fission is a prominent mechanism in neurodegenerative disorders such as Huntington disease.
- Parkin (*PARK2*) and PINK1 (*PARK3*) mutations are associated with autosomal recessive early-onset Parkinson disease (PD).
- Mitochondrial dysfunction is prominent in the pathogenesis of essentially all neurodegenerative disorders, including tauopathies and ALS.

REFERENCES

1. Milane L, Trivedi M, Singh A, Talekar M, Amiji M. Mitochondrial biology, targets, and drug delivery. J Control Release 2015;207:40–58.
2. Pfanner N, Warscheid B, Wiedemann N. Mitochondrial proteins: from biogenesis to functional networks. Nat Rev Mol Cell Biol 2019;20:267–284.
3. Glynn SE. Multifunctional mitochondrial AAA proteases. Front Mol Biosci 2017;4:34.
4. Levytskyy RM, Bohovych I, Khalimonchuk O. Metalloproteases of the inner mitochondrial membrane. Biochemistry 2017;56:4737–4746.
5. Steele TE, Glynn SE. Mitochondrial AAA proteases: a stairway to degradation. Mitochondrion 2019;49:121–127.
6. Tepikin AV. Mitochondrial junctions with cellular organelles: Ca(2+) signalling perspective. Pflugers Arch 2018;470:1181–1192.
7. Logan CV, Szabadkai G, Sharpe JA, et al. Loss-of-function mutations in MICU1 cause a brain and muscle disorder linked to primary alterations in mitochondrial calcium signaling. Nat Genet 2014;46:188–193.
8. Doghman-Bouguerra M, Lalli E. The ER-mitochondria couple: in life and death from steroidogenesis to tumorigenesis. Mol Cell Endocrinol 2017;441:176–184.
9. Issop L, Rone MB, Papadopoulos V. Organelle plasticity and interactions in cholesterol transport and steroid biosynthesis. Mol Cell Endocrinol 2013;371:34–46.
10. Awad AM, Bradley MC, Fernandez-Del-Rio L, Nag A, Tsui HS, Clarke CF. Coenzyme Q10 deficiencies: pathways in yeast and humans. Essays Biochem 2018;62:361–376.
11. Ward DM, Cloonan SM. Mitochondrial iron in human health and disease. Annu Rev Physiol 2018;81:453–482.
12. Cardenas-Rodriguez M, Chatzi A, Tokatlidis K. Iron-sulfur clusters: from metals through mitochondria biogenesis to disease. J Biol Inorg Chem 2018;23:509–520.
13. Picard M. Mitochondrial synapses: intracellular communication and signal integration. Trends Neurosci 2015;38:468–474.
14. Misgeld T, Schwarz TL. Mitostasis in neurons: maintaining mitochondria in an extended cellular architecture. Neuron 2017;96:651–666.

15. Tilokani L, Nagashima S, Paupe V, Prudent J. Mitochondrial dynamics: overview of molecular mechanisms. Essays Biochem 2018;62:341–360.
16. Barnhart EL. Mechanics of mitochondrial motility in neurons. Curr Opin Cell Biol 2016;38:90–99.
17. Panchal K, Tiwari AK. Mitochondrial dynamics, a key executioner in neurodegenerative diseases. Mitochondrion 2018;47:151–173.
18. Pareyson D, Saveri P, Sagnelli A, Piscosquito G. Mitochondrial dynamics and inherited peripheral nerve diseases. Neurosci Lett 2015;596:66–77.
19. Pickrell AM, Youle RJ. The roles of PINK1, parkin, and mitochondrial fidelity in Parkinson's disease. Neuron 2015;85:257–273.
20. Suomalainen A, Battersby BJ. Mitochondrial diseases: the contribution of organelle stress responses to pathology. Nat Rev Mol Cell Biol 2018;19:77–92.
21. Perez-Pinzon MA, Stetler RA, Fiskum G. Novel mitochondrial targets for neuroprotection. J Cereb Blood Flow Metab 2012;32:1362–1376.
22. Hayakawa K, Bruzzese M, Chou SH, Ning M, Ji X, Lo EH. Extracellular mitochondria for therapy and diagnosis in acute central nervous system injury. JAMA Neurol 2018;75:119–122.
23. Davis CH, Kim KY, Bushong EA, et al. Transcellular degradation of axonal mitochondria. Proc Natl Acad Sci U S A 2014;111:9633–9638.
24. Galluzzi L, Kepp O, Kroemer G. Mitochondria: master regulators of danger signalling. Nat Rev Mol Cell Biol 2012;13:780–788.
25. Burte F, Carelli V, Chinnery PF, Yu-Wai-Man P. Disturbed mitochondrial dynamics and neurodegenerative disorders. Nat Rev Neurol 2015;11:11–24.
26. Gorman GS, Chinnery PF, DiMauro S, et al. Mitochondrial diseases. Nat Rev Dis Primers 2016;2:16080.
27. Frazier AE, Thorburn DR, Compton AG. Mitochondrial energy generation disorders: genes, mechanisms and clues to pathology. J Biol Chem 2019;294:5386–5395.
28. Koopman WJ, Distelmaier F, Smeitink JA, Willems PH. OXPHOS mutations and neurodegeneration. EMBO J 2013;32:9–29.
29. Mayr JA, Haack TB, Freisinger P, et al. Spectrum of combined respiratory chain defects. J Inherit Metab Dis 2015;38:629–640.
30. McFarland R, Taylor RW, Turnbull DM. A neurological perspective on mitochondrial disease. Lancet Neurol 2010;9:829–840.
31. Murayama K, Shimura M, Liu Z, Okazaki Y, Ohtake A. Recent topics: the diagnosis, molecular genesis, and treatment of mitochondrial diseases. J Hum Genet 2019;64:113–125.
32. Nightingale H, Pfeffer G, Bargiela D, Horvath R, Chinnery PF. Emerging therapies for mitochondrial disorders. Brain 2016;139:1633–1648.
33. Schapira AH. Mitochondrial diseases. Lancet 2012;379:1825–1834.
34. Schon EA, Przedborski S. Mitochondria: the next (neurode) generation. Neuron 2011;70:1033–1053.
35. Craven L, Alston CL, Taylor RW, Turnbull DM. Recent advances in mitochondrial disease. Annu Rev Genomics Hum Genet 2017;18:257–275.
36. Olahova M, Ceccatelli Berti C, Collier JJ, et al. Molecular genetic investigations identify new clinical phenotypes associated with BCS1L-related mitochondrial disease. Hum Mol Genet 2019;28:3766–3776.
37. Finsterer J. Barth syndrome: mechanisms and management. Appl Clin Genet 2019;12:95–106.
38. Joshi AU, Ebert AE, Haileselassie B, Mochly-Rosen D. Drp1/Fis1-mediated mitochondrial fragmentation leads to lysosomal dysfunction in cardiac models of Huntington's disease. J Mol Cell Cardiol 2019;127:125–133.
39. Li C, Wang D, Wu W, et al. DLP1-dependent mitochondrial fragmentation and redistribution mediate prion-associated mitochondrial dysfunction and neuronal death. Aging Cell 2018;17:e12693.
40. Johri A, Beal MF. Mitochondrial dysfunction in neurodegenerative diseases. J Pharmacol Exp Ther 2012;342:619–630.
41. Perez MJ, Jara C, Quintanilla RA. Contribution of tau pathology to mitochondrial impairment in neurodegeneration. Front Neurosci 2018;12:441.
42. Kodavati M, Wang H, Hegde ML. Altered mitochondrial dynamics in motor neuron disease: an emerging perspective. Cells 2020;9:1065–1088.

12 Mechanisms of Cell Death and Axonal Degeneration

OVERVIEW

Cell death is defined as either irreversible membrane permeabilization or complete cell fragmentation. There are two major categories of cell death.[1,2] "Accidental" cell death occurs upon exposure to very harsh environment, such as shear forces that produce mechanical disassembly of cellular components, as occurs in traumatic injury. Cells undergoing accidental death release endogenous molecules known as damage-associated molecular patterns (DAMPs) that may have either cytotoxic or immunomodulatory effect. DAMPs can propagate the cytotoxic response elicited by traumatic injury either directly or upon involvement of the innate immune system, which triggers death of surrounding cells that survived the initial insult. The second and more common form of cell death is "regulated" cell death, which occurs in cells that experience moderate but unsolvable perturbation of homeostasis. Regulated cell death involves activation of different molecular machineries that are activated in the context of an adaptive response to cell stress that fails to restore homeostasis. Regulated cell death is typically triggered by DNA damage, accumulation of misfolded proteins in the endoplasmic reticulum (ER), or excessive production of reactive oxygen species (ROS). External stimuli such as activation of death receptors, including tumor necrosis factor receptors (TNFRs) can also trigger regulated cell death. A specific form of regulated cell death is "programmed" cell death, which occurs at predetermined points during development, in the course of immune responses, or during maintenance of adult tissue homeostasis. There are several mechanistically distinct variants of regulated cell death that may occur in different time-dependent combinations upon exposure to the initiating stimulus (Figure 12.1). Many such mechanisms primarily or secondarily involve the mitochondria. Axonal injuries produce Wallerian degeneration and formation of axonal spheroids via molecular mechanisms different from those involved in apoptosis or autophagy. The main aims of this chapter are to review the basic mechanisms of (1) cell death triggered by cellular stressors, (2) cell death triggered during inflammatory responses, (3) redox signaling and oxidative stress, (5) excitotoxicity, (6) axonal degeneration, and (7) neuronal and axonal senescence and its role in neurodegeneration. Understanding of the basic mechanism of cell death is relevant for development of neuroprotective approaches.

MORPHOLOGICAL FEATURES AND BASIC MECHANISMS OF REGULATED CELL DEATH AND AXONAL DEGENERATION

Regulated cell death involves two components, initiation and execution. Initiation refers to the signal transduction events that activate executioner mechanisms. Execution refers to the biochemical events that directly lead to cell death.

Morphological Aspects

The two main morphological types of cell death are apoptosis and necrosis. Apoptosis (meaning "falling off") is characterized by shrinkage of the cytoplasm, chromatin condensation initiated at the nuclear membrane (marginalization) and then involving the whole nucleus (pyknosis), nuclear fragmentation (karyorrhexis), and blebbing of the membrane with the formation of apoptotic bodies. Apoptotic cells retain plasma membrane integrity and, to some degree, metabolic activity. Apoptotic cell death is followed by the rapid clearance by macrophages or other cells with phagocytic activity. Necrosis manifests with a generalized swelling of the cytoplasm and organelles

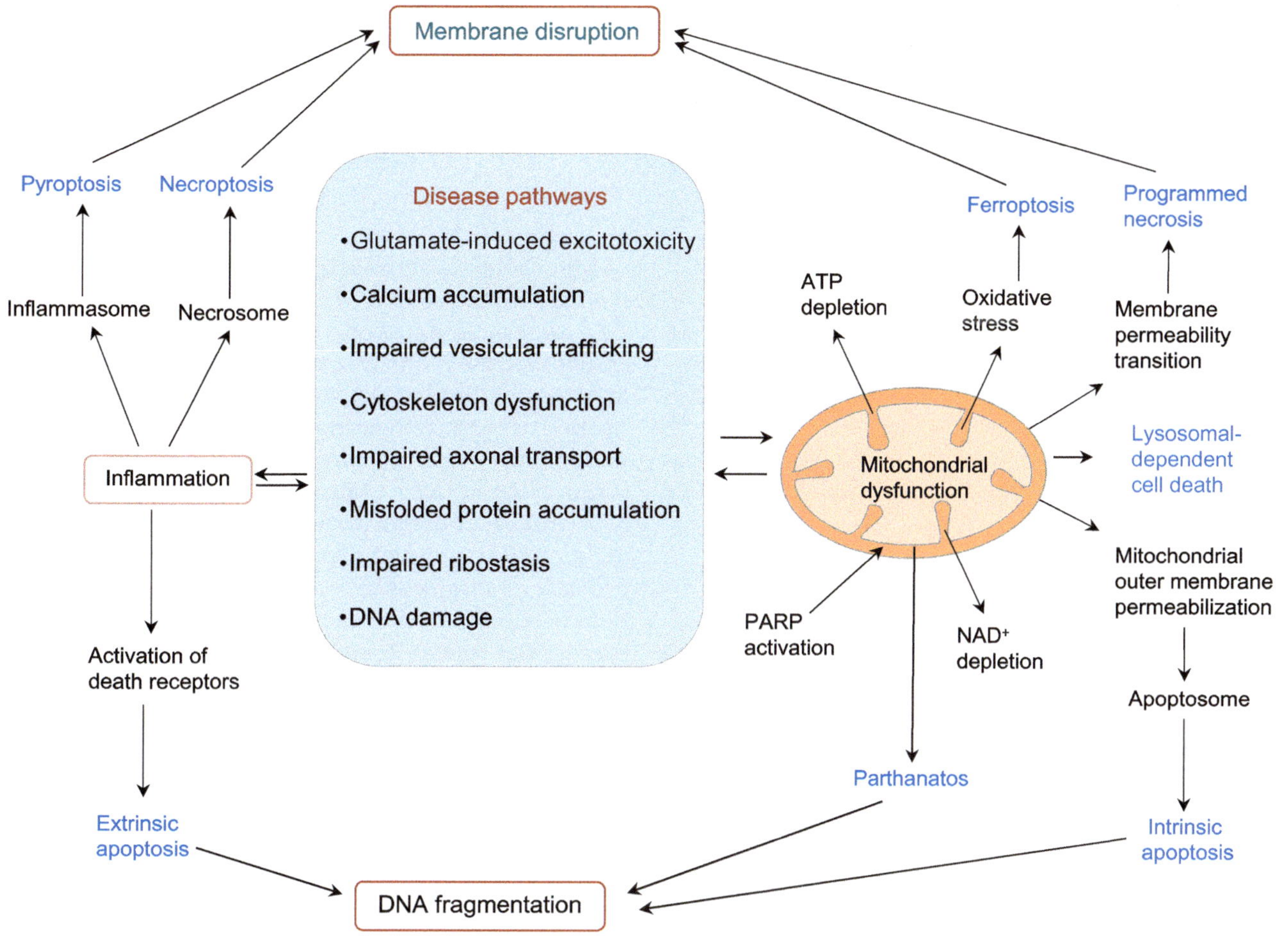

FIGURE 12.1 Mechanisms of regulated cell death.
The two main morphological types of cell death are apoptosis and necrosis. Many cell death mechanisms involve the mitochondria; they include intrinsic apoptosis; mitochondrial permeability transition-driven regulated necrosis and parthanatos. Ferroptosis is triggered by lipid peroxidation accelerated by intracellular iron, and like lysosomal-dependent cell death is triggered by membrane disturbances that can indirectly involve mitochondria. Regulated cell death can be triggered by exogenous stimuli during inflammation, such as activation of death receptors or pathogen molecular patterns that can trigger extrinsic apoptosis, necroptosis, and pyroptosis.

(oncosis), condensation of the chromatin in small and irregular patches, and dilatation of the nuclear membrane. Traumatic or ischemic injures that disconnect the neuronal cell body from the distal segment of the axon induce Wallerian degeneration, whereas genetic, degenerative, or inflammatory disorders lead to interruption of axonal transport and formation of large axonal swelling or spheroids. Dying-back axonopathy refers to the progressive distal-to-proximal axonal degeneration.

General Biochemical Mechanisms

The final common execution of the apoptotic death machinery is activation of cysteine proteases called caspases.[2] Major triggers of apoptosis are DNA damage, accumulation of misfolded proteins, activation of death receptors, or withdrawal of growth factors. Caspases are present in an inactive state (procaspases) and are activated by proteolytic cleavage. There are two main groups of caspases. Initiator caspases are activated as part of multiprotein complexes that vary according to the triggering stimulus. Once activated, initiator caspases cleave and activate the executioner caspases, which mediate the apoptotic death program, including DNA fragmentation. Necrosis typically occurs in the setting of mitochondrial failure, membrane lipid peroxidation, or formation of pore complexes in the plasma membrane. Events commonly involved in necrosis include disturbance in intracellular calcium (Ca^{2+}) homeostasis, oxidative stress, dissipation of mitochondrial potential, and impaired ATP production. Apoptosis and necrosis are not mutually exclusive forms of programmed cell and may occur sequentially in several conditions. For example, in ischemia, cells that are acutely deprived of ATP undergo necrotic cell death, whereas those exposed to lesser degree of ischemia and that have residual ATP stores may later undergo apoptosis. The key molecular mechanisms of Wallerian degeneration of axons converge on nicotinamide adenine dinucleotide (NAD^+) and involve a regulated axonal death program that leads to impaired axonal transport, mitochondrial dysfunction, increase in intra-axoplasmic Ca^{2+} and activation of proteases such as calpain.

REGULATED CELL DEATH TRIGGERED BY DISTURBANCES OF CELLULAR HOMEOSTASIS

The mitochondria is directly involved in cell death mechanisms triggered by disturbances of cell homeostasis, including intrinsic apoptosis, membrane transition pore-mediated necrosis, and parthanatos (Figure 12.2). Ferroptosis and lysosomal-dependent cell death are triggered by membrane disturbances that can also indirectly involve mitochondria.

Intrinsic Apoptosis

Intrinsic apoptosis is initiated by DNA damage, endoplasmic reticulum (ER) stress, reactive oxygen species (ROS) overload, and alteration in microtubule dynamics, among other triggers. The critical initial step is the irreversible and widespread mitochondrial outer membrane permeabilization (MOMP). This process is controlled by the antagonistic influence of antiapoptotic and proapoptotic members of the BCL2 (B-cell chronic lymphocytic leukemia/lymphoma 2) protein family. Antiapoptotic BCL2 family members, including BCL2 and BCL-XL (BCL2 like 1) and others, are normally inserted into the outer mitochondrial membrane and prevent the development of MOMP. Proapoptotic members, such as BAX (BCL2 associated X apoptosis regulator), BAK1 (BCL2 antagonist/killer 1) and BOK (BCL2 family apoptotic regulator) can form pores across the outer mitochondrial membrane, leading to MOMP in conditions of cell stress. Proapoptotic BH3-only proteins such as BIM (BCL2-interacting mediator of cell death) and BID (BH3-interacting domain death agonist) function as transducers of stress signaling. They transiently interact with and activate BAX and/or BAK, promoting their oligomerization in the outer mitochondrial membrane and the assembly of a lipidic pore that leads to MOMP. Mitochondrial outer membrane permeabilization allows release of apoptogenic factors that normally reside in the mitochondrial intermembrane space into the cytosol. One important example is cytochrome c, which in the cytosol binds to apoptotic peptidase-activating factor 1 (APAF1) and pro-caspase 9 (CASP9) in the presence of deoxyATP, leading to the formation of a supramolecular complex known as apoptosome. Within this complex, CASP9 becomes activated and catalyzes the proteolytic activation of the executioner caspases such as CASP3 (and CASP7). CASP3 elicits DNA fragmentation by inactivating a DNA fragmentation-inhibiting factor; and promotes formation of apoptotic bodies by triggering phosphatidylserine exposure from the inner to the outer membrane leaflet. A second apoptogenic factor released upon MOMP is the second mitochondrial activator of caspases (SMAC), which promotes apoptosis by binding to and inhibiting X-linked inhibitor of apoptosis (XIAP), a member of the protein family that counteracts apoptosis by physically blocking caspases.

Mitochondrial Permeability Transition-Driven Necrosis

Mitochondrial permeability transition-driven necrosis is typically initiated by severe oxidative stress and cytosolic Ca^{2+} overload. Mitochondrial permeability transition is the abrupt increase in the permeability of the inner mitochondrial membrane to small solutes, resulting in immediate dissipation of the mitochondrial membrane potential, massive water influx, osmotic organelle breakdown, and rapid drop of intracellular ATP availability. Mitochondrial permeability transition-driven necrosis results from the opening of the so-called permeability transition pore complex (PTPC), which is a supramolecular complex assembled at the junctions between the inner and the outer mitochondrial membranes. The composition and regulation of the PTPC are still incompletely defined. Cyclophilin D is required for induction of mitochondrial permeability transition, which may reflect its ability to control Ca^{2+} buffering of the mitochondria. Other proteins hypothesized to participate in the PTPC include the inorganic phosphate carrier, the inner mitochondrial membrane adenine nucleotide translocator, and the outer mitochondrial membrane voltage-dependent anion carrier. However, genetic studies indicate that these proteins are dispensable for PTPC formation. The role of the mitochondrial F_1F_0 ATPase within the PTPC is still incompletely established. Paraplegin, which is involved in mitochondrial protein quality control, may also be an essential component of the PTPC. Impaired activity of the inner mitochondrial membrane Ca^{2+} uniporter promotes mitochondrial Ca^{2+} overload and mitochondrial permeability transition-driven necrosis.

Parthanatos

Parthanatos is driven by the hyperactivation of poly (ADP-ribose) polymerase 1 (PARP1). PARP1 is a fundamental component of the DNA damage response machinery and utilizes NAD^+ and ATP to synthesize poly ADP-ribose (PAR) residues that can be added to a variety target proteins (PARylation). Parthanatos occurs in response to DNA damage, oxidative stress, hypoxia, hypoglycemia, inflammatory signals, and nitric oxide (NO). Excessive PARP1 activation elicits cytotoxic effects by several mechanisms. A major mechanism is depletion of both NAD^+ and ATP utilized for PAR synthesis, leading to eventual bioenergetic and redox collapse. Another important mechanism is accumulation of PAR polymers in the mitochondria and PARylation of a protein known as apoptosis-inducing factor mitochondria-associated 1 (AIF1). This promotes the release of AIF1 into the cytosol and its translocation into the nucleus, where it produces large-scale DNA fragmentation

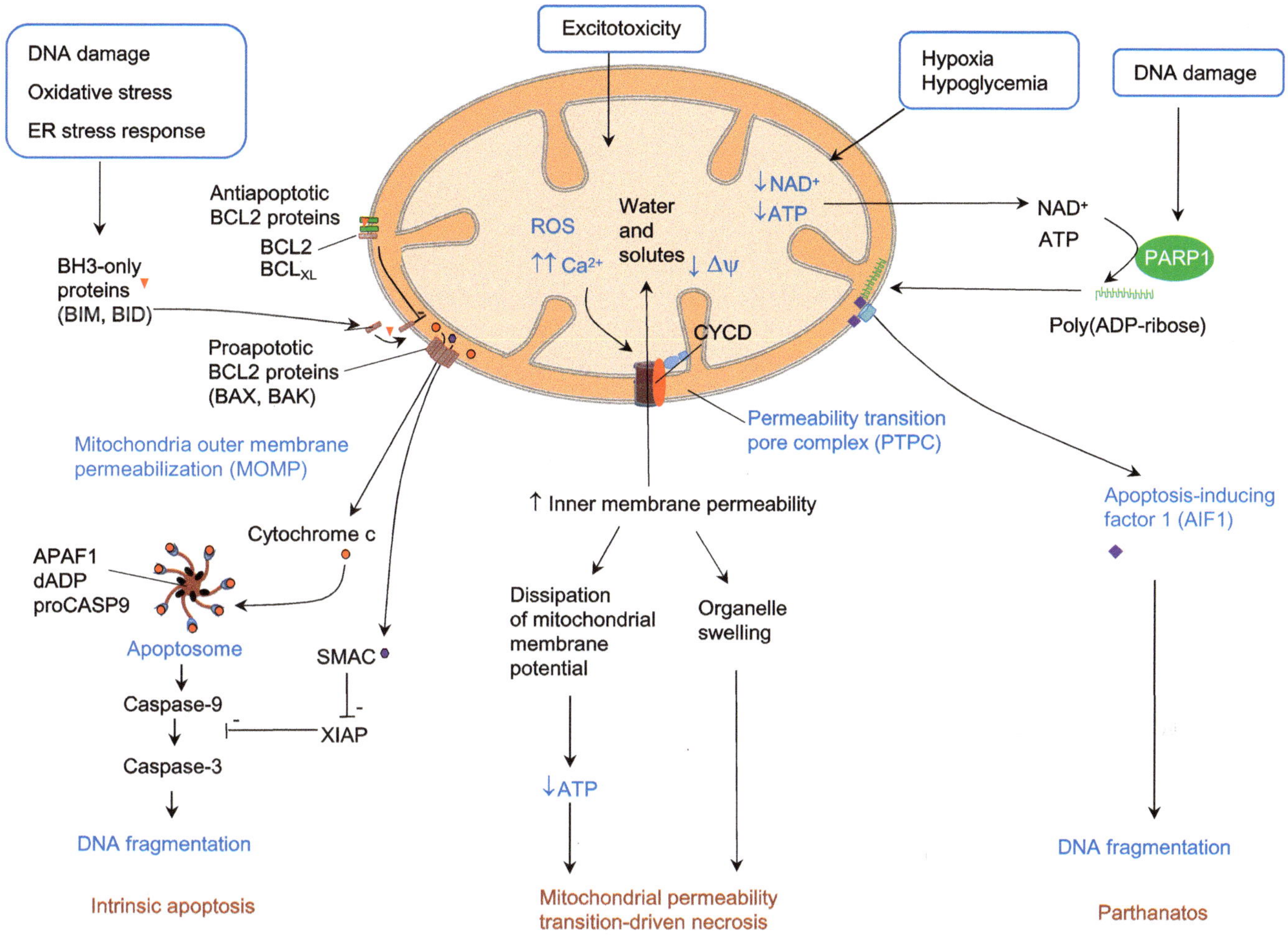

FIGURE 12.2 Role of the mitochondria in regulated cell death.

The mitochondria have a direct role in intrinsic apoptosis, membrane transition pore-mediated necrosis, and parthanatos. The critical step for intrinsic apoptosis is mitochondrial outer membrane permeabilization (MOMP), which is regulated by members of the BCL2 (B-cell chronic lymphocytic leukemia/lymphoma 2) protein family. Proapoptotic members, such as BCL2-associated X apoptosis regulator (BAX), BCL2 antagonist/killer 1 (BAK1), and BCL2 family apoptotic regulator (BOK), are able to form pores across the outer mitochondrial membrane, leading to MOMP. Proapoptotic BH3-only proteins such as BCL2-interacting mediator of cell death (BIM) and BH3-interacting domain death agonist (BID) activate the mitochondrial pools of BAX and/or BAK, promoting their assembly leading to MOMP. Anti-apoptotic BCL2 family members, including BCL2 and BCL2 like 1 (BCL-XL), prevent the development of MOMP in part by binding proapoptotic members of the BCL2 family. The processs of MOMP allow the release of releases proapoptotic mediators such as cytochrome c and second mitochondrial activator of caspases (SMAC). In the cytosol, cytochrome c binds to apoptotic peptidase-activating factor 1 (APAF1) and pro-caspase 9 (CASP9) in the presence of deoxyATP (dADP), forming a complex called apoptosome. Within this complex, CASP9 becomes activated and catalyzes the proteolytic activation of CASP3 and CASP7, which elicit DNA fragmentation and other features of apoptosis. Upon release from the mitochondria, SMAC promotes apoptosis by associating with and inhibiting X-linked inhibitor of apoptosis (XIAP), a member of the inhibitor of apoptosis protein IAP family that counteracts the apoptotic cascade by physically blocking caspases. Mitochondrial permeability transition-driven necrosis results from the opening of the so-called permeability transition pore complex (PTPC), which requires cyclophilin D (CYCD) activity. Parthanatos is driven by the hyperactivation of poly (ADP-ribose) (PAR) polymerase 1 (PARP1), which is involved in response to DNA damage and utilizes nicotinamide adenine nucleotide (NAD^+) and ATP to synthesize poly ADP-ribose. Excessive PARP1 activation elicits depletion of both NAD^+ and ATP and accumulation of polymers and PARylated proteins at the mitochondria. Binding of PAR polymers leads to release of a proapoptotic mitochondrial protein called apoptosis inducing factor mitochondria associated 1 (AIF1).

and chromatin condensation. Another protein involved in parthanatos is hexokinase 1, whose binding to PAR polymers inhibits glycolysis.

Ferroptosis

Ferroptosis is initiated by severe lipid peroxidation, which depends both on ROS generation and availability of free iron (Fe^{2+})[3] (Figure 12.3). The main endogenous inhibitor of ferroptosis is glutathione peroxidase 4 (GPx4), which utilizes glutathione (GSH) to reduce lipid hydroperoxides to lipid alcohols. Synthesis of GSH depends on the availability of cysteine in the cytosol, which requires the activity of the cystine/glutamate antiporter system xCT that allows influx of cystine (which is then reduced to cysteine in the cytosol) coupled with efflux of glutamate. Neuronal death caused by xCT inhibition may be in part mechanistically related to glutamate toxicity, or excitotoxicity, as excessive accumulation of extracellular glutamate impairs activity of the transporter. Ferroptosis involves the preferential oxidation of polyunsaturated fatty acids such as arachidonic acid. This process is regulated by the mutually antagonistic activity of lipoxygenases that catalyze lipid peroxidation and GPx4 that elicits reduction via GSH. Free intracellular iron may participate in ferroptosis by several mechanisms. For example, ferric (Fe^{3+}) iron may be reduced to its ferrous (Fe^{2+}) form via interaction with hydrogen peroxide (H_2O_2), leading to the formation of the highly oxidant hydroxyl radical (Fenton reaction) and nonenzymatic lipid peroxidation. Sequestration of intracellular iron by its binding to ferritin is thus a fundamental neuroprotective mechanism.

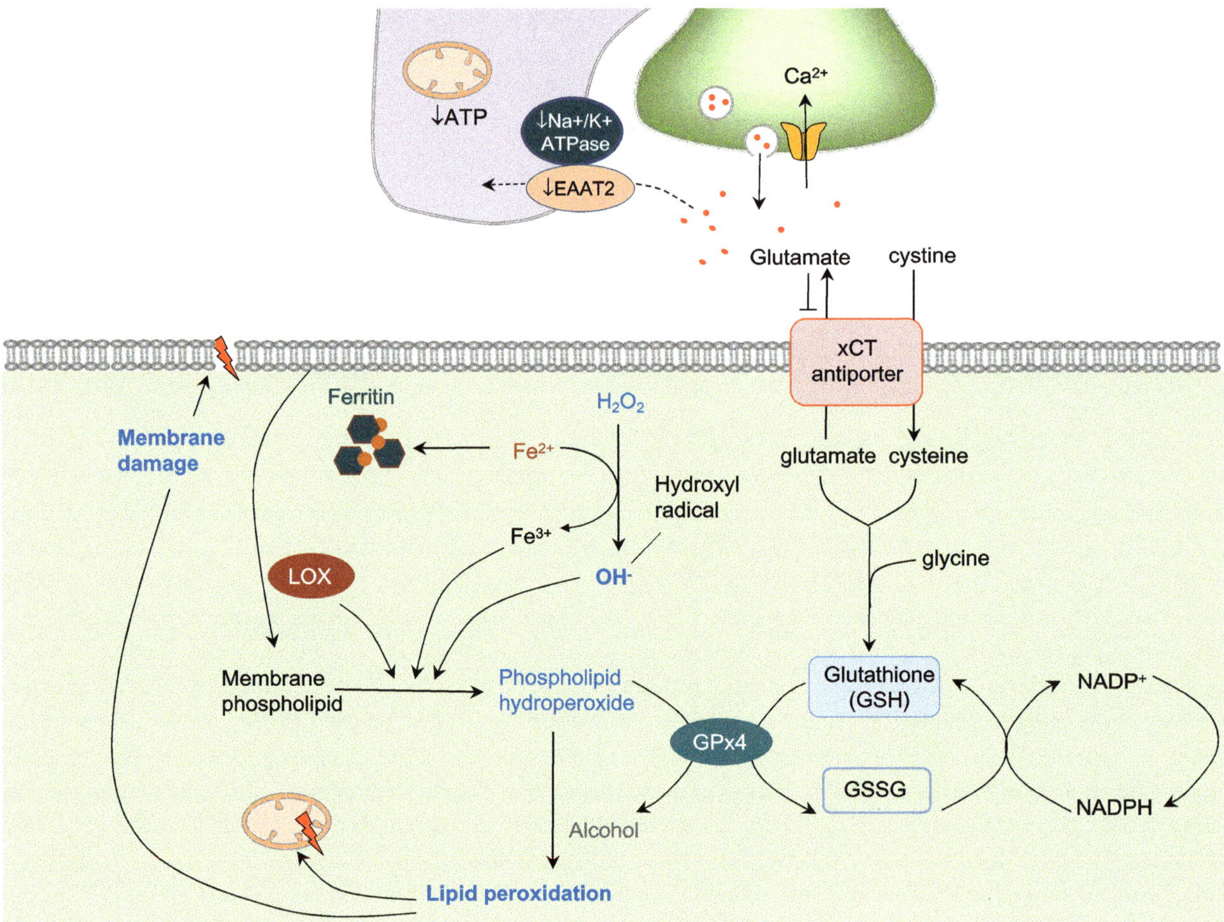

FIGURE 12.3 Mechanisms of ferroptosis.

Ferroptosis is initiated by severe lipid peroxidation and membrane disruption dependent on oxidative stress and iron (Fe) availability. Ferric (Fe^{3+}) iron may be reduced to its ferrous (Fe^{2+}) form via interaction with hydrogen peroxide (H_2O_2), leading to the formation of the highly oxidant hydroxyl radical (OH^-) and nonenzymatic lipid peroxidation. The main endogenous inhibitor of ferroptosis is glutathione (GSH) peroxidase 4 (GPx4), which limits lipid peroxidation by GSH-dependent reduction of lipid hydroperoxides. Synthesis of GSH depends on the activity of the cystine/glutamate antiporter system Xc (xCT). In the setting of energy failure, reduced activity of the astrocytic excitatory amino acid transporter (EAAT) leads to extracellular glutamate, preventing xCT activity and thus GSH synthesis. Sequestration of intracellular iron by its binding to ferritin protects against ferroptosis.

Lysosome-Dependent Cell Death

Lysosome-dependent cell death is initiated by perturbations resulting in the release of lysosomal contents such as cathepsin to the cytoplasm. In some circumstances, lysosomal membrane permeabilization may occur downstream of MOMP as a result of apoptotic signaling. In other settings it may involve direct BAX recruitment to the lysosomal membrane, followed by pore formation. ROS play a prominent causal role in lysosomal membrane permeabilization, both via H_2O_2-driven luminal production of hydroxyl radicals that destabilize the lysosomal membrane upon lipid peroxidation and via activation of lysosomal Ca^{2+} channels. Additional triggers of lysosomal membrane permeabilization are sphingosine and calpains. In the cytosol, cathepsins promote apoptosis by catalyzing the proteolytic activation or inactivation of several substrates, including BID, BAX, antiapoptotic BCL2 family members, and XIAP. Autophagy-dependent cell death relies on components of the autophagic machinery, discussed in a previous chapter of this book. Autolysis is a specific of autophagy-dependent cell death triggered by impairment of the plasma membrane Na^+/K^+ ATPase.

REGULATED CELL DEATH INDUCED BY INFLAMMATORY SIGNALS

Inflammatory and other environmental signals may trigger different forms of regulated cell death. They include extrinsic apoptosis, necroptosis, and pyroptosis (Figure 12.4).

Extrinsic Apoptosis

Extrinsic apoptosis is mostly driven by either of two types of plasma membrane receptors, death receptors and dependence receptors. Activation of death receptors, such as tumor necrosis factor receptor (TNFR) requires binding of a ligand. In contrast, activation of dependence receptors, such as low-affinity neurotrophin receptors, occurs when the level of their ligands drop below a specific threshold.

Ligand binding to death receptors, such as TNFR1 or FAS triggers assembly of dynamic multiprotein complexes that include adaptor proteins that provide molecular platforms for activation of CASP8 and other initiator caspases, triggering extrinsic apoptosis via downstream executioner caspases (Figure 12.5). In some cells, CASP8 elicits cleavage of BID, which provides a mechanism for mitochondrial-triggered (intrinsic) apoptosis. One such adaptor protein involved in CASP8 activation is receptor-interacting serine/threonine-protein kinase 1 (RIPK1). Deubiquitylation of RIPK1 favors CASP8 activity in the cytosol. Alternatively, TNFR1 activation may lead to survival and inflammatory signals. Upon recruitment by TRFR1 signaling, RIPK1 may undergo polyubiquitylation and serve as a scaffold for the sequential recruitment of several kinases. One downstream effect is to promote translocation of nuclear factor κ-light-chain-enhancer of activated B cells (NF-κB) to the nucleus, where it functions as a transcription factor that promotes inflammatory and cell survival responses.

Necroptosis

Necroptosis manifests with a necrotic morphology and is initiated by perturbations detected by death receptors such as TNFR1 or by pathogen recognition receptors such as toll-like receptors (TLRs). Necroptosis depends on the sequential activation of receptor-interacting-protein kinase 3 (RIPK3) and mixed-lineage kinase domain-like pseudokinase (MLKL). The activation of RIPK3 downstream of TNFR1 signal involves the formation of a complex called a necrosome. In the necrosome, RIPK1 and then RIPK3 undergo a series of phosphorylation events that lead to MLKL recruitment, phosphorylation, and activation, resulting in the formation of MLKL oligomers that translocate to the plasma membrane. At the plasma membrane MLKL oligomers trigger permeabilization and Ca^{2+} influx, formation of plasma membrane bubbles, activation of cell-surface proteases with shedding of plasma membrane-associated proteins, and formation of magnesium-permeant channels.

Pyroptosis and Inflammasome

Pyroptosis is triggered by signals that elicit innate immune responses. Cells of the innate immune system, including macrophages and microglia, utilize pattern recognition receptors that recognize pathogens or cellular danger signals. Some receptors, such as TLRs are expressed on the membrane surface, whereas others such as NLRs (nucleotide-binding oligomerization domain [NOD] and leucine-rich repeat-containing receptors) are expressed in the cytoplasm. Activation of these receptors stimulates the canonical inflammasome signaling.[4] The inflammasome consists of a multiprotein oligomer that promotes the maturation and secretion of pro-inflammatory cytokines such as IL-1β and IL-18. Upon activation of TLRs, a subset of NLRs named NLRP (NOD-, LRR-, and pyrin domain-containing) receptors assemble and oligomerize into an inflammasome. NLRP1 is expressed in neurons; NLRP3 is predominantly located in microglia. Several immune stimulatory molecular patterns may activate inflammasome formation. These include oligomeric and fibrillary forms of amyloid-β (Aβ), α-synuclein (α-SYN), and transactivation response (TAR) DNA-binding protein 43 (TDP-43). Once activated, the inflammasome forms a complex with an adaptor protein acting as a molecular platform that recruits pro-CASP1, which is then activated by autocatalysis. Activated CASP1 can elicit proteolytic cleavage of pro-IL-1β into IL-1β, cleavage of pro-IL-18 into IL-18 and induce IFN-γ and natural killer cell activation, DNA fragmentation, and cell pore formation. Once activated beyond a specific threshold, inflammatory caspases precipitate pyroptosis by catalyzing the proteolytic cleavage of gasdermin D. Gasdermin D then translocates to the inner leaflet of the plasma membrane, undergoes oligomerization and generates a pore leading to

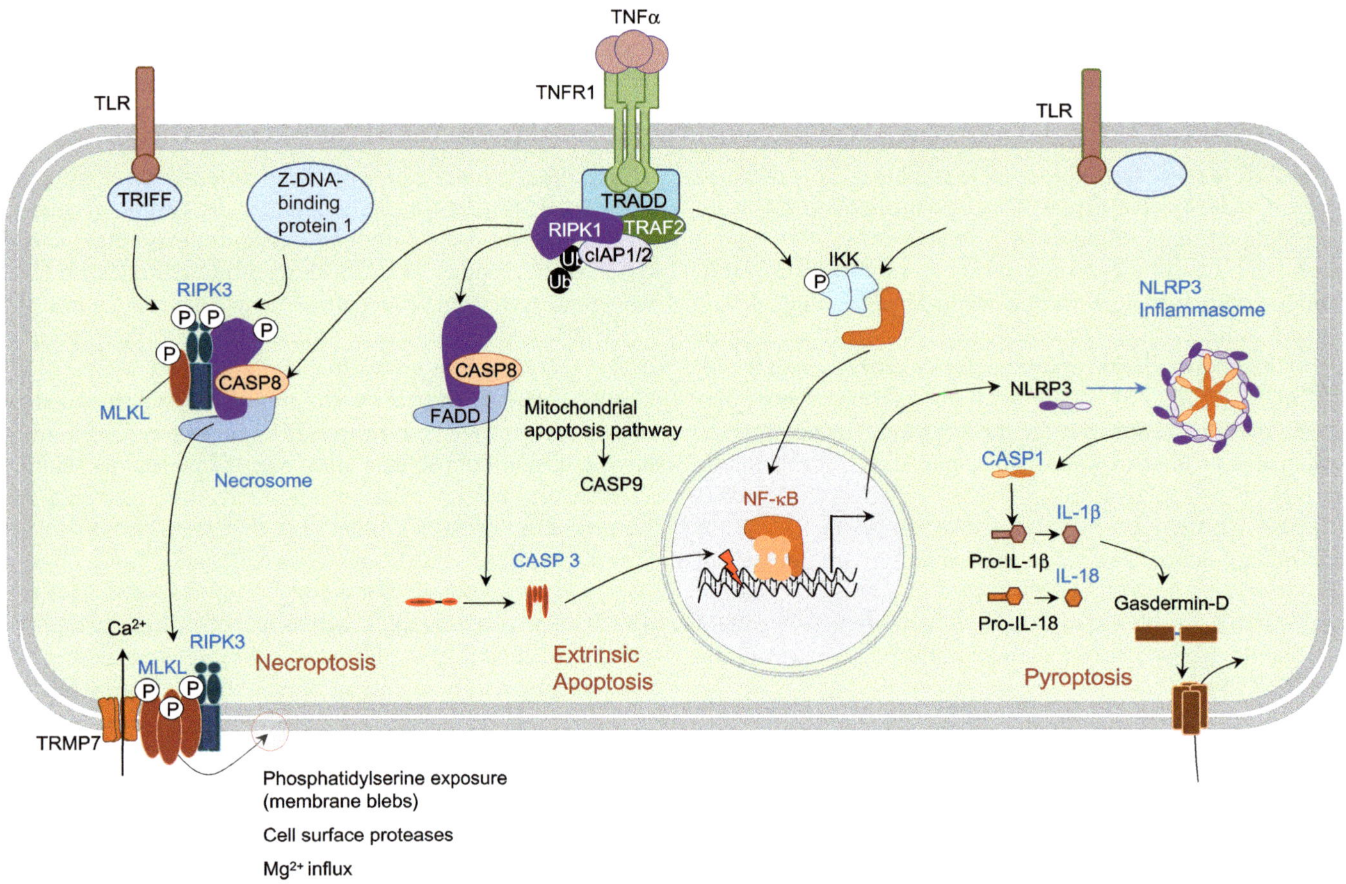

FIGURE 12.4 Mechanism of cell death triggered by inflammatory pathways.

Inflammatory and other environmental signals may trigger regulated cell death via extrinsic apoptosis, necroptosis, and pyroptosis. Activation of death receptors such as tumor necrosis factor (TNF) receptor superfamily member 1 (TNFR1) triggers extrinsic apoptosis by promoting the assembly of a dynamic multiprotein complex that includes TNFR1-associated via death receptor (TRADD), TNFR1-associated factors, the recaptor-interacting serine/threonine-protein kinase 1 (RIPK1), inhibitor of apoptosis (IAP), ubiquitin E3 ligases, and linear ubiquitin chain assembly complex. Deubiquitylation of RIPK1 favors its association with Fas-associated death domain (FADD) and caspase (CASP)8 in the cytosol, which drives extrinsic apoptosis via CASP3 and CASP7. TNFR1 receptor activation may lead to survival and inflammatory signals via polyubiquitylated RIPK1, which is the inhibitor of kappa B (IκB) kinase (IKK), thereby promoting dissociation of nuclear factor κB (NF-κB) and its translocation to the nucleus. Necroptosis is initiated by activation of death receptors such as TNFR1 or pathogen recognition receptors such as toll-like receptors (TLRs). It is mediated by receptor-interacting serine/threonine-protein kinase 3 (RIPK3), which phosphorylates and activates mixed-lineage kinase domains like pseudokinase (MLKL). MLKL oligomers translocate to the plasma membrane and Ca^{2+} influx, presumably via transient receptor potential cation channel subfamily M member 7 (TRPM7). Activation of RIPK3 downstream of TNFR1 involves the formation of a RIPK1- and RIPK3-containing signaling complex known as necrosome. Pyroptosis is triggered by activation of innate immune responses. Some receptors involved in these responses, such as TLRs, are expressed on the membrane surface, whereas others such as NLRs (nucleotide-binding oligomerization domain [NOD] and leucine-rich repeat-containing receptors), are expressed in the cytoplasm. Activation of these receptors stimulates the canonical inflammasome signaling. Once activated, the inflammasome forms a complex with an adaptor protein acting as a molecular platform that recruits pro-CASP1. Activated CASP1 elicits proteolytic cleavage and activation of proinflammatory cytokines such as interleukin (IL) 1β, and IL-18 to induce interferon (IFN)-γ and natural killer cell activation, DNA fragmentation, and cell pore formation, triggering pyroptosis. Inflammatory caspases also precipitate pyroptosis by cleavage of gasdermin D, which forms a pore responsible for rapid plasma membrane permeabilization, cell swelling, and lysis.

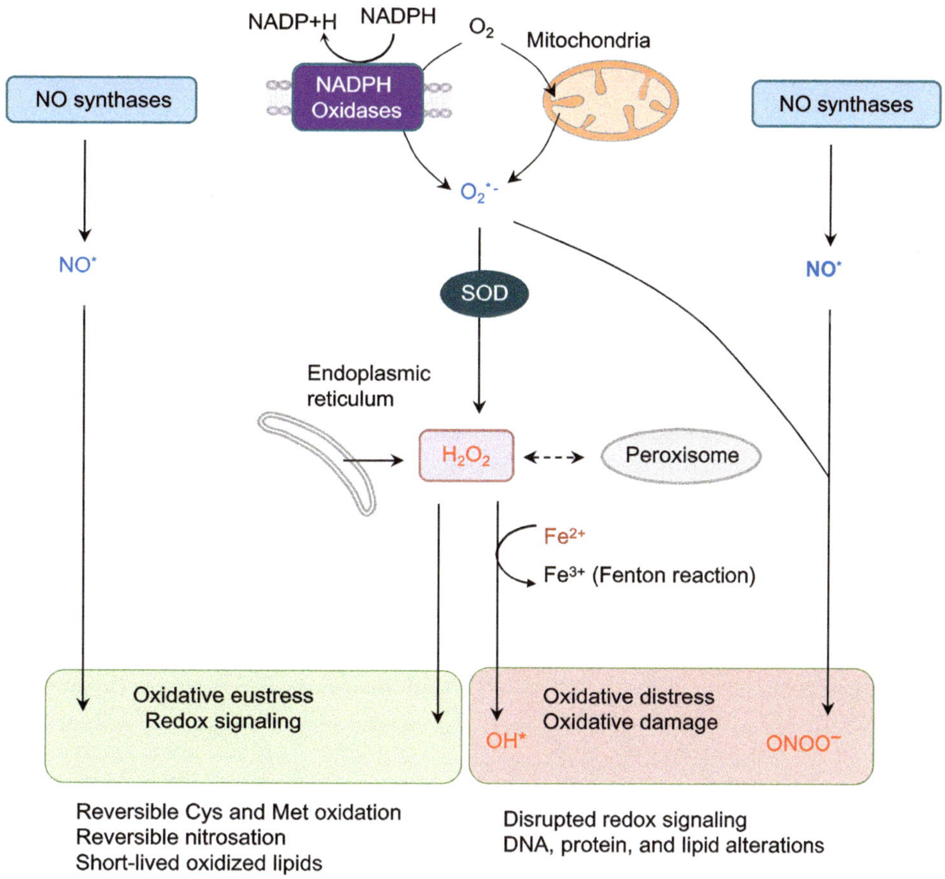

FIGURE 12.5 Signaling versus toxic effects of reactive oxygen and nitrogen species.
Hydrogen peroxide (H_2O_2) and nitric oxide (NO) have an important role both in redox signaling (oxidative eustress) and in oxidative damage (oxidative distress) The major sources of H_2O_2 via superoxide radical (O_2^-) formation are the mitochondria and NADPH oxidases (NOX). One important effect of O_2^- in mitochondria is the release of iron from iron-sulfur clusters of complexes I and II. This leads to both loss of energy production and the generation of hydroxyl radical (OH-) by Fenton reaction between excess H_2O_2 and Fe^{3+}, leading to membrane lipid peroxidation and ferroptosis. Nitric oxide is generated by nitric oxide synthases (NOSs). At high intracellular levels, NO reacts rapidly with O_2^- to form peroxynitrite ($ONOO^-$), which acts as a biological oxidant, affecting mitochondrial function and triggering cell death via oxidation and nitration reactions. Cys, cysteine, Met, methionine, NADPH, reduced nicotinamide adenine dinucleotide phosphate, SOD-1, superoxide dismutase 1.

rapid plasma membrane permeabilization, cell swelling, lysis, and release of inflammatory cytokines to recruit and activate immune cells.

REDOX SIGNALING AND OXIDATIVE STRESS

Redox biology depends primarily on the activity of redox switches that modify cysteine residues of a variety of proteins.[5] The so-called redox code depends on activation cycles involving superoxide ion (O_2^-) and H_2O_2 and the spatial location and temporal activation of systems that regulate redox signaling, such as the NAD^+/nicotinamide adenine dinucleotide phosphate (NADP) and the thiol systems, including GSH and thioredoxin. Whereas maintenance of a physiological level of oxidant challenge, or oxidative eustress, is essential for redox signaling, excessive oxidant challenge by ROS causes damage of biomolecules.[6]

Sources of Oxygen Species for Redox Signaling

The main sources of oxygen species are the mitochondria and microglia. Mitochondria produce O_2^- and H_2O_2 by two major mechanisms, mitochondrial inner membrane complexes I, II, and III and mitochondrial matrix and/or inner membrane–bound dehydrogenases. Approximately 1%–2% of molecular O_2 in mitochondria generates O_2^-, which rapidly undergoes enzymatic dismutation by superoxide dismutase (SOD)2, leading to production of H_2O_2. This reaction occurs primarily in matrix by action of manganese superoxide dismutase (SOD2); in the intramembrane space this reaction is catalyzed by copper-zinc SOD1. Hydrogen peroxide can diffuse across the lipid bilayer via aquaporins 3 and 8 (referred to as peroxiporins) to reach its targets at a distance. It is primarily metabolized in the cytosol by action of GPx and peroxiredoxins that require nicotinamide adenine dinucleotide phosphate (NADPH) as a cofactor. The second major source of H_2O_2 is the NADPH oxidase (NOX).

Role of Glial Cells

Microglia express the highest level of NOX2, and are thus a major source of H_2O_2 in the CNS.[7] Microglia also express a battery of antioxidant proteins that keep redox homeostasis and avoid excessive damage to macromolecules. For example, microglia express high levels of GSH and have the highest GPx activity in the brain. The GSH content of microglia decreases with increasing age, thus promoting an age-dependent increase in the vulnerability of microglia to oxidative stress.[7] Astrocytes also express high levels of antioxidant proteins and are thus critical for normal global redox balance in the CNS. They are the major source of GSH for neurons and oligodendrocytes.

Regulation of Redox Signaling

The two major systems involved in regulation of redox signaling are the NAD/NADP systems and the thiol systems, including GSH and the thioredoxin systems. The NAD/NADH system is involved in oxidative process in mitochondria and cytosol for catabolism, whereas the NADPH/NADP system drives reductive anabolism as well as oxidative reactions such as those mediated by NOX, nitric oxide synthases (NOS), and cytochrome P450-dependent hydroxylases. NADH and NADPH are interlinked by the ATP-regulated nicotinamide nucleotide transhydrogenase, which transfers electrons from NADH to $NADP^+$, thus backing up NADPH-related antioxidant defense. Since this reaction is reversible, under pathological metabolic demand NADPH is consumed to support NADH and ATP production thereby weakening antioxidant defense and promoting oxidative stress. The GSH and the thioredoxin systems catalyze the oxidation of free thiols (-SH) to disulfides (-S-S). Mitochondrial GSH accounts for 10%–15% of total cellular GSH. Thioredoxins reduce protein disulfides to free thiols by action of their respective thioredoxin reductases that utilize electrons provided by NADPH. Important substrates for thioredoxins are H_2O_2 and protein disulfide isomerases, which are involved in protein maturation in the ER. Once ROS are formed, powerful enzymatic systems, including SOD, catalase, and GPx directly counteract their oxidant effects. Nonenzymatic protection is provided by antioxidants such as α-tocopherol (vitamin E), or ascorbate (vitamin C) and carotenoids.

Molecular Redox Switches

Molecular redox switches control activation/deactivation cycles in redox signaling. The two master molecular switches are the transcription factors nuclear factor-E2-related factor (Nrf2) and NF-κB. In basal conditions, Nrf2 and NF-κB are present in an inactive state; in response to oxidative stress or other challenges of cell homeostasis they translocate to the nucleus where they function as transcriptional activators. Nrf2 is tethered to the outer mitochondrial membrane bound to Keap1 (Kelch-like ECH-associated protein 1), which promotes its rapid ubiquitination and degradation. Under oxidative or electrophilic stress, modifications of cysteinyl residues of Keap1 render it unable to promote ubiquitination Nrf2, allowing Nrf2 to accumulate in the nucleus. In the nucleus, Nrf2 forms a heterodimer with a small coactivator protein and binds to the antioxidant response element of genes encoding enzymes, transporters, and transcription factors involved in antioxidant responses, xenobiotic detoxication, mitochondrial biogenesis, and lipid metabolism, promoting their transcription. Nrf2 then becomes inactivated in the nucleus by acetylation and phosphorylation and undergoes either proteasome degradation or translocation back to the cytoplasm, where it again reassembles with Keap1. One important function of Nrf2 is to modulate mitochondrial function; it stimulates mitochondrial biogenesis and prevents the formation of the MOMP in response to cellular stress. Nuclear factor κB is a multisubunit transcription factor consisting of Rel and p50 heterodimers that can rapidly activate the expression of genes involved in inflammatory, immune, and survival responses. In an inactivated state, NF-κB is located in the cytosol coupled with the inhibitory protein IκB. A variety of extracellular signals activate IκB kinase, which phosphorylates IκB, leading to its dissociation from NF-κB, which then translocates to the nucleus. Oxidation by H_2O_2 also leads to NF-κB activation due to release of its binding to a subunit of IκB. NF-κB translocates to the nucleus, where it activates transcription of genes involved in inflammation, cell survival, and synaptic plasticity.

Oxidative Stress, Nitric Oxide, and Iron

Oxidative stress is the unbalanced or inappropriately localized oxidant production that can derange the redox signaling mechanism in an autocrine or paracrine manner (Figure 12.5). One important effect of O_2^- in mitochondria is the release of iron from iron-sulfur clusters of complexes I and II. This leads to both loss of energy production and the generation of hydroxyl radical (OH^-) by Fenton reaction between excess H_2O_2 and Fe^{3+}, resulting in membrane lipid peroxidation and ferroptosis. Nitric oxide is a reactive nitrogen species that participates both in normal redox signaling and oxidative stress. Inducible NOS is expressed primarily in inflammatory cells, is activated by proinflammatory cytokines, and may generate high NO levels for prolonged periods of time. At high intracellular levels, NO combines with oxidant molecules to form reactive nitrogen species that elicit posttranslational modifications of several target proteins. NO toxicity is potentiated by the concomitant excessive production of ROS, as NO reacts rapidly with O_2^- to form peroxynitrite ($ONOO^-$), which acts as a biological oxidant, affecting mitochondrial function and triggering cell death via oxidation and nitration reactions.[8] Oxidative stress may affect DNA, RNA, proteins, and lipids. DNA oxidation, particularly of guanine bases, is a major contributor to instability and decay of the genome. Accumulation of H_2O_2 in the ER affects protein maturation. Accumulation of unfolded proteins in the ER lumen activates the unfolded protein response. Biomarkers of oxidative stress include protein, advanced glycation end-products, 3-nitrotyrosine, malondialdehyde, 8-oxoguanine, and methionine sulfoxide. One of these

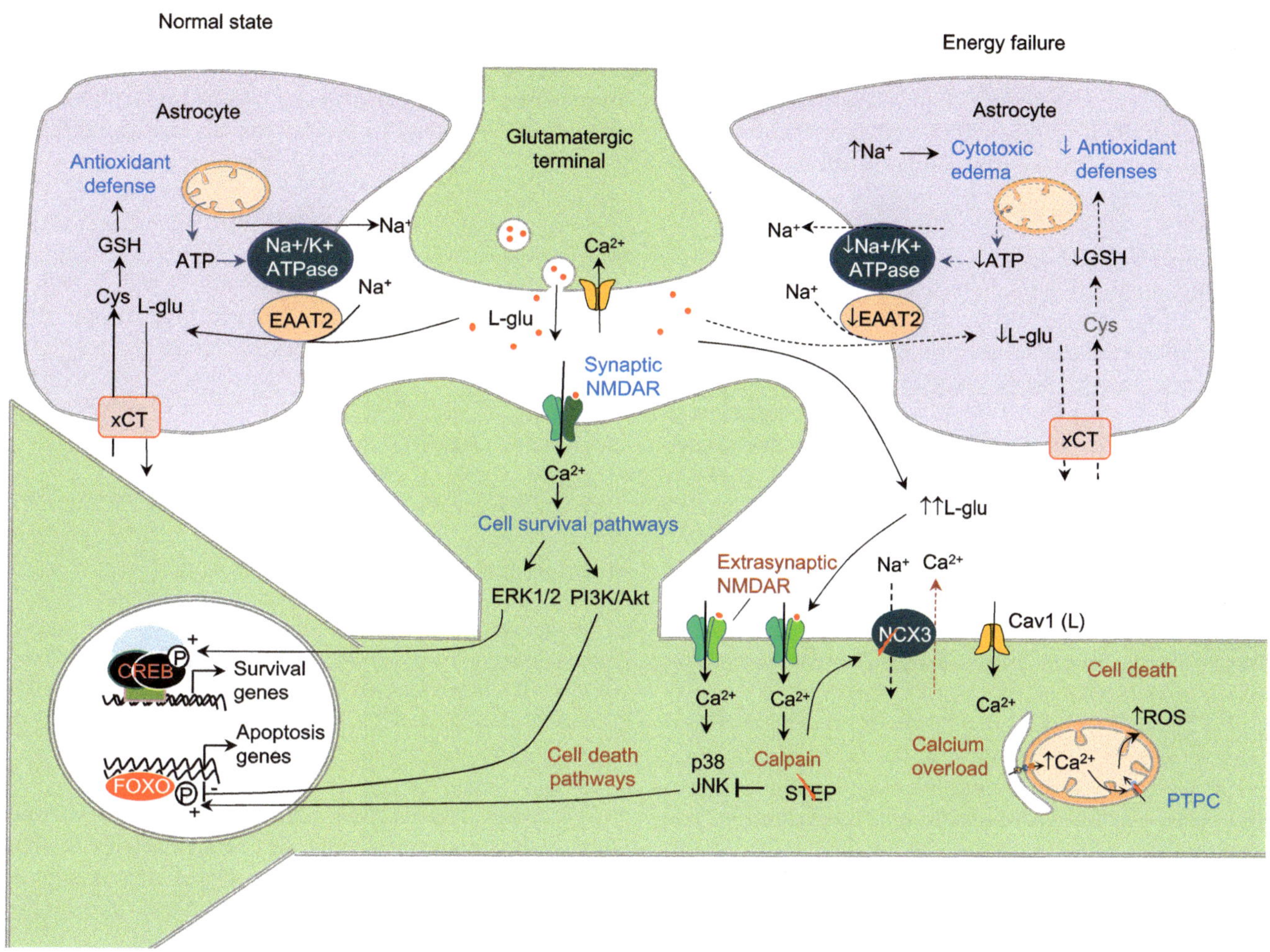

FIGURE 12.6 Mechanisms of excitotoxicity and calcium overload.

The classical mechanism of excitotoxicity is Ca^{2+} influx via N-methyl-D-aspartate receptors (NMDARs) in the setting of energy failure and ATP depletion affecting membrane pumps. Reduced levels of ATP, required to fuel the Na^+/K^+ ATPase, impair activity of astrocytic excitatory amino acid transporter 2 (EAAT 2), resulting in accumulation of glutamate, which activates both synaptic and extrasynaptic NMDARs, leading to massive Ca^{2+} influx via both NMDAR channels and voltage-gated Ca^{2+} channels activated by depolarization. The Na^+/Ca^{2+} exchanger (NCX) prevents excessive Ca^{2+} accumulation in the cytosol but becomes impaired by energy failure. Under conditions of high Ca^{2+} levels in the matrix, there is mitochondrial permeability transition pore complex (PTCP) formation, leading to regulated necrosis. The excessive extracellular glutamate prevents the normal function of the glutamate/cystine antiporter cXT, thereby decreasing synthesis of GSH and promoting oxidative stress, lipid peroxidation, and ferroptosis. Whereas activation of synaptic NMDARs triggers prosurvival pathways, including the PI3K (phosphoinositide 3 kinase)/AKT pathway and extracellular signal regulated kinase (ERK) pathway that elicit phosphorylation of CREB (cyclic AMP response element binding protein), activation of extrasynaptic NMDARs results in Ca^{2+} influx that triggers the production of several neuronal death complexes. Effects include excessive production of nitric oxide (NO). Calpains mediate NMDAR-triggered excitotoxicity by targeting NCX3 preventing Na^+/Ca^{2+} exchange leading to Ca^{2+} accumulation. STEP, striatal enriched phosphatase; JNK, Jun-N terminal kinase.

biomarkers is the length of telomeres, which decreases with oxidative stress.

EXCITOTOXICITY AND CALCIUM OVERLOAD

In conditions of energy failure such as hypoxia or ischemia, or in the setting of excessive excitatory synaptic activity, such as in seizures, there is accumulation of glutamate in the synaptic and extrasynaptic space, leading to Ca^{2+} mediated excitotoxicity[9,10] (Figure 12.6). Excitotoxicity is mechanistically linked to several cell death mechanisms, including mitochondrial permeability transition-driven necrosis and ferroptosis.

Mechanisms of Glutamate Accumulation

L-glutamate is the primary excitatory transmitter in the central nervous system and is rapidly released from excitatory synaptic terminals. Synaptic glutamate homeostasis depends on the activity of excitatory amino acid transporters (EAATs), primarily EAAT1 and EAAT2 present in astrocytes. The driving force for glutamate uptake is provided by the Na^+ gradient created by the Na^+/K^+ ATPase. This process prevents excessive glutamate in synapses; glutamate that escapes uptake may reach extrasynaptic sites. The removal of extracellular glutamate by the EAATs maintains the gradient necessary for the activity of xCT, which is critical for GSH production by allowing inward influx of cystine to the cytosol coupled with efflux of glutamate. In pathological conditions, impaired activity of the EATT coupled with upregulation of xCT results in excessive glutamate accumulation in the extracellular space, thereby decreasing intracellular levels of cysteine and thus GSH, promoting oxidative stress, lipid peroxidation, and ferroptosis.

Mechanisms of Calcium Overload

The classical mechanism of excitotoxicity is Ca^{2+} influx via N-methyl-D-aspartate receptors (NMDARs) in the setting of ATP depletion and impaired activity of the Na^+/K^+ ATPase. Inability to maintain Na^+ gradients leads to accumulation of intracellular Na^+; this not only impairs activity of the EAATs but also results in accumulation of intracellular Ca^{2+} via reverse activity of the Na^+/Ca^{2+} exchanger (NCX). In addition, oxidative and nitrosative stress enhance Ca^{2+} influx via the transient receptor potential channel TRPM7; and decreased extracellular pH activates the Ca^{2+} permeable acid sensitive cation channels. Excessive Ca^{2+} accumulation may lead to either necrotic or apoptotic cell death, depending of the severity of the initial insult and residual ATP reserve. One major consequence of Ca^{2+} overload is impairment of mitochondrial function. Accumulation of Ca^{2+} in the matrix triggers mitochondrial PTPC formation, membrane depolarization, impaired ATP production, and organelle swelling, which are typical of regulated necrosis.

Role of NMDARs in Neuronal Death

Activation of synaptic and extrasynaptic NMDARs have different downstream consequences on neuronal survival.[11,12] Whereas activation of synaptic NMDARs triggers prosurvival pathways, activation of extrasynaptic NMDARs typically results in Ca^{2+} influx that triggers the production of several neuronal death complexes.[13] One such complex results in excessive activation of neuronal NOS and production of NO, which can elicit oxidative and nitrosative stress via interactions with ROS. A second complex involves a transduction pathway that activates tumor suppressor p53, which triggers apoptosis. Important mediators of NMDAR-triggered excitotoxicity are the calpains, which are Ca^{2+}-activated cysteine proteases that cleave several proteins, including NCXs that regulate cytosolic Ca^{2+} level after glutamate-induced Ca^{2+} transients. Other targets are cytoskeletal proteins such as fodrin, which is involved in regulating and integrating neurotrophin and ephrin receptor signaling, and striatal enriched tyrosine phosphatase, which is involved in synaptic plasticity.[13]

AXONAL DEGENERATION

Axonal degeneration is a common feature of traumatic, ischemic, inflammatory, toxic, metabolic, genetic, and neurodegenerative disorders. Despite the wide diversity of initiating insults, the axonal death program results from the convergence of reduced NAD^+, impaired axonal transport, mitochondrial dysfunction, and increase in intraaxoplasmic Ca^{2+} leading to activation of calpain[14,15] (Figure 12.7).

Intrinsic Factors Promoting Axonal Survival or Self-Destruction

Wallerian degeneration following axonal transection consists of a latent phase followed by a catastrophic phase in which there is a sequential collapse of all of axonal structures. In parallel to Wallerian degeneration, the proximal axon segment undergoes resealing and retracts from the lesion site. Retrograde signaling along the proximal segment of the axon reaches the cell body, triggering either potentially reversible changes such as swelling, changes in nuclear location and fragmentation of intracellular organelles or eventually cell death. Axonal degeneration is an active and intrinsically regulated process. Studies in the *slow Wallerian degeneration* (*Wld*^{s}) mutant mice indicate that axons contain an intrinsic protective mechanism, and that Wallerian degeneration reflects the inability to deliver a putative natural inhibitor of the death program in the axon.[14,16–18] Axonal survival depends on activity of nicotinamide mononucleotide adenylyl transferases (NMNATs), which catalyze the synthesis of NAD^+ from nicotinamide mononucleotide and ATP. As a fundamental coenzyme, NAD^+ is involved in redox reactions required for ATP production; NAD^+ also has several signaling roles, including Ca^{2+} mobilization, and posttranslational protein modifications such

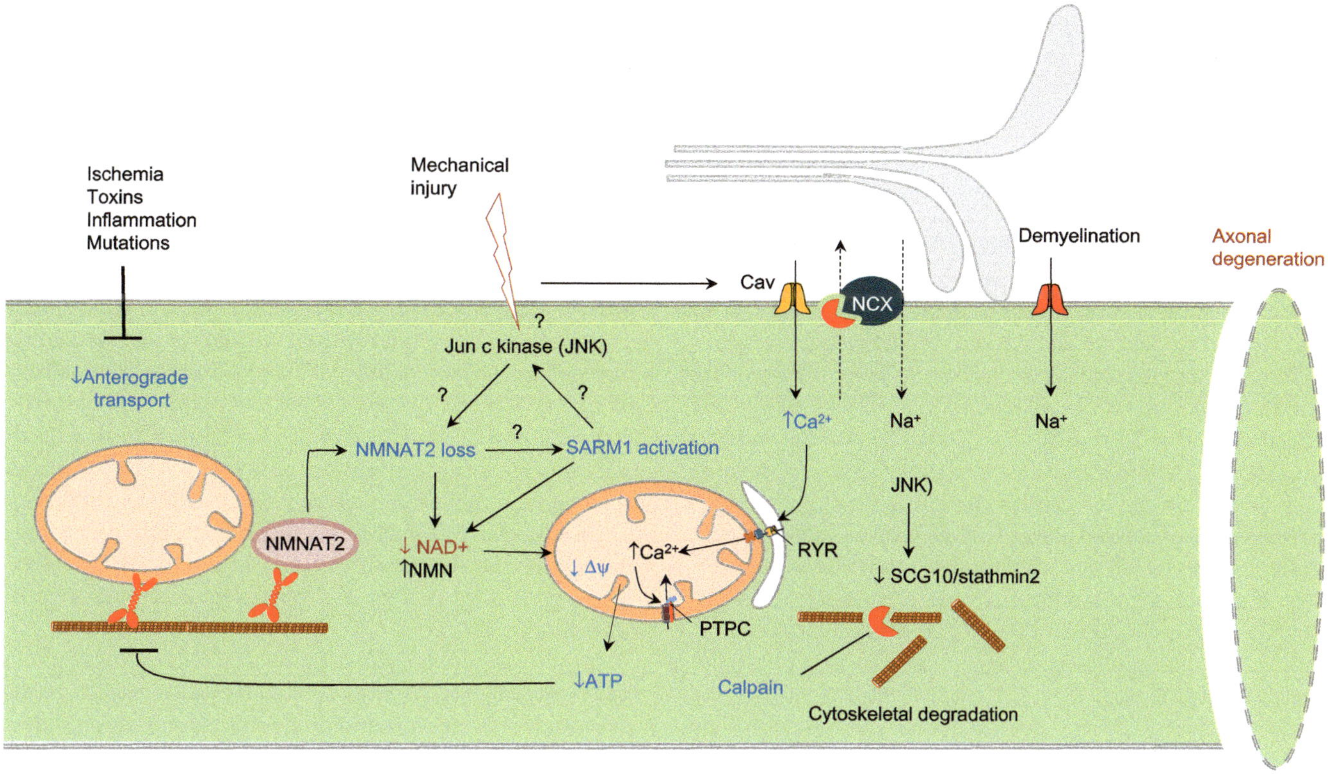

FIGURE 12.7 Mechanisms of axonal degeneration.
The axonal death program results from the convergence of reduced nicotinamide adenine dinucleotide (NAD^+), impaired axonal transport, mitochondrial dysfunction, and increase in intraaxoplasmic calcium (Ca^{2+}). Axonal survival depends on activity of nicotinamide mononucleotide adenylyl transferases (NMNATs). Axonal NMNAT1 protects axons from degeneration and may substitute for NMNAT2, which is the primary endogenous axon survival factor. Loss of NMNAT2 may result in activation of SARM1 (sterile α/armadillo/toll-interleukin receptor homolog domain-containing-1), which is required for axonal degeneration. Signaling via Jun-N-terminal kinase (JNK) affects the microtubule stability by targeting SCG10 (superior cervical ganglion 10) protein. Mitochondrial dysfunction leads to axonal damage via ATP depletion, impaired Ca^{2+} homeostasis, and generation of reactive oxygen species. Failure of the Na^+/K^+ ATPase leads to intra-axonal Na^+ accumulation and reversal of the Na^+/Ca^{2+} (NCX). Deleterious accumulation of Ca^{2+} can also result from influx via voltage-gated Ca^{2+} channels and release from intracellular stores in the endoplasmic reticulum (ER) via ryanodine receptors (RYRs). Calcium overload results in activation calpain, which degrades several structural proteins.

as PARylation and deacetylation catalyzed by sirtuins.[17] In axons, NMNAT2 is the primary endogenous survival factor and its levels are regulated by the balance between continuous anterograde transport from the cell body and local degradation.[19] NMNAT2 is a labile protein and its levels rapidly decrease following axon transection; NMNAT1 may protect axons by substituting for NMNAT2.[20] Studies in mutant models show that a protein known as SARM1 (sterile α/armadillo/toll-interleukin receptor homolog domain-containing-1) is required for axonal degeneration.[15] SARM1 contains a C-terminal toll-interleukin-1 receptor signaling domain that possesses intrinsic NAD^+ cleavage activity. SARM1 is normally present in the axon in an inactive state via interaction with NMNAT2. Axon injury results in a molecular rearrangement, dimerization, and activation of SARM1 triggering a downstream degenerative program that includes rapid NAD^+ loss, ATP depletion, cytoskeletal degradation, and axon destruction. For example, decreased NMNAT2 levels due to mitochondrial dysfunction or effect of drugs such as vincristine or bortezomib lead to SARM1 activation resulting in Ca^{2+} entry, calpain activation, and breakdown of the cytoskeleton, Loss of NMNAT2 in the distal axon also results in accumulation of its substrate NMN, which may be toxic for axons.[15] The breakdown of the axon releases neurofilament light chain (NfL), which can be detected in serum or CSF.

Signaling via mitogen-activated protein kinase and other kinases activated by injury converge into the Jun-N-terminal kinase (JNK); one of the targets of JNK is the microtubule-binding and -stabilizing protein stathmin 2. Phosphorylation by JNKs targets stathmin for degradation, leading to dismantling of the axon. Stathmin 2 is necessary for normal axonal outgrowth and regeneration; reduced stathmin 2 expression in motor neurons due to loss of TDP-43 function may contribute to the pathogenesis of amyotrophic lateral sclerosis (ALS) associated with *C9ORF72* mutation.[21]

Impaired Axonal Transport

Both physical injury and blockade of axonal transport trigger similar morphological patterns of axonal damage in a wide range disorders.[14,22] An almost universal finding in both Wallerian degeneration and dying-back axonopathies is axonal dystrophy, which is characterized by the presence of axonal spheroids or small axonal varicosities.[14] Spheroids appear as repeated swellings distributed in tandem in individual axons, which suggests a multifocal block of anterograde axonal transport resulting in a buildup of axoplasm.[14] The presence of axonal spheroids, as well as amyloid precursor protein (APP) accumulation in axons that maintain their morphological continuity, indicates that impaired axonal transport is an early event preceding axonal degeneration. The nodes of Ranvier and paranodes may be particularly vulnerable sites.[23]

Mitochondrial Dysfunction

Mitochondria are central sensors for stimuli that trigger axonal degeneration.[24] Axon injury depolarizes mitochondria and reduces the ATP content in the severed axon. Injury also impairs mitochondrial motility. Excessive Ca^{2+} entry causes depolarization of the mitochondrial inner membrane, reduced Ca^{2+} handling by the mitochondria, and dysfunction of the respiratory chain leading to excessive production of ROS.[24–27] High Ca^{2+} and ROS levels interact with each other to activate mitochondrial permeability transition and thus apoptosis.[28]

Axonal Calcium Overload

Deleterious accumulation of Ca^{2+} in the axon may result not only from reversal of the NCX but also from influx via voltage-gated Ca^{2+} channels and release from intracellular stores in the ER. Calcium-induced Ca^{2+} release via ryanodine receptors in the ER occurs in response to axonal depolarization and Ca^{2+} influx via voltage-gated channels present in discrete molecular nanocomplexes in the internodal axolemma.[26] These nanocomplexes also contain noninactivating Na^{+} channels and glutamate receptors that contribute to depolarization.[29] Severe ATP depletion impairs the function of the smooth endoplasmic reticulum Ca^{2+} ATPase, thereby impairing the ER Ca^{2+}-buffering activity. Calcium overload results in activation of cytotoxic downstream effectors, particularly the Ca^{2+} sensitive protease calpain and phospholipases.[30] Calpain degrades several targets in the axon, including cytoskeletal proteins such as actin, spectrin, tubulin, and neurofilament protein, and spectrin; transporters and ion channels; and all major myelin proteins.[25]

Diffuse Axonal Injury and Chronic Traumatic Encephalopathy

Diffuse axonal injury is the most common neuropathological consequence of closed traumatic brain injury (TBI).[31] Diffuse axonal injury reflects a progression from disruption in axonal transport leading to axonal swelling, followed by secondary disconnection, and finally Wallerian degeneration. The principal mechanical force responsible for diffuse axonal injury is rotational acceleration of the brain, which leads to cytoskeletal damage and subsequent depolymerization of microtubules from the break points. Anterogradely transported APP can be detected in damaged axons within 2 hours of injury and peaks in the initial 24 hours following injury. Even in severe TBI only a small percentage of axons, particularly the small diameter axons within a given tract undergo transport disruption. However, the remaining axons may suffer secondary pathophysiological changes that involve mitochondrial dysfunction, oxidative stress, lipid peroxidation, microglia activation, and neuroinflammation.[13]

Long-term axonal degeneration after TBI may have a role in development of AD-like neuropathological changes. In injured axons, APP co-accumulates with its cleaving enzymes involved in production of Aβ peptides. The abundant Aβ accumulation within axon bulbs and the eventual breakdown of injured axons may allow the expulsion and accumulation of Aβ into the parenchyma, where it can aggregate to form plaques.[31] Closed head trauma resulting in TBI significantly increases the risk of developing Alzheimer's disease (AD), Parkinson's disease (PD), and chronic traumatic encephalopathy (CTE), and perhaps sporadic amyotrophic lateral sclerosis (ALS). Following a moderate or severe concussion, or a series of mild blows to the head, the brain may undergo subtle pathophysiological changes. CTE is associated with brain atrophy, astrogliosis, loss of myelinated axons, microvascular injury, perivascular neuroinflammation, and phosphorylated tau protein pathology. Currently CTE is considered a tauopathy, characterized by a distinct perivascular accumulation of hyperphosphorylated tau in neurons and astrocytes within cerebral sulci.[32–35]

Studies in mouse models show that traumatic brain injury induced neuronal production of the toxic compound *cis*-phospho tau leading to degeneration via a process referred to as "cistauosis".[32] In CTE, astroglial tau pathology is composed of 4R-immunoreactive thorn-shaped astrocytes whereas neurofibrillary tangles contain both 3R and 4R tau.

AGE-RELATED CHANGES AFFECTING NEURON AND AXON SURVIVAL

Aging is major risk factor for neurodegenerative disorders. Several age-related processes contribute to neurodegeneration. They include, but are not limited to, reduced antioxidant defenses, oxidative stress leading to DNA damage, impaired DNA repair reduced motility of mitochondria and switch to a proinflammatory phenotype in glial cells.

Cellular Senescence

Cellular senescence refers to the process by which cells permanently lose their proliferative capacity but remain viable and metabolically active. Many factors can induce senescence, such as aging and cellular stress. Senescent cells exhibit specific morphological and phenotypic changes, including flattening, intracellular vacuolization, cellular and nuclear enlargement, altered chromatin structure, and resistance to apoptosis. At the biochemical level, cellular senescence is often characterized by increased lysosomal galactosidase β1 activity, inhibition of multiple cyclin-dependent kinases, and activation of p53 and other components of the response to DNA damage.[4] Senescent cells exhibit a unique secretory profile, termed the senescence-associated secretory profile (SASP), which includes a number of secreted proteins, primarily IL-1β and other pro-inflammatory cytokines such as IL-6 and IL-8, as well as mitogenic cytokines, chemokines, growth factors, and matrix metalloproteases. Formation of the inflammasome and IL-1 signaling in response to transforming growth factor-β family ligands can mediate the ability of senescent cells to induce senescence in neighboring cells through paracrine mechanisms. Microglia, astrocytes, and cells of the neurovascular unit can become senescent. Senescent astrocytes and microglia are typically found both in aging and in neurodegenerative diseases. Within the aged brain, glial cells change their response to various stimuli, with a key role for inflammasome-related signaling, including increase in IL-1β. This altered inflammatory response may predispose the brain to neurodegenerative conditions such as AD and PD, which are associated with inflammasome formation and IL-1β signaling.

Age-Related Axonal Loss

Normal aging is associated with extensive axonal loss.[37] In cerebral white matter there is average loss axonal loss of 10% per decade from the age of 20 to 80 years; axonal loss affects predominantly thinner fibers, which is consistent with age-related findings in peripheral nerves. Axons are particularly susceptible to the deleterious effects of oxidative stress; the threshold for mitochondrial membrane permeability transition decreases with age, which explains the age-related axonal degeneration that occurs in several neurodegenerative disorders. Some neurons such as spinal motor neurons and dopaminergic neurons of the substantia nigra undergo age-related compensatory changes, such as hypertrophy of cell bodies and processes to compensate for loss of neighboring neurons, thus allowing sprouting and reinnervation of their targets. This compensatory increase in axonal arborization may produce a metabolic stress that jeopardizes the survival of the axon. Axonal transport, including that of mitochondria, also decreases with age. These age-related axonal changes may interact with specific disease processes and promote axonal degeneration in several neurodegenerative disorders.

OXIDATIVE STRESS AND NEURODEGENERATION

The aging brain is uniquely vulnerable to oxidative and nitrosative damage.[38] Increasing evidence also implicates oxidative stress in the pathogenesis of AD, PD, ALS, Huntington disease (HD), and others.[39–43] For example, there is increasing evidence of astrocytic oxidative and nitrosative stress in PD pathogenesis.[39] Genes associated with PD pathogenesis, such as α-SYN synuclein, Parkin, and PTEN-induced kinase 1 (PINK1), regulate astrocytic function and may thus play an important role in mediating oxidative/nitrosative stress. Post-mortem analyses of PD patient brains, as well as experimental animal models, indicate that astrocyte activation and elevated levels of ROS/RNS are pathogenic features of PD. The presence of oxidative metabolites in PD patients has been correlated with the in vitro aggregation of α-SYN. The levels of oxidized α-SYN are elevated and those of antioxidants such as GSH, SOD, and catalase are reduced in the substantia nigra pars compacta in PD. Oxidative DNA lesions are also associated with dopaminergic neuronal loss in patients with Lewy body dementia. Astrocytic oxidative stress may be a consequence of aberrant ROS production resulting from mitochondrial dysfunction and dopamine metabolism in PD. For example, the vesicular transport and storage of dopamine are decreased in PD, leading to increased cytosolic dopamine, which can be oxidized to aldehyde products or form quinones or semiquinones that result in ROS production. Increased iron deposition is thought to predispose to oxidative stress.[8,44] There is iron deposition in neurons and glial cells in the substantia nigra pars compacta, which may predispose to α-SYN aggregation in PD.

In AD, there is accumulation of labile iron in Aβ plaques and tau tangles, while the neighboring cells express significant levels of ferritin and transferrin receptors. Iron increases translation of APP via an iron response element in the *APP* gene; APP in turn interacts with ferroportin, promoting iron influx to the cell. Tau promotes the export of neuronal iron by facilitating the trafficking of APP to the plasma membrane. Thus AD, PD, and tauopathies may all be associated with iron toxicity.

Several mechanisms, including excitotoxicity, mitochondrial dysfunction, ER stress, neuroinflammation, and oxidative stress may also contribute to neurodegeneration in ALS. Postmortem studies show evidence of oxidative damage to proteins, lipids, and RNA in this disorder. Gene mutations causing familial ALS, such as *SOD1* mutations result in abnormal aggregation on the mutant protein, indirectly triggering oxidative stress.[45] Familial ALS is associated with mutations in at least 20 genes, coding for proteins related to cell functions as diverse as RNA metabolism (*TARDBP, FUS/TLS, ATXN2, STX, ELPHNRNPA2/B1, ELP3, HNRNPA1, C9ORF72*), vesicle trafficking (*ALSIN, FIG4, OPTN, VABP, CHMP2B*), and proteasomal function (*UBQLN2, VCP*). Abnormal RNA metabolism causes mitochondrial damage and oxidative stress. Mutations affecting RNA-binding proteins such as TDP-43 or and FUS may have direct effect on the regulation of mRNAs coding for proteins involved in mitochondrial physiology. For example, ALS-related *TDP43* mutations alter the splicing of mRNA transcripts coding for Mtfr-1 (Mitochondrial fission regulator-1), an inner mitochondrial membrane protein involved in mitochondrial fission.

While the primary cause of HD is toxicity of the mutant *HTT*, protein misfolding, abnormal proteolysis, protein aggregation, transcriptional dysfunction, excitotoxic and oxidative stress, and glial activation have also been associated with neuronal death in HD.[46]

Mitochondrial dysfunction and oxidative stress provide targets for neuroprotective agents. Idebenone is a coenzyme Q analogue that has been approved for use in Friedreich ataxia[47] and may have beneficial effect by potentially bypassing defective complex I in other mitochondrial disorders such as Leber hereditary optic neuropathy and dominant optic atrophy. Edaravone is a scavenger of peroxyl radicals and peroxynitrite and was shown to reduce the rate of neurologic decline in a selected populations of patients with ALS.[48] Dimethyl fumarate, a drug used in multiple sclerosis, has potential neuroprotective and immunomodulatory effect both by inducing Nrf2/ and inhibiting NF-κB.[49]

KEY POINTS

- There are two major categories of cell death: accidental cell death occurs upon exposure to shear forces as in traumatic injury; regulated cell death involves molecular machineries that are potential targets for neuroprotection.
- The two main morphological types of cell death are apoptosis and necrosis.
- The final common execution of the apoptotic death machinery is activation of cysteine proteases called caspases.
- Necrosis is the manifestation of membrane fragmentation and typically occurs in the setting of mitochondrial failure, membrane lipid peroxidation, or formation of pore complexes in the plasma membrane.
- The mitochondria has a direct role in several cell death mechanisms, including intrinsic apoptosis, membrane transition pore-mediated necrosis, and parthanatos, and an indirect role in ferroptosis and lysosomal-dependent cell death.
- DNA damage or accumulation of misfolded proteins trigger intrinsic apoptosis.
- The initial event in intrinsic apoptosis is mitochondrial outer membrane permeabilization, which is controlled by the antagonistic influence of proapoptotic and antiapoptotic members of the BCL2 protein family.
- Mitochondrial outer membrane permeabilization allows release of cytochrome c, which is incorporated in a complex called apoptosome, leading to activation of caspase 3 responsible for DNA fragmentation.
- Mitochondrial permeability transition-driven necrosis results from the formation of a permeability transition pore complex triggered by severe oxidative stress and cytosolic Ca^{2+} overload and resulting in dissipation of the mitochondrial membrane potential, osmotic organelle breakdown, and rapid drop of ATP production.
- Parthanatos is driven by the hyperactivation of PARP1, resulting in depletion of both NAD^+ and ATP and release of an apoptosis-inducing factor from the mitochondria.
- Ferroptosis reflects severe lipid peroxidation in the setting of reflecting oxidative stress and availability of intracellular iron.
- Activation of death receptors such as tumor necrosis factor (TNF) receptor (TNFR) leads to the assembly of multiprotein complexes that trigger extrinsic apoptosis.
- Necroptosis is initiated by activation of either death receptors such as TNFR1 or toll-like receptors, resulting in the formation of a necrosome that affects cell membrane permeability.
- Pyroptosis is triggered during activation of innate immune responses leading to a formation of an inflammasome and release of proinflammatory cytokines.
- Reactive oxygen species, such as hydrogen peroxide, are involved both in normal redox signaling and in oxidative stress.
- The main sources of oxygen species are the mitochondrial respiratory chain and microglia.
- The two master molecular switches for redox signaling are the transcription factors nuclear factor-E2-related factor (Nrf2) and NF-κB.
- Oxidative stress may affect DNA, RNA, proteins, and lipids.
- Nitric oxide participates both in normal redox signaling and oxidative stress.
- At high intracellular levels, NO combines with superoxide to form peroxynitrite, promoting oxidative and nitrosative damage.
- Abnormal accumulation of glutamate leads to Ca^{2+}-mediated cell excitotoxicity.

- Axonal degeneration is an active and intrinsically regulated process that results from the reduced NAD^+, impaired axonal transport, mitochondrial dysfunction, increase in intraaxoplasmic Ca^{2+} and activation of calpains.
- Senescent cells, including astrocytes and microglia, exhibit a unique secretory profile, termed the senescence-associated secretory profile, which includes the release of pro-inflammatory cytokines that drive neurodegeneration.
- The aging brain is uniquely vulnerable to oxidative and nitrosative damage.
- Oxidative stress and mitochondrial dysfunction are key elements in in the pathogenesis of a neurodegenerative disorders.

REFERENCES

1. Galluzzi L, Bravo-San Pedro JM, Vitale I, et al. Essential versus accessory aspects of cell death: recommendations of the NCCD 2015. Cell Death Differ 2015;22:58–73.
2. Galluzzi L, Vitale I, Aaronson SA, et al. Molecular mechanisms of cell death: recommendations of the Nomenclature Committee on Cell Death 2018. Cell Death Differ 2018;25:486–541.
3. Doll S, Conrad M. Iron and ferroptosis: a still ill-defined liaison. IUBMB Life 2017;69:423–434.
4. Heneka MT, McManus RM, Latz E. Inflammasome signalling in brain function and neurodegenerative disease. Nat Rev Neurosci 2018;19:610–621.
5. Jones DP, Sies H. The redox code. Antioxid Redox Signal 2015;23:734–746.
6. Sies H, Berndt C, Jones DP. Oxidative stress. Annu Rev Biochem 2017;86:715–748.
7. Vilhardt F, Haslund-Vinding J, Jaquet V, McBean G. Microglia antioxidant systems and redox signalling. Br J Pharmacol 2017;174:1719–1732.
8. Liu C, Liang MC, Soong TW. Nitric oxide, iron and neurodegeneration. Front Neurosci 2019;13:114.
9. Bano D, Ankarcrona M. Beyond the critical point: an overview of excitotoxicity, calcium overload and the downstream consequences. Neurosci Lett 2018;663:79–85.
10. Wu QJ, Tymianski M. Targeting NMDA receptors in stroke: new hope in neuroprotection. Mol Brain 2018;11:15.
11. Brassai A, Suvanjeiev RG, Ban EG, Lakatos M. Role of synaptic and nonsynaptic glutamate receptors in ischaemia induced neurotoxicity. Brain Res Bull 2015;112:1–6.
12. Parsons MP, Raymond LA. Extrasynaptic NMDA receptor involvement in central nervous system disorders. Neuron 2014;82:279–293.
13. Lai TW, Zhang S, Wang YT. Excitotoxicity and stroke: identifying novel targets for neuroprotection. Prog Neurobiol 2014;115:157–188.
14. Coleman M. Axon degeneration mechanisms: commonality amid diversity. Nat Rev Neurosci 2005;6:889–898.
15. Ding C, Hammarlund M. Mechanisms of injury-induced axon degeneration. Curr Opin Neurobiol 2019;57:171–178.
16. Mack TG, Reiner M, Beirowski B, et al. Wallerian degeneration of injured axons and synapses is delayed by a Ube4b/NMNAT chimeric gene. Nat Neurosci 2001;4:1199–1206.
17. Conforti L, Gilley J, Coleman MP. Wallerian degeneration: an emerging axon death pathway linking injury and disease. Nat Rev Neurosci 2014;15:394–409.
18. Freeman MR. Signaling mechanisms regulating Wallerian degeneration. Curr Opin Neurobiol 2014;27:224–231.
19. Milde S, Gilley J, Coleman MP. Axonal trafficking of NMNAT2 and its roles in axon growth and survival in vivo. Bioarchitecture 2013;3:133–140.
20. Wang J, Zhai Q, Chen Y, et al. A local mechanism mediates NAD-dependent protection of axon degeneration. J Cell Biol 2005;170:349–355.
21. Klim JR, Williams LA, Limone F, et al. ALS-implicated protein TDP-43 sustains levels of STMN2, a mediator of motor neuron growth and repair. Nat Neurosci 2019;22:167–179.
22. Maday S, Twelvetrees AE, Moughamian AJ, Holzbaur EL. Axonal transport: cargo-specific mechanisms of motility and regulation. Neuron 2014;84:292–309.
23. Rasband MN, Tayler J, Kaga Y, et al. CNP is required for maintenance of axon-glia interactions at nodes of Ranvier in the CNS. Glia 2005;50:86–90.
24. Court FA, Coleman MP. Mitochondria as a central sensor for axonal degenerative stimuli. Trends Neurosci 2012;35:364–372.
25. Tsutsui S, Stys PK. Metabolic injury to axons and myelin. Exp Neurol 2013;246:26–34.
26. Stirling DP, Stys PK. Mechanisms of axonal injury: internodal nanocomplexes and calcium deregulation. Trends Mol Med 2010;16:160–170.
27. Mattson MP, Magnus T. Ageing and neuronal vulnerability. Nat Rev Neurosci 2006;7:278–294.
28. Zorov DB, Juhaszova M, Sollott SJ. Mitochondrial reactive oxygen species (ROS) and ROS-induced ROS release. Physiol Rev 2014;94:909–950.
29. Fern RF, Matute C, Stys PK. White matter injury: ischemic and nonischemic. Glia 2014;62:1780–1789.
30. Stys PK. General mechanisms of axonal damage and its prevention. J Neurol Sci 2005;233:3–13.
31. Johnson VE, Stewart W, Smith DH. Axonal pathology in traumatic brain injury. Exp Neurol 2013;246:35–43.
32. Albayram O, Kondo A, Mannix R, et al. Cis P-tau is induced in clinical and preclinical brain injury and contributes to post-injury sequelae. Nat Commun 2017;8:1000.
33. Arena JD, Smith DH, Lee EB, et al. Tau immunophenotypes in chronic traumatic encephalopathy recapitulate those of ageing and Alzheimer's disease. Brain 2020;143:1572–1587.
34. Falcon B, Zivanov J, Zhang W, et al. Novel tau filament fold in chronic traumatic encephalopathy encloses hydrophobic molecules. Nature 2019;568:420–423.
35. VanItallie TB. Traumatic brain injury (TBI) in collision sports: possible mechanisms of transformation into chronic traumatic encephalopathy (CTE). Metabolism 2019;100S:153943.
36. Lu KP, Kondo A, Albayram O, Herbert MK, Liu H, Zhou XZ. Potential of the antibody against cis-phosphorylated tau in the early diagnosis, treatment, and prevention of Alzheimer disease and brain injury. JAMA Neurol 2016;73:1356–1362.

37. Adalbert R, Coleman MP. Review: axon pathology in age-related neurodegenerative disorders. Neuropathol Appl Neurobiol 2013;39:90–108.
38. Liguori I, Russo G, Curcio F, et al. Oxidative stress, aging, and diseases. Clin Interv Aging 2018;13:757–772.
39. Rizor A, Pajarillo E, Johnson J, Aschner M, Lee E. Astrocytic oxidative/nitrosative stress contributes to Parkinson's disease pathogenesis: the dual role of reactive astrocytes. Antioxidants (Basel) 2019;8:265–284.
40. Ben Haim L, Carrillo-de Sauvage MA, Ceyzeriat K, Escartin C. Elusive roles for reactive astrocytes in neurodegenerative diseases. Front Cell Neurosci 2015;9:278.
41. Ferrer I, Martinez A, Blanco R, Dalfo E, Carmona M. Neuropathology of sporadic Parkinson disease before the appearance of parkinsonism: preclinical Parkinson disease. J Neural Transm (Vienna) 2011;118:821–839.
42. Niedzielska E, Smaga I, Gawlik M, et al. Oxidative stress in neurodegenerative diseases. Mol Neurobiol 2016;53:4094–4125.
43. Singh A, Kukreti R, Saso L, Kukreti S. Oxidative stress: a key modulator in neurodegenerative diseases. Molecules 2019;24:1583–1603.
44. Wang T, Xu SF, Fan YG, Li LB, Guo C. Iron pathophysiology in Alzheimer's diseases. Adv Exp Med Biol 2019;1173:67–104.
45. Bozzo F, Mirra A, Carri MT. Oxidative stress and mitochondrial damage in the pathogenesis of ALS: New perspectives. Neurosci Lett 2017;636:3–8.
46. Kumar A, Ratan RR. Oxidative stress and Huntington's disease: the good, the bad, and the ugly. J Huntingtons Dis 2016;5:217–237.
47. Clay A, Hearle P, Schadt K, Lynch DR. New developments in pharmacotherapy for Friedreich ataxia. Expert Opin Pharmacother 2019;20:1855–1867.
48. Writing G, Edaravone ALSSG. Safety and efficacy of edaravone in well defined patients with amyotrophic lateral sclerosis: a randomised, double-blind, placebo-controlled trial. Lancet Neurol 2017;16:505–512.
49. Lu MC, Ji JA, Jiang ZY, You QD. The Keap1-Nrf2-ARE pathway as a potential preventive and therapeutic target: an update. Med Res Rev 2016;36:924–963.

13 Growth Factors, Survival, and Regeneration

OVERVIEW

Neurotrophic or growth factors are soluble extracellular proteins that have a critical role in regulation of cell proliferation, growth, differentiation, and survival throughout life and have a major role in neural development, synaptic plasticity, and repair. There are several families of neurotrophic factors. Growth factors acting via tyrosine kinase receptors activate canonical downstream survival pathways. One important effector of survival pathways is the mechanistic (mammalian) target of rapamycin (mTOR), which promotes protein synthesis and inhibits both autophagy and apoptosis. Retrograde signaling following injury triggers profound changes in transcription and translation that drive axon growth. Hypoxia-inducible factors promote transcription of genes that promote angiogenesis, erythropoiesis, and glucose metabolism and are under inhibitory control by Von Hippel-Lindau (VHL) proteins. The activity of these growth-promoting pathways is negatively regulated by products of tumor suppressor genes. Loss of function mutations of genes controlling growth factors and hypoxia-inducible growth factor signaling are associated with hereditary tumor syndromes, some of them associated with seizures. Loss of neurotrophic signal is an important mechanism of neurodegeneration. Preclinical studies in experimental models indicate that neurotrophic factors exert neuroprotective effects in a wide variety of neurologic disorders. However, several variables, including the bioavailability of these factors in the CNS remain a therapeutic challenge and have so far limited the applicability of this approach to human neurologic disorders. The main aims of this chapter are to review: (1) the different families of growth factors and their signaling mechanism, (2) the role of neurotrophic factors in plasticity and survival in the nervous system, (3) the mechanisms of axonal repair after injury, (4) the factors mediating the response to hypoxia, (5) disorders resulting from dysregulated growth factor signaling, and (6) the growth factors as therapeutic targets in neurodegenerative disorders.

NEUROTROPHIC FACTORS

According to the "neurotrophic factor hypothesis," neurons innervating a particular target compete for a limited supply of target-derived trophic factors in order to match the density of innervation to the size of the target. For example, during development exuberant connectivity is pruned as the result of competition between axon terminals for trophic factors provided by potential postsynaptic targets. Neurotrophic factors also have multiple functions in the adult nervous system and act not only as target-derived retrograde signals but also as autocrine or paracrine signals between neurons and glial cells. Neurotrophic factors belong to different families of structurally related proteins that act via specific types of structurally related receptors in selected cell targets (Table 13.1).

Families of Neurotrophic Factors

The family of neurotrophins includes nerve growth factor (NGF), brain-derived neurotrophic factor (BDNF), and neurotrophins-3 (NT-3), NT-4, and NT-5.[1,2] Related molecules are members of the epidermal growth factor, fibroblast growth factor, and platelet-derived neurotrophic factor families. The neurotrophins are synthesized as precursors, or proneurotrophins, which are cleaved intracellularly to produce the mature proteins. These proteins form stable, noncovalent dimers that bind tyrosine kinase receptors known as neurotrophin receptors (NTFRs) or tropomyosin kinase (Trk) receptors. In addition to binding to their respective prosurvival tyrosine kinase receptors, neurotrophins also bind to the common, low-affinity p75^{NTR} receptor that responds to low levels of neurotrophins and has a predominantly proapoptotic effect. The overall level of neurotrophins and the functional interplay of signals generated by Trk and p75^{NTR} determine

TABLE 13.1 *Representative Families of Growth Factors, Their Receptors, and Targets*

Growth Factor (example)	Receptor	Targets (examples)
Nerve growth factor (NGF)	Tropomyosin kinase (Trk) A	Peptidergic DRG neurons Spinothalamic tract neurons Sympathetic neurons Basal forebrain cholinergic neurons
Brain-derived neurotrophic factor (BDNF)	TrkB	Neurons in cerebral cortex and, hippocampus Corticospinal tract Dopaminergic SNc neurons Trigeminal, petrosal nodose, vestibular, and cochlear ganglion neurons
Neurotrophin-3 (NT-3)	TrkC	Large proprioceptive DRG neurons Dorsal columns Hair cells Enteric neurons
Glial-derived neurotrophic factors GDNF, neurturin, artemin, and persephin	Ret and GFRα (GFRα1-4) heterodimer	Small nonpeptidergic DRG neurons Enteric neurons Parasympathetic neurons Midbrain dopaminergic neurons
Insulin-like growth factor-1 (IGF1) and 2 IGF2	IGF1-R and IGFR-2	Most neurons in developing brain Sensory organs Astrocytes Oligodendrocytes
Neuregulins	ErbB	Schwann cells Oligodendrocytes
Ephrins	EphA, EphB	Astrocytes Hippocampus Spinal cord
Ciliary neurotrophic factor, CNTF)	CNTFRα/gp130/LIFRβ tripartite receptor	Motor neurons Autonomic neurons Basal forebrain neurons Hippocampal neurons

DRG, dorsal root ganglion; IGFR, insulin-like growth factor receptor; LIF, leukemia inhibitory factor

the balance between cell survival and apoptosis during development. The insulin-like growth factor (IGF) family includes insulin, IGF1, and IGF2, and their effects are mediated by two types of receptors, IGF1 receptor (IGF1R) and IGF2 (IGF2R). There are several other families of growth factors that share final transduction mechanisms with neurotrophins. The glial-derived neurotrophic factor (GDNF) family includes GDNF, neurturin, artemin, and persephin. These growth factors form a complex with the GDNF family receptor alpha 1 (GFRα1) present in the neuronal membrane, and this complex binds to RET, a transmembrane receptor triggering an intracellular signaling cascade that promotes survival. The neuregulins (NRGs) are a family of proteins that act via the epidermal growth factor receptor tyrosine kinase ErbB. The Eph (erythropoietin-producing hepatocellular carcinoma) receptor tyrosine kinases bind ephrins on neighboring cells, generating cell contact-dependent bidirectional signals. Eph "forward" signaling depends on ephrin binding, which induces Eph receptor clustering, autophosphorylation, and activation; in the ephrin "reverse" signaling ephrins associate with transmembrane partners, such as the $p75^{NTR}$ neurotrophin receptor or the TrkB and RET receptor tyrosine kinases.[3]

The neurotrophic cytokines are related to the immune cytokine interleukin-6 (IL-6) and include ciliary neurotrophic factor (CNTF), leukemia inhibitory factor (LIF), and cardiotrophin-1. These neurotrophic cytokines act via a common receptor subunit, gp130, which forms a heterodimeric complex with the LIF receptor (LIFR) β. CNTF binds to a distinct subunit (CTNFR α) that forms a tripartite receptor to gp130 and LIFRβ.

Growth Factor Signaling via Tyrosine Kinase Receptors

Activation of neurotrophic factor receptors triggers several transduction cascades, including phosphorylation of transcription factors that regulate expression of several genes.[2] The prototypical growth signaling pathways are those triggered by activation of membrane tyrosine kinase receptors by members of the neurotrophin family, such as the TrkB receptor for BDNF (Figure 13.1).These receptors consist of an extracellular ligand-binding domain, a single transmembrane domain, and an intracellular tyrosine kinase domain. Upon binding of growth factors, these receptors undergo dimerization and *trans*-autophosphorylation at their tyrosine residues. Interaction of these phosphotyrosine residues with various adaptor molecules allows the recruitment of signal proteins to the membrane and initiates three main signal transduction pathways that modulate gene transcription and promote protein synthesis, vesicular trafficking, cell growth and differentiation, metabolism, and resistance to oxidative stress: the Ras-mitogen-activated kinase (MAPK), the phosphatidylinositol 3'kinase (PI3K)-AKT (protein kinase B) pathway, and the phospholipase Cγ (PLCγ) pathway. The Ras-MAPK pathway involves activation of the small GTP-binding protein Ras, which acts as a molecular switch transitioning between a GDP-bound inactive state and a GTP-bound active state. Binding of the growth factor to the tyrosine kinase receptor produces a switch from an inactive cytosolic Ras-GDP to an active membrane-bound Ras-GTP by action of a guanosine-exchanging factor that binds to phosphotyrosine residues of the receptors. Ras activates the MAPK pathway, which is a cytosolic signaling cascade that consists of sequential phosphorylation and activation of several serine/threonine protein kinases, including Raf, MAPK/extracellular signal receptor kinase (MEK) 1 and 2, and finally the extracellular signal-regulated kinases (ERKs)1/2. ERKs are the ultimate effectors of this pathway and target a large number of downstream cytosolic and nuclear molecules, including membrane proteins, other protein kinases, and transcription factors. One important target is the transcription factor CREB (cyclic adenylyl monophosphate responsive element binding protein). CREB phosphorylation downstream of growth factor signals allows the recruitment of the transcriptional coactivator CREB-binding protein, which promotes transcription of a large number of survival and synaptic plasticity genes. The second major survival pathway involves PI3K and eventually leads to membrane recruitment and activation of AKT which is a critical effector of neuronal growth and survival by phosphorylating several targets. The third major effector of growth factor signaling is PLCγ, leading to activation of protein kinase C, which phosphorylates NTFRs and stabilizes their interaction with neurotrophins. These cascades are also activated by other signals, including dehydroepiandrosterone (DHEA). This abundant steroid in humans interacts with and modulates a variety of membrane and intracellular receptors and induces the first step of the TrkA and TrkC receptors activation (phosphorylation at tyrosine residues).[4] This may provide a potential mechanism for the neuroprotective roles of DHEA or derivatives in neurodegenerative disorders such as motor neuron disease.[5]

Mammalian (Mechanistic) Target of Rapamycin: A Major Effector of Growth and Survival

The mechanistic (mammalian) target of rapamycin (mTOR) is a ubiquitously expressed serine threonine protein kinase that forms two functionally distinct multiprotein complexes, mTORC1 and mTORC2, and is a critical downstream effector of growth factor signaling (Figure 13.1).[6,7] The TORC1 kinase complex contains the regulatory scaffold protein Raptor (regulatory-associated protein of mTOR) and is inhibited by rapamycin. The mTORC1 pathway is activated by growth factors, excitatory synaptic activity, and amino acids, and is inhibited during starvation and cell stress. Activation of mTORC1 requires its binding to the small Ras-like GTPase Rheb (Ras homologous enriched in brain). In basal conditions, a functional complex formed by the tuberous sclerosis (TSC) proteins TSC1 (hamartin) and TSC2 (tuberin) stimulates Rheb GTPase activity, rendering an inactive Rheb-GDP complex that is unable to activate mTORC1. Growth factors, such as BDNF or IGF1, trigger inhibitory phosphorylation of TSC proteins and thus activate mTORC1 signaling. The two classical pathways for growth factor signaling activating mTORC1 are the PI3K-AKT and Ras-MEK-ERK pathways. The main effects of mTORC1 are activation of mRNA translation and protein synthesis, simulation of lipid synthesis, and inhibition of autophagy.[8] There is a reciprocal interaction between the mTORC1 and the adenosine monophosphate-activated kinase (AMPK) for regulating cellular metabolism, energy homeostasis, and cell growth.[8] AMPK is activated by a variety of cellular stressors that decrease ATP generation such as nutrient starvation, ischemia, and hypoxia. Under these conditions, AMPK phosphorylates many substrates that turn on alternative catabolic pathways. AMPK also phosphorylates TSC2 and activates the TSC, thereby attenuating the TORC1 pathway. However, in the setting of metabolic stress AMPK activates the mTORC2 axis as a promoter of cell survival.

Inhibition of Growth Factor Signaling by Tumor Suppressor Gene Products

Products of tumor suppressor genes inhibit several steps of the growth factor signaling pathway. For example, neurofibromin-1, a Ras GTPase-activating protein encoded by the *NF1* tumor suppressor gene, promotes the switch-off of Ras signaling. Phosphatase-tensin homolog (PTEN), encoded by the *PTEN* tumor-suppressor gene, inhibits the activity of the PI3K-AKT pathway. The basal activity of the complex formed by TSC1 and TSC2 stimulates Rheb

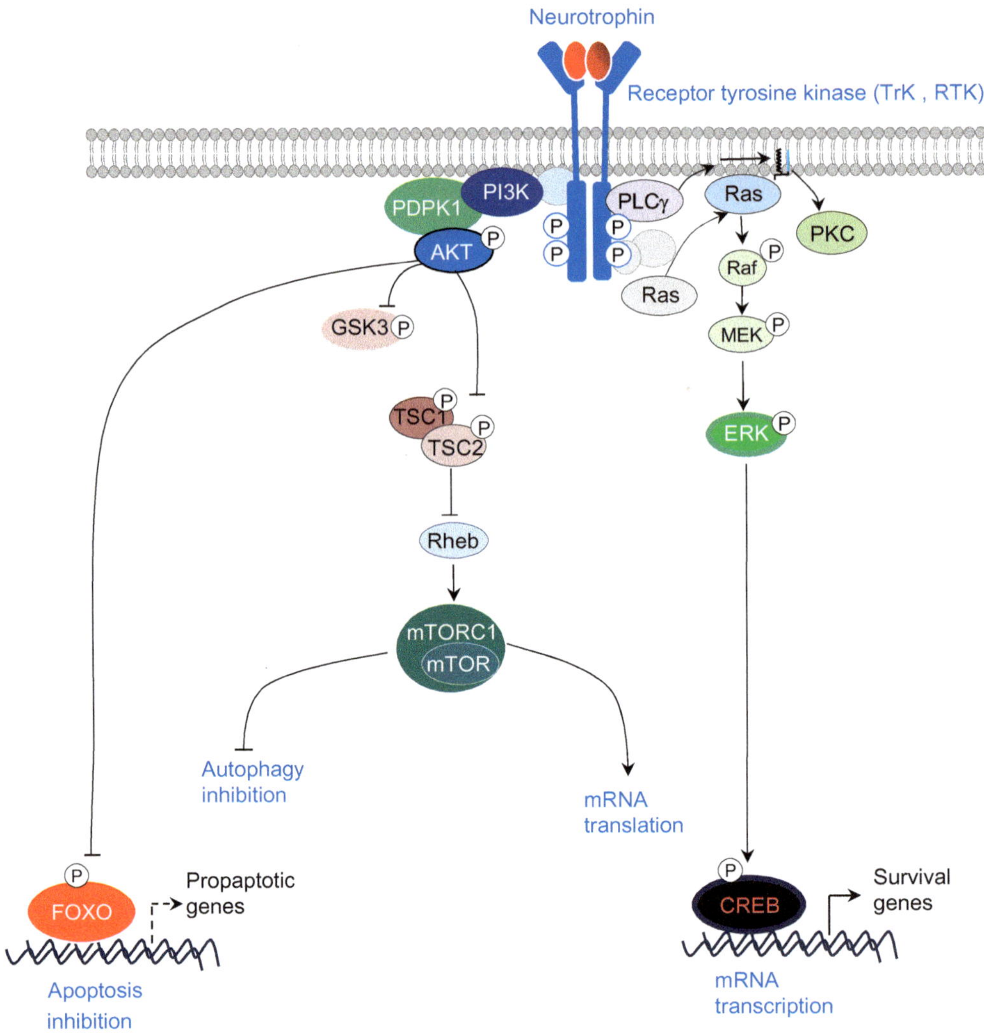

FIGURE 13.1 Growth factor signals.

The prototypical growth-signaling pathways are those triggered by neurotrophins acting via tyrosine kinase receptors. Upon binding of growth factors, these receptors undergo dimerization and *trans*-autophosphorylation. Interaction of their phosphotyrosine residues with various adaptor molecules allows membrane recruitment of signal proteins that initiates three main signal transduction pathways: Ras-mitogen activated kinase (MAPK); phosphatidylinositol 3'kinase (PI3K)-AKT (protein kinase B); and phospholipase Cγ (PLCγ). The Ras-MAPK pathway involves the small GTP-binding protein Ras, which activates the MAPK pathway. This involves a sequential phosphorylation cascade that includes the serine-threonine kinases Raf, MAPK/extracellular signal receptor kinase (MEK) 1 and 2, and the extracellular signal regulated kinases (ERKs) 1 and 2. ERK1/2 are the ultimate effectors and target a large number of downstream cytosolic and nuclear molecules. An important target is the transcription factor CREB (cyclic adenylyl monophosphate responsive binding element binding protein). The PI3K pathway leads to activation of phosphoinositide-dependent kinase 1 (PDPK1), leading to membrane recruitment, phosphorylation, and activation of AKT (protein kinase B). AKT is a critical effector of neuronal growth and survival by phosphorylating several targets, including the Bcl-2 family member BAD, glycogen synthase 3 kinase β (GSK3), and forehead box O (FOXO) family of transcriptional activators. The PLCγ pathway leads to activation of protein kinase C (PKC), which amplifies the cellular growth signal. A major effector of growth and survival pathways is mechanistic (mammalian) target of rapamycin (mTOR), which forms two functionally distinct multiprotein signaling complexes, mTOR complex 1 (mTORC1) and mTOR complex 2 (mTORC2) (not shown). Activation of mTORC1 requires the small Ras-like GTPase Rheb (Ras homologous enriched in brain). In basal conditions, a functional complex formed by the tuberous sclerosis (TSC) proteins TSC1 (hamartin) and TSC2 (tuberin) stimulates Rheb GTPase activity, rendering an inactive Rheb-GDP complex that is unable to activate mTORC1. Growth factors trigger inhibitory phosphorylation of TSC proteins and thus activate mTORC1 signaling.

GTPase activity and thus inhibits mTORC1 signaling. Mutations of the genes encoding these growth inhibitory proteins result in malformation of cortical development (typically associated with seizures) and predisposition to neoplasm, as discussed later in this chapter.

Signaling of Neurotrophic Cytokines

Cytokines such as CNTF may exert neurotrophic actions and promote axonal regeneration after injury. The effects of CNTF, as well other cytokines and interferons, involve the Janus kinase (JAK)-signal transducer of activator of transcription (STAT) pathwa.[9] Upon engagement by ligand, JAKs become activated and phosphorylate both each other and the intracellular tail of their receptors, thereby creating docking sites for latent STATs, which then directly bind DNA and regulate gene expression. There are different JAK and STAT isoforms. For example, STAT3 is expressed in neurons and mediates the effects of CNTF on axonal growth. Astrocytes express several STAT isoforms. For example activation of JAK-STAT1 and JAK-STAT3 promotes astrocytic production of expression of vascular endothelial growth factor (VEGF) in response to interleukin-17 released during hypoxia. The JAK-STAT signaling pathway has a crucial role in promoting astrogliogenesis during development; STAT3 also has an important role in the control of astrocyte reactivity, in response to injury.[10] JAK/STAT signaling regulates the transcription of the suppressor of cytokine signaling (SOCS), which provides a negative feedback, by inhibiting JAK and STAT activation and phosphorylation, and thereby signaling activated by cytokines and growth factors.[11]

NEUROTROPHIC SIGNALING FOR NEURONAL GROWTH, SURVIVAL, AND PLASTICITY

Neurotrophic factors may promote survival of selective neuronal or glial populations. The targets of growth factors may change during development or in response to synaptic activity or injury. Many growth factors act in combinatorial and sequential ways at different stages of growth and maturation of the cell. In some cases, they may be released at the synapses to produce fast modulation of postsynaptic responses and long-term structural changes in the postsynaptic cell.

Nerve Growth Factor as the Prototypical Retrograde Signal

Retrograde axonal transport of signaling endosomes is critical for the neurotrophic effects of some growth factors, such as NGF.[12] Signaling endosomes form during internalization of neurotrophins bound to their cognate tyrosine kinase (Trk) receptors. For example NGF-bound TrkA undergoes internalization via clathrin-dependent or caveolin-mediated endocytosis. Following internalization, the NGF-TrkA complex undergoes retrograde transport via signaling endosomes, including early (Rab5-positive) and late (Rab7-positive) endosomes.[12] Nerve growth factor, acting via TrkA (NTRK1) receptors is critical for survival of sympathetic ganglion neurons and small nociceptive peptidergic dorsal root ganglion (DRG) neurons. Mutations of the *NTRK1* gene encoding the NGF receptors produce hereditary sensory autonomic neuropathy type IV (HSAN-IV), an autosomal recessive disorder that usually begins in infancy and is characterized by anhidrosis, insensitivity to noxious stimuli leading to self-mutilating behavior, and intellectual disability[13] Mutation of the NGF gene produces a similar phenotype (HSAN-V).[14] Familial dysautonomia (HSAN-III) is associated with a germline loss-of-function mutation in the *Elp1* gene encoding a scaffolding protein within the nuclear Elongator protein complex that is essential for retrograde NGF-TrkA receptor signaling.[15] The NGF/TrkA signaling is also important for trophic support of basal forebrain cholinergic neurons. This system is particularly vulnerable to aging and is affected early in Alzheimer disease (AD).[16]

BDNF as the Prototype Growth Factor for Synaptic Plasticity

Brain-derived neurotrophic factor is the most ubiquitous member of the family of neurotrophins in the central nervous system and has a major role in activity-dependent synaptic plasticity.[17,18] It is produced "on demand" in response to neuronal activity from the precursor pro-BDNF that is transported and processed via the secretory pathway. The *BDNF* gene is complex, and its transcription is under epigenetic control by both DNA methylation and histone acetylation.[19,20] The methyl CpG-binding protein 2 (MeCP2) functions as transcriptional regulator of the *BDNF* gene. X-linked *MECP2* mutations are responsible for Rett syndrome. Synaptic activity promotes BDNF transcription by triggering neuronal depolarization, activation of glutamate N-methyl-D-aspartate receptors (NMDARs), and opening of L-type Ca^{2+} channels. The promoter region of some exons of the *BDNF* gene contains Ca^{2+} responsive elements that bind CREB. Activity dependent phosphorylation of CREB by calmodulin kinase IV, ERK 1/2, and other pathways triggered by neuronal activity promotes activation of the *BDNF* gene. Activity-dependent regulation of BDNF mRNA targeting and translation in dendrites is an important mechanism for fine-tuning of synaptic plasticity. For example, BDNF produced in cortical neurons is anterogradely transported to the striatum and supports survival of medium spiny neurons. The anterograde transport of BDNF depends on phosphorylated huntingtin.[21] BDNF may thus have a major role in the pathogenesis of Huntington disease (HD). Striatal medium spiny neurons are prone to degeneration in HD and depend on BDNF for their survival.[22] When BDNF binds to its receptors, the TrkB/BDNF receptor complex is endocytosed and trafficked to the cell body for downstream signal transduction. Huntingtin-associated protein 1

(HAP1), which is a huntingtin adaptor for axonal transport of vesicles along microtubules, also interacts with BDNF and its receptor, promoting endocytosis. Mature BDNF is stored and released from both axons and dendrites in response to excitatory synaptic activity.[23]

BDNF, acting via TrkB receptors, controls development and plasticity of neurons in the hippocampus, cerebral cortex, and striatum as well as those in the trigeminal, petrosal, nodoses, vestibular, and cochlear ganglia. BDNF-TrkB signaling promotes synaptic plasticity by activating the canonical Ras/MEK/ERK, PI3K/AKT, and PLCγ pathways.[24] Targets of phosphorylation by these pathways include CREB, mTOR, and actin-binding proteins.[25] Via these mechanisms BDNF promotes NMDAR-triggered long-term potentiation of glutamatergic synapses in the hippocampus and other cortical regions.[26,27] BDNF also promotes activity-dependent increase in the number and volume of dendritic spines via regulation Rho GTPases that facilitate actin-polymerization and stability.[28,29] BDNF also facilitates adult neurogenesis in the dentate gyrus of the hippocampus.[30] The effects of BDNF may also occur independently of TrkB receptor activation. BDNF also activates JAK-STAT3 signaling in neurons and elicits many changes in the transcriptome, altering expression of ion channels, receptors, and other modulators of cell excitability, synaptic plasticity, neurogenesis, and axonal remodeling.[31]

Insulin-Like Peptides

The insulin-like peptides IGF1 and IGF2 and their respective receptors, IGF1R and IGF2R, have a major role in cell differentiation in the nervous system.[32,33–35] They have higher expression during development than in then adult brain. IGF1 is produced by all cell types and is abundantly expressed in the neocortex, hippocampus, cerebellum, brainstem, hypothalamus, and spinal cord. IGF2 is the most abundant insulin-like peptide in the adult brain, with the highest levels of expression in the myelin sheaths, and in the choroid plexus, leptomeninges, and hypothalamus. Insulin is expressed in neural cells during development but not in the adult nervous system. Signaling by insulin-like peptides in the brain involves two mechanisms, paracrine, via local production of IGF1 and IGF2 in different brain cells; and endocrine, via movement of circulating insulin and IGF1 across the blood-brain barrier (BBB) and the blood-CSF barrier. Passage of circulating IGF1 across the BBB requires both the IGF1R and the low-density lipoprotein receptor-related protein 1. There is a synaptic activity-dependent uptake of serum IGF1 by neurons, which occurs in parallel with the activity-dependent increase in local blood flow.[36] The passage of circulating insulin and IGF1 across the blood-CSF barrier involves their constitutive transport by transcytosis also via the IGF1R and low-density lipoprotein receptor-related protein 1. IGF2 is directly synthesized by the choroid plexus. The function of IGF1 and IGF2 in the brain is regulated by their binding to IGF-binding proteins (IGFBPs), which are produced by neurons, glial cells, choroid epithelia, and cerebral blood vessels, and are widely expressed in the neocortex, hippocampus, cerebellum, and spinal cord. The biological actions of insulin-like peptides are mediated by three different types of receptors, with some functional overlap.[37] The effects of IGF1 and insulin are primarily mediated by IGF1R and involve the canonical PI3K/AKT and Ras/MEK/ERK pathways. IGF1 acts during all of the major phases of brain development. It promotes proliferation of neural precursor cells; acts as a prosurvival signal for developing neurons; facilitates subsequent neuronal differentiation, synaptogenesis, and network formation in the hippocampus, neocortex, and olfactory bulb; participates in the formation of the sensory organs of the eyes and ears; and promotes angiogenesis as well as maturation of astrocytes and oligodendrocytes. The importance of IGF1 signaling in human brain development is reflected by the phenotypes caused by congenital IGF1 deficiency (intrauterine and postnatal growth retardation, microcephaly, and sensorineural deafness) or *IGF1R* mutations (microcephaly and Moyamoya disease).[38]

GDNF Signaling in Neurons and Glia

In a healthy adult brain GDNF is exclusively expressed by neurons and exerts a paracrine effect complex with GFRα1, which may interact via either the RET tyrosine kinase receptor or via the neural cell adhesion molecule (NCAM).[39] RET is expressed in several neuron subtypes, including nigrostriatal dopaminergic neurons, motor neurons, enteric neurons, and sensory neurons. Both RET and GFRα1 are expressed in midbrain dopaminergic neurons from very early stages of their development. Evidence indicates that GDNF promotes growth and survival of dopaminergic nigrostriatal neurons and has a strong neuroprotective effect on adult dopaminergic cells.[40] Mice with constitutive RET activation have increased number of dopaminergic neurons in the substantia nigra pars compacta, associated with increased level of tyrosine hydroxylase and dopamine transporters, and increased level of dopamine in the striatum.[41] Gain-of-function mutations of *RET* cause multiple endocrine type 2 B (MEN2B). This is an uncommon autosomal dominant cancer syndrome characterized by young-onset axonal peripheral neuropathy with pes cavus associated with mucosal neuromas in the lips and tongue and Marfanoid habitus; these features are useful for early detection, as these patients are susceptible to medullary thyroid carcinoma, pheochromocytoma, and other neoplasms.[42] In addition to its neurotropic role on midbrain dopaminergic neuron survival, GDNF signal may have a role in synaptic formation in the hippocampus and in the development and maturation of several types of GABAergic neurons, including cerebellar Purkinje cells. GDNF also has a role in in the maintenance of functional properties of cellular elements of the BBB and blood-nerve barrier, including pericytes and endothelial cells. Neuroinflammation induces GDNF expression in activated astrocytes and microglia. GDNF secreted by astrocytes reduces the phagocytic activity and production of reactive oxygen species by activated microglia.

Neuroprotective Effects of Growth Factors

Many studies in experimental models indicate that growth factors such as BDNF and IGF1 may have neuroprotective effects in the setting of hypoxia/ischemia, traumatic brain or spinal cord injury, neuroinflammation, and neurodegenerative disorders such as Alzheimer disease (AD), Parkinson disease (PD), and amyotrophic lateral sclerosis (ALS).[43,44] These neuroprotective effects are primarily mediated by the PI3K/AKT/mTOR pathway, which inhibits apoptosis and autophagy. For example, AKT phosphorylates and inactivates several components of the machinery for apoptosis, such as Bcl-2 family member BAD; glycogen synthase 3 kinase β (GSK3), and Forehead box O family of transcriptional activators, while promoting expression of antiapoptotic BCL-2. Only few examples will be mentioned here. Hypoxic injury elicits upregulation of IGF1 and IGFR1 in neurons and astrocytes; IGF1 is neuroprotective in animal models of stroke and seizures. IGF1 also increases Aβ clearance and blocks the action of proinflammatory cytokines. BDNF released by microglia in the setting of neuroinflammation may also have neuroprotective action. GDNF has a strong neuroprotective effect on adult midbrain dopaminergic neurons.[40]

AXONAL REGENERATION

The process of axonal regeneration is complex, and requires the formation of a new growth cone, reorganization of the axonal cytoskeleton, transport of mRNA, proteins, mitochondria, and other materials, local translation of mRNAs, formation of new cell membranes, and insertion of cell surface molecules. Many studies on axonal regeneration have been performed in models of axonal transection of DRG neurons, spinal cord injury (SCI), and optic nerve transection.

Injury Signals Initiating Axonal Regeneration

Studies on DRG models showed that peripheral axotomy elicits a conditioning effect that switches DRG neurons into a growth state enabling both peripheral and central branch axon regeneration. This effect relies on a transcription-dependent program induced by the disruption of signals that are normally transported retrogradely to the nucleus after an axon reaches its target (Figure 13.2). In the normal state, this intrinsic neuronal growth program is suppressed by signals produced by the target itself.[45–51] One important retrograde signal is initiated by increased Ca^{2+} concentration at the site of injury. The breach of the axonal membrane triggers membrane depolarization, which activates Ca^{2+} influx via voltage-gated channels and initiates a Ca^{2+} wave that back-propagates along the axon to the cell body. Elevation of Ca^{2+} in activates protein kinase C-μ, which triggers nuclear export of histone deacetylase 5 (HDAC5); this promotes histone H3 acetylation and expression of regeneration-activating genes. In addition, HDAC5 undergoes anterograde transport in the axon and reduces levels of acetylated α-tubulin thereby promoting the formation of a dynamic growth cone tip.[52] The early wave of retrograde Ca^{2+} signaling is followed by a delayed phase of retrograde signaling mediated by macromolecular protein complexes that undergo retrograde transport to the nucleus via dynein/dynactin motors.[45] Increased levels of cyclic adenosine monophosphate (cAMP) triggers specific transcription factors and the activation of genes that are normally repressed by the target-derived negative signals. One important signal for local mRNA translation at the site of injury is upregulation of neurotrophic cytokines such as CNTF and interleukin-6. Upon binding to their receptors, these cytokines activate the JAK-STAT3 pathway; phosphorylated STAT3 is retrogradely transported from the site of injury to the nucleus via an importin complex that binds dynein/dynactin.[53] In the nucleus, STAT proteins dimerize and promote expression of repair-associated genes.[45] Members of the Krüppel-like family of transcription factors interact with activated STAT3 and inhibit JAK/STAT signaling. Another signaling pathway regulating axonal regeneration is the dual leucine zipper kinase–JUN amino terminal kinase pathway. This signaling has a dual effect on axonal growth, with positive or negative effect depending on the target.[11,45,48,54] One convergent mediator of axon regeneration is phosphorylated ERK, which is a transcriptional activator that is incorporated in its phosphorylated form within signaling complexes formed at the site of injury and then retrogradely transported to the soma to activate transcription. At the site of axonal injury there is local translation of vimentin, which binds to importin-β and forms a complex with phosphorylated ERK preventing its dephosphorylation in the cytosol and allowing its translocation to the nucleus.

Regulation of Axonal Repair

Several intracellular signaling proteins involved in regulation of cell proliferation, such as mTOR, promote axonal regeneration (Figure 13.3). Peripheral nerve axotomy activates the PI3K-AKT pathway, leading to upregulation of mTOR signaling.[46] AKT also phosphorylates and inhibits glycogen synthase kinase 3 β (GSK3 β), leading to disinhibition of a regeneration-associated transcription factor that mediates the growth-promoting effect of bone morphogenetic proteins.[47] Peripheral axotomy also triggers chromatin alterations and transcriptional activation via epigenetic mechanisms.[55]

Regulation of the cytoskeleton is an important mechanism controlling axonal regeneration (Figure 13.3). One important signaling pathway is mediated by the small GTPase RhoA, which acting via RhoA kinase (ROCK)

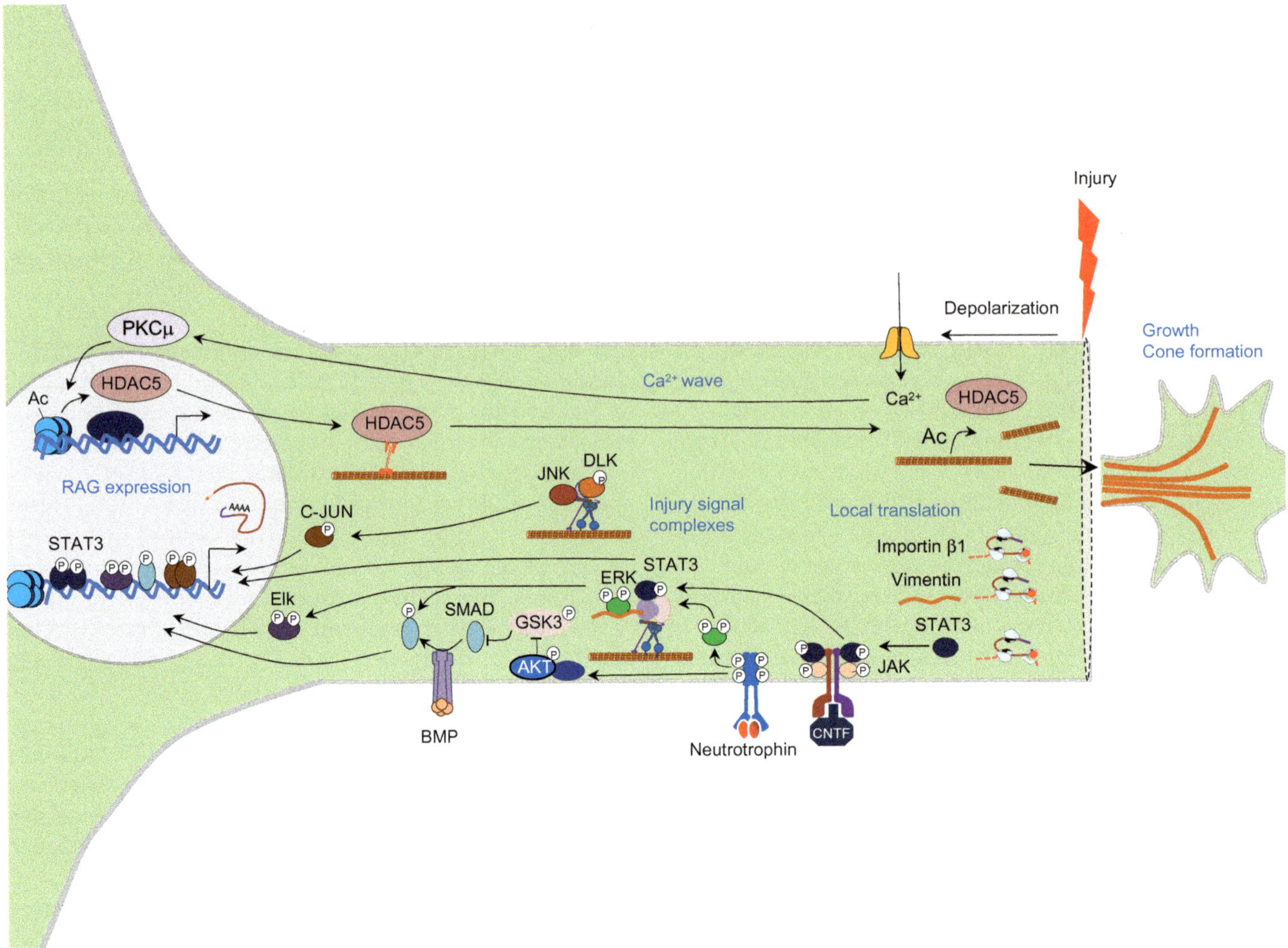

FIGURE 13.2 Signals initiating axonal regeneration.
Peripheral axotomy elicits activation of a transcription program for axonal regeneration. Increased Ca^{2+} concentration at the site of injury initiates a Ca^{2+} wave that back-propagates along the axon to the cell body, leading to activation of protein kinase C (PKC)-μ, which triggers export of histone deacetylase 5 (HDAC5) from the nucleus. This promotes activation of regeneration-genes (RAGs) whereas in the axon HDAC5 reduces levels of acetylated α-tubulin, promoting the formation of a dynamic growth cone tip for axonal regeneration. The early wave of retrograde Ca^{2+} signaling is followed by a delayed phase of retrograde signaling mediated by macromolecular protein complexes that undergo retrograde transport to the nucleus via dynein/dynactin motors. Axonal injury triggers local translation of mRNAs and retrograde transport of signals from injured axons to the nucleus. One important example is local upregulation of neurotrophic cytokines such ciliary neurotrophic factor (CNTF), which activates the transduction protein Janus kinase (JAK) resulting in phosphorylation of signal transducers and activators of transcription (STAT), such as STAT3.Phosphorylated STAT3 is retrogradely transported from the site of injury to the nucleus via interaction with the importin complex and the extracellular signal regulated kinase (ERK)within signaling complexes. Another retrograde signal involves dual leucine zipper kinase (DLK) and its downstream effector Jun N-terminal kinases (JNK), which activates STAT3 expression. Peripheral axotomy also activates the phosphatidylinositol 3' kinase (PI3K)/AKT pathway, which inhibits glycogen synthase kinase 3β (GSK3β), thereby disinhibiting the regeneration-associated transcription factor SMAD1, which mediates the effects of bone morphogenetic proteins (BMPs).

promotes actin depolymerization by activating cofilin, thereby preventing axonal growth. One mechanism by which GSK3β inhibits axonal regeneration is by phosphorylation and inhibition of the collapsin response mediator protein 2, which interacts with tubulin heterodimers in the growth cone controlling the rate of microtubule dynamics.

Myelin-Associated Inhibitors of Axonal Growth in the Central Nervous System

Whereas myelin debris after axon injury in the peripheral nervous system is rapidly cleared by Schwann cells, macrophages, and antibodies, it persists in the CNS. There are three prototypical myelin-derived inhibitory molecules in the CNS that inhibit axonal growth in vitro:

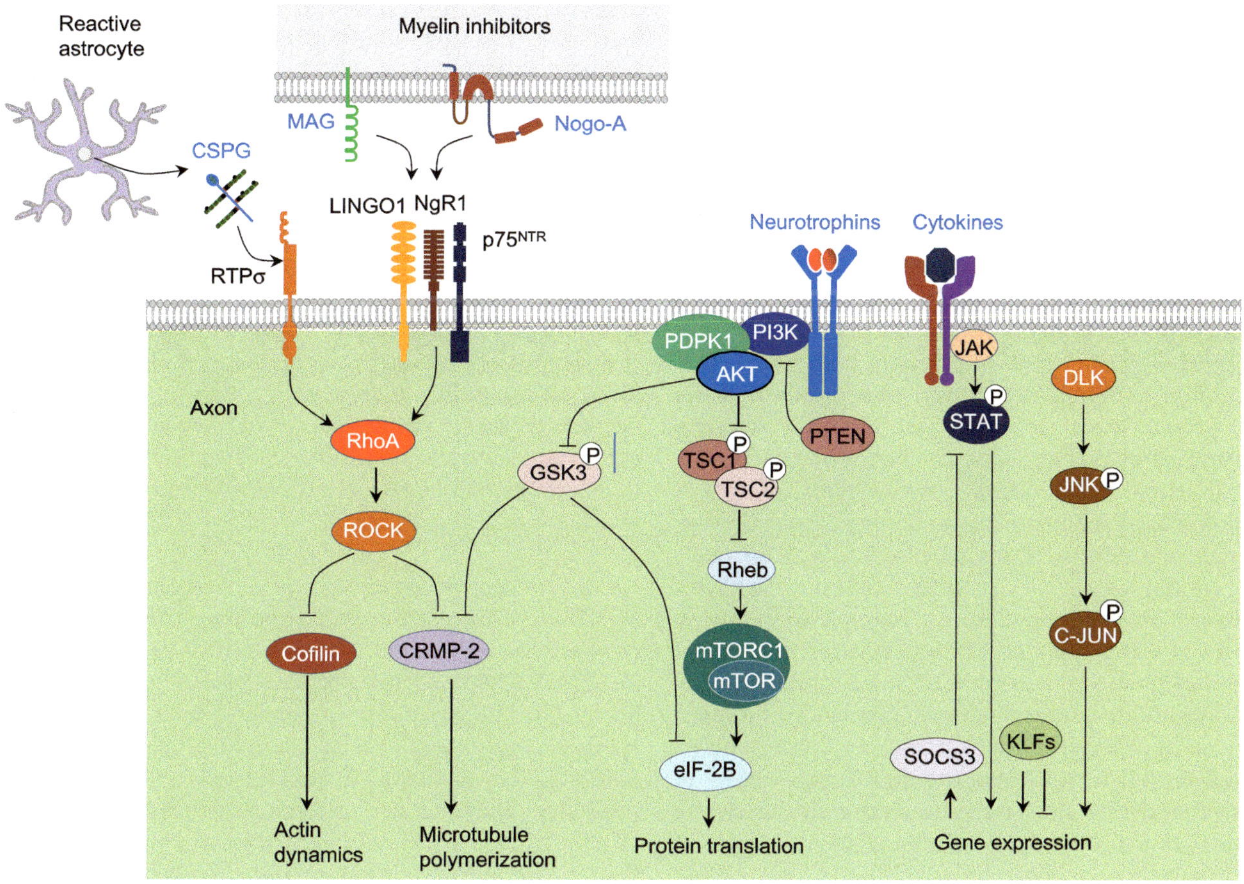

FIGURE 13.3 Regulation of axonal repair.

One important signaling pathway regulating axonal repair is mediated by the small GTPase RhoA, which via RhoA kinase (ROCK) promotes actin depolymerization via cofilin. Many of the extracellular signals inhibit axon regeneration in the CNS via this pathway. The prototype examples are myelin-derived inhibitory molecules such as myelin-associated glycoprotein (MAG), Nogo, and oligodendrocyte-myelin glycoprotein (not shown). These inhibitors bind common receptor/coreceptor complexes expressed on the axonal surface, including the; Nogo receptor (NgR) and its coreceptor p75 neurotrophin receptor ($p75^{NTR}$, also referred to as TROY) and the leucine-rich repeat and Ig domain-containing 1 (LINGO1). Reactive astrocytes secrete proteoglycans such as chondroitin sulfate proteoglycans (CSPGs) that trigger growth inhibitory signals via interactions with NgR1 and the receptor protein tyrosine phosphatase sigma (RTPϭ). Glycogen synthase kinase 3β (GSK3β) inhibits axonal regeneration by inhibition of the collapsin response mediator protein 2 (CRMP-2), which interacts with tubulin heterodimers in the growth cone. Downstream of growth factor signals, the phosphatidylinositol 3′ kinase (PI3K)–phosphoinositide-dependent kinase (PDPK1)–AKT pathway promotes axonal growth by inhibiting GSK3β and activating mammalian target of rapamycin complex 1 (mTORC1). Neurotrophic cytokines activate the transduction protein Janus kinase (JAK)–signal transducer and activator of transcription (STAT) pathway, promoting gene transcription. JAK/STAT signaling regulates the transcription of the suppressor of cytokine signaling (SOCS), which provides a negative feedback inhibiting JAK and STAT. Members of the Krüppel-like family of transcription factors (KLFs) physically interact with activated STAT3 and inhibit the JAK/STAT signaling and thus neurite growth. Another important signaling pathway regulating axonal regeneration is the dual leucine zipper kinase (DLK)–JUN amino terminal kinase (JNK) pathway. eIF-2E, eukaryotic translation initiation factor; Rheb, Ras homologous enriched in brain; TSC, tuberous sclerosis proteins TSC1 and TSC2.

myelin-associated glycoprotein (MAG), Nogo (NogoA, B, and C isoforms), and oligodendrocyte-myelin glycoprotein[48,56] (Figure 13.3). They bind common receptor/coreceptor complexes expressed on the axonal surface, formed by the Nogo receptor NgR1, its coreceptor 75^{NTR}, and the leucine-rich repeat and Ig domain-containing 1 (LINGO1). The final common mechanism by which these signals inhibit axonal growth is activation of RhoA and the RhoA-activated ROCK, which control actin dynamics via cofilin.[48,56]

Inhibitory Effect of Chondroitin Sulfate Proteoglycans and Ephrins

Following CNS injury, astrocytes become reactive and undergo hypertrophy and proliferation, leading to the formation of a glial scar at the lesion site creating a physical barrier to axonal growth. In addition, reactive astrocytes secrete proteoglycans, which are extracellular matrix proteins that contain sulfated glycosaminoglycan chains and inhibit axonal growth by various mechanisms. Glycosaminoglycan chains block the access of axons to growth-promoting adhesion molecules such as laminins and integrins, and trigger growth inhibitory signals via interactions with several surface receptors in axons, including NgR1, NgR3, and the receptor protein tyrosine phosphatase sigma.[7] Enzymatic degradation of glycosaminoglycan chains by chondroitinase or deletion of a chondroitin sulfate synthesizing enzyme, promotes axonal growth and functional recovery in experimental models of optic nerve and SCI. In pathological conditions such as multiple sclerosis, astrocytes may also inhibit remyelination, for example by releasing endothelin-1. Many Eph receptors and ephrins are upregulated after traumatic or ischemic CNS injury and negatively affect axon sprouting and other repair processes. Studies in experimental models show upregulation of EphA4 and its ligand ephrin-A3, which limits the regenerative ability of injured spinal cord axons. These inhibitory effects involve interactions of neuronal EphA4 with ephrin-A3/ephrin-B3 present in myelin and with ephrin-B2 in astrocytes, as well as EphA4 (and EphB3) promotion of reactive gliosis and neuroinflammation.[3] For example, there is upregulation of ephrins and Ephs in astrocytes in demyelinated areas in multiple sclerosis.[57]

HYPOXIA-INDUCED MEDIATORS

Cells have a rapid and efficient molecular response system that senses hypoxia and triggers an evolutionarily conserved pathway mediated by hypoxia-induced factors (HIFs).[58] These transcriptional regulators promote induction of several adaptive genes that facilitate oxygen supply and support anaerobic ATP production.

Hypoxia-Inducible Factor and Oxygen Sensing

Hypoxia-induced factors (HIFs) bind to canonical DNA sequences called hypoxia-regulated elements and activate the transcription of many genes that regulate cell metabolism, angiogenesis, vascular tone, and erythropoiesis (Figure 13.4). Transcriptional activation depends on the formation of a heterodimeric DNA-binding complex composed of one hypoxia-inducible HIFα-subunit (HIF1α or HIF2α) and a constitutive non-oxygen-responsive subunit HIF1β. The HIF pathway is regulated by oxygen-dependent posttranslational hydroxylation and inactivation of HIFα via oxygen-dependent enzymes, including prolyl hydroxylases and aspargyl hydroxylases.[59,60] These enzymes utilize molecular oxygen (O_2); require ferrous iron (Fe^{2+}), ascorbate, and α-ketoglutarate as cofactors; and catalyze the stepwise hydroxylation of HIFα during normoxia. In the presence of normal O_2 levels, hydroxylation of proline residues of HIF1α generates a binding site for the Von Hippel-Lindau (VHL) protein. Under normal tissue oxygen, VHL forms a complex that functions as a ubiquitin 3 ligase that promotes degradation of HIF1α and HIF2α by the proteasome.[61] Under hypoxic conditions, HIF1α escapes proteasomal destruction, accumulates in the cytosol, and translocates to the nucleus, where it forms a heteromeric complex with HIFβ and promotes transcription of hypoxia-inducible genes. Proinflammatory cytokines, such as tumor necrosis factor-α and interleukin-1β, may also induce HIF expression. Hypoxia also induces nuclear localization of the Repressor Element 1-Silencing Transcription factor (REST), which elicits gene repression.[62]

Mediators of the Hypoxia-Induced Response

HIF-dependent genes encode proteins that promote glycolysis, blood flow, and oxygen delivery to tissues. These include VEGF,[63] erythropoietin (EPO),[64] glucose transporter GLUT1, glycolytic enzymes, inducible nitric oxide synthase, and others[65] (Table 13.2). Members of the VEGF family are key regulators of angiogenesis and vascular permeability. They act via tyrosine kinase VEGF receptors (VEGFRs) and neuropilin receptors and promote proliferation, sprouting, migration, and survival of endothelial cells. VEGF-A also increases vascular permeability, causes vasodilatation via endothelial production of nitric oxide, promotes expression of several antiapoptotic proteins, and exerts neuroprotection against excitotoxicity in motor neurons.[66] Erythropoietin is a circulating glycoprotein whose principal function is to stimulate red blood cell production. Whereas the kidney produces around 90% of systemic EPO, its mRNA is constitutively expressed in the cortex and hippocampus of human brain. Neurons, astrocytes, microglia, and brain endothelial cells express EPO receptors, which are particularly abundant in the astrocyte foot processes surrounding capillaries. Erythropoietin promotes proliferation of astrocytes, differentiation of oligodendrocytes, and angiogenesis, and protects the BBB against VEGF-induced increased permeability.[67] Erythropoietin may also exert paracrine effects including neuroprotection, immunomodulation, and synaptic plasticity, as shown in experimental models of hypoxia and ischemia, head injury, and seizures. Potential neuroprotective effects of EPO include inhibition of glutamate release, inhibition of apoptosis, neurotrophic function, angiogenesis, decreased BBB permeability, and anti-inflammatory effects. EPO antagonizes the glutamate-induced increase in astrocyte water permeability dependent on aquaporin 4 channels and may thus reduce the risk of astrocyte swelling in stroke and other brain insults.[69] Many in vitro and in vivo studies have shown that prior exposure to noninjurious preconditioning hypoxic or ischemic stimuli transiently increases the resistance of the

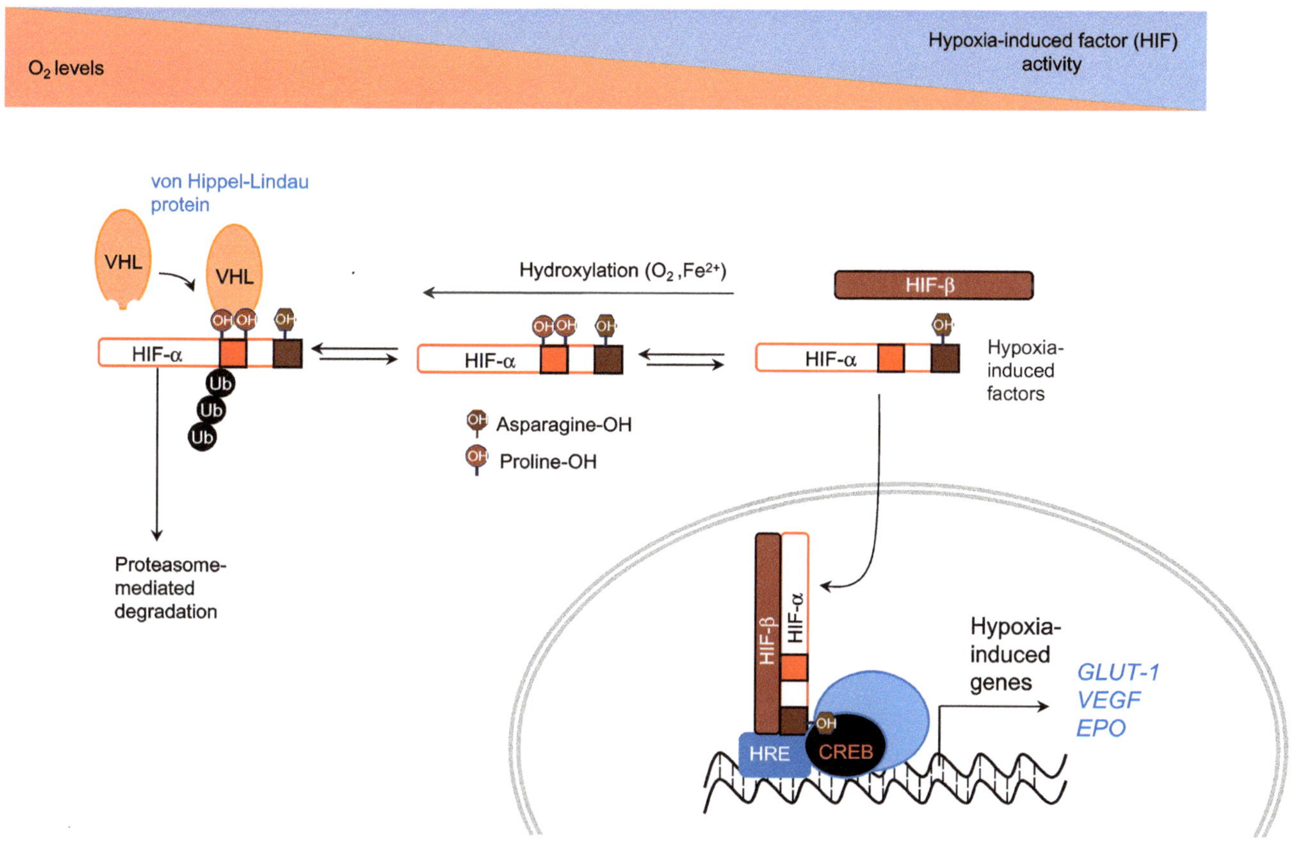

FIGURE 13.4 Hypoxia-inducible factor and oxygen sensing.

Cellular exposure to hypoxia results in altered gene expression in a range of physiologic and pathophysiologic states. Hypoxia-induced factors (HIFs) bind to canonical DNA sequences called hypoxia-regulated elements (HRE) and activate the transcription of many genes encoding proteins that regulate cell metabolism, angiogenesis, vascular tone, and erythropoiesis. Transcriptional activation depends on the formation of a heterodimeric DNA-binding complex composed of one hypoxia-inducible HIFα-subunit (HIF1α or HIF2α) and a constitutive non-oxygen-responsive subunit HIF1β. The HIF pathway is regulated by oxygen-dependent posttranslational hydroxylation and inactivation of HIFα via oxygen-dependent enzymes, including prolyl hydroxylases and aspargyl hydroxylases. In the presence of normal O_2 levels, hydroxylation of proline residues of HIF1α generates a binding site for the Von Hippel-Lindau (VHL) protein, which promotes degradation of HIF1α and HIF2α. Under hypoxic conditions, HIF1α escapes proteasomal destruction, accumulates in the cytosol, and translocates to the nucleus, where it forms a heteromeric complex with HIFβ. This complex binds to promoter or enhancer sequences of target genes including those encoding vascular endothelial growth factor (VEGF), erythropoietin (EPO), and glucose transporter GLUT1.

brain to ischemic injury. Whereas several mechanisms have been proposed for this neuroprotective effect, an important factor may be activation of HIF1-mediated responses.[68]

DISORDERS DUE TO EXCESSIVE GROWTH FACTOR SIGNALING

Mutations affecting products of tumor suppressor genes produce disorders that typically manifest with malformation of cortical development, seizures, and neoplasms both in the nervous system and in non-neural organs. A final common mechanism in many of these disorders is excessive mTOR signaling. As mentioned earlier in this chapter, tumor suppressor proteins inhibit several steps of the growth factor-mTOR signaling pathways. Neurofibromin 1, encoded by the *NF1* gene, switches off by Ras signaling downstream of growth factors. The TSC proteins TSC1 (hamartin) and TSC2 (tuberin) inhibit mTORC1 signaling. Inhibition of the PI3-AKT by PTEN encoded by the *PTEN* tumor-suppressor gene negatively regulates AKT, promotes TSC activity, and thus inhibits mTORC1 signaling.

TABLE 13.2 *Effectors of the Hypoxia-Induced Response*

Effector	Function
Glucose transporter 1	Glucose transport across the blood-brain barrier
Lactate-dehydrogenase 1	Conversion of pyruvate to lactate
Carbonic anhydrase	Formation of carbonic acid from CO_2 and water, leading to formation of HCO_3^- and H^+, which regulate pH
Adrenomedullin	Vasodilatation
β-adrenergic receptor	Vasodilatation
Vascular endothelial growth factor	Proliferation, sprouting, migration, and survival of endothelial cells Vasodilatation Increased vascular permeability Inhibition of apoptosis
Erythropoietin	Erythropoiesis Inhibition of apoptosis Angiogenesis Neurotrophic effect Inhibition of inflammation Reduction of BBB permeability Reduction of AQP4-mediated cellular edema

Neurofibromatosis Type 1 and Other RASopathies

Neurofibromatosis type 1 is the prototypical example of a group of neurodevelopmental disorders known as RASopathies, caused by germline mutations in genes that encode regulators of the Ras/MAPK pathway.[70,71] Whereas each RASopathy has a unique phenotype, many share overlapping characteristics, including craniofacial dysmorphology; neurocognitive impairment; cutaneous, musculoskeletal, and ocular abnormalities; cardiac malformations; and increased risk of nervous system and other neoplasms. Neurofibromatosis type 1 (NF1) is due to a mutation of the *NF1* gene, leading to haploinsufficiency of neurofibromin1.[72] The diagnosis of NF1 is based on the presence of two of the following features, café-au-lait maculae, intertriginous freckling, Lisch nodules in the iris, osseous abnormalities (including sphenoid dysplasia, pseudoarthrosis, or thinning of long bone cortex), plexiform neurofibromas, optic pathway glioma, and/or a first-degree relative with NF1. Other manifestations of NF1 include mild cognitive impairment, seizures, brain malformations, cardiac malformations, and vasculopathy such as Moyamoya disease. Pediatric patients are at risk of optic pathway glioma, neuroblastoma, rhabdomyosarcoma, and juvenile myelomonocytic leukemia; adult patients may develop malignant peripheral nerve tumors, pheochromocytoma, somatostatinomas, gastrointestinal stromal cell tumors, and breast cancer.[73] Selumetinib, an oral selective inhibitor of MAPK kinase (MEK) 1 and 2 has been shown to reduce the volume of plexiform neurofibromas in children with NF1.[74] Another RASopathies include the capillary malformation-arteriovenous (AV) malformation syndrome, Noonan syndrome, and Costello syndrome.[75] Neurofibromatosis type 2 (NF2) is not a RASopathy but is also an autosomal dominant disorder that increases risk of tumors in the central and peripheral nervous systems. NF2 is due to loss-of-function mutation of the *NF2* gene on chromosome 22 encoding a protein called merlin, which is a tumor suppressor that inhibits mitogenic receptors at the plasma membrane.[76] NF2 is most commonly associated with bilateral vestibular schwannomas; patients also have a predisposition to development of meningiomas, ependymomas, and peripheral, spinal, and cranial nerve schwannomas.[77]

Tuberous Sclerosis

The tuberous sclerosis complex (TSC) is an autosomal dominant disorder caused by loss-of-function mutations in either the *TSC1* (*hamartin*) or the *TSC2* (*tuberin*) genes. Most TSC mutations result in a truncated TSC1 or TSC2 protein, leading to hyperactivity of mTORC1 signaling.[78–80] Neuropathological findings in TSC include cortical tubers, subependymal nodules, and subependymal giant-cell astrocytomas. Tubers also form in the eyes, skin (facial angiofibromas), heart, kidneys (renal angiomyolipomas), and lung (pulmonary lymphangiomyomatosis). Epilepsy, behavioral disorders, and development delay are the most disabling features of TSC.[81] Seizures originate within or around the hamartoma, and in many patients resection of tubers provides good to excellent outcome. Everolimus, an inhibitor of the mTOR pathway, has been approved for treatment of partial-onset seizures in TSC patients.[81]

Focal Epilepsy Associated with Excessive mTOR Activation

In addition to TSC, other mutations leading to excessive mTOR signaling have been associated with focal malformations of cortical development subtypes associated with focal epilepsy. These disorders have been referred to as "mTORopathies."[82] Gain-of-function mutations of the *AKT3* gene encoding AKT produce hemimegalencephaly, which manifests with medically refractory epilepsy, intellectual delay, and contralateral hemiparesis. Mutations of the *DEPDC5* (disheveled, Egl-10, and pleckstrin domain-containing protein 5) gene, which encodes a member of the GATOR1 complex that prevents activation of the mTOR signaling by amino acids, have been associated with several forms of autosomal dominant focal epilepsy. These include autosomal dominant nocturnal frontal lobe epilepsy, familial temporal lobe epilepsy, familial focal epilepsy with variable foci, and benign epilepsy with centrotemporal spikes.[83]

PTEN Hamartoma Syndromes

Germline loss-of-function *PTEN* mutations have been associated with multiple syndromes encompassed under the umbrella or PTEN hamartoma tumor syndrome.[84] One relevant example is Lhermitte-Duclos disease, an hamartomatous overgrowth of the cerebellum with large neurons and producing unilateral cerebellar hypertrophy and widened cerebellar folia with a "tiger-striped" appearance on neuroimaging[84] About 10%–20% of individuals with autism spectrum disorder and macrocephaly harbor germline *PTEN* mutations, which produce a broad spectrum of neuropsychiatric phenotypes.

Von Hippel-Lindau Disease

Von Hippel-Lindau (VHL) disease is an autosomal dominant disorder due to loss-of-function mutations of the *VHL* gene on chromosome 3p25–26.[85] Mutation in VHL results in a state of "pseudohypoxia" with elevated HIF and subsequent activation of HIF-dependent genes, which in turn upregulate angiogenesis, increase cellular proliferation, and shift metabolism toward glycolysis. Typical manifestations include hemangioblastomas of the retina, cerebellum, and spinal cord; clear cell renal carcinoma; pheochromocytoma; and visceral cysts (especially in the kidney and pancreas). The rich vascularity of hemangioblastomas is due to overexpression of VEGF. Neoplastic cells are capable of extramedullary hematopoiesis and polycythemia due to EPO upregulation.

In addition to VHL disease, VEGF signaling is relevant in acquired neurologic disorders. For example, VEGF-induced angiogenesis is a typical feature of malignant gliomas as well as many other neoplasms and may reflect excessive HIF activity. Bevacizumab, a humanized monoclonal antibody against VEGF, and cediranib, a small molecule inhibitor of VEGFR, reduce the need for corticosteroids in patients with recurrent malignant glioma. Increased serum VEGF concentration is a feature of POEMS (polyneuropathy, organomegaly, endocrinopathy, M-protein, and skin changes), typically associated with underlying osteosclerotic myeloma with an IgG or IgA lambda paraprotein. VEGF increases microvascular permeability and may upregulate cytokines and matrix metalloproteinases that induce blood-nerve barrier breakdown and peripheral nerve demyelination; microangiopathy due to proliferative endothelial cells and occlusion due to hypercoagulability may also contribute to axonal damage in POEMS.

ROLE OF BDNF IN EPILEPSY

Epilepsy is associated with global transcriptional disturbances. For example, aberrant neurogenesis, mossy fiber sprouting, and hippocampal cell death contribute to neuronal circuit reorganization in mesial temporal sclerosis associated with temporal lobe epilepsy. A major mechanism for this altered brain plasticity is increased synthesis and release of BDNF, which elicits activity-dependent alterations in neuronal morphology and synaptogenesis promoting epileptogenesis via TrkB signaling.[86,87] For example, BDNF acting via TrkB promotes epileptogenesis in mouse models of traumatic brain injury and status epilepticus[88] and has an important role in aberrant axonal sprouting induced by transection of Schaffer collateral axons. In these models, inhibition of BDNF and TrkB signaling prevented epileptogenesis. The deleterious effects of BDNF/TrkB signaling are mediated by downstream PLCγ1 activation. The transcription inhibitory factor REST/NRSF (repressor element 1-silencing transcription factor/neuron-restrictive silencer factor) regulates expression of both BDNF and TrkB and could contribute to the prevention of TrkB activation and development of seizures, as shown in a kindling model of hippocampal seizures in rats.[89] In contrast, BDNF/TrkB signaling in the neocortex may have antiepileptic effects by activating local GABAergic interneurons. This indicates that the BDNF/TrkB pathway may have either deleterious effects by promoting axonal sprouting in medial temporal seizures or neuroprotective effects by promoting interneuron-mediated inhibition in neocortical seizures. BDNF may also affect epileptogenesis independently of the canonical TrkB signaling. BDNF activates JAK-STAT3 signaling in neurons and elicits many changes in the transcriptome, altering expression of epilepsy-related genes encoding ion channels, receptors, and other molecules regulating cell excitability, synaptic plasticity, neurogenesis, and axonal remodeling, including $GABA_A$ receptor subunits.[31]

NEUROTROPHIC FACTOR SIGNALING AS A THERAPEUTIC TARGET IN NEURODEGENERATION

Impaired Neurotrophic Factor Signaling in Neurodegenerative Disorders

Many studies in experimental models and in brain tissue obtained at autopsy show impaired growth factor signaling in a wide variety of disorders, including AD, HD, ALS, stroke, epilepsy, trauma, Rett syndrome, and fragile X syndrome.[90–102] Many such studies have been focused on impaired BDNF signaling. For example, studies in transgenic mice expressing mutant human amyloid precursor protein show reductions in BDNF mRNA and protein in the cerebral cortex; BDNF gene delivery or secretion by transplanted neural stem cells, or administration of a TrkB agonist, slowed entorhinal cortex and hippocampal atrophy and improved cognitive performance. Postmortem studies in patients with HD and studies in transgenic mice expressing human-mutated huntingtin show reduced BDNF mRNA and protein levels in the cerebral cortex, striatum, substantia nigra, and cerebellum. BDNF overexpression improved lifespan, motor performance, and corticostriatal connectivity and reduced loss of striatal neurons in mouse models of HD. Reduced expression of BDNF mRNA has been reported in the substantia nigra pars compacta in PD brains. Reduced BDNF production is closely associated with pathogenic mutations in α-synuclein in familial PD. Targeted BDNF deletion resulted in loss of dopaminergic neurons in the substantia nigra in PD mouse models. BDNF has also been reported to slow progression of motor neuron atrophy in an animal model of ALS; a truncated form of TrkB that is found in motor neurons and glia is involved in disease onset in an ALS mouse model.

In addition to BDNF, other neurotrophic factors have been implicated in neurodegenerative disorders. For example, it has been suggested that AD may be a state of resistance to the effects of insulin and IGF1.[99,100] Postmortem studies show downregulation of expression of insulin receptor, IGF1R, and the insulin receptor substrates IRS-1 and IRS-2 in AD.[101] Studies in transgenic mice indicate that full-length huntingtin influences IGF1 expression in the striatum; plasma IGF1 levels correlated with huntingtin levels in these transgenic animals. There are also reduced plasma IGF1 levels in mice overexpressing human α-synuclein. Mutant α-synuclein suppresses the IGF1-induced AKT activation. Experimental studies in stroke models suggest that tissue reorganization, axonal sprouting, expression of molecules involved in long-term potentiation, changes in excitatory/inhibitory balance, neurogenesis, gliogenesis, and angiogenesis all affect the possibility of repair and recovery of function, thus providing opportunity for therapeutic intervention.[102]

Use of Trophic Factors in Neurodegenerative Diseases

The promising results from preclinical studies in animals have prompted many studies to address the safety and possible efficacy of neurotrophic factors in neurodegenerative diseases.[103,104] Human studies have so far failed to show any clear clinical benefit of growth factor replacement therapy in these disorders. This has been primarily attributed to inadequate dosing and delivery. Furthermore, the majority of patients were enrolled in these clinical trials at relatively late stages of disease.[103,104] Trials with systemic administration were associated with dose-limiting side effects. For example recombinant human CNTF produced weight loss and anorexia in patients with ALS, and NGF produced local pain, hyperalgesia, and allodynia in patients with diabetic or HIV neuropathy. Intrathecal CNTF or BDNF resulted in headache, radicular pain, and lower limb paresthesia in ALS patients. Intraventricularly administered NGF showed no clear benefit in AD patients. Despite strong experimental evidence supporting neuroprotective effect of GDNF on midbrain dopaminergic neurons, intraputamenal GDNF administration to patients with moderately advanced PD did not show significant clinical improvements against placebo, although it significantly increased [18F] DOPA uptake throughout the entire putamen.[105] Ex vivo and in vivo gene therapy have also been used in clinical trials for neurodegenerative diseases. These include ex vivo *NGF* gene therapy for AD, in vivo therapy for AD using local administration of vector AAV2-NGF to the basal forebrain, and in vivo therapy for PD testing AAV2-neurturin and AAV2-GDNF. Autopsy data from these neurotrophic gene therapy trials in AD and PD show an ability of degenerating neurons to respond to the neurotrophic factor protein, but the response is much less robust than that observed in animal models. Mesenchymal stromal cells are multipotent cells that are being intensively explored as a potential neuroprotective approach in neurodegenerative diseases.[106] Preclinical and early clinical studies have focused in mesenchymal stromal cell therapy in ALS, PD, AD, and multiple system atrophy.[107]

Studies in experimental models show that local transplantation of human-derived neural progenitor cells engineered to secrete GDNF or other growth factors may be a potential approach to circumvent the technical limitations of other delivery systems. Transplantation of transgenic cells engineered to express the GDNF gene in the striatum of mice prior to administration of 1-methyl-4-phenyl-1,2,3,6-tetrahydropyridine (MPTP) reduced the deleterious effect of the neurotoxin on midbrain neurons.[108] In a rat model of ALS due to expression of mutant superoxide dismutase (SOD)1, human-derived progenitor cells engineered to produce GDNF and transplanted to the cerebral cortex matured into astrocytes, released GDNF, protected motor neurons, delayed disease pathology, and extended survival.[109]

KEY POINTS

- Neurotrophic factors and hypoxia-inducible factors participate in fundamental processes including growth, differentiation, survival, and plasticity in the nervous system.
- Neurotrophic factors include members of the neurotrophins family such as nerve growth factor (NGF) and brain-derived neurotrophic factor (BDNF), insulin-like growth factors, glial-derived neurotrophic factors (GDNFs), neuregulins, and neurotrophic cytokines such as ciliary neurotrophic factor (CNTF).
- Activation of tyrosine kinase receptors by neurotrophic factors trigger three downstream pathways, the Ras-mitogen activated kinase; the phosphatidylinositol 3'kinase-AKT (protein kinase B) pathway; and the phospholipase Cγ pathway.
- Activation of growth factor receptors promotes cell growth and differentiation and inhibits apoptosis and autophagy.
- The mechanistic (mammalian) target of rapamycin (mTOR) is a critical downstream effector of growth factor signaling.
- Products of tumor suppressor genes, such as neurofibromin-1 (NF1), tuberous sclerosis (TSC) proteins, and phosphatase-tensin homolog (PTEN) inhibit several components of the growth factor signaling pathways.
- NGF acting via TrkA (NTRK1) receptors acts as a retrograde signal critical for survival of sympathetic ganglion neurons, small dorsal root ganglion neurons, and basal forebrain cholinergic neurons.
- BDNF, acting via TrkB (NTRK2) receptors has a major role in activity-dependent synaptic plasticity.
- GDNF promotes growth and survival of dopaminergic nigrostriatal neurons and development of several types of GABAergic neurons, and enteric neurons.
- Growth factors have neuroprotective effects in the setting of hypoxia/ischemia, traumatic brain or spinal cord injury, neuroinflammation, and neurodegenerative disorders.
- Axonal injury triggers retrograde neurotrophic signaling to the nucleus to regulate transcription of genes involved in axonal repair.
- Regulation of the cytoskeleton is an important mechanism controlling axonal regeneration.
- Myelin-derived proteins inhibit axonal growth by promoting severing of actin.
- Sulfated glycosaminoglycan secreted by astrocytes and Eph-ephrins signaling are upregulated after injury and prevent axonal repair.
- Hypoxia triggers a pathway mediated by hypoxia-induced factors (HIFs) that activate transcription of genes encoding proteins that facilitate oxygen supply and anaerobic ATP production, such as vascular endothelial growth factor, erythropoietin, and glucose transporter 1.
- The HIF pathway is inhibited in normoxic conditions by the Von Hippel-Lindau (VHL) protein.
- Mutations impairing function of NF1 (neurofibromatosis type 1), TSC (tuberous sclerosis), and PTEN (PTEN hamartoma syndromes) manifest with malformation of cortical development, seizures, and neoplasms both in the nervous system and non-neural organs, reflecting excessive activation of the mTORC1 pathway.
- Von Hippel-Lindau (VHL) disease is due to elevated HIF signaling.
- Abnormal BDNF signal has an important role in temporal lobe and other forms of epilepsy.
- Impaired growth factor signaling is a common finding in experimental models of neurodevelopmental and neurodegenerative disorders.
- Transplantation of genetically engineered stem cells that make growth factors such as GDNF may provide benefit in disorders such as PD, as it may circumvent the technical limitations of other approaches.

REFERENCES

1. Schecterson LC, Bothwell M. Neurotrophin receptors: old friends with new partners. Dev Neurobiol 2010;70:332–338.
2. Mitre M, Mariga A, Chao MV. Neurotrophin signalling: novel insights into mechanisms and pathophysiology. Clin Sci (Lond) 2017;131:13–23.
3. Barquilla A, Pasquale EB. Eph receptors and ephrins: therapeutic opportunities. Annu Rev Pharmacol Toxicol 2015;55:465–487.
4. Pediaditakis I, Iliopoulos I, Theologidis I, et al. Dehydroepiandrosterone: an ancestral ligand of neurotrophin receptors. Endocrinology 2015;156:16–23.
5. Bennett JP, Jr., O'Brien LC, Brohawn DG. Pharmacological properties of microneurotrophin drugs developed for treatment of amyotrophic lateral sclerosis. Biochem Pharmacol 2016;117:68–77.
6. Liu GY, Sabatini DM. mTOR at the nexus of nutrition, growth, ageing and disease. Nat Rev Mol Cell Biol 2020;21:183–203.
7. Ryskalin L, Limanaqi F, Frati A, Busceti CL, Fornai F. mTOR-related brain dysfunctions in neuropsychiatric disorders. Int J Mol Sci 2018;19:2226–2255.
8. Inoki K, Kim J, Guan KL. AMPK and mTOR in cellular energy homeostasis and drug targets. Annu Rev Pharmacol Toxicol 2012;52:381–400.
9. O'Shea JJ, Schwartz DM, Villarino AV, Gadina M, McInnes IB, Laurence A. The JAK-STAT pathway: impact on human disease and therapeutic intervention. Annu Rev Med 2015;66:311–328.
10. Ceyzeriat K, Abjean L, Carrillo-de Sauvage MA, Ben Haim L, Escartin C. The complex STATes of astrocyte reactivity: How

are they controlled by the JAK-STAT3 pathway? Neuroscience 2016;330:205–218.
11. Sun F, He Z. Neuronal intrinsic barriers for axon regeneration in the adult CNS. Curr Opin Neurobiol 2010;20:510–518.
12. Spaulding EL, Burgess RW. Accumulating evidence for axonal translation in neuronal homeostasis. Front Neurosci 2017;11:312–319.
13. Altassan R, Saud HA, Masoodi TA, et al. Exome sequencing identifies novel NTRK1 mutations in patients with HSAN-IV phenotype. Am J Med Genet A 2017;173:1009–1016.
14. Carvalho OP, Thornton GK, Hertecant J, et al. A novel NGF mutation clarifies the molecular mechanism and extends the phenotypic spectrum of the HSAN5 neuropathy. J Med Genet 2011;48:131–135.
15. Li L, Gruner K, Tourtellotte WG. Retrograde nerve growth factor signaling abnormalities in familial dysautonomia. J Clin Invest 2020;130:2478–2487.
16. Parikh V, Howe WM, Welchko RM, et al. Diminished trkA receptor signaling reveals cholinergic-attentional vulnerability of aging. Eur J Neurosci 2013;37:278–293.
17. Park H, Poo MM. Neurotrophin regulation of neural circuit development and function. Nat Rev Neurosci 2013;14:7–23.
18. Miranda M, Morici JF, Zanoni MB, Bekinschtein P. Brain-derived neurotrophic factor: a key molecule for memory in the healthy and the pathological brain. Front Cell Neurosci 2019;13:363–388.
19. Zheng F, Zhou X, Moon C, Wang H. Regulation of brain-derived neurotrophic factor expression in neurons. Int J Physiol Pathophysiol Pharmacol 2012;4:188–200.
20. Karpova NN. Role of BDNF epigenetics in activity-dependent neuronal plasticity. Neuropharmacology 2014;76 Pt C:709–718.
21. Gauthier LR, Charrin BC, Borrell-Pages M, et al. Huntingtin controls neurotrophic support and survival of neurons by enhancing BDNF vesicular transport along microtubules. Cell 2004;118:127–138.
22. Ehinger Y, Bruyere J, Panayotis N, et al. Huntingtin phosphorylation governs BDNF homeostasis and improves the phenotype of Mecp2 knockout mice. EMBO Mol Med 2020;12:e10889.
23. Edelmann E, Lessmann V, Brigadski T. Pre- and postsynaptic twists in BDNF secretion and action in synaptic plasticity. Neuropharmacology 2014;76 Pt C:610–627.
24. Numakawa T, Suzuki S, Kumamaru E, Adachi N, Richards M, Kunugi H. BDNF function and intracellular signaling in neurons. Histol Histopathol 2010;25:237–258.
25. Leal G, Comprido D, Duarte CB. BDNF-induced local protein synthesis and synaptic plasticity. Neuropharmacology 2014;76 Pt C:639–656.
26. Cowansage KK, LeDoux JE, Monfils MH. Brain-derived neurotrophic factor: a dynamic gatekeeper of neural plasticity. Curr Mol Pharmacol 2010;3:12–29.
27. Panja D, Bramham CR. BDNF mechanisms in late LTP formation: a synthesis and breakdown. Neuropharmacology 2014;76 Pt C:664–676.
28. Ruiz CR, Shi J, Meffert MK. Transcript specificity in BDNF-regulated protein synthesis. Neuropharmacology 2014;76 Pt C:657–663.
29. Zagrebelsky M, Korte M. Form follows function: BDNF and its involvement in sculpting the function and structure of synapses. Neuropharmacology 2014;76 Pt C:628–638.
30. Bekinschtein P, Kent BA, Oomen CA, et al. Brain-derived neurotrophic factor interacts with adult-born immature cells in the dentate gyrus during consolidation of overlapping memories. Hippocampus 2014;24:905–911.
31. Hixson KM, Cogswell M, Brooks-Kayal AR, Russek SJ. Evidence for a non-canonical JAK/STAT signaling pathway in the synthesis of the brain's major ion channels and neurotransmitter receptors. BMC Genomics 2019;20:677.
32. Fernandez AM, Torres-Aleman I. The many faces of insulin-like peptide signalling in the brain. Nat Rev Neurosci 2012;13:225–239.
33. Russo VC, Gluckman PD, Feldman EL, Werther GA. The insulin-like growth factor system and its pleiotropic functions in brain. Endocr Rev 2005;26:916–943.
34. Cohen E, Dillin A. The insulin paradox: aging, proteotoxicity and neurodegeneration. Nat Rev Neurosci 2008;9:759–767.
35. Bibollet-Bahena O, Cui QL, Almazan G. The insulin-like growth factor-1 axis and its potential as a therapeutic target in central nervous system (CNS) disorders. Cent Nerv Syst Agents Med Chem 2009;9:95–109.
36. Nishijima T, Piriz J, Duflot S, et al. Neuronal activity drives localized blood-brain-barrier transport of serum insulin-like growth factor-I into the CNS. Neuron 2010;67:834–846.
37. Firth SM, Baxter RC. Cellular actions of the insulin-like growth factor binding proteins. Endocr Rev 2002;23:824–854.
38. Muller E, Dunstheimer D, Klammt J, et al. Clinical and functional characterization of a patient carrying a compound heterozygous pericentrin mutation and a heterozygous IGF1 receptor mutation. PLoS One 2012;7:e38220.
39. Ibanez CF, Andressoo JO. Biology of GDNF and its receptors—relevance for disorders of the central nervous system. Neurobiol Dis 2017;97:80–89.
40. Enterria-Morales D, Lopez-Lopez I, Lopez-Barneo J, d'Anglemont de Tassigny X. Role of glial cell line-derived neurotrophic factor in the maintenance of adult mesencephalic catecholaminergic neurons. Mov Disord 2020;35:565–576.
41. Mijatovic J, Piltonen M, Alberton P, Mannisto PT, Saarma M, Piepponen TP. Constitutive Ret signaling is protective for dopaminergic cell bodies but not for axonal terminals. Neurobiol Aging 2011;32:1486–1494.
42. Ramos-Levi AM, Diaz-Perez A, Sobrido MJ, et al. Axonal neuropathy, long limbs and bumpy tongue: think of MEN2B. Muscle Nerve 2012;46:961–964.
43. Chen A, Xiong LJ, Tong Y, Mao M. The neuroprotective roles of BDNF in hypoxic ischemic brain injury. Biomed Rep 2013;1:167–176.
44. Lu B, Nagappan G, Guan X, Nathan PJ, Wren P. BDNF-based synaptic repair as a disease-modifying strategy for neurodegenerative diseases. Nat Rev Neurosci 2013;14:401–416.
45. Rishal I, Fainzilber M. Axon-soma communication in neuronal injury. Nat Rev Neurosci 2014;15:32–42.
46. Park KK, Liu K, Hu Y, Kanter JL, He Z. PTEN/mTOR and axon regeneration. Exp Neurol 2010;223:45–50.
47. Zhong J, Zou H. BMP signaling in axon regeneration. Curr Opin Neurobiol 2014;27:127–134.
48. Chen M, Zheng B. Axon plasticity in the mammalian central nervous system after injury. Trends Neurosci 2014;37:583–593.
49. Lu Y, Belin S, He Z. Signaling regulations of neuronal regenerative ability. Curr Opin Neurobiol 2014;27:135–142.
50. Fawcett JW, Verhaagen J. Intrinsic determinants of axon regeneration. Dev Neurobiol 2018;78:890–897.

51. Curcio M, Bradke F. Axon regeneration in the central nervous system: facing the challenges from the inside. Annu Rev Cell Dev Biol 2018;34:495–521.
52. Cho Y, Sloutsky R, Naegle KM, Cavalli V. Injury-induced HDAC5 nuclear export is essential for axon regeneration. Cell 2013;155:894–908.
53. Lu Y, Belin S, He Z. Signaling regulations of neuronal regenerative ability. Curr Opin Neurobiol 2014;27:135–142.
54. Miller BR, Press C, Daniels RW, Sasaki Y, Milbrandt J, DiAntonio A. A dual leucine kinase-dependent axon self-destruction program promotes Wallerian degeneration. Nat Neurosci 2009;12:387–389.
55. Wahane S, Halawani D, Zhou X, Zou H. Epigenetic regulation of axon regeneration and glial activation in injury responses. Front Genet 2019;10:640.
56. Geoffroy CG, Zheng B. Myelin-associated inhibitors in axonal growth after CNS injury. Curr Opin Neurobiol 2014;27:31–38.
57. Sobel RA. Ephrin A receptors and ligands in lesions and normal-appearing white matter in multiple sclerosis. Brain Pathol 2005;15:35–45.
58. Kaelin WG, Jr., Ratcliffe PJ. Oxygen sensing by metazoans: the central role of the HIF hydroxylase pathway. Mol Cell 2008;30:393–402.
59. Kennel KB, Burmeister J, Schneider M, Taylor CT. The PHD1 oxygen sensor in health and disease. J Physiol 2018;596:3899–3913.
60. Strowitzki MJ, Cummins EP, Taylor CT. Protein hydroxylation by hypoxia-inducible factor (HIF) hydroxylases: unique or ubiquitous? Cells 2019;8.
61. Kaelin WG, Jr. The VHL tumor suppressor gene: insights into oxygen sensing and cancer. Trans Am Clin Climatol Assoc 2017;128:298–307.
62. Cavadas MA, Mesnieres M, Crifo B, et al. REST is a hypoxia-responsive transcriptional repressor. Sci Rep 2016;6:31355.
63. Testa U, Pannitteri G, Condorelli GL. Vascular endothelial growth factors in cardiovascular medicine. J Cardiovasc Med (Hagerstown) 2008;9:1190–1221.
64. Weidemann A, Johnson RS. Nonrenal regulation of EPO synthesis. Kidney Int 2009;75:682–688.
65. Gossage L, Eisen T, Maher ER. VHL, the story of a tumour suppressor gene. Nat Rev Cancer 2015;15:55–64.
66. Bogaert E, Van Damme P, Poesen K, et al. VEGF protects motor neurons against excitotoxicity by upregulation of GluR2. Neurobiol Aging 2010;31:2185–2191.
67. Rabie T, Marti HH. Brain protection by erythropoietin: a manifold task. Physiology (Bethesda) 2008;23:263–274.
68. Gidday JM. Extending injury- and disease-resistant CNS phenotypes by repetitive epigenetic conditioning. Front Neurol 2015;6:42.
69. Gunnarson E, Song Y, Kowalewski JM, et al. Erythropoietin modulation of astrocyte water permeability as a component of neuroprotection. Proc Natl Acad Sci U S A 2009;106:1602–1607.
70. Kim YE, Baek ST. Neurodevelopmental aspects of RASopathies. Mol Cells 2019;42:441–447.
71. Tajan M, Paccoud R, Branka S, Edouard T, Yart A. The RASopathy family: consequences of germline activation of the RAS/MAPK pathway. Endocr Rev 2018;39:676–700.
72. Plotkin SR, Wick A. Neurofibromatosis and schwannomatosis. Semin Neurol 2018;38:73–85.
73. Laycock-van Spyk S, Thomas N, Cooper DN, Upadhyaya M. Neurofibromatosis type 1-associated tumours: their somatic mutational spectrum and pathogenesis. Hum Genomics 2011;5:623–690.
74. Dombi E, Baldwin A, Marcus LJ, et al. Activity of selumetinib in neurofibromatosis type 1-related plexiform neurofibromas. N Engl J Med 2016;375:2550–2560.
75. Siegfried A, Cances C, Denuelle M, et al. Noonan syndrome, PTPN11 mutations, and brain tumors: a clinical report and review of the literature. Am J Med Genet A 2017;173:1061–1065.
76. Kim M, Kim S, Lee SH, et al. Merlin inhibits Wnt/beta-catenin signaling by blocking LRP6 phosphorylation. Cell Death Differ 2016;23:1638–1647.
77. Coy S, Rashid R, Stemmer-Rachamimov A, Santagata S. An update on the CNS manifestations of neurofibromatosis type 2. Acta Neuropathol 2019;139:643–665.
78. Huang J, Manning BD. The TSC1-TSC2 complex: a molecular switchboard controlling cell growth. Biochem J 2008;412:179–190.
79. Peron A, Northrup H. Tuberous sclerosis complex. Am J Med Genet C Semin Med Genet 2018;178:274–277.
80. Peron A, Au KS, Northrup H. Genetics, genomics, and genotype-phenotype correlations of TSC: insights for clinical practice. Am J Med Genet C Semin Med Genet 2018;178:281–290.
81. Canevini MP, Kotulska-Jozwiak K, Curatolo P, et al. Current concepts on epilepsy management in tuberous sclerosis complex. Am J Med Genet C Semin Med Genet 2018;178:299–308.
82. Crino PB. The mTOR signalling cascade: paving new roads to cure neurological disease. Nat Rev Neurol 2016;12:379–392.
83. Baldassari S, Picard F, Verbeek NE, et al. The landscape of epilepsy-related GATOR1 variants. Genet Med 2019;21:398–408.
84. Yehia L, Keel E, Eng C. The clinical spectrum of PTEN mutations. Annu Rev Med 2020;71:103–116.
85. Aronow ME, Wiley HE, Gaudric A, et al. Von Hippel-Lindau disease: update on pathogenesis and systemic aspects. Retina 2019;39:2243–2253.
86. Binder DK. The role of BDNF in epilepsy and other diseases of the mature nervous system. Adv Exp Med Biol 2004;548:34–56.
87. Heinrich C, Lahteinen S, Suzuki F, et al. Increase in BDNF-mediated TrkB signaling promotes epileptogenesis in a mouse model of mesial temporal lobe epilepsy. Neurobiol Dis 2011;42:35–47.
88. Lin TW, Harward SC, Huang YZ, McNamara JO. Targeting BDNF/TrkB pathways for preventing or suppressing epilepsy. Neuropharmacology 2020;167:107734.
89. Chmielewska N, Wawer A, Maciejak P, et al. The role of REST/NRSF, TrkB and BDNF in neurobiological mechanisms of different susceptibility to seizure in a PTZ model of epilepsy. Brain Res Bull 2020;158:108–115.
90. Zuccato C, Cattaneo E. Brain-derived neurotrophic factor in neurodegenerative diseases. Nat Rev Neurol 2009;5:311–322.
91. Weishaupt N, Blesch A, Fouad K. BDNF: the career of a multifaceted neurotrophin in spinal cord injury. Exp Neurol 2012;238:254–264.
92. Plotkin JL, Day M, Peterson JD, et al. Impaired TrkB receptor signaling underlies corticostriatal dysfunction in Huntington's disease. Neuron 2014;83:178–188.

93. Castren ML, Castren E. BDNF in fragile X syndrome. Neuropharmacology 2014;76 Pt C:729–736.
94. Nagahara AH, Merrill DA, Coppola G, et al. Neuroprotective effects of brain-derived neurotrophic factor in rodent and primate models of Alzheimer's disease. Nat Med 2009;15:331–337.
95. Nagahara AH, Mateling M, Kovacs I, et al. Early BDNF treatment ameliorates cell loss in the entorhinal cortex of APP transgenic mice. J Neurosci 2013;33:15596–15602.
96. Levivier M, Przedborski S, Bencsics C, Kang UJ. Intrastriatal implantation of fibroblasts genetically engineered to produce brain-derived neurotrophic factor prevents degeneration of dopaminergic neurons in a rat model of Parkinson's disease. J Neurosci 1995;15:7810–7820.
97. Frim DM, Uhler TA, Galpern WR, Beal MF, Breakefield XO, Isacson O. Implanted fibroblasts genetically engineered to produce brain-derived neurotrophic factor prevent 1-methyl-4-phenylpyridinium toxicity to dopaminergic neurons in the rat. Proc Natl Acad Sci U S A 1994;91:5104–5108.
98. Tsukahara T, Takeda M, Shimohama S, Ohara O, Hashimoto N. Effects of brain-derived neurotrophic factor on 1-methyl-4-phenyl-1,2,3,6-tetrahydropyridine-induced parkinsonism in monkeys. Neurosurgery 1995;37:733–739; discussion 739–741.
99. Craft S. Alzheimer disease: insulin resistance and AD: extending the translational path. Nat Rev Neurol 2012;8:360–362.
100. Neth BJ, Craft S. Insulin resistance and Alzheimer's disease: bioenergetic linkages. Front Aging Neurosci 2017;9:345.
101. Moloney AM, Griffin RJ, Timmons S, O'Connor R, Ravid R, O'Neill C. Defects in IGF-1 receptor, insulin receptor and IRS-1/2 in Alzheimer's disease indicate possible resistance to IGF-1 and insulin signalling. Neurobiol Aging 2010;31:224–243.
102. Carmichael ST. Emergent properties of neural repair: elemental biology to therapeutic concepts. Ann Neurol 2016;79:895–906.
103. Bartus RT, Johnson EM, Jr. Clinical tests of neurotrophic factors for human neurodegenerative diseases, part 1: Where have we been and what have we learned? Neurobiol Dis 2017;97:156–168.
104. Bartus RT, Johnson EM, Jr. Clinical tests of neurotrophic factors for human neurodegenerative diseases, part 2: Where do we stand and where must we go next? Neurobiol Dis 2017;97:169–178.
105. Whone AL, Boca M, Luz M, et al. Extended treatment with glial cell line-derived neurotrophic factor in Parkinson's disease. J Parkinsons Dis 2019;9:301–313.
106. Gage FH, Temple S. Neural stem cells: generating and regenerating the brain. Neuron 2013;80:588–601.
107. Staff NP, Jones DT, Singer W. Mesenchymal stromal cell therapies for neurodegenerative diseases. Mayo Clin Proc 2019;94:892–905.
108. Revishchin A, Moiseenko L, Kust N, et al. Effects of striatal transplantation of cells transfected with GDNF gene without pre- and pro-regions in mouse model of Parkinson's disease. BMC Neurosci 2016;17:34.
109. Thomsen GM, Avalos P, Ma AA, et al. Transplantation of neural progenitor cells expressing glial cell line-derived neurotrophic factor into the motor cortex as a strategy to treat amyotrophic lateral sclerosis. Stem Cells 2018;36:1122–1131.

Section II

Excitability, Signal Communication, and Plasticity

14 Ion Channels and Channelopathies

OVERVIEW

Initiation, conduction, and transmission of signals in the nervous system involve a complex interplay of a large variety of ion channels.[1] Ion channels are multimeric transmembrane proteins composed of several subunits surrounding a hydrophilic pore that allows the passive movement of ions down their concentration gradient (Figure 14.1). Ion channels vary in their ion selectivity, gating mechanism, threshold and kinetics of activation and inactivation, and distribution on the cell membrane. These properties are determined by the subunit composition, presence of auxiliary subunits, phosphorylation of channel proteins, and allosteric modulation by divalent ions or other molecules. Voltage-gated sodium (Na^+) channels are critical for generation and conduction of the action potential. Voltage-gated calcium (Ca^{2+}) channels promote membrane depolarization, trigger synaptic vesicle exocytosis, and mediate excitation-contraction coupling in skeletal muscle. Voltage-gated and other types of potassium (K^+) channels control neuronal excitability, duration and firing pattern of action potentials, and probability of neurotransmitter release. Neurotransmitter-gated channels (ionotropic receptors) mediate fast postsynaptic responses; cation channels trigger fast excitatory postsynaptic potentials, whereas chloride (Cl^-) channels trigger inhibitory postsynaptic potential in most adult neurons. Other channels such as hyperpolarization-gated, cyclic nucleotide-regulated (HCN) channels; transient receptor potential (TRP) channels; acid-sensing cation channels (ASICs); and anoctamin (ANO) channels are expressed in selective portion of neurons or axons, particularly nociceptors. Channelopathies affecting the central nervous system manifest with epilepsy, episodic ataxia, paroxysmal movement disorders, and hemiplegic migraine. Neuromuscular channelopathies produce neuromyotonia, myotonia, periodic paralysis, and myasthenic syndromes. Nociceptor channelopathies produce paroxysmal pain disorders or congenital insensitivity to pain. The aims of this chapter are to review (1) mechanisms by which ion channels affect neuronal electrophysiology, (2) role of different types of ion channel in shaping neuronal activity, and (3) examples of genetic and acquired channelopathies. The role of ionotropic receptors in synaptic transmission and their involvement in disease are discussed in other chapters of this book.

ELECTROPHYSIOLOGICAL BASES OF ION CHANNEL FUNCTION

Ion channels are transmembrane proteins consisting of several subunits forming a central pore. They are defined by their ion permeability, gating mechanism, and kinetics of activation and inactivation. Voltage-gated cation channels are activated by membrane depolarization and have different activation thresholds and kinetics of activation or inactivation. They are thus subclassified into subthreshold, low-threshold, or high-threshold channels and may carry fast inactivating, slow inactivating, or persistent currents. These properties depend on the amino acid composition of the channel subunits. Voltage-gated sodium (Na^+) and calcium (Ca^{2+}) channels promote membrane depolarization. They increase neuronal excitability and promote the generation of action potentials. Voltage-gated and other types of potassium (K^+) channels control neuronal excitability, duration and firing pattern of action potentials, and probability of neurotransmitter release. Neurotransmitter-gated cation channels may allow entry of Na^+, Ca^{2+}, or both and elicit

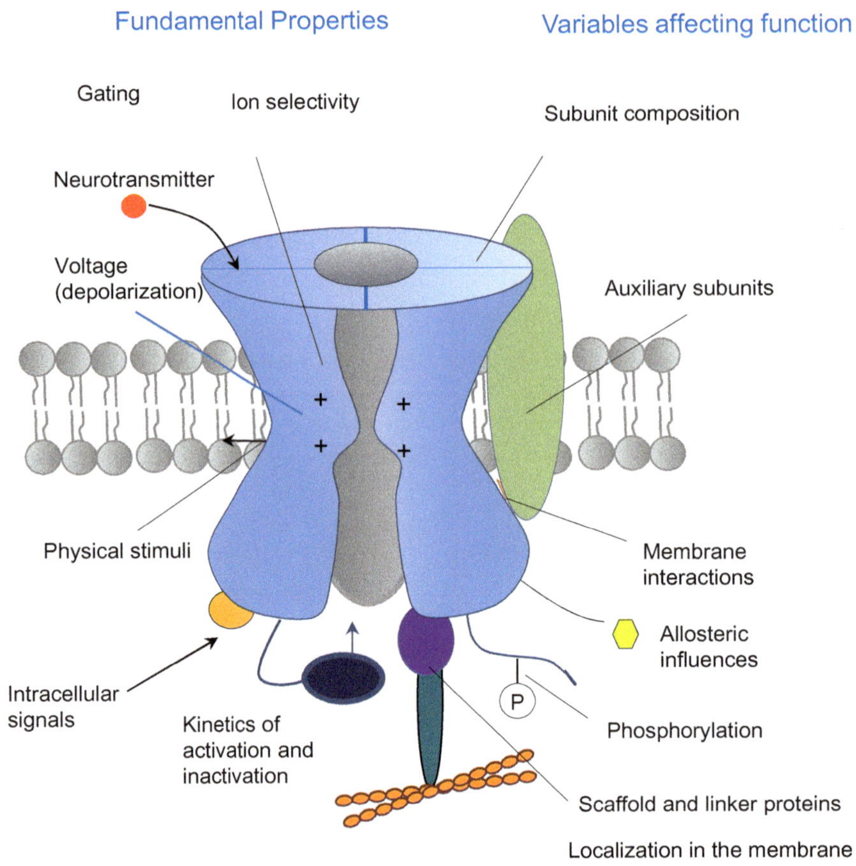

FIGURE 14.1 General features of ion channels.
Ion channels are multimeric transmembrane proteins composed of several subunits surrounding a hydrophilic pore. Ion channels vary in their ion selectivity, gating mechanism, threshold and kinetics of activation and inactivation, and distribution on the cell membrane. These properties are determined by the subunit composition, presence of auxiliary subunits, phosphorylation of channel proteins, and allosteric modulation by divalent ions or other molecules.

fast excitatory postsynaptic potentials. Neurotransmitter-gated chloride (Cl^-) channels typically produce inhibitory postsynaptic potentials in the adult nervous system but may also increase excitability is some cases. Several basic principles of cell physiology underlie the function of these ion channels.

Determinants of the Membrane Potential

The membrane potential (V_m) is determined by two major variables, the transmembrane ion concentration gradient and the weighted balance of electrical currents flowing through permeable ion channels (Figure 14.2). The transmembrane concentration gradient of a given ion determines the equilibrium potential of this ion (E_{ion}), which is the transmembrane voltage difference that exactly offsets the tendency of an ion to move down its concentration gradient and is calculated using the Nernst equation. The equilibrium potential for different ions varies according to the type of cell or axon and the species. The maintenance of the transmembrane Na^+ and K^+ gradient is critical to maintain cell excitability and depends on the activity of the Na^+/K^+-ATPase as well as the buffering of extracellular K^+ by astrocytes following synaptic activity. The transmembrane Cl^- gradient is determined by the opposing activities of the K-Cl cotransporter (KCCs) that extrudes Cl^- from the cell, and the Na-K-Cl cotransporters (NKCCs) that allows Cl^- influx into the cell.[2] The magnitude of ion flow through ion channels depends both on the state-dependent permeability (or electrical conductance) of the channel and the electrical driving potential. The driving potential is the difference between the membrane potential and the equilibrium potential of a particular ion. Since the membrane potential at a given time depends on the balanced influences of multiple ion channels, opening of a given ion channel moves the membrane potential toward the equilibrium potential of that ion, whereas closing the channel moves the membrane potential away from the equilibrium potential of the ion.

Resting Membrane Potential

The resting membrane potential (RMP) is the transmembrane voltage at which the movement of the various ions comes to a steady state. In most neurons it ranges between

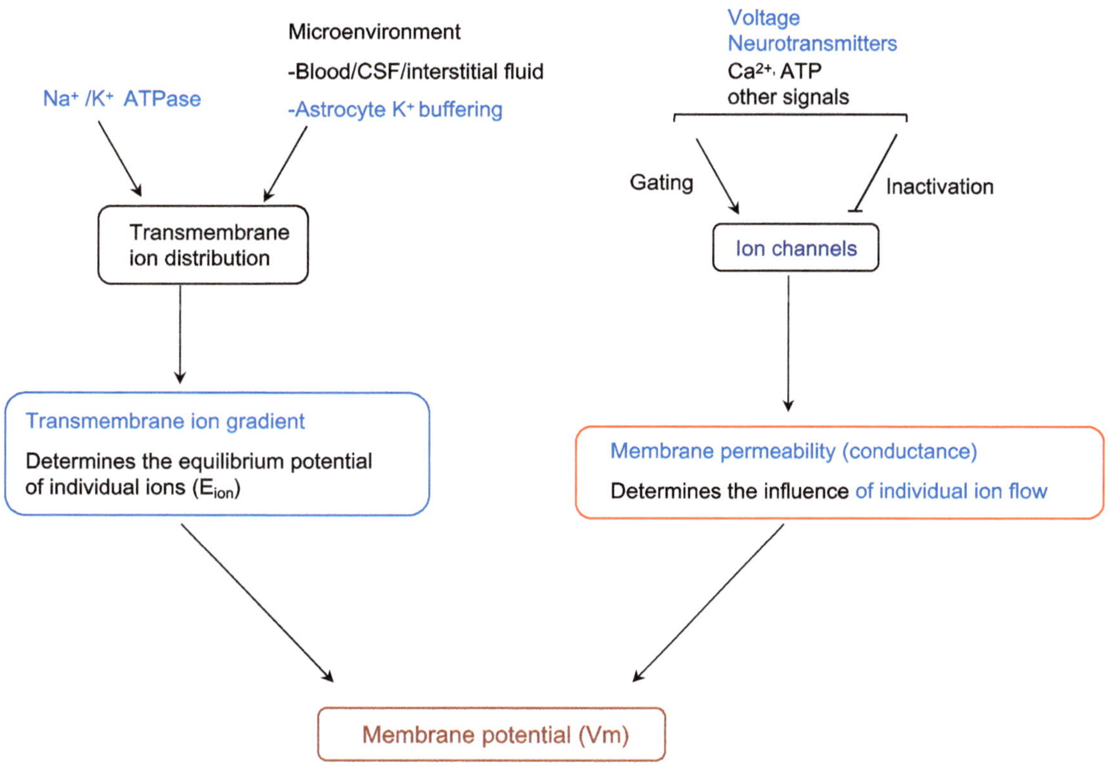

FIGURE 14.2 Determinants of the membrane potential.
The membrane potential (V_m) is determined by two major variables, the transmembrane ion concentration gradient and the weighted balance of electrical currents flowing through ion channels. The maintenance of the transmembrane Na^+ and K^+ gradient depends on the activity of the Na^+/K^+ ATPase as well as the buffering of extracellular K^+ by astrocytes. The magnitude of ion flow through ion channel depends both on the state-dependent permeability (or electrical conductance) of the channel and the electrical driving potential.

-60 and -80 mV. The value of the RMP determines both the spontaneous electrical activity and the responsiveness of the neuron to extrinsic inputs. Since at rest the membrane is much more permeable to K^+ than to Na^+, neuronal excitability is primarily determined by the transmembrane K^+ gradient, the relative permeability to K^+ and Na^+, and the activity of the Na^+/K^+ ATPase. This enzyme undergoes a phosphorylation-dephosphorylation cycle coupled with the transport of three Na^+ ions out of and two K^+ ions into the cell; thus the coupling of the pump is electronic and contributes approximately -10 mV to the RMP. The transmembrane potential at rest is also in part affected by the presence of negative charges on outer surface of the cell membrane, which are mostly due to the presence of polar glycosphingolipids. The electronegativity in the outer surface may reduce the activation threshold of Na^+ channels but is in part counteracted by binding of extracellular Ca^{2+}. This may explain why reduced levels of extracellular ionized Ca^{2+} increases excitability, as reflected, for example, by paresthesia or tetany.

Neuronal Excitability

Neuronal excitability is the probability to open the voltage-gated Na^+ channels responsible for initiation of the action potential. It depends on the difference between the RMP and the threshold depolarization required to open these channels. In most neurons, the membrane potential has spontaneous variations due to the activity of subthreshold ion channels. Neurotransmitters or sensory stimuli elicit a transient opening or closure of selective ion channels, resulting in local potentials that may either increase or decrease the probability to reach the threshold to trigger an action potential (Figure 14.3). Opening of Na^+ or Ca^{2+} channels results in an inward current that produces depolarization, thereby increasing neuronal excitability. In contrast, opening of K^+ channels elicits either an outward current (hyperpolarization) or stabilization of the membrane potential close to E_K, thereby reducing excitability. Closure of K^+ channels increases neuronal excitability. Since E_{Cl-} is close to the resting membrane potential, the direction of Cl^- flow and thus its effects on the membrane potential is determined by the activity of the Cl^--cation cotransporters KCC2 and NKCC1.

Action Potential

The action potential, or spike, communicates information rapidly from the peripheral receptor or dendrites to

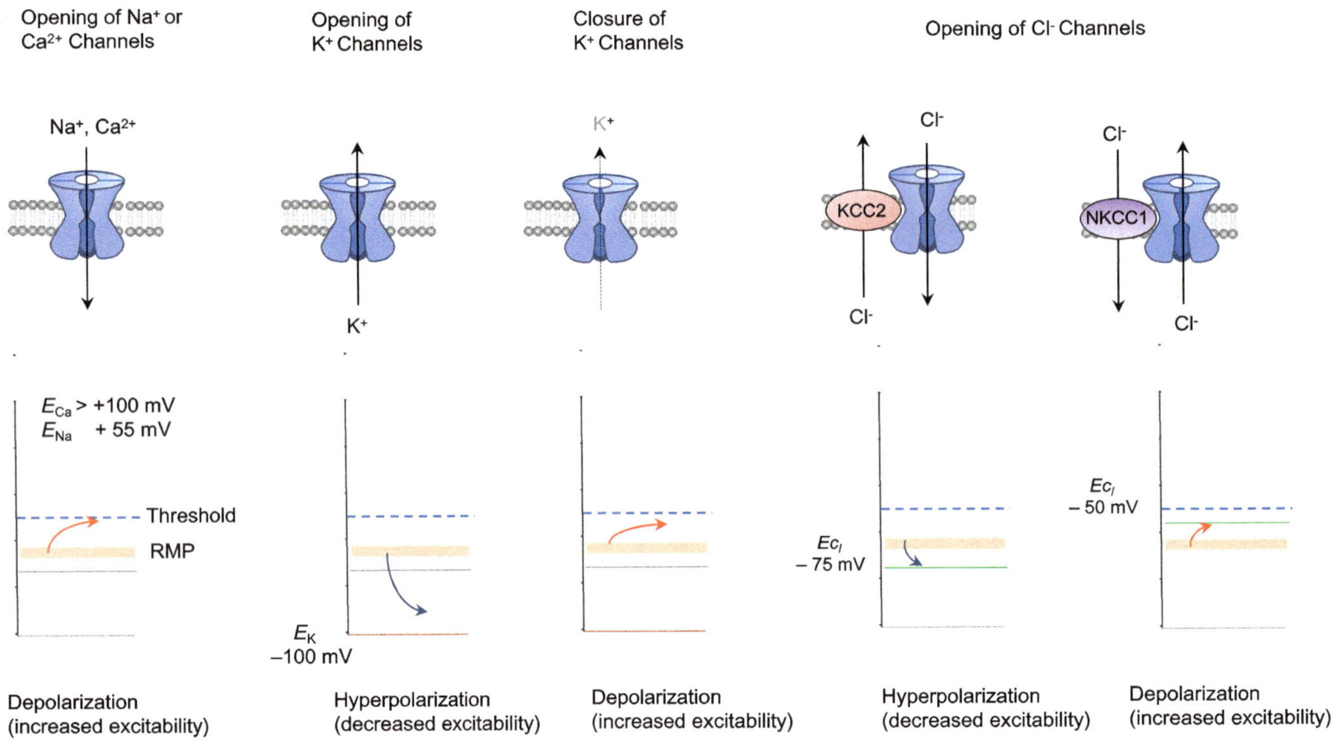

FIGURE 14.3 Effect of opening of ion channels on neuronal excitability.
Opening of Na^+ or Ca^{2+} channels elicits an inward current that produces depolarization, thereby increasing neuronal excitability. In contrast, opening of K^+ channels elicits either an outward current (hyperpolarization) or stabilization of the membrane potential close to E_K, thereby reducing excitability. Since E_{Cl-} is close to the resting membrane potential, the direction of Cl^- flow and thus its effects on the membrane potential is determined by the relative activity of the Cl^- cation cotransporters, KCC2 and NKCC1.

the soma or from the soma to the presynaptic axon terminal.[3,4] In most neurons, the membrane potential has spontaneous variations due to the interplay among activity of subthreshold Na^+, Ca^{2+}, and K^+ channels that are active in the absence of stimuli. The action potential is triggered when the membrane is depolarized approximately 10 mV from its resting potential (approximately -55 mV) and reaches threshold for opening of fast inactivating voltage-gated Na^+ channels. This elicits a rapid membrane depolarization, producing a fast Na^+ spike (approximately +55 mV), which is rapidly followed by channel inactivation. In some neurons, depolarization during the fast action potential promotes opening of voltage-gated Ca^{2+} channels (Figure 14.4). The threshold for action potential initiation is lowest at the axon initial segment (AIS), which contains a cluster of voltage-gated Na^+ channels. Repolarization of the action potential occurs via opening of a variety of voltage-gated K^+ channels as well as Ca^{2+}- and Na^+-activated K^+ channels. Repolarization is followed by an afterhyperpolarization via Ca^{2+} activated K^+ channels and, in some cells, an afterdepolarization. Conduction of the action potential is also mediated by fast inactivating Na^+ channels, whereas axon excitability is regulated by K^+ channels. The action potential is propagated along the axons and upon arriving to the presynaptic terminal triggers the opening of voltage-gated Ca^{2+} channels resulting in synchronous release of neurotransmitters from synaptic vesicles. The action potential may also be propagated back to the cell body and dendrites; the probability of action potential back-propagation is limited by a variety of voltage-gated K^+ channels.

General Structure of Voltage-Gated Ion Channels

Voltage-gated cation channels consist of a principal or α subunit that defines the different families of voltage-gated Na^+ (Na_v), Ca^{2+} (Ca_v), and K^+ (K_v) channels. This subunit contains a voltage sensor and forms the wall of the channel pore, and several auxiliary subunits that affect the kinetic properties and membrane expression of the channels. The basic pore-forming α subunit of voltage-gated K^+ channels (VGKC, K_v) consists of six transmembrane segments (S1–S6) that have a modular structure[1] (Figure 14.5). The S1–S4 module forms the selectivity filter and voltage sensor domain; the S4 segment contains positive charges (usually provided by arginine or lysine) that are important for voltage sensing. The S5–S6 segment forms a pore domain or module consisting of two helices and a reentrant loop (S5-P-S6) that forms the outer vestibule of the channel.

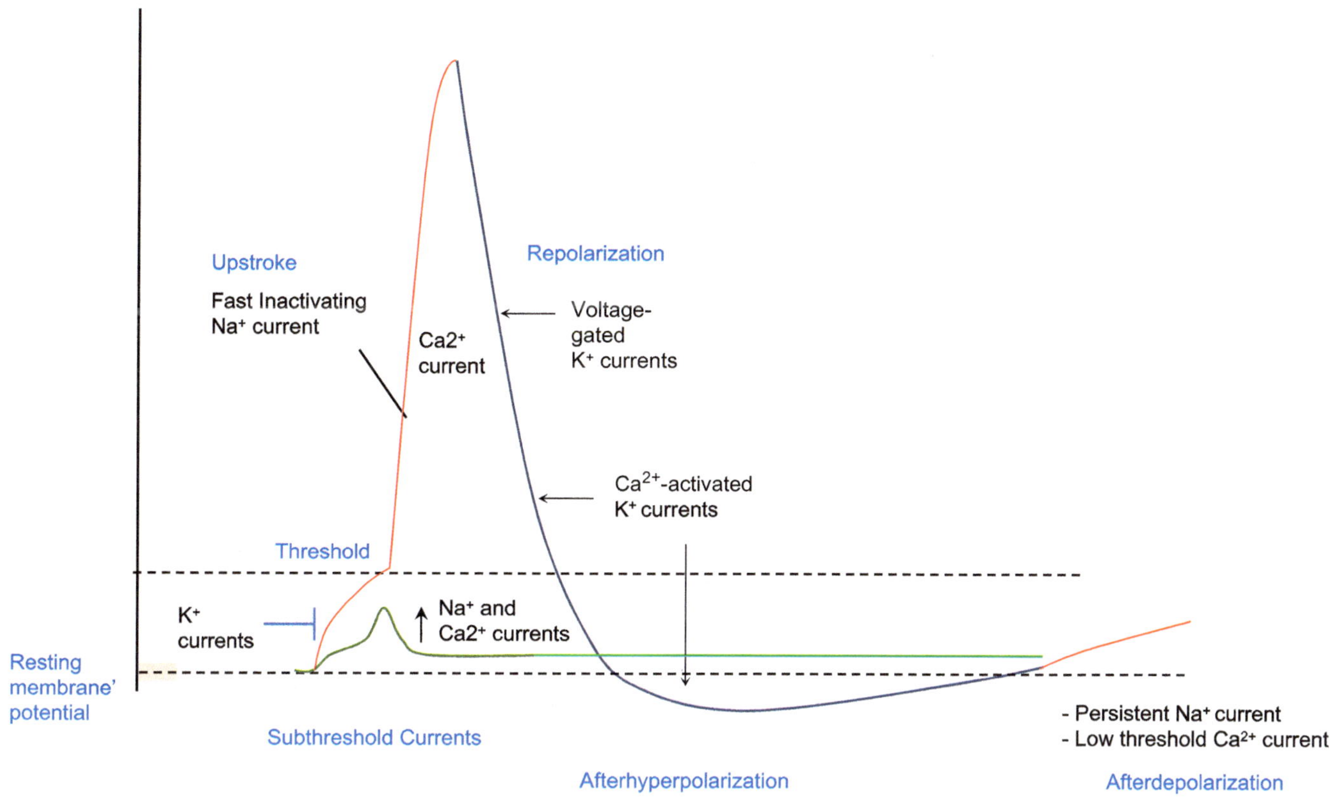

FIGURE 14.4 Channels involved in the action potential in neurons.
The resting membrane potential is primarily maintained by two-pore (K_{2P}) and inward-rectifying (K_{ir}) channels. There are subthreshold depolarizing currents, such as persistent Na^+ currents, and in some cases also currents via hyperpolarization-gated cyclic nucleotide-regulated (HCN) channels, and T-type (Ca_v3) Ca^{2+} channels. These depolarizing currents are counteracted by K^+ channels that are activated by subthreshold depolarizations, such as K_v1, K_v4, and K_v7 channels. The action potential is triggered when the membrane is depolarized approximately 10 mV, leading to opening of fast inactivating $Na_v1.1$, $Na_v1.2$, and $Na_v1.6$ channels. In some neurons, depolarization during the fast action potential promotes opening of voltage-gated Ca^{2+} channels, such as L-type (Ca_v2) channels. Repolarization of the action potential occurs via opening of a variety of voltage-gated K^+ channels, including K_v2 and, in case of fast spiking neurons, rapidly inactivating K_v3 channels as well large conductance (BK) and the slow conductance (SK) channels, which also elicit afterhyperpolarization. This is followed in some cells by an afterdepolarization.

Functional K_v channels consist of tetramers of this basic α subunit. The α subunit of voltage-gated Na^+ channels (VGSC, Na_v) and the α1 subunit of voltage-gated Ca^{2+} channels (VGCC, Ca_v) are arranged in four tandem domains (I–IV), each containing the basic S1–S4 voltage sensor module and the S5–S6 pore-forming module; these domains are linked together by intracellular loops connecting the S6 segment of the upstream domain to the S1 segment of the downstream domain. Most voltage-gated ion channels are part of macromolecular complexes and have auxiliary subunits that regulate surface expression and biophysical properties (gating, kinetics) of the channel and interact with scaffolding proteins.[5] The general four subunit structure surrounding a pore is shared by many types of ion channels, including other K^+ channels; and HCN, TRP, ASICs, and ANO channels.

VOLTAGE-GATED SODIUM CHANNELS

Voltage-gated sodium channels carry depolarizing currents that are critical to set subthreshold excitability, generation, repetitive firing, and conduction of the action potential, depolarization of the presynaptic terminal for Ca^{2+}-triggered neurotransmitter release, and excitation-contraction coupling in skeletal muscle.

Structure and Classification

Voltage-gated sodium channels consist of a principal α subunit that contains the voltage sensory and the pore domain and auxiliary β subunits. The intracellular loops provide the structural bases for channel inactivation and interaction with anchoring proteins such as ankyrin G

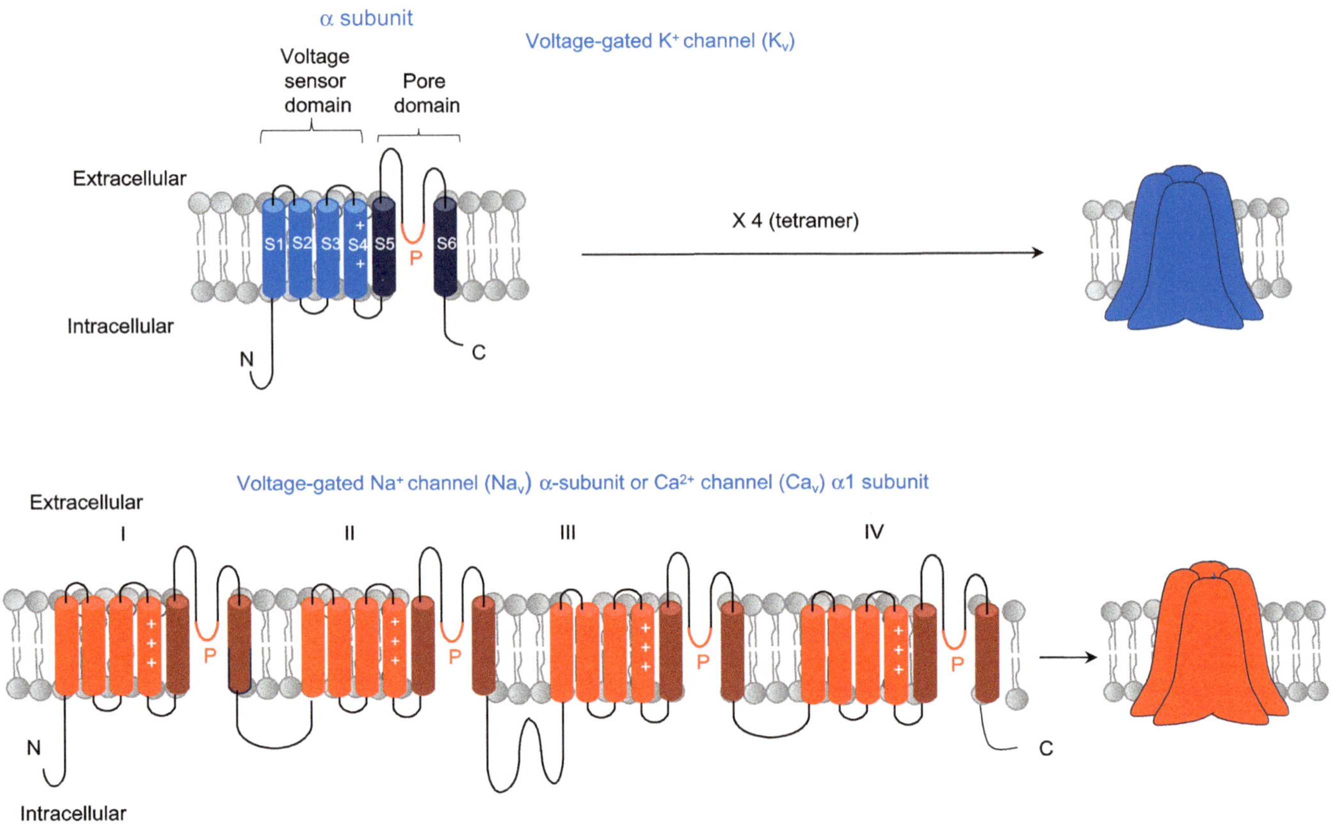

FIGURE 14.5 General structure of voltage-gated channels.

Voltage-gated cation channels consist of a principal or α subunit that contains a voltage sensor and forms the wall of the channel pore, and several auxiliary subunits that affect the kinetic properties and membrane expression of the channels. The basic pore-forming α subunit of voltage-gated K^+ channels consists of six transmembrane segments (S1–S6) that have a modular structure. The S1–S4 module forms the selectivity filter and voltage sensor domain; the S4 segment contains positive charges (usually provided by arginine or lysine) that are important for voltage sensing. The S5–S6 segment forms a pore domain consisting of two helices and a reentrant loop (S5-P-S6) that forms the outer vestibule of the channel that houses the ion selectivity filter. Functional K_v channels consist of tetramers of this basic α subunit. The α subunit of voltage-gated Na^+ channels and the α1 subunit of voltage-gated Ca^{2+} channels are arranged in four tandem domains (DI–DIV) each containing the basic S1–S4 voltage sensor module and the S5–S6 pore-forming module.

(Figure 14.6). These channels are classified according to their α subunits, which are encoded by 10 *SCNA* genes (Table 14.1).[6] The most abundant subunits in the mature CNS neurons are Na_v1.1, Na_v1.2, and Na_v1.6. The Na_v1.1 and Na_v1.2 subunits are primarily expressed in the cell body, soma and dendrites; Navl.1, Navl.2, and particularly Na_v1.6 are expressed in the AIS and nodes of Ranvier. Na_v1.3 is primarily expressed in the brain during early postnatal development; it only remains expressed in the adult sympathetic neurons, but becomes repressed in dorsal root ganglion (DRG) neurons following axonal injury. The Na_v1.7, Na_v1.8, and Na_v1.9 channels are expressed primarily in nociceptive dorsal root ganglion (DRG) neurons.[7,8] Na_v1.4 is the major sodium channel in adult skeletal muscle,[9] and Na_v1.5 in the heart. The auxiliary β subunits (Na_v β1–β4) are encoded by *SCNB* genes and affect the surface expression, threshold, and kinetics of channel activation and inactivation.

Function

The Na_v channels generate different types of Na^+ currents. The fast inactivating, transient Na^+ current is activated at threshold and is responsible for the spike of the action potential. This current is mediated by Na_v1.1, Na_v 1.2, and Na_v1.6 channels and is generated at the AIS and transmitted in myelinated axons at the nodes of Ranvier.[10] The other two Na^+ currents are activated at subthreshold or near-threshold membrane potential and regulate neuronal excitability and repetitive firing. The persistent Na^+ current amplifies subthreshold excitatory postsynaptic potentials and is generated in the proximal axon; the resurgent Na^+ current is activated during repolarization, may facilitate reexcitation during repetitive firing, and may be present throughout the axon. The Na_v1.7, Na_v1.8, and Na_v1.9 channels regulate excitability of unmyelinated nociceptive axons. In skeletal muscle, Na_v1.4 channels concentrated in

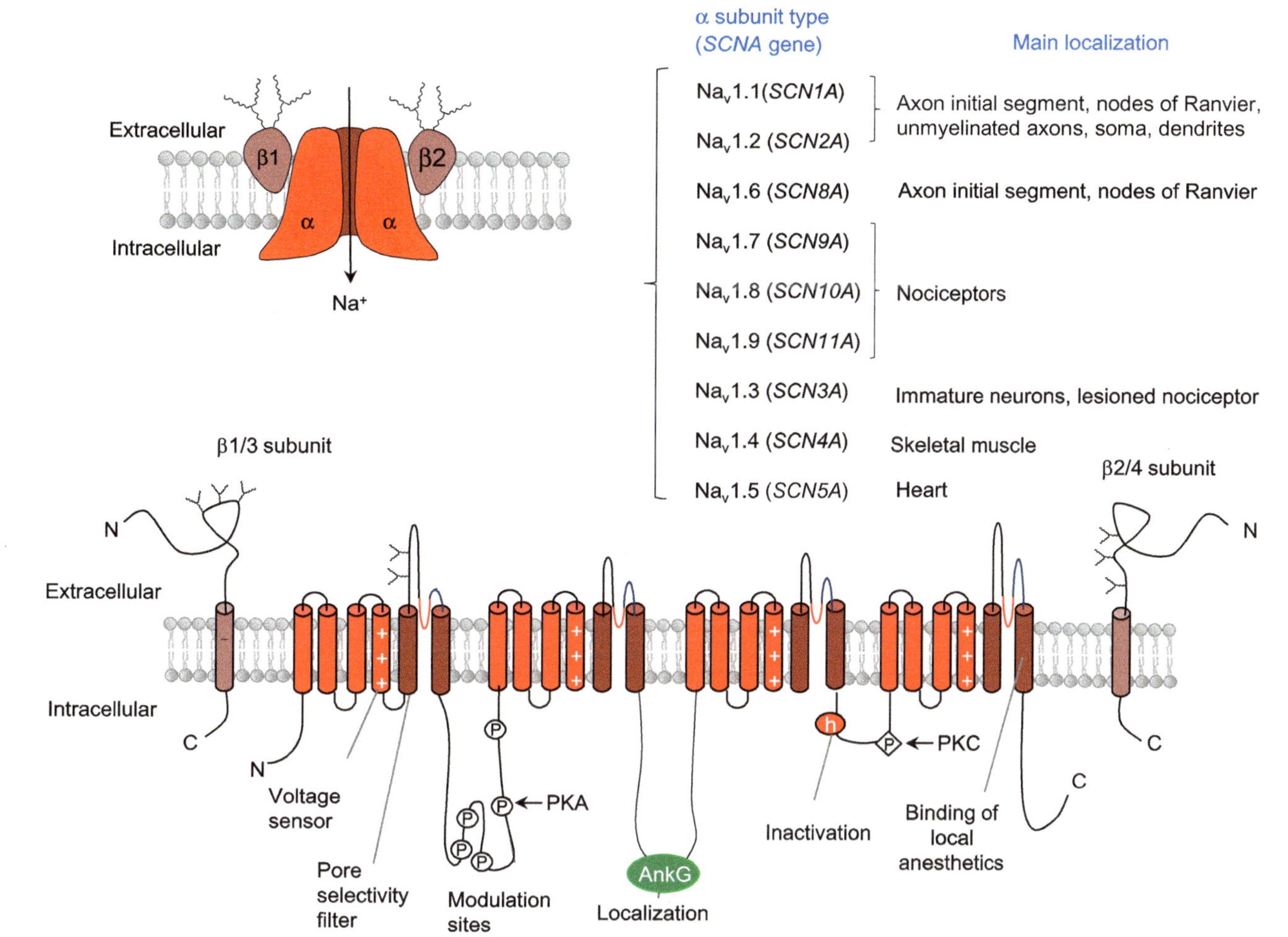

FIGURE 14.6 Structure and classification of voltage-gated sodium channels.
Voltage-gated sodium channels consist of a principal α subunit that contains the voltage sensory and the pore domain and auxiliary β subunits. The intracellular loops provide the structural bases for channel inactivation and interaction with anchoring proteins such as ankyrin G. These channels are classified according to their α subunits, encoded by 10 *SCNA* genes. The most abundant in the mature CNS neurons are $Na_v1.1$, $Na_v1.2$, and $Na_v1.6$. $Na_v1.3$ is primarily expressed during development. $Na_v1.7$, $Na_v1.8$, and $Na_v1.9$ channels are expressed primarily in nociceptive neurons. Auxiliary β subunits (Na_v β1–β4) a encoded by *SCNB* genes and affect the surface expression, threshold, and kinetics of the channel. AnkG, ankyrin G; PKA, protein kinase A; PKC, protein kinase C.

the depth of the junctional folds at the motor endplate are activated by the endplate potential mediated by nAChRs and mediate depolarization that triggers intracellular Ca^{2+} release and thus excitation-contraction coupling.

Voltage-gated Na^+ channels undergo both fast and slow inactivation. The classical "fast" inactivation occurs over the time course of milliseconds and limits the propensity of repetitive firing. Fast inactivation involves an inactivation gate in the domain cytoplasmic III–IV loop, the cytoplasmic end of the S5 and S6 segments at the inner mouth of the pore (the docking site for the inactivation gate) and the voltage sensors (S4 segment) of domain IV. Slow inactivation occurs over the course of seconds and occurs during prolonged intervals of depolarization or during sustained high-frequency bursts of action potentials and involves mechanisms different from those in fast inactivation.

VOLTAGE-GATED CALCIUM CHANNELS

Voltage-gated calcium channels are activated by membrane depolarization and allow Ca^{2+} influx that triggers a wide range of processes including cell depolarization, neurotransmitter release, muscle contraction, and gene transcription.[11–13]

Classification and Structure

The α1 subunit (encoded by *CACHNA1* genes) contains the voltage sensor and the pore motifs; their intracellular loops in combination with the amino and carboxyl termini provide hubs for channel regulation by a variety of signaling molecules and other molecular partners (Figure 14.7). According to their pore-forming α1 subunits, voltage-gated calcium channels are divided into three families Ca_v1 Ca_v2,

TABLE 14.1 *Types of Voltage-Gated Sodium Channels*

α subunit (gene)	Physiology	Distribution	Function
$Na_v1.1$ (*SCN1A*)	Low activation threshold, rapid kinetics of activation and inactivation Slow recovery from inactivation	Soma and dendrites Axon initial segment (AIS) of fast spiking GABAergic neurons	Initiation and conduction of the action potential (AP)
$Na_v1.2$ (*SCN2A*)	Low activation threshold, rapid kinetics of activation and inactivation Slow recovery from inactivation	Proximal portion of AIS of pyramidal neuron Unmyelinated axon	Initiation, conduction, and backpropagation of the AP
$Na_v1.6$ (*SCN8A*)	Lowest activation threshold, rapid kinetics of activation and inactivation	AIS in essentially all neurons Nodes of Ranvier Unmyelinated axons	Initiation and conduction of the AP Can produce resurgent currents
Nav1.3 (*SCN3A*)	Low activation threshold, rapid kinetics	Sympathetic neurons Upregulated in the sensory neurons after injury	Amplification of subthreshold inputs
$Na_v1.7$ (*SCN9A*)	Low activation threshold, fast kinetics	DRG neurons Sympathetic neurons Olfactory neurons	Contributes to the rising phase and amplifies subthreshold stimuli
$Na_v1.8$ (*SCN10A*)	High activation threshold, slow kinetics	Nociceptive DRG neurons	Major contributor to the rising phase of the AP Supports high-frequency firing
$Na_v1.9$ (*SCA11A*)	Low activation threshold Ultraslow kinetics	Nociceptive DRG neurons	Amplifies subthreshold stimuli
$Na_v1.4$(*SCN4A*)	Activated by depolarization via nAChRs Fast and slow inactivation	Depth of junctional folds and T-tubule system in skeletal muscle	Depolarization for intracellular Ca^{2+} release for excitation-contraction coupling
$Na_v1.5$(*SCN5A*)	Activated by depolarization via	Cardiac muscle	Depolarization

DRG, dorsal root ganglion; nAChR, nicotinic acetylcholine receptor

and Ca_v3 (Table 14.2). The Ca_v1 family or L-type channels (Ca_v1, Ca_v2, and Ca_v3) and the Ca_v2 family including $Ca_v2.1$ (P/Q-type), $Ca_v2.2$ (N-type), and $Ca_v2.3$ (R-type) channels, also contain a calcium-sensing site at their carboxyl-terminal domain that associates with calmodulin, which is critical to calcium-dependent inactivation of the channel in response to prolonged activation.[14] Both Ca_v1 and Ca_v2 family channels also contain auxiliary α2δ subunits encoded by four different genes, β subunits encoded by four different genes, and γ subunits encoded by nine different genes. The Ca_vα2δ subunits are attached to the extracellular leaflet of the plasma membrane via a glycophosphatidylinositol anchor, and their presence results in increased density of channels in the membrane surface. The β subunits are cytoplasmic adaptor proteins that associate with the α1 subunit and increase cell surface trafficking. There is only one γ subunit isoform (γ1) associated with the Ca_v1 and Ca_v2 channels. In contrast Ca_v3 (T-type) channels lack auxiliary subunits.

Functions

L-type (Ca_v1) channels have high-threshold, slow voltage-dependent gating and are sensitive to a number of different

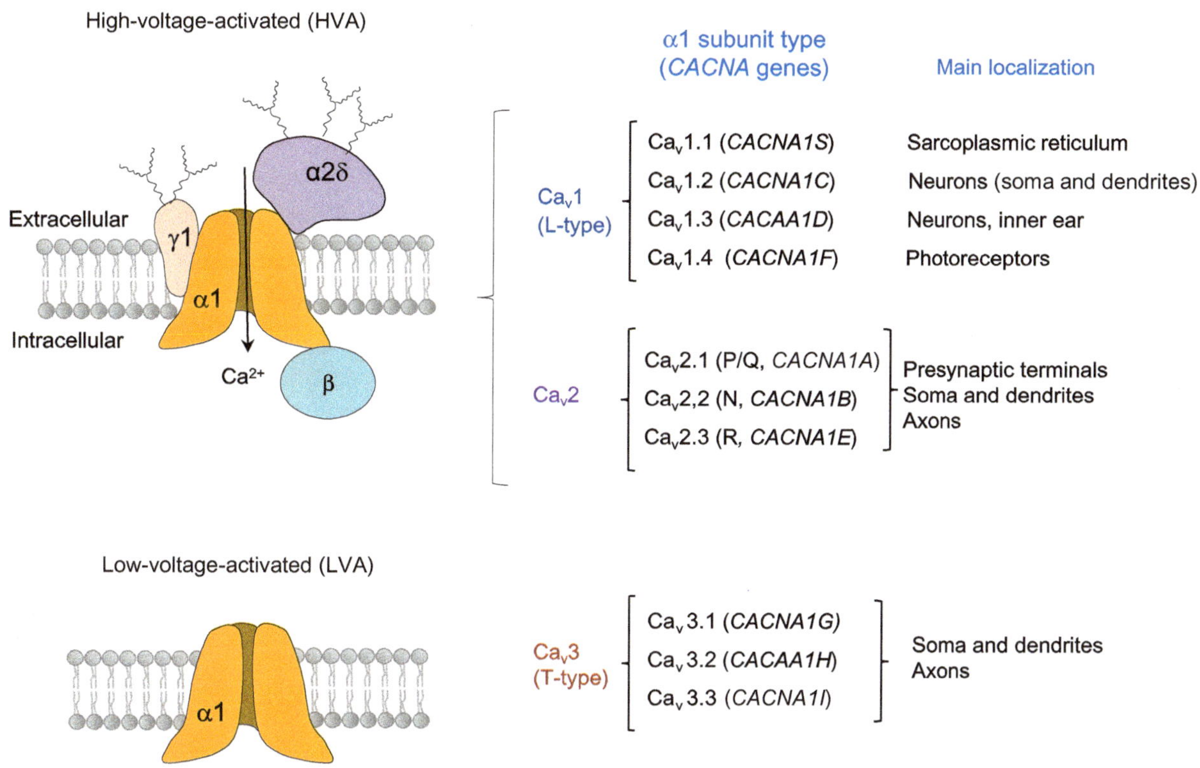

FIGURE 14.7 Structure, classification, and location of voltage-gated calcium channels.
Voltage-gated calcium channels consists of a principal α1 subunit (encoded by *CACHNA1* genes) that contains the voltage sensor and the pore motifs. According to their pore-forming α1 subunits, voltage-gated calcium channels are divided into three families. The Ca$_v$1 family (Ca$_v$1, Ca$_v$2, Ca$_v$3, and Ca$_v$4) conduct L-type currents and include a skeletal muscle isoform (Ca$_v$1.1) and three different neuronal isoforms (Ca$_v$1.2, Ca$_v$1.3, and Ca$_v$1.4). The Ca$_v$2 family includes Ca$_v$2.1 (P/Q-type), Ca$_v$2.2 (N-type), and Ca$_v$2.3 (R-type), which trigger neurotransmitter release from presynaptic terminals. The Ca$_v$3 channels (Ca$_v$3.1, Ca$_v$3.2, and Ca$_v$3.3) carry low-threshold T-type Ca^{2+} currents. The Ca$_v$1 and Ca$_v$2 channels also contain auxiliary α2δ subunits, β subunits, and γ1 subunits.

dihydropyridine antagonists and agonists such as verapamil, diltiazem, and nimodipine. The skeletal muscle isoform Ca$_v$1.1 (*CACANIS* gene) is located at the T-tubule system in skeletal muscles and interacts with ryanodine receptors in the sarcoplasmic reticulum to trigger excitation-contraction coupling. At postsynaptic sites, Ca$_v$1.2 channels form synaptic complexes at dendritic spines, dendritic shafts, and cell bodies with receptors, protein kinases, and protein phosphatases. These channels produce a slow depolarizing current and have a critical role in mechanisms of synaptic plasticity including local Ca^{2+} signaling and activation of transcription. Ca$_v$1.3 and Ca$_v$1.4 channels allow tonic release of L-glutamate at presynaptic ribbon synapses in cochlear hair cells and in photoreceptor terminals and are thus involved in sensory transduction.

The Ca$_v$2 family channels, particularly Ca$_v$2.1 (P/Q-type) and Ca$_v$2.2 (N-type) channels (are concentrated at active zones in presynaptic terminals where they trigger fast neurotransmitter release by exocytosis.[11] At active zones, these channels interact with a group of proteins that promote docking of synaptic vesicles in proximity to the channels for fast neurotransmitter release. These presynaptic mechanisms are described in the next chapter.

The Ca$_v$3 channels (Ca$_v$3.1, Ca$_v$3.2, and Ca$_v$3.3) carry low-threshold T-type Ca^{2+} currents.[12,15] Voltage-dependent opening of T-type channels occurs at comparatively negative membrane potentials and elicits membrane depolarization that increases opening probability of voltage-gated Na^+ channels and the propensity of cells to fire burst of action potentials. This is especially relevant in some CNS neurons including thalamic and hippocampal cells where T-type channels are abundant in dendrites to enhance subthreshold postsynaptic potentials and facilitate the propagation of the electrical signal to the cell body. Due to their fast recovery from inactivation T-type channels generate Ca^{2+} spikes after brief periods of hyperpolarization, which leads to the firing of rebound bursts of action potentials that support various forms of neuronal rhythmogenesis. T-channels also contribute to neuronal excitability by forming functional complexes with several types of voltage-activated and Ca^{2+}-activated K^+ channels. T-type channels also contribute to several forms of synaptic plasticity and participate in the low-threshold release of neurotransmitters and hormones due to their functional coupling with the vesicular release machinery.

TABLE 14.2 *Voltage-Gated Calcium Channels*

Family	Subfamilies (gene)	Distribution	Functions (example)
Ca_v1 (L-type)	$Ca_v1.1$ (*CACNA1S*)	T-transverse tubule	Excitation-contraction coupling
	$Ca_v1.2$ (*CACNA1C*)	Neurons	Slow depolarization Dendritic spikes Synaptic plasticity Neuronal circuit formation
	$Ca_v1.3$ (*CACNA1D*)	Neurons	Auditory hair cell transmission Pacemaking activity Slow depolarization Dendritic spikes Synaptic plasticity
	$Ca_v1.4$ (*CACNA1F*)	Neurons	Photoreceptor synaptic transmission
Ca_v2	$Ca_v2.1$ (P/Q-type) (*CACNA1A*)	Presynaptic terminals Neurons	Neurotransmitter release at glutamatergic synapses Neuromuscular transmission Purkinje cell physiology
	$Ca_v2.2$ (N-type) (*CACNA1B*)	Presynaptic terminals	Neurotransmitter release at nociceptive synapses
	$Ca_v2.3$ (R-type) (*CACNA1E*)	Presynaptic terminals	Neurotransmitter release
Ca_v3 (T-type)	$Ca_v3.1$ (*CACNA1G*) $Ca_v3.2$ (*CACNA1H*) $Ca_v3.3$ (*CACNA1I*)	Neurons Presynaptic terminal	Low-threshold spike for rhythmic burst firing Low-threshold neurotransmitter release

POTASSIUM CHANNELS

Potassium channels constitute the largest group of ion channels and include several types with distinct structure, subcellular localization, biophysical properties, modulation, and pharmacological profile. Due to their diverse gating properties and expression, potassium channels strongly affect many cellular functions. In general, they reduce membrane excitability and thus probability to generate an action potential; reduce duration and limit firing frequency of action potentials; mediate afterhyperpolarization preventing repetitive firing; and reduce probability of neurotransmitter release.

Classification and Structure

The classification of potassium channels into families is based on the primary amino acid sequence of the pore-containing α subunit, the number of transmembrane domains, and their mode of activation.[16] They are subdivided into superfamilies of channels consisting of six, four, or two transmembrane domains. Channels with six transmembrane domains include the voltage-gated K^+ channels (K_v), the Ca^{2+}-activated K^+ channels (K_{Ca}), and the Na^+-activated K^+ channels (K_{Na}) (Figure 14.8). Channels with four transmembrane domains include several types of two-pore channels (K_{2P}) or "leak" channels. Channels with two transmembrane domains comprise the inward-rectifying channels (K_{ir}) (Figure 14.9). Many potassium channels consist of heteromers of pore-forming α subunits and contain auxiliary β subunits that modulate the gating properties, inactivation, cell surface expression, and/or trafficking of the ion channel complex and may serve as binding sites for both endogenous and exogenous ligands. These features provide for an extreme diversity of potassium channels.

Voltage-Gated K^+ Channels (K_v)

The family of voltage-gated K^+ channels is the largest ion channel group and consists of 12 subfamilies.[17,18] These channels, together with K_{Ca} and K_{Na} channels have a fundamental role in the regulation of neuronal excitability[19] (Tables 14.3 and 14.4). All K_v are activated by depolarization and deactivated by repolarization. Inactivation occurs when the open channels is occluded by intracellular "ball domains," which can be part of the channel or of an accessory subunit. The K_v1 type channels (*KCNA* family) have a critical role in regulating the initiation and firing of the

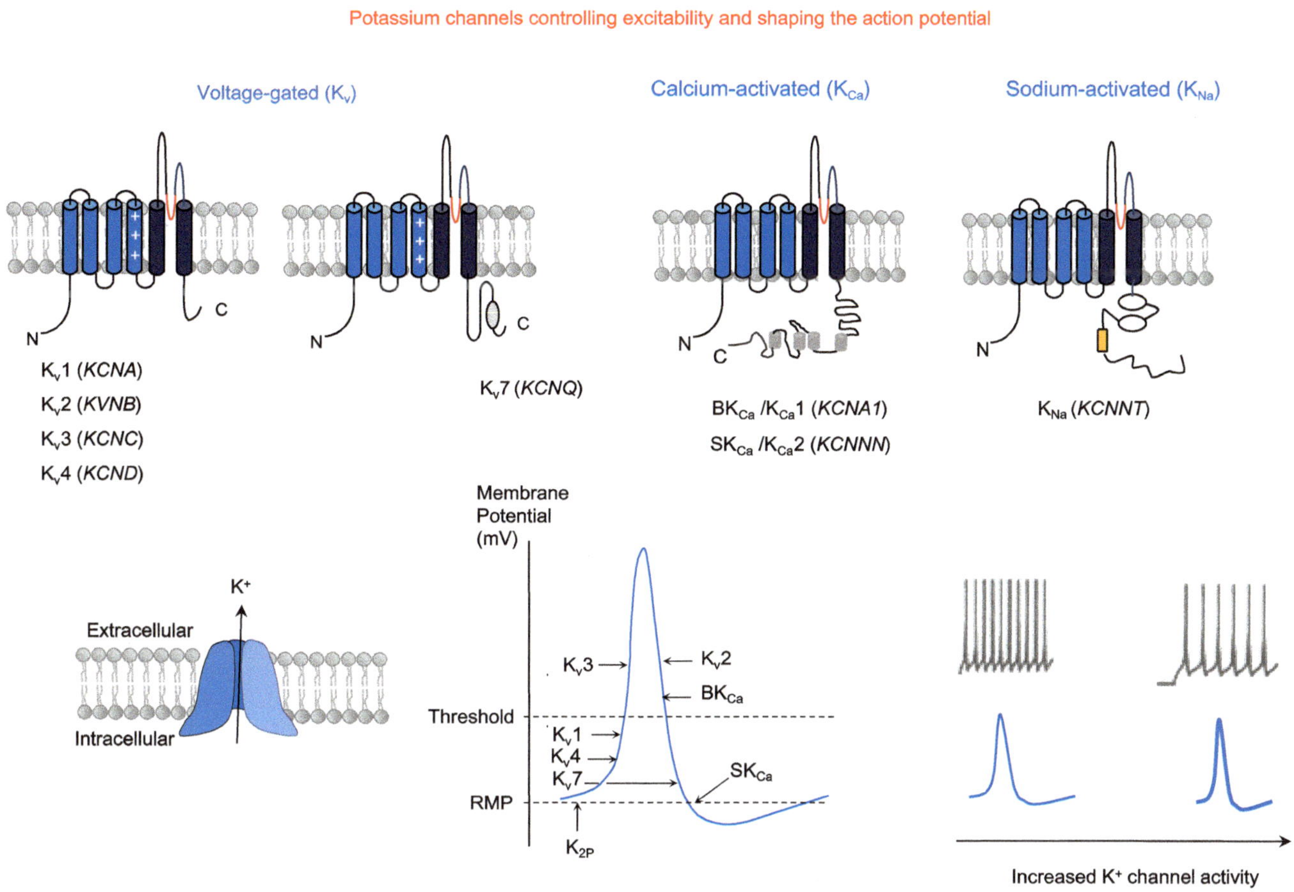

FIGURE 14.8 Voltage-gated and calcium-activated potassium channels.
Potassium channels with six transmembrane domains include the voltage-gated K^+ channels (K_v), the Ca^{2+}-activated K^+ channels (K_{Ca}), and the Na^+-activated K^+ channels (K_{Na}). The K_v1 channels mediate "delay" current (I_D), which delays the onset of the action potential. K_v2 channels mediate I_K currents responsible for repolarization. K_v3 channels have high threshold of activation and rapid kinetics. K_v4 channels are responsible for the subthreshold I_A current that regulates repetitive firing cells. K_v7 channels carry a low amplitude, slowly activating and inactivating M-current (I_M), which determines subthreshold neuronal excitability. The K_{Ca} channels include large conductance (BK_{Ca}) channels composed by K_{Ca}1.1 and they mediate fast afterhyperpolarization (AHP) that shortens the duration of the action potential. The low conductance (SK_{Ca}) channels consist of K_{Ca} 2.1–2.3 subunits and mediate slow AHP. The K_{Na} channels (*KCNT* family) are responsible for a delayed current that contributes to a long-lasting slow hyperpolarization.

action potential. K_v1.2 and K_v1.1 channels mediate a subthreshold "delay" (D) current (I_D) that delays the onset of the action potential, preventing repetitive firing. These channels are located in the AIS, the juxtaparanode and presynaptic terminals, and therefore negatively regulate axonal excitability, firing rates, and neurotransmitter release. The K_v2 channels (*KCNB* family) K_v2.1 and K_v2.2 have high threshold, slow activation, and slow inactivation and mediate a delayed rectifier (I_K) current responsible for repolarization of the action potential. These channels are located in the proximal dendrites, AIS, nodes of Ranvier, and presynaptic terminals and by shortening the duration of the action potential. This limits the frequency of repetitive firing prevents back-propagation of the action potential, and reduces probability of neurotransmitter release. The K_v3 channels (*KCNC* family) also have a high threshold of activation but have rapid kinetics of activation and inactivation; they accelerate repolarization and thus allow neurons to fire action potentials at high frequency. These channels are thus functionally important in fast-spiking GABAergic neurons, such as some cortical and hippocampal interneurons and cerebellar Purkinje cells.[20]

The K_v4 channels (*KCND* family) activate rapidly with small subthreshold depolarizations and rapidly inactivate; they are primarily responsible for the subthreshold A-type transient current (I_A) that regulates the spike timing and frequency in repetitive firing cells. These channels are primarily located in the soma and dendrites, and their function is strongly affected by interacting proteins, such as K^+ channel-interacting proteins (KChIPs) and the dipeptidyl

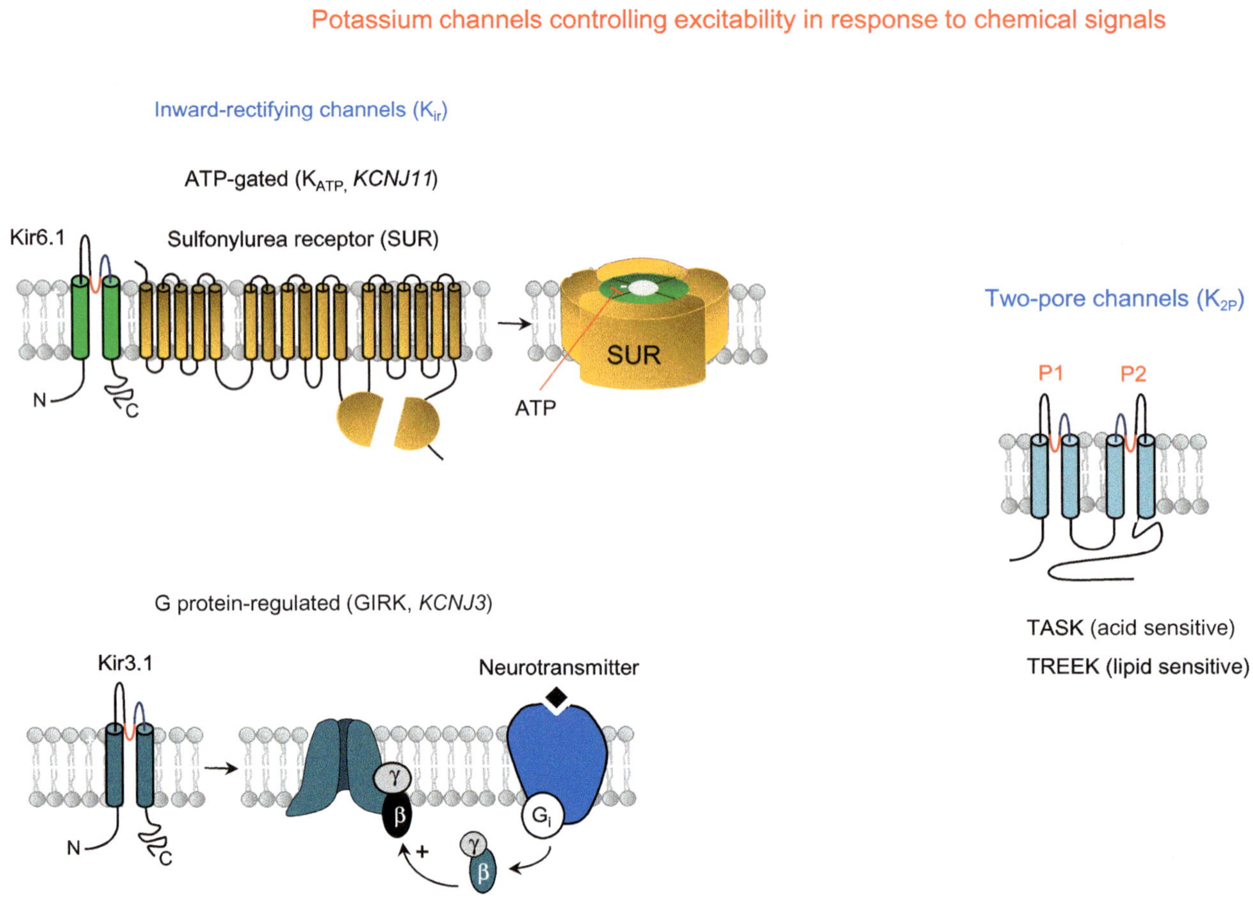

FIGURE 14.9 Inward-rectifying and two-pore potassium channels.
The inward-rectifying K^+ channels (K_{ir}) include several types that respond to different signals and mediate different functions. One typical example is the G protein-coupled inward-rectifying K^+ channels (GIRK, Ki_r3), which mediate effects of several inhibitory neuromodulators acting via G protein-coupled receptors (GPCRs) coupled to $Gi_{/o}$ signaling. The ATP-gated K^+ channel (K_{ATP}) consist of tetramers of $K_{ir}6$ subunits surrounded by four sulfonylurea receptor (SUR) subunits; they are tonically inhibited by ATP, and their activation in the setting of energy failure reduces neuronal activity and energy demands. The two-pore channels (K_{2P}), also known as "leak" or "background" channels function as integrators of diverse environmental signals affecting cell excitability, including extracellular pH, mechanical stress, and chemical mediators such as arachidonic acid, endocannabinoids, and volatile anesthetics. They include six families encoded by *KCNK* genes; examples are two-pore weak inward-rectifying K^+ channels (TWIKs); two-pore, acid-sensitive K^+ channels (TASKs); and the TWIK related channels (TREKs, TRESKs).

peptidase (DPP)-like proteins DPP6 (or DPPX) and DPP10 (DDPY). KChIPs are Ca^{2+}-binding proteins that interact with the intracellular N-terminal portion of the K_v4 subunits, preventing channel inactivation. DPP-like proteins are transmembrane proteins that associate with the channel core and, together with KChIPs, regulate surface channels expression and kinetics.[21–23] The K_v7 channels (*KCNQ* family) $K_v7.2$ (*KCNQ2*) and $K_v7.3$ (*KCNQ3*) form a molecular complex in neurons.[24] They have a low threshold of activation near RMP and carry a low-amplitude, slowly activating and inactivating current (M-current, $I_{M,}$ for muscarinic receptor-regulated) that stabilizes the resting membrane potential and has an important role in determining the subthreshold neuronal excitability. The K_v7 channels are enriched in the AIS and nodes of Ranvier, where they control the resting membrane potential, spiking threshold, firing frequency, and afterhyperpolarization after burst firing.[24] The K_v7 channel opener retigabine (ezogabine) reduces spiking and dampens network excitability but its side effects have preclude its use in epilepsy.

Calcium-Activated K^+ Channels (K_{Ca})

The calcium-activated K^+ channels (K_{Ca}) contain an intracellular Ca^{2+}-sensing domain and open in response to Ca^{2+} entering the cell via different types of Ca_v channels, with which that they are frequently colocalized and functionally coupled. The K_{Ca} channels include large conductance (BK, *KCNMA* gene) and small conductance (SK, *KCNN* gene) channels [25] (Table 14.4). The BK channels are activated by Ca^{2+} influx during the depolarization phase of

TABLE 14.3 *Voltage-Gated Potassium Channels*

Channel (gene)	Physiology (current)	Location	Function
K_v1 (*KCNA1*) K_v1.2 (*KCNA2*)	Delay (D) current (I_D) rapidly activated by subthreshold depolarization, slow inactivation	Widespread predominant in distal AIS and juxtaparanode	Delays onset of action potential (AP) Prevents repetitive firing Shortens AP duration
K_v2.1 (*KCNB*)	Delayed rectifying (I_K) current, high threshold and slow activation and inactivation	Somatodendritic	AP repolarization and afterhyperpolarization Controls AP duration and interspike interval during repetitive firing Prevents AP back-propagation
K_v 3.1-.3 (*KCNC*1-3)	High threshold of activation, fast activation and inactivation	Somatodendritic AIS Presynaptic terminal	Fast repolarization required for high-frequency firing
K_v4 (*KCND*)	Transient A-type (I_A), rapid activation, inactivation, and recovery from inactivation	Soma Distal dendrites	Attenuates AP back-propagation, regulates spike timing and frequency
K_v7.2 (*KCNQ2*) K_v7.3 (*KCNQ3*)	Muscarinic receptor-regulated (I_M) current Low threshold of activation near RMP Low amplitude, slowly activating and inactivating current	AIS Nodes of Ranvier	Stabilizes RMP Controls spiking threshold, firing frequency, and afterhyperpolarization

RMP, resting membrane potential

the action potential; they mediate a fast afterhyperpolarization (AHP) that shortens the width and thus duration of the action potential. This rapid repolarization promotes faster recovery of the voltage-gated Na^+ channels from inactivation; thus BK channel activation is typically associated with high firing frequency. The SK channels mediate slow AHP following the action potential. These channels are primarily responsible for spike frequency adaptation, which is a feedback mechanism that progressively reduces the firing frequency of action potentials in response to increase in intracellular calcium. The SK channels have a major role in regulating firing frequency of pacemaking cells, such as Purkinje cells and catecholaminergic brainstem neurons. The sodium-activated K^+ channels (K_{Na}) or Slack (sequence like a calcium-activated K^+ channel) channels (*KCNT* family) are also responsible for a delayed current that contributes to a long-lasting slow AHP that follows repetitive firing and thereby regulates neuronal excitability and adaptation.

Inward-Rectifying K^+ Channels (K_{ir})

The inward-rectifying K^+ channels (K_{ir}) are activated at membrane potentials more negative than the resting potential and support the flow of K^+ into the cell (hence their name "inward-rectifying"), pushing the membrane potential back to the resting potential.[26,27] These channels include several types that respond to different signals and mediate different functions. One typical examples is the G protein-coupled inward-rectifying K^+ channels (GIRK, K_{ir}3), which mediate effects of several inhibitory neuromodulators acting via G protein-coupled receptors (GPCRs) coupled to $G_{i/o}$ signaling. GIRK/K_{ir}3 channels form macromolecular complexes and are expressed primarily in the somatodendritic compartments. Direct interaction with $G_{i/o}$ $\beta\gamma$ subunits directly opens GIRK/K_{ir}3 channels, reducing cell excitability. The ATP-gated K channel (K_{ATP}) consists of tetramers of K_{ir}6 subunits surrounded by four sulfonylurea receptor (SUR) subunits. The K_{ATP} channels are molecular sensors that provide a link between cellular energy state and electrical excitability. They are tonically inhibited by ATP, and their activation in the setting of energy failure reduces neuronal activity and energy demands, leading to cell protective effects. Inward-rectifying K^+ channels also have a major role in maintenance of K^+ and volume homeostasis. In astrocytes, K_{ir}4.1 channels colocalize with the water channel aquaporin 4 and are important in buffering

TABLE 14.4 *Other Potassium-Affecting Neuronal Electrophysiology*

Channel (gene)	Physiology current)	Location	Function
BK_{Ca} ($K_{Ca}1$) (*KCNA1*)	Rapidly activated after Ca^{2+} influx	Somatodendritic Axons?	Fast repolarization and afterhyperpolarization (AHP) Allows high-frequency firing
SK ($K_{Ca}2$) 1-4 (*KCNN 1-4*)	Slowly activated after Ca^{2+} influx	Somatodendritic Axons?	Slow AHP Spike frequency adaptation
$K_{Na}1.1$ (*KCNT*)	Activated after Na+ influx	Somatodendritic	Contributes to repolarization
Kir6.1 (K_{ATP}) (*KCNJ11*)	Inward rectifying Inhibited by ATP forms a complex with SUR	Somatodendritic	Maintenance of resting membrane potential (RMP) Feedback mechanism that reduces cell excitability in the setting of energy failure
Kir3.1 (GIRK) (*KCNJ3*)	Inward rectifying Gated by $G_{i/o}$ protein βγ subunit	Somatodendritic	Reduces excitability in response to neurotransmitters acting via $G_{i/o}$-coupled receptors
Two-pore (2-P) channels (TASK, TREEK)	Activated by lipid mediators, acids, volume	Widespread	Leak current responsible for the RMP
Kir4.1 (KCNJ10)	Forms a complex with aquaporin 4	Astrocyte end foot process	Buffering of extracellular K+ and maintenance of cell volume

of extracellular K^+ increase and control of intracellular volume following neuronal activity.

Two-Pore ("Leak") K^+ Channels

The two-pore channels (K_{2P}) are also known as "leak" or "background " channels because they are constitutively open and provide for baseline resting K^+ currents that stabilize the RMP below firing threshold. These channels also modulate action potential duration and responsiveness to synaptic stimuli. Two-pore K^+ channels function as integrators of diverse environmental signals affecting cell excitability, including extracellular pH, mechanical stress, and chemical mediators such as arachidonic acid, endocannabinoids and volatile anesthetics. The K_{2P} channels include six families encoded by *KCNK* genes. Some representatives are the two-pore weak inward-rectifying K^+ channel (TWIK), two-pore, acid-sensitive K^+ channels (TASK), and the TWIK-related channels (TREK, TRESK).

OTHER CHANNELS REGULATING NEURONAL EXCITABILITY

There are several additional types of ion channels that regulate excitability and intracellular signaling. These channels have differential expression in neurons.

Hyperpolarization-Gated, Cyclic Nucleotide-Regulated (HCN) Channels

The hyperpolarization-gated, cyclic nucleotide-regulated (HCN) channels are activated by membrane hyperpolarization; in many cases activation is facilitated by direct interaction with cyclic nucleotides, such as cyclic adenosine monophosphate (cAMP).[28] The HCN channels are permeable to Na^+ and K^+ and are partially open at rest at voltages near the RMP. They provide a feedback mechanism that counteracts both membrane hyperpolarization and depolarization. When the cell is hyperpolarized, opening of HCN channels elicits current called I_h that brings the membrane potential near the resting membrane potential and toward the threshold for action potential generation. Because they antagonize both depolarization and hyperpolarization, HCN channels dampen the amplitude and duration of both excitatory and inhibitory postsynaptic potentials.

Channels in Sensory Receptors

Some types of ion channels have selective expression in subtypes of sensory receptors including nociceptors and mechanoreceptors. Some of these channels are expressed in intracellular organelles. The transient receptor potential (TRP) channels are nonselective cation channels with high permeability to Ca^{2+} and act as multimodal receptors. TRP channels include several families such as TRPV (vanilloid type), TRPA (ankyrin type), TRPM (melastatin type), and TRPC (canonical) channels. Different subtypes of TRP channels are expressed in small DRG nociceptive and chemoreceptive neurons, osmosensitive neural structures, astrocytes, and intracellular organelles such as lysosomes, as discussed in other chapters of this book. Channels of the Piezo family are critically involved in transduction of low-threshold tactile as well as proprioceptive stimuli. These channels consist of a trimer and form an ion pore that is directly gated by membrane stretch and is modulated by voltage. The acid-sensing ion channels (ASICs) are voltage-independent cation channels that are activated by acidic pH; they are primarily permeable to Na^+ and elicit cell depolarization, leading to secondary intracellular accumulation of Ca^{2+}. These channels are expressed in nociceptive terminals and can sense the acidic pH at synapses resulting from release of intravehicular content. Anoctamins (anion channels with eight transmembrane domains, ANO), also known as TMEM16 (transmembrane proteins with 16 domains) proteins, are activated by intracellular Ca^2 and participate in multiple cellular functions. Some anoctamins, such as ANO1 and ANO2, are prototypical Ca^{2+}-activated Cl^- channels. The direction of Cl^- flux through ANO and ANO2 channels depends on the intracellular Cl^- concentration.

Voltage-Dependent CIC-1 Channels

The voltage-dependent CIC-1 channels are primarily expressed in skeletal muscle, although they may also be expressed in the brain.[29] The CIC-1 channel is a dimer of two homologous subunits each forming a pore, allowing CIC-1 to function as a double-barrel channel. The CIC-1 channels regulate skeletal muscle excitability and are finely regulated by the metabolic states of the muscle, including ATP levels, redox state (NAD+/NADH ratio), acidification of exercising muscle, and modulation by protein kinase C. The majority of CIC-1 channels are located in the T-tubular system.

DISTRIBUTION AND CONTRIBUTION OF ION CHANNELS IN SHAPING OF NEURONAL ACTIVITY

The unique repertoire and distribution of ion channels in different compartments underlie the basic electrophysiological properties of neurons (Figure 14.10). Neurons receive a large number of excitatory and inhibitory synaptic influences, and the net result of their integration determines the probability of a neuron to generate an action potential. The action potential is initiated in the AIS and is conducted anterogradely along the axon; in myelinated axons, conduction is saltatory from one node of Ranvier to the next. The action potential eventually reaches the presynaptic terminal, where it triggers neurotransmitter release. In large neurons, such as pyramidal cells, the action potential may be back-propagated from the AIS to the somatodendritic compartment.

Dendritic Integration of Synaptic Inputs

Dendrites are the main receptive elements in neurons and integrate information from thousands of presynaptic inputs.[30,31] Excitatory glutamatergic synapses on many types of principal neurons in the CNS target the dendritic spines whereas inputs from different types of inhibitory neurons are targeted either to the distal dendrites to reduce local excitability or to the proximal somatodendritic compartment and AIS to influence the probability of generation of the action potential. The ability of a synaptic input to influence action potential generation at the AIS depends on how effectively the excitatory postsynaptic potential is transmitted by the dendrites. This depends both on the cable properties of the dendrite membrane and the presence of dendritic voltage-gated $Na_v1.2$ and Ca_v1 channels that can boost the effectiveness of distal synaptic inputs though the generation of local dendritic spikes. Dendritic spikes increase the probability of action potential generation and support active backpropagation of the action potential into the dendritic tree. Several potassium channels, K_v2, K_v4, and SK, dampen dendritic excitability and reduce the probability of back-propagation of the action potential from the AIS to the soma and dendrites. HCN channels, which are primarily located in the distal portion of the dendrites, act as an inhibitory brake that dampens dendritic excitability and amplitude of both excitatory and inhibitory postsynaptic potentials.

Axon Initial Segment and Regulation of Neuronal Excitability

All the excitatory and inhibitory inputs to the neuron are algebraically summed at the AIS, which is the site of initiation of the action potential.[32] The AIS has the highest density of sodium channels in the neuron. The $Na_v1.6$ channels have the lowest threshold for activation and cluster in a macromolecular complex in the distal portion of the AIS via interactions with the scaffolding protein ankyrin G.[33] The $Na_v1.1$ and $Na_v1.2$ channels are located in proximal portions of the AIS. $Na_v1.1$ channels support high-frequency firing of Purkinje cells or fast-spiking GABAergic neurons targeting the somatodendritic domain of cortical pyramidal cells. $Na_v1.2$ channels predominate in pyramidal neurons, axon terminals, and unmyelinated axons. The AIS also expresses abundant $K_v1.1$ and $K_v1.2$ channels that prevent repetitive firing and K_v7 channels that stabilize the resting membrane potential and control AIS responsiveness to subthreshold stimuli. However, fast-spiking GABAergic neurons express rapidly activating and inactivating K_v3 channels that allow high-frequency generation of action potentials.

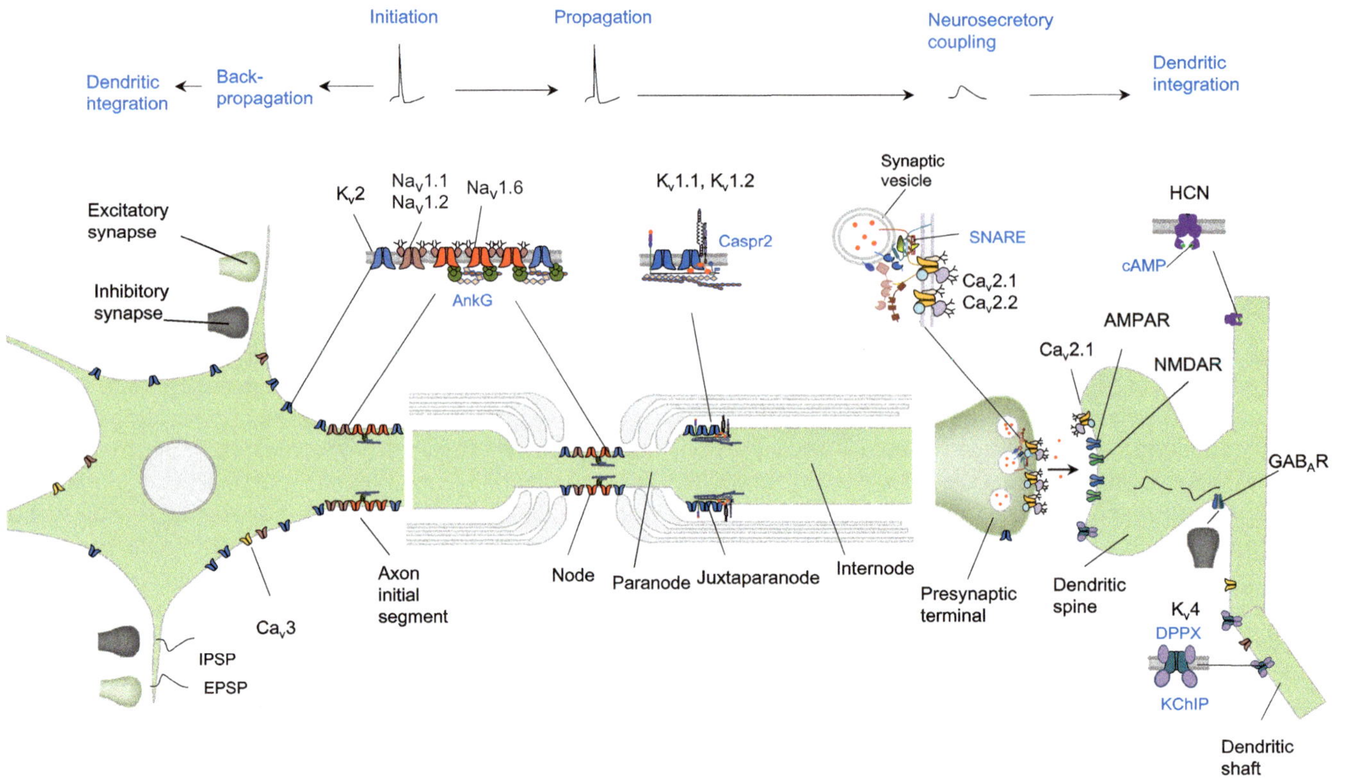

FIGURE 14.10 Distribution of representative ion channels in different neuronal domains.
Neurons receive a large number of excitatory and inhibitory synapses and the net result of the integration of excitatory postsynaptic potentials (EPSP) and inhibitory postsynaptic potentials (IPSP) determines the probability of a neuron to generate an action potential. Excitatory glutamatergic synapses onto principal neurons in the CNS target the dendritic spines, which contain and α-amino-3-hydroxy-5-methyl-4 isoxazole propionic acid receptors (AMPARs) and N-methyl-D-aspartate receptors (NMDARs). Inhibitory inputs, largely mediated by GABA via GABA$_A$ receptors (GABA$_A$Rs) are targeted to the distal dendrites or to the somatodendritic compartment. The action potential is initiated at the axon initial segment (AIS) and is conducted anterogradely along the axon; in myelinated axons, conduction is saltatory from one node of Ranvier to the next. Both the AIS and nodes of Ranvier contain a high density of sodium channels including Na$_V$1.1, Na$_V$1.2, and Na$_V$1., as well as K$_V$1.1, K$_V$1.2, and Kv7 channels. The Na$_V$1.6 and K$_V$7 channels cluster in a macromolecular complex in the distal portion of the AIS via interactions with the scaffolding protein ankyrin G (AnG). The nodes of Ranvier express K$_V$3.1 and K$_V$7.2/7.3 channels that dampen axonal excitability and reduce the probability of recitation of the axon. The paranode consists of noncompacted myelin and functions as a barrier that prevents invasion of K$_V$ channels from the juxtaparanode to the node. The juxtaparanode contains clustered K$_V$1.1 and K$_V$1.2 channels that have a major role in regulating axonal excitability, preventing back-propagation and repetitive firing. Clustering of paranodal K$_V$1.1 channels depends on the formation of a large macromolecular complex that includes auxiliary K$_V$β subunits and scaffolding molecules such as contactin-associated protein 2 (CASPR2). Upon arrival of the action potential, Ca^{2+} entering at presynaptic terminals via Ca$_V$2.1 (P-type) or Ca$_V$2.2 (N-type) channels clustered at active zones triggers exocytosis of neurotransmitter stored in synaptic vesicles. The presynaptic Ca^{2+} channel proteins interact with a group of proteins that promote docking of synaptic vesicles., including core proteins and SNARE proteins (for soluble NSF attachment receptor proteins). Several potassium channels dampen dendritic excitability and reduce the probability of backpropagation of the action potential from the AIS to the soma and dendrites. They include K$_V$2 channels, K$_V$4 channels forming a complex with K^+ channel interacting proteins (KChIPs), and the dipeptidyl peptidase (DPP)-like proteins. Hyperpolarization-gated, cyclic nucleotide regulated (HCN) channels bind cyclic adenosine monophosphate (cAMP) and act as an inhibitory brake that dampens dendritic excitability and amplitude of both EPSPs and IPSPs.

The coupling between Ca_v1, Ca_v2, and Ca_v3 with the Ca^{2+} activated K^+ channels BK and SK controlling AHP is also important in regulating pacemaker activity and firing frequency of neurons such as Purkinje cells, as described in other chapters of this book.

Conduction of the Action Potential in Myelinated Axons

In myelinated axons, the nodes of Ranvier are hot spots containing clustered $Na_v1.6$ and $Na_v1.2$ channels and are involved in propagation of the action potential. The nodes of Ranvier also express $K_v3.1$ and $K_v7.2/7.3$ channels that dampen axonal excitability and reduce the probability of reexcitation of the axon. The paranode consists of noncompacted myelin and functions as a barrier that prevents invasion of K_v channels from the juxtaparanode to the node. The juxtaparanode contains clustered $K_v1.1$ and $K_v1.2$ channels that have a major role in regulating axonal excitability, preventing back-propagation and repetitive firing. Clustering of paranodal $K_v1.1$ channels depends on the formation of a large macromolecular complex that includes auxiliary $K_v\beta$ subunits and scaffolding molecules such as contactin-associated protein 2 (CASPR2).

Control of Excitability of Unmyelinated Nociceptive Axons

In unmyelinated axons, the action potential is propagated by local circuits that depolarize the adjacent part of the membrane in a continuous sequential fashion; conduction of these action potentials is primarily supported by $Na_v1.2$ channels. Several sodium channels expressed in nociceptive afferents, including $Na_v1.7$, $Na_v1.8$, and $Na_v1.9$, control nociceptor excitability in response to both subthreshold and threshold stimuli. $Na_v1.7$ produces a low-threshold, rapidly activating and inactivating ramp current that boosts subthreshold stimuli to increase probability of action potential generation. $Na_v1.8$ is primarily responsible for the upstroke of the action potential in C-type nociceptive neurons and therefore supports repetitive firing in response to sustained depolarization. $Na_v1.9$ is activated at potentials close to RMP and produces a persistent Na^+ current that amplifies the response of nociceptors to subthreshold stimuli.

Synaptic Vesicle Exocytosis

Upon arrival of the action potential, Ca^{2+} entering a presynaptic terminal via $Ca_v2.1$ (P/Q-type) or $Ca_v2.2$ (N-type) channels triggers synaptic vesicle exocytosis and neurotransmitter release in less than a millisecond. The $Na_v1.2$ channels are primarily responsible for the depolarization that activates Ca_v2 channels at the presynaptic terminal. The probability of opening of Ca_v2 channels for exocytosis is decreased by influence of several types of K^+ channels that reduced membrane excitability, duration of the action potential, or both. The molecular bases of exocytosis are discussed in the next chapter.

CHANNELOPATHIES AND SYNAPTOPATHIES: GENERAL CONCEPTS

Channelopathies are episodic syndromes due to abnormal function of ion channels. Ion channels can be affected by genetic mutations, autoantibodies, or toxins affecting specific subunits or their interacting auxiliary or scaffold proteins.[9,34–36] Disorders affecting the interactions of ion channels with the presynaptic machinery for exocytosis, or the composition, expression, or gating of ionotropic receptors such as glutamate or GABA receptors may also produce episodic syndromes, which are referred to as synaptopathies. Missense mutations may cause channel gain-of-function or loss-of function by affecting open probability, voltage-dependence of activation, and/or surface expression. Dominant negative mechanisms are also common, as some channels are formed by different subunits encoded by both mutant and normal genes. Nonsense (truncation) mutations are almost always loss-of-function mutations. In the CNS, the effects of a mutation depend on whether its affects primarily excitatory or inhibitory neurons, resulting in hyperexcitable or hypoexcitable neuronal networks. Central channelopathies manifest with seizures,[37–39] episodic ataxia,[40] paroxysmal dyskinesia,[41,42] and hemiplegic migraine.[43,44] Some paroxysmal disorders mimicking channelopathies reflect presynaptic synaptopathies or glucose transport defects.[45] In the peripheral nervous system, the pathophysiology depends on whether the mutation makes the axons or muscle hypoexcitable or hyperexcitable. For example, nociceptor channelopathies associated with gain-of-function manifest with paroxysmal pain disorders whereas loss-of-function produces congenital insensitivity to pain.[8,36] Channelopathies resulting in muscle hyperexcitability manifest with myotonia. whereas muscle hypoexcitability manifests with periodic paralysis.[9] In channelopathies, episodes may be triggered by fever, fatigue, emotion, exercise, diet, or hormonal changes such as the menstrual cycle. Whereas channelopathies cause episodic dysfunction, some of them may eventually result in persistent damage of neurons, axons, or muscle. Paroxysmal manifestations, such as pain or muscle spasms, may also reflect abnormal axonal excitability in the setting of focal demyelination, as in the case of trigeminal neuralgia or painful spasms in multiple sclerosis. Immune channelopathies affecting voltage-gated channels, such as P/Q channels or proteins associated with voltage-gated K^+ channels may also manifest with epilepsy and ataxia, in general associated with other manifestations. A comprehensive review of channelopathies is beyond the scope of this chapter. Only some salient concepts will be emphasized here.

CHANNELOPATHIES ASSOCIATED WITH EPILEPSY

Ion channelopathies can result in excessive neuronal excitability or disrupt the balance between excitatory glutamatergic and inhibitory GABAergic transmission, leading to hypersynchronization of cortical networks and thus epileptogenesis. Many mutations resulting in epilepsy affect ion channels in the AIS.[37,46–49] The effects of these mutations largely depend on the whether they primarily affect the excitability of pyramidal neurons or that of inhibitory interneurons. Disruption of the balance between excitatory and inhibitory influences are associated with excessive Ca^{2+} influx via L-type ($Ca_v1.3$) channels in dendrites, resulting in paroxysmal depolarization shifts, which are abnormal fluctuations of the membrane voltage that outlast the depolarization of normal action potentials[48] Mutations affecting subunit expression, gating, and/or inactivation of ionotropic glutamate or $GABA_A$ receptors have also been linked to epilepsy, as discussed in other chapters of this book.

Sodium Channelopathies

Mutations in the sodium channels including *SCN1A*, *SCN1B*, *SCN2A*, *SCN3A*, *SCN8A*, and *SCN9A* are collectively responsible for a large proportion of cases of drug-resistant genetic epilepsies with onset in infancy and childhood (Table 14.5). *SCN1A*-related seizure disorders show remarkable phenotypic heterogeneity. The prototypes include generalized epilepsy with febrile seizures plus (GEFS+) and Dravet syndrome. The GFES+ phenotype ranges from simple febrile seizures to severe epileptic encephalopathies. *SCN1A* mutations have also been found to increase the risk for mesial temporal lobe epilepsy with hippocampal sclerosis and febrile seizures. The clinical phenotypes vary even among family members with the same pathogenic variant. Heterozygous loss-of-function mutations in *SCN1A* are responsible for the majority of cases of severe myoclonic epilepsy of infancy or Dravet syndrome. Studies in rodent models show that *SCN1A* mutations associated with Dravet syndrome impair function of $Na_v1.1$ channels in the AIS of inhibitory interneurons in the cerebral cortex, hippocampus, cerebellum, and thalamus, without affecting the function of excitatory neurons. Thus, sodium channel-blocking antiepileptic drugs (AEDs) such as carbamazepine, phenytoin, and lamotrigine, are usually ineffective and can even aggravate seizures and should be generally avoided in these patients. Alternative treatments include valproate, clobazam, stiripentol, cannabidiol, ketogenic diet, and fenfluramine. The $Na_v1.1$ channels are also expressed in the AIS of Purkinje cells, which accounts for ataxia observed in some patients. Mutations in *SCN2A* genes encoding $Na_v1.2$ channels have also been associated with a wide phenotype spectrum, which primarily includes three distinct disorders: infantile epileptic encephalopathy with developmental delay, benign familial infantile seizures, and autism spectrum disorder/intellectual disability.[50] Epileptic encephalopathy frequently presents with seizures in the neonatal period and includes Ohtahara syndrome (tonic seizures and burst suppression on the EEG), epilepsy of infancy with migrating focal seizures, and West syndrome (infantile spasms and hypsarrhythmia on EEG) later evolving to Lennox-Gastaut syndrome. Some children experience dystonia, chorea, or episodic ataxia. *SCN2A* mutations can cause gain-of-function, loss-of-function, or mixed effects, and this relates to both clinical phenotypes and response to treatment.[50] Missense variants associated with greater $Na_v1.2$ channel activity (gain-of-function) lead to either infantile epileptic encephalopathy or benign infantile seizures, while truncating or missense variants associated with diminished channel activity (loss-of-function) lead to autism spectrum disorder/intellectual disability. The threshold that distinguishes

TABLE 14.5 *Sodium Channelopathies Associated with Epilepsy*

Gene	Channel and Dysfunction	Phenotype
SCNA1	$Na_v1.1$ loss-of-function	Generalized epilepsy with febrile seizures plus (GEFS+) type 1 Severe myoclonic epilepsy of infancy (Dravet syndrome)
SCNA2	$Na_v1.2$ gain-of-function	Benign familial neonatal seizures (BFNS) Epileptic encephalopathies Dravet syndrome
	$Na_v1.2$ loss-of-function	Autism spectrum disorder/intellectual delay
SCNA8	$Na_v1.6$ gain-of-function	Epileptic encephalopathies
SCNB	Na_v β1 subunit loss-of-function	Generalized epilepsy with febrile seizures plus (GEFS+) type 2
SCNA3	$Na_v1.3$ gain-of-function	Cryptogenic partial epilepsy

infantile epileptic encephalopathy and benign infantile seizures may be related to the degree of compensation of neuronal excitability by $Na_v1.6$, which replaces $Na_v1.2$ at the AIS during maturation.[50] *SCN8A* mutations affecting $Na_v1.6$ channels are typically associated with severe epileptic encephalopathies with onset in the first 18 months of life and multiple seizure types. Movement disorders, cortical blindness, and startle and sleep problems may also be present. Most epilepsy-causing variants reported seem to have an activating effect on $Na_v1.6$ channel activity; therefore *SCN8A*-mutation-related seizures generally respond favorably to sodium channel-blocking AEDs. Mutations of the *SCN1B* gene encoding the accessory $Na_v\beta_1$ subunit expressed in the AIS have also been associated with different phenotypes, including GEFS+, Dravet syndrome, temporal lobe epilepsy, and nonfebrile absence seizures. These mutations may impair the ability to modulate Na_v channel gating.

Potassium Channelopathies

Potassium channels have a major role in both genetic and acquired forms of epilepsy[38,39] (Table 14.6). Whereas most mutations reflect K^+ channel loss-of-function, gain-of-function mutations may also paradoxically results in epileptogenesis.[39] Mutations of *KCNA1*, which codes for the $K_v1.1$ subunit, are typically linked to episodic ataxia type 1 (EA1) with neuromyotonia but may also manifest with seizures. This reflects the importance of $K_v1.1$ in regulating excitability at the AIS and juxtaparanode, and in reducing GABA release from basket cell synapses on Purkinje cells. Pathogenic variants of the *KCNA2* gene ($K_v1.2$ channel) and *KCNB1* ($K_v2.1$ channel) have been linked to epileptic encephalopathy. De novo mutations in the *KCNC1* gene encoding $K_v3.1$ results in progressive myoclonic epilepsy with ataxia. Mutations in *KCNQ2* and *KCNQ3*, which encode potassium channels $K_v7.2$ and $K_v7.3$, cause benign familial neonatal epilepsy (BFNE). This reflects loss-of-function with haploinsufficiency, resulting in subthreshold membrane depolarization and increased neuronal firing. Sequence variations of the *KCNQ2* and *KCNQ3* genes may also contribute to the etiology of common familial idiopathic epilepsy syndromes. In addition to benign familial neonatal seizures, *KCNQ2* mutations may also result in severe forms of epileptic encephalopathy. The electrophysiological changes associated with a majority of *KCNQ2* mutations in patients with encephalopathy are antagonized in vitro by the $K_v7.2$ and $K_v7.3$ opener retigabine (ezogabine). Whereas most of the identified KCNQ2 and KCNQ3 variants result in K_v7 loss-of-function, some variants elicit gain-of-function. In general, KCNQ2 gain-of-function mutations are associated with more severe seizure phenotype. This paradoxical effect suggests that these variants primarily dampen the excitability of

TABLE 14.6 *Potassium Channelopathies Associated with Epilepsy*

Gene	Channel dysfunction	Phenotype
KCNA1	$K_v1.1$ loss-of-function	Epilepsy associated with episodic ataxia (EA -1)
KCNA2	$K_v1.2$ gain- or loss-of-function	Epileptic encephalopathy
KCNB1	$K_v2.1$ loss-of-function	Epileptic encephalopathy
KCNC1	$K_v3.1$ loss-of-function	Progressive myoclonic epilepsy (PME) with ataxia
KCND2	$K_v4.2$ gain-of-function	Autism and intractable seizures
KCNQ2. *KCNQ3*	$K_v7.2$ or $K_v7.3$ loss-of-function	Benign familial neonatal convulsions (BFNC)
	$K_v7.2$ or $K_v7.3$ gain-of-function	Epileptic encephalopathy
KCNQ5	$K_v7.5$ gain-of-function	Epileptic encephalopathy
KCNMA1	BK_{Ca} gain-of-function	Generalized epilepsy with paroxysmal dyskinesia
KCNT1	Slack type Na^+-gated K^+ channel gain-of-function	Epilepsy of infancy with migrating focal seizures, West syndrome, Ohtahara syndrome, early myoclonic encephalopathy, focal epilepsy, multifocal epilepsy
KCNJ10	K_{ir} 4.1 in astrocyte loss-of-function	Epilepsy, ataxia, sensorineural hearing loss, and tubulopathy (EAST syndrome)
KCNJ11 *SUR1*	K_{ir} 6.2 loss-of-function SUR1 loss-of-function	Developmental delay, epilepsy, and neonatal diabetes (DEND syndrome)
KCTD7	K^+ channel tetramerization domain-7	Progressive myoclonic epilepsy Opsoclonus/myoclonus ataxia syndrome Infantile ceroid lipofuscinosis (CLCN14)

inhibitory interneurons. Gain-of-function mutations of the *KCNMA1* gene encoding the BK_{Ca} channel α subunit have been linked to generalized epilepsy and paroxysmal nonkinesigenic dyskinesia. The mutant BK_{Ca} channel has increased open-channel probability, which may lead to rapid repolarization allowing neurons to fire at a faster rate. Ethanol can directly activate the BK channel in vivo, and this may explain the observation that alcohol triggers dyskinesia in certain individuals. Autosomal dominant gain-of-function variants in *KCNT1*, which encodes the sodium activated-potassium channel $K_{Na}1.1$ have been associated with a wide spectrum of seizure disorders, including epilepsy of infancy with migrating focal seizures, West syndrome, Ohtahara syndrome, early myoclonic encephalopathy, focal epilepsy, and multifocal epilepsy and leukodystrophy. Seizures associated with *KCNT1*-related epilepsies are often severe and drug-resistant. These mutations are associated with increased channel function and may act similarly to BK mutations, accelerating repolarization and fast AHP, thereby limiting Na^+ channel inactivation, resulting in higher frequency firing. Quinidine, a partial antagonist of $K_{Na}1.1$ can attenuate the gain-of-function of the channel in vitro but the clinical response to this drug is variable. Some mutations affecting inward-rectifying K^+ channels are associated with epilepsy combined with systemic manifestations. For example, heterozygous activating mutations in the *KCNJ11* gene encoding the $K_{ir}6.2$ subunit of the K_{ATP} channel lead to developmental delay, epilepsy (including infantile spasms), and neonatal diabetes (DEND syndrome). These mutations decrease the ability of ATP to inhibit channel activity; this leads to an increase in the magnitude of the K_{ATP} current, pancreatic β-cell hyperpolarization, and reduced insulin secretion. Heterozygous gain-of-function *SUR1* mutations also causes DEND syndrome, by preventing the physical and functional interactions of SUR1 with the $K_{ir}6.2$ subunit. Loss-of-function mutations of the *KCNJ10* gene encoding the glial $K_{ir}4.1$ channel expressed in the astrocyte endfoot have been linked to a childhood syndrome comprising epilepsy, ataxia, sensorineural deafness, and tubulopathy (EAST syndrome). Finally, mutations affecting the *KCTD7* (potassium channel tetramerization domain-containing protein 7) produce progressive myoclonic epilepsy; opsoclonus/myoclonus/ataxia syndrome; and infantile-onset neuronal ceroid lipofuscinosis (CLN14). Whereas the function of the KCTD7 protein is largely unknown, its expression hyperpolarizes the membrane presumably by modulating K^+ channels and reduces cell excitability.

Calcium Channelopathies

In experimental models, gain-of-function of Ca_v3 (T)-channels or loss-of-function of $Ca_v2.1$ (P/Q) channels are associated with epilepsy.[15,51,52] However the precise role of voltage-gated calcium channel mutations in human epilepsy is still incompletely understood. Missense variants in the human *CACNA1H* gene encoding the $Ca_v3.2$ T-type channel subunit have been linked to a range of idiopathic genetic epilepsy syndromes including childhood absence, juvenile absence, juvenile myoclonic, and myoclonic astatic epilepsies as well as febrile seizures and temporal lobe epilepsy. Variants in the *CACNA1G* gene encoding $Ca_v3.1$ T-type channel subunits have been associated with both cerebellar ataxia and epilepsy. The *CACNA1G* gene can also act as a modifier of Dravet syndrome induced by defects in the sodium channel $Na_v1.2$, suggesting that *CACNA1G* mutations may also interact phenotypically with other genes, rather than being pathogenic per se. Mutations in the *CACNA1A* gene encoding the P/Q channel α1 subunit are typically associated with familial hemiplegic migraine type 1 (FHM1), episodic ataxia type 2 (EA2), and spinocerebellar ataxia type 6 (SCA6). Some patients with FHM1 or EA2 may also experience seizure, and a number of *CACN1A* mutations have been associated with different epilepsy syndromes. Variations of the *CACNB4* gene encoding the auxiliary β4 subunit of $Ca_v2.1$ channels have been associated with idiopathic generalized epilepsy and episodic ataxia.

PAROXYSMAL MOVEMENT DISORDERS

The paroxysmal movement disorders (PMDs) include episodic ataxias (EA) and the paroxysmal dyskinesias.[53–55] Like epilepsy, paroxysmal movement disorders may result from both channelopathies and synaptopathies. This is reflected by the frequent overlap of these three clinical manifestation in individual patients or within members of the same kindred.

Episodic Ataxias

Autosomal dominant episodic ataxias are characterized by recurrent episodes of cerebellar ataxia that are usually of short duration and often triggered by specific stimuli. The most common are EA1 and EA2. EA1is due to mutation of the *KCNA1* gene encoding $K_v1.1$ channels and is typically associated with myokymia. However, EA1 has a wider phenotype that includes visual blurring, diplopia, headaches, dyspnea, dysarthria, and nausea during the attacks. Epilepsy is a common comorbidity; other manifestations include intellectual disability, delayed motor milestones, progressive ataxia, neuromyotonia, and choreoathetosis. The attacks of EA1 can respond to acetazolamide and antiepileptic dugs. EA2 is the most common form of episodic ataxia and is due to mutation of the *CACNA1A* gene encoding the α1A subunit of $Ca_v2.1$ (P/Q) channels. Most *CACNA1A* mutations causing EA2 result in a truncated, nonfunctional protein. Findings in a mouse model suggest that the attacks of episodic ataxia may reflect reduced P/Q-type Ca^{2+} influx into presynaptic terminals at excitatory parallel-Purkinje cell synapses, abnormal intrinsic pacemaker firing of Purkinje neurons, or both. Between attacks patients with EA2 often have interictal downbeat nystagmus with other cerebellar ocular dysfunctions. These patients may develop slowly progressive ataxia and atrophy of the cerebellar vermis.[40,54] In EA2, acetazolamide or the nonselective potassium channel blocker 4-aminopyridine (4-AP) are effective. Other forms of episodic ataxia, such as EA5, caused by mutations in the *CACNB4* gene encoding the auxiliary β_4 subunit of Cav2.1, and EA6, caused by heterozygous mutations in *SLC1A3* encoding a subunit of a glial excitatory amino acid transporter, can also respond to acetazolamide. EA8 differs from the other episodic ataxias in that treatment is clonazepam.[54] Of note, paroxysmal attacks in multiple sclerosis or autoimmune CASPR2 encephalitis may also manifest with episodic ataxia.

Paroxysmal Dyskinesia

Many of the paroxysmal dyskinesias can be comorbid with other neurological disorders suggestive of an underlying channelopathy, such as epilepsy and migraine. The inherited forms often have an onset during childhood or adolescence with an autosomal dominant inheritance pattern. These disorders include four types: paroxysmal kinesigenic dyskinesia (PKD), paroxysmal nonkinesigenic dyskinesia (PNKD), and paroxysmal exercise-induced dyskinesia (PED). Paroxysmal hypnogenic dyskinesia is a variant of frontal lobe epilepsy now known as sleep-related hypermotor epilepsy. Whereas these disorders resemble channelopathies, PKD and PNKD reflect synaptopathies affecting proteins involved in control of exocytosis, as discussed in the next chapter. However, some paroxysmal dyskinesia may be associated with channelopathies. For example, mutations of the *SCN8A* gene have been found in families with infantile convulsions and paroxysmal choreoathetosis and benign familial infantile seizures. Mutations of the *KCNMA1* gene encodng the pore-forming α subunit of the BK channels are primarily associated with seizures, movement disorders, developmental delay, and intellectual disability. Gain-of-function *KCNMA1* mutations may also associate with PNKD and loss-of function with EA

NOCICEPTOR CHANNELOPATHIES

Different mutations of the *SCN9A* gene encoding $Na_v1.7$, the *SCN10A* gene encoding $Na_v1.8$,and the *SCN11A* gene encoding $Na_v1.9$ may result in channel gain-of-function or loss-of-function.[36,55] Gain-of-function mutations increase nociceptive dorsal root ganglion (DRG) neuron excitability and manifest with familial episodic pain syndromes or painful small fiber neuropathies; mutations resulting in channel loss-of-function result in congenital insensitivity to pain. These disorders are further discussed in chapter 34.

MUSCLE CHANNELOPATHIES

Muscle channelopathies provided the first insight into the mechanisms by which dysfunction of ion channels manifest with neurological abnormalities and they are still one of the best characterized in terms of their pathophysiology.[9] Only a few major concepts will be emphasized here.

Ion Channels in Skeletal Muscle and Excitation-Contraction Coupling

The sarcolemma of adult skeletal muscle fibers at rest has a high Cl^- conductance via ClC-1 channels. This Cl^- conductance produces a depolarizing current that is balanced at rest by a hyperpolarizing K^+ current via inward-rectifying K channels. Upon release of acetylcholine triggered by nerve stimulation, activation of nicotinic acetylcholine receptors (nAChRs) clustered at the junctional folds of the motor endplate triggers a depolarizing endplate potential that activates $Na_v1.4$ channels located at the depth of the folds. This results in a muscle action potential that is propagated along the surface of the sarcolemma and into the interior of the muscle fiber via the T-tubular system. Membrane repolarization involves both fast and slow inactivation of $Na_v1.4$ channels, followed by K^+ efflux via delayed rectifier channels. Potassium accumulation in the T-system causes a small, transient afterdepolarization at the end of the muscle contraction, but the high resting Cl^- conductance via ClC-1 channels prevents propagation of this depolarization along the sarcolemma.

Muscle channelopathies produce a spectrum ranging from muscle hyperexcitability, manifested as myotonia, or hypoexcitability, manifested as periodic paralysis[9,56–58] (Table 14.7).

Disorders Associated with Myotonia

Mutations of the *CLCN1* gene leading to partial or complete loss of ClC-1 channel function produce myotonia congenita.[29] This includes an autosomal dominant form (Thomsen disease) and more severe autosomal recessive form (Becker disease). Myotonia is characterized by muscle stiffness after a voluntary movement; it is worse after rest and improves with repetitive activity, what is known as warm-up phenomenon. The electrophysiological correlate is a burst of muscle action potentials that lasts a few seconds after the cessation of motor neuron activity and delays relaxation. The majority of mutations associated with myotonia congenita reduce channel expression or function. Myotonia in myotonic dystrophy types 1 and type 2, reflects impaired expression of functional ClC-1 due to impaired function of splicing of *ClC-1* mRNA.

Gain-of-function mutations of the *SCN4A* gene encoding $Na_v1.4$ produce several phenotypes. Most of these mutations disrupt fast inactivation of the channels. The excessive Na^+ influx may cause either excessive excitability, manifested with myotonia, or transient loss of excitability due to depolarization block, manifested with periodic paralysis. At one end of the spectrum is sodium channel myotonia, which includes several clinical subtypes according to severity and precipitating factors (e.g., potassium-aggravated myotonia). Paramyotonia congenita is a form of myotonia that is paradoxically worsened by repeated muscle activity

TABLE 14.7 *Muscle Channelopathies*

Gene	Channel Dysfunction	Phenotype
CLCN1	ClC-1 loss-of-function	Myotonia congenita: Thomsen disease (autosomal dominant) and Becker disease (autosomal recessive)
	Impaired ClC-1 expression due to mRNA splicing defect	Myotonic dystrophy types 1 and 2
SCN4A	$Na_v1.4$ gain-of-function	Potassium-aggravated myotonia Paramyotonia congenita Hyperkalemic periodic paralysis
	$Nav1._4$ loss-of-function	Hypokalemic periodic paralysis type 2 Sodium channel myasthenia
CACNA1S	$Ca_v1.1$ loss-of-function	Hypokalemic periodic paralysis type 1
KCNJ18	$K_{ir}6$ loss-of-function	Hypokalemic period paralysis
KCNJ12	$K_{ir}2.1$ loss-of-function	Anders-Tawil syndrome (hypokalemic periodic paralysis, long QT syndrome, neurocognitive and skeletal abnormalities)

or with muscle cooling; some patients may have episodes of periodic paralysis.

Disorders Associated with Periodic Paralysis

Gain-of-function *SCN4A* mutations are also linked to hyperkalemic periodic paralysis. This disorder is characterized by recurrent attacks of flaccid paralysis often associated with elevated serum K^+ (> 5mM) or precipitated by a K^+ challenge. Patients may have myotonia around the time of an episode of weakness. In hyperkalemic periodic paralysis, the incomplete $Na_v1.4$. channel inactivation results in as steady Na^+ influx that keeps the muscle fiber depolarized at about -45mV, where the channels are inactivated and the fibers are unable to generate and action potential. Hypokalemic periodic paralysis consists of recurrent episodes of weakness associated with low serum K^+ (< 3mM). Attacks are precipitated by oral load of carbohydrates, or K^+ loss by vomiting or diarrhea. About 60% of patients have a missense mutations in the *CACN1S* gene encoding the $Ca_v1.1$ channel expressed in the T-tubule system; 20% have a missense mutation in *SCN4A* gene encoding $Na_v1.4$ which is also highly expressed in this compartment. Mutations causing hypokalemic periodic paralysis result in substitutions of the arginine residues in S4 segments of the voltage sensor domain of the channels. These mutations result in a pore current that causes susceptibility to paradoxical depolarization in the setting of low K^+ and leads to loss-of-function of the channels.

Other Disorders

Sodium channel myasthenic syndrome is due to loss-of-function *SCNA4* missense mutation in the voltage sensor domain of the $Na_v1.4$ channel resulting in loss of muscle excitability downstream of activation of muscle nAChRs. Loss-of-function *SCN4A* mutations have also been linked to congenital myopathy. Some cases of hypokalemia periodic paralysis have been linked to mutations of genes encoding muscle inward-rectifying K^+ channels, including *KCNJ18* and *KCNJ2*. Mutations of the *KCNJ2* gene cause Andersen-Tawil syndrome, which is characterized by periodic paralysis (either hypo-or hyperkalemic), long QT syndrome, neurocognitive deficits, and skeletal dysmorphism.

AUTOIMMUNE VOLTAGE-GATED CHANNELOPATHIES

Autoimmune disorders may target proteins that are important for clustering of K_v channels into specific neuronal compartments. Autoantibodies against K_v channel complexes may occur in isolation, in the setting of a paraneoplastic disorder, particularly small cell lung carcinoma and thymoma, or in association with a coexisting autoimmune disorder. The K_v1 channels are clustered at the paranodes via interactions with CASPR2 and at presynaptic glutamatergic terminals via interactions mediated by the secreted scaffold protein LGI1, which forms transmembrane adhesion complexes, as discussed in the next chapter. The typical clinical manifestations associated with CASPR2 or LGI1 antibodies are limbic encephalitis, neuromyotonia, and Morvan syndrome. Voltage-gated potassium channelopathies affecting components of the K_v1 complex may also manifest with epilepsy associated with encephalitis, either in isolation or associated with other neurologic symptoms, and in some cases with neuropathic pain.[59–61] For example, a typical finding in LGI1 encephalitis is faciobrachial dystonic seizures that typically occur in the setting of limbic encephalitis. Paroxysmal pain and other manifestations of peripheral nerve excitability, and occasionally episodic ataxia, are characteristically associated with of CASPR2 antibodies. Autoimmune K_v1 channelopathies associated with encephalitis may lead to intractable seizures, which may occur in isolation.[60] The role of K_v1 impairment in the pathogenesis of seizures is still undetermined. Recognition of an autoimmune K^+ complex channelopathy as a cause of drug-resistant seizures may have clinical implications. A recent randomized double-blind placebo-controlled trial showed superiority of intravenous immunoglobulin (IVIG) over placebo in reducing seizure frequency in patients seropositive for LGI1 or CASPR2 antibodies.[62] Autoantibodies against dipeptidyl-peptidase-like protein-6 (DPPX), the regulatory subunit of somatodendritic $K_v4.2$ channels, produce limbic encephalitis with evidence of neuronal hyperexcitabiliy such as seizures, myoclonus, and tremor. The $K_v4.2$ channels are also present in the heart and enteric nervous system, where they regulate excitability. Consistent with this autoimmune DDPX encephalitis is commonly associated with cardiac arrhythmia and diarrhea. Other disorders are due to autoantibodies targeting presynaptic P/Q channels. Autoantibodies against the P/Q channels are classically associated with the Lambert-Eaton myasthenic syndrome reflecting a prominent role of these channels in acetylcholine release at the neuromuscular junction. These autoantibodies have also been associated with sporadic late-onset ataxia and paraneoplastic cerebellar degeneration.

ION CHANNELS AS TARGETS OF DRUGS AND TOXINS

Voltage-gated ion channels are major targets for drugs used in treatment of epilepsy, pain, some paroxysmal movement disorders, migraine, and psychiatric disorders (Table 14.8). Some neurotoxins also primarily target voltage-gated ion channels. One typical example is ciguatoxin, a dinoflagellate neurotoxin that activates voltage-gated Na^+ channels. Ciguatera fish poisoning is the most common seafood toxin poisoning and is characterized by gastrointestinal, cardiac, and neurologic symptoms including paresthesia, hypoesthesia, cold allodynia, and myalgia and in some

TABLE 14.8 *Voltage-Gated Ion Channels as a Therapeutic Target*

Drug	Mechanism	Therapeutic uses in neurology
Drugs affecting voltage-gated Na^+ channels		
Carbamazepine Oxcarbazepine Eslicarbazepine Phenytoin	Open channel blocker (fast-inactivated state)	Focal seizures Trigeminal neuralgia Paroxysmal kinesigenic dyskinesia
Lamotrigine	Open channel blocker (fast-inactivated state)	Focal seizures Primary generalized seizures Lennox-Gastaut syndrome Bipolar disorder Depression Migraine
Lacosamide	Open channel blocker (slow-inactivated state)	Focal seizures
Rufinamide	Prolongs inactive state	Lennox-Gastaut syndrome
Quinidine	Blocks voltage-gated Na^+ channels and Na^+-activated K^+ channels (K_{Na})	Slow channel myasthenic syndrome Epilepsy associated with gain-of-function *KCNT1* mutations
Drugs affecting voltage-gated Ca^{2+} channels		
Ethosuximide	T-channel blockade	Typical absence seizures
Gabapentin Pregabalin	Reduce expression of $\alpha 2\delta$ subunit of presynaptic P/Q and N- channels	Focal seizures Neuropathic pain Restless legs syndrome
Verapamil	L-type channel blocker	Cluster headache Migraine
Nimodipine	L-type channel blocker	Vasospasm prevention in SAH

cases headache, vertigo, ataxia, and impaired consciousness. The toxin may produce intramyelinic cytotoxic edema manifested by restricted diffusion on MRI and probably reflecting increased Na^+ influx in neurons and glial cells causing osmotic shift as well as hyperexcitability.[63,64]

KEY POINTS

- The unique repertoire and distribution of ion channels in different cell compartments underlie the basic electrophysiological properties of neurons.
- Voltage-gated channel properties are primarily determined by their subunit composition, and effected by phosphorylation, auxiliary subunits, and allosteric modulators.
- The membrane potential is determined both by the transmembrane ion concentration gradient and the weighted balance of electrical currents flowing through ion channels.
- The maintenance of the transmembrane Na^+ and K^+ gradient is critical to maintain cell excitability and depends on the activity of the Na^+/K^+ ATPase.
- Opening of Na^+ or Ca^{2+} channels results in an inward current that produces depolarization, thereby increasing neuronal excitability.
- Opening of K^+ channels elicits either an outward current (hyperpolarization) or stabilization of the membrane potential; closure of K^+ channels increases excitability.
- Voltage-gated cation channels consist of a principal or α subunit that contains a voltage sensor and forms the wall of the channel pore.
- Voltage-gated sodium channels are responsible for the initiation and conduction of the action potential.
- Voltage-gated calcium channels trigger a wide range of processes including neurotransmitter release, muscle contraction, and gene transcription.
- Potassium channels reduce membrane excitability, reduce duration and limit firing frequency of action potentials, prevent repetitive firing, and reduce probability of neurotransmitter release.
- Channelopathies are episodic syndromes caused by mutations, autoantibodies, or toxins affecting specific ion channel subunits or their interacting auxiliary or scaffold proteins.
- Mutations affecting sodium channel genes including *SCN1A*, *SCN1B*, *SCN2A*, *SCN3A*, *SCN8A*, and *SCN9A* are responsible for genetic epilepsies.
- Both loss-of-function and gain-of-function mutations affecting K^+ channels have been linked to various forms of epilepsy.
- Channelopathies are an important cause of paroxysmal movement disorders including episodic ataxias (EAs) and paroxysmal dyskinesias.
- The two most common autosomal dominant EAs are EA1 due to mutation of the *KCNA1* gene encoding $K_v1.1$ channels and EA2 due to mutation of the *CACNA1A* encoding the α1A subunit of $Ca_v2.1$ (P/Q) channels.
- Nociceptor channelopathies may manifest with paroxysmal pain disorders or congenital insensitivity to pain.
- Channelopathies resulting in muscle hyperexcitability manifest with myotonia, whereas muscle hypoexcitability manifests with periodic paralysis.
- Mutations of the *CLCN1* gene leading to partial or complete loss of CIC-1 channel function produce myotonia congenita.
- Gain-of-function mutations of the *SCN4A* gene encoding the $Na_v1.4$ channel produce sodium channel myotonia, paramyotonia congenita, or hyperkalemic periodic paralysis.
- Loss-of-function mutations in the *CACN1S* gene encoding the $Ca_v1.1$ channel or the *SCN4A* gene encoding $Na_v1.4$ produce hypokalemic periodic paralysis.
- Autoimmune voltage-gated potassium channelopathies commonly manifest with epilepsy, either in isolation or associated with encephalopathy, ataxia, and other neurologic symptoms.
- Antibodies against CASPR2 or LGI1 manifest with limbic encephalitis, neuromyotonia, sleep disorder, autoimmune epilepsy and neuropathic pain.
- Autoimmune encephalitis associated with LGI1 or CAPSR2 antibodies can cause drug-resistant seizures.
- Autoantibodies against dipeptidyl-peptidase-like protein-6 (DPPX) produce limbic encephalitis with seizures, myoclonus, tremor, cardiac arrhythmia, and diarrhea.
- Autoantibodies against the P/Q channels are associated with the Lambert-myasthenic syndrome, sporadic late-onset ataxia, and paraneoplastic cerebellar degeneration.

REFERENCES

1. Isacoff EY, Jan LY, Minor DL, Jr. Conduits of life's Spark: a perspective on ion channel research since the birth of neuron. Neuron 2013;80:658–674.
2. Blaesse P, Airaksinen MS, Rivera C, Kaila K. Cation-chloride cotransporters and neuronal function. Neuron 2009;61:820–838.
3. Baranauskas G. Ionic channel function in action potential generation: current perspective. Mol Neurobiol 2007;35:129–150.
4. Baranauskas G, Mukovskiy A, Wolf F, Volgushev M. The determinants of the onset dynamics of action potentials in a computational model. Neuroscience 2010;167:1070–1090.

5. Catterall WA, Perez-Reyes E, Snutch TP, Striessnig J. International Union of Pharmacology. XLVIII. Nomenclature and structure-function relationships of voltage-gated calcium channels. Pharmacol Rev 2005;57:411–425.
6. Goldin AL, Barchi RL, Caldwell JH, et al. Nomenclature of voltage-gated sodium channels. Neuron 2000;28:365–368.
7. Bennett DL, Clark AJ, Huang J, Waxman SG, Dib-Hajj SD. The role of voltage-gated sodium channels in pain signaling. Physiol Rev 2019;99:1079–1151.
8. Dib-Hajj SD, Waxman SG. Sodium channels in human pain disorders: genetics and pharmacogenomics. Annu Rev Neurosci 2019;42:87–106.
9. Cannon SC. Sodium channelopathies of skeletal muscle. Handb Exp Pharmacol 2018;246:309–330.
10. Lai HC, Jan LY. The distribution and targeting of neuronal voltage-gated ion channels. Nat Rev Neurosci 2006;7:548–562.
11. Nanou E, Catterall WA. Calcium channels, synaptic plasticity, and neuropsychiatric disease. Neuron 2018;98:466–481.
12. Zamponi GW, Striessnig J, Koschak A, Dolphin AC. The physiology, pathology, and pharmacology of voltage-gated calcium channels and their future therapeutic potential. Pharmacol Rev 2015;67:821–870.
13. Dolphin AC. Voltage-gated calcium channels and their auxiliary subunits: physiology and pathophysiology and pharmacology. J Physiol 2016;594:5369–5390.
14. Simms BA, Zamponi GW. Neuronal voltage-gated calcium channels: structure, function, and dysfunction. Neuron 2014;82:24–45.
15. Weiss N, Zamponi GW. Genetic T-type calcium channelopathies. J Med Genet 2019;57:1–10.
16. Goldstein SA, Bayliss DA, Kim D, Lesage F, Plant LD, Rajan S. International Union of Pharmacology. LV. Nomenclature and molecular relationships of two-P potassium channels. Pharmacol Rev 2005;57:527–540.
17. Gutman GA, Chandy KG, Grissmer S, et al. International Union of Pharmacology. LIII. Nomenclature and molecular relationships of voltage-gated potassium channels. Pharmacol Rev 2005;57:473–508.
18. Gonzalez C, Baez-Nieto D, Valencia I, et al. K(+) channels: function-structural overview. Compr Physiol 2012;2:2087–2149.
19. Johnston J, Forsythe ID, Kopp-Scheinpflug C. Going native: voltage-gated potassium channels controlling neuronal excitability. J Physiol 2010;588:3187–3200.
20. Kaczmarek LK, Zhang Y. Kv3 channels: enablers of rapid firing, neurotransmitter release, and neuronal endurance. Physiol Rev 2017;97:1431–1468.
21. Jensen CS, Rasmussen HB, Misonou H. Neuronal trafficking of voltage-gated potassium channels. Mol Cell Neurosci 2011;48:288–297.
22. Jerng HH, Pfaffinger PJ, Covarrubias M. Molecular physiology and modulation of somatodendritic A-type potassium channels. Mol Cell Neurosci 2004;27:343–369.
23. Jerng HH, Pfaffinger PJ. Modulatory mechanisms and multiple functions of somatodendritic A-type K (+) channel auxiliary subunits. Front Cell Neurosci 2014;8:82.
24. Greene DL, Hoshi N. Modulation of Kv7 channels and excitability in the brain. Cell Mol Life Sci 2017;74:495–508.
25. Contet C, Goulding SP, Kuljis DA, Barth AL. BK channels in the central nervous system. Int Rev Neurobiol 2016;128:281–342.
26. Butt AM, Kalsi A. Inwardly rectifying potassium channels (Kir) in central nervous system glia: a special role for Kir4.1 in glial functions. J Cell Mol Med 2006;10:33–44.
27. Kubo Y, Adelman JP, Clapham DE, et al. International Union of Pharmacology. LIV. Nomenclature and molecular relationships of inwardly rectifying potassium channels. Pharmacol Rev 2005;57:509–526.
28. Kase D, Imoto K. The role of HCN channels on membrane excitability in the nervous system. J Signal Transduct 2012;2012:619747.
29. Imbrici P, Altamura C, Pessia M, Mantegazza R, Desaphy JF, Camerino DC. ClC-1 chloride channels: state-of-the-art research and future challenges. Front Cell Neurosci 2015;9:156.
30. Stuart GJ, Spruston N. Dendritic integration: 60 years of progress. Nat Neurosci 2015;18:1713–1721.
31. Grienberger C, Chen X, Konnerth A. Dendritic function in vivo. Trends Neurosci 2015;38:45–54.
32. Kole MH, Stuart GJ. Signal processing in the axon initial segment. Neuron 2012;73:235–247.
33. Leterrier C, Brachet A, Fache MP, Dargent B. Voltage-gated sodium channel organization in neurons: protein interactions and trafficking pathways. Neurosci Lett 2010;486:92–100.
34. Bernard G, Shevell MI. Channelopathies: a review. Pediatr Neurol 2008;38:73–85.
35. Catterall WA, Kalume F, Oakley JC. NaV1.1 channels and epilepsy. J Physiol 2010;588:1849–1859.
36. Waxman SG, Dib-Hajj SD. The two sides of NaV1.7: painful and painless channelopathies. Neuron 2019;101:765–767.
37. Nolan D, Fink J. Genetics of epilepsy. Handb Clin Neurol 2018;148:467–491.
38. Kohling R, Wolfart J. Potassium channels in epilepsy. Cold Spring Harb Perspect Med 2016;6.
39. Niday Z, Tzingounis AV. Potassium channel gain of function in epilepsy: an unresolved paradox. Neuroscientist 2018;24:368–380.
40. Kipfer S, Strupp M. The clinical spectrum of autosomal-dominant episodic ataxias. Mov Disord Clin Pract 2014;1:285–290.
41. Bailey CS, Moldenhauer HJ, Park SM, Keros S, Meredith AL. KCNMA1-linked channelopathy. J Gen Physiol 2019;151:1173–1189.
42. Dhamija R, Goodkin HP, Bailey R, Chambers C, Brenton JN. A case of KCNQ2-associated movement disorder triggered by fever. J Child Neurol 2017;32:1123–1124.
43. Zarcone D, Corbetta S. Shared mechanisms of epilepsy, migraine and affective disorders. Neurol Sci 2017;38:73–76.
44. Lafreniere RG, Rouleau GA. Identification of novel genes involved in migraine. Headache 2012;52 Suppl 2:107–110.
45. Zhang XJ, Xu ZY, Wu YC, Tan EK. Paroxysmal movement disorders: recent advances and proposal of a classification system. Parkinsonism Relat Disord 2019;59:131–139.
46. Harty RC, Kim TH, Thomas EA, et al. Axon initial segment structural plasticity in animal models of genetic and acquired epilepsy. Epilepsy Res 2013;105:272–279.
47. Kubista H, Boehm S, Hotka M. The paroxysmal depolarization shift: reconsidering its role in epilepsy, epileptogenesis and beyond. Int J Mol Sci 2019;20.

48. Perucca P, Perucca E. Identifying mutations in epilepsy genes: impact on treatment selection. Epilepsy Res 2019;152:18–30.
49. Oyrer J, Maljevic S, Scheffer IE, Berkovic SF, Petrou S, Reid CA. Ion channels in genetic epilepsy: from genes and mechanisms to disease-targeted therapies. Pharmacol Rev 2018;70:142–173.
50. Sanders SJ, Campbell AJ, Cottrell JR, et al. Progress in understanding and treating SCN2A-mediated disorders. Trends Neurosci 2018;41:442–456.
51. Gambardella A, Labate A. The role of calcium channel mutations in human epilepsy. Prog Brain Res 2014;213:87–96.
52. Rajakulendran S, Hanna MG. The role of calcium channels in epilepsy. Cold Spring Harb Perspect Med 2016;6:a022723.
53. Xu Z, Lim CK, Tan LCS, Tan EK. Paroxysmal movement disorders: recent advances. Curr Neurol Neurosci Rep 2019;19:48.
54. Jen JC, Wan J. Episodic ataxias. Handb Clin Neurol 2018;155:205–215.
55. Waxman SG, Merkies ISJ, Gerrits MM, et al. Sodium channel genes in pain-related disorders: phenotype-genotype associations and recommendations for clinical use. Lancet Neurol 2014;13:1152–1160.
56. Phillips L, Trivedi JR. Skeletal muscle channelopathies. Neurotherapeutics 2018;15:954–965.
57. Statland JM, Fontaine B, Hanna MG, et al. Review of the diagnosis and treatment of periodic paralysis. Muscle Nerve 2018;57:522–530.
58. Sansone VA. The dystrophic and nondystrophic myotonias. Continuum (Minneap Minn) 2016;22:1889–1915.
59. Bien CG, Scheffer IE. Autoantibodies and epilepsy. Epilepsia 2011;52 Suppl 3:18–22.
60. Britton J. Autoimmune epilepsy. Handb Clin Neurol 2016;133:219–245.
61. Irani SR, Vincent A. Voltage-gated potassium channel-complex autoimmunity and associated clinical syndromes. Handb Clin Neurol 2016;133:185–197.
62. Dubey D, Britton J, McKeon A, et al. Randomized Placebo-controlled trial of intravenous immunoglobulin in autoimmune LGI1/CASPR2 epilepsy. Ann Neurol 2020;87:313–323.
63. Friedman MA, Fernandez M, Backer LC, et al. An updated review of ciguatera fish poisoning: clinical, epidemiological, environmental, and public health management. Mar Drugs 2017;15.
64. Yalachkov Y, Hildner M, Polomac N, Jahnke K, Wagner M, Baudrexel S. Cytotoxic edema affecting distinct fiber tracts in ciguatera fish poisoning. Neurology 2019;92:145–147.

15 Synaptic Transmission and Presynaptic Synaptopathies

OVERVIEW

Chemical synapses involve a presynaptic terminal, postsynaptic target, a synaptic cleft, and a surrounding glial cell (Figure 15.1). The presynaptic terminal harbors synaptic vesicles containing the chemical transmitters. Classical neurotransmitters such as amino acids, acetylcholine, and monoamines are stored in vesicles at the presynaptic terminals. Neuropeptides and growth factors synthesized in the cell bodies are stored in secretory granules and reach the presynaptic terminals via fast axonal transport. The presynaptic terminals contain active zones, which harbor clustered voltage-gated calcium (Ca^{2+}) channels that trigger fast neurotransmitter release. The postsynaptic targets, as well as the presynaptic terminals, contain different types of ionotropic and G protein-coupled receptors (GPCRs). The presynaptic and postsynaptic elements contain a large numbers of scaffold and adaptor proteins and are linked structurally and functionally by transsynaptic adhesion molecules. Synapses are enriched with mitochondria, which are critical to provide the energy required for synaptic events. Perisynaptic processes from astrocytes or Schwann cells ensheath the presynaptic and postsynaptic elements and participate in synaptic development, maintenance, and function. Chemical synaptic neurotransmission is bidirectional and involves several events. The presynaptic events include a neurotransmitter cycle and a synaptic vesicle cycle (Figure 15.2). The neurotransmitter cycle includes neurotransmitter synthesis, storage in synaptic vesicles, release by exocytosis, and reuptake from the synaptic cleft. The synaptic vesicle cycle includes trafficking, docking, priming of the synaptic vesicles at the presynaptic active zone, Ca^{2+}-dependent exocytosis, and recycling by endocytosis.[1] There is also a receptor cycle, described in the next chapter. Presynaptic events can be affected in genetic and immune synaptopathies and are an important target of drugs and toxins. The aims of this chapter are to review: (1) the general features of chemical synapses, (2) the events leading to exocytosis of synaptic vesicles, (3) the mechanisms of endocytosis at presynaptic terminals, and (4) examples of presynaptic synaptopathies.

HETEROGENEITY AND DYNAMICS OF CHEMICAL SYNAPSES

Synapses are communication nodes that connect neurons into vast networks, differentially process information encoded by the firing pattern of neurons, and exhibit plastic properties. The transformation of presynaptic neuronal activity into postsynaptic signals varies substantially among the thousands of input and output synapses on a single neuron on the basis of the properties and plasticity of the individual synapses. These events are further affected by modulatory inputs and diffusible signals.[2]

Synapse Formation and Elimination

Synapses are continuously formed and eliminated throughout life. Postnatally, an excess of synapses is produced, and 40%–50% of synapses are subsequently pruned during adolescence. Synapse formation involves multiple processes mediated by synaptic cell-adhesion molecules. They include initial establishment upon contact of an axon with a target cell, organization of synapse components into a canonical synaptic machinery, and specification of synapse properties characteristic of a given synapse.[3] Synapse specification and turnover are dynamic and depend on neuronal activity. Activity-dependent synaptic plasticity not only affects the strength of the synapse but may also switch its neurotransmitter type.[4] Synapse elimination, or "synaptic pruning" is a widespread process that may be intrinsic to neurons and is also at least in some cases, activity-dependent. Synaptic pruning involves activity of astrocytes and microglia.[5]

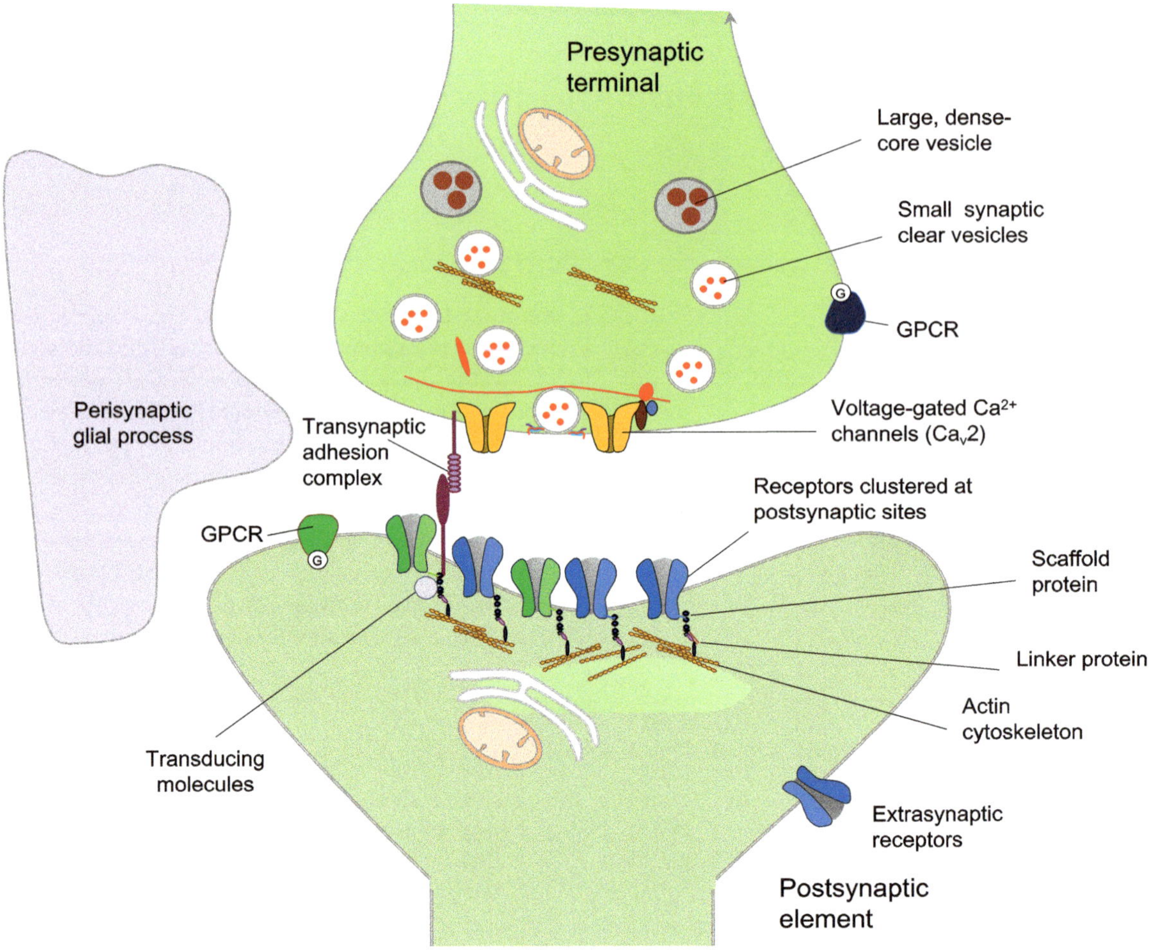

FIGURE 15.1 General organization of chemical synapses.
Chemical synapses involve a presynaptic terminal, postsynaptic target, a synaptic cleft, and surrounding glial cells. The presynaptic terminal harbors synaptic vesicles containing the chemical transmitters and active zones containing clustered voltage-gated calcium (Ca^{2+}) channels (Ca_v2) that trigger fast neurotransmitter release. The postsynaptic terminals, as well as the presynaptic terminals, contain different types of inotropic and G protein-coupled receptors (GPCRs). The presynaptic and postsynaptic elements contain a large numbers of scaffold and adaptor proteins and are linked structurally and functionally by transsynaptic adhesion molecule. Perisynaptic processes from astrocytes or Schwan cells ensheath the presynaptic and postsynaptic elements.

Structural Bases for Classical Neurotransmission

Classical neurotransmission is the fast and precise transmission of excitatory and inhibitory signals. It involves the rapid release of neurotransmitters from synaptic vesicles docked at presynaptic active zones containing clustered voltage-gated Ca^{2+} channels (Ca_v2) and their effects on ionotropic receptors clustered at postsynaptic sites. The efficacy of synaptic transmission requires complex interactions among presynaptic macromolecular complexes that allow the precise clustering of synaptic vesicles at presynaptic active zones. Transsynaptic interactions are critical for formation, specification, and plasticity of synapses; and postsynaptic macromolecular interactions allow clustering of postsynaptic receptors and their coupling with downstream signaling cascades.

Transsynaptic Interactions and Synaptic Function

The development, properties, and dynamics of synapses is controlled by diverse transsynaptic signaling molecules.[3] Presynaptic cell-adhesion molecules, particularly neurexins, constitute "hubs" that can interact with multiple classes of postsynaptic cell-adhesion molecules[3] (Figure 15.3). Important neurexin partners include neuroligins, cerebellins, latrophins, and dystroglycans.[6] Neurons express three major neuroligin isoforms that are targeted to

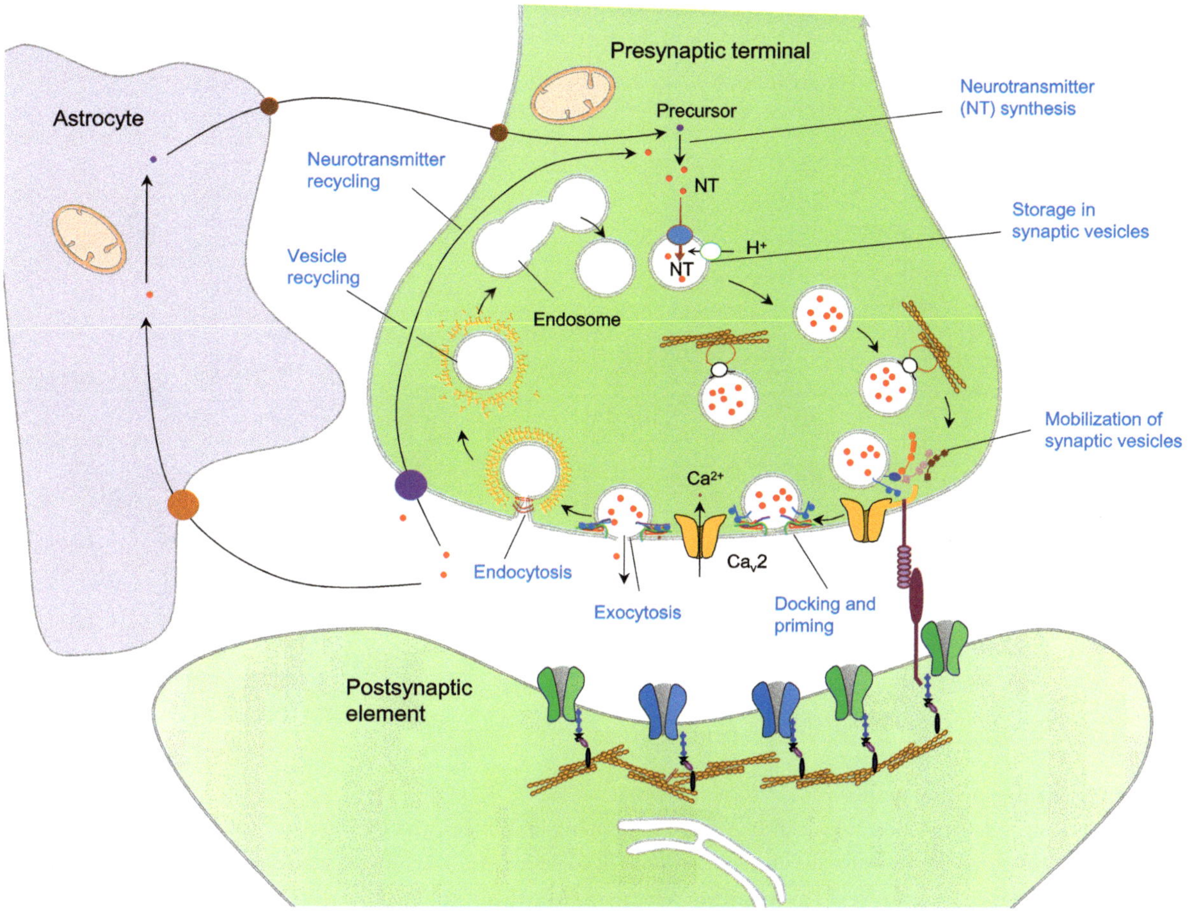

FIGURE 15.2 Presynaptic events in chemical neurotransmission.

The presynaptic events include a neurotransmitter cycle and a synaptic vesicle cycle. The neurotransmitter cycle include neurotransmitter synthesis, storage in synaptic vesicles, and release by exocytosis, and reuptake from the synaptic cleft. The synaptic vesicle cycle includes trafficking, docking, priming of the synaptic vesicles at the presynaptic active zone, Ca^{2+}-dependent exocytosis, and recycling of synaptic vesicles by endocytosis.

specific synapses, interact with scaffold proteins, and are required for the distribution of neurotransmitter receptors in postsynaptic specializations. Neuroligin 1 is expressed in excitatory synapses, and neuroligin 2 is present at inhibitory synapses.[6] Cerebellins are small secreted proteins that are broadly expressed throughout the brain.[7] They consist of an N-terminal cysteine-rich sequence and a C-terminal C1q-domain; the C1q domains assemble into trimers, and the cysteine-rich sequences dimerize the C1q-domain trimers into hexamers. Cerebellin 1 binds to the N-terminal domains of postsynaptic glutamate receptor subunits GluD1 (GluRδ1) and GluD2 (GluRδ2), which function as adhesion molecules instead of forming functional glutamate receptors.[8] For example, these interactions form trans-synaptic bridging complexes at the parallel fiber–Purkinje cell synapse in the cerebellum.[3] Latrophins are neurexin partners that bind α-latrotoxin (*Lactrodectus*–black widow spider venom); they may function as postsynaptic recognition molecules and recruit the toxin to synapses for its subsequent presynaptic insertion resulting in triggering of neurotransmitter release. This likely underlies manifestations of α-latrotoxin poisoning, including regional pain, diaphoresis, and fasciculations.[9] Dystroglycans bind not only neurexins but also laminin and other proteins and via interaction with intracellular dystrophin link the extracellular matrix to the intracellular cytoskeleton. Hypoglycosylation of α-dystroglycan has been associated with muscular dystrophy phenotypes and brain developmental abnormalities such as cobblestone lissencephaly, cerebellar cysts, pontine hypoplasia, and brainstem bowing.[10] Mutations in the *GMPPB* gene encoding a protein involved in dystroglycan glycosylation produce congenital myasthenic syndrome.[11]

One important example of a secreted molecular scaffold at excitatory synapses is leucine-rich, glioma-inactivated protein 1 (LGI1). This scaffold functions as a bridge between presynaptic and postsynaptic transmembrane proteins of the A Disintegrin and Metalloproteinase (ADAM) family. Via this mechanism, LGI1 functionally links presynaptic

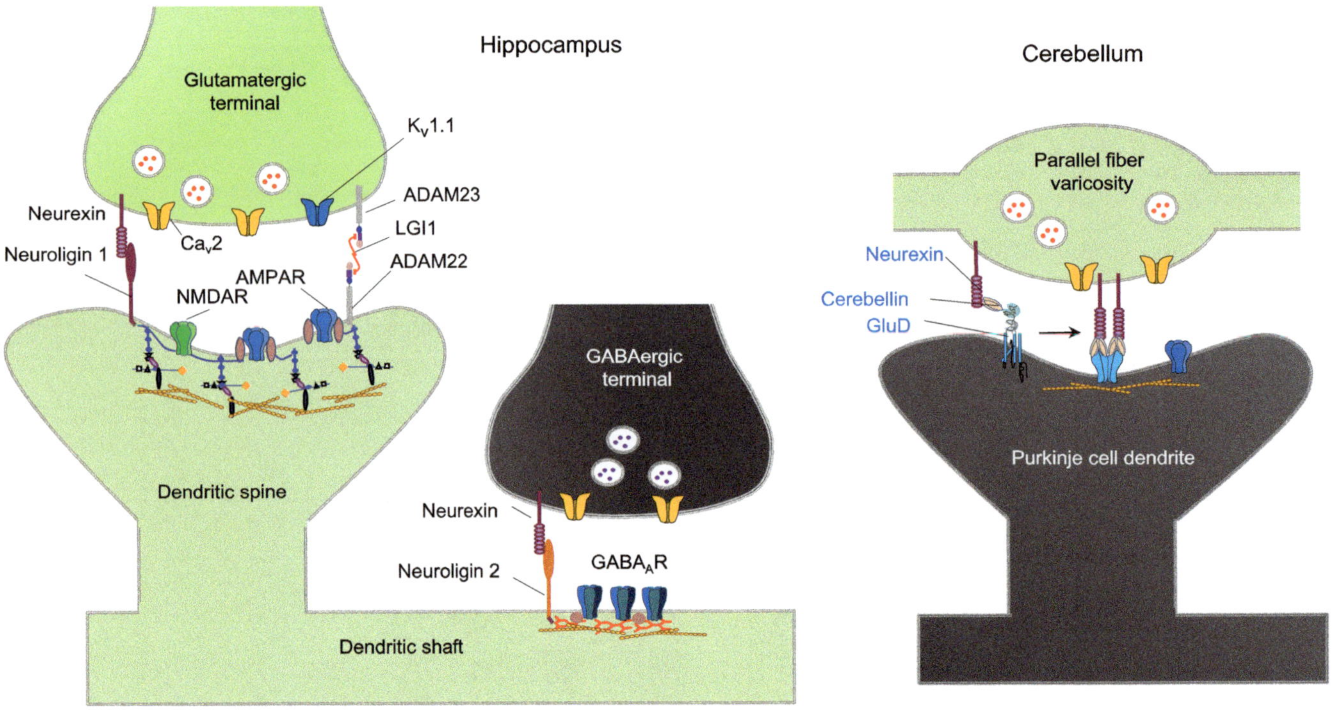

FIGURE 15.3 Transsynaptic adhesion interactions.
Several transsynaptic adhesion and signal molecules regulate the development, properties, and dynamics of synapses. Neurexins interact with multiple classes of postsynaptic cell-adhesion molecules such as neuroligin 1 expressed at excitatory synapses and neuroligin -2 at inhibitory synapses. Other neurexin partners are cerebellins, which are secreted proteins that interact with presynaptic neurexins and postsynaptic glutamate receptor subunits GluD1 (GluRδ1) and GluD2 (GluRδ2). Another secreted molecular scaffold at excitatory synapses is leucine-rich, glioma-inactivated protein 1 (LGI1), which functions as a bridge between presynaptic and postsynaptic transmembrane proteins of the A Disintegrin and Metalloproteinase (ADAM). LGI1 functionally links presynaptic voltage-gated K^+ channels (Kv1.1) associated with ADAM23 with postsynaptic, α-amino-3-hydroxy-5-methyl-4 isoxazole propionic acid receptors (AMPARs) associated with ADAM22.

voltage-gated K^+ channels ($K_v1.1$) associated with ADAM23 with postsynaptic, α-amino-3-hydroxy-5-methyl-4 isoxazole propionic acid receptors (AMPARs) associated with ADAM22.[12] *LGI1* gene mutations have been linked with temporal lobe epilepsy with auditory features,[12] and antibodies against LGI1 are a major mechanism of autoimmune epilepsy and limbic encephalitis.[13]

PRESYNAPTIC NEUROTRANSMITTER CYCLE

Amino acid neurotransmitters, acetylcholine, and monoamines are classical neurotransmitters synthesized in the presynaptic terminals and stored in synaptic vesicles. A single vesicle filled with neurotransmitter is the elementary unit (or "quantum") of synaptic transmission.[14] The presynaptic factors that determine quantal size include the amount of neurotransmitter availability in the cytosol depending on biosynthesis and recycling, vesicular storage mediated by vesicular neurotransmitter transporters and driven by the activity of the vacuolar (V) proton-ATPase (V-ATPase), and nonspecific leakage across the vesicle membrane.[15] Neuropeptides and growth factors are synthesized from mRNA in the cell body and then transported to the presynaptic terminal. In contrast, diffusible signals such endocannabinoids, prostaglandins, or nitric oxide are synthesized and released "on demand" without storage in synaptic vesicles, and may function as retrograde signals regulating neurotransmitter release and other functions.

Synthesis of Neurotransmitters

Neurotransmitters are synthesized from precursors via a critical enzymatic step. The biosynthetic steps vary according the neurotransmitter (Table 15.1). Both acetylcholine and L-glutamate are synthesized from intermediates of the Krebs cycle and are readily available. In inhibitory synapses, glutamic acid decarboxylase-65 (GAD-65) transforms L-glutamate into GABA. Dopamine, norepinephrine, serotonin, and histamine derive from essential dietary

TABLE 15.1 *Overview of Biosynthesis of Classical Neurotransmitters*

Neurotransmitter	Substrate (source)	Key Enzymatic Step(s)
L-glutamate	α-ketoglutarate Glutamine (astrocytes)	Glutamate dehydrogenase Glutaminase
GABA	L-glutamate	Glutamic acid decarboxylase (GAD)
Glycine		
Acetylcholine	Acetyl-CoA (mitochondria) and choline (reuptake)	Choline acetyltransferase (ChAT)
Dopamine	L-tyrosine (diet)	Tyrosine hydroxylase (TH)
Norepinephrine	L-tyrosine (diet)	Tyrosine hydroxylase (TH) Dopamine-β-hydroxylase (DBH)
Serotonin	L-tryptophan (diet)	Tryptophan hydroxylase (TPH)
Histamine	L-histidine (diet)	Histidine decarboxylase
Neuropeptides	mRNA in cell body	Peptidases

amino acids via specific, rate-limiting enzymatic steps. The mechanisms of biosynthesis of each these neurotransmitters will be discussed in other chapters of this book.

Vacuolar (V)-ATPase and+ Storage of Neurotransmitters

Transport of the cytoplasmic neurotransmitter into the synaptic vesicle involves the exchange with luminal H^+ and depends on a H^+ electrochemical gradient produced by the vacuolar (V)-ATPase[16] (Figure 15.4). The large electrochemical proton gradient generated by the V-ATPases (with pH around 5.5 inside the vesicles) provides the energy used by specific vesicular transporters to accumulate neurotransmitters within synaptic vesicles. The V-ATPase is composed of two domains, a peripheral V1 domain that catalyzes ATP hydrolysis and an integral membrane V0 domain that translocates H^+. The membrane V0 domain also participates in vesicular membrane fusion.[16] Intracellular chloride channels may function as Cl^-/H^+ exchangers and have an important role in vesicle acidification.

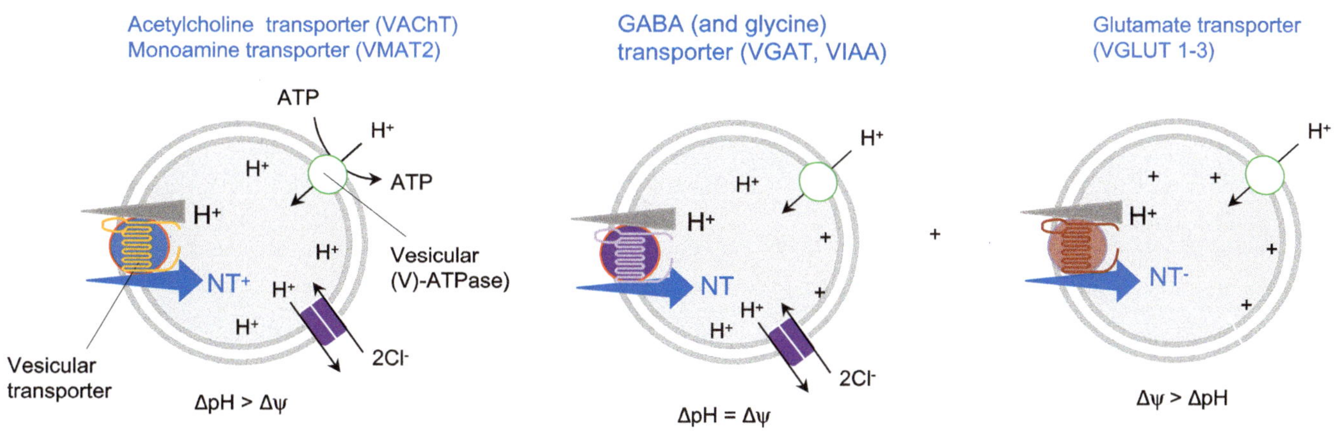

FIGURE 15.4 Mechanism of vesicular storage of classical neurotransmitters.
Transport of the cytoplasmic neurotransmitter (NT) into the synaptic vesicle involves the exchange with luminal H^+ and depends on a H^+ electrochemical gradient produced by the vacuolar (V)-ATPase. Intracellular chloride channels may function as Cl^-/H^+ exchangers and have an important role in vesicle acidification. The vesicular acetylcholine transporter (VChAT) and the vesicular monoamine transporters (VMAT1 and VMAT2) are driven by the H^+ chemical gradient (ΔpH) across the vesicular membrane. The vesicular GABA transporter (VGAT), which is also involved in vesicular storage of glycine depends on both the chemical and the electrical gradient (Δψ). The vesicular glutamate transporters (VGLUT 1–3) are driven primarily by the electrical gradient across the vesicular membrane.

TABLE 15.2 *Vesicular Neurotransmitter Transporters*

Vesicular Neurotransmitter Transporter	Gene Family	Location	Ion Coupling
VMAT2	*SLC18*	Monoaminergic neurons	Monoamine ↔ 2H+
VAChT	*SLC18*	Cholinergic neurons	Acetylcholine ↔ 2H+
VGAT/VIAAT	*SLC32*	Inhibitory neurons	GABA/glycine ↔ nH+
VGLUT1 VGLUT2	*SLC17*	Glutamatergic neurons	Glutamate ↔ nH+ Cl^--dependent
VGLUT3	*SLC17*	Nonglutamatergic neurons	Glutamate ↔ nH+ Cl^--dependent

VMAT2: vesicular monoamine transporter 2; VAChT: vesicular ACh transporter; VGAT: vesicular GABA and glycine (Gly) transporter, also known as VIAAT, vesicular inhibitory amino acid transporter; VGLUT, vesicular glutamate transporter

Vesicular Neurotransmitter Transporters

There are three families of vesicular neurotransmitter transporters functionally coupled to the V-ATPase (Table 15.2). One family includes the vesicular acetylcholine transporter (VChAT) and the vesicular monoamine transporters (VMAT1 and VMAT2). The second includes the vesicular GABA transporter (VGAT), which is also involved in vesicular storage of glycine and is thus also referred to as vesicular inhibitory amino acid transporter (VIAAT). The third family includes the vesicular glutamate transporters (VGLUT 1–3). Vesicular acetylcholine or monoamine transport, which involves the exchange of protonated cytosolic transmitter for two lumenal H^+, depends more on the chemical gradient. Transport of glutamate involves the movement of both H^+ and a positive charge, and depends more on the electrical gradient. Transport of GABA with no net charge involves the movement of equal number of H^+ and charge. Within the vesicle, neurotransmitters may be costored with ATP, synthetic enzymes, or ions.

Recycling of Neurotransmitters

The high rates of firing by many neurons would deplete the terminal of vesicular stores. This is prevented in the case of most neurotransmitters by recycling after exocytosis, either directly back into the nerve terminal or indirectly via astrocytes (Table 15.3). Neurotransmitter recycling is important not only for termination of the synaptic effects of neurotransmitter but also to increase their availability in

TABLE 15.3 *Plasma Membrane Transporters*

Plasma Membrane Neurotransmitter Transporter	Gene Family	Location	Ion Coupling
DAT	*SLC6*	Dopaminergic neurons	2 Na^+:1 Cl-: DA
NET	*SLC6*	Noradrenergic neurons	1Na^+:1Cl^-: NE
SERT	*SLC62*	Serotonergic neurons	1Na^+:1Cl^-: 5-HT ↔ 1K^+
GAT-1, GAT-2	*SLC6*	GABAergic neurons Astrocytes	2Na^+:1Cl^-: GABA
GLYT1	*SLC6*	Astrocytes	2Na^+:1Cl^-: glycine
GLYT21	*SLC6*	Glycinergic neurons	2Na^+:1Cl^-: glycine
CHT	*SLC5*	Cholinergic neurons	Na^+ dependent
EAAT1, EATT2	*SLC1*	Astrocytes	3Na^+:1H^+: glutamate ↔ 1K^+
EAAT3	*SLC1*	Neurons (dendrites)	3Na^+:1H^+: glutamate ↔ 1K^+ Chloride conductance
EAAT4	*SLC1*	Purkinje cells	Chloride conductance
EAAT5	*SLC1*	Retina	Chloride conductance

NET, norepinephrine (NE) transporter; DAT, dopamine (DA) transporter; GAT, GABA transporter; GlyT, glycine (Gly) transporter; EAAT, excitatory amino acid transporter; CHT, choline transporter the cytosol for storage into vesicles. In the case of catecholamines, serotonin, GABA, and glycine reuptake occurs primarily into the nerve terminal and is mediated by a family of plasma membrane transporters dependent on cotransport of both Na^+ and Cl^-. In the case of acetylcholine, hydrolysis by acetylcholinesterase terminates signaling, and the product choline is then recycled into the nerve terminal via a Na^+-dependent choline transporter present in a subset of synaptic vesicles.[17] In contrast, glutamate is taken up by excitatory amino acid transporters (EAATs) 1 and 2 expressed on astrocytes and converted to glutamine which is transferred back to excitatory and inhibitory neurons by the sequential action of glial and then neuronal transporters. GABA and glycine also undergo astrocytic uptake.

CALCIUM-TRIGGERED EXOCYTOSIS

Synaptic vesicle exocytosis is restricted to active zones containing clustered voltage-gated Ca^{2+} channels of the Ca_v2 family. This process involves the interaction among a large group of evolutionarily conserved proteins (Table

TABLE 15.4 *Major Proteins Involved in Synaptic Vesicle Exocytosis*

Process	Protein	Function
Organization of the core active zone	RIM (Rab-interacting protein)	Required for synaptic vesicle docking and priming Interactions with Rab3 and Rab 27 in synaptic vesicles as well as with Munc13, and Ca_v2 channels. Involved in long-term presynaptic plasticity
	RIM-BP	Interacts with both RIM and Ca_v2 channels
	Munc-13	Renders synaptic vesicles competent for fusion by maintaining the open state of syntaxin
	α-liprins	Link the RIM/RIM-BP/Munc 13 complex to a receptor phosphoprotein phosphatase that acts as an adhesion molecule.
	ELKs	Interact with α-liprins and with presynaptic scaffolds
	Bassoon/Piccolo	Guide synaptic vesicles from the reserve pool to the active zones
Transsynaptic adhesion interactions	Neurexin	Interacts with postsynaptic neuroligins, cerebellins, and other partners
Vesicular mobilization	Synapsin	Tethers synaptic vesicles to the acting cytoskeleton. Its phosphorylation promotes synaptic vesicle mobilization.
Docking, fusion, and exocytosis	Syntaxin	Presynaptic membrane SNARE protein
	SNAP-25	Presynaptic membrane SNARE protein
	Synaptobrevin/VAMP	Synaptic vesicle SNARE protein
	Munc-18	Maintains the closed form of syntaxin, then further promotes assembly and fusion
	Complexin	Controls zippering of the SNARE complex
	Synaptotagmin	Ca^{2+} sensor protein. Binds to both SNARE and the presynaptic membrane and triggers fusion.
Other presynaptic vesicle proteins	SV2	Synaptic vesicle glycoprotein involved in multiple functions. Interacts with synaptotagmin. Target of levetiracetam.
	Synaptophysin	Release site clearance Prevents exocytosis
Disassembly of SNARE complexes	N-ethylmaleimide-sensitive factor (NSF)	ATPase that disassembles the cis-SNARE complex
	SNAP (soluble NSF attachment protein)	Adaptor for NSF disassembly to the SNARE complex

15.4). Active zones are surrounded by a perisynaptic zone that is the site of synaptic vesicle endocytosis. Upon arrival of the action potential, the synaptic vesicles fuse and release neurotransmitter either in a time-locked or delayed manner. The time-locked, synchronous release transmits fast and reliable excitatory or inhibitory signals. Delayed asynchronous release modulates the efficacy of neurotransmission, network synchronicity, and plasticity. Synaptic vesicles can also fuse spontaneously in the absence of action potentials, affecting formation and strength of synaptic connections.[18]

Functional Pools of Synaptic Vesicles

Synaptic vesicles are organized in four different pools at the presynaptic terminal: a rapid releasable pool, a recycling pool, a reserve pool, and a resting pool. The rapid releasable pool is docked and ready to fuse upon Ca^{2+} influx at the active zone and mediates synchronous transmission.[19,20] Synaptic vesicles in the reserve pool are linked to the actin cytoskeleton via synapsin 1, a vesicular membrane ATPase. In response to phosphorylation triggered by cyclic adenosine monophosphate (cAMP) activated protein kinase A or Ca^{2+} synapsin 1 dissociates from the synaptic vesicles and allows their mobilization toward the presynaptic active zone.

Presynaptic Active Zone

Presynaptic active zones are the sites of docking and priming of the synaptic vesicles and contain a group of core and associated proteins. The core complex consists of five conserved proteins: Rab-3 interacting molecule (RIM); RIM-binding protein; mammalian uncoordinated -13 (Munc13); α-liprin, and CAST/ELKS proteins.[19] RIM is a multiple-domain protein that is a central organizer of the active zones; it interacts both with Rab3 (or Rab27) located in the vesicle membrane and with Munc13, a core active zone protein that primes the fusion machinery for exocytosis. In addition, RIM together with RIM-binding protein recruits the Ca_v2 channels to the active zones. CAST/ELKS proteins are positive regulators of exocytosis, controlling organization in the presynaptic terminal in part via interactions with α-liprins. In addition to the core complex, active zones also contain two large homologous proteins, Piccolo and Bassoon, whose main function may be to guide synaptic vesicles from the reserve pool to the active zone. Once loaded with the neurotransmitter and mobilized synaptic vesicles undergo docking (attachment) at the presynaptic active zones followed by their priming (preparation) for Ca^{2+}-triggered exocytosis.

Presynaptic Machinery for Exocytosis

The mechanisms of fast synchronous exocytosis has been well characterized[21] (Figure 15.5). Synchronous fusion is mediated by the canonical mechanism mediated by the neuronal SNARE (for soluble NSF attachment protein receptor) complex, which includes the synaptic vesicle synaptobrevin 2 (also known as vesicle-associated membrane protein, VAMP), the presynaptic plasma membrane syntaxin-1 and SNAP-25 (synaptosomal-associated protein-25), and the neuronal Ca^{2+}-sensing proteins called synaptotagmins.[19,21] Synaptobrevin, syntaxin, and SNAP-25 form a transcomplex that involves a progressive zippering of their four α-helices (one from synaptobrevin, one from syntaxin, and two from SNAP25, which forces the fusing membranes into close proximity. The SNARE complex for exocytosis is a target of botulinum and tetanus toxins.

Prior to SNARE-complex formation, syntaxin-1 is present in a closed conformation via its association with the protein Munc18-1. When the closed conformation of syntaxin-1 "opens" in preparation to fusion and SNARE complexes formation, Munc18-1 remains attached and interacts with the SNARE complex to promote the formation of the fusion pore. During an action potential, Ca^{2+} entering a presynaptic terminal triggers synaptic vesicle exocytosis and neurotransmitter release in less than a millisecond.[21] This process requires the vesicular synaptotagmins and the cytoplasmic complexins. Synaptotagmins are anchored to synaptic vesicles and are the primary Ca^{2+} sensors for exocytosis.[22,23] At resting state, synaptotagmin clamps the SNARE complex. Upon Ca^{2+} influx following an action potential, synaptotagmin binds both to syntaxin in the SNARE complex and to acidic phospholipids in the plasma membrane and triggers fusion of the synaptic vesicle. Synaptotagmins 1, 2, and 9 are primarily involved in fast, synchronous neurotransmitter release. Complexins bind to a groove on the surface of the SNARE complex and inhibit spontaneous release while facilitating synchronous, evoked release.[21] Synaptotagmin 7 binds Ca^{2+} with high sensitivity and slow kinetics, and mainly functions to mediate the slow phase of exocytosis, or asynchronous release.[24] In the final step of exocytosis, the synaptic vesicle membrane fuses with the plasma membrane; the two lipid bilayers merge at the contact site. Then a fusion pore opens and then expands, leading to complete membrane fusion and complete release of the vesicular content. The transmembrane V0 component of the V-ATPase interacts with synaptobrevin and syntaxin-1 and may be involved in formation of the fusion pore, independently of proton translocation.[16] After fusion, the SNARE complexes, now in the *cis* position, need to be disassembled by the ATPase N-ethylmaleimide-sensitive factor (NSF), which binds to SNARE complexes via the adaptor soluble NSF-attachment proteins (SNAP) proteins, completing the cycle.

Synaptic vesicles may also fuse and recycle spontaneously in the absence of action potentials.[25] This involves noncanonical SNAREs and different types of Ca^{2+} sensors, such as Doc-2 proteins.[26,27] Spontaneous release is reflected by the presence of miniature postsynaptic potentials (such as the miniature endplate potential at the neuromuscular junction).

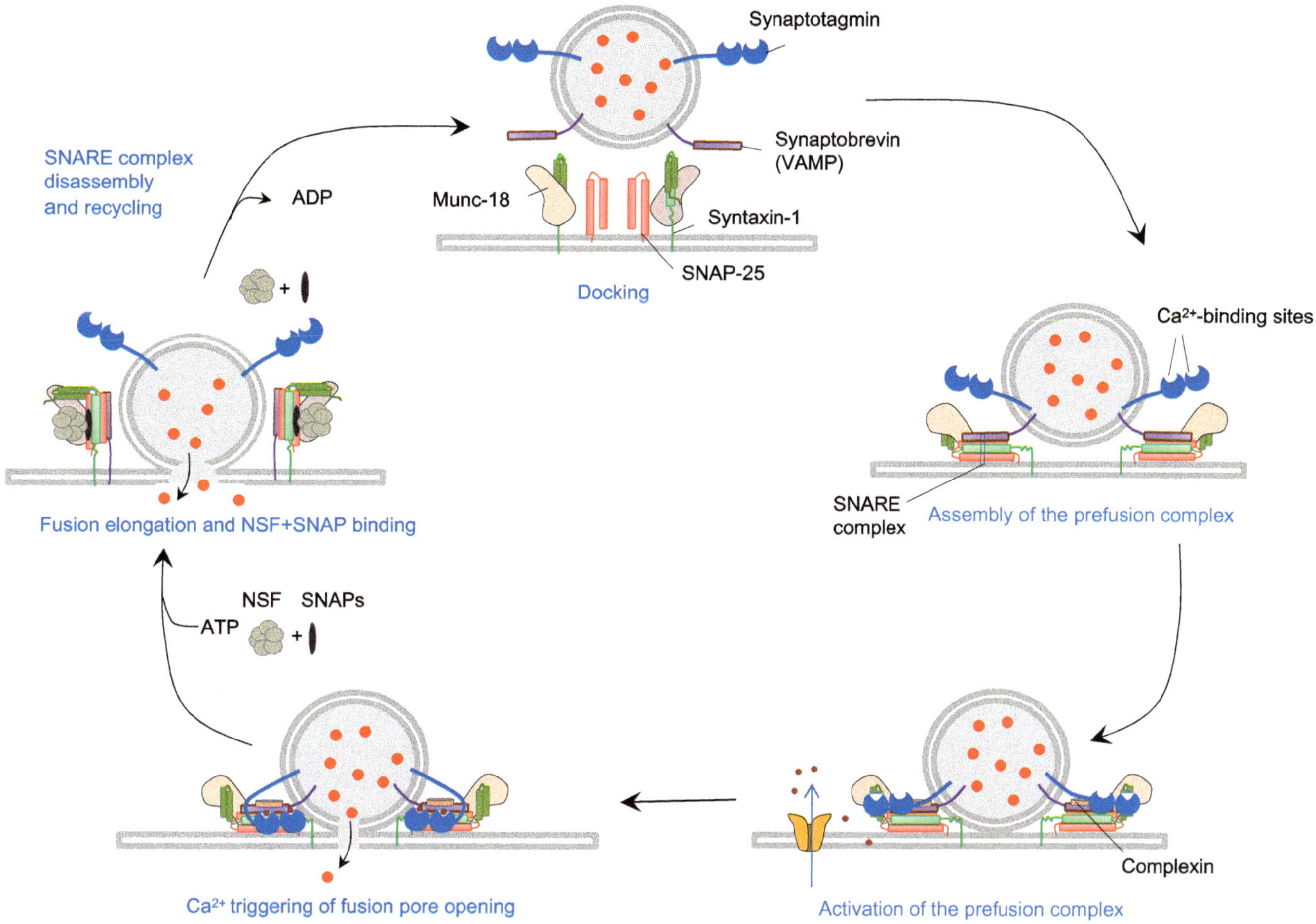

FIGURE 15.5 Machinery for fast synaptic vesicle exocytosis.
Synchronous fusion of synaptic vesicles is mediated by the canonical mechanism mediated by neuronal SNARE (for soluble NSF attachment protein receptor) complex, which includes the synaptic vesicle synaptobrevin 2 (also known as vesicle-associated membrane protein, VAMP) and the presynaptic plasma membrane syntaxin-1 and SNAP-25 (synaptosomal associated protein-25), and by the neuronal Ca^{2+}-sensing proteins called synaptotagmins. Synaptobrevin, syntaxin, and SNAP-25 form a transcomplex that involves a progressive zippering of their four α-helices, which forces the fusing membranes into close proximity. Prior to SNARE-complex formation, syntaxin-1 is present in a closed conformation via its association with the protein Munc 18-1, which remains attached to the SNARE complex. Synaptotagmins are anchored to synaptic vesicles by a single transmembrane region, contain two Ca^{2+}-binding domains, and are the primary Ca^{2+} sensors for exocytosis. Complexins bind to a groove on the surface of the SNARE complex formed by the helices of syntaxin and synaptobrevin. During an action potential, Ca^{2+} entering a presynaptic terminal triggers synaptic vesicle exocytosis. Synaptotagmin 1 triggers fast, synchronous neurotransmitter release in response to local Ca^{2+} influx via Ca_v2 channels. Following exocytosis, the SNARE complexes are disassembled by the ATPase N-ethylmaleimide-sensitive factor (NSF), which binds to SNARE complexes via the adaptor soluble NSF-attachment proteins (SNAP) proteins, completing the cycle.

Proteins Regulating Exocytosis

Proline repeat-rich transmembrane protein 2 (PRRT2) negatively regulates exocytosis by interacting with proteins of the fusion machinery, particularly SNAP25 and synaptotagmin 1 (in excitatory synapses) or synaptotagmin 2 (in inhibitory synapses). PRRT2 may also interact with postsynaptic targets, including the GluA1 subunit of AMPA receptors and is a negative modulator of $Na_v1.2$ and $Na_v1.6$ channels in the axon initial segment. Overall, the effects of PPRT2 appear to reduce CNS excitability.[28] In contrast, synaptic vesicle glycoprotein 2 (SV2) promotes several steps leading to exocytosis. SV2 forms large molecular complexes with other vesicular proteins, anchoring them into their appropriate orientation to enable efficient association with vesicular fusion machinery and making them more responsive to Ca^{2+} via its interactions with synaptotagmin. SV2 is the molecular target of the antiepileptic drug levetiracetam. Upon vesicular fusion, the luminal domain of SV2 becomes the extracellular domain and is free to interact with extracellular proteins. For example, SV2 participates in an activity-dependent interaction with laminin-1, which may slow vesicular recycling. SV2 may also function as a transporter for botulinum and tetanus neurotoxins, which thereby hijack endocytosis into the presynaptic neuron. Synaptophysins and synaptogyrins are a family of widely expressed synaptic vesicle membrane proteins. Synaptophysin interacts with synaptobrevin but its role in exocytosis is yet to be precisely defined. Studies in knockout mice suggest that synaptophysin modulates exocytosis, primarily by inhibition.

REGULATION OF PRESYNAPTIC CALCIUM CHANNELS

Presynaptic Ca^{2+} channels have three main functions: they interact with core active zone proteins and SNARE proteins bringing docked synaptic vesicles close to the source of Ca^{2+} entry, allow fast and spatially focused Ca^{2+} entry for rapid and synchronous neurotransmitter release, and respond to residual Ca^{2+} in nerve terminals to mediate multiple forms of short-term synaptic plasticity. Neurotransmitter release is proportional to the third or fourth power of Ca^{2+} influx. Therefore, regulation of Ca_v2 channels is a major mechanism to regulate exocytosis.[29,30] Calcium-dependent neurotransmitter release occurs in two phases, a fast synchronous (phasic) and a slow asynchronous (tonic) component. The fast synchronous release, driven by the Ca^{2+} current activated by the action potential, produces a large, fast postsynaptic response. The slower asynchronous component results from residual Ca^{2+} remaining in the terminal after an action potential, and provides a basic level of neurotransmitter release at many synapses.

Structure of Presynaptic Ca^{2+} Channels

The presynaptic voltage-gated Ca^{2+} channels include P/Q ($Ca_v2.1$), N ($Ca_v2.2$), and less frequently R ($Ca_v2.3$) channels. The P/Q-type channels predominate at central glutamatergic synapses and at the neuromuscular junction; the N-type channels predominate in peripheral synapses. These channels consist of an α_1 subunit with a four homologous domains (I–IV); each domain consists of six-transmembrane α-helices (S1–S6), with the S1–S4 module forming the voltage sensor module and a membrane-associated P loop between S5 and S6 forming the channel pore. Unique to presynaptic Ca_v2 channels, the intracellular loop between domains II and III contains the synaptic *pro*tein *int*eraction (*synprint*) site that allows the interactions of Ca_v2 channels with SNARE proteins. The large carboxy (C)-terminal intracellular loop contains a calcium sensor domain (CaS) that binds calmodulin (CaM) and other neuronal Ca^{2+} sensor proteins. The Caβ subunit interacts with intracellular molecules that regulate Ca_v2 channel activity. The $\alpha_2\delta$ subunit complex of the channel enhances the forward trafficking and insertion of the α_1 subunit into the presynaptic terminal and is the target of the inhibitory effects of gabapentin and pregabalin on neurotransmitter release.

Influences Regulating Presynaptic Ca^{2+} Channels

There are several influences that regulate the activity of presynaptic Ca_v2 channels.[30] The major influence is feedback inhibitory modulation in response to increases in intracellular Ca^{2+}; this involves CaM and related neuron-specific Ca^{2+}-sensing proteins such as calcium-binding protein 1 (CaBP1) and neuronal calcium sensor 1 (NCS1). For example, there is a Ca^{2+}/CaM-dependent inactivation of $Ca_v2.1$ channels in response to global Ca^{2+} elevations at axon terminals. CaBP1-1 also causes rapid inactivation, whereas NCS1 facilitates synaptic activity by reducing Ca^{2+}-dependent inactivation of $Ca_v2.1$currents.

Presynaptic Ca_v2 channels are also regulated by proteins involved in exocytosis. At the resting state associated with low Ca^{2+} concentrations, syntaxin-1 and SNAP25 bind the *synprint* site of Ca_v2 channels, inhibiting channel opening. Higher Ca^{2+} concentrations associated with exocytosis relieve this inhibitory effect by triggering phosphorylation of the *synprint site* by protein kinase C (PKC) or $Ca2^{+}$/CaM kinase II (CaMKII). The activity of Ca_v2 channels is also affected by their interactions with proteins of the active zone core complex. The interaction of RIM with the C-terminal cytoplasmic tails of Ca_v2 channels is essential for recruiting Ca^{2+} channels to the presynaptic active zone and determines channel density and synaptic vesicle docking at this region. Activation of GPCRs coupled to G_i/G_o signaling reduce the magnitude of presynaptic Ca^{2+} currents. Important examples of such G_i/G_o coupled receptors include $GABA_B$, opioid, and endocannabinoid CB1 receptors. This inhibitory effect is mediated by the Gβγ subunits, which bind directly to the Ca_v2 α1 subunits at multiple sites, increasing their activation threshold.

MECHANISMS OF PRESYNAPTIC PLASTICITY

Plasticity at the presynaptic terminal can increase or decrease the strength of a synaptic signal and thus alter the size of a postsynaptic response.[19,29] Many mechanisms contribute to short-term and long-term plasticity.

Effects of Calcium-Binding Proteins

A basic mechanism of short-term presynaptic plasticity is the interplay among the buildup of residual Ca^{2+} after the action potential, the local availability of Ca^{2+} buffers, and the size of the readily releasable pool of vesicles. Calcium entering the active zone via Ca_v2 channels is buffered quickly, so that Ca^{2+} transients last less than 1 millisecond. Parvalbumin, calbindin, and related calcium-binding proteins are expressed at high levels in many types of presynaptic terminals, where they control Ca^{2+} transients, participate in Ca^{2+}-signaling pathways, protect against Ca^{2+} overload, and participate in mechanisms of short-term presynaptic plasticity.[31] During repeated action potentials (especially at frequencies of >10 Hz), residual Ca^{2+} accumulates as Ca^{2+} buffers become saturated, resulting in an increase of the release probability and thus presynaptic facilitation. However, this facilitation is rate-limited by the availability of readily releasable pool of synaptic vesicles. Another major mechanism of short-term plasticity at the active zone is mediated by the Ca^{2+}-dependent modulation of presynaptic Ca^{2+} channels.

Effects of Active Zone Proteins, G Proteins, and Phosphorylation

Presynaptic plasticity also involves proteins that regulate the docking and fusion machinery, such as Munc13 and synaptotagmin-7, which directly or indirectly interact with the Ca_v2 channels. Active zone proteins also participate in long-term presynaptic plasticity. For example, the amount of RIM1α available for RIM/Rab3 interactions is important for both long-term potentiation and long-term depression of neurotransmitter release. Activation of presynaptic GPCRs does not only directly affect Ca_v2 channels but also controls the availability of synaptic vesicles. For example activation of presynaptic GPCRs coupled to the G_s-cAMP-dependent PKA pathway may have a positive modulatory effect by phosphorylating synapsin, thereby detaching synaptic vesicles from their tethering to the actin cytoskeleton and promoting their mobilization to the active zone. Calmodulin kinase II is the most prominent Ca^{2+}/CaM-dependent regulator of presynaptic function. In its autophosphorylated form, CaMKII binds to the α1 subunit of $Ca_v.2$ channels and enhances their activity by slowing inactivation; CAMKII also phosphorylates synapsin thus regulating trafficking of synaptic vesicles. Release of calcium from intracellular stores may also contribute to presynaptic plasticity.[32] The synaptic boutons contain endoplasmic reticulum (ER) harboring ryanodine receptors (RYRs), which are calcium-activated channels that mediate Ca^{2+} release from this organelle. Calcium influx via voltage-gated channels in response to an action potential elicits a highly localized RYR-dependent release of Ca^{2+} from the ER at active synapses. This intracellular Ca^{2+} spark may also contribute to spontaneous transmitter release. In contrast, high frequency and prolonged stimuli produce net loading, rather than depletion, of ER Ca^{2+} stores, suggesting that under these more intense stimulation conditions the dominant function of the ER is to sequester cytosolic Ca^{2+} within the bouton.

ENDOCYTOSIS AT PRESYNAPTIC TERMINALS

Endocytosis retrieves the fused synaptic vesicle components from the neuronal surface and is tightly coupled to exocytosis. This coupling is necessary to sustain a high rate of neurotransmission without depleting the recycling vesicle pools and to prevent the unlimited expansion of presynapse plasma membrane. Following exocytosis, synaptobrevin and synaptotagmin are resorted and preassembled in membrane patches, constituting a "readily retrievable pool" for endocytosis outside of the active zone. This involves control of localization and dynamics of synaptic vesicle proteins during partition from sites of fusion (active zone) to sites of endocytosis (periactive zone).

Mechanisms of Endocytosis

Several modes of endocytosis operate to ensure a sufficient and precise vesicle-recycling rate during neurotransmission.[18] Clathrin-mediated endocytosis is the best-characterized endocytic pathway and the predominant route of vesicle retrieval. This process includes four major steps: clathrin coat recruitment, vesicle budding, vesicle fission, and vesicle uncoating; these processes involve sequential recruitment of endocytic proteins, eventually leading to fission of endocytic vesicles by action of dynamin[33,34] (Figure 15.6) (Table 15.5). At presynaptic membranes, clathrin-mediated endocytosis is initiated by the recruitment of the adaptor protein 2 complex, which interacts with the synaptic vesicle protein SV2 and vesicular neurotransmitter transporters. The sequential stages of endocytosis involve the sequential recruitment, assembly, and disassembly of protein scaffolds that bind acidic membrane phospholipids and stabilize or induce membrane curvature to produce clathrin-coated pits. They include endophilin A, synaptojanin-1, and amphiphysin. Amphiphysin is a scaffold protein that recruits dynamin, which elicits fission of the membrane and separation of the vesicle. This process is followed by disassembly of the clathrin coat dependent on the heat shock protein called heat shock cognate 70 and its cofactor auxilin (DCJ6), a heat shock protein 40 cochaperone (Figure 15.6).

There are other mechanisms of endocytosis. Ultrafast endocytosis occurs after brief neuronal activity both at the neuromuscular junction and central synapses. In this process, membranes rapidly invaginate to form large endocytic vesicles. This process may share mechanisms with clathrin-mediated endocytosis as it requires synaptojanin-1 and endophilin A and dynamin.[35] The kiss-and-run mode of endocytosis involves a reversal of the exocytotic fusion; in this mode synaptic vesicles that released their contents through a transient fusion pore are retrieved rapidly without full collapse into the plasma membrane. Intense bursts of neuronal activity trigger activity-dependent bulk endocytosis, which internalizes a large area of plasma membrane and forms an endosome-like endocytic structure that is finally converted into a releasable synaptic vesicle. This process depends on the transient activation of the Ca^{2+}-dependent phosphatase calcineurin, and rapid actin-dependent invagination leading to the formation of a bulk endosome. Synaptic vesicle proteins such as VAMP2, synaptophysin,

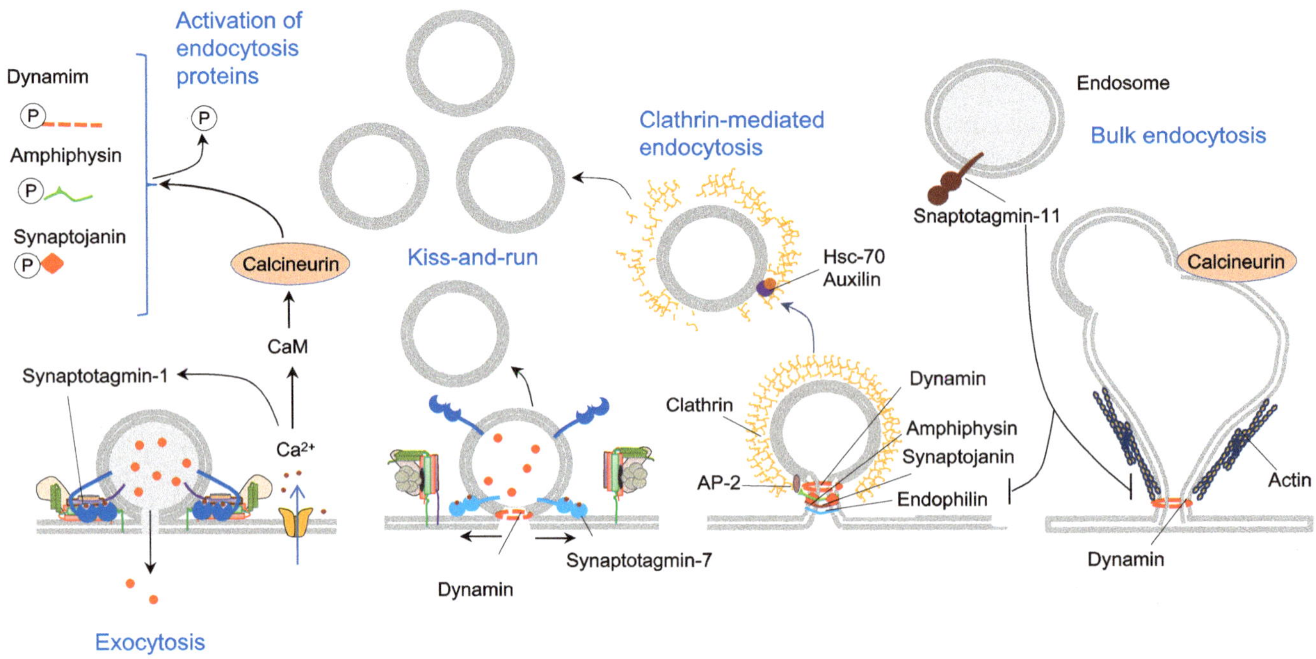

FIGURE 15.6 Coupling of exocytosis and endocytosis.
Endocytosis retrieves the fused synaptic vesicle components from the neuronal surface and is tightly coupled to exocytosis. There are several forms of endocytosis. The kiss-and-run mode of endocytosis involves a reversal of the exocytic fusion. Clathrin-mediated endocytosis is a relatively slow process that includes four major steps: clathrin coat recruitment, vesicle budding, vesicle fission, and vesicle uncoating; these processes involve sequential recruitment of endocytic proteins, eventually leading to fission of endocytic vesicles by action of dynamin. Coat recruitment is by the adaptor protein 2 (AP2) complex. The sequential stages of endocytosis involve the sequential recruitment of endophilin A, synaptojanin-1, and amphiphysin. Dynamin elicits fission of the membrane and separation of the vesicle, which is followed by disassembly of the clathrin coat dependent on the heat shock protein called heat shock cognate-70 (Hsc70) and its cofactor the heat shock protein 40 cochaperone auxilin. Activity-dependent bulk endocytosis forms an endosome-like endocytic structure that is finally converted into a releasable synaptic vesicle. The tight coupling between exocytosis and endocytosis involves calmodulin (CaM), synaptotagmins, SNARE proteins, and synaptophysin. CaM is involved in most forms of endocytosis by a mechanism mediated by the phosphatase calcineurin, which dephosphorylates endocytic proteins such as synaptojanin, amphiphysin, and dynamin.

and glutamate transporters are retrieved by activity-dependent bulk endocytosis.

Coupling Between Endocytosis and Exocytosis

The tight coupling between endocytosis and exocytosis is critical for the maintenance of presynaptic structural integrity and function (Figure 15.6). Following exocytosis, endocytosis occurs immediately to retrieve synaptic vesicle membrane and fusion machinery for local recycling.

The transient elevation in cytosolic Ca^{2+} following opening of Ca_v2 channels triggers and accelerates both clathrin-dependent and clathrin-independent endocytosis. Among the Ca^{2+} sensors that initiate and mediate Ca^{2+}-dependent endocytosis, CaM is involved in most forms of endocytosis by a mechanism mediated by the phosphatase calcineurin, which dephosphorylates endocytic proteins known as dephosphins.[36] Dephosphins include synaptojanin, amphiphysin, and dynamin, which are constitutively phosphorylated and in an inactive conformation in resting nerve terminals. During synaptic activity, these dephosphins undergo rapid dephosphorylation by the Ca^{2+}/CaM -activated calcineurin and drive endocytosis via their enhanced binding to other endocytic factors. Synaptotagmin 11 has also been proposed to be a major Ca^{2+}-sensing protein that promotes clathrin-mediated endocytosis following exocytosis. Synaptotagmin 11, unlike other synaptotagmins, does not bind Ca^{2+} but resides in vesicles that resemble recycling endosomes and inhibits both clathrin-mediated and bulk endocytosis and thus vesicle recycling. Synaptotagmin 11 may function as a clamp protein to ensure the precise coupling and balance of endocytosis to exocytosis during neurotransmission.[37]

Role of Proteins and Phospholipids in the Synaptic Vesicle Cycle

All steps of the synaptic vesicle cycle involve complex protein–protein and protein–lipid interactions. Many proteins involved in exocytosis and endocytosis contain a

TABLE 15.5 *Major Proteins Involved in Synaptic Vesicle Endocytosis and Recycling*

Process	Protein	Function
Clathrin coat proteins and adaptors	Clathrin heavy and light chain	Clathrin lattice
	AP2	Clathrin adaptor for several proteins of vesicle membrane
	AP180/CALM	Specific clathrin adaptor for synaptobrevin
	Epsin	Clathrin adaptor specific for ubiquitylated membrane proteins
	Stonin	Specific clathrin adaptor for synaptotagmin
BAR domain-containing proteins generate/sense membrane curvature	Endophilin	Coordinates curvature acquisition with fission and uncoating via interactions with synaptojanin and dynamin
	Amphiphysin	Scaffold protein that interacts with clathrin, AP2, dynamin, synaptojanin, endophilin, and actin-binding proteins coordinating curvature acquisition with fission
	FCho	Key nucleator for endocytic clathrin-coated pits
	Syndapin	Coordinates endocytosis with actin nucleation via interaction with dynamin, synaptojanin, and N-WASP
Phosphoinositide metabolism	Synaptojanin 1	Phosphatidylinositol (4,5) diphosphate (PIP2) phosphatase, which couples fission of clathrin-coated vesicles to shedding of the adaptors during uncoating
	Phosphatidylinositol kinase 1 γ	Major PIP2-synthesizing enzyme at the plasma membrane
Scaffolding	Intersectin	Coordinates the recruitment of multiple endocytic factors
Membrane fission	Dynamin	GTPase responsible for membrane fission
Clathrin lattice disassembly	Hsc70	Heats shock protein 70 ATPase that triggers disassembly of clathrin cages
	Auxilin (DJA6)	Hsp40 cochaperone that recruits Hsc70 to clathrin-coated vesicles

high proportion of charged residues with few hydrophobic amino acids; this allows them to interact both with multiple proteins and with lipid membranes. Synapses are enriched in cholesterol and phospholipids. Negatively charged membrane phospholipids, particularly phosphatidylinositol phosphates located in the cytosolic face of the membrane, function at multiple steps of the synaptic vesicle cycle. The polar heads of these phospholipids are binding sites for proteins and organize both transmembrane proteins and peripheral membrane proteins that cycle between a cytosolic and a membrane-bound state. Phospholipids are therefore key to both exocytosis and endocytosis and couple these two processes.

Role of α-Synuclein

Alpha-synuclein (α-SYN) is abundant at presynaptic terminals and interacts with synaptic vesicles to modulate membrane remodeling and vesicle recycling at nerve terminals.[38] Alpha-synuclein binds to synaptic vesicles via interactions in its amphipathic α-helix conformation with negatively charged membrane lipids. Alpha-synuclein facilitates SNARE assembly by simultaneously binding to synaptobrevin and to membrane phospholipids. It also functions as a molecular chaperone that prevents the accumulation of unfolded or partly folded SNARE protein molecules, which are prone to nonspecific interactions. Alpha-synuclein may cooperate with cysteine string protein-α (CSPα, DNAJ5) to maintain SNARE complex assembly. Via its interactions with both synaptobrevin and negatively charged lipids, α-SYN promotes vesicle clustering. Thus, α-SYN regulates the trafficking of synaptic vesicles in distal reserve pool, controls the amount of vesicles docked at the synapses for neurotransmitter release, and participates in mechanisms of docking and priming of synaptic vesicles. Alpha-synuclein may also act at early steps of vesicular endocytosis before dynamin.

PRESYNAPTIC SYNAPTOPATHIES

Paroxysmal Disorders Caused by PRRT2 and PNKD Mutations

Mutations in the *PRRT2* gene are a leading cause of a wide and evolving spectrum of paroxysmal diseases.[39] They include paroxysmal kinesigenic dyskinesia (PKD), benign familial infantile epilepsy (BFIE), paroxysmal kinesigenic dyskinesia with infantile convulsions, and hemiplegic migraine.[39] The vast majority of mutations lead to happloinsufficency and reduction of PRRT2 activity. This results in dysregulated neurotransmitter release and neuronal excitability, leading to paroxysmal movement disorders and seizure phenotypes. PRRT2 has both pre- and postsynaptic function.[40] Presynaptically, PRRT2 prevents the formation of SNARE complexes. PRRT2 also reduces neuronal excitability by reducing membrane expression and activity of $Na_v1.2$ and $Na_v1.6$ channels in the axonal initial segment.[41] These pathophysiological mechanisms relate to similar syndromes caused by mutations in ion channels located in the axon initial segment, including benign familial neonatal seizures (*KCNQ2/KCNQ3* mutations), benign familial neonatal-infantile seizures (*SCN2A* mutations), and benign familial infantile seizures and paroxysmal kinesigenic choreoathetosis (*SCN8A* mutations).[42] The paroxysmal attacks in PKD are frequent, short-duration attacks of dystonia or choreoathetosis precipitated by voluntary movements such as standing from a sitting position, or transition from standing to walking; they may be preceded by paresthesia or crawling sensation in the affected limb. The episodes are often well controlled with Na^+ channel blockers such as carbamazepine. In contrast, paroxysmal nonkinesigenic dyskinesia (PNKD) is characterized by attacks triggered by alcohol, coffee, or strong emotions. The attacks are longer than those in PKD (from 10 min to 1 h or up to 12 h) but are much less frequent and may occur only a few times a year. In some cases PNKD also reflects a presynaptic synaptopathy. It has been linked to loss-of- function mutations of the *PNKD* gene encoding the PNKD protein that self-oligomerizes and interacts with RIM1 and RIM2 and normally inhibits exocytosis.[43] *PNKD* mutations have also been associated with other phenotypes, including episodic ataxia, familial hemiplegic migraine, and Tourette syndrome.[44]

SNAREopathies

Mutations in genes encoding proteins involved in SNARE-mediated exocytosis result in several phenotypes. Most reported mutations are heterozygous de novo missense or loss-of function mutations and manifest with a wide range of neurodevelopment disorders leading to intellectual disability, autism, speech and language difficulties, seizures, ataxia, hyperkinesia, or myasthenic syndrome.[45] Most described cases are due to *MUNC18/STXBP1* (syntaxin-binding protein 1) mutations; others have been linked to mutations of *STX1A* (syntaxin 1A), *STX1B*, *SNPA25*, *VAMP2* (synaptobrevin), *MUNC13A*, *RIMS1* (RIM active zone protein), *SYT1 (*synaptotagmin 1), and *CPLX1* (complexin1). Some mutations such as those affecting *MUNC18/STXBP1* have been associated with severe epilepsy phenotypes, including West syndrome, Dravet syndrome, and Lennox-Gastaut syndrome; others may produce less severe epilepsy, and some have not yet been linked to seizures. Several SNAREopathies such as those due to *STX1B* mutations are associated with ataxia or hyperkinetic movement disorders. Other mutations such as *VAMP1* (synaptobrevin), *SYT2* (synaptotagmin 2), and *MUNC13A* may produce congenital myasthenic syndrome.[46] For example, synaptotagmin-2 myasthenia is associated with weakness and areflexia, low-amplitude compound muscle potential, and great facilitation by exercise. *RIMS1* mutations also produce rod-cone dystrophy and *SYT1* mutations produce strabismus and nystagmus.[45] Missense mutations in *SYT1* gene produce variable phenotypes that include infantile hypotonia, congenital ophthalmic abnormalities, childhood-onset hyperkinetic movement disorders, motor stereotypies, developmental delay of varying severity, sleep disturbances, and episodic agitation.[47] Some of the identified heterozygous missense mutations resulted in synaptotagmin localization at synaptic terminals or impaired endocytic retrieval and trafficking, resulting in slowed exocytic release following sustained action potential stimulation.[47]

Disorders of Endocytosis

The fundamental role of clathrin-mediated endocytosis in synaptic function is reflected by the consequences of mutations affecting critical proteins in this process.[48] Mutations of the *SYNJ1* gene encoding the phosphoinositide phosphatase synaptojanin[49] or the *DCAJ6* gene encoding tyrosine protein phosphatase auxilin[50] have been linked to inherited forms of Parkinson disease (PD). The *SYT-11* gene encoding synaptotagmin 11 is a PD risk gene.[51] Synaptotagmin-11 inhibits endocytosis and thus vesicle pool replenishment and thus dopamine release. PARKIN, an E3 ubiquitin ligase whose mutations are linked to familial recessive and sporadic early-onset PD triggers synaptotagmin 11 ubiquitination; PARKIN deficiency induces synaptotagmin-11 accumulation and PD-like neurotoxicity in mouse models.[52]

Manifestations of CACNA1A Mutations

Mutations affecting the *CACNA1A* gene encoding the Cav2.1 (P/Q) channel have been linked to various phenotypes.[53] Gain-of-function *CACNA1* mutations cause familial hemiplegic migraine type 1 (FHM1). In this disorder, activity of $Ca_v2.1$ channels is permanently facilitated and causes a greater increase in excitatory than in inhibitory synapses.[54] This imbalance leads to cortical spreading depression, a wave of synchronized depolarization that causes the aura associated with FHM migraine attacks. In contrast, loss-of-function *CACNA1A* mutations cause episodic ataxia type 2 (EA2). These mutations cause reduced

$Ca_v2.1$ channel function by multiple mechanisms.[55] Loss of $Ca_v2.1$ channel function leads to impaired pacemaker activity and eventually death of cerebellar Purkinje cells. Expansion of the CAG repeat in *CACNA1A* codons encoding the C-terminal portion of $Ca_v1.2$ cause spinocerebellar ataxia type 6 (SCA6). In this disorder alternative splicing and posttranslational processing of $Ca_v2.1$ leads to cleavage of the C-terminal tail and release of the polyglutamine repeat segments, which accumulate in the cytosol and are also transported to the cell nucleus, where they may disrupt gene expression.

Presynaptic Targets of Antibodies and Toxins

As mentioned earlier in this chapter, the multiple effects of gabapentin and pregabalin in disorders such as neuropathic pain and restless legs syndrome (and to a lesser extent seizures) reflect their ability to reduce presynaptic Ca^{2+} function by decreasing the post-Golgi trafficking and surface expression of both the $\alpha_2\delta$ and α_1 subunits. Levetiracetam, which is widely used for treatment of seizures and myoclonus, targets SV2.[56] Autoantibodies against the presynaptic Cav2.1 (P/Q) channels are associated with the Lambert-Eaton myasthenic syndrome, which can occur in the setting of small-cell lung carcinoma. Antibodies against the scaffold protein amphiphysin, which is involved in the endocytic pathway, are typically associated with stiff-man-like syndrome in patients with small-cell lung carcinoma or breast cancer. Antibodies against neurexin-1 are associated with limbic encephalitis. Antibodies against presynaptic proteins such as septin 5 and the synaptic vesicle coat protein AP3B2 (adaptor protein-3, neuronal form-B2) have been linked to rapidly progressive autoimmune cerebellar ataxia.[57,58] Septins are cytoskeletal GTP-binding proteins that regulate exocytosis by providing a membrane-associated scaffold for vesicular SNAREs such as SNAP 25. The neuron-restricted AP3B2 isoform of adaptor protein 3 (AP-3) directs proteins from endosomes to synaptic vesicles. Ataxia associated with AP3B2 IgG has both several and sensory component due to commonly associated myeloneuropathy.[58]

Clostridial toxins, such as tetanus neurotoxin and botulinum neurotoxins (A–G) are metalloproteases that target SNARE proteins. The binding domain of these toxins interacts both with complex gangliosides (such as GT1b) located in the outer leaflet of the membrane and with the intraluminal domain of SV2 or synaptotagmin, which are transiently exposed to the synaptic cleft during exocytosis. The anchored toxin then undergoes endocytosis during vesicle recycling; acidification of the vesicle lumen triggers membrane insertion of the translocation domain of the neurotoxin, and then translocation of the enzymatically active light chain hydrolase domain to target specific SNARE proteins. Tetanus toxin and botulinum toxins B and D target synaptobrevin; botulinum toxins A and E target SNAP-25; and botulinum toxin C targets syntaxin. After being internalized in motor neurons, tetanus toxin undergoes transcytosis into inhibitory interneurons and blocks the release of GABA or glycine in the brainstem or spinal cord, whereas botulinum toxins blocks acetylcholine release at the neuromuscular junction and release of neuropeptides from nociceptive afferents. Both types of clostridial toxins can undergo fast retrograde axonal transport to more proximal sites in the central nervous system.

KEY POINTS

- Chemical synapses allow precise and bidirectional information in the nervous system.
- The presynaptic terminal harbors synaptic vesicles containing the chemical transmitters.
- Classical neurotransmitters are synthesized locally and stored in vesicles at the presynaptic terminals.
- Neuropeptides and growth factors synthesized in the cell bodies are stored in secretory granules and reach the presynaptic terminals via fast axonal transport.
- The presynaptic terminals contain active zones, which harbor clustered voltage-gated calcium (Ca^{2+}) channels (Ca_v2 family) that trigger fast neurotransmitter release.
- The presynaptic and postsynaptic elements contain a large number of scaffold and adaptor proteins and are linked structurally and functionally by transsynaptic adhesion molecules.
- Perisynaptic processes from astrocytes or Schwann cells ensheath the presynaptic and postsynaptic elements and participate in synaptic development, maintenance, and function.
- Synapses are continuously formed and eliminated throughout life in an activity-dependent manner in response to neuronal activity.
- The efficacy of synaptic transmission depends on complex molecular interactions at the presynaptic, transsynaptic, and postsynaptic levels.
- The classical neurotransmitters, L-glutamate, GABA, acetylcholine, and monoamines, are synthesized in the presynaptic terminals and stored in synaptic vesicles.
- A single vesicle filled with neurotransmitter is the elementary unit (or "quantum") of synaptic transmission.
- Neurotransmitters are synthesized from precursors via a critical enzymatic step.
- Storage of neurotransmitter into the synaptic vesicle requires specific vesicular transporters driven by the vacuolar (V)-ATPase.
- Neurotransmitter recycling is important both to terminate their synaptic effects and to increase their availability in the cytosol for storage into vesicles.
- Synaptic vesicle exocytosis is restricted to active zones containing clustered voltage-gated Ca^{2+} channels of the Ca_v2 family.

- Presynaptic active zones are the sites of docking and priming of the synaptic vesicles for rapid neurotransmitter release and contain core and associated proteins that recruit Ca_v2 channels close to the synaptic vesicles, participate in priming of synaptic vesicles, and mediate presynaptic plasticity.
- Synchronous fusion of synaptic vesicles depends on a canonical mechanism mediated by neuronal SNARE complex, which involves the interactions between synaptic vesicle synaptobrevin 2 and the presynaptic plasma membrane syntaxin-1 and SNAP-25.
- The SNARE complex for exocytosis is a target of botulinum and tetanus toxins.
- Synaptotagmins are Ca^{2+} sensors that are critical for the last steps of exocytosis.
- Proline repeat-rich transmembrane protein 2 (PRRT2) negatively regulates exocytosis.
- Synaptic vesicle glycoprotein 2 (SV2) facilitates exocytosis and is the target of inhibition by levetiracetam.
- Presynaptic Ca_v2 channels (P/Q and N-channels) allow fast and spatially focused Ca^{2+} influx for rapid and synchronous neurotransmitter release and mediate multiple forms of short-term synaptic plasticity.
- The $\alpha_2\delta$ subunit complex of the Cav2 channels enhances the forward trafficking and insertion of the α_1 subunit into the presynaptic terminal; this process is inhibited by gabapentin or pregabalin.
- Endocytosis retrieves the fused synaptic vesicle components from the neuronal surface and is tightly coupled to exocytosis.
- Alpha-synuclein (α-SYN) binds to synaptic vesicle, facilitates SNARE assembly, and functions as a molecular chaperone.
- Mutations in the *PRRT2* gene cause a spectrum of paroxysmal diseases including paroxysmal kinesigenic dyskinesia, benign familial infantile epilepsy, and hemiplegic migraine.
- Mutations affecting proteins of the SNARE complex or associated proteins (SNAREopathies) manifest with variable phenotypes that include intellectual disability, autism, speech and language difficulties, seizures, ataxia, hyperkinesia, or myasthenic syndrome.
- Mutations of the *SYNJ1* gene encoding synaptojanin and the *DCAJ6* gene tyrosine protein phosphatase auxilin have been linked to inherited forms of Parkinson disease; the *SYT-11* gene encoding synaptotagmin 11 is a Parkinson disease risk gene.

REFERENCES

1. Wu LG, Hamid E, Shin W, Chiang HC. Exocytosis and endocytosis: modes, functions, and coupling mechanisms. Annu Rev Physiol 2014;76:301–331.
2. Patzke C, Brockmann MM, Dai J, et al. Neuromodulator signaling bidirectionally controls vesicle numbers in human synapses. Cell 2019;179:498–513 e422.
3. Sudhof TC. Synaptic neurexin complexes: a molecular code for the logic of neural circuits. Cell 2017;171:745–769.
4. Spitzer NC. Neurotransmitter switching in the developing and adult brain. Annu Rev Neurosci 2017;40:1–19.
5. Neniskyte U, Gross CT. Errant gardeners: glial-cell-dependent synaptic pruning and neurodevelopmental disorders. Nat Rev Neurosci 2017;18:658–670.
6. Chanda S, Hale WD, Zhang B, Wernig M, Sudhof TC. Unique versus redundant functions of neuroligin genes in shaping excitatory and inhibitory synapse properties. J Neurosci 2017;37:6816–6836.
7. Seigneur E, Sudhof TC. Cerebellins are differentially expressed in selective subsets of neurons throughout the brain. J Comp Neurol 2017;525:3286–3311.
8. Yuzaki M. Two classes of secreted synaptic organizers in the central nervous system. Annu Rev Physiol 2018;80:243–262.
9. Isbister GK, Fan HW. Spider bite. Lancet 2011;378:2039–2047.
10. Brun BN, Mockler SR, Laubscher KM, et al. Comparison of brain MRI findings with language and motor function in the dystroglycanopathies. Neurology 2017;88:623–629.
11. Rodriguez Cruz PM, Palace J, Beeson D. The neuromuscular junction and wide heterogeneity of congenital myasthenic syndromes. Int J Mol Sci 2018;19.
12. Yamagata A, Fukai S. Insights into the mechanisms of epilepsy from structural biology of LGI1-ADAM22. Cell Mol Life Sci 2020;77:267–274.
13. Britton JW, Dalmau J. Recognizing autoimmune encephalitis as a cause of seizures: treating cause and not effect. Neurology 2019;92:877–878.
14. Katz B, Miledi R. Estimates of quantal content during "chemical potentiation" of transmitter release. Proc R Soc Lond B Biol Sci 1979;205:369–378.
15. Edwards RH. The neurotransmitter cycle and quantal size. Neuron 2007;55:835–858.
16. Morel N, Poea-Guyon S. The membrane domain of vacuolar H(+)ATPase: a crucial player in neurotransmitter exocytotic release. Cell Mol Life Sci 2015;72:2561–2573.
17. Haga T. Molecular properties of the high-affinity choline transporter CHT1. J Biochem 2014;156:181–194.
18. Chanaday NL, Cousin MA, Milosevic I, Watanabe S, Morgan JR. The synaptic vesicle cycle revisited: new insights into the modes and mechanisms. J Neurosci 2019;39:8209–8216.
19. Sudhof TC. The presynaptic active zone. Neuron 2012;75:11–25.
20. Neher E, Brose N. Dynamically primed synaptic vesicle states: key to understand synaptic short-term plasticity. Neuron 2018;100:1283–1291.
21. Sudhof TC. Neurotransmitter release: the last millisecond in the life of a synaptic vesicle. Neuron 2013;80:675–690.
22. Sudhof TC. Calcium control of neurotransmitter release. Cold Spring Harb Perspect Biol 2012;4:a011353.
23. Burgoyne RD, Helassa N, McCue HV, Haynes LP. Calcium sensors in neuronal function and dysfunction. Cold Spring Harb Perspect Biol 2019;11:a035154.
24. MacDougall DD, Lin Z, Chon NL, et al. The high-affinity calcium sensor synaptotagmin-7 serves multiple roles in regulated exocytosis. J Gen Physiol 2018;150:783–807.

25. Kavalali ET. The mechanisms and functions of spontaneous neurotransmitter release. Nat Rev Neurosci 2015;16:5–16.
26. Ramirez DMO, Crawford DC, Chanaday NL, Trauterman B, Monteggia LM, Kavalali ET. Loss of Doc2-dependent spontaneous neurotransmission augments glutamatergic synaptic strength. J Neurosci 2017;37:6224–6230.
27. Courtney NA, Briguglio JS, Bradberry MM, Greer C, Chapman ER. Excitatory and inhibitory neurons utilize different Ca(2+) sensors and sources to regulate spontaneous release. Neuron 2018;98:977–991 e975.
28. Lerche H. Synaptic or ion channel modifier? PRRT2 is a chameleon-like regulator of neuronal excitability. Brain 2018;141:938–941.
29. Nanou E, Catterall WA. Calcium channels, synaptic plasticity, and neuropsychiatric disease. Neuron 2018;98:466–481.
30. Mochida S. Presynaptic calcium channels. Int J Mol Sci 2019;20.
31. Elies J, Yanez M, Pereira TMC, Gil-Longo J, MacDougall DA, Campos-Toimil M. An update to calcium binding proteins. Adv Exp Med Biol 2020;1131:183–213.
32. Padamsey Z, Foster WJ, Emptage NJ. Intracellular Ca(2+) release and synaptic plasticity: a tale of many stores. Neuroscientist 2019;25:208–226.
33. Saheki Y, De Camilli P. Synaptic vesicle endocytosis. Cold Spring Harb Perspect Biol 2012;4:a005645.
34. Azarnia Tehran D, Kuijpers M, Haucke V. Presynaptic endocytic factors in autophagy and neurodegeneration. Curr Opin Neurobiol 2018;48:153–159.
35. Watanabe S, Mamer LE, Raychaudhuri S, et al. Synaptojanin and endophilin mediate neck formation during ultrafast endocytosis. Neuron 2018;98:1184–1197 e1186.
36. Cousin MA, Robinson PJ. The dephosphins: dephosphorylation by calcineurin triggers synaptic vesicle endocytosis. Trends Neurosci 2001;24:659–665.
37. Xie Z, Long J, Liu J, Chai Z, Kang X, Wang C. Molecular mechanisms for the coupling of endocytosis to exocytosis in neurons. Front Mol Neurosci 2017;10:47.
38. Huang M, Wang B, Li X, Fu C, Wang C, Kang X. Alpha-synuclein: a multifunctional player in exocytosis, endocytosis, and vesicle recycling. Front Neurosci 2019;13:28.
39. Ebrahimi-Fakhari D, Saffari A, Westenberger A, Klein C. The evolving spectrum of PRRT2-associated paroxysmal diseases. Brain 2015;138:3476–3495.
40. Valtorta F, Benfenati F, Zara F, Meldolesi J. PRRT2: from paroxysmal disorders to regulation of synaptic function. Trends Neurosci 2016;39:668–679.
41. Fruscione F, Valente P, Sterlini B, et al. PRRT2 controls neuronal excitability by negatively modulating Na+ channel 1.2/1.6 activity. Brain 2018;141:1000–1016.
42. Gardella E, Becker F, Moller RS, et al. Benign infantile seizures and paroxysmal dyskinesia caused by an SCN8A mutation. Ann Neurol 2016;79:428–436.
43. Shen Y, Ge WP, Li Y, et al. Protein mutated in paroxysmal dyskinesia interacts with the active zone protein RIM and suppresses synaptic vesicle exocytosis. Proc Natl Acad Sci U S A 2015;112:2935–2941.
44. Sun N, Nasello C, Deng L, et al. The PNKD gene is associated with Tourette disorder or tic disorder in a multiplex family. Mol Psychiatry 2018;23:1487–1495.
45. Verhage M, Sorensen JB. SNAREopathies: diversity in mechanisms and symptoms. Neuron 2020;107:22–37.
46. Engel AG. Congenital myasthenic syndromes in 2018. Curr Neurol Neurosci Rep 2018;18:46.
47. Baker K, Gordon SL, Melland H, et al. SYT1-associated neurodevelopmental disorder: a case series. Brain 2018;141:2576–2591.
48. Murdoch JD, Rostosky CM, Gowrisankaran S, et al. Endophilin-A deficiency induces the Foxo3a-Fbxo32 network in the brain and causes dysregulation of autophagy and the ubiquitin-proteasome system. Cell Rep 2016;17:1071–1086.
49. Krebs CE, Karkheiran S, Powell JC, et al. The Sac1 domain of SYNJ1 identified mutated in a family with early-onset progressive Parkinsonism with generalized seizures. Hum Mutat 2013;34:1200–1207.
50. Edvardson S, Cinnamon Y, Ta-Shma A, et al. A deleterious mutation in DNAJC6 encoding the neuronal-specific clathrin-uncoating co-chaperone auxilin, is associated with juvenile parkinsonism. PLoS One 2012;7:e36458.
51. Shimojo M, Madara J, Pankow S, et al. Synaptotagmin-11 mediates a vesicle trafficking pathway that is essential for development and synaptic plasticity. Genes Dev 2019;33:365–376.
52. Wang C, Kang X, Zhou L, et al. Synaptotagmin-11 is a critical mediator of parkin-linked neurotoxicity and Parkinson's disease-like pathology. Nat Commun 2018;9:81.
53. Rajakulendran S, Kaski D, Hanna MG. Neuronal P/Q-type calcium channel dysfunction in inherited disorders of the CNS. Nat Rev Neurol 2012;8:86–96.
54. Vecchia D, Tottene A, van den Maagdenberg AM, Pietrobon D. Abnormal cortical synaptic transmission in CaV2.1 knockin mice with the S218L missense mutation which causes a severe familial hemiplegic migraine syndrome in humans. Front Cell Neurosci 2015;9:8.
55. Dorgans K, Salvi J, Bertaso F, et al. Characterization of the dominant inheritance mechanism of episodic ataxia type 2. Neurobiol Dis 2017;106:110–123.
56. Stout KA, Dunn AR, Hoffman C, Miller GW. The synaptic vesicle glycoprotein 2: structure, function, and disease relevance. ACS Chem Neurosci 2019;10:3927–3938.
57. Honorat JA, Lopez-Chiriboga AS, Kryzer T, et al. Autoimmune septin-5 cerebellar ataxia. Neurol Neuroimmunol Neuroinflamm 2018;5:e474.
58. Honorat JA, Lopez-Chiriboga AS, Kryzer T, et al. Autoimmune gait disturbance accompanying adaptor protein-3B2-IgG. Neurology 2019;93:e954–e963.

16 Neurotransmission, Neuromodulation, and Plasticity

OVERVIEW

Neurons communicate with each other largely via chemical synapses. Several chemical signals mediate cell–cell interactions in the nervous system (Table 16.1). Many neurons contain and release more than one neurotransmitter.[1,2] Neurochemical signals released at synapses or by perisynaptic processes of glial cells produce three fundamental effects on their target: classical neurotransmission, neuromodulation, and plasticity (Figure 16.1). Classical neurotransmission is the rapid, precise transmission of excitatory or inhibitory signals between cells and is typically mediated by ionotropic receptors. Neuromodulation refers to the mechanisms by which neurochemical signals influence the efficacy of synaptic transmission and is mediated largely by G protein-coupled receptors (GCPRs), also known as metabotropic receptors. In many cases, the same neurotransmitter may exert several effects acting via different receptor subtypes. Synaptic plasticity refers to the activity-dependent changes in the efficacy of excitatory or inhibitory neurotransmission. They include long-term potentiation (LTP) and long-term depression (LTD) and may affect glutamatergic or GABAergic transmission via presynaptic or postsynaptic mechanisms. Synaptic plasticity may be triggered by calcium (Ca^{2+}) influx via ionotropic receptors, second-messenger cascades triggered by GPCRs, retrograde signals from the postsynaptic targets, and effects of growth factors and cytokines. These signals initiate transduction cascades triggering changes in the state of phosphorylation of a wide range of target proteins, resulting in ionotropic receptor recycling, local mRNA translation at dendritic spines, activation of transcription of target genes, and dynamic changes in the actin cytoskeleton leading to dendritic remodeling. Whereas synaptic plasticity is a fundamental mechanism for development of appropriate connectivity in the CNS and use-dependent learning and adaptation, abnormal plasticity is a fundamental mechanism in neurologic disorders such as epilepsy, chronic pain, levodopa-induced dyskinesia, cerebellar ataxia, Alzheimer disease, and intellectual disability/autism spectrum. The aims of this chapter are to briefly review (1) the main features of classical neurotransmission, (2) the function of GPCRs in neuromodulation, (3) the roles of cotransmitters and retrograde signals, and (4) the general mechanisms of synaptic plasticity.

CLASSICAL NEUROTRANSMISSION

Classical neurotransmission is the mechanism for fast, precise point relay and local processing of excitatory or inhibitory information in the nervous system. In the CNS, excitatory transmission is primarily mediated by L-glutamate, whereas the main inhibitory neurotransmitter is GABA. Glycine, together with GABA, is a major neurotransmitter of local inhibitory circuits in the brainstem and spinal cord. Acetylcholine (ACh) mediates fast neurotransmission at the neuromuscular junction and autonomic ganglia. Classical neurotransmission requires the rapid Ca^{2+}-triggered release of neurotransmitters from synaptic vesicles docked at presynaptic active zones, and is mediated by ionotropic receptors clustered at postsynaptic sites facing the presynaptic active zone; the apposition between presynaptic and postsynaptic sites involves transsynaptic adhesion molecules.

Ionotropic Receptor Families

Inotropic receptors are neurotransmitter-gated channels. Based on their structure, they are subdivided into three families (Figure 16.2). The cysteine loop-rich family is characterized by abundant cysteine residues and disulfide bonds in their large extracellular amino (N-) terminal domain. This family includes the nicotinic acetyl choline receptors (nAChRs) which are permeable to Na^+ and Ca^{2+}; the $GABA_A$ receptors and the glycine receptors, which are permeable to Cl^- (and bicarbonate); and the serotonin 5-hydroxytryptamine (5-HT)3 receptors, which are Ca^{2+}

TABLE 16.1 *Signal Molecules in the Nervous System*

Signal	Examples
Amino acids	Glutamate, GABA, glycine
Acetylcholine	N/A
Monoamines	Dopamine, norepinephrine, serotonin, histamine
Neuropeptides	Substance P, enkephalins, calcitonin gene-related peptide, somatostatin, vasoactive intestinal polypeptide, neuropeptide Y
Purines	ATP, adenosine
Lipid mediators	Endocannabinoids, prostaglandin E2
Trophic factors	Brain-derived neurotrophic factor, nerve growth factor, glial-derived neurotrophic factor
Cytokines and chemokines	Tumor necrosis factor-α, interleukin-1 β, ciliary neurotrophic factor
Gases	Nitric oxide, carbon monoxide
Extracellular matrix proteins	Laminin, thrombospondin

channels. All receptors of this family are pentamers formed by various combinations of subunits.[3,4] The second large family is that of ionotropic glutamate receptors and includes the α-amino-3-hydroxy-5-methyl-4 isoxazole propionic acid receptors (AMPARs), N-methyl-D-aspartate receptors (NMDARs) and kainate receptors (KARs). These receptors are permeable to Na^+, Ca^{2+}, or both, according to the receptor subtype. Ionotropic glutamate receptors are formed by combinations of four subunits.[5] The third family comprises the purinergic P2x receptors, which assemble in trimers, are primarily permeable to Ca^{2+}, and are activated by ATP.

Fast Synaptic Transmission

Activation of nAChRs, ionotropic glutamate receptors (primarily AMPARs and NMDARs), and serotonin 5-HT3 receptors triggers influx of Na^+ and Ca^{2+}, eliciting fast excitatory postsynaptic potentials (EPSPs). In contrast, activation of $GABA_A$ or glycine receptors elicits Cl^- influx in most adult neurons, resulting in membrane hyperpolarization and fast inhibitory postsynaptic potentials (IPSPs). However, the synaptic effects of the GABA and glycine receptors depends on the direction of Cl^- movement across the channels, which is determined by the transmembrane Cl^- gradient, determined by activity of the cation-chloride cotransporters.[6]

Scaffold Proteins and Clustering of Ionotropic Receptors

The efficacy of classical neurotransmission depends on the precise apposition of presynaptic release zones and postsynaptic receptors clustered at the site of neurotransmitter release. This requires structural interactions mediated by transsynaptic adhesion molecules, and binding of postsynaptic receptors to scaffold proteins, forming macromolecular complexes that interact with transsynaptic adhesion molecules, actin cytoskeleton, and downstream signaling molecules.[7,8] There are three classical examples of scaffold proteins that are critical for clustering of ionotropic receptors (Figure 16.3). Postsynaptic density protein of 95 kDa (PSD-95) is the major scaffold protein for clustering of ionotropic glutamate at excitatory synapses on dendritic spines. PSD-95 contains several functional domains that mediate interactions between glutamate receptor subunits and linker proteins, signal molecules, and transsynaptic adhesion molecules such as neuroligin 1. Gephyrin is the central scaffold protein required for clustering of $GABA_A$ and glycine receptors at inhibitory synapses.[9] Gephyrin interacts with specific subunits of these receptors, with neuroligin-2, and with the cytoskeleton. Rapsyn stabilizes the nAChRs at the neuromuscular junction. The precise apposition of the nAChRs clustered at the level of junctional folds and the presynaptic active zones involves the binding of agrin secreted by motor neuron terminals to low-density lipoprotein receptor-related protein 4; this results in activation of muscle-specific kinase (MUSK) and downstream of kinase-7 (Dock 7), followed by recruitment of rapsyn.[10]

Recycling of Ionotropic Receptors

The different subunits of ionotropic receptors, such as the AMPAR and $GABA_AR$, are synthesized and assembled in the endoplasmic reticulum (ER) and then enter the vesicular secretory pathway.[11] Assembled receptors undergo continuous trafficking between intercellular, extrasynaptic, and postsynaptic sites as they constantly switch between mobile and immobile states in the membrane (Figure 16.4). Receptor dynamics reflects the interplay between their lateral diffusion and their reversible binding to scaffolding proteins. Newly synthesized receptors are inserted in the membrane by constitutive exocytosis, undergo lateral diffusion to reach the synapse, become localized and stabilized at the postsynaptic membrane, and then undergo recycling by

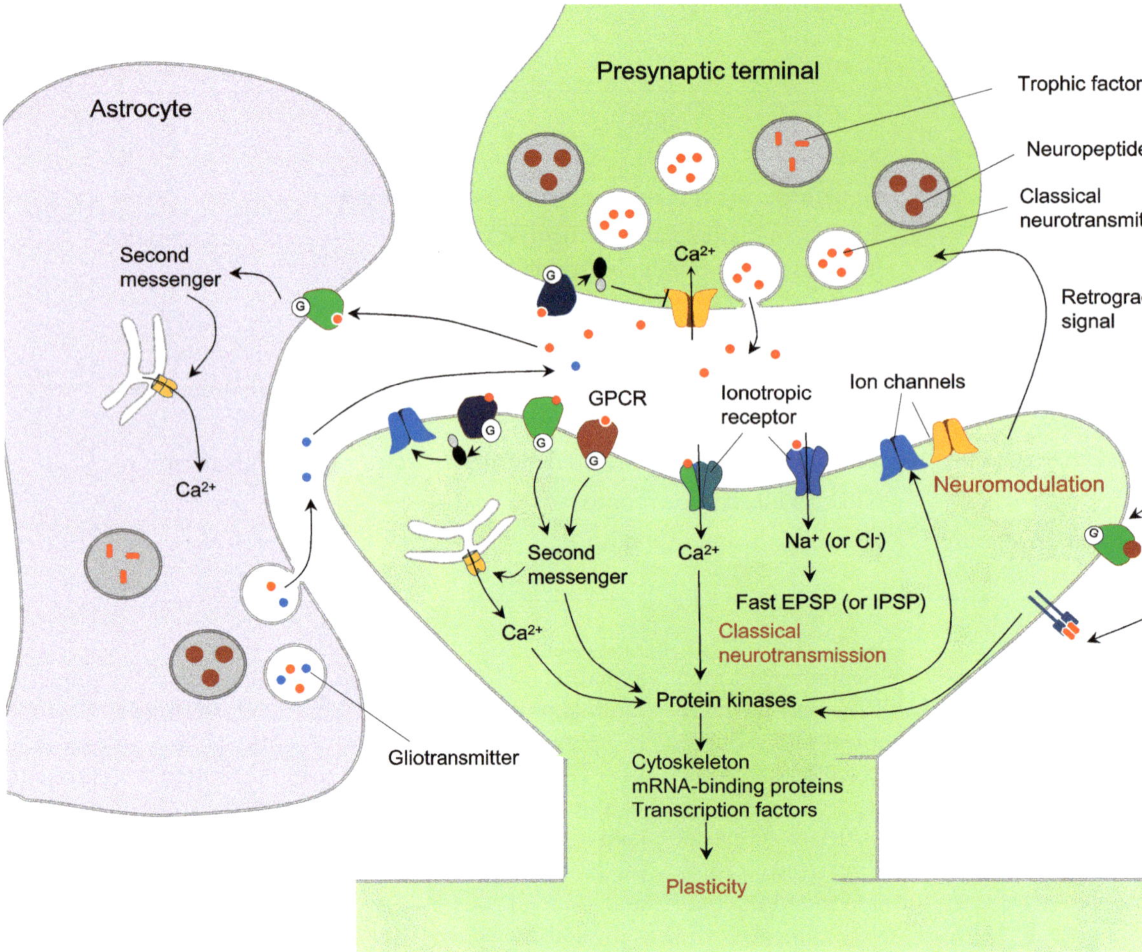

FIGURE 16.1 Overview of signaling in the central nervous system.
Chemical synapses are sites of bidirectional communication and involve a presynaptic terminal, postsynaptic target, and surrounding astrocytic process. Presynaptic terminals contain vesicles containing classical neurotransmitters and secretory granules containing neuropeptides or trophic factors. Classical neurotransmission involves the rapid release of neurotransmitters triggered by opening of voltage-gated calcium channels at presynaptic active zones and is mediated by neurotransmitter-gated cation (Na^+, Ca^+) or Cl^- channels, which respectively trigger fast excitatory postsynaptic potentials (EPSPs) or inhibitory postsynaptic potentials (IPSPs). Neuromodulation occurs at both postsynaptic and presynaptic levels via G protein-coupled receptors (GPCRs), which affect the function of ion channels via second-messenger-triggered phosphorylation or direct protein–protein interactions. Presynaptic modulation affects the availability of synaptic vesicles and activation of presynaptic voltage-gated Ca^{2+} channels. Postsynaptic modulation depends on the opening probability of potassium (K^+) channels. Many chemical signals diffuse from the synapse to the extracellular space to act on extrasynaptic receptors located at a distance from the release sites by a mechanism known as volume transmission. These signals also participate in reciprocal interactions between neurons and astrocytes. Synaptic plasticity may be triggered by Ca^{2+} influx via ionotropic receptors, second-messenger cascades triggered by GPCRs, retrograde signals from the postsynaptic targets, and effects of growth factors and cytokines.

endocytosis. Receptors that do not interact with their scaffold remain located outside the synapse, becoming extrasynaptic receptors, and are activated by neurotransmitters that have spilled over from the synapse upon escaping reuptake. The number of ionotropic receptors at the postsynaptic membrane is tightly regulated by phosphorylation of receptor subunits, which controls their relative rates of exocytosis and endocytosis.

Calcium Influx and Downstream Signals for Synaptic Modulation and Plasticity

Activation of ionotropic glutamate receptors triggers influx of Ca^{2+}, which has profound downstream effects on synaptic function. Calcium influx occurs both via NMDARs and through voltage-gated Ca^{2+} channels activated by depolarization. Calcium binds to calmodulin (CaM), which is a fundamental mediator of synaptic plasticity

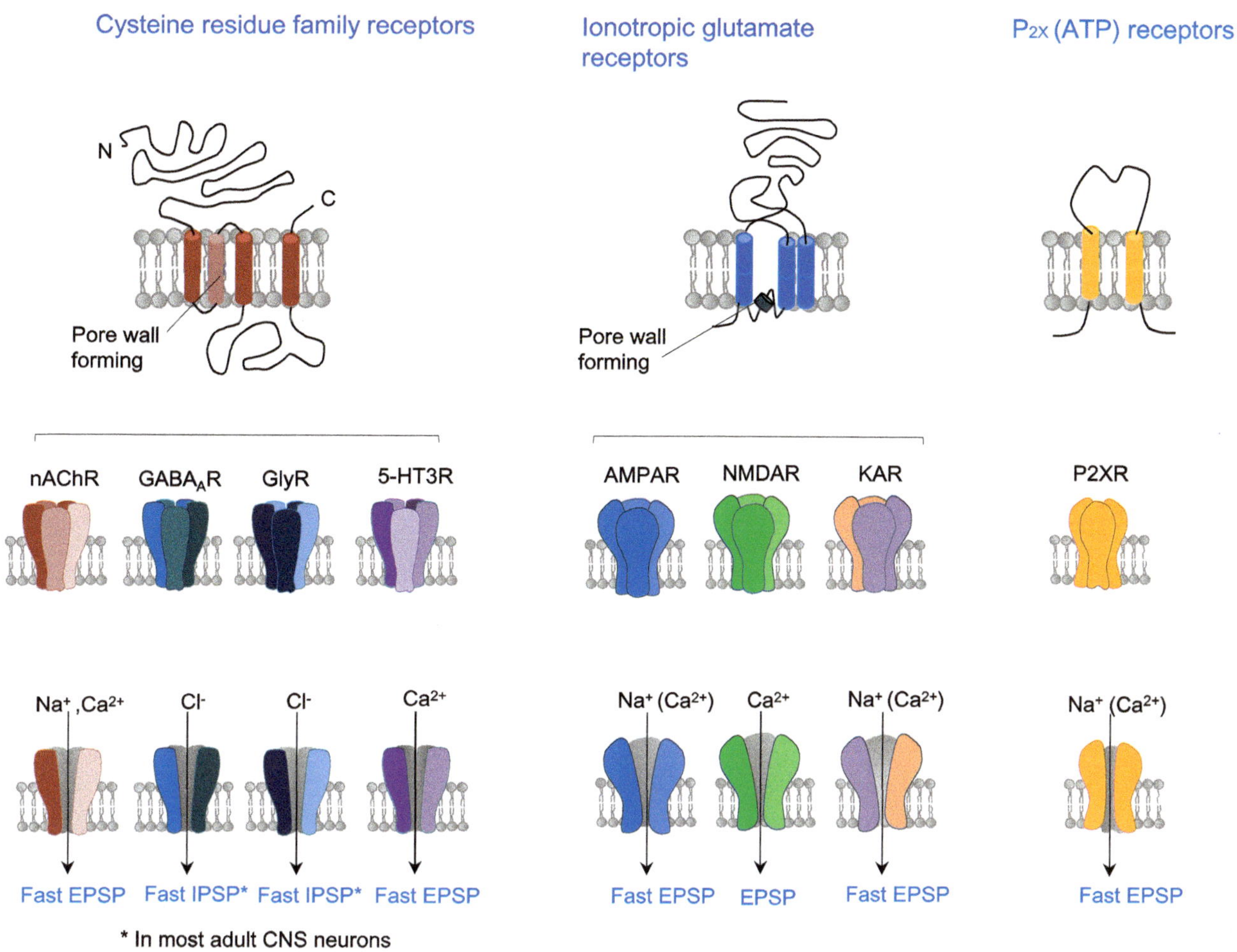

FIGURE 16.2 Structure and effects of ionotropic receptors.
Ionotropic receptors are subdivided into three families. The cysteine loop-rich family includes the nicotinic acetyl choline receptors (nAChRs), which are permeable to Na^+ and Ca^{2+}; the $GABA_A$ receptor and the glycine receptors, which are permeable to Cl^- (and bicarbonate); and the serotonin 5-hydroxytryptamine $(5\text{-HT})_3$ receptors, which are Ca^{2+} channels. The second family is that of the ionotropic glutamate receptors, which include the AMPA (α-amino-3-hydroxy-5-methyl-4 isoxazole propionic acid) receptors (AMPARs), kainate receptors (KARs), and NMDA (N-methyl-D-aspartate), receptors which are permeable to Na^+, Ca^{2+}, or both according to the receptor subtype. The third family comprises the purinergic P2x receptors, which assemble in trimers, are primarily permeable to Ca^{2+}, and are activated by ATP. Activation of nAChRs, ionotropic glutamate receptors (primarily AMPAR and NMDARs), and serotonin 5-HT3 receptors triggers influx of Na^+ and Ca^{2+}, eliciting fast excitatory postsynaptic potentials (EPSPs). In contrast, activation of $GABA_A$ receptors or glycine receptors elicits Cl^- influx in most adult neurons, resulting in membrane hyperpolarization or fast inhibitory postsynaptic potentials (IPSPs).

and modulation. According to the magnitude of the Ca^{2+} signal, CaM may activate CaM kinase (CaMK) II, leading to protein phosphorylation, or the phosphatase calcineurin, leading to protein dephosphorylation. Calcium also mediates a crosstalk between different signal transduction pathways downstream of GPCR activation.

NEUROMODULATION

Neuromodulation refers to the mechanisms by which neurochemical signals influence the efficacy of synaptic transmission. Presynaptic modulation affects the probability of neurotransmitter release, which depends on the availability of synaptic vesicles at release zones and the state of activity of presynaptic $Ca_v2.1$ (P/Q-type) and $Ca_v2.2$ (N-type) voltage-gated Ca^{2+} channels. Postsynaptic modulation determines the responsiveness of the postsynaptic target to excitatory or inhibitory signals and depends on the opening probability of potassium (K^+) channels that control cell excitability. Both presynaptic and postsynaptic modulations are mediated by GPCRs. Activation of GPCRs affects the function of Na^+, Ca^{2+}, or K^+ channels either via second-messenger-triggered phosphorylation or

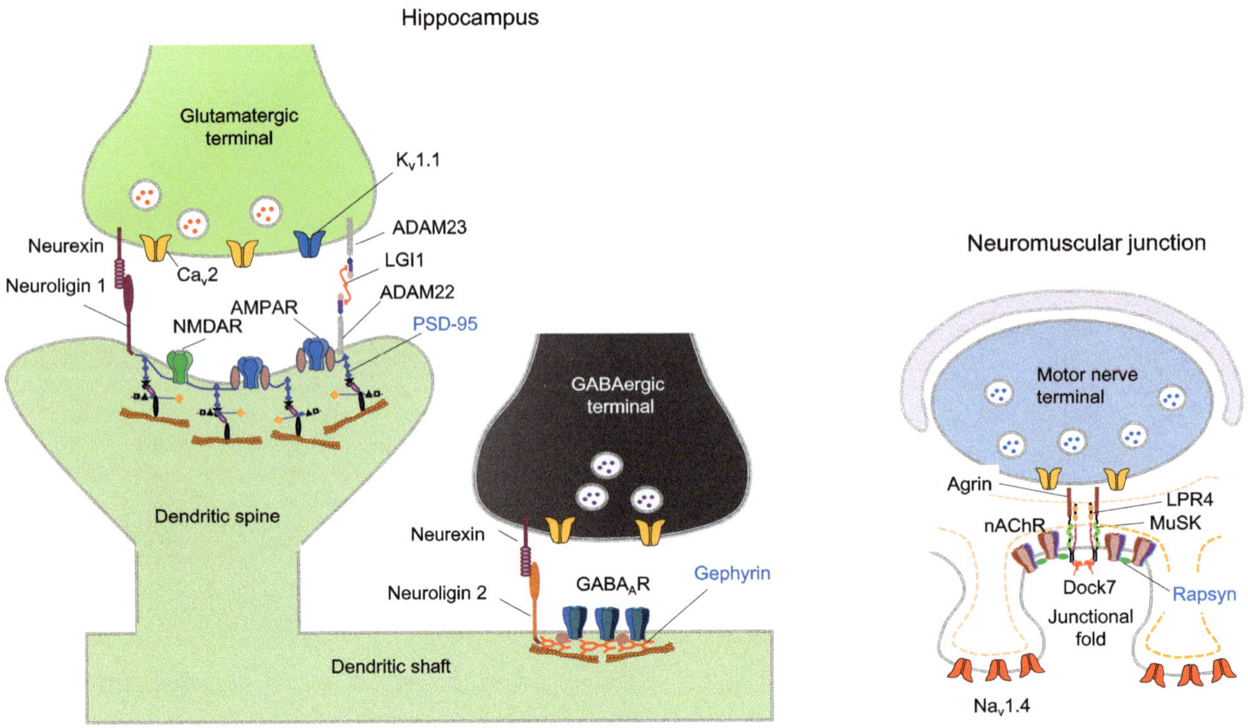

FIGURE 16.3 Clustering of postsynaptic ionotropic receptors.
The efficacy of classical neurotransmission depends on the precise apposition of presynaptic release zones and postsynaptic receptors. Postsynaptic density protein of 95 kDa (PSD 95) is the major scaffold protein in excitatory synapses. Gephyrin is the central scaffold required for clustering of $GABA_A$ and glycine receptors at inhibitory synapses. At the neuromuscular junction, the precise apposition of the nAChRs clustered at the level of junctional folds and the presynaptic active zones involve the adhesion the extracellular matrix protein agrin secreted by a motor neuron terminals, its binding to low-density lipoprotein receptor-related protein 4 (LRP4), activation of muscle specific kinase MUSK) and downstream of kinase-7 (Dock 7), and recruitment ofrapsyn.

via direct protein–protein interactions at the level of the membrane.

Neuromodulatory Signals

Several chemical signals released from neurons and glial cells have modulatory effect at presynaptic and postsynaptic levels, acting via many subtypes of GPCRs. They include glutamate and GABA via their respective metabotropic receptors; acetylcholine via muscarinic receptors; monoamines; neuropeptides; purines; and lipid mediators (Table 16.2). There is both divergence and convergence of neuromodulatory signals. A single neurotransmitter may exert different effects via different GPCR subtypes. Different neurotransmitters, acting via their respective GPCR, may exert similar cellular effects via common G protein-triggered downstream signal transduction cascades (Table 16.3). Postsynaptic neurons may release chemical signals that provides a retrograde message affecting the release of neurotransmitter from the presynaptic terminal. These signals include nitric oxide (NO), endocannabinoids, arachidonic acid and prostaglandins, growth factors, cytokines, and steroids. Neurotransmitters that escape reuptake or hydrolysis at the synaptic cleft may diffuse via the extracellular fluid to affect extrasynaptic receptors located at a distance from their site of release. Via this mechanism, known as volume transmission, neurochemical signals participate in coordination of neuronal networks, reciprocal paracrine neuron–glia and glia–glia interactions among astrocytes, oligodendrocytes, and microglia, and control of local metabolism and cerebral blood flow.

Downstream Transduction for Neuromodulation

As GPCRs for many neurotransmitters share similar downstream signal transduction pathways, the selectivity of neurotransmitter action is largely determined by the distribution of receptors and the type of target cells (Figure 16.5). GPCRs coupled to $G\alpha_s/G\alpha_{olf}$ family proteins stimulate membrane-bound adenylyl cyclase, leading to production of cyclic adenosine monophosphate (cAMP), which directly modulates hyperpolarization-gated cation channels and activates protein kinase A (PKA), which targets membrane receptors, ion channels, cytoskeletal proteins, phosphatase inhibitors, and transcription factors. Several neurotransmitter receptors influence synaptic excitability

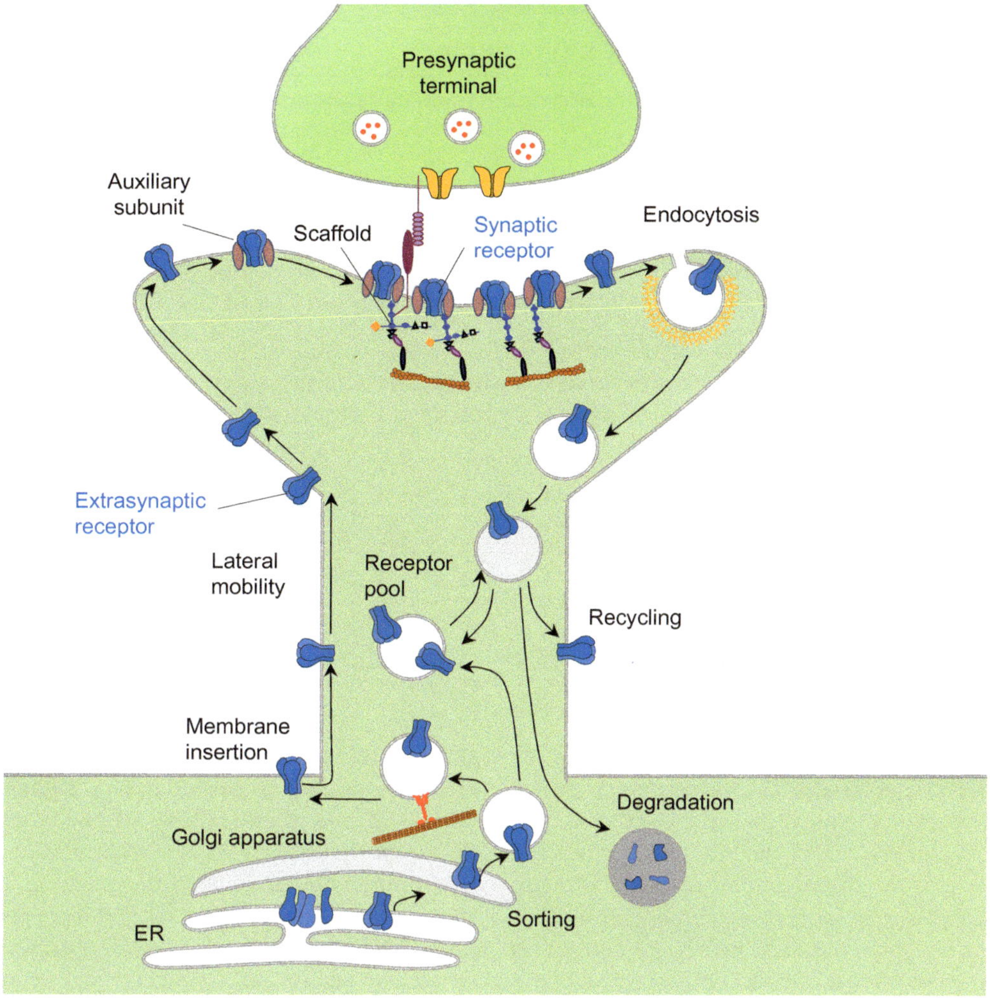

FIGURE 16.4 Recycling of ionotropic receptors.
The different subunits of ionotropic receptors are synthesized and assembled in the endoplasmic reticulum (ER) and then enter the vesicular secretory pathway. Newly synthesized receptors are inserted in the membrane by constitutive exocytosis, undergo lateral diffusion to reach the synapse, are localized and stabilized at the postsynaptic membrane, and are recycled via endocytosis. Receptors are stabilized at synaptic sites via interactions with scaffold proteins, either directly or via accessory subunits. The number of ionotropic receptors at the postsynaptic membrane is tightly regulated by phosphorylation of receptor subunits, which controls their relative rates of exocytosis and endocytosis, which may occur via clathrin-mediated and other mechanisms. Once in the endosomes, receptors may be recycled back or targeted for degradation by the lysosomes.

and plasticity via this pathway (Table 16.3). Typical examples are the dopamine the D1 receptor (D1R) and the norepinephrine β adrenergic receptor. Ligand binding to GPCRs coupled to $G\alpha_{i/o}$ leads to inhibition of adenylyl cyclase via the $G\alpha_{i/o}$ subunit and dissociation of the βγ subunit complex, which directly interacts with membrane ion channels. The major effects are activation of G protein-activated inward-rectifying K^+ channels (GIRKs), leading to reduced neuronal excitability, and inhibition of presynaptic voltage-gated Ca^{2+} channels, resulting in inhibition of neurotransmitter release (Figure 16.5). Some important examples are $GABA_B$, muscarinic M2, dopamine D2, norepinephrine α2, serotonin 5-HT1, opioid, and cannabinoid CB1 receptors (Table 16.3). Activation of receptors coupled to G_q family proteins leads to activation of phospholipase C (PLC), which hydrolyzes membrane phosphatidylinositol 4,5 bisphosphate (PIP2), yielding diacylglycerol (DAG) and inositol triphosphate (IP_3) (Figure 16.5). Since PIP2 is important for function of K^+ channels, activation of this pathway typically reduces K^+ currents and increase cell excitability. Inositol triphosphate binds to IP_3 receptors (IP_3R, ITPR) in the ER, leading to Ca^{2+} release; DAG together with Ca^{2+} activates protein kinase C (PKC), which acts on several targets and has a major role

TABLE 16.2 *Examples of G protein-Coupled Receptors*

Neurotransmitter/Other Signal	GPCR Type/Family
L-glutamate	Metabotropic glutamate receptors (mGluRs) types I, II, III
GABA	$GABA_B$
Acetylcholine	Muscarinic (M), M1 and M2
Dopamine	D1 and D2
Norepinephrine	α (alpha)1, α2, $\beta_{1\text{-}3}$
Serotonin	5-hydroxytryptamine (5-HT)1, 5-HT2, 5-HT4–7
Histamine	H1, H2, H3
Neuropeptides	Several, according to the neuropeptide; e.g., neurokinin 1 (substance P), mu opioid receptors, Y2 (neuropeptide Y), etc.
Purines	A1 and A2 (adenosine) P2Y (ATP)
Endocannabinoids	CB1, CB2

in synaptic plasticity. Diacylglycerol is also a substrate for synthesis of endocannabinoids.

Receptor Mosaics

Whereas GPCRs in general act as monomers, metabotropic glutamate receptors (mGluRs) and $GABA_B$ receptors are obligatory dimers; one of the monomers binds the neurotransmitter and the other couples to the G protein. Many types of GPCRs may form heterodimers with other receptors or form receptor mosaics, which are defined as the assembly of receptors that interact both physically and functionally, so that one receptor modulates via allosteric mechanisms the features of another receptor (s) of the assembly.[12–17] One important example is that of dopamine receptors. Whereas D1Rs are coupled to $G_{s/olf}$ signaling and D2 receptors (D2Rs) with $G_{i/o}$ signaling, the D1R/D2R heterodimer is coupled to $G_{q/11}$ signaling. The interactions within heteromers may also be antagonistic. For example, in the case of D2R/adenosine $A2_A$ receptor ($A2_AR$) heterodimers in neurons of the striatum, the downstream effects of dopamine acting via D2Rs coupled to $G_{i/o}$ inhibition of the adenylyl cyclase–cAMP pathway is antagonized by those of adenosine, acting via $A2_A$Rs coupled to $G_{s/olf}$ signaling activating this pathway.

TABLE 16.3 *Signaling Mechanisms of G Protein-Coupled Receptors*

G Protein	$G\alpha_s$/ $G\alpha_{olf}$	$G\alpha_i$/ $G\alpha_o$	$G\alpha_q$
Transduction	Adenylyl cyclase (AC)-cyclic AMP Protein kinase A-PKA	Inhibition of AC GIRK K^+ channel activation Ca_v2 inhibition	Phospholipase C/DAG/ IP_3 Inhibition of Kir Protein kinase C Intracellular Ca^{2+}
Receptor subtype (examples)	Dopamine D1 Adrenergic β Serotonin 5HT4–7 Histamine H2 Adenosine A2 Vasopressin V2 Calcitonin receptor-like receptor (CALCRL)	Dopamine D2 Adrenergic α2 Serotonin 5HT1 Histamine H3 Adenosine A1 Muscarinic M2 $GABA_B$ mGluR II, III Opioid CB1 cannabinoid Neuropeptide Y	Adrenergic α1 Serotonin 5HT2 Histamine H1 Muscarinic M1 mGluR 1, mGluR5 Neurokinin 1 Orexin 1 Vasopressin V1 Oxytocin

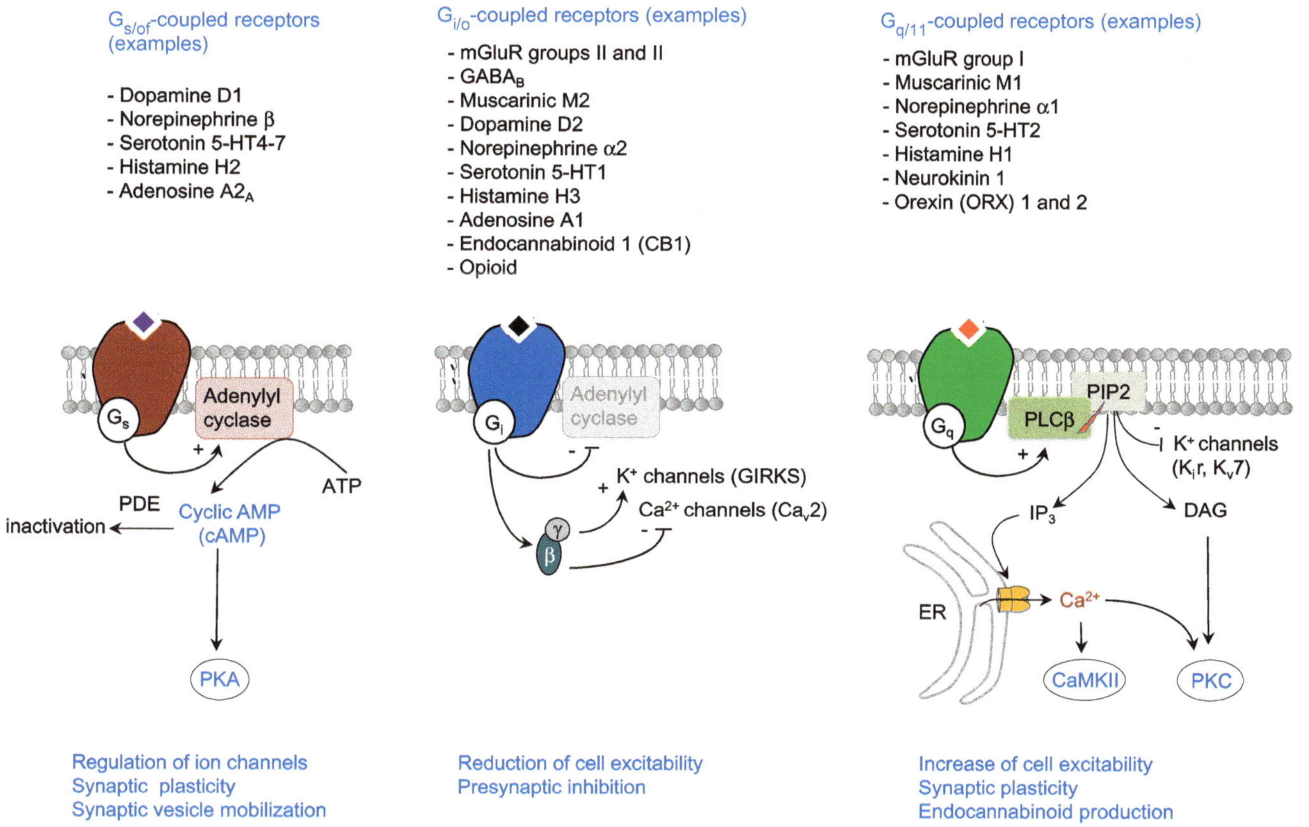

FIGURE 16.5 Canonical transduction cascades form G protein-coupled receptors.
A single neurotransmitter may trigger different signaling cascades acting via different G protein-coupled receptors (GPCRs); several neurotransmitters may trigger similar downstream transduction signals via GPCRs coupled to the same class of G protein. Proteins of the $G\alpha_s$ family, including $G\alpha_s$ and $G\alpha_{olf}$, stimulate membrane-bound adenylyl cyclase, which catalyzes the formation of cyclic adenosine monophosphate (cAMP) from ATP. The major downstream signal is protein kinase A (PKA), which phosphorylates several targets. Cyclic AMP also binds to and modulates cyclic nucleotide-gated channels. The cAMP signal is terminated by its hydrolysis by cAMP phosphodiesterases (PDEs). Ligand binding to GPCRs coupled to $G\alpha_{i/o}$ leads to inhibition of adenylyl cyclase via the $G\alpha_{i/o}$ subunit and dissociation of the βγ subunit complex, which directly activate G protein-activated inward-rectifying K^+ channels (GIRKs), leading to reduced neuronal excitability and inhibition of presynaptic voltage-gated Ca^{2+} channels, resulting in inhibition of neurotransmitter release. Activation of receptors coupled to G_q family proteins leads to activation of phospholipase C (PLC), which hydrolyzes membrane phosphatidylinositol 4,5 bisphosphate (PIP2), yielding diacylglycerol (DAG) and inositol triphosphate (IP_3) Since PIP2 is important for function of K^+ channels activation of this pathway typically results in reduced K^+ currents and increased cell excitability. Inositol triphosphate binds to IP3 receptors (IP_3R, ITPR) in the endoplasmic reticulum (ER), leading to Ca^{2+} release; DAG together with Ca^{2+} activates protein kinase C (PKC), which acts on several targets and has a major role in synaptic plasticity.

Non-G-Protein-Mediated Effects of G Protein-Coupled Receptors

GPCRs may trigger signal transduction cascades independently of their interactions with G proteins. Upon phosphorylation by GPCR kinases, the GPCR dissociates from the G protein and recruits the scaffold protein β-arrestin, which recruits signaling complexes to mediate non-G-protein-mediated signaling. For example, activation of D2Rs promotes long-term depression of glutamatergic synapses via a noncanonical transduction pathway that involves β2-arrestin and activation of the protein phosphatase calcineurin, which leads to inhibition of PKA and its downstream signaling pathways.

Cotransmitters and Retrograde Signals for Neuromodulation

Neurons frequently produce more than one neuromodulatory signal.[1] Important examples are neuropeptides synthesized in the cell body, stored in secretory vesicles, and reaching the synaptic terminal via axon transport, and signals such as endocannabinoids or NO that are produced locally on demand at the presynaptic terminal, are not stored in vesicles, and can diffuse retrogradely to exert presynaptic modulation. ATP may function as a classical transmitter released from synaptic or other vesicles and is a precursor of adenosine, which acts as a synaptic modulator. Many cotransmitters and local signals participate in reciprocal neuron–glia interactions as well as interactions between different types of glial cells. These signals also have vasoactive effects, thereby contributing to local control of cerebral blood flow.

NEUROPEPTIDES

Neuropeptides are abundant in the central and peripheral nervous systems.[18] Central peptidergic neurons are organized into two main systems: diffuse projection systems from the hypothalamus, amygdala, and brainstem, and local or short projection neurons located throughout the central nervous system. In the periphery, neuropeptides are abundant in a subpopulation of small dorsal root ganglion neurons and in autonomic neurons.

Neuropeptide Signaling

Neuropeptides are members of several families. Unlike classical neurotransmitters, neuropeptides are synthesized in the cell bodies from messenger RNA (mRNA) as precursors (prepropeptides), undergo posttranslational modification within the ER and Golgi apparatus, and are transported in large dense vesicles to the synaptic terminal by fast anterograde axonal transport (Figure 16.6). The release of neuropeptides is not restricted to active zones, but is also triggered by large Ca^{2+} influx primarily via channels distributed throughout the presynaptic terminal. In many central and peripheral neurons, neuropeptides coexist with classical neurotransmitters (such as GABA or monoamines). In these neurons, the pattern of presynaptic synaptic activity determines the relative proportion of classical neurotransmitter and neuropeptide released; low-frequency firing releases the classical neurotransmitter and high-frequency burst firing releases both the classical neurotransmitter and the neuropeptide. This is referred to as frequency-dependent chemical coding. Neuropeptides act via postsynaptic, presynaptic, and extrasynaptic GPCRs, and their action is terminated by hydrolysis by extracellular

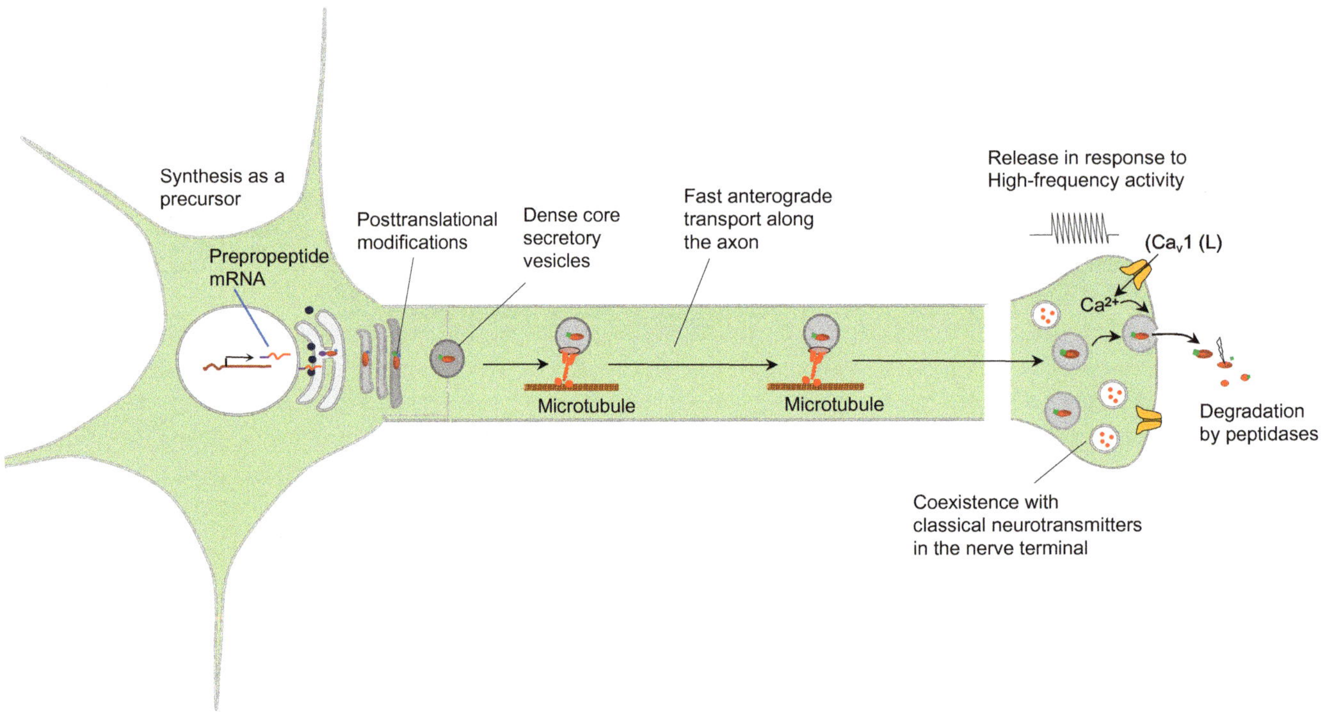

FIGURE 16.6 Main features of neuropeptides as neurotransmitters.
Neuropeptides are synthesized in the cell bodies from messenger RNA (mRNA) as precursors (prepropeptides), undergo posttranslational modification within the endoplasmic reticulum and Golgi apparatus, and are transported in large dense vesicles to the synaptic terminal by fast anterograde axonal transport. The release of neuropeptides is not restricted to active zones, but is also triggered by large Ca^{2+} influx via channels distributed throughout the presynaptic terminal. In many central and peripheral neurons, neuropeptides coexist with classical neurotransmitters. In these neurons, low-frequency firing releases the classical neurotransmitter and high-frequency burst firing releases both the classical neurotransmitter the neuropeptide. Neuropeptides act via postsynaptic, presynaptic, and extrasynaptic GPCRs, and their action is terminated by hydrolysis by extracellular peptidases.

peptidases. Several neuropeptides exert profound neuromodulatory action in the nervous system. Many of these neuropeptides affect glial cells and blood vessels (Table 16.4). A comprehensive review of neuropeptide systems is beyond the scope of this chapter, and only few examples will be emphasized here.

Calcitonin Gene-Related Peptide

Calcitonin gene related peptide (CGRP) derives from the calcitonin–CGRP gene (*CALCA*) precursor, follows the secretory pathway, and following its release is degraded by metalloproteinase. CGRP is expressed in a subgroup of neurons in the dorsal root ganglion, trigeminal, and vagal ganglia that respond to noxious, thermal, or visceral input. CGRP is also present in ascending pathways from the parabrachial nuclear complex to the thalamus, basal forebrain, and amygdala. The CGRP receptor is a heterodimeric complex formed by the GPCR calcitonin receptor-like receptor (CALCRL), which is coupled to G_s-cAMP-PKA signaling and receptor activity-modifying protein 1 (RAMP1), which affects receptor pharmacology and cell trafficking.[19] The CGRP receptor complex also includes two cytoplasmic proteins (receptor component protein) that associate with the CALCRL–RAMP1 heterodimer to mediate signal transduction. CGRP can also be released antidromically in the periphery, eliciting vasodilatation as a component of neurogenic inflammation and is thus involved in the pathophysiology of inflammatory and neuropathic pain. Release of CGRP both at the trigeminovascular junction and at the dura is a major mechanism of migraine. Presynaptic 5-$HT1_B$/

TABLE 16.4 *Representative Neuropeptide Systems*

Neuropeptide	Distribution	Receptor (G protein)	Main function (s)
Opioids (β endorphin, enkephalin, dynorphin)	Hypothalamus Forebrain, brainstem, spinal and peripheral autonomic and pain modulatory systems	μ (mu, MOR) δ (delta, DOR) and κ (kappa, KOR) Coupled to Gi/o	Supraspinal and spinal inhibitory pain modulation Autonomic and endocrine control
Somatostatin	Hypothalamus GABAergic interneurons	Coupled to Gi/o	Synaptic inhibition Inhibits release of GH and other hormones
Neuropeptide Y	Hypothalamus GABAergic interneurons Sympathetic noradrenergic terminals Amygdala	Y1, Y2, Y3 Coupled to Gi/o	Increases appetite Sympathoexcitation Anxiolytic
Substance P	Primary nociceptive and visceroceptive afferents	Neurokinin 1 (NK1) Coupled to Gq/11	Thermal pain Visceral sensation Pain plasticity Increased motoneuron excitability
Calcitonin gene-related peptide	Primary nociceptive and visceroceptive afferents Central nociceptive, visceroceptive, and arousal pathways	CALCRL-RAMP1 Coupled to Gs	Vasodilation Pain sensitization Arousal Appetite suppression
Orexin (hypocretin)	Lateral hypothalamus	ORX1 and ORX Coupled to Gq/11	Maintenance of arousal Stress response Motivation
Oxytocin	Hypothalamic magnocellular and parvicellular neurons	OXT Couple to Gq/11	Social behavior Milk ejection
Arginine vasopressin (antidiuretic hormone)	Hypothalamic magnocellular and parvicellular neurons	V1 (coupled to Gq/11) V2 (coupled to Gs)	Antidiuresis Increases blood pressure Stress response Circadian regulation

5-HT1$_D$ receptors (targeted by the classical triptans) and 5-HT1$_F$ receptor (targeted by lasmiditan) reduce CGRP release and are thus used for treatment of acute migraine attacks. Several small-molecule antagonists of the CGRP receptor complex, collectively referred to as gepants, potently and selectively block CGRP responses and are effective in patients with migraine. They include olcegepant, telcagepant, and ubrogepant. Anti-CGRP antibodies, such as galcanezumab, eptinezumab, and fremanezumab proved effective for the prevention of episodic and chronic migraine. Erenumab is a human monoclonal antibody against a fusion protein of the extracellular domains of human CALCRL and RAMP1 and is also an effective prophylactic therapy for episodic and chronic migraine.[19] Brainstem inputs to the forebrain have relevance for mechanisms of pain modulation and are also relevant to the pathophysiology of migraine.[20,21] In addition, CGRP inputs from the parabrachial nucleus have an important role in satiety,[22] and those to the basal forebrain mediate hypercapnia-induced arousal.[23]

Substance P

Substance P is a major neuropeptide cotransmitter in a subpopulation of primary nociceptive neurons projecting to the dorsal horn and autonomic and enteric ganglia. In the CNS, substance P is also distributed in several brainstem and forebrain areas, including a subpopulation of projection neurons in the striatum, amygdala, hippocampus, and medullary raphe. Substance P elicits both postsynaptic and presynaptic excitation via neurokinin-1 receptors (NK1Rs) coupled to G_q signaling, resulting in depolarization and intracellular Ca^{2+} release. The NK1R is expressed in many areas of the CNS, including lamina 1 nociceptive spinothalamic neurons in the dorsal horn and striatum, and may also function as an autoreceptor. Substance P acting via NK1R in spinothalamic neurons has a major role in promoting synaptic plasticity resulting in central sensitization. In the periphery, substance P also activates the Mas-related GPCR (Mrgrp)X2 in mast cells leading to release of proinflammatory cytokines. Experimental studies indicate that substance P acting via NK1R may have a role in epileptogenesis, in part by promoting glutamatergic neurotransmission.[24]

Endogenous Opioids

Endogenous opioids consists of three families: proopiomelanocortin (POMC), which is the precursor of β-endorphin; preproenkephalin, which is the precursor of leucine- and methionine-enkephalins; and preprodynorphin, which is the precursor of dynorphins.[25] Neurons synthesizing POMC are restricted to the arcuate (infundibular) nucleus of the hypothalamus and project mostly to limbic and brainstem regions. Other opioids are expressed, to different extents, in local neurons at multiple levels of the CNS, including the components of the pain modulatory, reward, and autonomic systems. The opioid receptor family includes the mu receptor (μ receptor, MOR), delta receptor (δ receptor, DOR), and kappa receptor (κ receptor, KOR). These receptors are expressed primarily in the cerebral cortex, limbic system, brainstem, and spinal cord, particularly the dorsal horn and primary sensory afferents. These receptors are coupled to $G_{i/o}$ signaling and elicit pre- and postsynaptic inhibition. In some areas, such as the periaqueductal gray involved in central pain modulation and ventral tegmental area involved in reward responses, opioids target local GABAergic neurons, thereby disinhibiting projection neurons. This underlies the central mechanism of opioid-triggered analgesia and addictive behavior.

Other Peptides with Potential Relevance in Neurologic Disorders

Oxytocin (OXT) and arginine vasopressin (AVP) function both as circulating hormones and as neuropeptides in the central nervous system. Circulating AVP has a major role in mechanisms of water homeostasis and blood pressure control and OXT in parturition and lactation. Both OXT and AVP have been referred to as "social" neuropeptides as they have a highly conserved role as mediators of complex social cognition and interactions in both animals and humans. OXT also exerts anxiolytic and antidepressant effects whereas AVP promotes anxiety and stress response. Oxytocin appears to improve social aspects of cognition and behavioral symptoms in individuals with frontotemporal dementia.[26] In addition, AVP produced in this suprachiasmatic nucleus has a major role in circadian regulation. Neuropeptide tyrosine (neuropeptide Y, NPY) is widely expressed in the central and peripheral nervous systems and has been shown to have a role in numerous physiological processes, including modulation of cortical excitability, circadian rhythms, stress response and emotion, pain processing, food intake, and cardiovascular function. NPY has been implicated in mechanisms of epilepsy, pain and analgesia, anxiety, and depression. All NPY receptors (Y1–Y5) are $G_{i/o}$ coupled inhibitory receptors. There is upregulation of NPY expression in the dorsal root ganglion following peripheral nerve injury. Both Y1R and Y2R are expressed in nociceptive peptidergic afferents and in interneurons in the dorsal horn and may have an antinociceptive effect.[27] Neuropeptide Y is expressed in a subpopulation of GABAergic interneurons in the hippocampus and neocortex. There is upregulation of NPY receptors in experimental models on epilepsy. Intrahippocamapal administration of recombinant adeno-associated viral vectors encoding NPY and Y2 receptor genes reduced seizure frequency in a model of medial temporal lobe seizures.[28]

RETROGRADE SIGNALS

Endocannabinoids

Endocannabinoids derive from membrane phospholipids and are released on demand in response to increase in intracellular Ca^{2+} in the soma and dendrites. Triggers include depolarization or glutamatergic inputs acting via GPCRs coupled to $G_{q/11}$ signaling and activation of PLC leading to production of DAG and IP_3.[29] The two major endocannabinoids in the nervous system are 2-arachydonoyl glycerol (2-AG) and N-arachidonoyl ethanolamine (anandamide) (Figure 16.7). In the CNS, these endocannabinoids primarily act via presynaptic cannabinoid type 1 receptors (CB1Rs) coupled to $G_{i/o}$ inhibitory signaling. For example, 2-AG synthesized and released in response to activation of group I metabotropic glutamate receptors (mGluRs) functions as a retrograde messenger that inhibits neurotransmitter release via presynaptic CB1Rs in both GABAergic and glutamatergic synapses. At glutamatergic synapses the negative feedback mediated by 2AG may act as a "synaptic circuit breaker." Endocannabinoids also act via CB1Rs in astrocytes and oligodendrocytes and cannabinoid type 2 receptors (CB2Rs) that are primarily expressed in microglia but also very scarcely in neurons. In addition to CB1R and CB2Rs, anandamide is a full agonist of transient receptor potential vanilloid type 1 (TRPV1) channels and thus participates in nociceptive processing as well as rapid signaling and synaptic plasticity. The endocannabinoid system has been implicated in wide range of disorders,

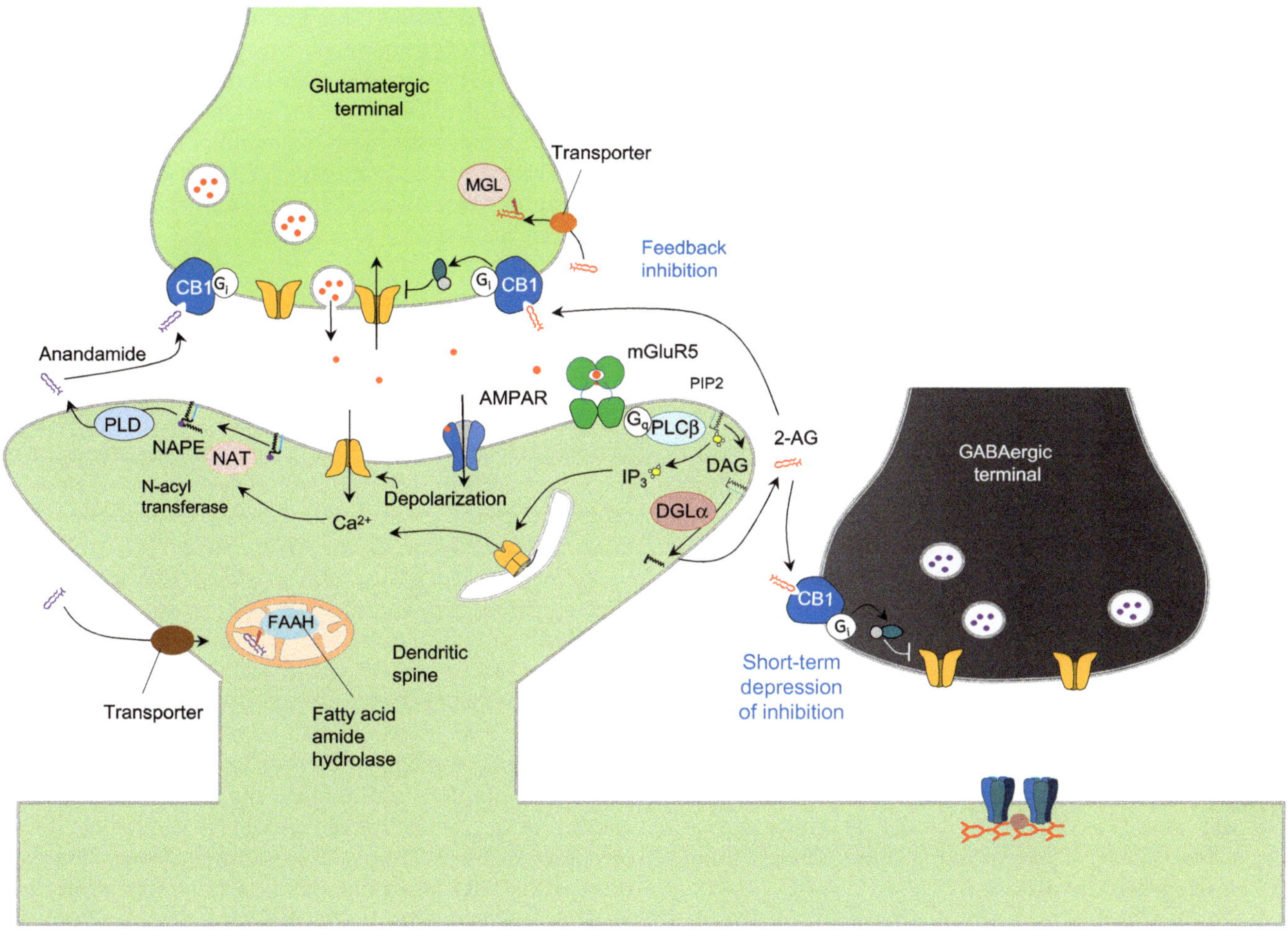

FIGURE 16.7 Endocannabinoid signaling.
Endocannabinoids derive from membrane phospholipids and are released in response to increase in intracellular Ca^{2+} or activation of G protein-coupled receptors that activate phospholipase, leading to production of diacylglycerol (DAG) and inositol triphosphate (IP_3). The two major endocannabinoids in the nervous system are 2-arachydonoyl glycerol (2-AG), synthesized from DAG via the DAG lipase, and N-arachidonoyl ethanolamine (anandamide), synthesized by a pathway that involves the action of N-acetyltransferase with formation of N-acetyl phosphatidyl ethanolamine (NAPE) and its hydrolysis by phospholipase D (PLD). Following release, 2-AG is transported into neurons and subsequently inactivated by the enzyme monoacylglycerol lipase located at the presynaptic membrane. Anandamide is transported into postsynaptic terminals and undergoes hydrolysis by a fatty acid amide hydrolase (FAAH) located in mitochondria and other organelles in dendritic spines. In the CNS endocannabinoids primarily act via cannabinoid type 1 receptors (CB1Rs) coupled to $G_{i/o}$ inhibitory signaling.

including neurodegenerative disorders such as Parkinson disease, multiple sclerosis, seizures, glioma, and others. Cannabidiol, the major nonpsychoactive cannabis ingredient does not act via CB1Rs or CB2Rs but has many other potential mechanisms of action, including modulation of intracellular Ca^{2+} via its effects on a variety of ion channels and transporters. Cannabidiol may enhance GABA activity and is approved for treatment of seizures in Lennox-Gastaut syndrome and Dravet syndrome.

Nitric Oxide

Nitric oxide is a gaseous neurotransmitter that may have physiological, neuroprotective, or deleterious actions depending on the site, concentration, and duration of its effects.[30] Nitric oxide is produced from L-arginine by the nitric oxide synthase (NOS), which includes neuronal, endothelial, and inducible isoforms. Neuronal and endothelial NOS are constitutively expressed and generate low levels of NO for short periods of time; inducible NOS is activated by proinflammatory cytokines, and may generate high NO levels for prolonged periods of time. The primary trigger of NO production in the CNS is Ca^{2+} influx via NMDARs, which form a functional macromolecular complex with nNOS and CaM at the postsynaptic density (Figure 16.8). Nitric oxide reacts with other radicals such as superoxide ions and lipid radicals and activates cytosolic guanylyl cyclase, leading to the formation of cGMP, which activates both protein kinase G (PKG) and cyclic nucleotide-gated channels. Downstream effects of PKG include inhibition of Ca^{2+} release from intracellular stores and regulation of downstream protein kinases, phosphodiesterases, ion channels, and transcription factors. By these mechanisms, NO acts as an activity-dependent retrograde signal that is important for plasticity of both glutamatergic and GABAergic synapses. Nitric oxide has potent vasodilator action and has a major role in coupling between neuronal activity and local blood flow (functional hyperemia). Under physiological conditions, mild activation of NMDARs located at postsynaptic sites drives the production of physiological levels of NO, sufficient to maintain normal synaptic plasticity and survival. In contrast, excessive activation of extrasynaptic NMDARs results in excessive production of NO, contributing to the pathophysiology of neurodegenerative diseases.

PURINES

Adenosine triphosphate (ATP) and its metabolite adenosine may act both as neurotransmitters and neuromodulators in the central and peripheral nervous systems.[1]

ATP as a Neurotransmitter and Paracrine Signal

ATP is incorporated into synaptic and secretory vesicles via a chloride-dependent vesicular nucleotide transporter. In some synaptic terminals ATP can be co-stored and co-released with other neurotransmitters. ATP is also released from astrocytes and mediates their interactions with neurons, with other astrocytes, and with microglia. The effects of ATP are mediated by ionotropic P2X and metabotropic P2Y receptors. The P2X receptors are cation channels that trigger fast Ca^{2+} influx in target cells. The P2Y receptors include two subgroups, one is coupled to $G_{q/11}$ signaling activating intracellular Ca^{2+} and a second subgroup is coupled to $G_{i/o}$, signaling and modulating ion channel activity. Glial cells express both P2X and P2Y receptors, which have an important role in activation of astrocytes and microglia, and promote oligodendrocyte-mediated myelination. In the CNS, ATP has a major signaling role. For example, ATP released from active neurons activates microglial cells promoting synaptic pruning; ATP released from astrocytes acts as an important paracrine signal within the astrocyte network. Presynaptic P2X receptors facilitate release of several neurotransmitters. In the periphery, ATP is released by distension of visceral organs and via P2X receptors has a major role in transduction of visceral signals, including pain. ATP is also an important cotransmitter in enteric cholinergic and sympathetic noradrenergic neurons.

Adenosine as a Neuromodulator

After release, ATP undergoes rapid enzymatic degradation by ectonucleotidases, leading to the production of extracellular adenosine. Metabolic stress triggers ATP hydrolysis to adenosine monophosphate, which is converted to adenosine by action of the 5'nucleotidase; adenosine is then released from cells by facilitated diffusion via nucleoside transporters. The primary route of adenosine metabolism is adenosine kinase, which is expressed primarily in astrocytes. Adenosine exerts widespread modulatory effects via four types of adenosine (A) receptors; the most abundant and physiologically relevant are A1 receptors (A1R) and $A2_A$ receptors ($A2_A$Rs). The A1Rs are coupled to G_i and mediate presynaptic and postsynaptic inhibitory effects. These receptors mediate several effects of adenosine, including antiepileptic effect, neuroprotection, sleep induction, and pain modulation. The $A2_A$Rs receptors are coupled to $G_{s/olf}$ and stimulate cAMP-PKA signaling. These receptors are abundant in the striatum and form heterodimers with D2Rs in a subpopulation of striatal projection neurons, antagonizing the effects of dopamine. Both A1 and A2A receptors are also expressed in astrocytes and microglia, where they regulate proliferation and production of inflammatory cytokines.

NEUROSTEROIDS

Neurosteroids (neuroactive steroids) are synthesized in the nervous system, both in neurons and glial cells, primarily astrocytes. They have a major role in development, plasticity, and neuroprotection.

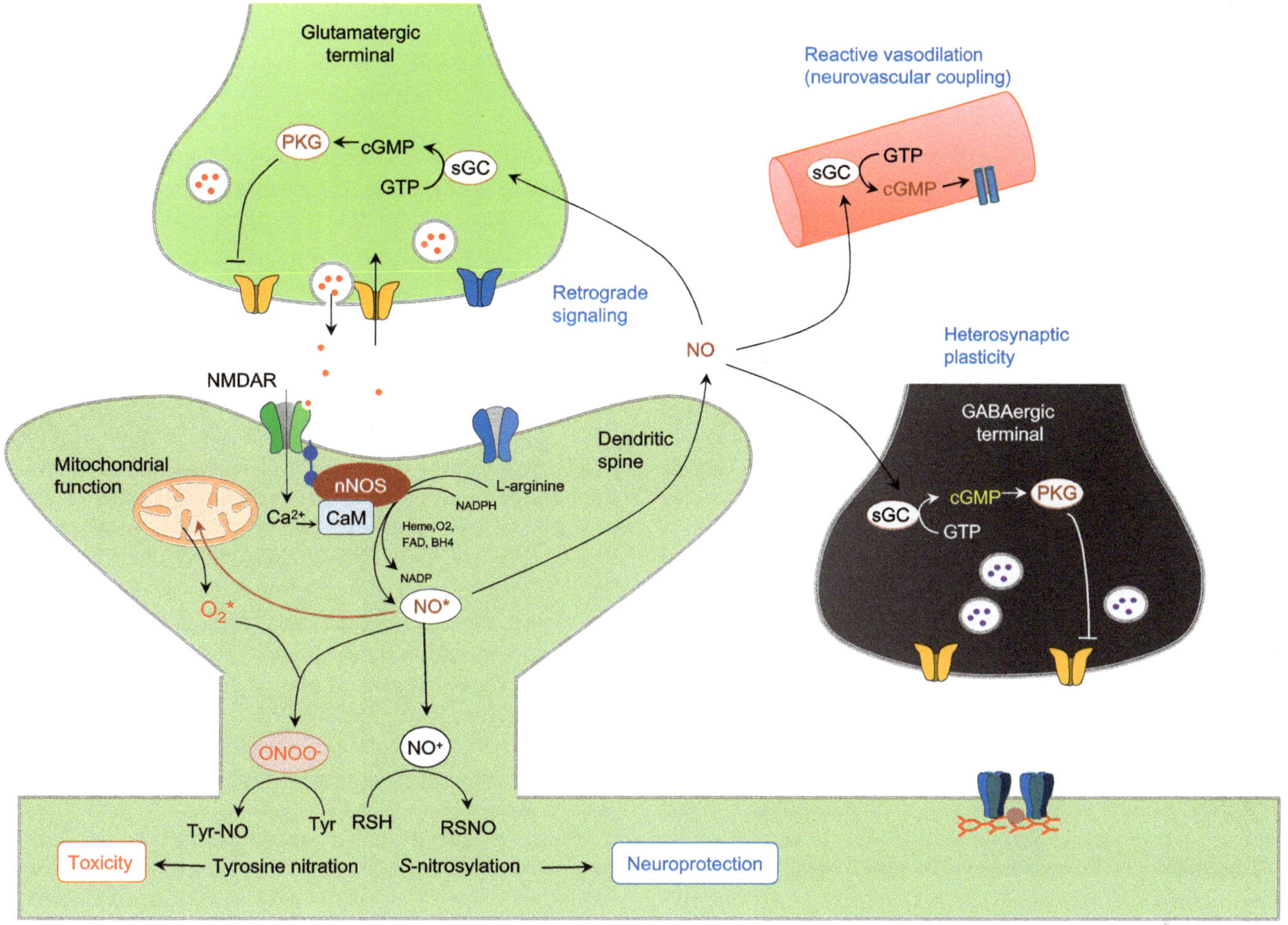

FIGURE 16.8 Nitric oxide signaling.

Nitric oxide (NO) is produced from L-arginine by the nitric oxide synthase (NOS), which includes neuronal, endothelial, and inducible isoforms. The primary trigger of NO production in neurons is Ca^{2+} influx via N-methyl-D-aspartate receptors (NMDARs), which form a functional macromolecular complex with NOS and calmodulin (CaM). NO diffuses into cells and activates cytosolic guanylyl cyclase, sGC resulting in formation of cyclic guanylyl monophosphate (cGMP) and activation of protein kinase G (PKG). Via this mechanism, NO functions both as a retrograde neuromodulator and potent vasodilator. Many effects of NO are mediated by protein S-nitrosylation via its conversion to nitrosonium cation (NO^+) and regulate the function of multiple proteins. At high intracellular levels, NO may also react rapidly with a superoxide radical (O_2^-) to produce peroxynitrite ($ONOO^-$), which elicits multiple neurotoxic effects via nitration of tyrosine residues of proteins.

Source of Neurosteroids in the CNS

Steroidogenesis in the CNS is regulated independently of that in endocrine organs. This process occurs primarily in mitochondria, and involves the steroidogenic acute regulatory protein and a translocator protein that transports cholesterol from the outer to the inner mitochondrial membrane; at this level the cytochrome P450 cholesterol side chain cleavage enzyme transforms cholesterol into pregnenolone. Pregnenolone is then transferred to the ER, where it is converted to allopregnanolone and other steroids thorough a series of consecutive steps. Pregnenolone is hydroxylated to dehydroepiandrosterone (DHE), which is then sequentially metabolized to testosterone; the p450 aromatase transforms testosterone into estradiol. Both neuronal activity and injury promote estradiol synthesis in the brain by increasing activity of presynaptic aromatase; the activity-induced presynaptic production and release of estradiol has been referred to as "synaptocrine" signaling.

Mechanisms of Action and Effects of Neurosteroids in the CNS

Neurosteroids exert paracrine and autocrine effects both via genomic and nongenomic mechanisms.[31] For example, the effects of estradiol are mediated by the estradiol receptors ERα and ERβ, which belong to the steroid/thyroid hormone superfamily of nuclear receptors. In the basal state, these receptors are found as monomers that associate with heat shock protein 90 in the cytoplasm. Binding of estradiol triggers their phosphorylation, dissociation from the heat shock protein, dimerization, and translocation to the nucleus. In the nucleus, the estrogen receptors interact with estrogen response elements on regulatory sequences of target genes. The nongenomic effects are rapid and involve direct effects on membrane receptors. For example, ERα and ERβ receptors present in lipid rafts interact with other receptors and participate in a crosstalk mechanism via shared downstream signaling pathways, including survival pathways downstream of growth factor signaling. Furthermore, DHE may directly activate growth factors signaling via interaction with tyrosine kinase receptors[32] and have several downstream effects via estrogen, sigma 1, and other receptors.[33] Activation of membrane steroid receptors may also elicit rapid changes via direct interactions with ion channels. Estrogens and DHEA also act via a distinct type of GPCR (GPER1), which may mediate neuroprotective effects, for example, in the setting cerebral ischemia.[34]

Activation of membrane estrogen receptors elicits rapid changes in intrinsic neuronal excitability via protein kinase-dependent phosphorylation of membrane ion channels and ionotropic receptors. For example, allopregnanolone is a potent positive allosteric modulator of extrasynaptic $GABA_A$ receptors responsible for tonic GABAergic inhibition in the central nervous system. Brain levels of allopregnanolone increase in response to drugs that increase GABAergic transmission, including alcohol, γ-hydroxybutyrate, and diazepam. Fluctuations in the circulating levels of progesterone and allopregnanolone during the menstrual cycle are believed to underlie catamenial epilepsy. However, in a multicenter, double-blind, phase III clinical trial, progesterone treatment did not suppress catamenial seizures. Studies in experimental epilepsy models show reduced expression of neurosteroid-sensitive delta subunit-containing $GABA_A$Rs, which may explain the negative results of clinical trials.[35]

In contrast, estradiol and DHEA are negative noncompetitive modulators of the $GABA_A$ receptors and positive modulators of NMDAR receptors. Activation of membrane estrogen receptors may also elicit rapid changes in intrinsic neuronal excitability via protein kinase-dependent phosphorylation of membrane ion channels. Via their genomic and multiple extragenomic mechanisms, neurosteroids have a major role in functional and structural plasticity in the nervous system. Via their interaction with growth factor signaling cascades neurosteroids also contribute to neuroprotection. For example, evidence from animal models supports a neuroprotective role of estradiol in the setting of traumatic, hypoxic, or ischemic injury, seizures, and neurodegeneration. Estrogen-triggered neuroprotection involves several mechanisms, including activation of survival pathways, stimulation of mitochondrial biogenesis, preservation of energy metabolism, and increase expression of antioxidant enzymes.

SYNAPTIC PLASTICITY

Neuronal activity triggers plastic changes in synapses that affect the efficacy of information processing, connectivity, and structure of the CNS. Plasticity occurs during normal development, throughout life, and in response to injury.

General Concepts

The two prototypical forms of synaptic plasticity are long-term potentiation (LTP) and long-term depression (LTD). Synaptic plasticity may affect excitatory glutamatergic or inhibitory GABAergic synapses and may be triggered and maintained by either presynaptic or postsynaptic mechanisms. Presynaptic plasticity affects the probability of neurotransmitter release by altering the availability of synaptic vesicles at presynaptic active zones or the activity of presynaptic Ca_v2 channels. Postsynaptic plasticity includes induction and maintenance states that critically depend on changes in phosphorylation of receptors, transcription factors, mRNA-binding proteins, and actin-binding proteins. The mechanisms of synaptic plasticity have been primary studied in the hippocampus, cerebellum, and striatum and are discussed in other more detail in the next chapter. Briefly, the two final common mechanisms involved in synaptic plasticity are intracellular Ca^{2+} transients and protein phosphorylation triggered by neurotransmitters or neurotrophic factors such as brain-derived neurotrophic factor (BDNF) (Figure 16.9).

Induction of LTP or LTD

Induction of LTP or LTD results from changes in the phosphorylation state of ionotropic receptor subunits, which may lead to either increased membrane expression or internalization of the receptor depending on the type and activity of the synapse.[36] The prototypical example of LTP of excitatory synapses is NMDAR-induced LTP at the synapse between CA3 Schaffer collateral terminals and CA1 pyramidal neurons in the hippocampus.[36–38] Activation of NMDARs leads to a large influx of Ca^{2+} and activation of CaM kinase II (CaMKII), which phosphorylates an AMPAR subunit, thus promoting AMPAR insertion at postsynaptic sites. In contrast, induction of LTD at excitatory synapses involves internalization of AMPARs, reducing synaptic efficacy. LTD may occur in response to activation of NMDARs or type I mGluRs, and has been primarily studied in the hippocampus and the cerebellum. For example, at the CA3 to CA1 synapse in the hippocampus, low-level NMDAR stimulation triggers CaM activation of calcineurin, which dephosphorylates a subunit of the AMPAR subunits promoting its internalization by endocytosis. Hippocampal mGluR5-triggered LTD involves several downstream

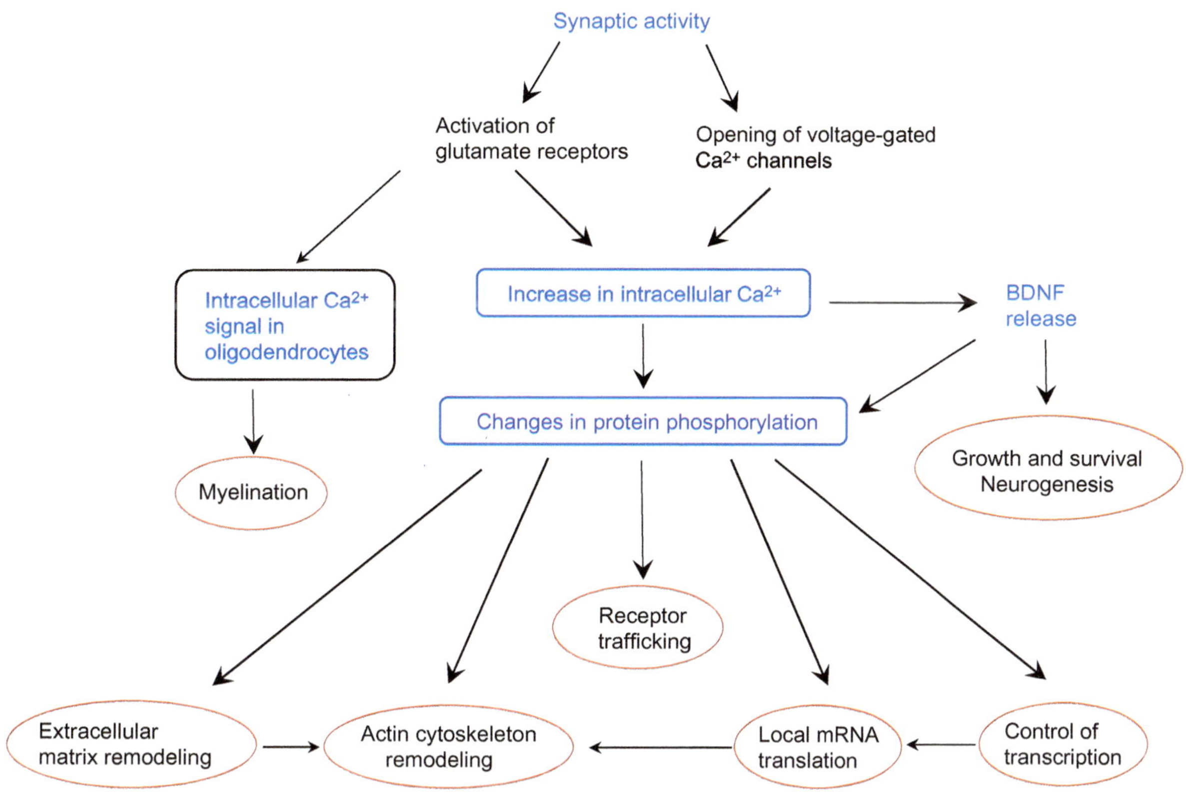

FIGURE 16.9 Overview of mechanisms of use-dependent synaptic plasticity.
Use-dependent synaptic plasticity is triggered primarily by activation of glutamate receptors and/or calcium (Ca^{2+}) influx via voltage-gated channels. The downstream mechanisms are intracellular Ca^{2+} transients and changes in protein phosphorylation. Synaptic plasticity is promoted by neurotrophic factors, primarily brain-derived neurotrophic factor (BDNF). Induction of synaptic plasticity involves changes in the phosphorylation state of ionotropic receptor subunits. Maintenance of synaptic plasticity involves changes of phosphorylation of transcription factors and activation of local mRNA translation. Structural plasticity results from dynamic changes of the actin cytoskeleton and interactions with the extracellular matrix. Activity of astrocytes and microglia are fundamental additional contributors to synaptic plasticity (not shown). Use-dependent plasticity also includes changes in axon myelination by oligodendrocytes and adult neurogenesis in the dentate gyrus.

signals that are independent of G proteins. Induction of LTD in the parallel fiber–Purkinje cells synapse involves mGluR1, triggering a large increase in intracellular Ca^{2+}, and activation of PKC, which phosphorylates a subunit of AMPARs leading to its internalization. GABAergic synapses are also highly plastic.

Maintenance of LTP by Translation and Transcriptional Mechanisms

Maintenance of LTP requires phosphorylation pathways that promote both gene transcription and local mRNA translation of synaptic proteins. Transcriptional activation critically depends on phosphorylation of the cAMP response element-binding protein (CREB), which promotes transcription of several glutamatergic synapse proteins. Synaptic activity also promotes the formation of several signal-containing synaptonuclear complexes that are translocated to the nucleus and elicit CREB phosphorylation. The resulting mRNAs are transported in association with mRNA-binding proteins, such as fragile X mental retardation protein (FMRP), which inhibit mRNA translation until arrival to the active dendrites. At this level, several activity-dependent mechanisms, particularly phosphorylation of FMRP and other inhibitory mRNA-binding proteins, leads to their dissociation from mRNAs and thus "unmasking" mRNA allowing its access to the translation machinery.[39] Protein synthesis is promoted by mechanistic (mammalian) target of rapamycin (mTOR).

Remodeling of the Dendritic Cytoskeleton

Activity-dependent dendritic growth and maturation involves remodeling of the actin cytoskeleton via regulation of actin-depolymerizing proteins such as cofilin and interactions among dendrites, astrocytes, and extracellular matrix.[40-43] Excitatory synaptic activity promotes transcription and release of BDNF, which activates mTORC1-mediated and other phosphorylation pathways that increase protein and lipid biosynthesis, inhibit autophagy, and promote actin cytoskeletal remodeling.[43] Transsynaptic cell adhesion molecules such as neuroligin 1 organize synapse formation and control synapse morphology, receptor function, and synaptic elimination.

Role of the Extracellular Matrix in Synaptic Development, Maintenance, and Plasticity

The extracellular matrix (ECM) constitutes 10%–20% of the brain volume. The ECM forms the basement membrane around blood vessels, thus contributing to maintenance of the integrity of the blood-brain barrier; forms a diffuse matrix in the interstitium of the brain parenchyma; and is condensed around a subset of neurons forming structures known as perineuronal nets.[40,44] Components of the ECM, including molecules secreted by astrocytes, have an important role in synaptic plasticity. The major components of the ECM are glycosaminoglycans, primarily hyaluronic acid, which provides the scaffold for attachment of proteoglycans such as chondroitin sulfate and heparan sulfate proteoglycans. Adhesion molecules such as integrins and dystroglycans form a structural and functional link between the ECM and both the intracellular cytoskeleton and signal transduction pathways.

Perineuronal nets are composed of ECM molecules that organize in lattice-like structures that enwrap the perikaryon, dendrites, and axon initial segments of specific subsets of neurons in the mature CNS. Perineuronal nets have an important role in regulating plasticity both during development and in the adult brain. They are particularly abundant around highly active neurons, including fast-spiking GABAergic interneurons that innervate the cell bodies and proximal segments of the axon of pyramidal cells and excitatory burst neurons and onmipause neurons in the oculomotor system. The formation of perineuronal nets depends on synaptic activity and has a critical role during development, where they stabilize synaptic connectivity after the so-called "critical period" for formation of use-dependent synaptic connections. Perineuronal nets form a barrier that prevents lateral diffusion of membrane receptors at postsynaptic sites and may also prevent inappropriate crosstalk between neurotransmitters, promote local ion homeostasis, and play a protective role. Loss of perineuronal nets surrounding brainstem saccadic burst neurons may explain the selective saccadic palsy reported following cardiac surgery.[45]

The interactions between pre- and postsynaptic neuronal elements with astroglial processes and ECM for formation and plasticity of chemical synapses have led to the concept of "tetrapartite synapase."[46] Several extracellular secreted scaffolding molecules drive synaptogenesis. They include astrocyte-secreted thrombospondins, neuronal pentraxins, and cerebellins. Synapse maturation involves signaling mediated by reelin and integrin ligands. Activity-dependent activation of extracellular proteases, such as matrix metalloproteinase 9, is important for control of synaptic remodeling through localized degradation of perisynaptic ECM and generation of proteolytic fragments that induce synaptic plasticity.[46] Reelin is a large ECM protein that has a major role in neurogenesis, neuronal polarization and migration during development, and synaptic plasticity in the adult brain. Dysfunctions in reelin signaling are associated with brain lamination defects such as lissencephaly, but also have been implicated in neurodegeneration. Reelin signaling involves a core signal transduction pathway that eventually affects both the dynamics of actin and microtubules and membrane trafficking.[47] Changes in reelin levels in the CSF have been proposed as a potential early biomarker in some forms of dementia.[48]

Glia–Neuron Interactions and Synaptic Plasticity

Astrocytes have a major role in development and maintenance of synapses. They release ECM proteins, growth factors, cytokines, and extracellular proteases that contribute to synaptic plasticity. Astrocytes sense excitatory synaptic activity and may contribute to synaptic plasticity via release of mediators known as gliotransmitters. Release of glutamate and ATP from active synapses triggers Ca^{2+} transients in astrocytes, which in turn release glutamate, ATP, D-serine, GABA, and other signals that may either increase or decrease excitatory or inhibitory neurotransmission. Both astrocytes and microglia participate in elimination of redundant or senescent synapses via phagocytosis and activation of the complement pathway.[49] Microglia express the complement receptor CR3 that is activated by C1q associated with senescent synapses; this increases the number of phagocytic microglia and thereby promotes synaptic pruning.[50] In normal conditions, processes from microglial cells make brief, repetitive contacts with synapses and then rapidly retract. The dynamic structural interactions between the microglial processes and dendritic spines respond to synaptic activity and depend on signals from neurons and astrocytes, particularly gradient concentrations of ATP, acting via $P2Y_{12}$ receptors in microglia.[51,52] Microglial–synaptic interactions participate in control of synaptic plasticity in the adult brain as mediators of synaptic scaling, which regulates the strength of excitatory synapses in response to changes in activity.

NEUROTRANSMISSION, NEUROMODULATION, AND PLASTICITY AS DISEASE TARGETS

Essentially all neurologic disorders, either directly or indirectly, are associated with disturbed synaptic transmission, modulation, or plasticity. The identification of the molecular mechanisms involved in these processes has provided the basis for pharmacological and in some cases genetic approaches for treatment. For example, abnormal NMDAR-triggered plasticity underlies cognitive and behavioral manifestations of neurodevelopmental disorders such as intellectual delay and autism spectrum disorders,[53] neurodegenerative disorders such as Alzheimer disease,[54,55] and autoimmune limbic encephalitis.[56] The mechanisms of synaptic plasticity involved in LTP may be abnormally activated, leading to abnormal cell excitability. Typical examples are central sensitization underlying chronic pain,[57] levodopa-induced dyskinesia,[58] fragile X mental retardation syndrome,[59] and epilepsy.[60,61] Genetic or acquired disorders affecting different components of specific signal transduction pathways may manifest with overlapping phenotypes. One typical example is hyperkinetic movement disorders due to mutations affecting the G_{olf}–adenylyl cyclase–cAMP–PKA pathway downstream of D1R signaling in medium spiny neurons in the striatum.[62,63] These include disorders linked to mutations in the *GNAL* (guanine nucleotide-binding protein subunit alpha L) gene encoding the stimulatory α subunit of $G\alpha_{olf}$, *ADCY5* encoding adenylyl cyclase 5, and *PDE10A* encoding phosphodiesterase 10. Elderly persons with *PDE10A* mutations may develop levodopa-responsive parkinsonism; autoantibodies against PDE10 have been associated with paraneoplastic hyperkinetic movement disorders; in some cases the clinical manifestations were unmasked by the use of immune checkpoint inhibitors to treat the underlying malignancy.[64]

Another example of disorders affecting different components of a signal transduction pathway are genetic or autoimmune disorders causing cerebellar ataxia by disrupting the mGluR1–IP_3R–PKC pathway involved in LTD at the parallel fiber–Purkinje cell synapse.[65,66] These include hereditary spinocerebellar ataxias due to mutations of the *GRM1* gene encoding mGluR1, the *ITPR1* gene encoding the IP_3R1, or the *PRKCG* gene encoding PKCγ. Similarly, autoantibodies against different components of this pathway have been associated with autoimmune ataxia. The typical example is paraneoplastic ataxia associated with mGluR1 autoantibodies in patients with Hodgkin lymphoma. Downstream components of this pathway are also target of autoimmune attack.

KEY POINTS

- Neurochemical signals include excitatory and inhibitory amino acids, acetylcholine, monoamines, neuropeptides, purines, lipid mediators, nitric oxide, growth factors, cytokines, and extracellular matrix proteins.
- Many neurons and glial cells release more than one neurochemical signal.
- A single neurotransmitter may exert different effects via different receptor subtypes.
- Classical neurotransmission is the rapid, precise transmission of excitatory or inhibitory signals and is largely mediated by ionotropic receptors.
- Neuromodulation affects the probability of neurotransmitter release by presynaptic terminals or responsiveness of the postsynaptic cells to the neurotransmitter and is mediated by G protein-coupled receptors (GPCRs).
- Synaptic plasticity is the use-dependent change in efficacy of excitatory or inhibitory signals, eventually associated with changes in dendritic structure and connectivity.
- Inotropic receptors are neurotransmitter-gated cation (Na^+, Ca^+) or Cl^- channels and belong to different families.
- Activation of nAChRs, ionotropic glutamate receptors, 5-HT3. and P2X receptors allows influx in Na^+, Ca^{2+}, or both and elicit fast postsynaptic excitation.
- Activation of $GABA_A$Rs and glycine receptors increases influx of Cl- and triggers fast postsynaptic inhibition in most adult neurons; in immature neurons, in some adult neurons, and in some pathological conditions they allow efflux of K^+ and depolarization.
- The efficacy of classical neurotransmission depends on the precise apposition of presynaptic release zones and postsynaptic receptors.
- Postsynaptic scaffold proteins include postsynaptic density protein of 95 kDa (PSD 95) in excitatory glutamatergic synapses, gephyrin in inhibitory synapses, and rapsyn at the neuromuscular junction.
- Assembled ionotropic receptors undergo activity-dependent trafficking between intercellular, extrasynaptic, and postsynaptic sites.
- Presynaptic modulation affects the probability of neurotransmitter release.
- Postsynaptic modulation determines the responsiveness of the postsynaptic target to excitatory or inhibitory signals.
- Both presynaptic and postsynaptic modulations are mediated by GPCRs, which may form receptor mosaics with other types of GPCRS.
- Neuropeptides are potent neuromodulators that frequently coexist with other neurotransmitters.
- Calcitonin gene-related peptide (CGRP) has a major role in the pathophysiology of migraine and is also involved in appetite suppression and hypercapnic-induced arousal.
- Substance P has a major role in promoting synaptic plasticity resulting in central sensitization as a mechanism of chronic pain.
- Endogenous opioids have major roles in analgesia, addiction, autonomic control, and other functions via both direct and indirect mechanisms.
- Endocannabinoids derive from membrane phospholipids, are released on demand, and primarily act as retrograde messengers eliciting presynaptic inhibition.
- Nitric oxide is a diffusible messenger that affects neurotransmitter release and elicits vasodilation.

- Adenosine triphosphate (ATP) and its metabolite adenosine may act both as neurotransmitters and as neuromodulators in the central and peripheral nervous systems.
- Neurosteroids exert their effects both via genomic mechanisms acting as transcription factors and via interactions with membrane receptors.
- Synaptic plasticity may affect excitatory or inhibitory synapses and may be both triggered and maintained by presynaptic and postsynaptic mechanisms.
- The two common mechanisms involved in synaptic plasticity are intracellular Ca^{2+} transients and protein phosphorylation.
- Induction of LTP or LTD results from activity-dependent changes in phosphorylation of ionotropic receptor subunits, which may affect their membrane expression.
- Maintenance of synaptic plasticity involves changes of phosphorylation of transcription factors and activation of local mRNA translation at selected synapses.
- Structural plasticity results from dynamic changes of the actin cytoskeleton in dendrites.
- Extracellular matrix (ECM) proteins secreted from astrocytes and neurons have a major role in formation, maturation, and activity-dependent plasticity of synapses.
- Astrocytes and microglia participate in activity-dependent pruning of dendritic processes during development, synaptic plasticity, and pathological conditions.
- Abnormal plasticity of glutamatergic synapses is a fundamental disease mechanism of intellectual delay and autism spectrum disorders, Alzheimer disease, autoimmune limbic encephalitis, chronic pain, levodopa-induced dyskinesia. and epilepsy.
- Genetic or acquired disorders affecting components of specific signal transduction pathways may manifest with overlapping phenotypes.

REFERENCES

1. Burnstock G. Cotransmission in the autonomic nervous system. Handb Clin Neurol 2013;117:23–35.
2. Hnasko TS, Edwards RH. Neurotransmitter corelease: mechanism and physiological role. Annu Rev Physiol 2012;74:225–243.
3. Madsen KK, Hansen GH, Danielsen EM, Schousboe A. The subcellular localization of GABA transporters and its implication for seizure management. Neurochem Res 2015;40:410–419.
4. Hernandez CC, Macdonald RL. A structural look at $GABA_A$ receptor mutations linked to epilepsy syndromes. Brain Res 2019;1714:234–247.
5. Greger IH, Watson JF, Cull-Candy SG. Structural and functional architecture of AMPA-type glutamate receptors and their auxiliary proteins. Neuron 2017;94:713–730.
6. Kahle KT, Staley KJ, Nahed BV, et al. Roles of the cation-chloride cotransporters in neurological disease. Nat Clin Pract Neurol 2008;4:490–503.
7. Zhu J, Shang Y, Zhang M. Mechanistic basis of MAGUK-organized complexes in synaptic development and signalling. Nat Rev Neurosci 2016;17:209–223.
8. Gorlewicz A, Kaczmarek L. Pathophysiology of trans-synaptic adhesion molecules: implications for epilepsy. Front Cell Dev Biol 2018;6:119.
9. Alvarez FJ. Gephyrin and the regulation of synaptic strength and dynamics at glycinergic inhibitory synapses. Brain Res Bull 2017;129:50–65.
10. Burden SJ, Huijbers MG, Remedio L. Fundamental molecules and mechanisms for forming and maintaining neuromuscular synapses. Int J Mol Sci 2018;19.
11. Henley JM, Wilkinson KA. Synaptic AMPA receptor composition in development, plasticity and disease. Nat Rev Neurosci 2016;17:337–350.
12. Fuxe K, Marcellino D, Borroto-Escuela DO, et al. The changing world of G protein-coupled receptors: from monomers to dimers and receptor mosaics with allosteric receptor-receptor interactions. J Recept Signal Transduct Res 2010;30:272–283.
13. Agnati LF, Guidolin D, Vilardaga JP, Ciruela F, Fuxe K. On the expanding terminology in the GPCR field: the meaning of receptor mosaics and receptor heteromers. J Recept Signal Transduct Res 2010;30:287–303.
14. Fuxe K, Borroto-Escuela DO, Marcellino D, et al. GPCR heteromers and their allosteric receptor-receptor interactions. Curr Med Chem 2012;19:356–363.
15. Perreault ML, Hasbi A, O'Dowd BF, George SR. Heteromeric dopamine receptor signaling complexes: emerging neurobiology and disease relevance. Neuropsychopharmacology 2014;39:156–168.
16. Khelashvili G, Dorff K, Shan J, et al. GPCR-OKB: the G protein coupled receptor oligomer knowledge base. Bioinformatics 2010;26:1804–1805.
17. Przydzial MJ, Bhhatarai B, Koleti A, Vempati U, Schurer SC. GPCR ontology: development and application of a G protein-coupled receptor pharmacology knowledge framework. Bioinformatics 2013;29:3211–3219.
18. van den Pol AN. Neuropeptide transmission in brain circuits. Neuron 2012;76:98–115.
19. Edvinsson L, Haanes KA, Warfvinge K, Krause DN. CGRP as the target of new migraine therapies—successful translation from bench to clinic. Nat Rev Neurol 2018;14:338–350.
20. Goadsby PJ, Holland PR, Martins-Oliveira M, Hoffmann J, Schankin C, Akerman S. Pathophysiology of migraine: a disorder of sensory processing. Physiol Rev 2017;97:553–622.
21. Holland PR, Saengjaroentham C, Vila-Pueyo M. The role of the brainstem in migraine: potential brainstem effects of CGRP and CGRP receptor activation in animal models. Cephalalgia 2019;39:390–402.
22. Campos CA, Bowen AJ, Schwartz MW, Palmiter RD. Parabrachial CGRP neurons control meal termination. Cell Metab 2016;23:811–820.
23. Saper CB, Kaur S. Brain circuitry for arousal from apnea. Cold Spring Harb Symp Quant Biol 2018;83:63–69.
24. Chi G, Huang Z, Li X, Zhang K, Li G. Substance P regulation in epilepsy. Curr Neuropharmacol 2018;16:43–50.
25. Bodnar RJ. Endogenous opiates and behavior: 2017. Peptides 2020;124:170223.

26. Tampi RR, Maksimowski M, Ahmed M, Tampi DJ. Oxytocin for frontotemporal dementia: a systematic review. Ther Adv Psychopharmacol 2017;7:48–53.
27. Diaz-delCastillo M, Woldbye DPD, Heegaard AM. Neuropeptide Y and its involvement in chronic pain. Neuroscience 2018;387:162–169.
28. Ledri LN, Melin E, Christiansen SH, et al. Translational approach for gene therapy in epilepsy: model system and unilateral overexpression of neuropeptide Y and Y2 receptors. Neurobiol Dis 2016;86:52–61.
29. Joshi N, Onaivi ES. Endocannabinoid system components: overview and tissue distribution. Adv Exp Med Biol 2019;1162:1–12.
30. Nakamura T, Lipton SA. Protein S-nitrosylation as a therapeutic target for neurodegenerative diseases. Trends Pharmacol Sci 2016;37:73–84.
31. Tuem KB, Atey TM. Neuroactive steroids: receptor interactions and responses. Front Neurol 2017;8:442.
32. Pediaditakis I, Iliopoulos I, Theologidis I, et al. Dehydroepiandrosterone: an ancestral ligand of neurotrophin receptors. Endocrinology 2015;156:16–23.
33. Clark BJ, Prough RA, Klinge CM. Mechanisms of action of dehydroepiandrosterone. Vitam Horm 2018;108:29–73.
34. Bai N, Zhang Q, Zhang W, et al. G-protein-coupled estrogen receptor activation upregulates interleukin-1 receptor antagonist in the hippocampus after global cerebral ischemia: implications for neuronal self-defense. J Neuroinflammation 2020;17:45.
35. Joshi S, Kapur J. Neurosteroid regulation of GABAA receptors: a role in catamenial epilepsy. Brain Res 2019;1703:31–40.
36. Nicoll RA. A brief history of long-term potentiation. Neuron 2017;93:281–290.
37. Greer PL, Greenberg ME. From synapse to nucleus: calcium-dependent gene transcription in the control of synapse development and function. Neuron 2008;59:846–860.
38. Saura CA, Cardinaux JR. Emerging roles of CREB-regulated transcription coactivators in brain physiology and pathology. Trends Neurosci 2017;40:720–733.
39. Glock C, Heumuller M, Schuman EM. mRNA transport & local translation in neurons. Curr Opin Neurobiol 2017;45:169–177.
40. Song I, Dityatev A. Crosstalk between glia, extracellular matrix and neurons. Brain Res Bull 2018;136:101–108.
41. Luscher C, Malenka RC. NMDA receptor-dependent long-term potentiation and long-term depression (LTP/LTD). Cold Spring Harb Perspect Biol 2012;4:a005710.
42. Petratos S, Li QX, George AJ, et al. The beta-amyloid protein of Alzheimer's disease increases neuronal CRMP-2 phosphorylation by a Rho-GTP mechanism. Brain 2008;131:90–108.
43. Perluigi M, Di Domenico F, Butterfield DA. mTOR signaling in aging and neurodegeneration: at the crossroad between metabolism dysfunction and impairment of autophagy. Neurobiol Dis 2015;84:39–49.
44. Testa D, Prochiantz A, Di Nardo AA. Perineuronal nets in brain physiology and disease. Semin Cell Dev Biol 2019;89:125–135.
45. Eggers SD, Horn AK, Roeber S, et al. Saccadic palsy following cardiac surgery: possible role of perineuronal nets. PLoS One 2015;10:e0132075.
46. Ferrer-Ferrer M, Dityatev A. Shaping synapses by the neural extracellular matrix. Front Neuroanat 2018;12:40.
47. Santana J, Marzolo MP. The functions of reelin in membrane trafficking and cytoskeletal dynamics: implications for neuronal migration, polarization and differentiation. Biochem J 2017;474:3137–3165.
48. Lidon L, Urrea L, Llorens F, et al. Disease-specific changes in reelin protein and mRNA in neurodegenerative diseases. Cells 2020;9:1252–1270.
49. Jung YJ, Chung WS. Phagocytic roles of glial cells in healthy and diseased brains. Biomol Ther (Seoul) 2018;26:350–357.
50. Hong S, Beja-Glasser VF, Nfonoyim BM, et al. Complement and microglia mediate early synapse loss in Alzheimer mouse models. Science 2016;352:712–716.
51. Wake H, Moorhouse AJ, Miyamoto A, Nabekura J. Microglia: actively surveying and shaping neuronal circuit structure and function. Trends Neurosci 2013;36:209–217.
52. Tremblay ME. The role of microglia at synapses in the healthy CNS: novel insights from recent imaging studies. Neuron Glia Biol 2011;7:67–76.
53. Ebrahimi-Fakhari D, Sahin M. Autism and the synapse: emerging mechanisms and mechanism-based therapies. Curr Opin Neurol 2015;28:91–102.
54. Pozueta J, Lefort R, Shelanski ML. Synaptic changes in Alzheimer's disease and its models. Neuroscience 2013;251:51–65.
55. De Strooper B, Karran E. The cellular phase of Alzheimer's disease. Cell 2016;164:603–615.
56. Dalmau J, Armangue T, Planaguma J, et al. An update on anti-NMDA receptor encephalitis for neurologists and psychiatrists: mechanisms and models. Lancet Neurol 2019;18:1045–1057.
57. Alles SRA, Smith PA. Etiology and pharmacology of neuropathic pain. Pharmacol Rev 2018;70:315–347.
58. Espay AJ, Morgante F, Merola A, et al. Levodopa-induced dyskinesia in Parkinson disease: current and evolving concepts. Ann Neurol 2018;84:797–811.
59. Westmark CJ. Fragile X and APP: a decade in review, a vision for the future. Mol Neurobiol 2019;56:3904–3921.
60. Avanzini G, Forcelli PA, Gale K. Are there really "epileptogenic" mechanisms or only corruptions of "normal" plasticity? Adv Exp Med Biol 2014;813:95–107.
61. Bockaert J, Marin P. mTOR in brain physiology and pathologies. Physiol Rev 2015;95:1157–1187.
62. Lohmann K, Klein C. Update on the genetics of dystonia. Curr Neurol Neurosci Rep 2017;17:26.
63. Niccolini F, Mencacci NE, Yousaf T, et al. PDE10A and ADCY5 mutations linked to molecular and microstructural basal ganglia pathology. Mov Disord 2018;33:1961–1965.
64. Zekeridou A, Kryzer T, Guo Y, et al. Phosphodiesterase 10A IgG: a novel biomarker of paraneoplastic neurologic autoimmunity. Neurology 2019;93:e815–e822.
65. Paulson HL, Shakkottai VG, Clark HB, Orr HT. Polyglutamine spinocerebellar ataxias—from genes to potential treatments. Nat Rev Neurosci 2017;18:613–626.
66. Jarius S, Wildemann B. "Medusa-head ataxia": the expanding spectrum of Purkinje cell antibodies in autoimmune cerebellar ataxia. Part 1: Anti-mGluR1, anti-Homer-3, anti-Sj/ITPR1 and anti-CARP VIII. J Neuroinflammation 2015;12:166.

17 Glutamatergic Transmission and Synaptopathies

OVERVIEW

L-glutamate is the primary excitatory neurotransmitter in projection neurons of the adult nervous system (CNS). These projection neurons include all pyramidal neurons of the cerebral cortex, hippocampus, and amygdala; thalamic neurons; relay neurons in all sensory and cerebellar afferent pathways; and neurons in subthalamic nucleus and cerebellar nuclei (Figure 17.1). In many neurons, glutamatergic synapses are primarily targeted to dendritic spines, whereas GABAergic synapses typically target dendritic shafts as well as the cell body. Glutamatergic inputs relay fast excitation between projection cells and activate local interneurons, thereby shaping local circuits and network activity. Glutamate also mediates neuron–astrocyte interactions and promotes myelination by oligodendrocytes. These multiple functions depend on ionotropic and metabotropic receptors. Glutamate receptors are located at postsynaptic densities (PSDs) in dendritic spines or at surrounding perisynaptic areas. The PSD contains scaffold proteins such as PSD-95 that are critical for clustering and functional interactions of glutamate receptors with downstream transduction pathways, actin cytoskeleton, and transsynaptic complexes. Glutamatergic synapses are surrounded by perisynaptic astrocytic processes forming "tripartite" synapses. Astrocytes are critical for uptake and metabolism of glutamate, respond to synaptic signals, and release signals that affect excitatory synaptic transmission and modulate excitatory synaptic activity. Glutamatergic synapses are highly plastic and undergo activity-dependent long-term potentiation (LTP) or long-term depression (LTD). Abnormal plasticity of glutamatergic synapses is a major disease mechanism in intellectual disability, autism, and Alzheimer disease. Glutamate receptors and their transduction pathways can be affected by mutations resulting in seizures or cerebellar ataxia and are a major disease target in autoimmune encephalitis.

The aims of this chapter are to review: (1) the mechanisms regulating L-glutamate levels at synapses, (2) the structure and dynamic regulation of glutamate receptors, (3) the effects of glutamatergic transmission in information transfer and network activity, (4) different forms of plasticity of glutamatergic synapses, and (5) examples of genetic, immune, and degenerative disorders affecting glutamatergic activity.

PRESYNAPTIC EVENTS IN GLUTAMATERGIC TRANSMISSION

The concentrations of L-glutamate at synaptic and extrasynaptic sites are finely regulated by different mechanisms of biosynthesis and reuptake (Figure 17.2).

Biosynthesis and Storage

Brain glutamate derives from two major sources: glucose metabolism (Krebs cycle) via transamination of α-ketoglutarate in the mitochondria, and glutamine derived from astrocytes by action of mitochondrial phosphate-activated glutaminase. The trafficking of glutamate and glutamine between neurons and astrocytes is called the glutamate-glutamine cycle.[1,2] Glutamate is translocated into synaptic vesicles by the action of vesicular glutamate transporters (VGLUTs 1-3, *SLC17* family) driven by the H^+-dependent electrochemical gradient across the vesicle membrane created by a vacuolar-type ATPase.[3] VGLUT1 and VGLUT2 are selectively expressed in distinct populations

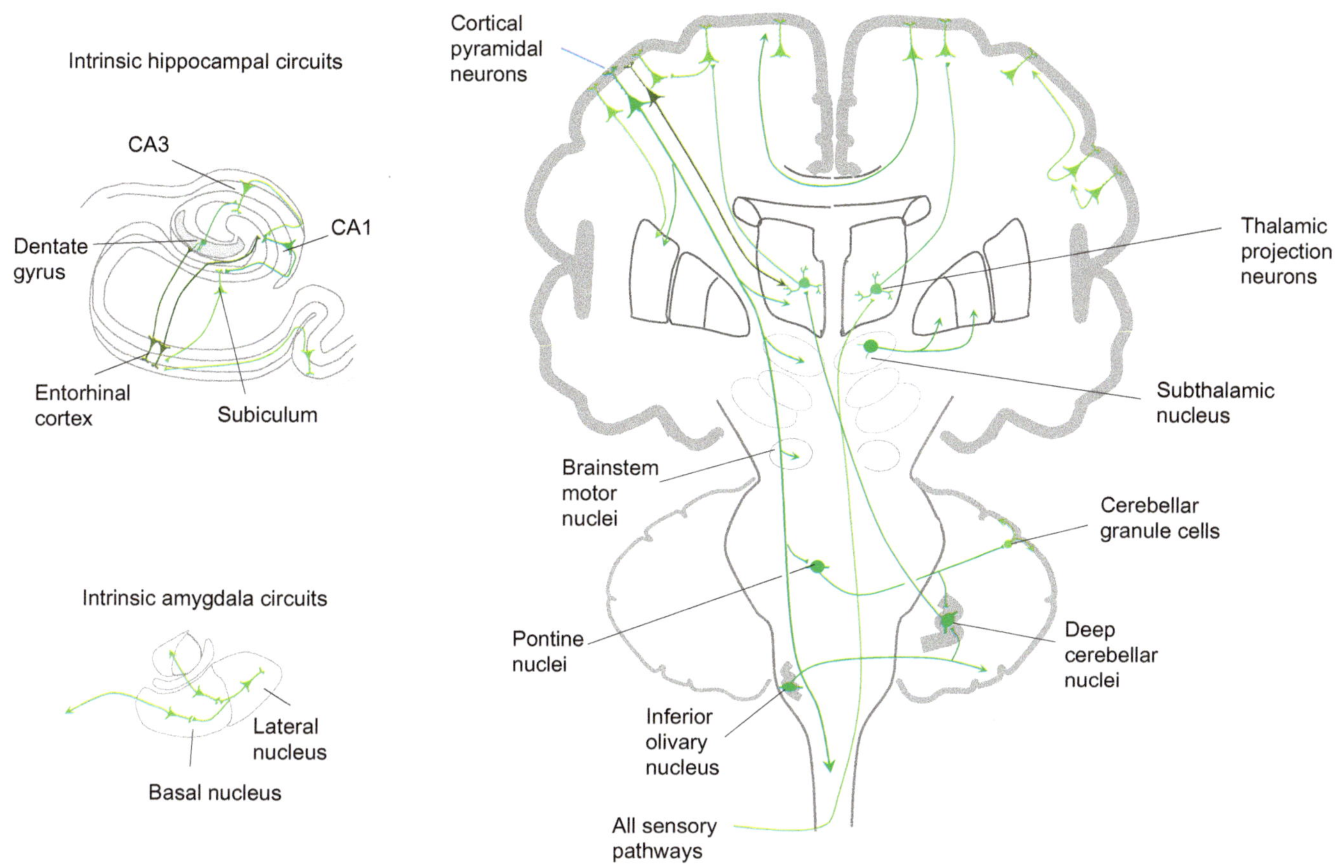

FIGURE 17.1 Distribution of glutamatergic and pathways.
L-glutamate is the primary excitatory neurotransmitter in projection neurons of the adult nervous system (CNS). They include all pyramidal neurons of the cerebral cortex, hippocampus, and amygdala; thalamic neurons; relay neurons in all sensory and cerebellar afferent pathways; and neurons in subthalamic nucleus and cerebellar nuclei.

of glutamatergic neurons; VGLUT3 is in both glutamatergic and nonglutamatergic neurons, as well as in astrocytes. In some glutamatergic terminals, such as mossy fiber terminals in the hippocampus, L-glutamate is co-stored with zinc (Zn^{2+}), which accumulates in the synaptic vesicle via the ZnT3 transporter and exerts important regulatory function on glutamatergic transmission.[4]

Synaptic Glutamate Transporters

The removal of glutamate from the synaptic cleft is critical to regulate synaptic and network excitability and avoid excitotoxicity. Removal occurs via the excitatory amino acid transporters (EAATs, *SLC1* family). They include EAAT1 and EAAT2, expressed in astrocytes, and EAATs 3, 4, and 5, expressed in neurons.[5–7] Astrocytic EAAT2 is the most important membrane glutamate transporter in the adult CNS. The driving force for glutamate uptake is provided by the Na^+ gradient created by the Na^+/K^+ ATPase. Astrocytic EAAT1 and EAAT2 prevent the potentially toxic accumulation of glutamate in synapses and provide glutamate as the substrate for synthesis of glutamine. These EAATs are physically and functionally coupled to the Na^+/K^+ ATPase, glutamine transporters, glucose transporters, and glycolytic enzymes, forming a supramolecular functional assembly termed as "glutamosome."[7] This functional coupling is bidirectional; many of these systems are both regulated by glutamate transport and provide the fuel to support glutamate uptake.[8] EAAT1 and EAAT2 are also expressed in astrocyte endfeet surrounding brain capillaries, in close association with the water channels aquaporin 4, and $K_{ir}4.1$ channels; this suggests a coupling among the mechanisms regulating activity-dependent glutamate uptake, cell volume, and K^+ homeostasis in the CNS.[9] EAAT3 is predominantly located postsynaptically at perisynaptic sites on dendritic spines in glutamatergic, GABAergic, and dopaminergic neurons, and contributes to buffer glutamate and regulates its effects on extrasynaptic ionotropic and metabotropic receptors. EAAT3 can also control neuronal activity through a negative feedback on excitatory neurotransmission by regulating the synthesis of GABA at inhibitory terminals. EAAT4 is highly expressed in Purkinje cells, and EAAT5 is expressed in retinal bipolar cells. EAATs may also function of glutamate-activated chloride channels; for example, EAAT5 mediates glutamate-activated chloride

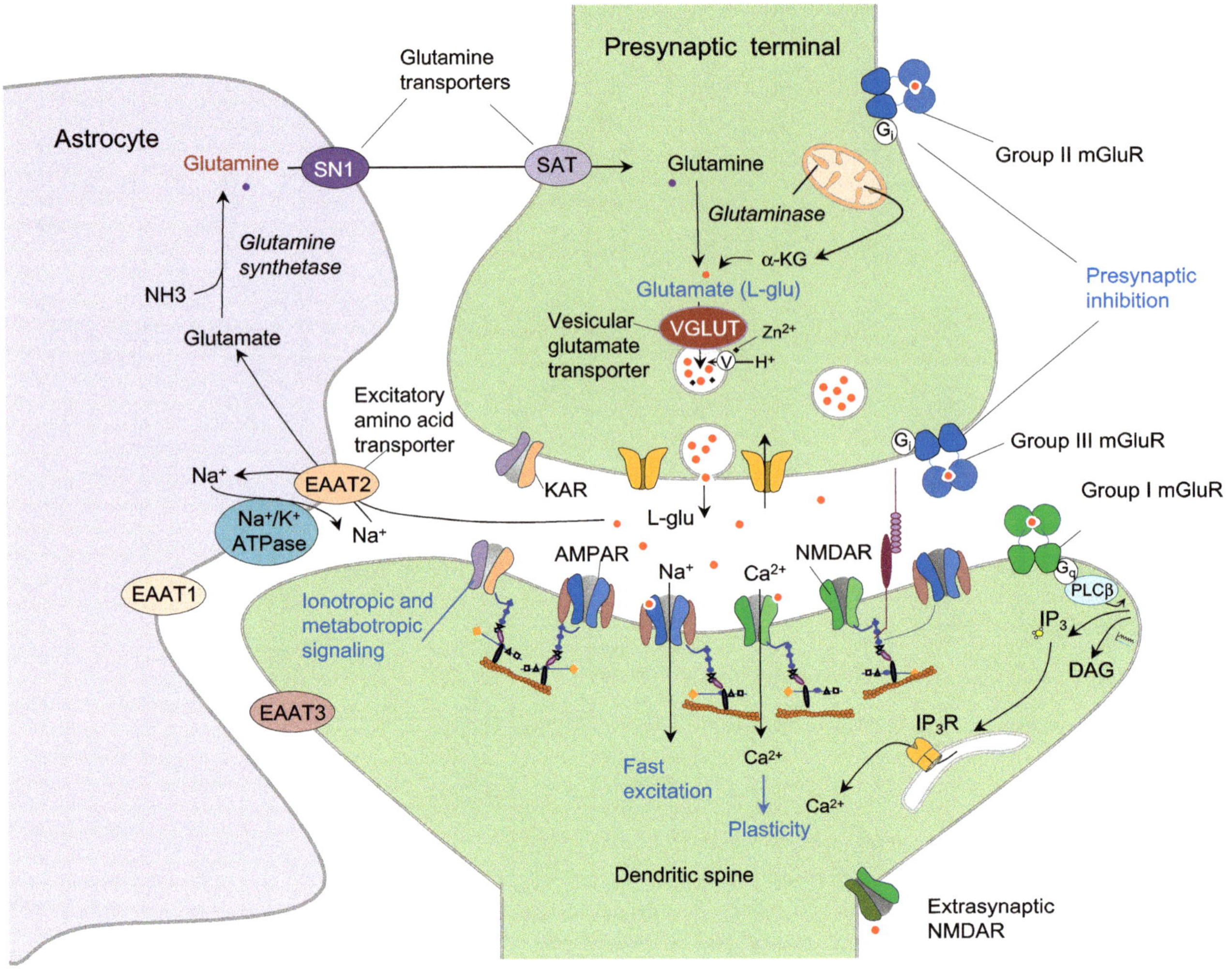

FIGURE 17.2 Main events in glutamatergic neurotransmission.

Synaptic glutamate derives from α-ketoglutarate and glutamine derived from astrocytes by action of glutaminase. Glutamate is translocated into synaptic vesicles by the vesicular glutamate transporters (VGLUTs) driven by the vacuolar-type ATPase (V) and in some glutamatergic terminals is co-stored with zinc (Zn^{2+}). The excitatory amino acid transporters (EAATs), primarily astrocytic EAAT2, remove glutamate from the synaptic cleft and require the Na^+ gradient created by the Na^+/K^+ ATPase. In astrocytes, glutamate is used for synthesis of glutamine by glutamine synthetase with utilization of ammonia (NH_3). Glutamine is exported from the astrocytes via the N transporter SN1 and then incorporated into neurons via the system A transporter (SAT). The synaptic effects of glutamate are mediated by α-amino-3-hydroxy-5-methyl-4 isoxazole propionic acid receptors (AMPARs), kainate receptors (KARs), and N-methyl-D-aspartate receptors (NMDARs), which are cation channels, and by different types of metabotropic glutamate receptors (mGluRs). The AMPARs are responsible for fast transmission of excitatory signals. NMDARs and postsynaptic group I mGluRs are involved in synaptic plasticity. Presynaptic group II and group III mGluRs inhibit neurotransmitter release. KAR may be located both pre- and postsynaptically and mediates noncanonical G protein signaling. DAG, diacylglycerol; IP_3, inositol triphosphate; PKC, protein kinase C, PLC, phospholipase C.

conductances that affect light responses in bipolar cells. Several factors modulate EAAT activity. Short-term modulation includes regulation of trafficking and posttranslational modifications, particularly phosphorylation, which controls surface expression of the transporters via their interaction with scaffold proteins. Expression of EAATs may also be regulated by the level of the promoter region of DNA or by alternative mRNA splicing of transcripts.[10]

Neuron–Astrocyte Interactions and Glutamate-Glutamine Cycle

The bidirectional interaction between neurons and astrocytes is critical for maintenance of glutamate availability for both excitatory and inhibitory synapses. Astrocytic EAAT1 and EAAT2 provide glutamate as the substrate for synthesis of glutamine via a process mediated by glutamine synthetase that utilizes ammonia (NH_3) and ATP. Astrocytic synthesis of glutamine is the major mechanism of ammonia detoxification in the brain. Glutamine is exported from the astrocytes via the N transporter SN1, and is then incorporated into neurons via system A transporters (SATs). After transfer from glia, glutamine undergoes conversion by the neuronal glutaminase in the mitochondria back to glutamate. Whereas this process is important to maintain glutamate availability in excitatory synapses, it is particularly critical in inhibitory synapses, where L-glutamate is the substrate for the synthesis of GABA. Glutamate uptake via EAATs requires the activity of the Na^+/K^+ ATPase to maintain the Na^+ gradient necessary for glutamate transport. Both this process and synthesis of glutamine consume ATP, and the reduction of the ATP:ADP ratio promotes glycolysis and production of lactate in astrocytes. Astrocytic derived lactate is shuttled back to neurons to support energy metabolism during synaptic activity.

IONOTROPIC GLUTAMATE RECEPTORS

The ionotropic glutamate receptors include three families: α-amino-3-hydroxy-5-methyl-4 isoxazole propionic acid receptors (AMPARs), kainate receptors (KARs), and N-methyl-D-aspartate receptors (NMDARs). All these receptors are cation channels with similar general structure and distribution but differ in some of their properties.[11]

General Structure

All ionotropic glutamate receptors assemble as tetramers of four intertwined subunits. Each subunit consists of four different modules or domains: an extracellular amino-(N) terminal domain (ATD), a ligand-binding domain, a common pore-forming transmembrane domain, and an intracellular carboxy (C)-terminal domain. The large ATD is involved in subunit assembly and allosteric modulation. The ligand-binding domain forms a structure that adopts a clamshell-like conformation containing the agonist-binding pocket. The transmembrane domain consists of three transmembrane helices (M1, M3, and M4) and a membrane reentrant loop (M2) that lines the inner cavity of the pore. The C-terminal domain is the site of posttranslational modification, primarily phosphorylation, and mediates protein–protein interactions that influence receptor trafficking, anchoring, and activation of signal molecules. The expression pattern of different ionotropic glutamate receptor subtypes varies in different brain regions, but their expression is widespread, with individual cells typically expressing multiple subtypes.[12]

AMPA Receptors

The AMPARs consist of several combinations of GluA1–4 subunits encoded by *GRIA* genes.[13,14] Most AMPAR tetramers contain GluA1 subunits with either GluA2 or GluA3. The GluA2 subunit is modified posttranscriptionally by RNA editing at the glutamine-arginine (Q/R) site located at the apex of the reentrant loop of M2 (Figure 17.3). The presence of edited GluA2 renders the AMPAR ion channel impermeable to calcium (Ca^{2+}). Most AMPARs contain an edited GluA2 subunit and only carry fast Na^+-mediated currents. Those containing either unedited GluA2 subunits or combinations of GluA1 with either GluA3 or GluA4 subunits are Ca^{2+} permeable. The overall architecture of AMPAR consists of a receptor core and a receptor periphery. The core includes the tetrameric combinations of GluA1–4 subunits and auxiliary subunits, including the transmembrane AMPA receptor regulatory proteins (TARPs).[15] Auxiliary subunits have a major influence on AMPAR synaptic stabilization, kinetics, conductance, and block by polyamines. For example, TARPs such as stargazin serve as anchors for AMPAR stabilization at the postsynaptic density. The C-terminal domain of the GluA1 and GluA2 subunits are targets of phosphorylation by calmodulin kinase II (CaMKII), protein kinase A (PKA), and protein kinase C (PKC) and by dephosphorylation by calcineurin. The phosphorylation state of GluA1 or GluA2 critically controls the expression of AMPARs at the synaptic membrane and regulates induction of synaptic plasticity. For example, phosphorylation of GluA1 by CAMKII or PKA facilitates GluA2 insertion in the synaptic membrane, whereas its dephosphorization by calcineurin promotes receptor internalization. The C-terminal domain also interacts with several proteins that affect trafficking, targeting, synaptic localization, stabilization, endocytosis, and function of AMPARs.

NMDA Receptors

The NMDARs are formed by various assemblies of subunits encoded by three *GRN* genes.[16] The GluN1 (formerly NR1) subunit is encoded by a single gene with different alternative spliced isoforms. There are four different subtypes of GluN2 (formerly NR2) subunits and two subtypes of GluN3 (formerly NR3) subunits. Most NMDARs are formed by two GluN1 and two GluN2 subunits (Figure 17.4). GluN1 is an obligatory subunit and binds the cotransmitter glycine (or, alternatively, D-serine). The GluN2 subunit binds the agonist L-glutamate and is the major determinant of the distribution, kinetics, and modulation of NMDARs. The most common GluN2 isoforms are GluN2A and GluN2B. In the adult central nervous system, GluN2A-containing NMDARs are located at synaptic sites and are activated by glutamate released to the synaptic cleft. Extrasynaptic NMDARs containing GluN2B are located at the neck of the dendritic spines and dendritic shaft and are activated by ambient levels of glutamate, resulting from either spillover of synaptic glutamate that escaped astrocytic uptake via EAATs, or glutamate release by astrocytes.[17] GluN2B-containing NMDARs also predominate during development. The GluN2 subunits can be replaced by GluN3 subunits, which bind glycine or D-serine.[16,18]

The NMDAR has several unique features (Figure 17.5). They include the requirement of binding of both glycine

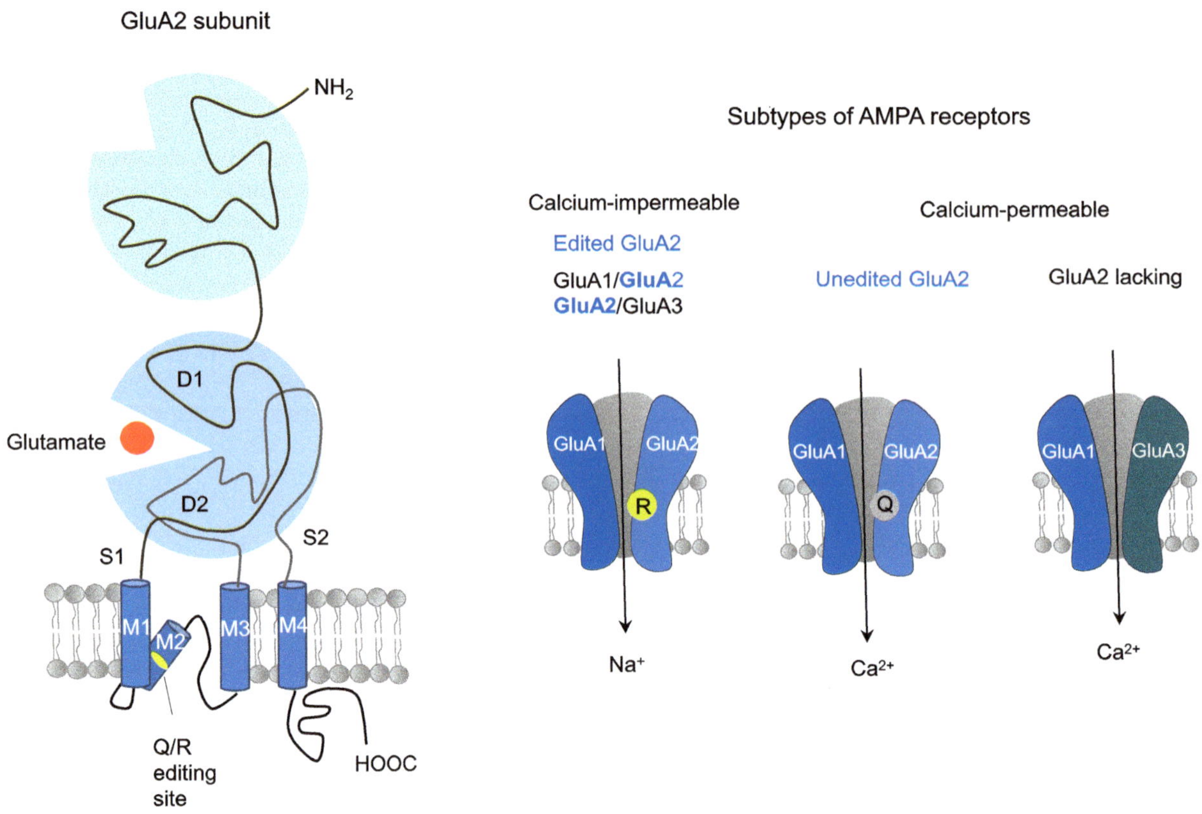

FIGURE 17.3 Heterogeneity of AMPA receptors.
Ionotropic glutamate receptors assemble as tetramers consisting of four intertwined subunits. Each subunit has a large extracellular amino-terminal domain, a ligand-binding domain, a pore-forming transmembrane domain, and an intracellular carboxy terminal domain. The ligand-binding domain adopts a clamshell-like conformation with two lobes containing the agonist-binding pocket. The transmembrane domain consists of three transmembrane helices (M1, M3, and M4) and a membrane reentrant loop (M2) that lines the inner cavity of the pore. The C-terminal domain is the site of posttranslational modification such as phosphorylation and mediates protein–protein interactions. The α-amino-3-hydroxy-5-methyl-4 isoxazole propionic acid receptors (AMPARs) consist of several combinations of GluA1-4 subunits; most AMPAR tetramers contain GluA1 subunits with either GluA2 or GluA3 subunits. The GluA2 subunit is modified post-transcription by RNA editing at the glutamine-arginine (Q/R) site located at the apex of the reentrant loop of M2 The presence of edited GluA2 renders the AMPAR ion channel impermeable to calcium Ca^{2+}.

(or D-serine) to the GluN1 and glutamate to the GluN2 subunits for its activation; highly permeability to Ca^{2+}; voltage-dependent block of its channel by magnesium (Mg^{2+}); slow kinetics of inactivation; and presence of several modulatory sites. At resting state, extracellular Mg^{2+} causes an open channel block by permeating the pore and preventing the passage of Ca^{2+} ions. Depolarization removes the Mg^{2+} blockade, allowing Ca^{2+} flow. The type of GluN2 subunit is the major determinant of receptor conductance, kinetics, and sensitivity to voltage-dependent Mg^{2+} blockade. The NMDAR has several allosteric modulatory sites; these include a polyamine site, allosteric sites for divalent cations such as Zn^{2+} and copper (Cu^{2+}), a proton (H^+)-sensitive site, and a redox modulatory site. Endogenous polyamines may produce either stimulation or inhibition of NMDAR currents depending on the subunit composition. Zinc elicits a voltage-dependent inhibition; this effect may be physiologically relevant, as Zn^{2+} is co-released with glutamate by exocytosis in some brain regions. The NMDARs are also inhibited by protons acting at the redox modulatory site located in the extracellular domain. Nitric oxide (NO) reacts with critical cysteine residues at the redox modulatory sites of the receptor producing S-nitrosylation, which reduces the affinity of the glycine modulatory site and thus inhibits NMDAR currents.[19] Prion protein (PrP^c) is a widely expressed cuproprotein that interacts with many channels and receptors, including NMDARs. Copper bound to PrP^c oxidizes NO to nitrosyl ion, thereby promoting S-nitrosylation of extracellular thiol residues of GluN1 and GluN2A subunits, decreasing steady state activation of NMDARs.[19,20] The intracellular C-terminus of NMDAR subunits contains phosphorylation sites that regulate both membrane expression and function of the receptor.

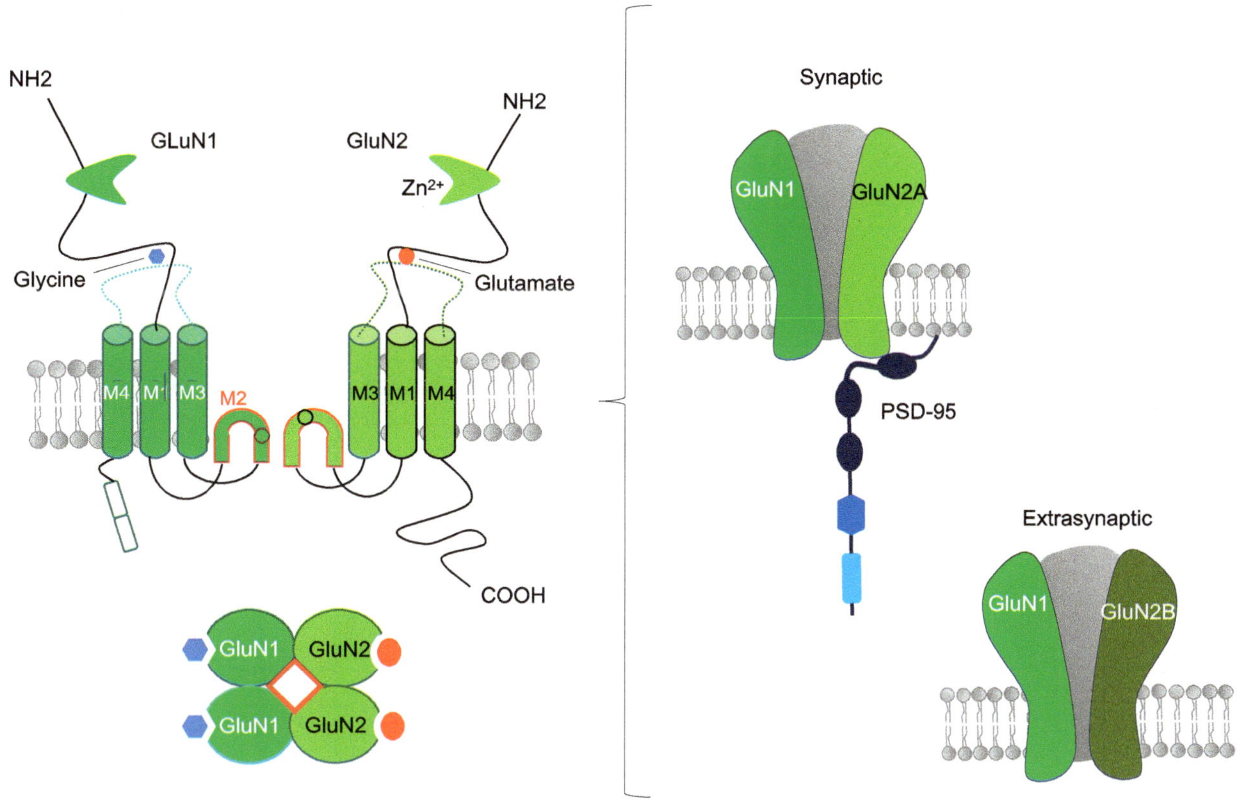

FIGURE 17.4 Structure of NMDA receptors.
Most N-methyl-D-aspartate receptors (NMDARs) are heterotetramers of two GluN1 and two GluN2 subunits. GluN1 is an obligatory subunit and binds the cotransmitter glycine (or, alternatively, D-serine). The GluN2 subunit binds the agonist L-glutamate. In the adult central nervous system, GluN2A-containing NMDARS are located at synaptic sites at the neck of the dendritic spines and dendritic shaft. PSD-95, postsynaptic density protein of 95 kDa.

Kainate Receptors

The KARs consist of combinations of GluK1-5 subunits forming homo- or heterotetrameric receptors.[21] These receptors are expressed both postsynaptically and presynaptically where they contribute to excitatory synaptic transmission and modulate network excitability by regulating neurotransmitter release.[22] The KARs function both as ionotropic and metabotropic receptors. They elicit fast influx of Na^+ resulting in fast excitation, and are also coupled to G protein signaling that activates PKC and inhibits Ca^{2+} activated K^+ currents, thereby increasing neuronal excitability and neurotransmitter release at some synapses. Presynaptic KARs may elicit either inhibition or facilitation of release of glutamate or GABA, depending on the type of neurons and glutamate concentration.

METABOTROPIC GLUTAMATE RECEPTORS

The metabotropic glutamate receptors (mGluRs) are GPCRs that exist as obligatory dimers of two subunits. One of the subunits binds glutamate, whereas the second subunit couples the receptor with the G protein. Metabotropic glutamate receptors differ structurally from other GPCRs by the presence of a large extracellular ligand-binding domain that is linked to the transmembrane domain via a cysteine-rich domain. There are eight mGluRs, which are divided into group I, II, or III subfamilies based on sequence homologies and their preferred G_α protein-signaling partners. These receptors also defer in their cellular distribution and functions (Figure 17.6).

Group I mGluRs

Group I receptors include mGluR1 and mGluR5, which are primarily located postsynaptically in the neuronal soma and dendrites at the periphery of postsynaptic densities. The mGluR1 is abundantly expressed in Purkinje cells, whereas mGluR5 is expressed in both neurons and astrocytes of the cerebral cortex, striatum, and spinal cord. Group I mGluRs are primarily coupled to G_q, and activate phospholipase C (PLC) signaling, leading to hydrolysis of membrane phosphatidylinositol 4,5 bisphosphate with production

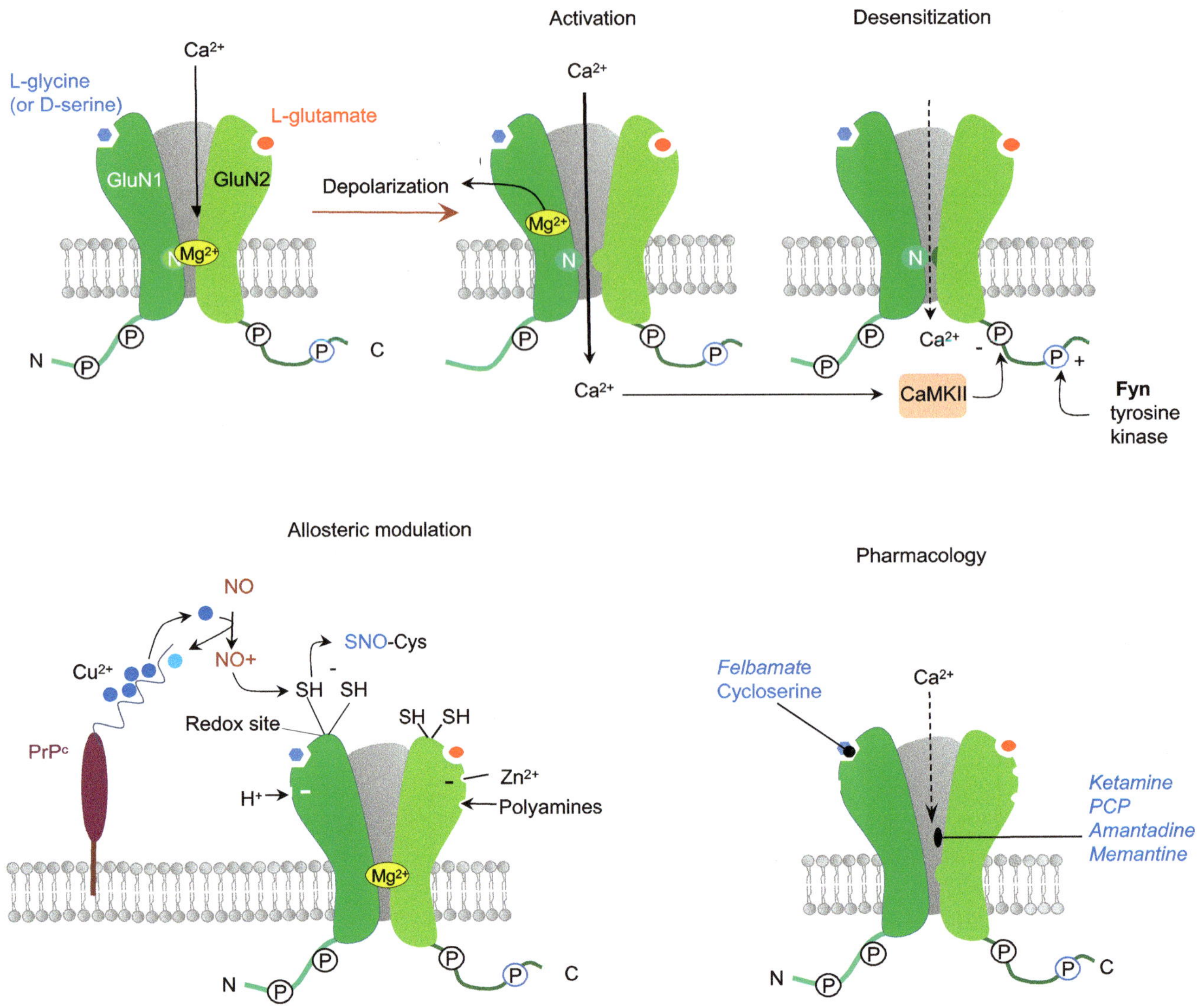

FIGURE 17.5 Activation and modulation of NMDARs.
The N-methyl-D-aspartate receptor (NMDAR) requires binding of both glycine (or D-serine) to the GluN1 and glutamate to the GluN2 subunits for activation. At resting state, extracellular Mg^{2+} causes an open channel block by permeating the pore and preventing the passage of Ca^{2+} ions. Depolarization removes the Mg^{2+} blockade allowing Ca^{2+} flow. The intracellular C-terminus of NMDAR subunits contains phosphorylation sites for protein kinase (PKC), PKA, CaMKII, and the tyrosine kinase Fyn. The NMDAR has several allosteric modulatory sites; these include a polyamine site, allosteric sites for divalent cations such as Zn^{2+} and copper (Cu^{2+}), a proton (H^+)-sensitive site, and a redox modulatory site. Nitric oxide (NO) reacts with critical cysteine residues at the redox modulatory sites of the receptor, producing S-nitrosylation, which reduces the affinity of the glycine modulatory site and thus inhibits NMDAR currents. Prion protein (PrP^c) reduces the affinity of the GluN1 subunit for glycine. Copper bound to PrP^c also oxidizes NO to nitrosyl ion, thereby promoting S-nitrosylation of extracellular thiol residues of GluN1 and GluN2A subunits.

of diacylglycerol (DAG) and inositol triphosphate (IP_3). Diacylglycerol, together with Ca^{2+} activates PKC and serves as a precursor for synthesis of endocannabinoids. Inositol triphosphate acts via IP_3 receptors (IP_3R, ITPR) in the endoplasmic reticulum (ER) and triggers Ca^{2+} release. Group I mGluRs also potentiate L-type Ca^{2+} channels and inhibit K^+ channels. In addition, group I mGluRs may activate noncanonical transduction cascades including those mediated by p38 mitogen-activated protein kinase (MAPK) and extracellular signal-regulated kinase (ERK).

Group II and Group III mGluRs

Group II receptors (mGluR 2 and mGluR3) and group III receptors (mGluR4, mGluR6, mGluR7 and mGluR8)

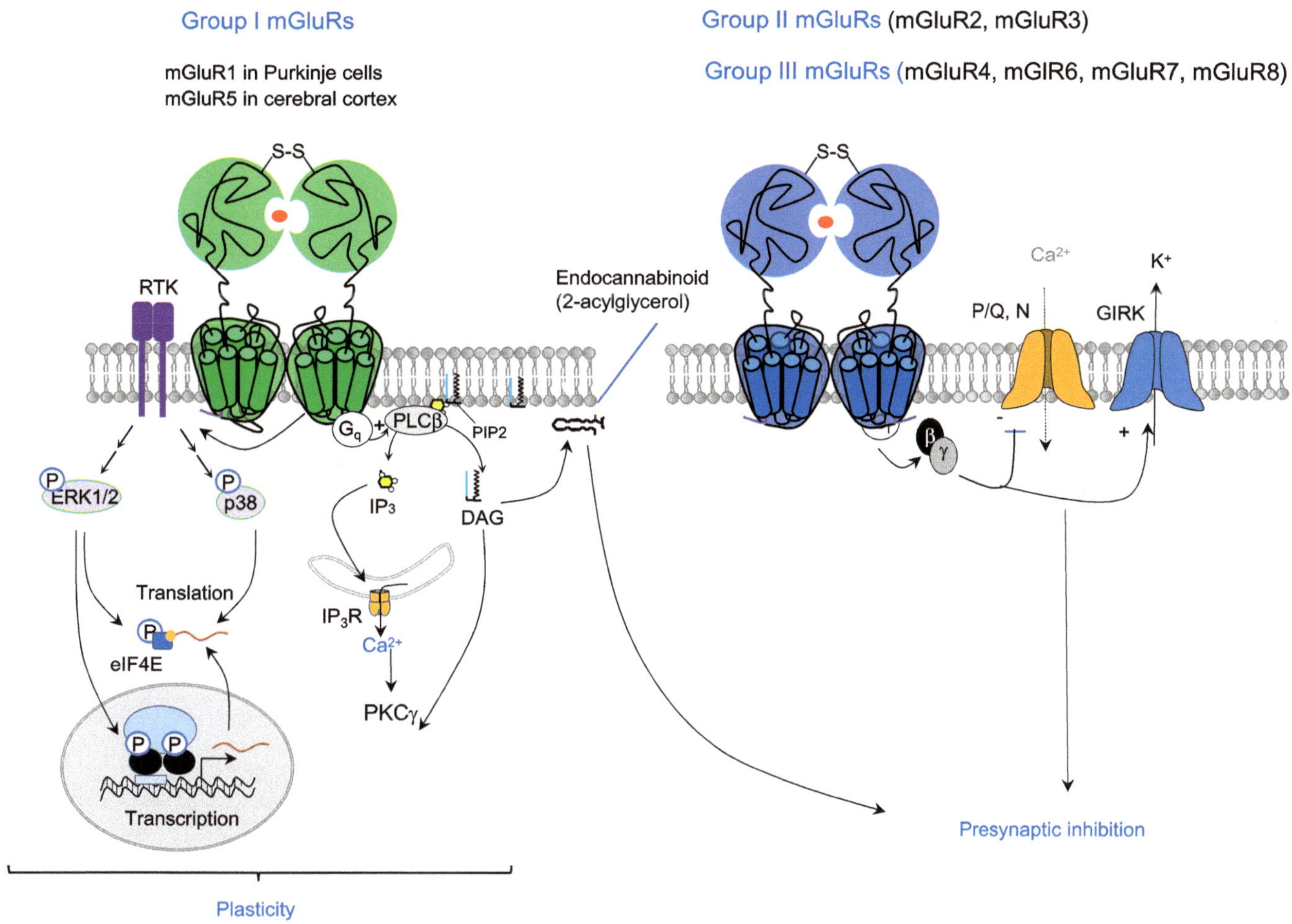

FIGURE 17.6 Signal transduction of metabotropic glutamate receptors.
The metabotropic glutamate receptors (mGluRs) exist as obligatory dimers of two subunits; one binds glutamate and the second couples the receptor with the G protein. Group I receptors mGluRs are primarily coupled to G_q, and activate phospholipase C (PLC) signaling leading to hydrolysis of membrane phosphatidylinositol 4,5 bisphosphate (PIP2) with production of diacylglycerol (DAG) and inositol triphosphate (IP_3). Diacylglycerol together with Ca^{2+} activates protein kinase C (PKC). Group I mGluRs coupled to G_q may also activate via p38 mitogen-activated protein kinase and extracellular signal regulated kinase (ERK). Group II receptors (mGluR 2 and mGluR3) and group III receptors (mGluR4, mGluR6, mGluR7 and mGluR8) are coupled to $G\alpha_{i/o}$ and therefore inhibit adenylyl cyclase; and via the βγ subunit they activate K^+ currents via G-protein-coupled inward-rectifying K^+ channels (GIRK) and inhibit presynaptic Ca_v2 channels.

are located primarily presynaptically. With the exception of mGluR6, which is primarily expressed in retinal ON bipolar cells, mGluRs are widely expressed throughout the nervous system. Group II mGluRs are primarily located at the preterminal portions of the axons and may be activated by spillover of glutamate from the same or a distant synapse. In general, group-III mGluRs are located close to presynaptic active zones and may act as inhibitory autoreceptors. Group II and group III mGluRs are coupled to $G\alpha_{i/o}$ and therefore inhibit adenylyl cyclase; and via the βγ subunit they activate K^+ currents via G protein-coupled inward-rectifying K^+ channels (GIRK) and inhibit presynaptic Ca_v2 channels. Group II and group III mGluRs inhibit release of glutamate as well as that of GABA or other neurotransmitters. Activation of mGluR5 in astrocytes leads to release in intracellular Ca^{2+} that initiates a Ca^{2+} wave that propagates throughout the astrocyte syncytial network.

POSTSYNAPTIC DENSITY AND INTERACTIONS OF GLUTAMATE RECEPTORS

Glutamate receptors form macromolecular complexes with a wide variety of auxiliary, scaffolding, adaptor, anchoring, cytoskeletal, and signal proteins that regulate receptor trafficking, synaptic localization, stabilization, and endocytosis.[23,24]

Molecular Structure of the Postsynaptic Density

Glutamatergic synapses in many CNS neurons are made on dendritic spines at the postsynaptic densities (PSDs) containing clustered AMPA and NMDA receptors (Figure 17.7). The PSD is a multiprotein complex that consists of scaffolding and linker proteins, adhesion molecules, and signal proteins.[23] The major scaffold protein is PSD-95, which binds glutamate receptor subunits and contains several functional domains that provide for its interactions with linker proteins, signal molecules, and adhesion molecules. One important PSD scaffold is SHANK, a multidomain protein that indirectly interacts with PSD-95 via an associated protein and forms a key postsynaptic network that provides a direct link between membrane receptors, cell adhesion molecules, and the actin cytoskeleton, thus facilitating effective activity-dependent dendritic remodeling. There is a functional interaction between NMDAR-mediated Ca^{2+}

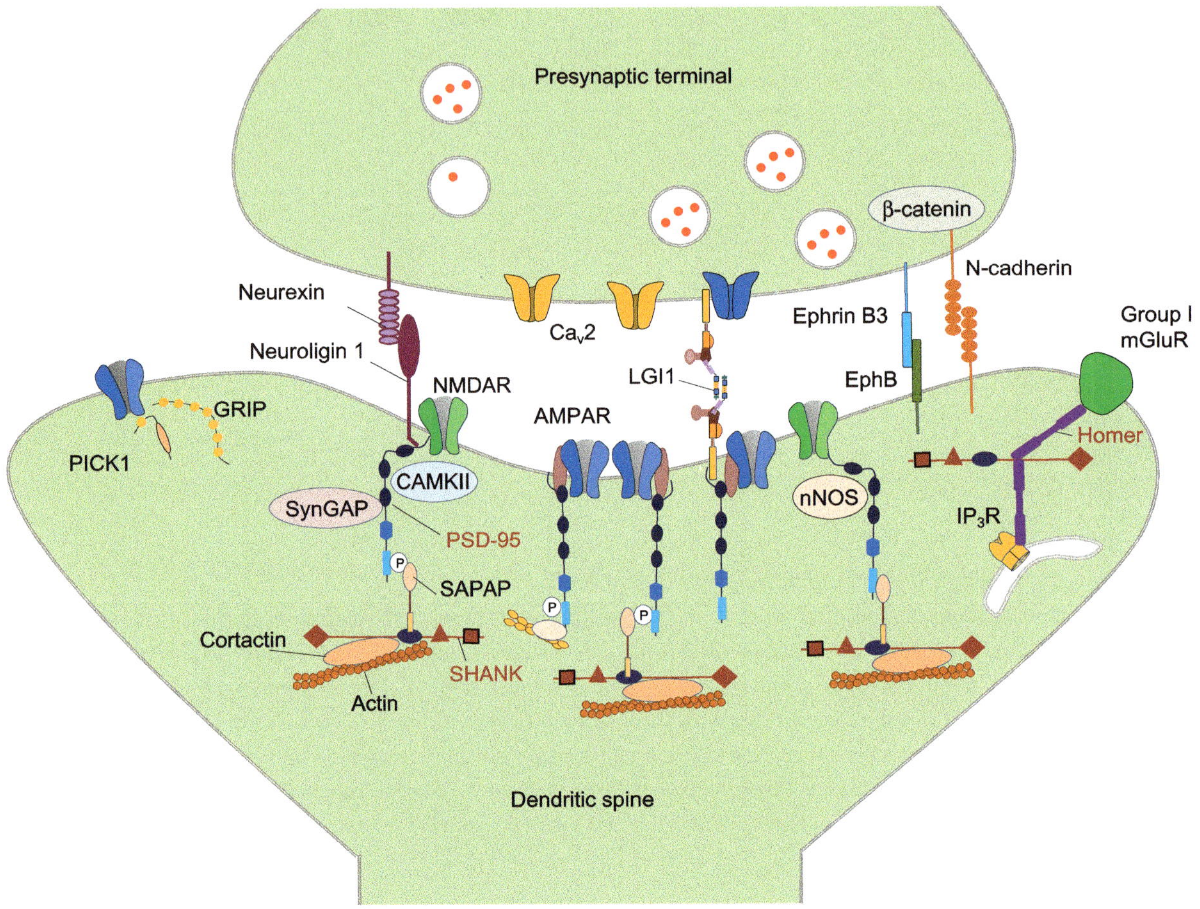

FIGURE 17.7 Organization of the postsynaptic density at excitatory synapses.

The postsynaptic density (PSD) is a multiprotein complex that consists of scaffolding and linker proteins, adhesion molecules, and signal proteins. The major scaffold is PSD 95, which provides for the interactions between glutamate receptors and linker proteins, signal molecules, and adhesion molecules. SHANK provides a direct link between membrane receptors, cell adhesion molecules, and the actin cytoskeleton and forms a network that includes synaptic-associated protein 90/PSD95-associated protein (SAPAP) and the linker protein cortactin. PSD 95 couples N-methyl-D-aspartate receptors (NMDARs) with calmodulin kinase II (CaMKII), neuronal nitric oxide synthase (nNOS), and synaptic Ras GTPase-activating protein (synGAP). Homer allows the functional interaction between group I mGluRs with NMDAR via interactions with the inositol triphosphate receptor (IP_3R) in the endoplasmic reticulum. Transsynaptic interactions mediated by neuroligin 1 and neurexin, ephrin B receptor (EphB) and ephrin B3, cadherins, and those involving secreted bridging proteins such as leucine-rich glioma-inactivated-1 protein (LGI1) contribute to the development, stabilization, and plasticity of glutamatergic synapses. PSD-95 provides a link between these complexes and α-amino-3-hydroxy-5-methyl-4 isoxazole propionic acid receptor (AMPAR) and NMDAR subunits.

influx and group I mGluR-triggered Ca^{2+} release from the ER; this interaction is mediated by the scaffold protein Homer, which binds to PSD-95 via SHANK and with the IP_3R receptor in the ER. PSD-95 also couples NMDARs with downstream signal transduction proteins, such as CaMKII, nitric oxide synthase, and synaptic Ras GTPase-activating protein 1 (SynGAP1). SynGAP suppresses Ras/ERK activity in dendritic spines and limits protein translation and AMPAR exocytosis. Several transsynaptic cell adhesion molecular complexes and secreted synaptic organizers have a major role in development, stabilization, maintenance, and plasticity of glutamatergic synapses.[25] The typical example is the complex formed by postsynaptic neuroligin 1 and presynaptic neurexins.[26,27] Ephrin B3 is a bidirectional signaling protein that binds both to PSD-95 and to the EphB tyrosine kinase. Leucine-rich, glioma-inactivated protein 1 (LGI1) is a secreted scaffold that creates a transsynaptic structure that allows clustering of AMPARs in the synapse.[28] LGI1 functions as a bridge between A disintegrin and metalloproteinase 22 (ADAM-22), which is anchored to the postsynaptic membrane by interactions with PSD-95, and presynaptic ADAM-23, which interacts with voltage-gated K^+ channels.

The fundamental role of the macromolecular organization of the PSD in development and plasticity of glutamatergic synapses explains the consequences of mutations affecting proteins in this complex. Mutations affecting *SHANK*, *SYGAP*, *NRX1* (neurexin 1), *NRX2* (neurexin 2), and *NLG1* (neuroligin 1) constitute a major disease pathway for intellectual disability and autism spectrum disorders.[29–32]

Localization and Trafficking of Ionotropic Glutamate Receptors

Ionotropic glutamate receptor subunits are synthesized and assembled in the ER and then enter the vesicular secretory pathway.[33] Assembled receptors undergo continuous trafficking between intercellular, extrasynaptic, and postsynaptic sites as they constantly switch between mobile and immobile states in the membrane. This dynamics is determined by the interplay between their lateral diffusion and their reversible binding via their C-terminal domains to PSD-95 or other scaffolding proteins. Receptors that do not interact with PSD-95 or with other postsynaptic density scaffolds remain located outside the synapse and are activated by glutamate that spills over from the synapse. The number of ionotropic receptors at the postsynaptic membrane is tightly regulated by phosphorylation of receptor subunits, which controls their relative rates of exocytosis and endocytosis. The regulation of AMPAR availability via phosphorylation of GluA1 or GluA2 subunits is a fundamental mechanism for induction of synaptic plasticity. Phosphorylation of the AMPAR auxiliary subunit stargazin promotes the interaction of the AMPARs with PSD-95, thus stabilizing these receptors at the postsynaptic membrane.[15]

SYNAPTIC AND NETWORK EFFECTS OF GLUTAMATERGIC SIGNALING

The expression of inotropic and metabotropic glutamate receptors is widespread and highly overlapping throughout nearly all brain regions. Both types of receptors are found in both excitatory glutamatergic and inhibitory GABAergic interneurons, with distinct patterns of distribution for different receptor subtypes. The wide range of receptor subtype distribution greatly increases the range of glutamatergic receptor signaling and crosstalk.[11] For example, KARs and some AMPARs and NMDARs are located not only postsynaptically but also extra or presynaptically.[34,35] In addition to their primarily presynaptic localization, group II and III mGluRs may also be expressed postsynaptically, whereas group I mGluRs may also be present in presynaptic terminals.

Fast Excitation of Principal Neurons and Interneurons

In most mature CNS neurons, AMPARs express edited GluA2 subunits and are therefore primarily permeable to Na^+ and mediate fast excitatory postsynaptic potentials. The rapid activation and inactivation of GluA2-containing AMPARs allows the transmission of high-frequency presynaptic inputs and moment-to-moment excitatory signaling in the CNS. The co-localization of AMPARs with NMDARs at the PSD provides for their functional coupling with each other. The depolarizing actions of AMPARs promote the removal of the Mg^{2+} block of the NMDAR receptor pore, allowing influx of Ca^{2+} at dendrites. In the cerebral cortex both types of receptors are expressed in pyramidal neurons and in fast-spiking GABAergic interneurons. These interneurons have a critical role in regulating pyramidal cell excitability and network oscillations in the cerebral cortex. The expression of Ca^{2+} permeable AMPARs results in a rapid time course of excitatory postsynaptic currents in these interneurons, allowing them to provide temporally precise control of network activity.

Metabotropic Glutamate Receptors and Modulation of Excitability

Metabotropic glutamate receptors control neuronal excitability by modulating ion channels. Activation of group I mGluRs typically induces depolarization in most neurons by either opening Ca^{2+} channels such as transient receptor potential (TRP) channels, or by inhibiting K^+ channels. However, increase in intracellular Ca^{2+} in response to mGluR1 signaling can also activate Ca^{2+}-activated K^+ channels to produce hyperpolarization. There is also an interaction between NMDARs that allow Ca^{2+} influx and group I mGluRs that trigger Ca^{2+} release from the ER; this potentiates the ability of NMDARs and type I mGluRs to increase intracellular Ca^2 and CaMKII signaling.[11] Protein kinase C in dendrites may function as a coincidence detector that is activated by signals triggered by both group I mGluRs and

NMDARs and shares downstream targets with CaMKII. In addition to their acute effects, glutamate receptors can affect cellular function over longer timescales through regulation of transcription and local mRNA translation via both Ca^{2+}-dependent and Ca^{2+}-independent control of phosphorylation of transcription factors and mRNA-binding proteins.[36] Activation of group II and III mGluRs typically produces hyperpolarization via activation of K^+ channels and inhibits presynaptic Ca_v2 channels. Thus, these $G_{i/o}$-coupled mGluRs provide a feedback inhibition that opposes inotropic glutamatergic receptor-mediated excitation.

PLASTICITY AT GLUTAMATERGIC SYNAPSES

Plasticity of glutamatergic synapses may occur via presynaptic or postsynaptic mechanisms. The mechanisms of postsynaptic LTP or LTD in these synapses have been primarily studied in the hippocampus (Figure 17.8).

NMDAR-Triggered LTP Induction in the Hippocampus

The classical example of synaptic plasticity is NMDAR-triggered LTP (NMDA-LTP) at the synapses from CA3 Schaffer collaterals on CA1 pyramidal neurons of the hippocampus.[36,37] Activation of synaptic NMDARs results in a large influx of Ca^{2+}, which activates calmodulin (CaM) and initiates CaMKII-dependent signaling cascades.[38] CaMKII phosphorylates both the GluA1 subunit and scaffold proteins, thereby promoting AMPAR insertion at postsynaptic sites. By this mechanism, "silent" synapses lacking AMPARs can be converted into active synapses.[38] Transsynaptic adhesion interactions involving neuroligin-1 (and its presynaptic partner neurexin) or the EphB-ephrin B3 complex promote NMDAR-induced LTP in the hippocampus.[26]

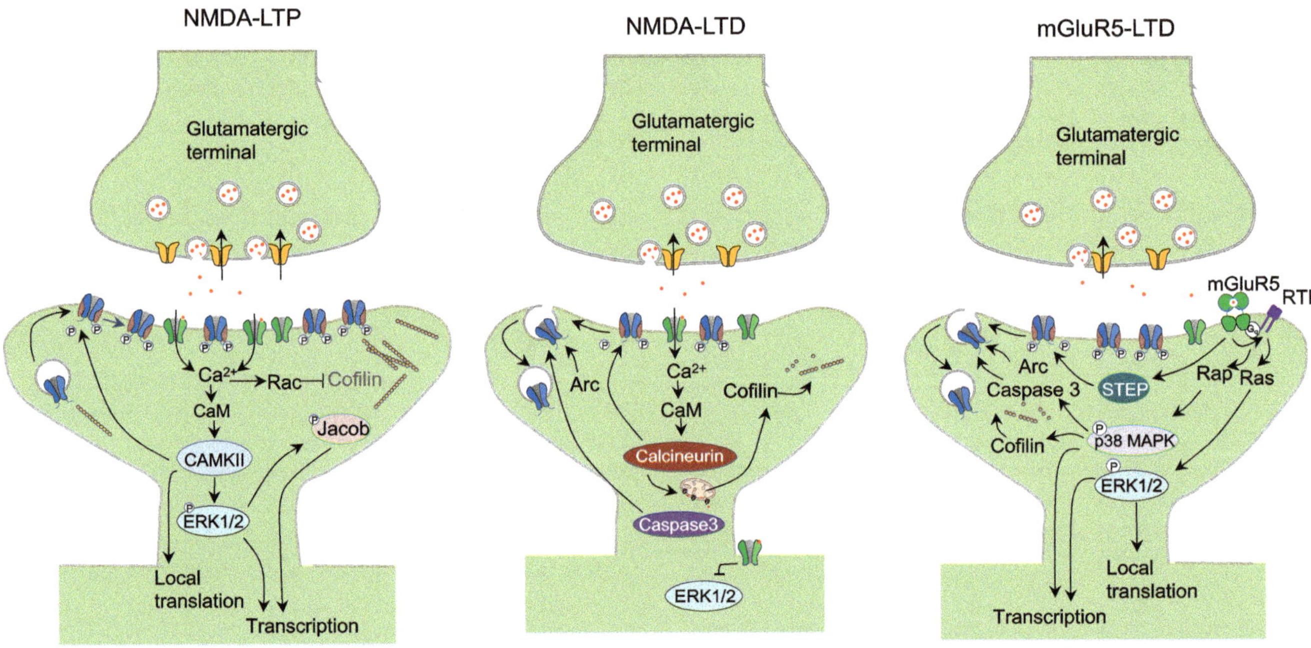

FIGURE 17.8 Induction of synaptic plasticity in the hippocampus.
Activation of N-methyl-D-aspartate receptors (NMDARs) triggers either long-term potentiation (LTP) or long-term depression (LTD) at the synapses from CA3 Schaffer collateral on CA1 pyramidal neurons of the hippocampus. A large influx of Ca^{2+} via synaptic NMDARs activates calmodulin (CaM), leading to CaM kinase II (CaMKII)-mediated phosphorylation of the GluA1 subunit of α-amino-3-hydroxy-5-methyl-4 isoxazole propionic acid receptors (AMPARs), increasing their insertion at postsynaptic sites. Ca^{2+} also activates Rac (Ras-related C3 botulinum toxin substratel), a small RhoGTPase that triggers downstream signaling cascades that lead to inhibition of cofilin promoting formation and maintenance of dendritic spines. Activation of NMDARs by low levels of glutamate may trigger LTD via CaM activation of calcineurin, which dephosphorylates the GluA1 subunit promoting internalization of AMPARs from the synapses. Calcineurin also triggers activation of caspase-3, which contributes to reduced expression of AMPAR at synapses. Activation of type 5 metabotropic glutamate receptors (mGluR5) elicits LTD via noncanonical G_q protein-activated pathways involving p38 mitogen-activated protein kinase (MAPK) and extracellular signal-regulated kinase (ERK). These signals activate the activity-regulated cytoskeleton-associated protein (Arc), which promotes endocytosis of AMPARs remodeling of the actin cytoskeleton by the cofilin. Both p38 MAPK and ERK promote transcription of striatum-enriched tyrosine phosphatase (STEP), which dephosphorylates tyrosine residues on the GluA2 subunit promoting its internalization.

Maintenance of functional and structural plasticity after induction of LTP requires changes in transcription and local translation of mRNA, actin cytoskeleton remodeling, and changes in transsynaptic adhesion interactions. Increase in intracellular Ca^{2+} has a major role in all these processes[39] (Figure 17.9). Calcium influx into the postsynaptic neuron via L-type voltage-gated Ca^{2+} channels or NMDAR activates CaMKII calmodulin-dependent kinase kinase (CaMKK), ERK 1/2 and other signaling molecules critical for maintenance of use-dependent synaptic plasticity. The canonical mechanism for activity-dependent regulation of mRNA transcription is phosphorylation of the cyclic AMP and calcium-activated regulatory element-binding protein (CREB) by several kinases. These include CAMKIV downstream of Ca^{2+} influx and CAMKII-CaMKK signaling and phosphorylated ERK downstream of signaling by NMDARs and brain-derived neurotrophic factor (BDNF) tyrosine kinase receptors. Phosphorylated CREB recruits CREB-binding protein, leading to transcriptional activation of immediate early genes encoding transcription factors such as c-Fos and c-Jun, and several synaptic proteins such GluA2 subunits, CaMKII, BDNF, and activity-regulated cytoskeleton-associated protein (Arc).[40] In addition to this canonical Ca^{2+}-dependent pathway, synaptic activity promotes the formation of several signal-containing synaptonuclear complexes that are translocated to the nucleus to regulate transcription.[41–43] One typical example is Jacob, which is phosphorylated by ERK in response to activation of synaptic NMDARs and forms a complex that is translocated to the nucleus via importins. Other examples include

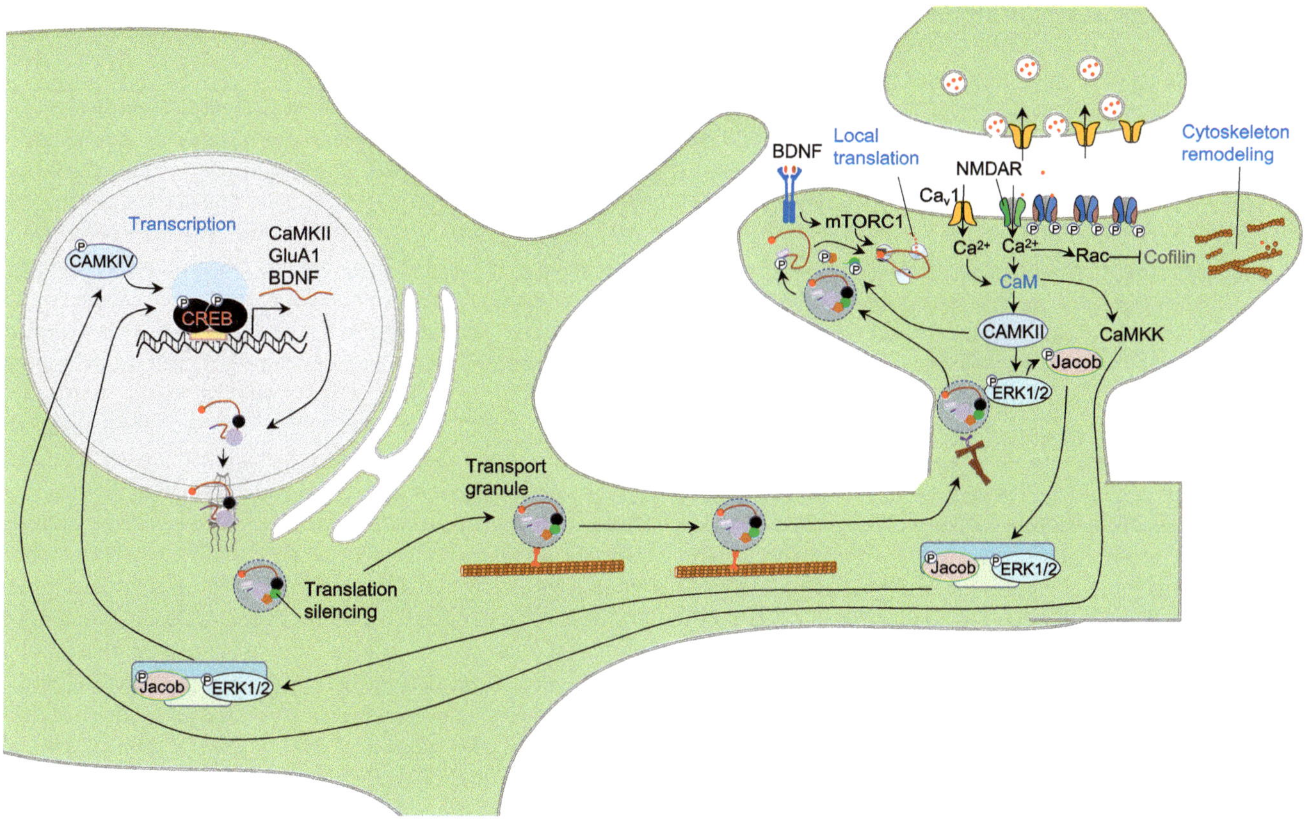

FIGURE 17.9 Maintenance of plasticity at glutamatergic synapses.
Calcium influx into the postsynaptic neuron via L-type voltage-gated Ca^{2+} channels, NMDARs, and in some cases Ca^{2+}-permeable AMPARs, activates CaMKII, calmodulin-dependent kinase kinase (CaMKK), extracellular signal-regulated kinase (ERK) 1/2, and other signaling molecules critical for maintenance of use-dependent synaptic plasticity. Phosphorylation of the cyclic AMP and calcium-activated regulatory element-binding protein (CREB) activates the transcription of immediate early genes encoding synaptic proteins. Synaptic activity also promotes the formation of several signal-containing synaptonuclear complexes such as the one involving Jacob, which is translocated to the nucleus via importins. After transcription, mRNAs encoding synaptic proteins are incorporated into mRNA transport granules in association with several mRNA-binding proteins. At the level of active dendrites, phosphorylation of mRNA-binding proteins and activation of mechanistic (mammalian) target of rapamycin complex 1 (mTORC1) downstream of BDNF and NMDAR signaling promotes local protein synthesis and dendritic cytoskeleton remodeling.

CREB transcriptional coactivator 1 and the amyloid precursor protein (APP) intracellular domain-associated protein-1 (AIDA-1).[41,42,44]

Maintenance of LTP also requires activity-dependent translation of mRNA at active dendritic sites. The mRNAs encoding synaptic proteins are incorporated into transport granules in association with several mRNA-binding proteins, such as fragile X mental retardation protein (FMRP), which prevent mRNA translation. At active dendrites, several activity-dependent mechanisms lead to "unmasking" mRNA, allowing its access to the translation machinery at the active synaptic spines.[45] One example is phosphorylation of FMRP, leading to its dissociation from the mRNA. Local protein synthesis is promoted by mechanistic (mammalian) target of rapamycin (mTOR) downstream of BDNF and NMDAR signaling.

The structural correlate of synaptic plasticity is dendritic growth and maturation, which requires remodeling of the actin cytoskeleton. This dynamic process involves the regulation of the actin-depolymerizing protein cofilin.[46] LTP of glutamatergic synapses relies on accumulation of F-actin in dendritic spines. Both Ca^{2+} influx via NMDARs and BDNF receptor signaling activate the small Rho GTPases Rac (Ras-related C3 botulinum toxin substrate1) and Cdc42 (cell division cycle 42), which triggers downstream phosphorylation and inhibition of the actin-severing protein cofilin, promoting formation and maintenance of dendritic spines. Oher actin-binding proteins such as CaMKII and Debrin stabilize the actin cytoskeleton in dendritic spines.

NMDAR-Triggered LTD in the Hippocampus

Activation of either synaptic or extrasynaptic NMDARs by low levels of glutamate may trigger LTD in the hippocampus (NMDA-LTD)[36,37] (Figure 17.8). In the case of synaptic NMDARs, induction of LTD involves CaM activation of the phosphatase calcineurin, which dephosphorylates the GluA1 subunit and triggers internalization of AMPARs from the synapses. Calcineurin also acts via the mitochondria to trigger nonapoptotic activation of caspase-3, which contributes to reduced expression of AMPAR at synapses.[47] When synaptic activity is low CaMKII phosphorylates Arc, which is recruited to the presynaptic membrane, interacts with actin, and promotes clathrin-mediated endocytosis of AMPARs. Another mediator of NMDA-LTD is glycogen synthase kinase3β (GSK3β) which in its basal unphosphorylated state constitutively promotes AMPAR endocytosis.[48] BDNF activation of AKT leads to inhibitory phosphorylation GSK3β, thus preventing LTD. In contrast, caspase-3 cleaves AKT, thereby promoting GSK3β activity and AMPAR endocytosis. NMDAR-LTD is a physiological mechanism used to eliminate synapses during development.[49] LTD is associated with F-actin loss and shrinkage of dendritic spines. This is thought to involve Ca^{2+} activation of calcineurin, which in turn activates cofilin. Gelsolin, one of the most potent actin-severing factors, may also have a potentially important role in this process.[50]

Metabotropic mGluR5 Receptor-Triggered LTD in the Hippocampus

Activation of mGluR5 receptors may elicit LTD in the hippocampus via either presynaptic or postsynaptic mechanisms. The postsynaptic mechanisms are complex and involve noncanonical pathways[51,52] (Figure 17.8). For example, mGluR5-coupled G_q protein activates receptor tyrosine kinases and downstream signaling via p38 MAPK and ERK. These signals activate Arc, resulting both in cytoskeleton remodeling via cofilin and clathrin-dependent endocytosis of AMPARs. Both p38 MAPK and ERK also promote transcription of several proteins that promote LTD. One example is the striatum-enriched tyrosine phosphatase (STEP), which dephosphorylates tyrosine residues on the GluA2 subunit promoting its internalization.[53] In addition, both p38 MAPK and STEP promote activation of caspase 3, which contributes to AMPAR internalization and dendritic remodeling.[54,55] Other pathways involved in mGluR5-triggered LTD involves the calcium-triggered activation of the protease calpain-1.[56]

Synaptic Homeostatic Plasticity (Synaptic Scaling)

Synaptic homeostatic plasticity, also known as synaptic scaling, is the mechanism that maintains synaptic weight in different portions of the dendrites, thereby preventing excessive excitation or inhibition of neurons. In response to repetitive firing of the presynaptic neuron, active synapses with high probability of neurotransmitter release show LTD rather than LTP. In contrast, less active synapses are more likely to undergo LTP in response to repetitive activation. Synaptic scaling resulting from the balanced increase or decrease in AMPAR expression in different portions of the dendrite keeps the firing of neurons at the target level. The number of receptors at each synapse is scaled up or down thus maintaining the relative ratio between the synapses; this allows restoration of target activity while preserving the changes elicited by LTP or LTD at the individual synapses. Metaplasticity refers to changes in the ability of synapses to undergo plasticity after a previous synaptic or modulatory event, sometimes called "priming." The prototypic form of metaplasticity is depotentiation, which is a form of LTD that can only be induced following the induction of LTP. Another form of metaplasticity occurs when prior activation of NMDARs can inhibit the subsequent induction of NMDAR-LTP.

Metabotropic mGluR1 Receptor-Triggered LTD in the Cerebellum

Another important example of plasticity of glutamatergic synapses is LTD at the parallel fiber-Purkinje cell synapse in the cerebellum. This process is induced by concomitant activation of mGluR1 receptors in dendritic spines and large increase in dendritic Ca^{2+} triggered by climbing fiber inputs.[57] This mechanism is important for error-signal-based learning in the cerebellum. Activation of mGluR1 receptors triggers the PLCβ cascade leading to production of DAG and IP_3; this results in Ca^{2+} release from the ER via the IP_3R and activation of PKCα. Phosphorylation of GluA2 subunit of the AMPAR by PKCα promotes AMPAR internalization in the dendritic spines of the Purkinje cell, resetting its tonic firing in response to parallel fiber input.

GLUTAMATE RECEPTORS SIGNALS RELATED TO SURVIVAL AND NEURODEGENERATION

The role of synaptic and extrasynaptic NMDARs and their interactions with normal membrane PrP^c and APP has multiple potential implications in mechanisms of neurotoxicity and neurodegeneration.

Downstream Effects of Synaptic and Extrasynaptic NMDA Receptors

Synaptic and extrasynaptic NMDARs trigger different downstream transducing cascades that have opposite effects on cell survival. In general, synaptic NMDARs are neuroprotective by activating downstream signals that lead to CREB phosphorylation and transcription of survival genes, such as those encoding BDNF, and suppression of death genes. In contrast, activation of extrasynaptic NMDARs may initiate cell death pathways by shutting-off the CREB signaling.[58] Extrasynaptic NMDARs may also trigger nuclear import of the pro-death transcription factors and excessive accumulation of Ca^{2+}, which triggers activation of the protease calpain and other downstream cascades leading to cell injury.[58] However, some evidence indicates that the canonical dichotomy between synaptic and extrasynaptic NMDAR effects on survival has may be an oversimplification.[17]

Interactions of Glutamate Receptors with Prion Proteins and Amyloid Precursor Protein

Prion protein is a widely expressed cuproprotein that is particularly abundant in synaptic membranes, where it is concentrated at cholesterol-enriched lipid rafts.[59] PrP^c interacts with many channels and receptors, including NMDAR, AMPAR, Ca_v1 (L) channels, and mGluR5. In its copper-bound state, PrP^c may have neuroprotective effects against NMDAR-triggered toxicity by interacting with the GluN1 subunit, reducing its affinity for glycine and thus increasing NMDAR desensitization. Copper bound to PrP^c also promotes S-nitrosylation of extracellular thiol residues of GluN1 and GluN2A subunits, decreasing steady state activation of NMDARs.[19,20]

Amyloid precursor protein is localized at postsynaptic densities and has an important role in neuronal survival, synaptogenesis, and synaptic plasticity.[60] Synaptic activity promotes APP processing and generation of amyloid-β peptide (Aβ) via β- and γ-secretase. Aβ may sustain LTP, for example, by regulating vesicular release of glutamate via presynaptic α7 nicotinic receptors.[61] Oligomeric Aβ interacts with a wide range of molecular components located both at the postsynaptic densities and at extrasynaptic sites, including NMDARs, mGluR5, PrP^c, calcium channels, and adhesion molecules such as ephrin and EphB2 receptors.[62] These interactions trigger several downstream cascades regulating synaptic plasticity, cell survival, oxidative stress, actin remodeling, and vesicular trafficking.

Some critical mediators required for maintenance of LTP, such as cAMP, promote expression of the gene encoding APP and increase production of Aβ.[63] The APP intracellular domain associated protein-1 (AIDA-1) facilitates GluN2B transport from the ER to synapses and provides a potential link among NMDAR expression, synaptic plasticity, and Aβ production.[41,42,64]

GLUTAMATERGIC SYNAPTIC PATHOLOGY IN ALZHEIMER DISEASE

Impaired synaptic plasticity and dendritic loss in the excitatory glutamatergic synapses in the hippocampus are early events in Alzheimer disease (AD). Accumulation of soluble Aβ oligomers disrupts LTP and promotes LTD (Figure 17.10). Whereas at early stages the synaptic changes elicited by Aβ oligomers are reversible, later in the disease they are rendered irreversible by associated tau-related neuropathology.[65–69] However, several mouse models show that the presence of Aβ enhances tau hyperphosphorylation-associated neuropathology throughout the disease course.[66]

Role of NMDARs and mGuR5

Many of the effects of Aβ oligomers leading to synaptic loss are thought to be mediated by extrasynaptic NMDARs and largely reflect altered Ca^{2+} dynamics in dendrites and dendritic spines. Effector mechanisms include activation of calcineurin, translocation of cofilin into the mitochondria, and initiation of the intrinsic apoptosis cascade via caspase-3 activation.[70–72] Extrasynaptic NMDARs also elicit p38MAPK triggered cascades, calpain activation, and downregulation of CREB signaling. Nuclear translocation of unphosphorylated Jacob may also shut-off CREB mediated plasticity and neuroprotection signals.

Interaction of Aβ oligomers with mGluR5 receptors and PrP^c also promote LTD in the hippocampus.[73–76] The downstream cascades are similar to those involved in normal mGluR5-triggered LTD and include p38 MAPK, Jun-terminal kinases, cyclin-dependent kinase 5, STEP, caspase 3, and GSK3β, resulting in AMPAR internalization. Toxic Aβ1–42 oligomers increase cholesterol concentration at synapses, thereby promoting the formation of $A\beta/PrP^c$ complexes that interact with mGluR5 to activate the Fyn tyrosine kinase, leading to activating phosphorylation of the GluN2B subunit of the NMDAR. These oligomers also bind copper, thereby its promoting effect on NO-mediated nitrosylation and inhibition of the NMDAR.[74]

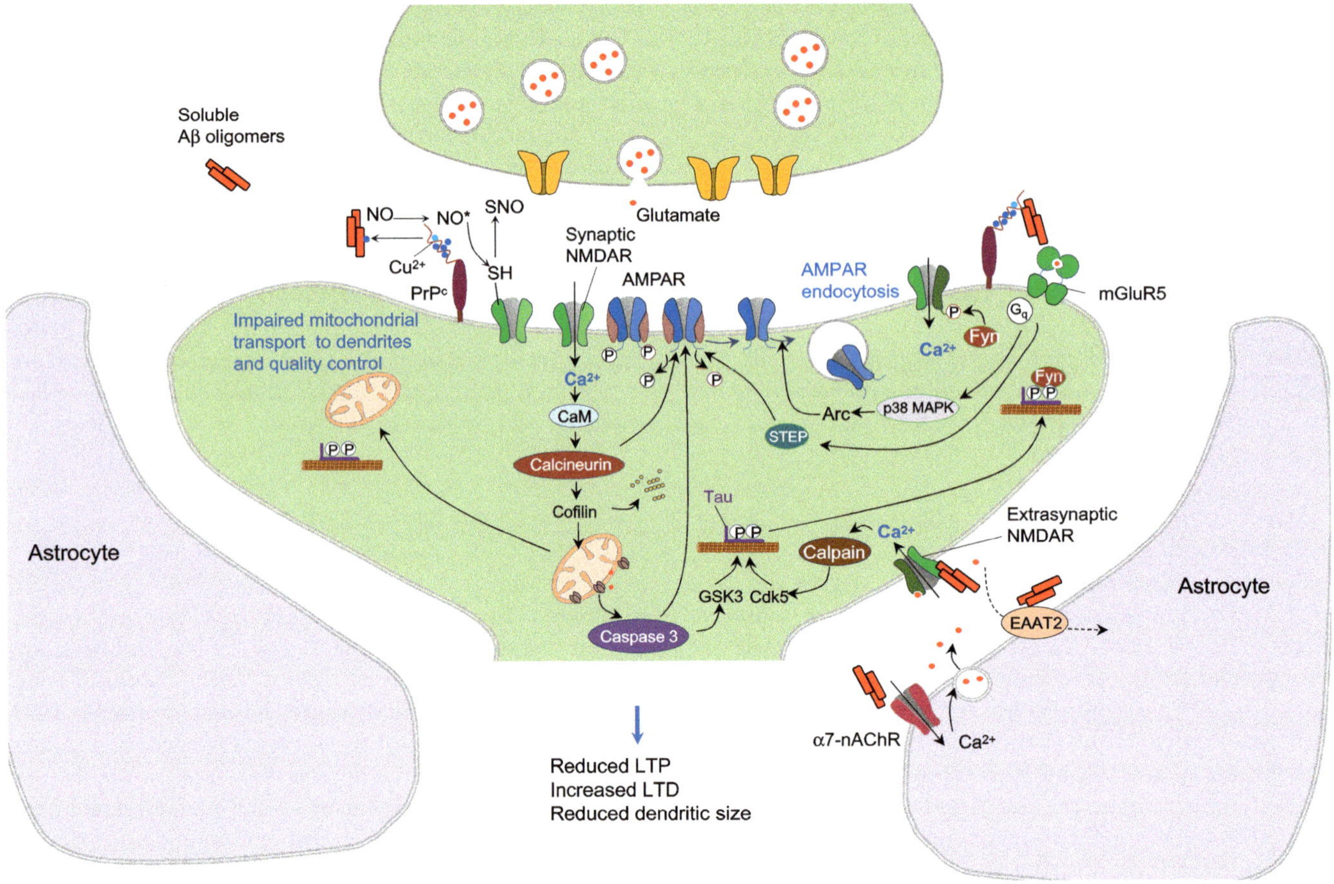

FIGURE 17.10 Glutamatergic synaptic toxicity in Alzheimer disease.
Accumulation of soluble amyloid β (Aβ) oligomers disrupts long-term potentiation (LTP) and promotes long-term depression (LTD) at glutamatergic synapses in Alzheimer disease. Activation of extrasynaptic N-methyl-D-aspartate receptors (NMDARs) leads to altered Ca^{2+} dynamics with activation of calcineurin, translocation of cofilin into the mitochondria, and initiation of the intrinsic apoptosis cascade via caspase-3 activation. Interaction of Aβ oligomers with mGluR5 receptors and prion protein (PrP^c) also prevents LTP and promotes LTD. The downstream cascades include p38 mitogen activated kinase (p38 MAPK), striatum-enriched tyrosine phosphatase (STEP), and caspase 3-induced internalization of α-amino-3-hydroxy-5-methyl-4 isoxazole propionic acid receptors (AMPARs). Toxic Aβ1-42 oligomers promote the formation of Aβ/PrP^c complexes that interact with mGluR5 to activate the Fyn tyrosine kinase, leading to activation of NMDARs. Activation of extrasynaptic NMDARs and mGluR5 by Aβ oligomers triggers tau-mediated neuropathology cyclin-dependent kinase 5 (CdK5) and glycogen synthase kinase 3 β (GSK-3β) that elicit tau phosphorylation leading to impaired microtubule-based dendritic transport and mitochondrial dysfunction. Aβ oligomers induce glutamate release from astrocytes via α7 nicotinic receptors and inhibit its uptake by excitatory amino acid transporters (EATTs). There is increased activity of astrocytes and microglia in elimination of senescent synapses via phagocytosis in AD.

Interactions of Aβ with Tau

Studies in experimental models show that there are complex interactions between Aβ and tau in regulation of synaptic plasticity, neuronal excitability and network oscillations.[66] These interactions affect tau phosphorylation, dynamics, and distribution and potentiate toxicity at the levels of dendritic spines and mitochondria. Neuronal hyperactivity enhances tau secretion from neurons, and secreted tau can be internalized by recipient cells, where it subsequently seeds additional tau.

Aβ can thus induce tau oligomer aggregation and seeding. Tau acts synergistically with Aβ to impair LTP and promote synaptic loss. Tau is expressed in the postsynaptic density, where it regulates NMDAR-mediated synaptic plasticity and toxicity.[77] Activation of extrasynaptic NMDARs by Aβ oligomers increases tau mRNA and protein levels as well as tau phosphorylation at synapses. Several downstream kinases activated by Aβ/mGluR5 interactions, including cyclin-dependent kinase 5 and GSK3β elicit tau phosphorylation. This promotes interaction of hyperphosphorylated tau with Fyn and targets Fyn to dendrites, where it phosphorylates the GluN2B, leading to excitotoxic cascades.[78] Tau hyperphosphorylation also leads to impaired microtubule-based dendritic transport, resulting in reduced glutamate receptor trafficking and synaptic anchoring.[79] Tau also acts synergistically with Aβ to impair mitochondrial function and ATP synthesis and enhance production of reactive oxygen species. This may result in DNA damage contributing to downregulation of several survival and synaptic genes eventually leading to accelerated neuronal hypoexcitability. PrP^c is upregulated in AD and may participate in Aβ–tau synergy; binding of soluble Aβ or tau to PrP^c may impair synaptic plasticity and promote seeding of abnormal tau.

Contribution of Astrocytes and Microglia

Astrocytes and microglia contribute to early synaptic dysfunction and loss in AD independently of inflammation.[80] Aβ induces glutamate release from astrocytes via α7 nicotinic receptors and inhibits its uptake via EAATs; this may contribute to glutamate spillover with excessive activation of extrasynaptic NMDARs.[81] There is increased activity of astrocytes and microglia in elimination of senescent synapses via phagocytosis in AD. Aβ upregulates nuclear factor κB expression and release of the C3 component of complement from astrocytes; C3 acts on C3a receptors in neurons to disrupt dendritic morphology.[82] Microglia express the complement receptor CR3 that is activated by C1q associated with senescent synapses; this increases the number of phagocytic microglia and thereby promotes synaptic pruning.[83] Cytokines released by glial cells may also contribute to synaptic dysfunction in AD. For example, tumor necrosis α promotes AMPAR internalization in hippocampal neurons, leading to impaired LTP.[84]

AUTOIMMUNE GLUTAMATERGIC SYNAPTOPATHIES

Several forms of autoimmune encephalitis are due to autoantibodies directed against glutamate receptors or adhesion molecules that organize the postsynaptic density. The most typical manifestation is limbic encephalitis with prominent memory impairment and seizures.[85–89]

NMDAR Encephalitis

NMDAR encephalitis is caused by IgG autoantibodies against the GluN1 subunit of the receptor. These autoantibodies induce internalization and downregulation of the NMDAR by affecting its interaction with ephrin B3, an important stabilizing regulator of PSD-95.[90] By reducing surface expression of NMDARs, these autoantibodies interfere with induction of LTP in the hippocampus and may also potentially impair local GABAergic interneurons controlling network synchronization. NMDAR encephalitis is characterized by rapid onset of abnormal behaviors, psychosis, cognitive dysfunction, seizures, and movement disorders (such as catatonia in adults and chorea in children); this is followed by reduced level of consciousness, and then autonomic dysfunction and central hypoventilation. A characteristic feature is the presence of a delta-brush pattern on the electroencephalogram. Anti-NMDAR encephalitis is paraneoplastic in a substantial portion of young women with ovarian teratoma, which also expresses NMDARs. Patients may develop NMDAR encephalitis following herpes simplex type 1 or other viral infections or as consequence of treatment with immune checkpoint inhibitors in patients with cancer.

AMPAR Encephalitis

AMPAR encephalitis is due to autoantibodies against the GluA subunits of the receptor. As in the case of anti-NMDAR encephalitis, these autoantibodies cause internalization of AMPARs and reduced excitatory synaptic transmission.[91] Manifestations of AMPAR receptor encephalitis include confusion, executive dysfunction, psychosis, seizures, and sometimes rapidly progressive encephalopathy. Neoplasms (particularly small-cell lung carcinoma, breast carcinoma, or thymoma) may be present in more than half of the cases, in general associated with other membrane and onconeural antibodies.

LGI1 Encephalitis

LGI1 encephalitis has typical features of limbic encephalitis and may present with characteristic faciobrachial dystonic or other types of seizures. In the hippocampus of mice, LGI1 antibodies decreased the levels of both presynaptic Kv1.1 and postsynaptic AMPAR clusters, resulting in increased presynaptic glutamate release and enhancement of glutamatergic synaptic transmission. These effects suggest that the autoantibodies disturb the transsynaptic linkage through the LGI1–ADAM22/23 assembly by inhibiting the interaction between LGI1 and both ADAM22 and ADAM23. There is a degree of phenotype overlap between LGI11 antibody-associated disorders and those associated with antibodies against contactin associated-protein related 2 (CASPR2), which is another antigenic component the K_v1 complex.[92] Whereas faciobrachial dystonic seizures reliably indicate LGI1 encephalitis, neuropathic pain and neuromyotonia reflecting peripheral nerve hyperexcitability are more common with CASPR2 antibodies.[92]

Antibodies Affecting Group I mGluRs

Autoimmune disorders due to autoantibodies against group I mGluRs is commonly associated with Hodgkin lymphoma. The primary manifestation of antibodies disrupting mGluR1 signaling in Purkinje cells is cerebellar ataxia.[93,94] These antibodies target different components of the mGluR1–IP_3R–PKC pathway involved in LTD at the parallel fiber-Purkinje cell synapse. The term "medusa-head ataxia" refers to the characteristic somatodendritic immunocytochemical staining of antibodies targeting antigens involved in these mGluR1/calcium pathways. They include anti-mGluR1, anti-Homer protein homolog 3, anti-IP3R (ITPR), and anti-PKC γ.[95–97] For example, mGluR1 antibodies impair Purkinje cell activity and cerebellar LTD, and chronically lead to Purkinje cell loss. Mutations of many of these proteins underlie several forms of spinocerebellar ataxia. For example, mutations of the *GRM1* gene encoding mGluR1 produce a form of autosomal recessive cerebellar ataxia; mutations of the *ITPR1* causes spinocerebellar ataxia (SCA) 15–16; and mutations of the *PRKCG* gene cause SCA14.[98,99] In contrast, antibodies against mGluR5 cause an encephalitis with marked cognitive and behavioral changes.[100]

EPILEPSY SYNDROMES

Epilepsy is a manifestation of a network disorder reflecting imbalance between excitation and inhibition. Experimental and clinic evidence indicates AMPARs, NMDARs, and KARs participate in this process. Perampanel is a selective blocker of AMPA receptors showing efficacy in treating various epileptic disorders.[101,102] Recent evidence in experimental models show that GluA1-mediated plasticity initiated by seizures leads to expression of Ca^{2+}-permeable AMPAR-mediated transmission in the CA1 area of the hippocampus in status epilepticus and provides a therapeutic target in this condition.[103]

Mutations of the Genes Encoding NMDAR Subunits

Familial *GRIN2A* mutations affecting the GluN2A subunit have been linked with epilepsy-aphasia syndromes.[104,105] They include benign centrotemporal epilepsy of childhood, continuous spike and wave during sleep syndrome, and Landau-Kleffner syndrome. Some of these mutation produce gain-of-function of the channel, while others result in haploinsufficiency and loss-of-function of NMDARs.[106] These complex effects would likely cause an imbalance between excitation and inhibition of neuronal circuits. De novo mutations of the *GRIN1* gene (encoding GluN1 and the *GRIN2B* gene encoding GluN2B mutations have been linked to epileptic encephalopathies.[107]

Autosomal Dominant Temporal Lobe Epilepsy

Mutations of the *LGI1* causes autosomal dominant temporal lobe epilepsy with auditory features.[108] Most of are missense mutations that cause LGI1 proteins to be misfolded and degraded in the ER. In experimental models, loss of LGI1 or ADA22 prevents AMPAR stabilization at synapses and reduce AMPAR-mediated currents increasing susceptibility to epilepsy.[109]

INTELLECTUAL DISABILITY AND AUTISM SPECTRUM DISORDERS

Effects of genetic mutations and studies in animal models indicate the presence of two common disease pathways for developmental intellectual disability and autism spectrum disorders. One involves aberrant mRNA translation of synaptic proteins. Examples include loss-of-function mutations affecting proteins that normally inhibit translation through the mTOR signaling pathway, such as tuberous sclerosis complex proteins (*TSC 1*, *TSC2*) proteins, neurofibromin 1 (*NF1*), and phosphatase tensin homolog (*PTEN*). Aberrant mRNA processing also occurs with mutations affecting proteins directly involved in inhibiting mRNA translation at the synapse, such as fragile X mental retardation protein (*FMRP*). All these abnormalities elicit downstream effects that alter synaptic plasticity. The second major pathway reflects abnormal excitation/inhibition balance in the CNS. This occurs with mutations of several genes encoding transsynaptic adhesion molecules, scaffold proteins, and other PSD associated proteins.[29] They include mutations affecting *NRX1*, *NRX2*, *NLG1*,[30] *SHANK1-3*,[31] and *SYNGAP*.[32] For example, heterozygous loss-of-function variants in *SYNGAP1* cause autosomal mental retardation type 5, characterized by cognitive impairment, severely impaired language, behavioral deficits, epilepsy, autism spectrum disorder, and attention deficit hyperactivity disorder.[32] Reduced SynGAP protein levels may result in excessive excitation in neural circuits and impaired synaptic plasticity. *SHANK1*, *SHANK2*, and *SHANK3* mutations account for ~1% of patients with autism spectrum disorders. Deletions within *NRXN1* have been associated with intellectual disability, developmental delay, speech and language delay, autism spectrum disorders, schizophrenia, and epilepsy.

KEY POINTS

- L-glutamate is the primary excitatory neurotransmitter in projection neurons of the adult nervous system (CNS).
- Glutamatergic inputs relay fast excitation between projection cells and activate local inhibitory interneurons, thereby shaping local circuits and network activity.
- Glutamate is also a key neuromodulator of synapse and circuit function, mediates neuron–astrocyte interactions, and promotes myelination by oligodendrocytes.
- The removal of glutamate from the synaptic cleft via astrocytic excitatory amino acid transporters (EAATs) is critical to prevent excitotoxicity.
- Astrocytic EAATs (EAAT1 and EAAT2) provide glutamate as the substrate for synthesis of glutamine.

- Inotropic glutamate receptors are ligand-gated cation channels and include AMPA, kainate, and NMDA receptors.
- The AMPARs are the primary receptors responsible for fast excitatory transmission, and most are permeable to Na^+ but not to Ca^{2+} given the presence of an edited GluA2 subunit.
- Activation of NMDARs requires glutamate binding, membrane depolarization to remove the Mg^{2+} blockade of the Ca^{2+} channel, and obligatory binding of glycine (or D-serine).
- Group I metabotropic glutamate receptors (mGluR1 and mGluR5) are primarily located postsynaptically and have a major role in synaptic plasticity.
- Group II receptors (mGluR 2 and mGluR3) and group III receptors (mGluR4, mGluR6, mGluR7 and mGluR8) produce presynaptic inhibition.
- Glutamate receptors form macromolecular complexes with a wide variety of auxiliary, scaffolding, adaptor, anchoring, cytoskeletal, and signaling proteins.
- Assembled receptors undergo continuous trafficking between intercellular, extrasynaptic, and postsynaptic sites.
- The number of ionotropic receptors at the postsynaptic membrane is tightly regulated by phosphorylation of receptor subunits.
- NMDAR-triggered synaptic LTP in the hippocampus involves CaMKII-dependent phosphorylation of GluA1 subunit with insertion of AMPARs at postsynaptic sites and is maintained by CREB activated transcription and local mRNA translation of synaptic proteins as well as remodeling of dendritic spines.
- NMDAR-triggered LTD in the hippocampus involves activation of calcineurin, which dephosphorylates the GluA1 subunit.
- mGluR5 receptors triggered LTD in the hippocampus involves noncanonical pathways.
- Synaptic homeostatic plasticity, or synaptic scaling, maintains synaptic weight in different portions of the dendrites.
- In general, activation of synaptic NMDARs triggers neuroprotective signals whereas that of extrasynaptic NMDARs triggers cell injury.
- Prion protein (PrP^c) may have a potential neuroprotective role in preventing excessive NMDAR activation.
- Amyloid precursor protein (APP) is localized to postsynaptic densities and has an important role in neuronal survival, synaptogenesis, and synaptic plasticity.
- Synaptic activity promotes APP processing and generation of amyloid-β peptide (Aβ) via β- and γ-secretase.
- Interactions between Aβ and tau impair synaptic plasticity and promote dendritic loss in glutamatergic synapses in Alzheimer disease.
- Autoantibodies directed against NMDARs or AMPARs or adhesion transsynaptic adhesion molecules such as LGI1 molecules produce limbic encephalitis with prominent memory impairment and seizures.
- Mutations or autoimmune disorders affecting mGluR1s or their downstream signaling cascades produce cerebellar ataxia.
- *LGI1* mutations gene causes autosomal dominant temporal lobe epilepsy; *GRIN2A* mutations produce epilepsy-aphasia syndromes; and *GRIN1* mutations have been linked to epileptic encephalopathies.
- Mutations of genes encoding proteins involved in the macromolecular organization and signaling at the PSD are a major cause of intellectual disability and autism spectrum disorders.

REFERENCES

1. Hayashi MK. Structure-function relationship of transporters in the glutamate-glutamine cycle of the central nervous system. Int J Mol Sci 2018;19.
2. Eid T, Gruenbaum SE, Dhaher R, Lee TW, Zhou Y, Danbolt NC. The glutamate-glutamine cycle in epilepsy. Adv Neurobiol 2016;13:351–400.
3. Omote H, Miyaji T, Hiasa M, Juge N, Moriyama Y. Structure, function, and drug interactions of neurotransmitter transporters in the postgenomic era. Annu Rev Pharmacol Toxicol 2016;56:385–402.
4. McAllister BB, Dyck RH. Zinc transporter 3 (ZnT3) and vesicular zinc in central nervous system function. Neurosci Biobehav Rev 2017;80:329–350.
5. Jensen AA, Fahlke C, Bjorn-Yoshimoto WE, Bunch L. Excitatory amino acid transporters: recent insights into molecular mechanisms, novel modes of modulation and new therapeutic possibilities. Curr Opin Pharmacol 2015;20:116–123.
6. Rose CR, Ziemens D, Untiet V, Fahlke C. Molecular and cellular physiology of sodium-dependent glutamate transporters. Brain Res Bull 2018;136:3–16.
7. Gegelashvili G, Bjerrum OJ. Glutamate transport system as a key constituent of glutamosome: molecular pathology and pharmacological modulation in chronic pain. Neuropharmacology 2019;161:107623.
8. Robinson MB, Jackson JG. Astroglial glutamate transporters coordinate excitatory signaling and brain energetics. Neurochem Int 2016;98:56–71.
9. Hinson SR, Clift IC, Luo N, Kryzer TJ, Lennon VA. Autoantibody-induced internalization of CNS AQP4 water channel and EAAT2 glutamate transporter requires astrocytic Fc receptor. Proc Natl Acad Sci U S A 2017;114:5491–5496.
10. Martinez-Lozada Z, Guillem AM, Robinson MB. Transcriptional regulation of glutamate transporters: from extracellular signals to transcription factors. Adv Pharmacol 2016;76:103–145.

11. Reiner A, Levitz J. Glutamatergic signaling in the central nervous system: ionotropic and metabotropic receptors in concert. Neuron 2018;98:1080–1098.
12. Hadzic M, Jack A, Wahle P. Ionotropic glutamate receptors: which ones, when, and where in the mammalian neocortex. J Comp Neurol 2017;525:976–1033.
13. Schwenk J, Baehrens D, Haupt A, et al. Regional diversity and developmental dynamics of the AMPA-receptor proteome in the mammalian brain. Neuron 2014;84:41–54.
14. Greger IH, Watson JF, Cull-Candy SG. Structural and functional architecture of AMPA-type glutamate receptors and their auxiliary proteins. Neuron 2017;94:713–730.
15. Jackson AC, Nicoll RA. The expanding social network of ionotropic glutamate receptors: TARPs and other transmembrane auxiliary subunits. Neuron 2011;70:178–199.
16. Paoletti P, Bellone C, Zhou Q. NMDA receptor subunit diversity: impact on receptor properties, synaptic plasticity and disease. Nat Rev Neurosci 2013;14:383–400.
17. Papouin T, Oliet SH. Organization, control and function of extrasynaptic NMDA receptors. Philos Trans R Soc Lond B Biol Sci 2014;369:20130601.
18. Stroebel D, Casado M, Paoletti P. Triheteromeric NMDA receptors: from structure to synaptic physiology. Curr Opin Physiol 2018;2:1–12.
19. Huang S, Chen L, Bladen C, Stys PK, Zamponi GW. Differential modulation of NMDA and AMPA receptors by cellular prion protein and copper ions. Mol Brain 2018;11:62.
20. Stys PK, You H, Zamponi GW. Copper-dependent regulation of NMDA receptors by cellular prion protein: implications for neurodegenerative disorders. J Physiol 2012;590:1357–1368.
21. Mollerud S, Frydenvang K, Pickering DS, Kastrup JS. Lessons from crystal structures of kainate receptors. Neuropharmacology 2017;112:16–28.
22. Contractor A, Mulle C, Swanson GT. Kainate receptors coming of age: milestones of two decades of research. Trends Neurosci 2011;34:154–163.
23. Zhu J, Shang Y, Zhang M. Mechanistic basis of MAGUK-organized complexes in synaptic development and signalling. Nat Rev Neurosci 2016;17:209–223.
24. Biederer T, Kaeser PS, Blanpied TA. Transcellular nanoalignment of synaptic function. Neuron 2017;96:680–696.
25. Gorlewicz A, Kaczmarek L. Pathophysiology of trans-synaptic adhesion molecules: implications for epilepsy. Front Cell Dev Biol 2018;6:119.
26. Wu X, Morishita WK, Riley AM, Hale WD, Sudhof TC, Malenka RC. Neuroligin-1 signaling controls LTP and NMDA receptors by distinct molecular pathways. Neuron 2019;102:621–635 e623.
27. Sudhof TC. Synaptic neurexin complexes: a molecular code for the logic of neural circuits. Cell 2017;171:745–769.
28. Yamagata A, Fukai S. Insights into the mechanisms of epilepsy from structural biology of LGI1-ADAM22. Cell Mol Life Sci 2020;77:267–274.
29. Huguet G, Ey E, Bourgeron T. The genetic landscapes of autism spectrum disorders. Annu Rev Genomics Hum Genet 2013;14:191–213.
30. Mackowiak M, Mordalska P, Wedzony K. Neuroligins, synapse balance and neuropsychiatric disorders. Pharmacol Rep 2014;66:830–835.
31. Lee SE, Kim JA, Chang S. nArgBP2-SAPAP-SHANK, the core postsynaptic triad associated with psychiatric disorders. Exp Mol Med 2018;50:2.
32. Weldon M, Kilinc M, Lloyd Holder J, Jr., Rumbaugh G. The first international conference on SYNGAP1-related brain disorders: a stakeholder meeting of families, researchers, clinicians, and regulators. J Neurodev Disord 2018;10:6.
33. Henley JM, Wilkinson KA. Synaptic AMPA receptor composition in development, plasticity and disease. Nat Rev Neurosci 2016;17:337–350.
34. Valbuena S, Lerma J. Non-canonical signaling, the hidden life of ligand-gated ion channels. Neuron 2016;92:316–329.
35. Bouvier G, Larsen RS, Rodriguez-Moreno A, Paulsen O, Sjostrom PJ. Towards resolving the presynaptic NMDA receptor debate. Curr Opin Neurobiol 2018;51:1–7.
36. Nicoll RA. A brief history of long-term potentiation. Neuron 2017;93:281–290.
37. Luscher C, Malenka RC. NMDA receptor-dependent long-term potentiation and long-term depression (LTP/LTD). Cold Spring Harb Perspect Biol 2012;4.
38. Herring BE, Nicoll RA. Long-term potentiation: from CaMKII to AMPA receptor trafficking. Annu Rev Physiol 2016;78:351–365.
39. Puri BK. Calcium signaling and gene expression. Adv Exp Med Biol 2020;1131:537–545.
40. Bading H. Nuclear calcium signalling in the regulation of brain function. Nat Rev Neurosci 2013;14:593–608.
41. Herbst WA, Martin KC. Regulated transport of signaling proteins from synapse to nucleus. Curr Opin Neurobiol 2017;45:78–84.
42. Marcello E, Di Luca M, Gardoni F. Synapse-to-nucleus communication: from developmental disorders to Alzheimer's disease. Curr Opin Neurobiol 2018;48:160–166.
43. Parra-Damas A, Saura CA. Synapse-to-nucleus signaling in neurodegenerative and neuropsychiatric disorders. Biol Psychiatry 2019;86:87–96.
44. Saura CA, Cardinaux JR. Emerging roles of CREB-regulated transcription coactivators in brain physiology and pathology. Trends Neurosci 2017;40:720–733.
45. Glock C, Heumuller M, Schuman EM. mRNA transport & local translation in neurons. Curr Opin Neurobiol 2017;45:169–177.
46. Petratos S, Li QX, George AJ, et al. The beta-amyloid protein of Alzheimer's disease increases neuronal CRMP-2 phosphorylation by a Rho-GTP mechanism. Brain 2008;131:90–108.
47. Jiao S, Li Z. Nonapoptotic function of BAD and BAX in long-term depression of synaptic transmission. Neuron 2011;70:758–772.
48. Bradley CA, Peineau S, Taghibiglou C, et al. A pivotal role of GSK-3 in synaptic plasticity. Front Mol Neurosci 2012;5:13.
49. Collingridge GL, Peineau S, Howland JG, Wang YT. Long-term depression in the CNS. Nat Rev Neurosci 2010;11:459–473.
50. Hlushchenko I, Koskinen M, Hotulainen P. Dendritic spine actin dynamics in neuronal maturation and synaptic plasticity. Cytoskeleton (Hoboken) 2016;73:435–441.
51. Izumi Y, Zorumski CF. NMDA receptors, mGluR5, and endocannabinoids are involved in a cascade leading to hippocampal long-term depression. Neuropsychopharmacology 2012;37:609–617.

52. Sanderson TM, Hogg EL, Collingridge GL, Correa SA. Hippocampal metabotropic glutamate receptor long-term depression in health and disease: focus on mitogen-activated protein kinase pathways. J Neurochem 2016;139 Suppl 2:200–214.
53. Gladding CM, Fitzjohn SM, Molnar E. Metabotropic glutamate receptor-mediated long-term depression: molecular mechanisms. Pharmacol Rev 2009;61:395–412.
54. Chen X, Lin R, Chang L, et al. Enhancement of long-term depression by soluble amyloid beta protein in rat hippocampus is mediated by metabotropic glutamate receptor and involves activation of p38MAPK, STEP and caspase-3. Neuroscience 2013;253:435–443.
55. Unsain N, Barker PA. New views on the misconstrued: executioner caspases and their diverse non-apoptotic roles. Neuron 2015;88:461–474.
56. Zhu G, Briz V, Seinfeld J, Liu Y, Bi X, Baudry M. Calpain-1 deletion impairs mGluR-dependent LTD and fear memory extinction. Sci Rep 2017;7:42788.
57. Hoxha E, Tempia F, Lippiello P, Miniaci MC. Modulation, plasticity and pathophysiology of the parallel fiber-Purkinje cell synapse. Front Synaptic Neurosci 2016;8:35.
58. Hardingham GE, Bading H. Synaptic versus extrasynaptic NMDA receptor signalling: implications for neurodegenerative disorders. Nat Rev Neurosci 2010;11:682–696.
59. Wulf MA, Senatore A, Aguzzi A. The biological function of the cellular prion protein: an update. BMC Biol 2017;15:34.
60. Selkoe DJ. Normal and abnormal biology of the beta-amyloid precursor protein. Annu Rev Neurosci 1994;17:489–517.
61. Lazarevic V, Fienko S, Andres-Alonso M, et al. Physiological concentrations of amyloid beta regulate recycling of synaptic vesicles via alpha7 acetylcholine receptor and CDK5/calcineurin signaling. Front Mol Neurosci 2017;10:221.
62. Pozueta J, Lefort R, Shelanski ML. Synaptic changes in Alzheimer's disease and its models. Neuroscience 2013;251:51–65.
63. Ricciarelli R, Fedele E. cAMP, cGMP and amyloid beta: three ideal partners for memory formation. Trends Neurosci 2018;41:255–266.
64. Tindi JO, Chavez AE, Cvejic S, Calvo-Ochoa E, Castillo PE, Jordan BA. ANKS1B gene product AIDA-1 controls hippocampal synaptic transmission by regulating GluN2B subunit localization. J Neurosci 2015;35:8986–8996.
65. Selkoe DJ. Soluble oligomers of the amyloid beta-protein impair synaptic plasticity and behavior. Behav Brain Res 2008;192:106–113.
66. Busche MA, Hyman BT. Synergy between amyloid-β and tau in Alzheimer's disease. Nature Neuroscience 2020;23:1183–1193.
67. Ma T, Klann E. Amyloid beta: linking synaptic plasticity failure to memory disruption in Alzheimer's disease. J Neurochem 2012;120 Suppl 1:140–148.
68. Tu S, Okamoto S, Lipton SA, Xu H. Oligomeric abeta-induced synaptic dysfunction in Alzheimer's disease. Mol Neurodegener 2014;9:48.
69. De Strooper B, Karran E. The cellular phase of Alzheimer's disease. Cell 2016;164:603–615.
70. Tackenberg C, Grinschgl S, Trutzel A, et al. NMDA receptor subunit composition determines beta-amyloid-induced neurodegeneration and synaptic loss. Cell Death Dis 2013;4:e608.
71. Li S, Jin M, Koeglsperger T, Shepardson NE, Shankar GM, Selkoe DJ. Soluble abeta oligomers inhibit long-term potentiation through a mechanism involving excessive activation of extrasynaptic NR2B-containing NMDA receptors. J Neurosci 2011;31:6627–6638.
72. Sun XY, Tuo QZ, Liuyang ZY, et al. Extrasynaptic NMDA receptor-induced tau overexpression mediates neuronal death through suppressing survival signaling ERK phosphorylation. Cell Death Dis 2016;7:e2449.
73. Freir DB, Nicoll AJ, Klyubin I, et al. Interaction between prion protein and toxic amyloid beta assemblies can be therapeutically targeted at multiple sites. Nat Commun 2011;2:336.
74. You H, Tsutsui S, Hameed S, et al. Abeta neurotoxicity depends on interactions between copper ions, prion protein, and N-methyl-D-aspartate receptors. Proc Natl Acad Sci U S A 2012;109:1737–1742.
75. Um JW, Kaufman AC, Kostylev M, et al. Metabotropic glutamate receptor 5 is a coreceptor for Alzheimer abeta oligomer bound to cellular prion protein. Neuron 2013;79:887–902.
76. Hu NW, Nicoll AJ, Zhang D, et al. mGlu5 receptors and cellular prion protein mediate amyloid-beta-facilitated synaptic long-term depression in vivo. Nat Commun 2014;5:3374.
77. Hoover BR, Reed MN, Su J, et al. Tau mislocalization to dendritic spines mediates synaptic dysfunction independently of neurodegeneration. Neuron 2010;68:1067–1081.
78. Ittner LM, Gotz J. Amyloid-beta and tau--a toxic pas de deux in Alzheimer's disease. Nat Rev Neurosci 2011;12:65–72.
79. Brandt R, Bakota L. Microtubule dynamics and the neurodegenerative triad of Alzheimer's disease: The hidden connection. J Neurochem 2017;143:409–417.
80. Thuraisingham RA. Examining the role of microglia and astroglia during the pathogenesis of Alzheimer's disease via the Puri-Li model. J Mol Neurosci 2017;62:363–367.
81. Talantova M, Sanz-Blasco S, Zhang X, et al. Abeta induces astrocytic glutamate release, extrasynaptic NMDA receptor activation, and synaptic loss. Proc Natl Acad Sci U S A 2013;110:E2518–2527.
82. Lian H, Yang L, Cole A, et al. NFkappaB-activated astroglial release of complement C3 compromises neuronal morphology and function associated with Alzheimer's disease. Neuron 2015;85:101–115.
83. Hong S, Beja-Glasser VF, Nfonoyim BM, et al. Complement and microglia mediate early synapse loss in Alzheimer mouse models. Science 2016;352:712–716.
84. Samidurai M, Ramasamy VS, Jo J. beta-amyloid inhibits hippocampal LTP through TNFR/IKK/NF-kappaB pathway. Neurol Res 2018;40:268–276.
85. Dalmau J. NMDA receptor encephalitis and other antibody-mediated disorders of the synapse: the 2016 Cotzias lecture. Neurology 2016;87:2471–2482.
86. Geis C, Planaguma J, Carreno M, Graus F, Dalmau J. Autoimmune seizures and epilepsy. J Clin Invest 2019;129:926–940.
87. Huda S, Wong SH, Pettingill P, O'Connell D, Vincent A, Steiger M. An 11-year retrospective experience of antibodies against the voltage-gated potassium channel (VGKC) complex from a tertiary neurological centre. J Neurol 2015;262:418–424.
88. Irani SR, Gelfand JM, Al-Diwani A, Vincent A. Cell-surface central nervous system autoantibodies: clinical relevance and emerging paradigms. Ann Neurol 2014;76:168–184.

89. Scotton WJ, Karim A, Jacob S. Glutamate receptor antibodies in autoimmune central nervous system disease: basic mechanisms, clinical features, and antibody detection. Methods Mol Biol 2019;1941:225–255.
90. Gleichman AJ, Spruce LA, Dalmau J, Seeholzer SH, Lynch DR. Anti-NMDA receptor encephalitis antibody binding is dependent on amino acid identity of a small region within the GluN1 amino terminal domain. J Neurosci 2012;32:11082–11094.
91. Gleichman AJ, Panzer JA, Baumann BH, Dalmau J, Lynch DR. Antigenic and mechanistic characterization of anti-AMPA receptor encephalitis. Ann Clin Transl Neurol 2014;1:180–189.
92. Binks SNM, Klein CJ, Waters P, Pittock SJ, Irani SR. LGI1, CASPR2 and related antibodies: a molecular evolution of the phenotypes. J Neurol Neurosurg Psychiatry 2018;89:526–534.
93. Lopez-Chiriboga AS, Komorowski L, Kumpfel T, et al. Metabotropic glutamate receptor type 1 autoimmunity: clinical features and treatment outcomes. Neurology 2016;86:1009–1013.
94. Gollion C, Dupouy J, Roberts M, et al. Reversible myoclonus-ataxia encephalitis related to anti-mGLUR1 autoantibodies. Mov Disord 2019;34:438–439.
95. Jarius S, Wildemann B. "Medusa-head ataxia": the expanding spectrum of Purkinje cell antibodies in autoimmune cerebellar ataxia. Part 1: Anti-mGluR1, anti-Homer-3, anti-Sj/ITPR1 and anti-CARP VIII. J Neuroinflammation 2015;12:166.
96. Jarius S, Wildemann B. "Medusa head ataxia": the expanding spectrum of Purkinje cell antibodies in autoimmune cerebellar ataxia. Part 2: Anti-PKC-gamma, anti-GluR-delta2, anti-Ca/ARHGAP26 and anti-VGCC. J Neuroinflammation 2015;12:167.
97. Jarius S, Wildemann B. "Medusa head ataxia": the expanding spectrum of Purkinje cell antibodies in autoimmune cerebellar ataxia. Part 3: Anti-Yo/CDR2, anti-Nb/AP3B2, PCA-2, anti-Tr/DNER, other antibodies, diagnostic pitfalls, summary and outlook. J Neuroinflammation 2015;12:168.
98. Paulson HL, Shakkottai VG, Clark HB, Orr HT. Polyglutamine spinocerebellar ataxias—from genes to potential treatments. Nat Rev Neurosci 2017;18:613–626.
99. Brown SA, Loew LM. Integration of modeling with experimental and clinical findings synthesizes and refines the central role of inositol 1,4,5-trisphosphate receptor 1 in spinocerebellar ataxia. Front Neurosci 2014;8:453.
100. Lancaster E, Martinez-Hernandez E, Titulaer MJ, et al. Antibodies to metabotropic glutamate receptor 5 in the Ophelia syndrome. Neurology 2011;77:1698–1701.
101. Abril Jaramillo J, Estevez Maria JC, Giron Ubeda JM, et al. Effectiveness and safety of perampanel as early add-on treatment in patients with epilepsy and focal seizures in the routine clinical practice: Spain prospective study (PERADON). Epilepsy Behav 2020;102:106655.
102. Lai MC, Tzeng RC, Huang CW, Wu SN. The novel direct modulatory effects of perampanel, an antagonist of AMPA receptors, on voltage-gated sodium and m-type potassium currents. Biomolecules 2019;9:638–656.
103. Adotevi N, Lewczuk E, Sun H, et al. alpha-Amino-3-Hydroxy-5-Methyl-4-Isoxazolepropionic Acid Receptor Plasticity Sustains Severe, Fatal Status Epilepticus. Ann Neurol 2020;87:84–96.
104. Perucca P, Perucca E. Identifying mutations in epilepsy genes: impact on treatment selection. Epilepsy Res 2019;152:18–30.
105. Yang X, Qian P, Xu X, et al. GRIN2A mutations in epilepsy-aphasia spectrum disorders. Brain Dev 2018;40:205–210.
106. Sibarov DA, Bruneau N, Antonov SM, Szepetowski P, Burnashev N, Giniatullin R. Functional properties of human NMDA receptors associated with epilepsy-related mutations of GluN2A subunit. Front Cell Neurosci 2017;11:155.
107. Smigiel R, Kostrzewa G, Kosinska J, et al. Further evidence for GRIN2B mutation as the cause of severe epileptic encephalopathy. Am J Med Genet A 2016;170:3265–3270.
108. Ottman R, Winawer MR, Kalachikov S, et al. LGI1 mutations in autosomal dominant partial epilepsy with auditory features. Neurology 2004;62:1120–1126.
109. Lovero KL, Fukata Y, Granger AJ, Fukata M, Nicoll RA. The LGI1-ADAM22 protein complex directs synapse maturation through regulation of PSD-95 function. Proc Natl Acad Sci U S A 2015;112:E4129–4137.

18 Inhibitory Amino Acid Neurotransmission and Synaptopathies

OVERVIEW

GABA is the most abundant inhibitory neurotransmitter in the CNS. It is the primary neurotransmitter of local circuit neurons (interneurons) at all levels of the neuraxis from the forebrain to the spinal cord. GABA is also the primary transmitter in neurons in the reticular thalamic nucleus, striatum, globus pallidus, Purkinje cells and other local and projection neurons of the hypothalamus and brainstem (Figure 18.1). Synthesis of GABA is coupled with the glutamate-glutamine cycle, and thus critically depends on neuron–astrocyte interactions. The inhibitory effects of GABA are mediated by $GABA_A$ receptors ($GABA_A$Rs), which are chloride (Cl^-) channels involved in fast inhibition, and $GABA_B$ receptors ($GABA_B$Rs), which are G protein-coupled receptors (GPCRs) involved in slower postsynaptic and presynaptic inhibition. GABAergic transmission is critical for determining neuronal excitability and shaping activity of cortical networks for cognitive processing and has a central role in gating thalamocortical interactions, sleep-wake cycle, basal ganglia output for action selection, and cerebellar learning and timing functions. Glycine, either alone or together with GABA, is a major inhibitory neurotransmitter of local circuit and commissural inhibitory neurons in the brainstem and spinal cord, including those controlling pain processing and motor output. Glycine exerts fast inhibition via glycine receptors. The fast inhibitory effects of GABA and glycine critically depend on the transcellular Cl^- gradient, which is controlled by chloride-cation cotransporters. Genetic, autoimmune, or toxic disorders affecting GABAergic or glycinergic transmission result in seizures and other manifestations of excessive CNS excitability such as rigidity and myoclonus. The GABAergic system is a major pharmacological target for management of these and other disorders including insomnia, pain, spasticity, and anxiety. The main aims of this chapter are to review (1) the basic mechanisms of GABAergic transmission; (2) the functional heterogeneity of $GABA_A$Rs; (3) the effects of $GABA_B$Rs; (4) the functions of glycine as an inhibitory transmission; (5) examples of inhibitory circuits and their function; and (6) examples of neurologic disorders due to impaired inhibitory transmission.

PRESYNAPTIC EVENTS IN GABAERGIC NEUROTRANSMISSION

Biosynthesis and Storage

GABA is synthesized from L-glutamate by action of the glutamic acid decarboxylase (GAD), which requires pyridoxal phosphate as a cofactor[1,2] (Figure 18.2). There are two GAD isoforms encoded by different genes; GAD67 is primarily responsible for baseline synthesis of GABA whereas GAD65 promotes replenishment of GABA into synaptic vesicles during increased GABAergic activity. GABA is stored in synaptic vesicles via the vesicular GABA transporter (VGAT) that is functionally coupled to the vacuolar proton (H^+) ATPase. This transporter also mediates vesicular storage of glycine, and is therefore also referred to as vesicular inhibitory amino acid transporter (VIAAT).[3]

Uptake and Metabolism

GABA is released by exocytosis and undergoes uptake in neurons and astrocytes via the Na/Cl^--dependent GABA

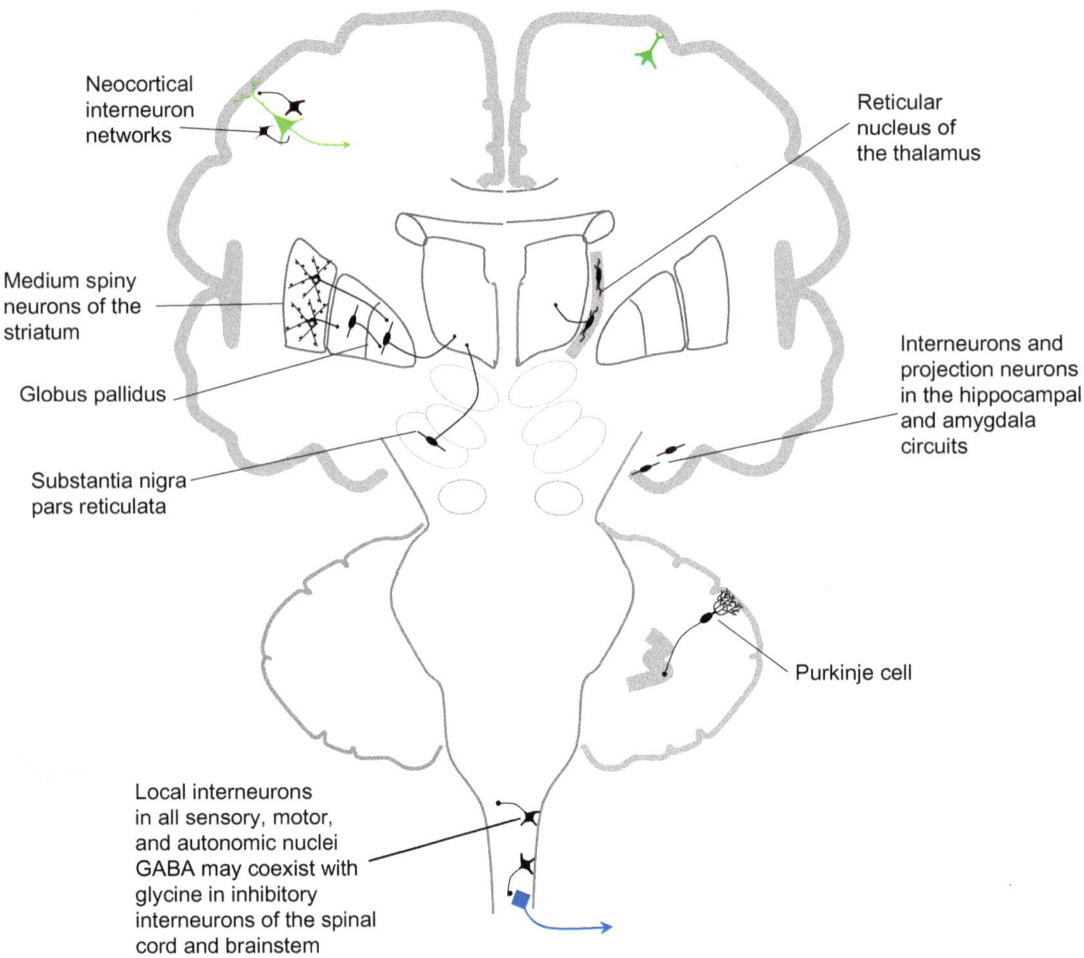

FIGURE 18.1 Main groups of GABAergic neurons in the central nervous system.
The main groups of GABAergic neurons in the central nervous include local circuit neurons (interneurons) at all levels of the neuraxis from the forebrain to the spinal cord; neurons in the reticular thalamic nucleus, striatum, globus pallidus and Purkinje cells; and other local and projection neurons of the hypothalamus and brainstem.

transporters (GAT).[4,5] GAT1 is expressed perisynaptically and regulates GABA levels near synapses, thereby modulating the magnitude of inhibitory GABAergic responses. GAT3 is expressed in astrocytes and limits the diffusion of GABA toward extrasynaptic regions.[6] GAT is the target of the antiepileptic drug tiagabine.[7]

After uptake, GABA is catabolized in the mitochondrial matrix by GABA transaminase (GABA-T) to succinic semialdehyde (SSA).[8] GABA-T is inhibited by the antiepileptic drug vigabatrin. Succinic semialdehyde undergoes oxidation to succinate by the succinic semialdehyde dehydrogenase (SSADH) to succinic acid, which enters the Krebs cycle to produce α-ketoglutarate for the resynthesis of glutamate. Alternatively, SSA can also undergo reduction by succinic semialdehyde reductase to yield γ-hydroxybutyrate (GHB), which is also formed in GABAergic terminals and may function as a neurotransmitter.[9] Succinic semialdehyde dehydrogenase deficiency is a neurometabolic disorder associated with accumulation of both GABA and GHB.[10]

$GABA_A$ RECEPTORS

Structure

The $GABA_A$Rs are chloride (Cl^-) channels that belong to the cysteine (Cys) loop family ligand-gated ion channels (Figure 18.3). Like other members of this family, $GABA_A$Rs are heteropentamers, consisting of different combinations of five subunits forming a structural scaffold composed of two amino (N)-terminal extracellular ligand-binding domains, five pore-forming transmembrane domains, and the intracellular M3-M4 cytoplasmic domain. The $GABA_A$Rs are formed by different combinations of α, β, γ, δ, and θ subunits, each comprising several subtypes.[11–13] Most $GABA_A$Rs contain 2 α subunits (α_1, α_2, α_3, or α_5) combined with 2 β and either γ or δ subunits.[14,15] The $GABA_A$R has three structural cores. The extracellular region, encompassing the N-terminal domains of the different subunits encloses binding sites for agonists, antagonists, and benzodiazepines (BZPs). The two GABA binding sites are at the interface between β and α subunits, while the canonical

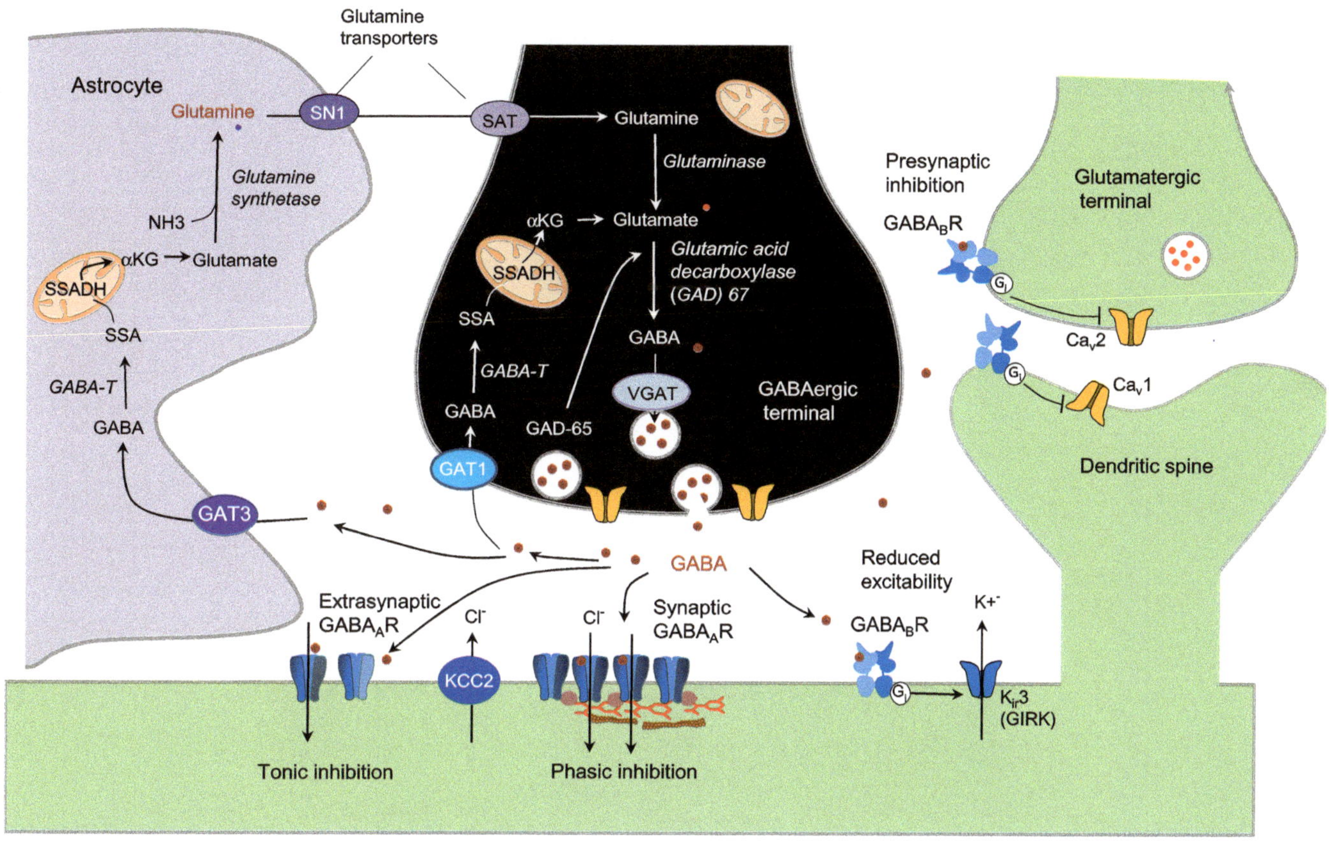

FIGURE 18.2 Main steps in GABAergic neurotransmission.
GABA is synthesized from L-glutamate by action of the glutamic acid decarboxylase (GAD), which requires pyridoxal phosphate (PAL) as a cofactor. GAD67 is responsible for baseline synthesis of GABA whereas GAD65 promotes replenishment of GABA. GABA is stored in synaptic vesicles via the vesicular GABA transporter (VGAT). GABA is released by exocytosis and undergoes uptake in neurons and astrocytes via the GAT1, which is expressed perisynaptically and mediate GAT3 expressed in astrocytes. After uptake, GABA is catabolized by GABA transaminase (GABA-T) to succinic semialdehyde (SSA) followed by oxidation to succinate succinic semialdehyde dehydrogenase (SSADH) to succinic acid, which enters the Krebs cycle to produce α-ketoglutarate for the resynthesis of glutamate. The inhibitory effects of GABA are mediated by GABA$_A$ receptors (GABA$_A$Rs), which are chloride (Cl$^-$) channels that mediate fast inhibition. Synaptic GABA$_A$Rs mediate phasic inhibition and extrasynaptic GABA$_A$Rs. The second type of GABA receptors are GABA$_B$ receptors (GABA$_B$Rs), which are G protein-coupled receptors involved in slower postsynaptic and presynaptic inhibition.

high-affinity binding site for BZPs is at the α/γ interface. This site also binds non-BZP compounds such as the antagonist flumazenil. The pore domain is formed by four transmembrane α-helices (M1, M2, M3, M4), where residues of the M2 transmembrane α-helix demarcate the channel pore. The intracellular M3-M4 loop domain is a variable-length region that contains key binding sites for regulatory proteins. GABA binding at the β/α interface induces rotation of the N-terminal extracellular domain, which transduces conformational alterations in the transmembrane domain described as a "lock-and-pull" interaction.

Synaptic Effects and Role of Cation-Chloride Cotransporters

GABA binding to GABA$_A$Rs opens their intrinsic Cl$^-$ channel; this brings the membrane potential toward the Cl$^-$ equilibrium potential, which depends on the transmembrane Cl$^-$ gradient and determines the direction of Cl-flow through the channel and thus the consequences of GABA$_A$R activation (Figure 18.4). The glycine receptors (GlyRs) are also Cl$^-$ channels and their synaptic effect also depends on the transmembrane Cl$^-$ gradient. The transmembrane Cl $^-$gradient is determined by the opposing activity of 2 Cl$^-$-cation cotransporters.[16] The predominant cotransporter in mature neurons is the K–Cl cotransporter 2 (KCC2), which extrudes Cl$^-$ from neurons maintaining a higher Cl$^-$ concentration in the extracellular than in the intracellular space. Thus, in neurons expressing KCC2, activation of GABA$_A$R (or GlyR) allows Cl$^-$ influx. This leads to postsynaptic inhibition either by hyperpolarization (fast inhibitory postsynaptic potential) or by reduced membrane resistance and thus amplitude of the excitatory postsynaptic potential

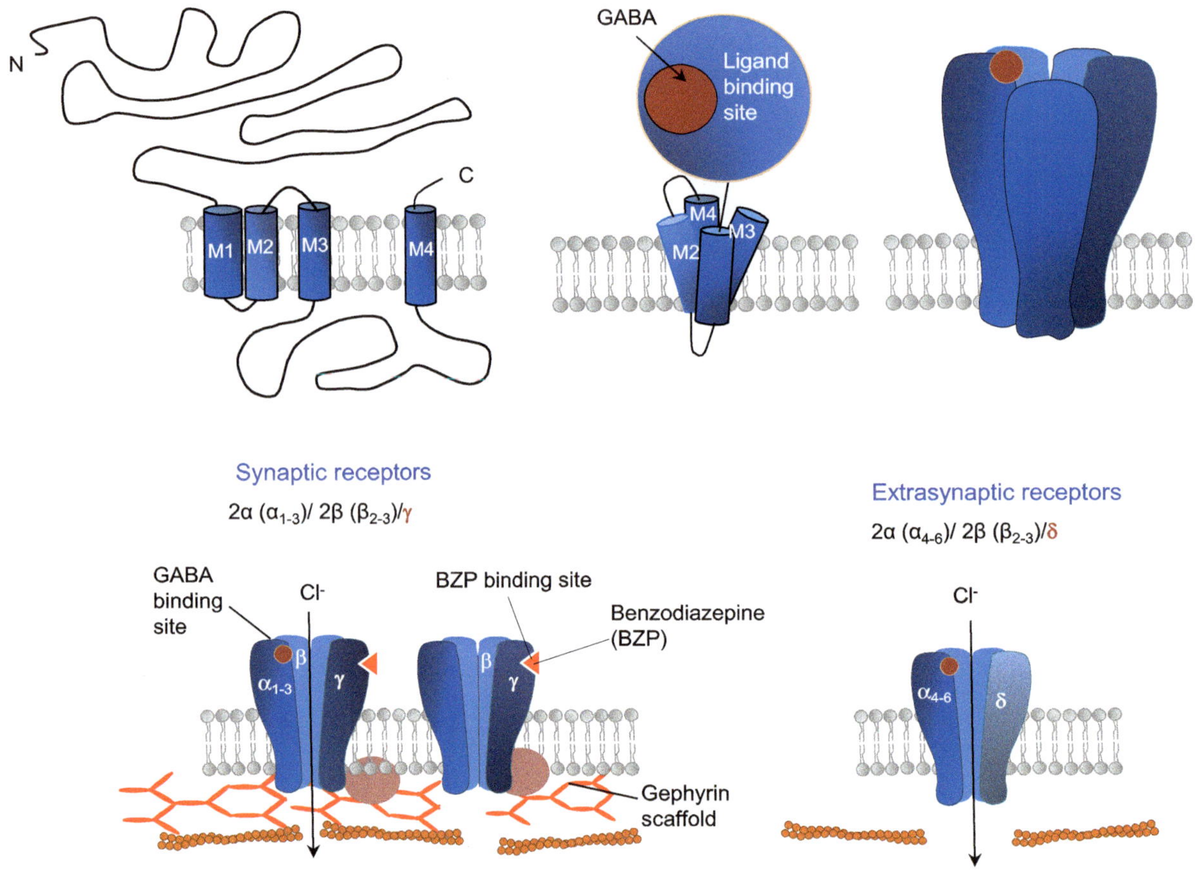

FIGURE 18.3 Structure of $GABA_A$Rs.

The $GABA_A$Rs are chloride (Cl^-) channels that are heteropentames, consisting of different combinations of five subunits forming a structural scaffold composed of two amino (N)-terminal extracellular ligand-binding domains, five pore-forming transmembrane domains, and the intracellular M3-M4 cytoplasmic domain. The $GABA_A$Rs are formed by different combinations of α, β, γ, δ, and θ subunits, each comprising several subtypes. Most $GABA_A$Rs contain 2 α subunits (α_1, α_2, α_3, or α_5) combined with 2 β and either γ or δ subunits. The $GABA_A$R has three structural cores. The extracellular region, encompassing the N-terminal domains of the different subunits encloses binding sites for agonists, antagonists, and benzodiazepines (BZDs). The two GABA binding sites are at the interface between β and α subunits, while the canonical high-affinity binding site for BZDs is at the α/γ interface. The pore domain is formed by four transmembrane α-helices (M1, M2, M3, M4), where residues of the M2 transmembrane α-helix demarcate the channel pore.

("shunt" inhibition). In contrast, immature neurons and some mature CNS neurons express the Na^+-potassium (K^+)-2 Cl^- cotransporter 1 (NKCC1), which mediates Cl^- influx maintaining a higher intracellular than extracellular Cl^- concentration.[17] In this case, opening of the $GABA_A$R (or GlyR) channel allows efflux of Cl^- and elicits depolarization. The depolarizing effects of GABA (and glycine) are important for development of neuronal circuits. Thus, the precise balance between KCC2 and NKCC1 determines the driving force and direction of Cl^- flow upon opening of the $GABA_A$R (or GlyR) channel. In some mature synapses, such as axo-axonal synapses on the axon initial segment of pyramidal neurons, $GABA_A$R activation may exert a depolarizing effect due to low KCC2 expression. KCC2 downregulation in the setting of ischemia, status epilepticus, or microglial activation of the dorsal horn, reduces efficacy of GABAergic inhibition.[18–20] Reduced KCC2 expression is in part due to brain-derived neurotrophic factor (BDNF) signaling.[21]

Synaptic Versus Extrasynaptic $GABA_A$Rs: Phasic and Tonic Inhibition

$GABA_A$Rs are distributed at both postsynaptic and extrasynaptic sites (Figure 18.5).[22–24] Synaptic $GABA_A$Rs contain α1–α3 and β2 or β3 subunits, together with γ2 subunits. The γ2 subunit is critical for clustering of the receptors at post synaptic sites by interaction with the scaffold protein gephyrin. The γ2 subunits also contain the BZP binding site.[25] The type of α subunit of synaptic $GABA_A$Rs determines the pharmacological effects of these drugs. The α1 subunit is involved in sedation, amnesia, and part of the

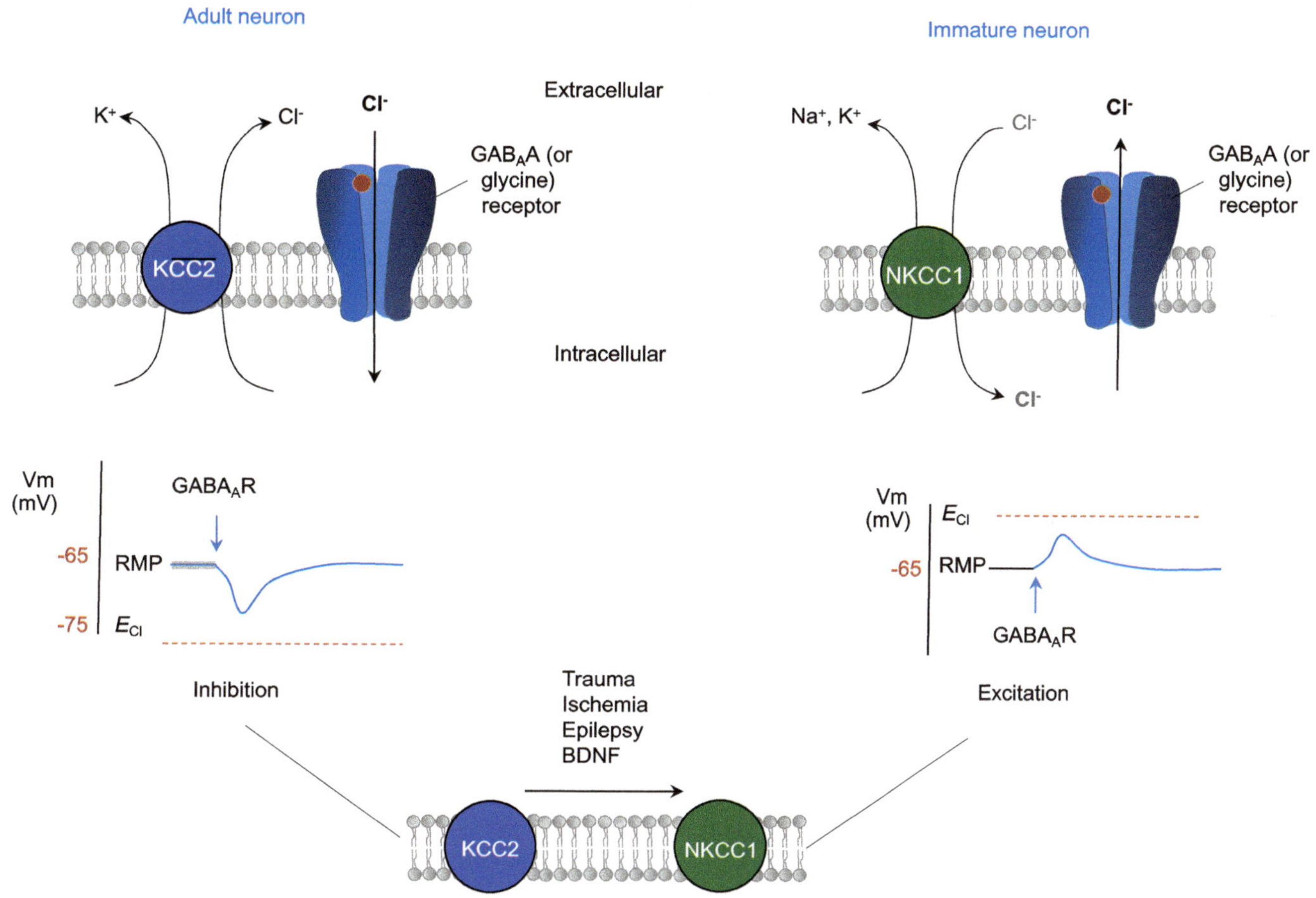

FIGURE 18.4 Synaptic effects of $GABA_A$Rs and role of cation-chloride cotransporters.
GABA binding to $GABA_A$Rs opens their intrinsic Cl^- channel; this brings the membrane potential toward the Cl^- equilibrium potential, which depends on the transmembrane Cl^- gradient and determines the direction of Cl-flow through the channel. The transmembrane Cl^- gradient is determined by the opposing activity of the K–Cl cotransporter 2 (KCC2), which predominates in the adult CNS and extrudes Cl^- from neurons; in neurons expressing KCC2, $GABA_A$R activation allows Cl^- influx, leading to postsynaptic inhibition. In contrast, immature neurons during development and some mature CNS neurons primarily express the Na^+-potassium (K^+)-2 Cl^- cotransporter 1 (NKCC1), which mediates Cl^- influx and maintains a higher intracellular an extracellular Cl^- concentration. In this case, opening of the $GABA_A$R channel allows efflux of Cl^- and elicits depolarization. Several pathological conditions reduce the efficacy of GABAergic inhibition by reducing KCC2 and increasing NKCC1 activity.

anticonvulsant effect of $GABA_A$Rs. For example, the actions of zolpidem and eszopiclone utilized for sleep induction depend on the presence of α1 subunits in the receptors.[26] In contrast, α2 subunits mediate the anxiolytic, muscle relaxant, and some of the anticonvulsant effects of $GABA_A$Rs. For example, clobazam, which is used for treatment of seizures in Lennox-Gastaut syndrome has greater affinity for α2 subunit containing receptors.[27] Extrasynaptic receptors contain α4 or α6 subunits combined with δ subunits instead of γ2 subunits and are not sensitive to BZPs.

GABA exerts two types of inhibitory influence of its targets, phasic and tonic. Phasic inhibition is triggered by GABA released at synapses and acting on γ_2 subunit-containing $GABA_A$Rs clustered at the postsynaptic membrane. Fast GABAergic inhibition generates rapid onset and short duration inhibitory postsynaptic potentials and is critical for control of network interactions in the cerebral cortex. Tonic inhibition is initiated by "ambient" levels of extracellular GABA that has escaped presynaptic reuptake and is mediated by extrasynaptic $GABA_A$Rs. Tonic GABAergic inhibition regulates cell excitability and frequency of discharge in response to excitatory inputs.

Allosteric Modulation of $GABA_A$Rs

The $GABA_A$R contains multiple allosteric binding sites[28] (Figure 18.6). Benzodiazepines bind at the α/γ2 interface of synaptic $GABA_A$Rs and function as positive modulators by increasing the probability of Cl^- channel opening.[25] Barbiturates and neuroactive steroids enhance $GABA_A$R currents by increasing the average duration or

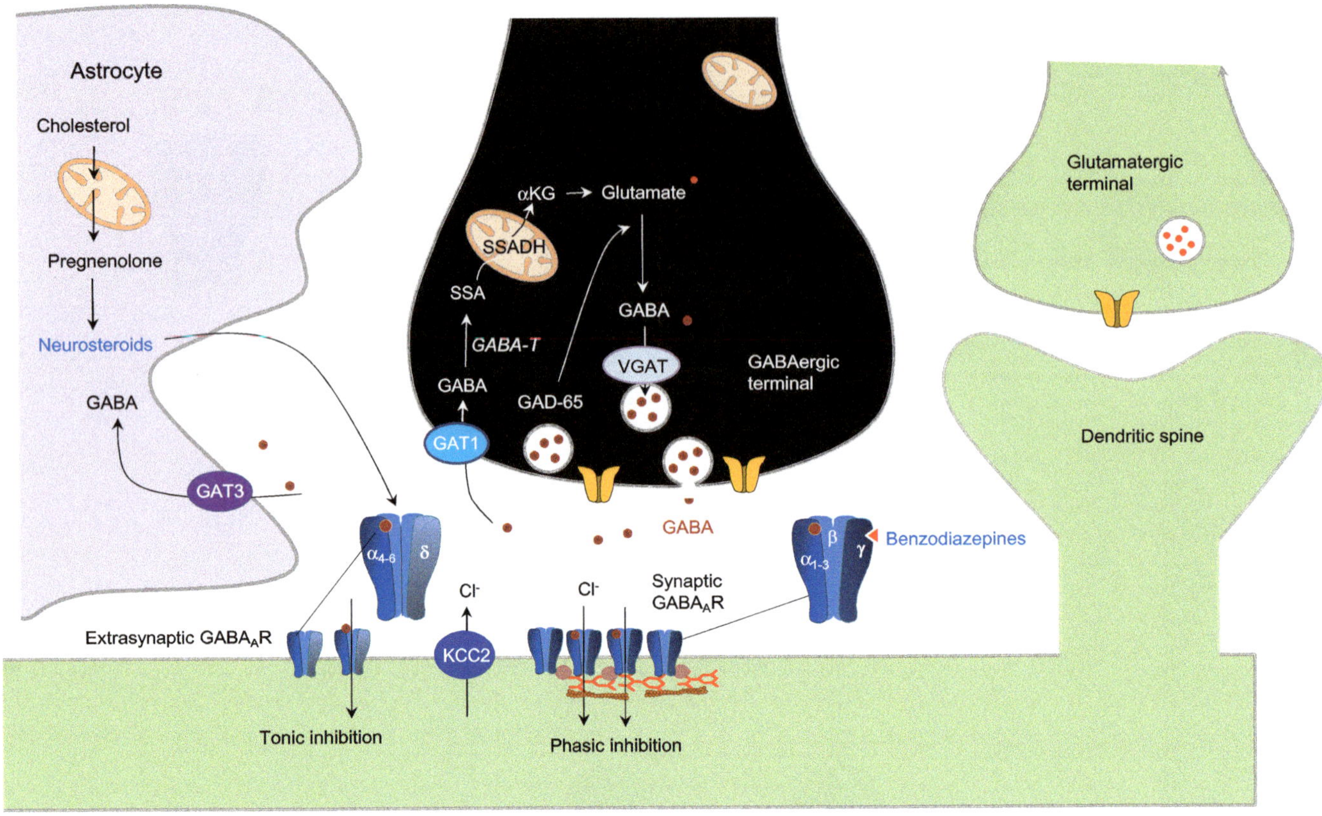

FIGURE 18.5 Synaptic versus extrasynaptic $GABA_A$Rs: phasic and tonic inhibition.
Synaptic $GABA_A$ receptors contain α1–α3 and β2 or β3 subunits, together with γ2 subunits and are clustered at postsynaptic sites by interaction with the scaffold protein gephyrin. These receptors are allosterically activated by BZPs and related drugs. Extrasynaptic receptors contain α4 or α6 subunits combined with δ subunits instead of γ2 subunits and are not sensitive to BZPs. GABA exerts phasic inhibition via $GABA_A$Rs clustered at the postsynaptic membrane. Tonic inhibition is initiated by "ambient" levels of extracellular GABA that has escaped presynaptic reuptake and is mediated by extrasynaptic $GABA_A$ receptors. Neurosteroids secreted from astrocytes promote tonic GABAergic inhibition.

the Cl^- channel receptor opening. General anesthetics, such as etomidate and volatile anesthetics, as well as neuroactive steroids such as progesterone and allopregnanolone,[29] bind to critical residues in the transmembrane portion of the β subunit of the receptor. Reduced levels of progesterone relative to estradiol, which has a proconvulsant effect by facilitating N-methyl-D aspartate receptor (NMDAR) activity, are thought to be responsible for catamenial epilepsy. Certain subtypes of extrasynaptic $GABA_A$Rs involved in tonic inhibition are positively modulated by ethanol, which appears to bind to an extracellular portion of the δ subunit. Beta-lactam antibiotics, such as penicillin, imipenem, and some cephalosporins, may act as competitive or noncompetitive $GABA_A$R blockers. Penicillin is an open channel blocker; cefepime and ceftriaxone are only weak $GABA_A$R blockers but in the setting of renal insufficiency or altered ionic environment they may become a clinically relevant $GABA_A$R antagonists producing underlying encephalopathy associated with seizures.[30]

Organization of the GABAergic Inhibitory Synapses

The central scaffold element of inhibitory synapses is gephyrin.[31,32] Gephyrin is involved both in the development of inhibitory synapse and in clustering of $GABA_A$ and GlyRs. One important feature of inhibitory synapses is the presence of regulators of small GTPases, including the guanine nucleotide exchange factor collybistin, which binds to phospholipids in the endosome membranes and recruits gephyrin from intracellular stores. Autoantibodies against gephyrin produce a stiff-man-like syndrome;[33] mutations of the of the *ARHGEF9* encoding collybistin produce intellectual disability and seizures.[34] This emphasizes the clinical relevance of gephyrin scaffolds in organizing inhibitory synapses.

Transsynaptic adhesion molecules in inhibitory synapses, such as neuroligin-2 and neuroligin-3, bind presynaptic neurexins and promote gephyrin clustering. Dystroglycans link the extracellular matrix to the cytoskeleton and also

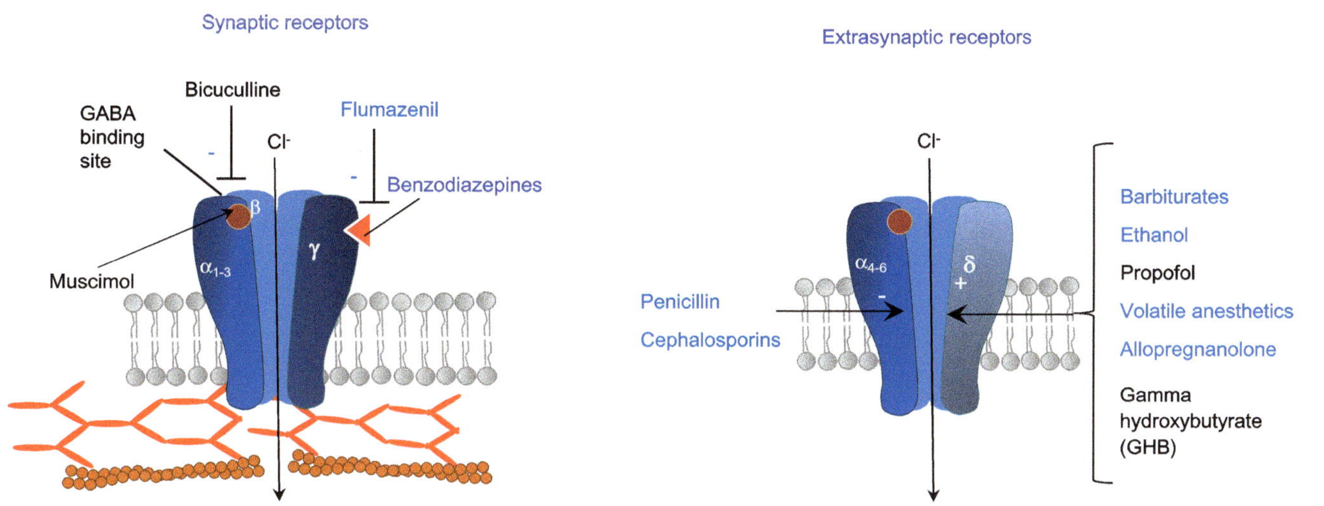

FIGURE 18.6 Allosteric modulation of $GABA_A$Rs.
The $GABA_A$ receptor contains multiple allosteric binding sites.[28] Benzodiazepines bind at the α/γ2 interface synaptic $GABA_A$Rs and function as positive modulators by increasing the probability of Cl^- channel opening. Barbiturates and neuroactive steroids enhance $GABA_A$R currents by increasing the average duration or the Cl^- channel receptor opening. General anesthetics, such as etomidate and volatile anesthetics, as well as neuroactive steroids such as allopregnenolone,[29] bind to critical residue in the transmembrane portion of the β subunit of the receptor. Certain subtypes of extrasynaptic $GABA_A$Rs involved in tonic inhibition are positively modulated by ethanol, which appears to bind to an extracellular portion of the δ subunit. Beta-lactam antibiotics, such as penicillin, imipenem, and some cephalosporins, may act as competitive or noncompetitive $GABA_A$R blockers. Penicillin is an open channel blocker; cefepime and ceftriaxone are only weak $GABA_A$R receptor blockers.

bind to presynaptic neurexins in some inhibitory synapses, where they may be involved in homeostatic plasticity. This may explain the frequent association of muscular dystrophy associated with dystroglycan mutations with epilepsy and cognitive impairment.[35]

$GABA_A$R Trafficking

$GABA_A$Rs undergo regulated trafficking.[36] They are assembled within the endoplasmic reticulum (ER) and are then transported to the Golgi apparatus. In the ER, unassembled receptor subunits are subjected to polyubiquitination that targets them for proteasomal degradation. Inside the Golgi, $GABA_A$Rs bind to $GABA_A$R associated protein (GABARAP), which is involved and autophagy and vesicular transport and interacts with the γ2 subunit, facilitating $GABA_A$R transport to the plasma membrane.[36,37] Once in the membrane, $GABA_A$Rs are very dynamic, exchanging between synaptic and extrasynaptic locations. The accumulation of the receptors at the inhibitory synapses is regulated by gephyrin. $GABA_A$R endocytosis occurs mainly via clathrin- and dynamin-dependent mechanisms. A sequence motif in the β3 subunit includes a major phosphorylation site that is important for $GABA_A$R internalization and is targeted by protein kinase A (PKA) and protein kinase C (PKC), which inhibit $GABA_A$R internalization. N-methyl-D-aspartate receptor signaling may control the stability of synaptic $GABA_A$R via calcineurin-mediated dephosphorylation of the receptors. The internalized $GABA_A$R may be rapidly recycled back to the neuronal plasma membrane or targeted for lysosomal degradation. The interaction of $GABA_A$R β1–β3 subunits with huntingtin-associated protein 1 (HAP1) determines whether endocytosed $GABA_A$Rs are recycled to the surface and thus determines the availability of $GABA_A$R at synapses; this may have relevance in Huntington disease.[38]

Plasticity of GABAergic Synapses

GABAergic synapses are highly plastic, both presynaptically and postsynaptically.[39] $GABA_A$Rs are typically located at the axon initial segment, soma, and dendritic shafts of pyramidal cells in the cerebral cortex. There is an activity-dependent phosphorylation of both $GABA_AR$ and gephyrin by calmodulin kinase II (CaMKII), which has a major role in long-term potentiation of GABAergic synapses. For example, calcium influx in response to activation of NMDARs triggers a CaMKII mediated phosphorylation of the β3 subunit of the $GABA_AR$ leading to synaptic clustering of the receptor. GABAergic synapses also undergo heterosynaptic plasticity through retrograde signals released in response to glutamatergic inputs (Figure 18.7). For example, activation of metabotropic glutamate receptors (mGluR5), triggers production and release of the endocannabinoids, which act as a retrograde transmitters reducing GABA release via presynaptic cannabinoid-1 (CB1) receptors[40]. Activation of NMDARs in excitatory synapses at the granular cell layer of the cerebellum elicits release of nitric oxide, which functions as a retrograde messenger to regulate efficacy of GABAergic connections between Golgi cells and granule cells.[41]

$GABA_B$ RECEPTORS

Structure and Dynamics

The $GABA_BRs$ are GPCRs that mediate slow inhibitory transmission.[42] These receptors are obligatory heterodimers of two subunits, $GABA_{B1}$ and $GABA_{B2}$.[43] The $GABA_{B1}$ subunit binds GABA or other ligands such as baclofen whereas the $GABA_{B2}$ couples with the $G_{i/o}$ protein (Figure 18.8). There are two main isoforms of the $GABA_{B1}$ subunit: $GABA_{B1a}$, found predominantly in the presynaptic terminal, and $GABA_{B1b}$, associated with the postsynaptic terminal. These isoforms differ by the presence of two modules called sushi

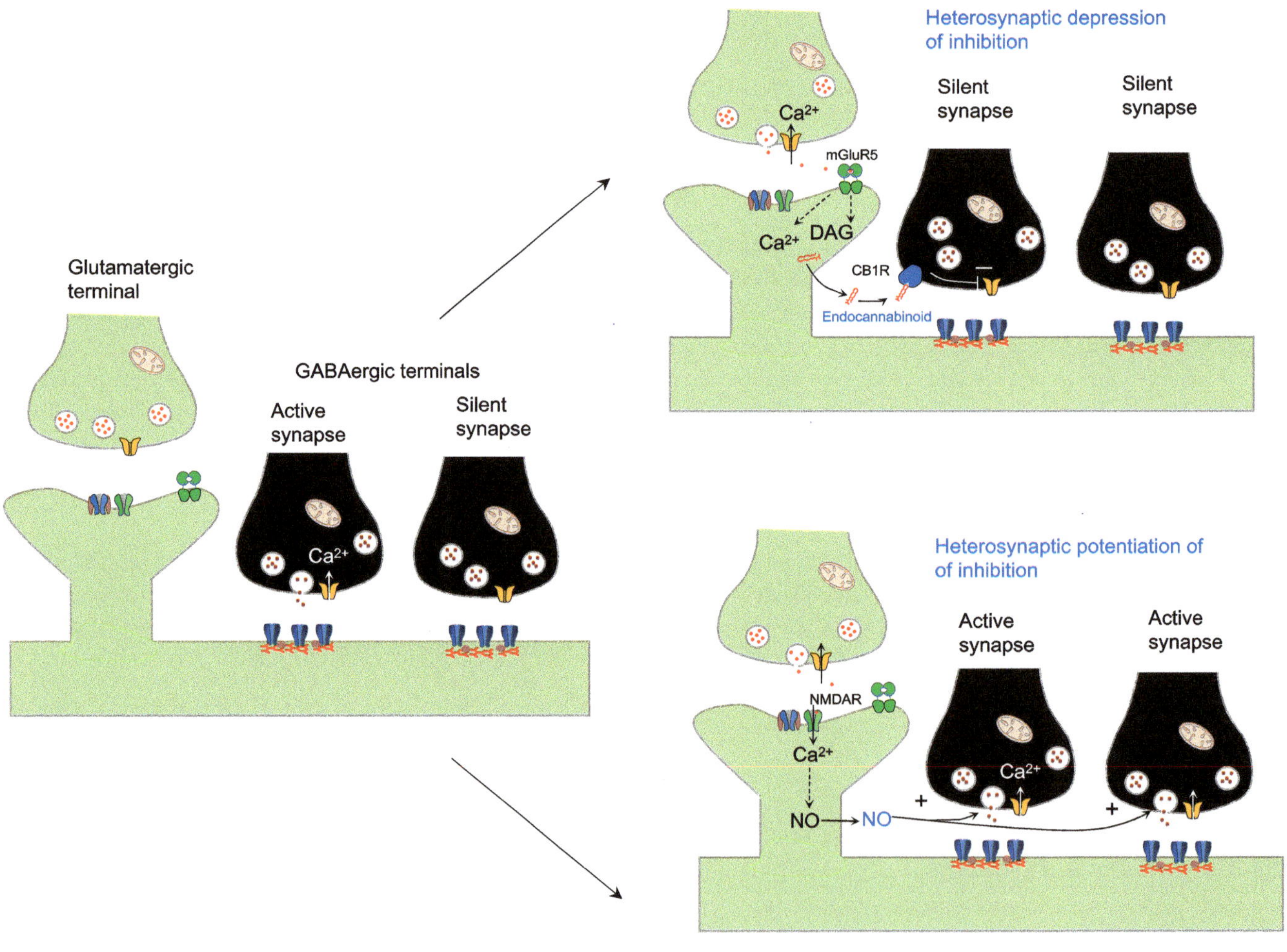

FIGURE 18.7 Heterosynaptic plasticity of GABAergic neurotransmission.
GABAergic synapses undergo heterosynaptic inhibition or potentiation through retrograde signals released in response to glutamatergic inputs. For example, activation of metabotropic glutamate receptors (mGluR5) elicits production and release of endocannabinoids, which inhibit release of GABA via presynaptic cannabinoid-1 (CB1) receptors thus reducing GABAergic inhibition. In contrast, activation of NMDAR may elicit release of nitric oxide (NO), which may elicit potentiation of GABAergic transmission.

domains in the N-terminus of $GABA_{B1a}$. The sushi domains bind several proteins, including amyloid precursor protein (APP). Binding of the soluble form of APP to this domain of $GABA_{B1a}$ may be necessary for vesicular trafficking of $GABA_BRs$ to axon terminals.[44] Vesicular kinesin-1 adaptors bind to both the extracellular domain $GABA_{B1a}$ and APP and with kinesin-1 motor, thereby contributing to axonal $GABA_BR$ targeting. The $GABA_BR$ is susceptible to allosteric modification by extracellular Ca^{2+}; binding of Ca^{2+} to the $GABA_{B1}$ subunit increases its affinity for GABA and enhances G protein activation. The intracellular domain of $GABA_BR$ controls the surface expression of the intact receptor. The $GABA_{B1}$ subunit is only transported to the cell surface when it is chaperoned by $GABA_{B2}$ in a heterodimeric pair. An ER protein functions as a gatekeeper that binds to and traps $GABA_B1$ subunit within the ER; $GABA_{B1}$ exits the ER only after $GABA_{B2}$ displaces this gatekeeper protein. The $GABA_{B1}$ cytoplasmic tail contains internalization and ER retention signals that reduce or eliminate $GABA_{B1}$ expression on the cell surface.

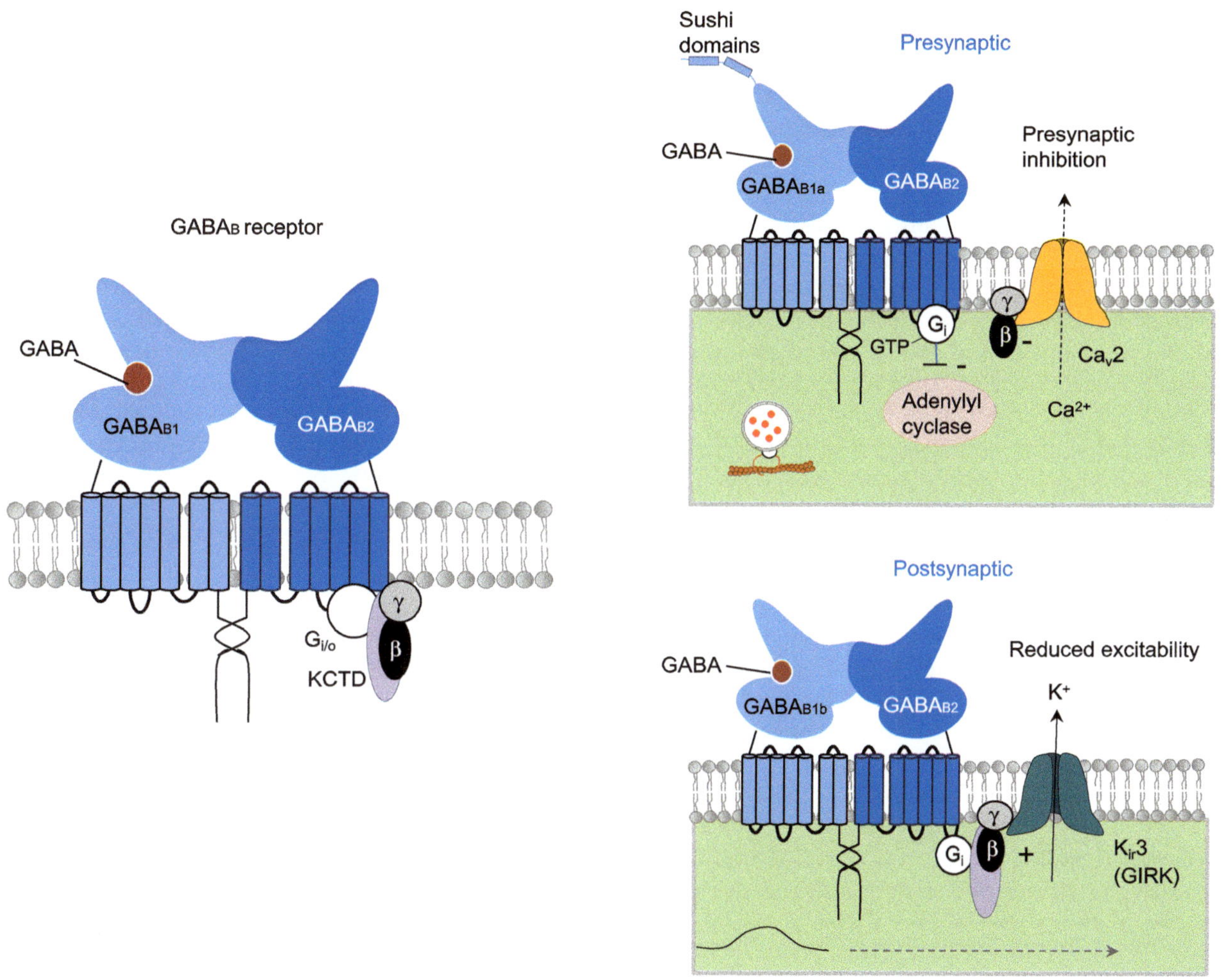

FIGURE 18.8 Structure of and effects of $GABA_BRs$.
The $GABA_BRs$ are obligatory heterodimers of two subunits, $GABA_{B1}$ and $GABA_{B2}$. The $GABA_{B1}$ subunit binds GABA or other ligands such as baclofen; the $GABA_{B2}$ subunit couples with the $G_{i/o}$ proteins. Each $GABA_BR$ subunit consists of three domains: an N-terminal extracellular domain, a seven-helix transmembrane domain, and a cytoplasmic tail. The extracellular portions of the $GABA_{B1}$ and $GABA_{B2}$ subunits each harbor a module containing two domains or lobes that undergo conformational changes upon ligand binding. The $GABA_{B1a}$ subunit is found predominantly in the presynaptic terminal, $GABA_{B1b}$ is associated with the postsynaptic terminal. $GABA_{B1a}$ contains two modules called sushi domain. The main signaling effects of $GABA_BRs$ are inhibition of adenylyl cyclase via the $G_{i/o}$ α subunit, and inhibition of presynaptic Ca_v2 (N-and P/Q- type) Ca^{2+} channels and activation of G protein-activated inward-rectifying Kir3-type K^+ channels (GIRKs) via the Gβγ subunits. The decrease in cAMP production and inhibition of Ca_v2 channels dampens neurotransmitter release. Postsynaptic $GABA_BRs$ activate Kir3 channels in the dendrites of most neurons, which hyperpolarizes the membrane and shunts excitatory neurotransmission.

Effects of $GABA_B$ Receptors

The $GABA_B$Rs are coupled to $G_{i/o}$ signaling and elicit presynaptic and postsynaptic inhibition. Mechanism include inhibition of adenylyl cyclase via the $G\alpha_{i/o}$ subunit and direct membrane interactions of the $G\beta\gamma$ subunit, which inhibits presynaptic Ca_v2 (N-and P/Q- type) Ca^{2+} channels and activates G protein activated inward-rectifying Kir3-type K^+ channels (GIRKs). The decrease in cAMP production, together with inhibition of Ca_v2 channels dampens neurotransmitter release at glutamatergic, GABAergic, and other synaptic terminals. Postsynaptic $GABA_B$Rs activate Kir3 channels in the dendrites of most neurons, which hyperpolarize the membrane and shunt excitatory neurotransmission. $GABA_B$Rs form a functional complex with a subfamily of the potassium channel tetramerization-domain (KCTD) proteins that bind to the intracellular domain of $GABA_{B2}$, and act as auxiliary subunits that expedite agonist-dependent receptor activation by pre-anchoring the G protein to the $GABA_B$ receptor.[43,45] The KCTD proteins interact with the $G\beta\gamma$ subunits and not only accelerate receptor signaling but also induce receptor desensitization by activity-dependent uncoupling of the $G\beta\gamma$ subunits from effector K^+ channels. KCTD proteins also scaffold effector channels such as N-type $Ca2^+$ channels and hyperpolarization-activated cyclic nucleotide-gated channels and other proteins to the $GABA_B$R. The transient receptor potential vanilloid 1 (TRPV1) channels also associate with the $GABA_B$Rs; activation of $GABA_B$Rs reverts the sensitized state of TRPV1 channels in the setting of inflammation or axonal injury. Additional proteins of the $GABA_B$R interactome are neuroligin-3, synaptotagmin-11, calnexin, and others.[43] These complex interactions are characteristic of GPCRs.[46]

The $GABA_B$Rs are distributed both in the CNS and peripheral nervous system, including autonomic ganglia and visceral organs. Within the CNS, they are predominantly localized to neurons, with their largest density in the cerebral cortex, thalamic nuclei, cerebellum, and amygdala. The intimate association of $GABA_B$Rs with glutamatergic synapses at pre- and postsynaptic locations provides for a tight coupling between synaptic excitation and inhibition. Most $GABA_B$ Rs are located distant from GABA release sites but have high affinity for GABA. Presynaptic $GABA_B$Rs on excitatory terminals may be tonically activated by ambient levels of GABA and prevent neurotransmitter release both by inhibiting voltage-sensitive Ca^{2+}-channels and lowering presynaptic levels of cAMP and thus recruitment of synaptic vesicles during sustained activity. Postsynaptic $GABA_B$Rs located on dendritic shafts and spines sense GABA spilling over from neighboring GABAergic synapses. In dendritic spines, $GABA_B$Rs counteract the excitatory synaptic currents elicited by glutamate and prevent long-term potentiation of glutamatergic synapses by reducing L-channel activation and promoting voltage-sensitive magnesium block of NMDARs. In dendritic shafts $GABA_B$Rs reduce the probability for dendritic depolarization to reach the axon hillock and generate an action potential. In addition to their effects on individual synapses, $GABA_B$ Rs modulate the oscillatory activity of cortical and thalamic neural networks. For example, $GABA_B$Rs have an important role in mechanisms of volume transmission in the cerebral cortex by mediating the inhibitory effects of neurogliaform cells on populations of pyramidal neurons. In the thalamus, they mediate the effects of reticular thalamic neurons in generating burst firing in thalamocortical neurons. Presynaptic $GABA_B$Rs have a major role in reducing transmission from primary afferents in the spinal cord.

Gamma-Hydroxybutyric Acid as an Endogenous $GABA_B$R Agonist

Gamma-hydroxybutyric acid (GHB, 4-hydroxybutyrate) is both a precursor and a degradation product of GABA. It is produced from SSA by action of succinic semialdehyde reductase and can be converted back to GABA.[47] GHB may localize with GABA in some inhibitory synaptic terminals, incorporate into vesicles via the VIAAT, be released by exocytosis, and undergo presynaptic uptake. At physiological concentrations, GHB may act via its own GPCR to inhibit presynaptic Ca_v2 channels and neurotransmitter release. However, many of the pharmacological and clinical effects of exogenously administered GHB are probably mediated via the $GABA_B$Rs, where GHB might act as a weak agonist.[9] Important targets of GHB are the thalamocortical circuits involved both in the sleep-wake cycle and susceptibility to generalized seizures.[48,49]

GLYCINE AS A NEUROTRANSMITTER

Glycine is the primary neurotransmitter of many inhibitory interneurons in the motor and sensory nuclei of the spinal cord and brainstem (Figure 18.9).

Synthesis and Uptake

Glycine is the precursor to the one-carbon pool of folic acid intermediates that are fundamental to many synthetic reactions. Glycine is metabolized by the glycine cleavage system, a mitochondrial multienzyme system that includes a glycine decarboxylase encoded by the *GLDC* gene. Loss-of-function *GLDC* mutations cause nonketotic hyperglycinemia.[50] Glycine is incorporated into synaptic vesicles via the VIAAT that also mediates vesicular uptake of GABA; this explains the frequent colocalization and co-release of glycine and GABA in inhibitory terminals in the spinal cord and brainstem. The glycine levels at synapses are controlled by two high-affinity Na^+/Cl^--dependent transporters glycine transporters, GlyT1 (SLC6A9) and GlyT2 (SLC6A5). GlyT1 is expressed in astrocytic processes ensheathing glycinergic and in some glutamatergic terminals; its main role is to decrease the levels of glycine at glycinergic synapses. Loss-of-function mutation of the *SLC6A9/GLYT1* gene causes a severe neonatal encephalopathy with hypotonia and respiratory depression.[51] In contrast, GlyT2 is expressed

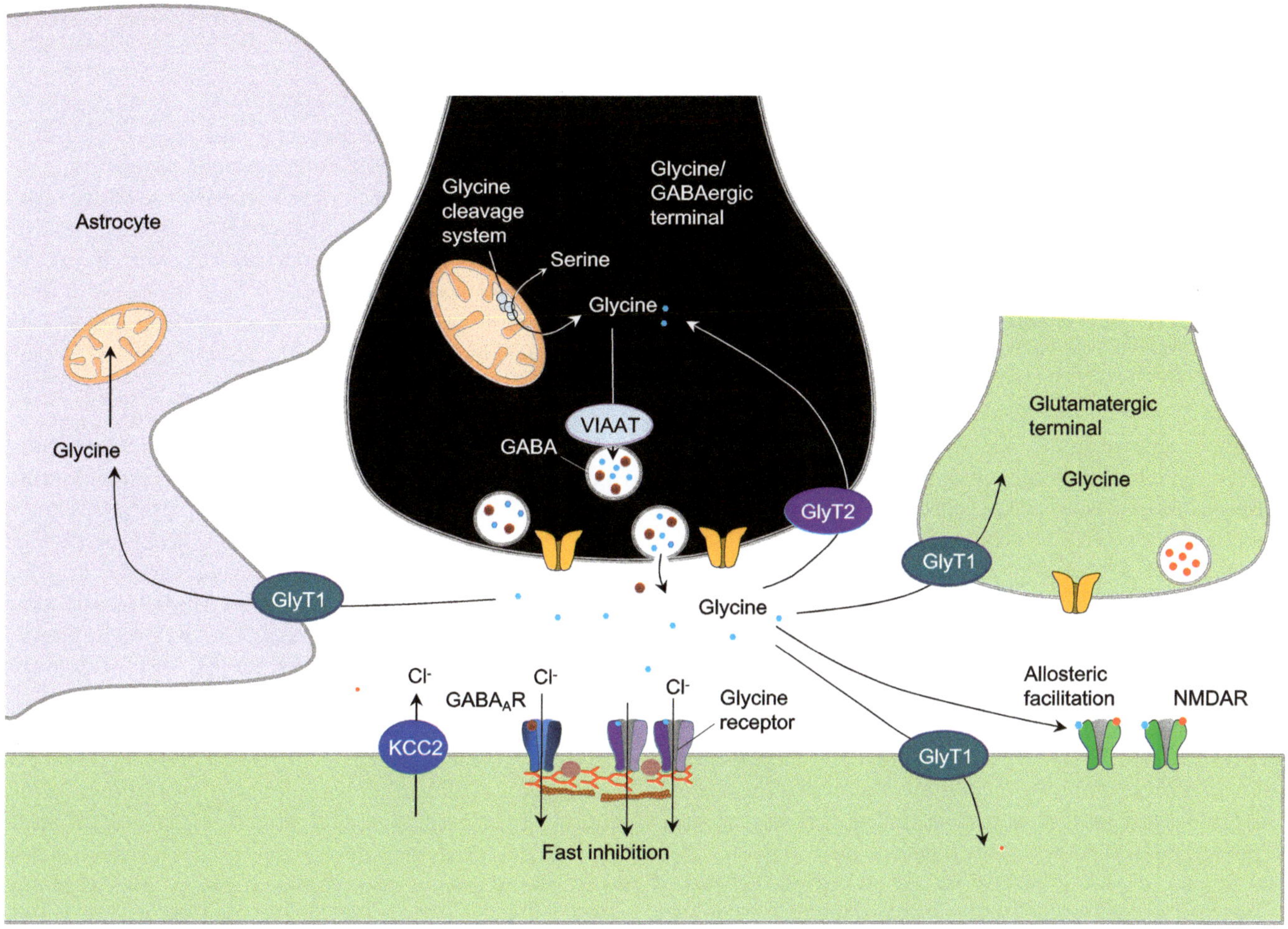

FIGURE 18.9 Glycinergic neurotransmission.
Glycine is produced by the mitochondrial glycine cleavage system and is incorporated into synaptic vesicles via the vesicular inhibitory amino acid transporter (VIAAT) that also mediates vesicular uptake of GABA, which explains the frequent colocalization and co-release of glycine and GABA. The concentration of glycine at synapses is controlled by two high-affinity Na^+/Cl^- dependent transporters glycine transporters (GlyTs), GlyT1 is expressed in astrocytic processes and its main role is to decrease the levels of glycine at glycinergic synapses, whereas GlyT2 is expressed at presynaptic terminals of glycinergic neurons and replenishes the glycine pool. Glycine receptors (GlyRs) form Cl^- channels, and their postsynaptic clustering at mature synapses critically depends on their interactions with gephyrin. In addition to its function as a fast inhibitory neurotransmitter, glycine is also an obligatory coagonist required for activation of N-methyl-D-aspartate receptors (NMDARs).

at presynaptic terminals of glycinergic neurons and its primary role is to replenish of the presynaptic glycine pool to refill synaptic vesicles. Mutations of the *SC6A5/GLYT2* gene cause impaired glycinergic inhibition and cause familial hyperekplexia.[52]

The regulation of glycine fluxes in the CNS via GlyT1 and GlyT2 may involve cooperation of diverse neutral amino acid transporters expressed in neurons and in astrocytes.[4]

Glycine Receptors

Glycine receptors (GlyRs) are pentamers formed by the association of any of four α subunit subtypes (α1–α4, encoded by the *GLRA*1–4 genes) and a β subunit (encoded by a single *GLRB* gene), with a putative 2α:3β stoichiometry.[53] Receptors containing α1 subunits are the predominant population in the postnatal and adult human brainstem and spinal cord. Like the $GABA_A$Rs, GlyRs form Cl^- channels and their postsynaptic clustering at mature synapses critically depends on their interactions with gephyrin.[31,33] Gephyrin has a large degree of variation and regulation by splice variants, posttranslational modifications, intracellular trafficking, and interactions with the underlying cytoskeleton. These mechanisms define the size and number of gephyrin scaffolds and the numbers and proportions of glycine and $GABA_A$ receptors contained within the inhibitory postsynaptic densities. Activation of the GlyRs requires binding of glycine to two to three sites at their α/β interfaces for full activation. These receptors can also be activated by D-alanine and taurine, and are selectively blocked by the competitive antagonist strychnine. Binding of glycine to the GlyR elicits opening of the Cl^- channel; this effect is similar to that of GABA acting on $GABA_A$Rs. In both cases, the resulting change in membrane potential elicited depends on the transmembrane Cl^- concentration, which is determined by the activity KCC2.

Mixed Glycine-GABA Cotransmission

Many interneurons in the spinal cord and brainstem, as well as cerebellar Golgi cells, express both glycine and GABA and function as mixed inhibitory interneurons. For example, glycine/GABA cotransmission in the spinal cord and brainstem provides for a wide range of time courses of postsynaptic inhibition at single synapses; GlyR-mediated responses are faster than those mediated by $GABA_A$Rs. Mixed inhibitory neurons may perform cotransmission at some of their synapses, pure glycinergic or GABAergic inhibition at others, or both.

Glycine and GABA mediate the effects of different types of inhibitory interneurons in the ventral horn of the spinal cord and thus have a major role in regulation of segmental reflexes, muscle tone, and central pattern generation for locomotion. Glycinergic inhibition of brainstem and spinal motoneurons may be responsible for muscle atonia during REM sleep.[54] There is also colocalization of glycine and GABA in neurons and synaptic terminals in the superficial dorsal horn (lamina I–II), where glycine and GABA have a critical role in inhibiting excitatory interneurons and thus nociceptive circuits.[55]

Synaptic Crosstalk Between Glycine and Glutamate

In addition to its function as a fast inhibitory neurotransmitter, glycine is also an obligatory coagonist required for activation of NMDARs[56] (Figure 18.9). Glycine released from glycinergic terminals might reach nearby glutamatergic synapses by spillover and may have an important role in regulating NMDAR-mediated synaptic plasticity and network interactions. Reciprocally, glutamate may allosterically potentiate GlyR-mediated currents, suggesting a functional crosstalk between glycine and glutamate providing a rapid homeostatic control mechanism for neuronal excitability. The endogenous amino acid D-serine released from astrocytes may substitute for glycine at the costimulatory site in the NMDAR. The NMDAR subunits GluN3A and GluN3B are glycine-binding and can assemble with the GluN1 subunit to form unconventional receptors activated by glycine alone.[57] These receptors may participate in mechanisms of excitotoxicity injury.[58]

FUNCTIONS OF INHIBITORY NEUROTRANSMISSION

Inhibitory interneurons target different domains of principal cells and other interneurons and exert effects both at the levels of single cells and neuronal networks.[59,60] At a single cell level, GABA (or glycine) elicits selective filtering of synaptic excitation and modulates the threshold of action potential (spike) generation and the timing, tuning, and bursting of spikes in target cells.[60] At the network level, selective inhibition allows the coordination of transient interactions among the principal cells to form cooperative assemblies, which is required for routing of information across networks in the form of brain oscillations.[61]

There is high diversity of GABAergic interneurons, which differ in their developmental origin, target domains, neurochemical composition, and activity patterns.[62] For example, cortical GABAergic interneurons have been divided into several subgroups according to their targets. A group of neurons targets the soma, proximal dendrites, and axon initial segment and powerfully controls the precise timing of pyramidal cells spikes, coordinating their synchrony within local networks. A second group targets specific dendritic domains of principal cells and control local processing of synaptic inputs. A third group of interneurons specifically contacts other interneurons, resulting in disinhibition of the principal cells. Finally, there is a group of long-range GABAergic interneurons whose axons span two or more anatomical brain regions; in some cases axon collaterals even cross the hemispheric midline and/or innervate subcortical structures. There are relevant examples of GABAergic neurons that project within specific functional circuits. They include neurons of the reticular thalamic nucleus targeting thalamic relay nuclei; Purkinje cells targeting the deep cerebellar nuclei; and projection neurons of the striatum and the globus pallidus.

Inhibitory Control Motifs

Inhibitory interneurons control excitability of principal cells by several circuit motifs, including feedforward inhibition, feedback inhibition, lateral inhibition, and presynaptic inhibition (Figure 18.10). In feedforward inhibition, excitatory afferents that target the principal cells also target dedicated GABAergic interneurons that project to the same principal cell. Feedforward inhibition may affect dendrites or proximal portions of the neurons. Feedforward inhibition at the soma or the axonal initial segment can arrive before the membrane of principal cells reaches threshold and thus prevents the initiation of an action potential. Feedback or recurrent inhibition requires that the principal neuron in a given circuit discharges first and recruits a postsynaptic inhibitory neuron, whose feedback action can prevent further discharges of the principal cells. A related form of inhibition is lateral inhibition, in which the excited interneuron suppresses the activity of principal cells different than those

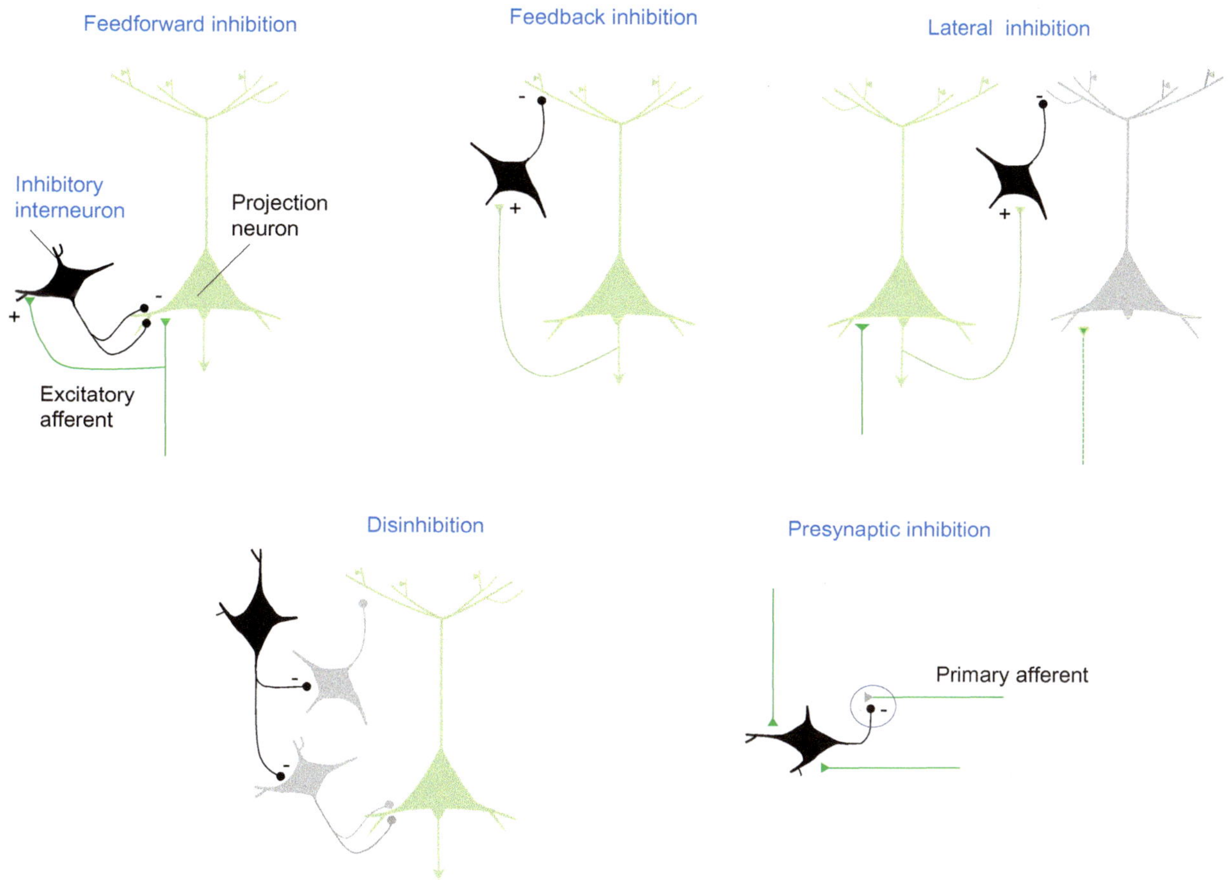

FIGURE 18.10 Inhibitory motifs in the central nervous system.
Inhibitory interneurons control excitability of principal cells by feedforward inhibition, feedback inhibition, lateral inhibition, and presynaptic inhibition. In feedforward inhibition, excitatory afferents that target various dendritic domains of the principal cells also target dedicated GABAergic interneurons, which in turn target the same domains as the excitatory afferents. Feedback or recurrent inhibition requires that the principal neuron in a given circuit discharges first and recruits a postsynaptic inhibitory neuron, whose feedback action can prevent further discharges of the principal cells. In lateral inhibition, the excited interneuron suppresses the activity of principal cells different than those that gave rise to the interneuron excitation. Disinhibition is mediated by GABAergic interneurons that target other interneurons, which results in disinhibition of the principal cells. Presynaptic inhibition involves GABAergic axo-axonic synapses on primary afferents; in these afferents $GABA_AR$ activation elicits efflux of Cl^- and reduces the opening probability of presynaptic calcium channels.

that gave rise to the interneuron excitation. Lateral inhibition is the fundamental mechanism of selection of neuronal groups and competition between different neuronal assemblies and is critical for shaping receptive fields of sensory neurons. Disinhibition is mediated by GABAergic interneurons that target other interneurons; such interactions can mediate disinhibition of the principal cells and induce network synchrony. Presynaptic inhibition is a prominent mechanism for control of segmental reflexes and interneuron activity in the spinal cord. It involves GABAergic axo-axonic synapses on primary afferents; in these afferents $GABA_AR$ activation elicits efflux of Cl^- and thus depolarization, which reduces the opening probability of presynaptic Ca_V2 channels in response to an incoming action potential.[63]

Role of GABAergic Neurons in Shaping Neuronal Network Oscillations

The mutual connectivity and interactions between principal cells and inhibitory interneurons shape the spatial and temporal features of their firing patterns and maintain a balance between excitation and inhibition, which allows proper dynamics in neuronal networks. Interneuron networks are the backbone of many brain oscillations, as they provide rhythm-based timed inhibition to principal cells. Once a collective oscillatory pattern arises, the rhythmic inhibitory volleys provide temporally coordinated alternating periods of reduced and enhanced excitability to the principal cells. This constrains the windows of opportunity for the discharge of principal cells, leading to their synchronization at different frequencies and over multiple time scales, from milliseconds to seconds. This leads to the creation of transiently active neuronal ensembles that underlie numerous operations of the brain,[64] as discussed in other chapters of this book.

PATHOPHYSIOLOGICAL MECHANISMS OF IMPAIRED INHIBITION

Impaired inhibitory neurotransmission in the CNS manifests with increased cell excitability, abnormal network activity, and frequently both. Mechanisms of impaired inhibition include decreased availability of GABA or glycine; reduced activity of inhibitory neurons; loss of surface expression of GABA or glycine receptors due to retention in the ER, degradation, or impaired clustering at the postsynaptic density; abnormal gating of the $GABA_AR$ or GlyR Cl^- channel; and reduced efficacy of inhibition due to downregulation of KCC2 transporters. These abnormalities may result from mutations, autoantibodies, or other mechanisms. For example, reduced availability of GABA may occur in the setting of pyridoxine deficiency leading to reduced GAD activity,[65] whereas reduced availability of glycine may occur in the setting of GlyT2 deficiency.[52] Reduced activity of GABAergic neurons due to loss-of-function mutations affecting the $Na_v1.1$ channel in their axon initial segment occurs in Dravet syndrome.[66] Many genetic and immune disorders affect postsynaptic mechanisms of inhibition. Mutations affecting $GABA_AR$ subunits result in reduced availability of receptors at synapses or abnormal gating of their ion channels. Autoantibodies against $GABA_AR$, $GABA_BR$, or GlyR may lead to receptor internalization or blockade. Downregulation of KCC2 transporters affect the direction of Cl^- flow via $GABA_AR$ and GlyR reducing the efficacy of inhibition or rendering the activity of these receptors excitatory. Thus, impaired inhibitory transmission may result in encephalopathy, seizures, muscle stiffness, and neuropathic pain.[13,36,67–78] Only some examples will be briefly reviewed here.

AUTOIMMUNE SYNAPTOPATHIES AFFECTING INHIBITORY NEUROTRANSMISSION

A large number of neuropsychiatric diseases are linked to specific antineuronal autoantibodies targeting synaptic proteins involved in inhibitory neurotransmission.[71–77] Most of these antibodies are directly pathogenic by downregulating synaptic proteins, activating complement or antagonizing ligand binding. Patients with autoantibodies against inhibitory synapses commonly develop seizures, limbic encephalitis, or signs of peripheral hyperexcitability.

$GABA_AR$ Antibodies

Patients with $GABA_AR$ antibodies have prominent seizures that are often refractory to standard antiseizure medications,[72] but are typically immunotherapy responsive. GAD65 antibody coexists in approximately 50% of cases. Other symptoms include behavioral changes, cognitive impairment, reduced levels of consciousness or focal neurological signs including dyskinesias and aphasia, associated with cortical and subcortical MRI abnormalities and CSF pleocytosis. About one-quarter of patients may have an underlying tumor, often a thymoma.[72] Autoantibodies against $GABA_ARs$ mainly target extracellular epitopes of the $\alpha1$, $\beta3$, and $\gamma2$ subunits, leading to reduced expression and density of synaptic and extrasynaptic $GABA_ARs$ or reduced surface $GABA_AR$ membrane expression.

$GABA_BR$ Antibodies

Patients with antibodies against the $GABA_BRs$ commonly present with seizures in the setting of limbic encephalitis. This disorder is commonly associated with an underlying malignancy, in most cases small cell lung cancer. Seizures occur early and can be resistant to treatment. In the cases described patient[71] antibodies were of the IgG1 isotype and targeted the extracellular domain of the $GABA_B1$ subunit containing the binding site for GABA. In cultured $GABA_BR$-expressing rat hippocampal neurons, human $GABA_BR$ antibodies did not deplete the levels of $GABA_BRs$ at the cell surface, but antagonized the blocking effect of the $GABA_BR$ agonist baclofen[71].

GAD65 Antibodies

Antibodies against GAD65, which mediates GABA synthesis, are typically associated with stiff man syndrome, also referred to as stiff-person syndrome (SPS, initially described as stiff man syndrome).[73,74] These autoantibodies may coexist with other autoantibodies in the setting of paraneoplastic disorders. The presence of GAD65 autoantibodies has also been associated with cerebellar ataxia, epilepsy, oculomotor dysfunction, and limbic and extralimbic encephalitis.[75,76] Classical SPS usually starts insidiously with axial muscle stiffness that progresses to involve the proximal and then the distal part of the limbs and even the cranial muscles; in other cases stiffness may start in the lower limbs and then involve the axial muscles. Stiffness is due to cocontractions of agonist and antagonist muscles and may have diurnal fluctuations. Episodic painful muscle spasms are usually precipitated by auditory, tactile, or emotional stimuli and can be accompanied sympathetic hyperactivity manifested with hypertension, tachycardia, diaphoresis, and hyperthermia that may lead to sudden death. Variants of SPS include stiff-limb syndrome, stiff-trunk, and jerking-SPS associated with prominent spontaneous or stimulus-sensitive myoclonus. Cerebellar ataxia is one of the most common manifestations associated with GAD65 antibodies, with a prevalence similar to SPS. In about 25%

of cases, the cerebellar syndrome may be preceded by transient brainstem dysfunction called "brainstem attacks." Drug-resistant focal epilepsy may also coexist with anti-GAD cerebellar ataxia. Neuroimaging studies usually show normal or mild to moderate cerebellar atrophy in 57% of cases; pathological studies show selective loss of Purkinje cells. Limbic encephalitis can also be associated with elevated serum GAD65 antibodies; these patients are typically younger and present with seizures more commonly that those with encephalitis associated with antibodies against K^+ channel complex proteins. Pharmacoresistant chronic epilepsy, as well as epilepsia partialis continua and status epilepticus may be present in patients with positive GAD65 antibodies without evidence of active brain inflammation in the MRI. Oculomotor dysfunction, nystagmus (particularly downbeat nystagmus), and opsoclonus have also been associated with GAD65 antibodies, either in isolation or associated with other syndromes. These autoantibodies may coexist with other autoantibodies in the setting of paraneoplastic disorders.[75] Small-cell lung cancer, followed by thymoma and breast cancer are the neoplasms most commonly associated with GAD65 antibodies. As GAD65 is an intracellular antigen, the mechanism pathogenicity is less clear and the response to immunotherapy less predictable than in disorders associated with antibodies against surface proteins.[75]

Glycine Receptor (GlyR) Autoantibodies

Patients with antibodies against GlyRs show signs of CNS hyperexcitability, which may manifest as hyperekplexia, seizures, stiff-person syndrome, or progressive encephalomyelitis with rigidity and myoclonus (PERM).[77] This disorder is characterized by muscle stiffness, superimposed spasms, myoclonus, and brainstem dysfunction such as oculomotor abnormalities, dysphagia, and gait ataxia. Other prominent manifestations include seizures, hypersomnia, behavioral changes, sympathetic hyperactivity, corticospinal signs, and somatosensory abnormalities indicating a clinical picture of diffuse encephalomyelitis. Isolated cases of limbic encephalitis or hypersomnia also occur. Tumors are found in approximately 5% of cases, including thymoma, small-cell lung cancer, and Hodgkin lymphoma. Whereas PERM is mostly related to GlyR antibodies, GAD65 antibodies are detected in about 20% of cases.

Amphiphysin Autoantibodies

Amphiphysin is an adaptor protein that interacts with other proteins involved in clathrin-mediated endocytosis and recycling of synaptic vesicles. Though expressed at both excitatory and inhibitory synapses, amphiphysin is more critical to sustained transmitter release from subpopulations of inhibitory cells that discharge at high frequencies. Amphiphysin autoantibodies account for approximately 5% of patients with SPS spectrum disorders, though phenotypically there are differences from classical SPS. The phenotype includes stiffness limited to the limbs, and motor hyperactivity predominantly affecting the arms and neck muscles. The clinical presentation is typically that of a myeloneuropathy, with both stiffness and spasms (upper motor neuron) and radiculoneuropathic symptoms (pain) and signs and EMG findings. This occurs as a paraneoplastic disorder in the setting of an underlying malignancy, in particular breast cancer and small-cell lung carcinoma. Electrophysiological studies in animal passively immunized with amphiphysin autoantibodies animals show markedly decreased presynaptic inhibition and reduced presynaptic vesicle pool.

GENETIC EPILEPSY SYNDROMES ASSOCIATED WITH $GABA_A$R MUTATIONS

Genetic epileptic syndromes are often monogenic (familial or sporadic). Genetic epilepsy syndromes, account for 30%–50% of epilepsy. They vary in severity from relatively mild childhood absence epilepsy to very severe epileptic encephalopathies such as infantile spasms and Lennox-Gastaut syndrome. Different mutations in the same gene can produce mild epilepsy or severe epileptic encephalopathy with associated cognitive impairment and developmental delay.

Phenotypic Variability

Missense and nonsense mutations in *GABR* genes encoding subunits of $GABA_A$Rs (*GABRA1*, *GABRA2*, *GABRA5*, *GABRA6*, *GABRB1*, *GABRB2*, *GABRB3*, *GABRD*, and *GABRG2*) are found in cases of both monogenic autosomal dominant familial and de novo genetic epilepsy syndromes.[13] More than 60 de novo mutations in *GABRA1*, *GABRA2*, *GABRA5*, *GABRB1*, *GABRB2*, *GABRB3*, and *GABRG2* have been found in cases with broad phenotypic range of epileptic encephalopathies, which include Ohtahara syndrome, infantile spasms, myoclonic astatic epilepsy, Lennox-Gastaut syndrome, early onset epileptic encephalopathy, and Dravet syndrome.[13,67,68]

Pathogenic Mechanisms

Monogenic *GABR* mutations have been subdivided into six classes; five of them include mutations that reduce subunit expression and others reduce receptor function by impairing channel gating. Impaired subunit expression may be due to impaired transcription or translation; misfolding and degradation; truncation and retention in the ER with or without a dominant negative effect on other subunits; or ER retention of functional receptors.[13]

Mutations mapped to different *GABR* genes may share common mechanisms of dysfunction if they occur at the same receptor structural domains. The severity of the channel dysfunction correlates structurally with the location of the mutation in the $GABA_A$ receptor.

De novo and familial $GABA_AR$ missense mutations are distributed along its three well-defined structural cores. Depending on the location, these mutations cause perturbations coupled to channel opening, impairing the receptor "lock-and-pull" mechanism, ultimately contributing to a specific epilepsy phenotype. Mutations located at the extracellular β/α interface and at the coupling junction region are linked to direct changes in channel opening and are more deleterious than mutations at the α/β or γ/β interfaces, which are indirectly coupled to channel gating. Mutations located in the pore domain are usually more deleterious than mutations in the intracellular loop, which are rarely deleterious. Many mutations causing severe epileptic encephalopathies occur at highly homologous residues of $GABA_AR$ subunits, indicating that the pore domain is a hot spot causing the epilepsies.

OTHER PEDIATRIC DISORDERS OF GABA OR GLYCINE NEUROTRANSMISSION

Disorders of GABA or Glycine Metabolism

Several genetic disorders affect different steps of GABA or glycine metabolism. They frequently start in infancy. Some disorders are treatable. For example, pyridoxine-dependent epilepsies are autosomal recessive disorders with neonatal onset characterized by seizures that are unresponsive to conventional antiepileptic drugs.[65] Cases due to mutations of the *ALDH7A1* gene encoding α-aminoadipic-semialdehyde dehydrogenase or *PROSC* gene encoding a pyridoxal-5-phosphate binding protein respond to pyridoxine replacement; a similar syndrome due to mutations in the *PNPO* gene encoding pyridoxal-5'-phosphate oxidase enzyme responds to pyridoxal-5-phosphate but not to pyridoxine administration.

Succinic semialdehyde dehydrogenase deficiency (GHB aciduria) is an autosomal recessive disorder due to a mutation affecting the *SSADH* (*ALDH5A1*, aldehyde dehydrogenase 5 family, member A1) gene, resulting in impaired conversion of SSA to succinic acid and accumulation of both GHB and GABA.[47] SSADH deficiency has considerable phenotypic heterogeneity with predominance of neurologic and psychiatric manifestations, including developmental language delay, hypotonia, hyporeflexia, ataxia, inattention, hyperactivity, sleep disturbances, hyperkinetic movement disorders, and different types of generalized seizures. MRI shows cerebral and cerebellar (particularly vermian) atrophy and enhanced T2 signal in the globus pallidus, subcortical white matter, dentate nucleus, and substantia nigra. There is marked elevation of GBH and to a lesser extent GABA and reduced level of glutamine in the CSF.

Therapeutic approaches to reduce GHB levels in SSADH deficiency include vigabatrin, which inhibits GABA transaminase, and taurine, which may act as an antagonist of $GABA_BRs$.

Mutations of the *ABAT* gene encoding GABA-transaminase result in increased GABA levels in the brain detected on magnetic resonance spectroscopy. This disorder manifests with drowsiness, epileptic encephalopathy, developmental delay, paroxysmal dyskinesia, nonprogressive ataxia, or cortical visual impairment. MRI shows secondary hypomyelination in the internal capsule and brainstem tegmentum and thalamic hyperintensities. The diagnosis of GABA-T deficiency has potential therapeutic implications as GABAergic agonists are potentially harmful whereas the BZP receptor antagonist flumazenil may improve neurologic function.[78,79]

As mentioned earlier, nonketotic hyperglycinemia (NKH), also known as glycine encephalopathy, is an autosomal recessive disorder linked to mutations of the *GLDC* (glycine decarboxylase) causing a deficiency in the glycine cleavage system.[50] This disorder affects term neonates within the first or second day of life and manifests with progressive lethargy, severe seizures associated with hypsarrhythmia or burst-suppression pattern on EEG; myoclonic jerks, hiccupping, and severe hypotonia. NKH may also manifest in older children with intermittent choreoathetosis.

Glycine transporter 1 encephalopathy (glycine encephalopathy with normal serum glycine, GLYT1 transporter dysfunction) is caused by mutations in the *SLC6A9* gene.[51] This disorder is characterized by neonatal onset respiratory failure severe hypotonia that progressed to hypertonicity, and startle-like responses. Additional characteristics included dysmorphic features and musculoskeletal abnormalities, and abnormal antenatal findings. There are elevated levels of glycine in CSF and elevated CSF to plasma glycine ratio.

Hereditary Hyperekplexia

Hereditary hyperekplexia, or human startle disease, is a paroxysmal motor disorder caused by a defect of glycinergic inhibition of motor neurons.[70] Hyperekplexia is characterized by an exaggerated startle reflex in response to tactile or acoustic stimuli. This disorder first manifests as neonatal hypertonia, followed in some cases by episodes of life-threatening apnea. Mental development usually is normal. Hereditary hyperekplexia is genetically heterogeneous. Missense and nonsense mutations in the *GLRA1* gene encoding the GlyR α1 subunit are the primary cause. Missense, nonsense, and frameshift mutations have also been identified in the glycine transporter GlyT2 gene (*SLC6A5*) demonstrating a presynaptic component to this disease. Other rare mutations have been identified in the genes encoding the GlyR β subunit (*GLRB*), collybistin (*ARHGEF9*), and gephyrin (*GPHN*)—all of which are postsynaptic proteins involved in orchestrating glycinergic neurotransmission.[70]

TABLE 18.1 *GABAergic Transmission as a Therapeutic Target*

Target	Mechanism	Drug	Therapeutic Use
GABA transporter	Inhibition	Tiagabine	Focal seizures (exacerbates typical absence)
GABA-transaminase	Inhibition	Vigabatrin	Infantile spasms
Synaptic $GABA_A$ receptor ($GABA_AR$)	Allosteric agonist of of all γ2-containing benzodiazepine receptors)	Clonazepam Lorazepam Diazepam Midazolam Alprazolam	Myoclonus Status epilepticus Spasticity Anxiety
	Allosteric agonist of α1-containing receptors	Zolpidem Eszopiclone	Insomnia
	Benzodiazepine (BZP) receptor antagonist	Flumazenil	BZP overdose Endozepine stupor
Extrasynaptic $GABA_A$ R	Allosteric facilitation	Propofol Volatile anesthetics	Status epilepticus General anesthesia
All $GABA_ARs$	Cl^- channel opening	Clobazam	Lennox-Gastaut syndrome
$GABA_BR$	Agonist	Baclofen	Spasticity Dystonia Pain (trigeminal neuralgia)
	Agonist	γ-hydroxybutyrate	Insomnia Narcolepsy Alcohol withdrawal

INHIBITORY NEUROTRANSMISSION AS A THERAPEUTIC TARGET

The GABAergic system has been a major target for management of neurologic and psychiatric disorders (Table 18.1). For example, BZPs that are positive allosteric modulators of synaptic (γ2 subunit-containing) $GABA_ARs$ and are used for treatment of epilepsy (e.g., lorazepam for status epileptics), myoclonus (clonazepam), spasticity, stiff man syndrome, and anxiety. Agonists of α1 subunit containing $GABA_ARs$ (such as zolpidem or eszopiclone) are used for insomnia. Clobazam is a nonselective $GABA_AR$ agonist used for treatment of Lennox-Gastaut syndrome. Stripentol directly interacts with $GABA_ARs$ and is approved used for treatment of Dravet syndrome. Other antiepileptic drugs that increase GABAergic transmission include the GABA-T inhibitor vigabatrin used for infantile spasms, and the GAT inhibitor tiagabine, which is rarely used for focal seizures. In contrast, flumazenil, a BZP receptor antagonist, is used in cases of BZP intoxication, hepatic encephalopathy, and a rare disorder known as endozepine stupor. A $GABA_BR$ agonist baclofen is used for treatment of spasticity, dystonia, and painful disorders such as trigeminal neuralgia. Gamma hydroxybutyrate is used for treatment of narcolepsy.

KEY POINTS

- GABA is the main inhibitory neurotransmitter in the CNS; glycine, together with GABA, is critical in inhibitory circuits of the brainstem and spinal cord.
- GABA is synthesized from L-glutamate by action of the glutamic acid decarboxylase (GAD), which requires pyridoxal phosphate as a cofactor.
- Pyridoxine deficiency impairs the first step of GABA synthesis and produces neonatal seizures.
- Storage of GABA (and glycine) in synaptic vesicles depends on the vesicular GABA transporter (VGAT, vesicular inhibitory amino acid transporter, VIAAT).
- GABA undergoes uptake in neurons and astrocytes via GABA transporters (GAT).
- After uptake, GABA is catabolized in the mitochondrial matrix by GABA transaminase (GABA-T).

- The inhibitory effects of GABA are mediated by $GABA_A$ receptors ($GABA_ARs$), which are chloride (Cl^-) channels and $GABA_B$ receptors ($GABA_BRs$), which are GPCRs.
- The effects of $GABA_AR$ (and GlyR) activation depend on the transcellular Cl^- gradient, which is controlled by the antagonistic influence of the chloride-cation cotransporters KCC2 and NKCC1.
- In most adult neurons, which express KCC2, $GABA_A$ (or glycine) receptor activation elicits influx of Cl- resulting in fast inhibitory potential.
- KCC2 downregulation in the setting of ischemia, status epilepticus, or microglial activation reduces efficacy of GABAergic inhibition.
- Synaptic $GABA_ARs$ contain α1–α3, β, and γ2 subunits; are clustered as postsynaptic sites by interactions with gephyrin; are sensitive to benzodiazepines (BZPs); and mediate phasic GABAergic inhibition.
- Extrasynaptic $GABA_ARs$ contain α4 or α6 subunits combined with δ subunits and are not sensitive to BZPs but to alcohol and general anesthetics, and mediate tonic GABAergic inhibition.
- Benzodiazepines, barbiturates, allopregnanolone, general anesthetics, and ethanol are positive modulators of $GABA_ARs$.
- Penicillin, imipenem, and some cephalosporins are $GABA_AR$ antagonists.
- Gephyrin is the central scaffold element of inhibitory GABAergic and glycinergic synapses.
- $GABA_ARs$ undergo dynamic trafficking to and retrieval from the synapse in response to synaptic activity.
- There is activity-dependent plasticity of GABAergic synapses.
- $GABA_BRs$ mediate both presynaptic and postsynaptic inhibition via activation of K^+ channels and inhibition of presynaptic Ca^{2+} channels.
- Gamma-hydroxybutyric acid (GHB, 4-hydroxybutyrate) is both a precursor and a degradation product of GABA and is an agonist of $GABA_BR$.
- Glycine is the primary neurotransmitter of many inhibitory interneurons in the motor and sensory nuclei of the spinal cord and brainstem.
- Glycine is frequently colocalized and co-released with GABA.
- The concentration of glycine at synapses is controlled by GlyT1, expressed in astrocytic processes, and GlyT2, expressed at presynaptic glycinergic terminals.
- Glycine receptors (GlyRs) are chloride channels that elicit fast inhibitory transmission in adult neurons.
- Inhibitory interneurons control excitability of principal cells by, feedforward inhibition, feedback inhibition, lateral inhibition, and presynaptic inhibition.
- The mutual connectivity and interactions between principal cells and inhibitory interneurons provide the basis for brain oscillations.
- Impaired inhibitory neurotransmission in the CNS manifests with increased excitability, abnormal network activity, and frequently both.
- Disorders due to $GABA_AR$ or $GABA_BRs$ antibodies manifest with prominent seizures often refractory to standard antiseizure medication and may indicate an underlying neoplasm.
- Antibodies against GAD65 are typically associated with stiff man syndrome, may coexist with other autoantibodies in the setting of paraneoplastic disorders, and may be also produce cerebellar ataxia, epilepsy, and oculomotor dysfunction.
- Antibodies against GlyRs produce CNS hyperexcitability, which may manifest as hyperekplexia, seizures, stiff-person syndrome, or progressive encephalomyelitis with rigidity and myoclonus.
- Amphiphysin antibodies produce a myeloneuropathy, with both stiffness and spasms (upper motor neuron) and radiculoneuropathic symptoms (pain).
- Genetic epilepsy syndromes associated with missense and nonsense mutations in *GABR* genes encoding subunits of $GABA_ARs$ are found in cases of both monogenic autosomal dominant familial and de novo genetic epilepsy syndromes.
- Mutations affecting GABAergic of glycinergic transmission underlie several childhood neurologic disorders.
- The GABAergic system is a major target for management of neurologic and psychiatric disorders.

REFERENCES

1. Modi JP, Prentice H, Wu JY. Regulation of GABA neurotransmission by glutamic acid decarboxylase (GAD). Curr Pharm Des 2015;21:4939–4942.
2. Wilson MP, Plecko B, Mills PB, Clayton PT. Disorders affecting vitamin B6 metabolism. J Inherit Metab Dis 2019;42:629–646.
3. Aubrey KR, Supplisson S. Heterogeneous signaling at GABA and glycine co-releasing terminals. Front Synaptic Neurosci 2018;10:40.
4. Zafar S, Jabeen I. Structure, FUNCTION, AND MODULATION of gamma-aminobutyric acid transporter 1 (GAT1) in neurological disorders: a pharmacoinformatic prospective. Front Chem 2018;6:397.
5. Madsen KK, Hansen GH, Danielsen EM, Schousboe A. The subcellular localization of GABA transporters and its implication for seizure management. Neurochem Res 2015;40:410–419.
6. Lie MEK, Al-Khawaja A, Damgaard M, et al. Glial GABA transporters as modulators of inhibitory signalling in epilepsy and stroke. Adv Neurobiol 2017;16:137–167.
7. Schousboe A, Wellendorph P, Frolund B, Clausen RP, Krogsgaard-Larsen P. Astrocytic GABA transporters:

pharmacological properties and targets for antiepileptic drugs. Adv Neurobiol 2017;16:283–296.
8. Ravasz D, Kacso G, Fodor V, Horvath K, Adam-Vizi V, Chinopoulos C. Catabolism of GABA, succinic semialdehyde or gamma-hydroxybutyrate through the GABA shunt impair mitochondrial substrate-level phosphorylation. Neurochem Int 2017;109:41–53.
9. Bay T, Eghorn LF, Klein AB, Wellendorph P. GHB receptor targets in the CNS: focus on high-affinity binding sites. Biochem Pharmacol 2014;87:220–228.
10. Vogel KR, Ainslie GR, Walters DC, et al. Succinic semialdehyde dehydrogenase deficiency, a disorder of GABA metabolism: an update on pharmacological and enzyme-replacement therapeutic strategies. J Inherit Metab Dis 2018;41:699–708.
11. Hibbs RE, Gouaux E. Principles of activation and permeation in an anion-selective Cys-loop receptor. Nature 2011;474:54–60.
12. Scott S, Aricescu AR. A structural perspective on $GABA_A$ receptor pharmacology. Curr Opin Struct Biol 2019;54:189–197.
13. Hernandez CC, Macdonald RL. A structural look at GABAA receptor mutations linked to epilepsy syndromes. Brain Res 2019;1714:234–247.
14. Laverty D, Desai R, Uchanski T, et al. Cryo-EM structure of the human alpha1beta3gamma2 GABAA receptor in a lipid bilayer. Nature 2019;565:516–520.
15. Masiulis S, Desai R, Uchanski T, et al. GABAA receptor signalling mechanisms revealed by structural pharmacology. Nature 2019;565:454–459.
16. Ben-Ari Y, Khalilov I, Kahle KT, Cherubini E. The GABA excitatory/inhibitory shift in brain maturation and neurological disorders. Neuroscientist 2012;18:467–486.
17. Watanabe M, Fukuda A. Development and regulation of chloride homeostasis in the central nervous system. Front Cell Neurosci 2015;9:371.
18. Akita T, Fukuda A. Intracellular Cl(-) dysregulation causing and caused by pathogenic neuronal activity. Pflugers Arch 2020;472(7):977–987.
19. Liu R, Wang J, Liang S, Zhang G, Yang X. Role of NKCC1 and KCC2 in epilepsy: from expression to function. Front Neurol 2019;10:1407.
20. Martin-Aragon Baudel MA, Poole AV, Darlison MG. Chloride co-transporters as possible therapeutic targets for stroke. J Neurochem 2017;140:195–209.
21. Lee-Hotta S, Uchiyama Y, Kametaka S. Role of the BDNF-TrkB pathway in KCC2 regulation and rehabilitation following neuronal injury: a mini review. Neurochem Int 2019;128:32–38.
22. Farrant M, Nusser Z. Variations on an inhibitory theme: phasic and tonic activation of GABA(A) receptors. Nat Rev Neurosci 2005;6:215–229.
23. McBain CJ, Kittler J, Luscher B, Mody I, Orser BA. GABAergic signaling in health and disease. Neuropharmacology 2015;88:1.
24. Brickley SG, Mody I. Extrasynaptic GABA(A) receptors: their function in the CNS and implications for disease. Neuron 2012;73:23–34.
25. Sigel E, Ernst M. The benzodiazepine binding sites of GABAA receptors. Trends Pharmacol Sci 2018;39:659–671.
26. Che Has AT, Absalom N, van Nieuwenhuijzen PS, Clarkson AN, Ahring PK, Chebib M. Zolpidem is a potent stoichiometry-selective modulator of alpha1beta3 GABAA receptors: evidence of a novel benzodiazepine site in the alpha1-alpha1 interface. Sci Rep 2016;6:28674.
27. Jensen HS, Nichol K, Lee D, Ebert B. Clobazam and its active metabolite N-desmethylclobazam display significantly greater affinities for alpha(2)- versus alpha(1)-GABA(A)-receptor complexes. PLoS One 2014;9:e88456.
28. Olsen RW. GABAA receptor: positive and negative allosteric modulators. Neuropharmacology 2018;136:10–22.
29. Tuem KB, Atey TM. Neuroactive steroids: receptor interactions and responses. Front Neurol 2017;8:442.
30. Triplett JD, Lawn ND, Chan J, Dunne JW. Cephalosporin-related neurotoxicity: metabolic encephalopathy or non-convulsive status epilepticus? J Clin Neurosci 2019;67:163–166.
31. Kasaragod VB, Schindelin H. Structure-function relationships of glycine and $GABA_A$ receptors and their interplay with the scaffolding protein gephyrin. Front Mol Neurosci 2018;11:317.
32. Pizzarelli R, Griguoli M, Zacchi P, et al. Tuning GABAergic inhibition: gephyrin molecular organization and functions. Neuroscience 2019;439:125–136.
33. Butler MH, Hayashi A, Ohkoshi N, et al. Autoimmunity to gephyrin in stiff-man syndrome. Neuron 2000;26:307–312.
34. Yao R, Zhang Y, Liu J, et al. Clinical and molecular characterization of three novel ARHGEF9 mutations in patients with developmental delay and epilepsy. J Mol Neurosci 2020;70:908–915.
35. Contreras A, Hines DJ, Hines RM. Molecular specialization of GABAergic synapses on the soma and axon in cortical and hippocampal circuit function and dysfunction. Front Mol Neurosci 2019;12:154.
36. Mele M, Costa RO, Duarte CB. Alterations in $GABA_A$-receptor trafficking and synaptic dysfunction in brain disorders. Front Cell Neurosci 2019;13:77.
37. Schaaf MB, Keulers TG, Vooijs MA, Rouschop KM. LC3/GABARAP family proteins: autophagy-(un)related functions. FASEB J 2016;30:3961–3978.
38. Yuen EY, Wei J, Zhong P, Yan Z. Disrupted GABAAR trafficking and synaptic inhibition in a mouse model of Huntington's disease. Neurobiol Dis 2012;46:497–502.
39. Barberis A. Postsynaptic plasticity of GABAergic synapses. Neuropharmacology 2019;169:107643.
40. Kim HH, Park JM, Lee SH, Ho WK. Association of mGluR-dependent LTD of excitatory synapses with endocannabinoid-dependent LTD of inhibitory synapses leads to EPSP to spike potentiation in CA1 pyramidal neurons. J Neurosci 2019;39:224–237.
41. Mapelli J, Gandolfi D, Vilella A, Zoli M, Bigiani A. Heterosynaptic GABAergic plasticity bidirectionally driven by the activity of pre- and postsynaptic NMDA receptors. Proc Natl Acad Sci U S A 2016;113:9898–9903.
42. Bowery NG. Historical perspective and emergence of the GABAB receptor. Adv Pharmacol 2010;58:1–18.
43. Fritzius T, Bettler B. The organizing principle of GABAB receptor complexes: physiological and pharmacological implications. Basic Clin Pharmacol Toxicol 2019;126(Suppl 6):25–34.
44. Rice HC, de Malmazet D, Schreurs A, et al. Secreted amyloid-beta precursor protein functions as a GABABR1a ligand to modulate synaptic transmission. Science 2019;363(6423):eaao4827.
45. Frangaj A, Fan QR. Structural biology of GABAB receptor. Neuropharmacology 2018;136:68–79.

46. Dunn HA, Orlandi C, Martemyanov KA. Beyond the ligand: extracellular and transcellular G protein-coupled receptor complexes in physiology and pharmacology. Pharmacol Rev 2019;71:503–519.
47. Menduti G, Biamino E, Vittorini R, et al. Succinic semialdehyde dehydrogenase deficiency: the combination of a novel ALDH5A1 gene mutation and a missense SNP strongly affects SSADH enzyme activity and stability. Mol Genet Metab 2018;124:210–215.
48. Venzi M, Di Giovanni G, Crunelli V. A critical evaluation of the gamma-hydroxybutyrate (GHB) model of absence seizures. CNS Neurosci Ther 2015;21:123–140.
49. Xu XM, Wei YD, Liu Y, Li ZX. Gamma-hydroxybutyrate (GHB) for narcolepsy in adults: an updated systematic review and meta-analysis. Sleep Med 2019;64:62–70.
50. Bravo-Alonso I, Navarrete R, Arribas-Carreira L, et al. Nonketotic hyperglycinemia: Functional assessment of missense variants in GLDC to understand phenotypes of the disease. Hum Mutat 2017;38:678–691.
51. Alfallaj R, Alfadhel M. Glycine transporter 1 encephalopathy from biochemical pathway to clinical disease: review. Child Neurol Open 2019;6:2329048X19831486.
52. Dafsari HS, Kawalia A, Sprute R, et al. Novel mutations in SLC6A5 with benign course in hyperekplexia. Cold Spring Harb Mol Case Stud 2019;5.
53. Lynch JW, Zhang Y, Talwar S, Estrada-Mondragon A. Glycine receptor drug discovery. Adv Pharmacol 2017;79:225–253.
54. Krenzer M, Anaclet C, Vetrivelan R, et al. Brainstem and spinal cord circuitry regulating REM sleep and muscle atonia. PLoS One 2011;6:e24998.
55. Imlach WL. New approaches to target glycinergic neurotransmission for the treatment of chronic pain. Pharmacol Res 2017;116:93–99.
56. Zafra F, Ibanez I, Bartolome-Martin D, Piniella D, Arribas-Blazquez M, Gimenez C. Glycine transporters and its coupling with NMDA receptors. Adv Neurobiol 2017;16:55–83.
57. Grand T, Abi Gerges S, David M, Diana MA, Paoletti P. Unmasking GluN1/GluN3A excitatory glycine NMDA receptors. Nat Commun 2018;9:4769.
58. Pachernegg S, Strutz-Seebohm N, Hollmann M. GluN3 subunit-containing NMDA receptors: not just one-trick ponies. Trends Neurosci 2012;35:240–249.
59. Tremblay R, Lee S, Rudy B. GABAergic interneurons in the neocortex: from cellular properties to circuits. Neuron 2016;91:260–292.
60. Roux L, Buzsaki G. Tasks for inhibitory interneurons in intact brain circuits. Neuropharmacology 2015;88:10–23.
61. Engin E, Benham RS, Rudolph U. An emerging circuit pharmacology of GABAA receptors. Trends Pharmacol Sci 2018;39:710–732.
62. DeFelipe J, Lopez-Cruz PL, Benavides-Piccione R, et al. New insights into the classification and nomenclature of cortical GABAergic interneurons. Nat Rev Neurosci 2013;14:202–216.
63. Cote MP, Murray LM, Knikou M. Spinal control of locomotion: individual neurons, their circuits and functions. Front Physiol 2018;9:784.
64. Buzsaki G. Neural syntax: cell assemblies, synapsembles, and readers. Neuron 2010;68:362–385.
65. Mastrangelo M. Actual insights into treatable inborn errors of metabolism causing epilepsy. J Pediatr Neurosci 2018;13:13–23.
66. Yamagata T, Raveau M, Kobayashi K, et al. CRISPR/dCas9-based Scn1a gene activation in inhibitory neurons ameliorates epileptic and behavioral phenotypes of Dravet syndrome model mice. Neurobiol Dis 2020;141:104954.
67. Maljevic S, Moller RS, Reid CA, et al. Spectrum of GABAA receptor variants in epilepsy. Curr Opin Neurol 2019;32:183–190.
68. Kahle KT, Khanna AR, Duan J, Staley KJ, Delpire E, Poduri A. The KCC2 Cotransporter and Human Epilepsy: Getting Excited About Inhibition. Neuroscientist 2016;22:555–562.
69. Malaspina P, Roullet JB, Pearl PL, Ainslie GR, Vogel KR, Gibson KM. Succinic semialdehyde dehydrogenase deficiency (SSADHD): pathophysiological complexity and multifactorial trait associations in a rare monogenic disorder of GABA metabolism. Neurochem Int 2016;99:72–84.
70. Davies JS, Chung SK, Thomas RH, et al. The glycinergic system in human startle disease: a genetic screening approach. Front Mol Neurosci 2010;3:8.
71. Dalmau J, Graus F. Antibody-mediated encephalitis. N Engl J Med 2018;378:840–851.
72. Spatola M, Petit-Pedrol M, Simabukuro MM, et al. Investigations in GABAA receptor antibody-associated encephalitis. Neurology 2017;88:1012–1020.
73. El-Abassi R, Soliman MY, Villemarette-Pittman N, England JD. SPS: understanding the complexity. J Neurol Sci 2019;404:137–149.
74. Baizabal-Carvallo JF. The neurological syndromes associated with glutamic acid decarboxylase antibodies. J Autoimmun 2019;101:35–47.
75. McKeon A, Tracy JA. GAD65 neurological autoimmunity. Muscle Nerve 2017;56:15–27.
76. Arino H, Hoftberger R, Gresa-Arribas N, et al. Paraneoplastic neurological syndromes and glutamic acid decarboxylase antibodies. JAMA Neurol 2015;72:874–881.
77. Hinson SR, Lopez-Chiriboga AS, Bower JH, et al. Glycine receptor modulating antibody predicting treatable stiff-person spectrum disorders. Neurol Neuroimmunol Neuroinflamm 2018;5:e438.
78. Koenig MK, Hodgeman R, Riviello JJ, et al. Phenotype of GABA-transaminase deficiency. Neurology 2017;88:1919–1924.
79. Koenig MK, Bonnen PE. Metabolomics profile in ABAT deficiency pre- and post-treatment. JIMD Rep 2019;43:13–17.

19 Cholinergic Transmission

OVERVIEW

Cholinergic neurons are widely distributed in the central and peripheral nervous systems (Figure 19.1). The two major cholinergic groups in the central nervous system (CNS) are located in the basal forebrain and the mesopontine tegmentum (Figure 19.2). There are also local cholinergic interneurons in the striatum and in other brain areas. Acetylcholine (ACh) is the primary neurotransmitter of cranial and spinal motor neurons, preganglionic autonomic neurons, many parasympathetic ganglion and enteric neurons, and sympathetic neurons innervating the sweat glands. Synaptic availability of ACh is controlled by its synthesis by choline acetyltransferase (ChAT) and by its rapid hydrolysis by acetylcholinesterase (AChE). The effects of ACh are mediated by nicotinic ACh receptors (nAChRs), which are cation channels that mediate fast excitatory action, and several types of muscarinic (M) receptors, which are G protein-coupled receptors. Cholinergic activity in the CNS is critical for directed attention, encoding of episodic memories, and thalamocortical arousal, and contributes to action selection and switching. Normal cholinergic activity is also critical to maintain the safety margin of neuromuscular transmission and autonomic control of visceral organs. Cholinergic neurotransmission can be affected by degenerative, genetic, immune, or toxic mechanisms. Impaired cholinergic activity in the CNS has been linked to attention and memory disturbances in Alzheimer disease (AD) and Lewy body disorders. Impaired cholinergic neurotransmission at the neuromuscular junction (NMJ) occurs as a consequence of genetic and autoimmune myasthenic disorders. Impaired ganglionic cholinergic transmission is a prominent manifestation of autoimmune autonomic ganglionopathy. The aims of this chapter are to review (1) the presynaptic and postsynaptic events in cholinergic transmission and cholinergic pharmacology; (2) the anatomy and main functions of cholinergic neurons; and (3) examples of disorders affecting the cholinergic system.

CHOLINERGIC NEUROTRANSMISSION

Biosynthesis, Storage, Release, and Metabolism of Acetylcholine

Acetylcholine is synthesized from acetyl coenzyme A and choline by the action of ChAT, which is present in the synaptic terminals bound to the membrane of synaptic vesicles (Figure 19.3).[1] The rate of ACh biosynthesis primarily depends on availability of choline. The main source of choline is recycling after ACh hydrolysis. Choline is incorporated into presynaptic terminals via a specific, high-affinity Na^+/ATP-dependent transporter choline transporter 1 (ChT1, SLC5), which colocalizes with ChAT in synaptic vesicles and is translocated to the plasma membranes in response to neuronal activity. An additional source of choline is metabolism of phosphatidylcholine present in neuronal membranes. The mitochondrial enzyme carnitine acetyltransferase may also contribute to the synthesis of ACh. Acetylcholine is incorporated into synaptic vesicles via the vesicular ACh transporter (VAChT), which is driven by the proton gradient dependent on the vesicular (V)-ATPase and is released at presynaptic active zones. The synaptic effects of ACh are rapidly terminated by its hydrolysis by AChE. This enzyme is present both in neurons and in the basal lamina at the NMJ, and exists in several molecular forms. In the periphery ACh is typically released in excess in close apposition to its postsynaptic target in the skeletal muscle and autonomic ganglia; despite rapid hydrolysis by AChE, remaining levels of ACh are sufficient to elicit fast and robust excitation of these targets. In the brain, ACh release can be both fast, transient, and focally restricted, or slow and tonic exerting neuromodulatory effects via mechanisms of volume transmission.[1,2] Acetylcholine exerts its effects via two families of receptors, nicotinic and muscarinic.

Nicotinic Receptors

The nAChRs are ligand-gated nonselective cation channels of the cysteine residue family. Functional nAChRs are

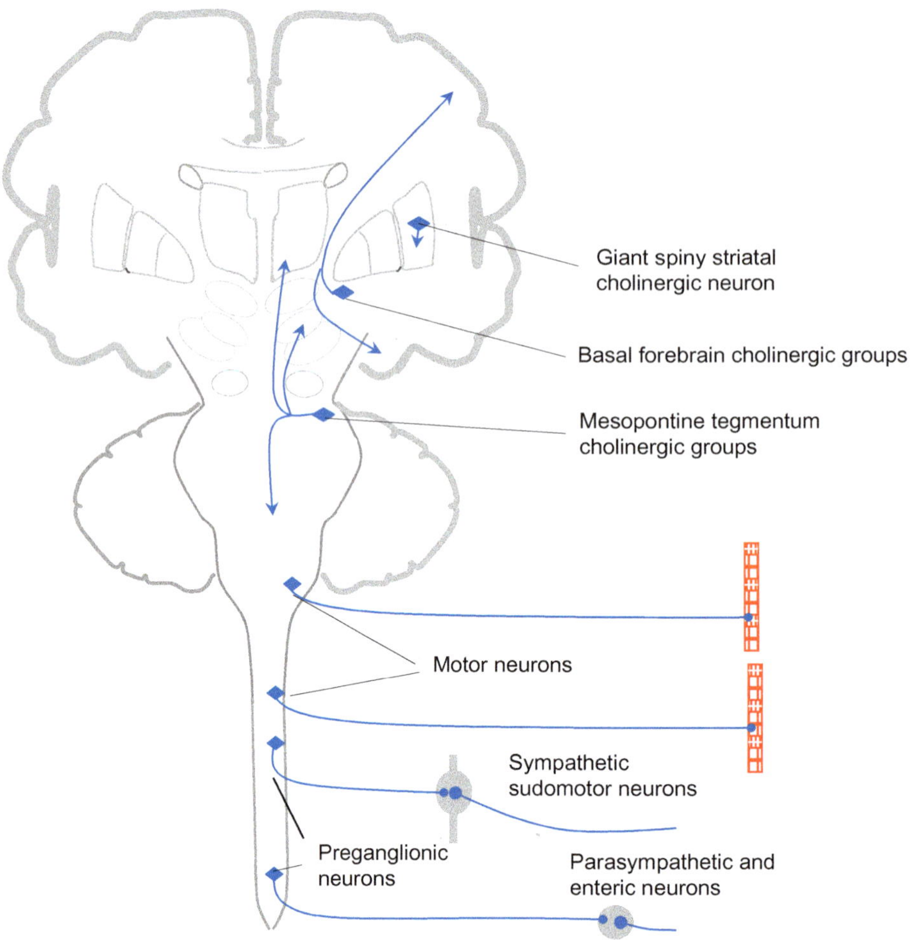

FIGURE 19.1 Distribution of cholinergic neurons.
Cholinergic neurons are widely distributed in the central and peripheral nervous system. The two major cholinergic systems in the CNS are located in the basal forebrain and the mesopontine tegmentum. There are also local cholinergic interneurons in the striatum and in other brain areas. Acetylcholine (ACh) is the primary neurotransmitter of cranial and spinal motor neurons, preganglionic autonomic neurons, many parasympathetic ganglion and enteric neurons, and sympathetic neurons innervating the sweat glands.

pentamers composed of various combinations of subunits, each consisting of a large amino (N)-terminal extracellular domain, four transmembrane α-helical domains (M1–M4) with the pore formed by M2, and an intracellular domain containing binding sites for cytoskeletal and regulatory proteins such as protein kinases. There are two main subtypes of nAChRs, muscle type and neuronal type (Figure 19.4). Muscle-type nAChRs have a fixed stoichiometry, consisting of two α1, one β1, one δ, and either one ε-subunit in adult innervated muscle or one γ-subunit in fetal or non-innervated muscle.[3] The neuronal nAChRs consist of various combinations of α (α2–α10) and β (β2–β4) subunits. In general, the stoichiometry of neuronal nAChRs is two α and three β subunits. The majority of high-affinity nAChRs in the brain are of the α4/β2 subtype. Some subunits, such as the α7, α8, and α9 subunits, form functional homo-oligomers or heteromers.[4] Ganglionic nAChRs are composed of α3/β4 subunits.[5]

The ACh binding site in all nAChRs is located at the interface between the α and the non-α subunits. Binding of ACh produces large conformational changes in the α subunits that open the cation channel, resulting in rapid membrane depolarization. The conductance and kinetics of the channel critically depend on its subunit composition. The type of α subunit and receptor composition also determine both the affinity to ACh and the relative permeability to Ca^{2+} with respect to Na^{+}. Among neuronal nAChRs, the most common α4β2 receptor has high agonist affinity and low Ca^{2+} conductance; in contrast the α7 containing receptors have low agonist affinity but high Ca^{2+} conductance.[6] Presynaptic α7 containing nAChRs may increase neurotransmitter release.[1] The adult-type muscle nAChR (α2/β1/δ/ε) is also highly permeable to Ca^{2+}, which predisposes to toxicity by Ca^{2+} which could predispose to development of endplate myopathy in some congenital myasthenic syndromes (CMS).[7]

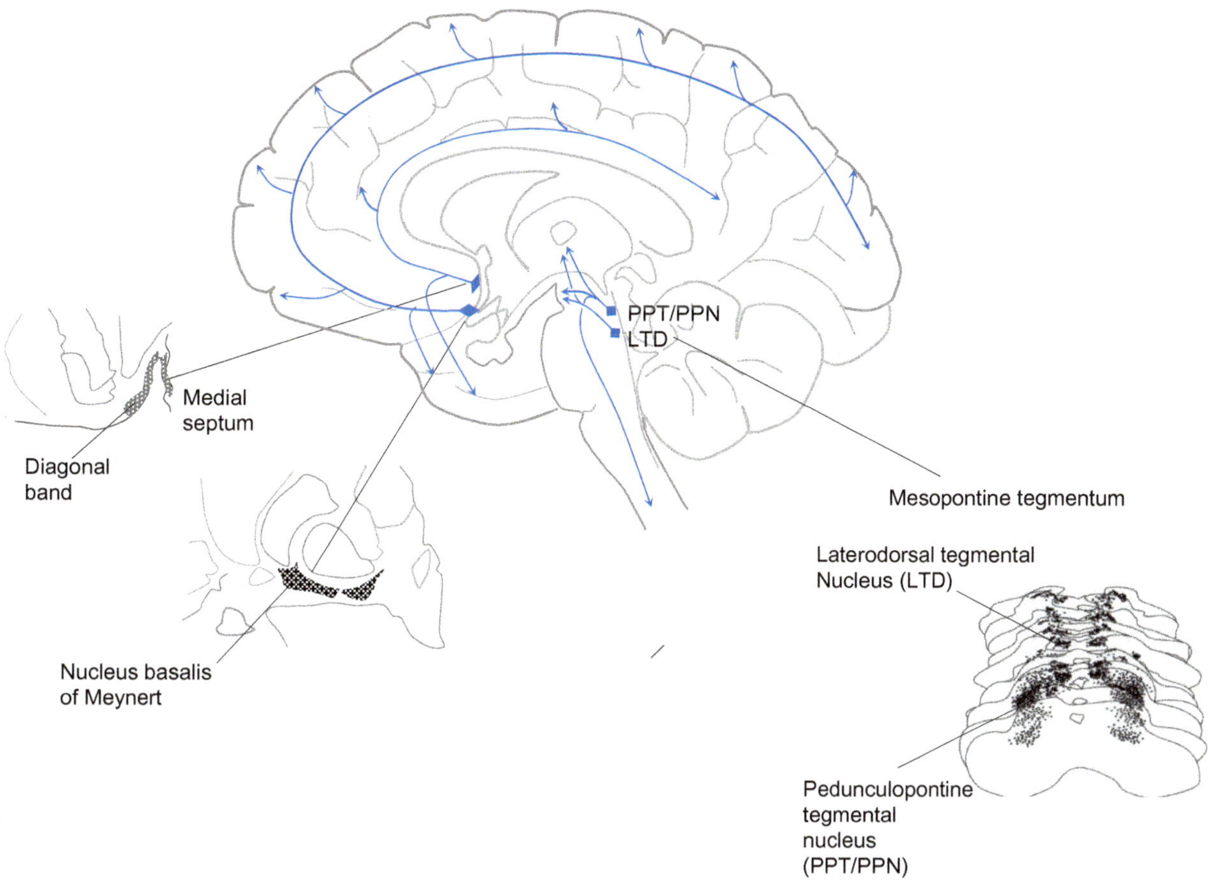

FIGURE 19.2 Major cholinergic groups in the central nervous system.
The two major groups of cholinergic CNS neurons are located in the basal forebrain and mesopontine tegmentum. The basal forebrain cholinergic system includes the medial septum, diagonal band of Broca, and the basal magnocellular complex that includes nucleus basalis of Meynert (NBM). The medial septum and diagonal band project primarily to the hippocampus, parahippocampus, and midline cortical areas; the NBM innervates the neocortex, amygdala, and thalamus. The mesopontine cholinergic column includes the pedunculopontine tegmental nucleus (PPT, PPN) and the laterodorsal tegmental nucleus (LDT). These nuclei provide ascending projections that innervate the thalamus, and give off collaterals to the hypothalamus, basal forebrain, and cerebral cortex.

Nicotinic AChRs contain various allosteric sites. Calcium potentiates channel function, increasing opening frequency by binding to a site in the extracellular N-terminal domain in proximity to the ACh binding site. The nAChRs also have binding sites for noncompetitive blockers, such as ethanol, barbiturates, local anesthetics, chlorpromazine, phencyclidine, and steroids. Phosphorylation by protein kinase A (PKA), protein kinase C (PKC), and protein tyrosine kinases regulates assembly, clustering, function, degrees of desensitization, and degradation rate of the receptor. Long-term or repeated exposure to ACh causes desensitization of the nAChR. Onset is slow and recovery is rapid, as ACh dissociates rapidly from the nicotinic receptor.

Muscarinic Receptors

Muscarinic ACh receptors are G protein-coupled receptors, which are divided into two main families: M1-type (including M1, M3, and M5) and M2-type (M2 and M4) (Figure 19.5). M1-type receptors are located postsynaptically and have excitatory function. They are coupled to $G_{q/11}$ and activate phospholipase C (PLC), leading to hydrolysis of membrane phosphatidylinositol diphosphate (PIP_2) and formation of inositol triphosphate (IP_3) and diacylglycerol (DAG). Hydrolysis of PIP_2 decreases activity of several types of K^+ channels, including Kir3 and Kv7 (M-type) channels, resulting in membrane depolarization. Inositol triphosphate triggers Ca^{2+} release from the endoplasmic reticulum (ER) and together with DAG activates PKC. Calcium also activates calmodulin-dependent cascades, including calmodulin kinase II and calcineurin. Activation of PKC leads to stimulation of phospholipase D, which hydrolyzes phosphatidylcholine and contributes to a second increase in DAG. The M2-type receptors mediate inhibitory action, both presynaptically and postsynaptically.

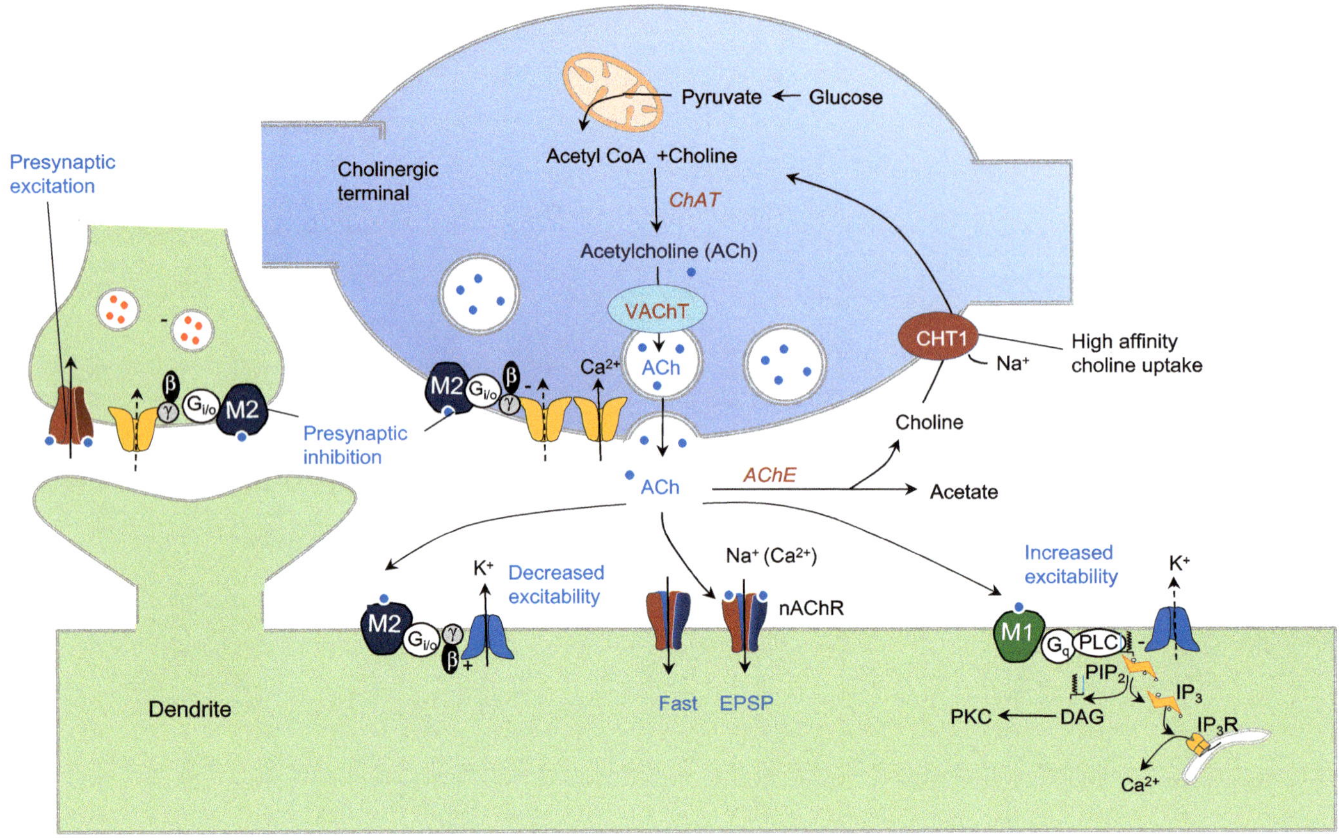

FIGURE 19.3 Main steps of cholinergic neurotransmission.
Acetylcholine is synthesized from acetyl coenzyme A and choline by the action of choline acetyltransferase (ChAT), which is present in the synaptic terminals bound to the membrane of synaptic vesicles. Acetylcholine is incorporated into synaptic vesicles via the vesicular ACh transporter (VChAT), which is driven by the proton gradient dependent on the vesicular (V)-ATPase. Acetylcholine is released at presynaptic active zones and its effects are rapidly terminated by its hydrolysis by acetylcholinesterase (AChE). Choline is incorporated into presynaptic terminals via a specific, high-affinity Na^+/ATP-dependent transporter choline transporter 1 (ChT1). Acetylcholine exerts its effects via two families of receptors, nicotinic and muscarinic. The nicotinic ACh receptors (nAChRs) are cation channels that trigger rapid membrane depolarization resulting in excitation of the postsynaptic target or increase in neurotransmitter release. The muscarinic ACh receptors are G protein-coupled receptors and are divided into two main families: M1-type and M2-type. In general, M1-type receptors are located postsynaptically and have excitatory function. They are coupled to $G_{q/11}$ and activate phospholipase C (PLC), leading to hydrolysis of membrane phosphatidylinositol diphosphate (PIP_2) and formation of inositol triphosphate (IP_3) and diacylglycerol (DAG). Hydrolysis of PIP_2 results in decreased K^+ permeability and membrane depolarization. Inositol triphosphate triggers Ca^{2+} release from the endoplasmic reticulum, which together with DAG activates PKC. The M2-type receptors are coupled to $Gi_{/o}$ and their transducing mechanisms include inhibition of adenylate cyclase via the Gα subunit and, via direct membrane effect of the β/γ subunits, activation of G protein-activated inward-rectifying K^+ channels (GIRKs) and inhibition of presynaptic N and P/Q channels.

They are coupled to $G_{i/o}$ signaling, and their transducing mechanisms include inhibition of adenylyl cyclase via the Gα subunit, activation of G protein-activated inward-rectifying K^+ channels (GIRKs), and inhibition of presynaptic N and P/Q channels via direct membrane effect of the β/γ subunits. Postsynaptic M2 receptors trigger slow hyperpolarization and reduce excitability and firing frequency of the target neurons, whereas presynaptic M2 receptors inhibit neurotransmitter release and may also act as inhibitory autoreceptors.

Pharmacology of Cholinergic Transmission

Cholinergic neurotransmission is an important target of therapeutic drugs and toxins.

Drugs that inhibit AChE activity, or cholinesterase inhibitors, increase synaptic availability of ACh, which promotes its effects via nicotinic and muscarinic receptors. Pyridostigmine and neostigmine, which do not cross the blood-brain barrier (BBB), increase ACh availability at the NMJ, autonomic ganglia, and peripheral cholinergic neuroeffector junctions. Centrally acting AChE inhibitors

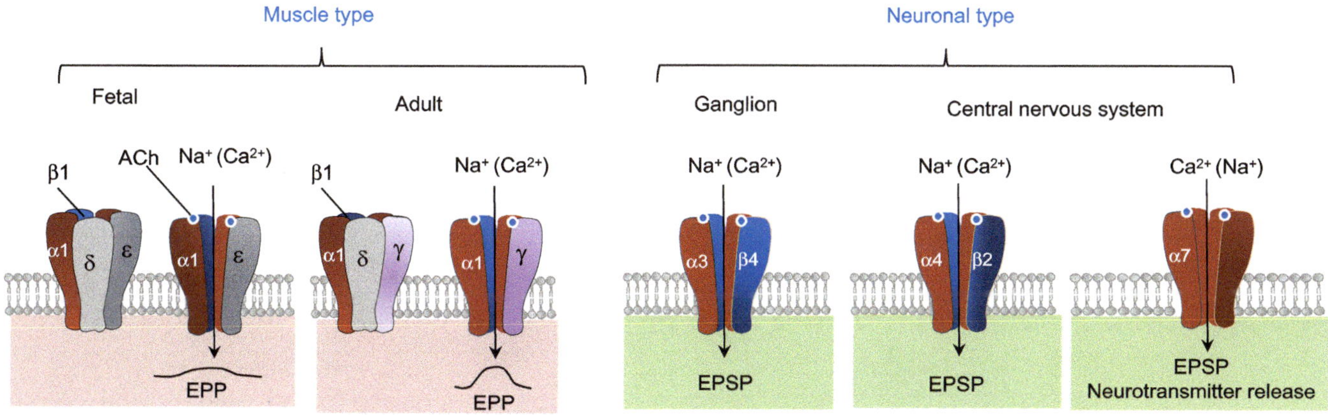

FIGURE 19.4 Nicotinic receptors.
The nicotinic ACh receptors (nAChRs) are ligand-gated pentameric nonselective cation channels composed of various combination of subunits, each consisting of a large amino-terminal extracellular domain, four transmembrane α-helical domains (M1–M4) with the pore formed by M2, and an intracellular domain containing binding sites for cytoskeletal and regulatory proteins such as protein kinases. There are two main subtypes of neuronal nAChRs, muscle type and neuronal type. Muscle nAChRs are pentamers with a fixed stoichiometry, consisting of two α1, one β1, one δ, and either one ε subunit (in adult innervated muscle) or one γ subunit (in fetal or noninnervated muscle). The neuronal nAChRs consist of various combinations of α (α2–α10) and β (β2–β4) subunits. In general, the stoichiometry is two α and three β subunits. The majority of high-affinity nAChRs in the brain are of the α4/β2 subtype. Some subunits, such as the α7, α8, and α9 subunits, form functional homo-oligomers or heteromers.

include donepezil and rivastigmine. Irreversible AChE inhibitors include the organophosphate agents such as those used as insecticides or in chemical warfare such as soman or sarin.

The main agonist of the neuronal nAChRs is nicotine, which readily crosses the BBB. In the brain nAChRs undergo upregulation upon long-term exposure to nicotine, which may reflect receptor desensitization after chronic exposure. Varenicline is a partial agonist of the α4β2 receptor with a maximal effect ~50% that of nicotine. This action relieves nicotine withdrawal symptoms, including craving, and blocks the effects of nicotine on the receptor, thereby diminishing its rewarding action via the dopaminergic system. L-type Ca^{2+} channel antagonists such as nifedipine and nimodipine may block the agonist-induced activation of nAChRs. In contrast, the AChE inhibitor galantamine promotes channel opening.

Several compounds also act as agonists or antagonists of muscarinic receptors. Typical agonists include pilocarpine and methacholine. The typical muscarinic receptor blocker is atropine, which does not readily cross the BBB; scopolamine is another natural alkaloid that crosses the BBB and inhibits central cholinergic transmission. Muscarinic receptors are also blocked by several drugs used for treatment of neurologic and psychiatric disorders. Important examples include amitriptyline, doxepin, chlorpromazine, diphenhydramine, and trihexyphenidyl. Neither of these muscarinic receptor agonists or antagonists has selectivity for M1- or M2-type receptors. Several groups of drugs may act as allosteric modulators of the muscarinic receptors. These include neuromuscular blockers, reactivators of cholinesterase, antiarrhythmic agents, spasmolytics, and local anesthetics. Most modulators decelerate the rate of association and dissociation of the ligand to the receptor.

BASAL FOREBRAIN CHOLINERGIC SYSTEM

Anatomical Organization

The basal forebrain cholinergic system comprises the medial septum, diagonal band of Broca, and the basal magnocellular complex that includes nucleus basalis of Meynert (NBM)[8] (Figure 19.2). The medial septum and diagonal band project primarily to the hippocampus, parahippocampus, and midline cortical areas including the cingulate gyrus; the NBM innervates the neocortex, amygdala, and thalamus. Specific subsectors of cholinergic neurons innervate separate portions of the neocortex; this allows a modality-selective control of regional cortical activation.[9] A characteristic of the cholinergic neurons of the basal forebrain is their dependence on nerve growth factor.[10]

Basal Forebrain Cholinergic System and Cognition

The basal forebrain cholinergic system is critically involved in mechanisms of attention, arousal, memory, and emotion (Figure 19.6). Basal forebrain cholinergic neurons are active during wakefulness, particularly in active states, progressively reduce their activity during non-REM sleep, and become again active during REM sleep. The location of both nicotinic and muscarinic receptors at presynaptic, postsynaptic,

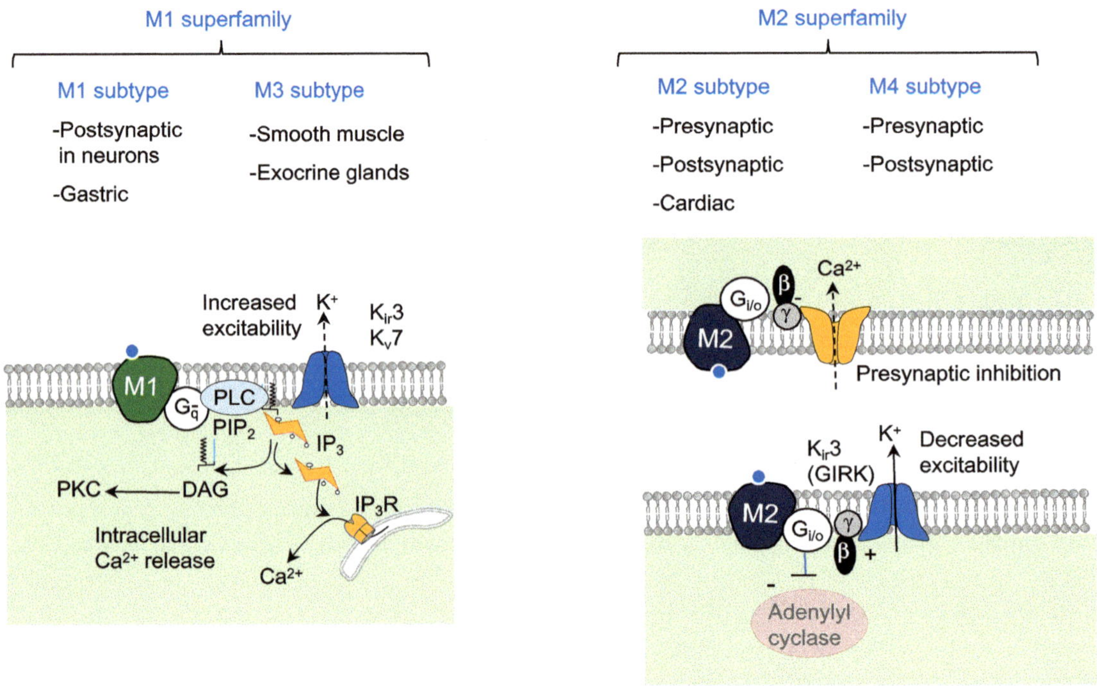

FIGURE 19.5 Muscarinic receptors.
Muscarinic ACh receptors (mAChRs) are G protein-coupled receptors and are divided into two main families: M1-type (including M1, M3, and M5) and M2-type (M2 and M4). In general, M1-type receptors are located postsynaptically and have excitatory function and M2-type receptors are inhibitory both presynaptically and postsynaptically. The M1-type receptors are coupled to $G_{q/11}$ and activate phospholipase C (PLC) leading to hydrolysis of membrane phosphatidylinositol diphosphate (PIP_2) and formation of inositol triphosphate (IP_3) and diacylglycerol (DAG). Hydrolysis of PIP_2 results in decreased K^+ channel permeability and membrane depolarization. Inositol triphosphate triggers Ca^{2+} release from the endoplasmic reticulum and together with DAG activates PKC. Calcium also activates calmodulin-dependent cascades, including calmodulin kinase II and calcineurin. The M2-type receptors are coupled to $Gi_{/o}$ signaling and their transducing mechanisms include inhibition of adenylate cyclase via the Gα subunit and, via direct membrane effect of the β/γ subunits, activation of G protein-activated inward-rectifying K^+ channels (GIRKs), and inhibition of presynaptic N and P/Q channels. Thus, postsynaptic M2 receptors trigger slow hyperpolarization and reduce excitability and firing frequency of the target neurons, whereas, presynaptic M2 receptors inhibit neurotransmitter release. Presynaptic M2 receptors in cholinergic neurons act as inhibitory autoreceptors.

and extrasynaptic sites provides the basis for multiple types of cholinergic signaling by these neurons. The presence of both spatially specific rapid ACh release (cholinergic "transients") and slower and spatially broader tonic ACh release may reflect the existence of two functionally distinct types of cholinergic neurons that support two different aspects of information processing.[11] A fast, localized ACh release may have a major role in attention and sensory processing, whereas tonic ACh release over broad cortical areas may modulate global cortical arousal in a brain-state-dependent manner.[2]

In primary cortical sensory areas, cholinergic activity enhances responses to attended stimuli, increasing signal-to-noise ratio by promoting responses triggered by thalamic inputs while reducing background intracortical noise. This involves M1-mediated increases in pyramidal cell excitability; presynaptic nAChR-mediated increase in glutamate release from thalamocortical afferents; M1- and nAChR-mediated activation of GABAergic neurons involved in lateral inhibition; and presynaptic M2 receptor-mediated inhibition of glutamate release from recurrent cortico-cortical connections. Acetylcholine also exerts profound network effects via modulation canonical microcircuits consisting of different subtypes of GABAergic interneurons. As discussed in other chapters of this book, ACh promotes local fast (gamma) and desynchronization of background cortical activity preventing slow oscillations.

Cholinergic signaling in the lateral prefrontal cortex is important for top-down modulation of attention and working memory. Cholinergic neurons of NBM, either directly or via cortical GABAergic interneurons, also promote cerebral vasodilation in response to sensory stimuli.[12] Cholinergic neurons in the medial septum projecting the hippocampus have a major role in generation of theta rhythm, which is critical for encoding of new memories. Reduced levels of ACh during NREM sleep promote memory consolidation.

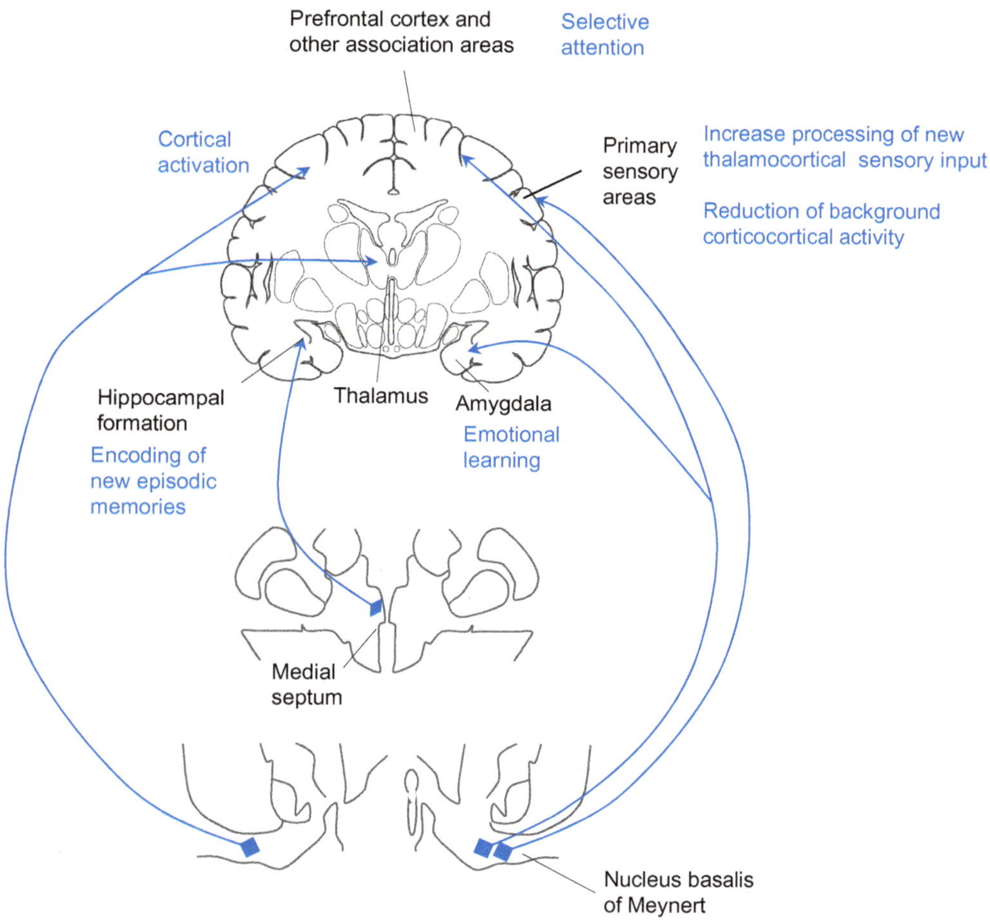

FIGURE 19.6 Functions of the basal forebrain cholinergic system.
The basal forebrain cholinergic system is critically involved in mechanisms of attention, arousal, memory, and emotion. In primary cortical sensory areas, cholinergic activity enhances responses to attended stimuli, increasing signal-to-noise ratio by promoting responses triggered by thalamic inputs while reducing background intracortical noise. ACh promotes local fast (gamma) oscillations desynchronization of background cortical activity preventing slow oscillations. Cholinergic signaling in the lateral prefrontal cortex is important for top-down modulation of attention and working memory. Cholinergic neurons in the medial septum projecting the hippocampus have a major role in generation of theta rhythm, which is critical for encoding of new memories. Reduced levels of ACh during NREM sleep promote memory consolidation.

Involvement in Neurodegenerative Disorders

Alzheimer disease and Lewy body disorders such as Parkinson disease (PD) and Lewy body dementia (LBD) are characterized by impaired cholinergic signaling associated with disturbances in attention and memory performance. Basal forebrain cholinergic neurons are particularly susceptible to accumulation of hyperphosphorylated tau and neurofibrillary degeneration in AD.[13] There is early involvement of the cholinergic system in AD starting at preclinical or mild cognitive impairment stages of disease, as reflected by reduced AChE activity in the cerebral cortex, loss of presynaptic α4β2 and α7 nAChRs and M2 presynaptic receptors, loss of postsynaptic α7 nAChRs, and dysfunction of postsynaptic M1 receptors.[14–17] Whereas loss of episodic memory is the hallmark of the most common amnestic form of AD, there is also impaired attention; cholinergic denervation in the left hemisphere has been associated with the primary progressive aphasia variant of AD.[18] Loss of cholinergic NBM neurons may affect attention and memory processing by several mechanisms, including impaired synaptic plasticity and abnormal network oscillations. Cholinergic NBM neurons provide local innervation of cerebral vessels and participate in neurovascular coupling in response to sensory stimulation; therefore loss of activity-dependent functional hyperemia can contribute to AD pathophysiology.[12] In experimental AD models, stimulation of α7 nAChRs and M1 receptors has neuroprotective effects against amyloid β (Aβ) toxicity, including stimulation of survival pathways inhibiting apoptosis, inhibition of glycogen synthase kinase 3 and thus tau phosphorylation, activation of anti-inflammatory pathways, and facilitation of anti-amyloidogenic processing of amyloid precursor protein (APP).[17,19] The endosome/lysosome pathway is disrupted early in the course of AD and may contribute to the pathogenesis of cholinergic impairment.[20] The *APOEε4* allele is associated with deficits of compensatory sprouting of cholinergic axons in the hippocampus.[21] Several studies provide some support for the early and continuous use of cholinesterase inhibitors in amnestic MCI and AD.[15,17,22–24] Impaired cortical and subcortical cholinergic activity is also a prominent feature of Lewy body disorders. There is involvement of the NBM and cholinergic denervation of the thalamus and cerebral cortex in both PD and LBD.[25–27] Cholinesterase inhibitors may be even more effective in improving cognitive manifestations in dementia with Lewy bodies than in AD.[28]

MESOPONTINE TEGMENTAL CHOLINERGIC GROUPS

Anatomical Organization

The mesopontine cholinergic column includes two groups: pedunculopontine tegmental nucleus (PPT/PPN) and the laterodorsal tegmental nucleus (LDT) (Figure 19.2). These nuclei provide ascending projections that innervate the thalamus, and give off collaterals to the hypothalamus, basal forebrain, and cerebral cortex. The main target is the thalamus. Both the PPT/PPN and the LDT also provide inputs to midbrain dopaminergic neurons; the PPT/PPN also provides inputs to the basal ganglia and superior colliculus. Descending inputs from the PPT/PPN reach the brainstem reticular formation and spinal cord.

Control of Arousal, Reward Responses, and Motor Function

Like basal forebrain neurons, mesopontine cholinergic neurons have a tonic level of activity during wakefulness and further increase their activity during REM sleep. The presence of cholinergic as well as glutamatergic and GABAergic neurons allows the PPT/PPN to function as a master switch for behavioral state control and action selection (Figure 19.7). Cholinergic inputs to the thalamus have a major role in cortical activation associated with arousal states. Acetylcholine increases tonic activity of thalamocortical relay neurons via nAChRs and M1 receptors, while inhibiting via M2 receptors, the GABAergic neurons of the reticular nucleus of the thalamus that promote burst firing of these thalamocortical cells. The cholinergic mesopontine neurons are "REM-on" neurons and promote REM sleep events. Cholinergic PPT/PPN neurons are also a critical component of the basal ganglia circuits. They promote reward-based action selection via excitatory inputs to midbrain dopaminergic neurons, mediated by nAChRs. Via their descending projections to the medullary reticular formation and spinal cord, the PPT/PPN neurons also have a major role in regulating muscle tone, particularly during locomotion.[2,29]

Involvement in Parkinsonian Syndromes

There is marked loss of cholinergic PPT/PPN neurons in several parkinsonian disorders, including PD, LBD, multiple system atrophy (MSA), and progressive supranuclear palsy (PSP). These disorders, particularly MSA and PSP, are characterized by prominent postural instability and gait disturbance. The PPT/PPN provides cholinergic input to the basal ganglia and midbrain dopaminergic neurons involved in action selection and motor control, as well as both cholinergic and glutamatergic inputs to medullary reticulospinal neurons innervating the spinal locomotor pattern generator and controlling muscle tone. However, the role of cholinergic input in gait control and muscle tone has remained elusive. The loss of cholinergic PPT/PPN neurons in PD brains correlates with the degree of gait difficulties. Loss of cholinergic PPT/PPN output may affect gait by several mechanisms, including reducing the ability to regulate muscle tone via descending pathways or loss of ascending projections to the thalamus affecting integration of sensory with attentional signals for postural control.[30]

A positron emission tomography study using a ligand for the VAChT showed that there is loss of cholinergic innervation in the visual thalamus, limbic cortex, and caudate nucleus in patients with history of fall or freezing of gait.[31] Loss of cholinergic innervation in the right visual thalamus, including the pulvinar involved in a visuospatial attention, was more marked in patients with history of falls, whereas cholinergic denervation in the caudate was associated with freezing of gait.[31] Loss of cholinergic innervation in the amygdala and hippocampal formation in PD patients with freezing of gait may reflect degeneration of the more rostral basal forebrain cholinergic neurons, whereas decreased frontal cholinergic innervation in a patient with history of falls might reflect a preferential loss of populations of more cholinergic groups.

A typical feature of synucleinopathies such as PD, LBD, and MSA is REM sleep behavior disorder (RBD), which is characterized by loss of normal muscle atonia during REM sleep. The role of PPT/PPN neuronal loss in this manifestation RBD remains to be established.

MEDIUM SPINY CHOLINERGIC NEURONS OF THE STRIATUM

The striatum has a small but important population of large aspiny cholinergic interneurons that have a major role in regulating the activity of the striatal projection neurons and local GABAergic interneurons, both directly and via interactions with dopamine. These cholinergic interneurons have a tonic activity primarily modulated by presynaptic M2 inhibitory autoreceptors. Tonic release of ACh increases the signal-to-noise ratio in the striatum via presynaptic M2/M4 receptors-mediated inhibition release of glutamate from both cortical and thalamic afferents. In response to an alerting stimulus a short burst of activity of

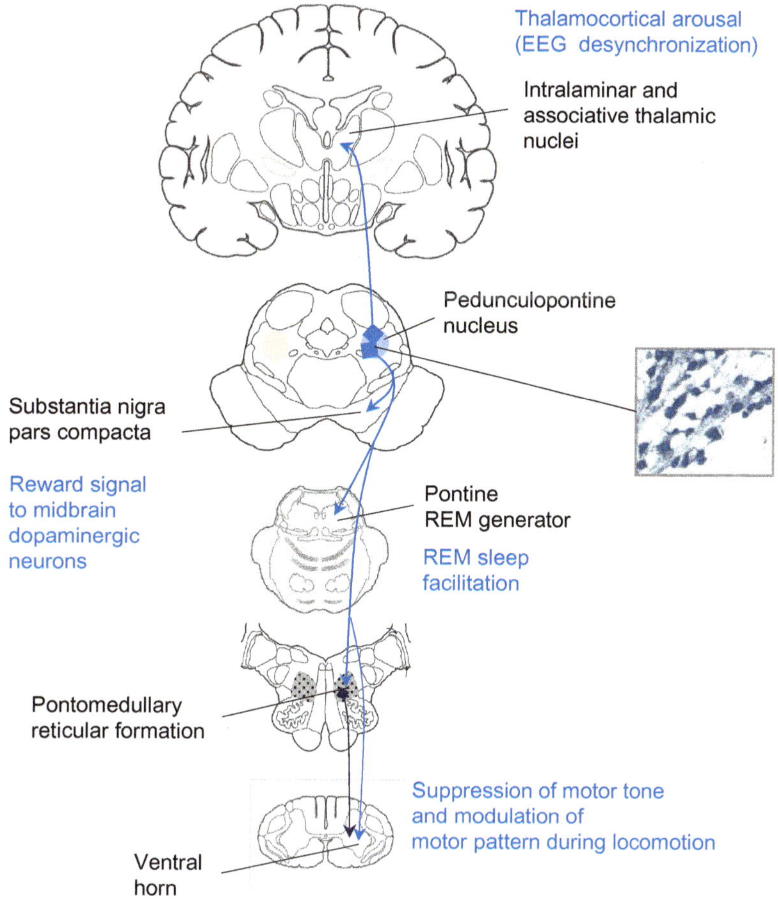

FIGURE 19.7 Functions of the pedunculopontine nucleus.
Mesopontine cholinergic neurons, including those in the pedunculopontine tegmental nucleus (PPT/PPN), have a tonic level of activity during wakefulness and further increase their activity during REM sleep. The presence of cholinergic as well as glutamatergic and GABAergic neurons allows the PPT/PPN to function as a master switch for behavioral state control and action selection. Cholinergic inputs to the thalamus have a major role in cortical activation associated with arousal states. The cholinergic mesopontine neurons are "REM-on" neurons and promote REM sleep events. Cholinergic PPT/PPN neurons promote reward-based action selection via excitatory inputs to midbrain dopaminergic neurons. Via their descending projections to the medullary reticular formation and spinal cord, the PPT/PPN neurons also have a major role in regulating muscle tone, particularly during locomotion.

these cholinergic interneurons stops ongoing motor actions and activates local release of dopamine via nicotinic and M5 receptors in dopaminergic terminals. Dopamine then elicits a pause in the activity of cholinergic interneuron activity, followed by secondary burst resulting from ACh release and inhibition of the previous action. Impaired cholinergic/dopaminergic interactions may contribute to movement disorders such as dystonia and tics. The role of ACh in the striatum and its interactions with dopamine are discussed in chapter 34.

MOTOR NEURONS AND NEUROMUSCULAR TRANSMISSION

Motor neurons located in motor nuclei of the brainstem and in lamina IX of the ventral horn innervate skeletal muscles of their corresponding motor unit at the NMJ. These neurons include both γ-motor neurons that innervate the muscle spindles and α-motor neurons that innervate the extradural fibers.

Neuromuscular Transmission and Determinants of Its Safety Margin

The NMJ is the best characterized cholinergic synapse[3] (Figure 19.8). Muscle nAChRs are clustered at the junctional folds of the NMJ or motor plate. Adult-type (ε-subunit-containing) have shorter mean open times and larger single channel cation conductances than fetal-type (γ-subunit-containing) nAChRs. About 20% of extraocular muscle fibers are multi-innervated fibers that express both adult- and fetal-type nAChRs. At rest, there is a spontaneous, random quantal release of ACh at most motor nerve terminals. A single quantum is the ACh content of an individual

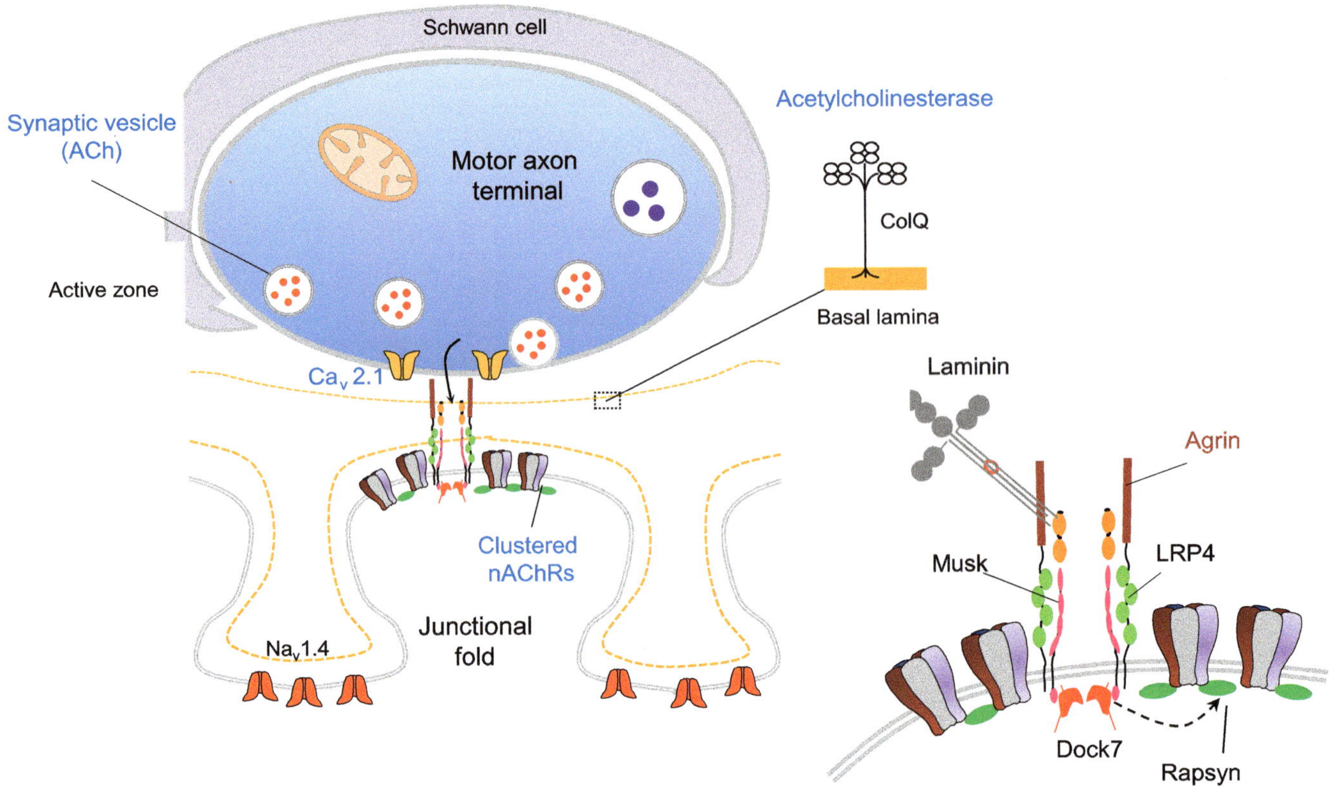

FIGURE 19.8 General organization of the neuromuscular junction.
At the neuromuscular junction (NMJ), muscle nicotinic acetylcholine receptors (nAChRs) are clustered at the junctional folds. The highly efficient synaptic transmission at the NMJ depends on the precise apposition of the nAChRs clustered at the level of junctional folds and the presynaptic active zones. Fundamental molecules involved in the organization and maintenance of the NMJ and clustering of the nAChRs at the junctional folds are agrin, low-density lipoprotein receptor-related protein 4 (LRP4), muscle-specific kinase (MuSK), downstream of kinase-7 (Dok-7), and rapsyn. Agrin is secreted by motor nerve terminals and its tethered to the synaptic basal lamina. Agrin binds LRP4; this receptor binds MuSK and promotes its membrane clustering and kinase activity. MuSK is a central scaffold that orchestrates all steps of NMJ formation in part by phosphorylating Dok-7. Rapsyn binds to the intracellular loop between the M3 and M4 domains on the nAChRs and stabilizes these receptors in the junctional folds.

vesicle; and quantal release elicits opening of 1,000 to 2,000 nAChR channels, producing a small (≈1 mV), subthreshold muscle fiber depolarization, called a miniature endplate potential. A single nerve impulse causes the rapid release of 20 to 200 quanta, which produces a large depolarization of the muscle fiber, the endplate potential (EPP). At the NMJ, ACh is released via P/Q-type (Cav2.1) Ca^{2+} channels clustered at the presynaptic active zones. The EPP activates Na_v1.4 channels located in the depths of the junctional folds, triggering an action potential that propagates the depolarization beyond the endplate to initiate excitation-contraction coupling. The difference between the amplitude of the depolarization caused by the EPP and the depolarization required to activate Na_v1.4 is the safety margin of neuromuscular transmission. At the NMJ, the effects of ACh are rapidly terminated by action of AChE located in the junctional cleft. This AChE isoform is composed of catalytic subunits forming a tetramer, and a structural subunit COLQ composed of three identical strands that anchors the complex to the synaptic basal lamina. The three factors that determine the safety margin of neuromuscular transmission are the number of ACh molecules per synaptic vesicle; the quantal release of ACh; and the efficacy of individual quanta. The effects of ACh in turn depend on the functional state of AChE, the number and functional properties of the nAChRs, and the cable properties of the muscle membrane.[32] There are several presynaptic factors that influence the safety margin, including the nerve terminal size and thus the density of active zones and pattern of nerve activity. During repetitive high-frequency (50–100 Hz) activity there is an initial increase, or facilitation, of ACh release, due to persistently increased Ca^{2+} concentrations at the nerve terminal. This is followed by a decrease, or depression, due to the reduction of the rapidly releasable pool of vesicles docked at the active zones. Quantal release may also be modulated on a timescale of seconds to minutes by presynaptic receptors. Fast-twitch muscle fibers need a higher safety margin because they operate at a higher firing frequency than slow-twitch fibers.

Molecular Organization of the Neuromuscular Junction

The highly efficient synaptic transmission at the NMJ depends on the precise apposition of the nAChRs clustered at the level of junctional folds and the presynaptic active zones (Figure 19.8). The development of the NMJ requires extensive communication among the presynaptic motor neurons, postsynaptic muscle fibers, and Schwann cells surrounding the synapse.[33] Fundamental molecules involved in the organization and maintenance of the NMJ and clustering of the nAChRs at the junctional folds are agrin, low-density lipoprotein receptor-related protein 4 (LRP4), muscle specific kinase (MuSK), downstream of kinase-7 (Dok-7), and rapsyn.[34] Agrin is a glycoprotein that is secreted by motor nerve terminals into the synaptic cleft and contains a laminin-binding motif that allows its tethering to the synaptic basal lamina. Agrin binds LRP4; this receptor binds MusK and promotes its membrane clustering and kinase activity. MuSK is a tyrosine kinase that functions as a central scaffold that orchestrates all steps of NMJ formation in part by phosphorylating Dok-7, a key adaptor protein that maintains MuSK tyrosine phosphorylation, undergoes dimerization, and promotes recruitment of two further adapters. MuSK also activates the small Ras-GTPases involved in actin remodeling necessary for clustering of nAChRs. Rapsyn binds to the intracellular loop between the M3 and M4 domains on the nAChRs and stabilizes these receptors in the junctional folds by binding to α-actinin and other scaffold proteins.[34]

Continuous coordination of synaptic growth, in relation to muscle size, also requires the release of a retrograde signal mediated by bone morphogenetic protein. Micro RNAs have a major role in motoneuron development, function, survival, and regeneration after injury.[35]

Congenital Myasthenic Syndromes

Congenital myasthenic syndromes (CMS) are classified based on the location and function of the affected protein.[32] Presynaptic CMS reflect decreased store of ACh quanta available for release and may be caused by mutations that directly affect ACh availability, including endplate ChAT deficiency and defects in VAChT. These disorders are characterized by sudden episodes of apnea triggered by fever or other stressors against a background of variable myasthenic symptoms, such as poor feeding, since birth. Other group of presynaptic CMS affects proteins regulating the formation of SNARE complexes required for synaptic vesicle docking and fusion. These include synaptobrevin-1 myasthenia, SNAP25B deficiency, synaptotagmin-2 myasthenia, and Munc13-1 myasthenia. Synaptotagmin-2 myasthenia affects the presynaptic Ca^{2+} sensor protein for exocytosis and therefore resembles the Lambert-Eaton myasthenic syndrome (LEMS) in that it is associated with weakness and areflexia, low amplitude compound muscle potential, and great facilitation by exercise. In addition to myasthenia, Munc 3-1 mutations may predispose to seizures and impair development of mature neurons, leading to microcephaly.[32] The prototype CMS involving synaptic space proteins is endplate AChE deficiency due to *ColQ* mutations affecting its structural subunit. Deficiency of AChE prolongs the EPP, which outlasts the absolute refractory period of the muscle fiber and generates a second (or repetitive) action potential after a single stimulus. Cholinergic hyperactivity can lead to Ca^{2+} influx that damages the junctional folds with loss of nAChRs. Therefore, weakness worsens with treatment with pyridostigmine or 3,4-diaminopyridine (3,4-DAP). This disorder can be improved by ephedrine or albuterol. Other CMS due to mutations of proteins in the synaptic space are laminin β2 myasthenia (*LAMB2* mutations), laminin α5 myasthenia (*LAMA5* mutations), and collagen 13A myasthenia (*COL13A1*). These disorders affect development of and pre- and postsynaptic interactions at the NMJ. Postsynaptic CMS may occur as a consequence of mutations that affect the availability or function of nAChRs, or impair development and maintenance of the NMJ. Approximately one-half of CMS result from mutations of nAChR subunit genes that reduce the expression or alter the kinetic properties of the receptor. Most mutations causing decreased expression of the nAChR reside in the ε subunit, as fetal δ subunit partially compensate for the low or absent ε subunit. Most patients respond to cholinesterase inhibitors or 3,4-DAP, which increase the number of quanta released by nerve impulse; albuterol has an additional benefit effect. Kinetic mutations of the nAChRs include recessive loss-of-function mutations that shorten the openings of the nAChR channel and cause fast-channel syndromes, and dominant gain-of-function mutations that prolong the opening of the channels and cause slow-channel syndromes. Mutations causing fast-channel syndromes decrease endplate currents and symptoms respond to pyridostigmine in combination with 3,4-DAP. In contrast, dominant gain-of-function mutations causing slow-channel syndromes prolong the opening rate and decrease the ion channel closing rate, or increase the affinity of nAChR affinity for ACh, so the channel opens repeatedly during a single ACh occupancy generating repetitive action potentials. This allows excessive Ca^{2+} influx resulting in progressive depolarization block at physiological rates of stimulation and eventual degeneration of junctional folds and loss of nAChRs. Therefore, symptoms are worsened by cholinergic blockers but gradually respond to long-lived open channel blockers such as quinidine or fluoxetine.[32]

A second group of postsynaptic disorders are due to mutations that affect endplate development and maintenance, such as defects in agrin, LRP4, MuSK, Dok-7, or rapsyn. Mutations of Dok-7 are a common cause of CMS, producing primarily limb-girdle weakness and occasional mild ptosis and facial weakness. Like the case of AChE deficiency as slow-channel syndrome, pyridostigmine and 3,4-DAP aggravate the symptoms; therapy with adrenergic agonists such as ephedrine or albuterol is effective. Mutations in rapsyn cause endplate nAChR deficiency;

many patients respond to cholinergic therapy or become stable or occasionally become asymptomatic. Sodium channel myasthenia is associated with *SCN4A* mutations producing loss-of-function of the $Na_v1.4$ channels at the endplate, rendering them inexcitable. Myasthenic symptoms in this disorder may be associated with episodes of hypokalemic periodic paralysis. There are several CMS due to congenital defects in *N*- or *O*-glycosylation; these disorders affect limb girdle muscles that often display tubular aggegates.[32]

Autoimmune Neuromuscular Transmission Defects

Autoimmune myasthenia gravis (MG) is primarily due to nAChR autoantibodies but has also been linked to other autoantibodies.[36] Most autoantibodies are IgG1 or IgG3 isotype and directed to epitopes located around a loop of amino acids on the α1 subunit; this results in loss of functional nAChRs. Mechanisms include simplification of the postsynaptic membrane resulting in complement-mediated lysis of the NMJ; accelerated internalization and degradation of nAChRs caused by cross-linkage by specific IgG; and to a lesser extent blockade of the nAChRs. About 50% of patients with pure ocular and 15% of patients with generalized MG have negative nAChR autoantibodies. Antibodies to MuSK are present in about 70% of myasthenic patients lacking nAChR antibodies. MuSK antibodies lead to declustering of nAChRs, thereby destabilizing the NMJ. MusK MG is characterized by predominant involvement of cranial and bulbar muscles and higher risk of respiratory crises compared to patients with nAChR MG. Facial atrophy, particular in the tongue muscles is a particular feature. A small number of antibodies target other proteins, including those regulating NMJ organization, such as LRP4 and rapsyn, or cytoplasmic muscle proteins such as titin, myosin, and actin and ryanodine receptor. Anti-titin antibodies have been strongly associated with the development of thymomas. The Lambert-Eaton myasthenic syndrome is caused by a presynaptic defect in neuromuscular transmission due to autoantibodies against the P/Q-type ($Ca_v2.1$) voltage-gated Ca^{2+} channels, typically associated with small cell lung carcinoma in more than 50% of cases.

AUTONOMIC CHOLINERGIC NEUROTRANSMISSION

Preganglionic Neurons

The sympathetic preganglionic neurons are primarily distributed in the intermediolateral cell column located in lamina VII of the intermediate spinal gray matter between the T1 and L1 (or L2) segments. The cranial preganglionic parasympathetic neurons occupy general visceral efferent column of the brainstem and project via the oculomotor, facial, glossopharyngeal, and vagus nerves. Sacral preganglionic parasympathetic neurons are located in the sacral preganglionic nucleus at S1–S3 levels. Peripheral cholinergic neurons are located in autonomic and enteric ganglia. Most neurons of parasympathetic ganglia and enteric nervous system utilize ACh as their primary neurotransmitter. There is a unique population of sympathetic ganglia cholinergic neurons that innervate the sweat glands.

Cholinergic Neurotransmission in the Autonomic Nervous System

Acetylcholine is a fundamental neurotransmitter in the autonomic nervous system (Figure 19.9). The cholinergic input from preganglionic neurons to the autonomic or enteric ganglia is mediated by the ganglion-type nAChRs, which consist of α_3 and β_4 subunits.[5] Activation of these receptors elicits fast excitation of ganglion neurons, which allows the rapid transmission of preganglionic inputs to the autonomic targets. Acetylcholine also mediates slow excitatory transmission in autonomic ganglia via M1 receptors and, in some cases, may also activate M4 receptors that reduce of the response to nAChR to subsequent stimulations.

The effects of many parasympathetic and enteric neurons, as well as sympathetic sudomotor neurons on their targets are mediated by muscarinic receptors. Their excitatory effects are mediated by M1-like receptors, primarily M3 receptors. These receptors mediate visceral smooth muscle contraction, exocrine gland secretion, and endothelial nitric oxide production and thus vasodilation. They are responsible for contraction of the pupil sphincter and ciliary muscle; bronchial constriction; and esophageal peristalsis, gastric emptying, propulsion of the intestinal content, and defecation and contraction of the bladder detrusor (micturition). The M3 receptors also mediate parasympathetic activation of lacrimal, salivary, gastrointestinal, and sexual organ secretion, as well as sympathetically triggered activation of sweat gland secretion. In contrast, M2 receptors mediate inhibitory actions of ACh on the autonomic targets. In the heart, postsynaptic M2 receptors directly activate K^+ channels and reduce the rate of spontaneous depolarization of the sinus node, resulting in reduction of heart rate and decreased atrioventricular conduction. Presynaptic M2 receptors inhibit release of norepinephrine from sympathetic terminals. Via this mechanism, M2 receptors mediate some of the antagonistic interactions between the parasympathetic and sympathetic systems at some target organs such as the heart and the bladder.

Autoimmune Autonomic Ganglionopathy

Autoantibodies specific for the ganglionic nAChR produce autoimmune autonomic ganglionopathy (AAG).[5] About 50% of patients with AAG have high levels of these antibodies. This disorder typically has an acute or subacute course, but other cases show a slow insidious onset, which can suggest the diagnosis of a neurodegenerative autonomic disorder. Characteristic features of AAG include orthostatic hypotension and lower gastrointestinal symptoms (constipation) in 70% of patients. Prominent cholinergic failure

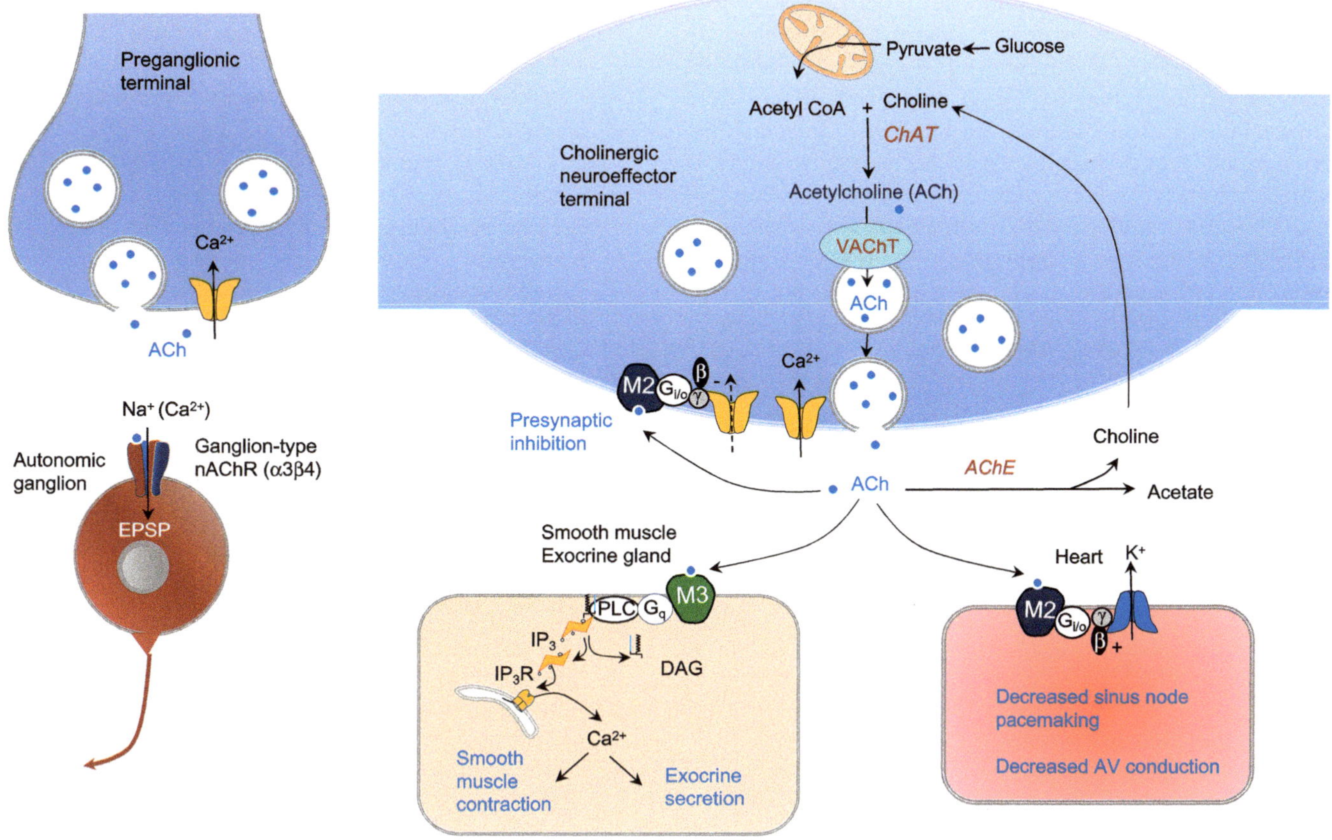

FIGURE 19.9 Cholinergic autonomic neurotransmission.
The cholinergic input from preganglionic neurons to the autonomic or enteric ganglia is mediated by the ganglion-type nAChRs, which consist of α_3 and β_4 subunits. Activation of these receptors elicits fast excitation of ganglion neurons, which allows the rapid transmission of preganglionic inputs to the autonomic targets. Acetylcholine also mediates slow excitatory transmission in autonomic ganglia via M1 receptors and, in some cases, may also activate M4 receptors that reduce the response of nAChR to subsequent stimulation. The effects of many parasympathetic and enteric neurons, as well as sympathetic sudomotor neurons on their targets, are mediated by muscarinic receptors. Their excitatory effects are mediated by M1-like receptors, primarily M3 receptors. These receptors mediate visceral smooth muscle contraction, exocrine gland secretion, and endothelial nitric oxide production and thus vasodilation. They are responsible for contraction of the pupil sphincter and ciliary muscle; bronchial constriction; esophageal peristalsis, gastric emptying, propulsion of the intestinal content, and defecation and contraction of the bladder detrusor (micturition). The M3 receptors also mediate parasympathetic activation of lacrimal, salivary, gastrointestinal, and sexual organ secretion, as well as sympathetically triggered activation of sweat gland secretion. In contrast, M2 receptors mediate inhibitory actions of ACh on the autonomic targets. In the heart, postsynaptic M2 receptors directly activate K^+ channels and reduce the rate of spontaneous depolarization of the sinus node, resulting in reduction of heart rate and decreased atrioventricular conduction. Presynaptic M2 receptors inhibit release of norepinephrine from sympathetic terminals. Via this mechanism, M2 receptors mediate some of the antagonistic interactions between the parasympathetic and sympathetic systems at some target organs such as the heart and the bladder.

(dry mouth and dry eyes, urinary retention, and impaired pupil responses) are also commonly present and help differentiate AAG from peripheral autonomic neuropathy or neurodegenerative disorders. Ganglionic AChR antibody levels correlate with disease severity.[5] Autonomic cholinergic neurotransmission is also typically affected in LEMS due to impaired ACh release at the autonomic ganglia and peripheral effects caused by P/Q channel autoantibodies. These patients typically experience impaired salivation and sweating, erectile dysfunction, and other manifestations of autonomic cholinergic failure.

Manifestations of Impaired Cholinergic Autonomic Transmission

Many drugs used for treatment of neurologic and psychiatric conditions, such as depression, psychosis, insomnia, vertigo, and dystonia, have collateral side effects due to their effect of blocking muscarinic receptors. They include anhidrosis, blurred vision, dry mouth, constipation, and urinary retention. Strong muscarinic receptor blockers include amitriptyline, doxepin, trihexyphenydil, benztropine, and chlorpromazine. Drugs that produce moderate muscarinic blockade include nortriptyline, mirtazapine, promethazine, and clozapine. Anticholinergic toxicity primarily reflects blockade of muscarinic receptors in the CNS and PNS and manifests with confusional state (delirium), tachycardia, mydriasis, hyperthermia (due to impaired sweating), constipation, and urinary retention. Botulinum toxin impairs activity of SNARE proteins required for ACh release, resulting both in weakness due to impaired neuromuscular transmission and manifestations of autonomic cholinergic failure. In contrast, excessive cholinergic activity, as occurs as a consequence of AChE inhibition (for example by organophosphates) manifests with excessive activation of muscle nAChRs (fasciculations) and autonomic muscarinic receptors (excessive sections, bradycardia, abdominal cramps, diarrhea).

KEY POINTS

- Cholinergic neurons include the basal forebrain cholinergic group; the mesopontine tegmental group; large aspiny neurons of the striatum; motor neurons innervating skeletal muscle (motoneurons): preganglionic autonomic neurons; sudomotor sympathetic neurons and a large proportion of parasympathetic and enteric neurons.
- Acetylcholine is by action of choline acetyltransferase (ChAT) and incorporated into synaptic vesicles via the vesicular ACh transporter (VChAT).
- The effects of ACh are rapidly terminated by its hydrolysis by acetylcholinesterase (AChE).
- ACh exerts its effects via nicotinic (nAChRs) and muscarinic (M) receptors.
- The nicotinic ACh receptors (nAChRs) mediate fast excitation in the central nervous system, skeletal muscle, and autonomic ganglia.
- Muscarinic ACh receptors include excitatory M1-type (including M1, M3, and M5) and inhibitory M2-type (M2 and M4) receptors.
- Several therapeutic drugs affect cholinergic transmission, including AChE inhibitors, muscarinic agonists, and muscarinic antagonists.
- The basal forebrain cholinergic system includes the nucleus basalis of Meynert (NBM), medial septum, and diagonal band of Broca.
- The basal forebrain cholinergic system is critically involved in mechanisms of attention, arousal, memory, and emotion.
- Basal forebrain cholinergic neurons are active during wakefulness, reduce their activity during non-REM sleep, and become again active during REM sleep.
- Cholinergic signaling in primary cortical sensory areas enhances responses to attended stimuli while reducing background activity
- Cholinergic signaling in the lateral prefrontal cortex is important for top-down modulation of attention and working memory.
- Cholinergic inputs from the medial septum to the hippocampus are critical for encoding of new memories
- The mesopontine cholinergic column includes the pedunculopontine tegmental nucleus (PPT/PPN) and the laterodorsal tegmental nucleus (LDT).
- Cholinergic mesopontine neurons are active during wakefulness and REM sleep and decrease their activity during non-REM sleep.
- Cholinergic inputs from the PPT/PPN to the thalamus promote thalamocortical arousal.
- Mesopontine cholinergic inputs to midbrain dopaminergic neurons promote reward-based action selection.
- Impaired cholinergic transmission in the neocortex, hippocampus, and thalamus is a fundamental mechanism for cognitive impairment in Alzheimer disease and Lewy body disorders.
- Giant aspiny cholinergic neurons in the striatum regulate basal ganglia circuits, both directly and via interactions with midbrain dopaminergic inputs.
- The organization and maintenance of the NMJ and clustering of the nAChRs requires agrin, low-density lipoprotein receptor-related protein 4 (LRP4), muscle specific kinase (MuSK), downstream of kinase-7 (Dok-7), and rapsyn.
- Congenital myasthenic syndromes may be manifestations of disorders affecting ACh synthesis or release by exocytosis, degradation by AChE, the kinesics of nAChRs, or molecular organization and maintenance of the NMJ.
- The cholinergic input from preganglionic neurons to the autonomic or enteric ganglia is mediated by the ganglion-type nAChRs, which consist of α_3 and β_4 subunits.
- Antibodies against ganglionic nicotinic ACh receptors cause autoimmune autonomic neuropathy, characterized by sympathetic, parasympathetic, and enteric nervous system failure.
- Many drugs used for treatment of neurologic disorders block cholinergic receptors and have side effect such as constipation, urinary retention, lack of sweating, dry mouth, and dry eyes.
- Intoxication with cholinesterase inhibitors produces increase secretions, bronchoconstriction, bradycardia, fasciculations, and eventually paralysis.
- Anticholinergic toxicity manifests with confusional state, hyperthermia, mydriasis, tachycardia, urinary retention, and constipation.

REFERENCES

1. Ballinger EC, Ananth M, Talmage DA, Role LW. Basal forebrain cholinergic circuits and signaling in cognition and cognitive decline. Neuron 2016;91:1199–1218.
2. Picciotto MR, Higley MJ, Mineur YS. Acetylcholine as a neuromodulator: cholinergic signaling shapes nervous system function and behavior. Neuron 2012;76:116–129.
3. Engel AG. The neuromuscular junction. Handb Clin Neurol 2008;91:103–148.
4. Gotti C, Zoli M, Clementi F. Brain nicotinic acetylcholine receptors: native subtypes and their relevance. Trends Pharmacol Sci 2006;27:482–491.
5. Vernino S, Hopkins S, Wang Z. Autonomic ganglia, acetylcholine receptor antibodies, and autoimmune ganglionopathy. Auton Neurosci 2009;146:3–7.
6. Dani JA. Neuronal nicotinic acetylcholine receptor structure and function and response to nicotine. Int Rev Neurobiol 2015;124:3–19.
7. Fucile S, Sucapane A, Grassi F, Eusebi F, Engel AG. The human adult subtype ACh receptor channel has high Ca2+ permeability and predisposes to endplate Ca2+ overloading. J Physiol 2006;573:35–43.
8. Mesulam MM. The cholinergic innervation of the human cerebral cortex. Prog Brain Res 2004;145:67–78.
9. Zaborszky L, Gombkoto P, Varsanyi P, et al. Specific basal forebrain-cortical cholinergic circuits coordinate cognitive operations. J Neurosci 2018;38:9446–9458.
10. Cuello AC, Bruno MA, Bell KF. NGF-cholinergic dependency in brain aging, MCI and Alzheimer's disease. Curr Alzheimer Res 2007;4:351–358.
11. Sarter M, Kim Y. Interpreting chemical neurotransmission in vivo: techniques, time scales, and theories. ACS Chem Neurosci 2015;6:8–10.
12. Lecrux C, Bourourou M, Hamel E. How reliable is cerebral blood flow to map changes in neuronal activity? Auton Neurosci 2019;217:71–79.
13. Mesulam MM. Cholinergic circuitry of the human nucleus basalis and its fate in Alzheimer's disease. J Comp Neurol 2013;521:4124–4144.
14. Schmitz TW, Nathan Spreng R, Alzheimer's disease neuroimaging I. Basal forebrain degeneration precedes and predicts the cortical spread of Alzheimer's pathology. Nat Commun 2016;7:13249.
15. Richter N, Beckers N, Onur OA, et al. Effect of cholinergic treatment depends on cholinergic integrity in early Alzheimer's disease. Brain 2018;141:903–915.
16. Jiang S, Li Y, Zhang C, et al. M1 muscarinic acetylcholine receptor in Alzheimer's disease. Neurosci Bull 2014;30:295–307.
17. Hampel H, Mesulam MM, Cuello AC, et al. The cholinergic system in the pathophysiology and treatment of Alzheimer's disease. Brain 2018;141:1917–1933.
18. Mesulam MM, Lalehzari N, Rahmani F, et al. Cortical cholinergic denervation in primary progressive aphasia with Alzheimer pathology. Neurology 2019;92:e1580–e1588.
19. Hascup KN, Hascup ER. Soluble amyloid-beta42 stimulates glutamate release through activation of the alpha7 nicotinic acetylcholine receptor. J Alzheimers Dis 2016;53:337–347.
20. Xu W, Weissmiller AM, White JA, 2nd, et al. Amyloid precursor protein-mediated endocytic pathway disruption induces axonal dysfunction and neurodegeneration. J Clin Invest 2016;126:1815–1833.
21. Bott JB, Heraud C, Cosquer B, et al. APOE-sensitive cholinergic sprouting compensates for hippocampal dysfunctions due to reduced entorhinal input. J Neurosci 2016;36:10472–10486.
22. Cavedo E, Grothe MJ, Colliot O, et al. Reduced basal forebrain atrophy progression in a randomized Donepezil trial in prodromal Alzheimer's disease. Sci Rep 2017;7:11706.
23. Dubois B, Chupin M, Hampel H, et al. Donepezil decreases annual rate of hippocampal atrophy in suspected prodromal Alzheimer's disease. Alzheimers Dement 2015;11:1041–1049.
24. Van Beek AH, Claassen JA. The cerebrovascular role of the cholinergic neural system in Alzheimer's disease. Behav Brain Res 2011;221:537–542.
25. Muller ML, Bohnen NI, Kotagal V, et al. Clinical markers for identifying cholinergic deficits in Parkinson's disease. Mov Disord 2015;30:269–273.
26. Bohnen NI, Kanel P, Muller M. Molecular imaging of the cholinergic system in Parkinson's disease. Int Rev Neurobiol 2018;141:211–250.
27. Klein JC, Eggers C, Kalbe E, et al. Neurotransmitter changes in dementia with Lewy bodies and Parkinson disease dementia in vivo. Neurology 2010;74:885–892.
28. Weintraub D, Somogyi M, Meng X. Rivastigmine in Alzheimer's disease and Parkinson's disease dementia: an ADAS-cog factor analysis. Am J Alzheimers Dis Other Demen 2011;26:443–449.
29. Gut NK, Winn P. The pedunculopontine tegmental nucleus-A functional hypothesis from the comparative literature. Mov Disord 2016;31:615–624.
30. Snijders AH, Takakusaki K, Debu B, et al. Physiology of freezing of gait. Ann Neurol 2016;80:644–659.
31. Bohnen NI, Kanel P, Zhou Z, et al. Cholinergic system changes of falls and freezing of gait in Parkinson's disease. Ann Neurol 2019;85:538–549.
32. Engel AG. Congenital myasthenic syndromes in 2018. Curr Neurol Neurosci Rep 2018;18:46.
33. Maggio S, Ceccaroli P, Polidori E, Cioccoloni A, Stocchi V, Guescini M. Signal exchange through extracellular vesicles in neuromuscular junction establishment and maintenance: from physiology to pathology. Int J Mol Sci 2019;20:2804–2820.
34. Burden SJ, Huijbers MG, Remedio L. Fundamental molecules and mechanisms for forming and maintaining neuromuscular synapses. Int J Mol Sci 2018;19:490–509.
35. Hawley ZCE, Campos-Melo D, Droppelmann CA, Strong MJ. MotomiRs: miRNAs in motor neuron function and disease. Front Mol Neurosci 2017;10:127.
36. Paz ML, Barrantes FJ. Autoimmune attack of the neuromuscular junction in myasthenia gravis: nicotinic acetylcholine receptors and other targets. ACS Chem Neurosci 2019;10:2186–2194.

20 Monoaminergic Systems

OVERVIEW

The central monoaminergic systems consist of neurons in restricted areas of the brainstem and hypothalamus that project to widespread areas and exert a global control of neuronal excitability that is fundamental for behavioral arousal, attention, motivation, and stress responses. These monoaminergic systems include dopamine (DA)-synthesizing neurons of the substantia nigra pars compact (SNc) and ventral tegmental area (VTA); norepinephrine (NE)-synthesizing neurons of the locus coeruleus (LC) and NE- and epinephrine-synthesizing neurons in the ventrolateral medulla; serotonin (5-hydroxytryptamine, 5-HT)-synthesizing neurons the rostral and caudal raphe nuclei; and histamine (HA)-synthesizing neurons of the tuberomammillary nucleus (TMN) of the hypothalamus (Figure 20.1). In the periphery NE is the primary neurotransmitter of sympathetic neurons. Monoaminergic systems have several features in common (Table 20.1). Monoamine neurotransmitters are synthesized from essential amino acids by action of rate-limiting enzymes and are incorporated into synaptic vesicles via a common vesicular monoamine transporter. They are released from highly arborized varicose axons and may act both via synaptic and volume transmission mechanisms. They all act via several subtypes of G protein-coupled receptors (GPCRs), with the exception of the 5-HT3 receptor. They all undergo presynaptic reuptake via partially selective membrane transporters, except for HA. Monoaminergic neurons have slow tonic activity during wakefulness, decrease their activity in non-REM sleep, and become silent during REM sleep. They respond with increasing firing to behavioral relevant stimuli. Monoaminergic systems promote arousal and attention, modulate emotion and memory, and regulate excitability of segmental motor, nociceptive, and autonomic processes (Figure 20.2). The monoaminergic system have a major role in a wide range of neurologic and psychiatric disorders and provide a major target for pharmacological therapy. The aims of this chapter are to review (1) the distribution and central monoaminergic neurons, (2) the main steps in metabolism of monoamine neurotransmitters, (3) the receptors mediating their effects, (4) the overall functions of these systems, and (5) the clinical manifestation of disorders affecting monoamine metabolism.

GENERAL FEATURES OF MONOAMINERGIC NEUROTRANSMISSION

Several steps of synthesis and metabolism are shared among different systems and are affected in genetic monoamine neurotransmitter disorders[1] (Figure 20.3) (Table 20.2).

Biosynthesis

Monoamine neurotransmitters derive from essential aromatic amino acids provided by the diet (i.e., L-tyrosine, L-tryptophan, and L-histidine), which undergo facilitated transport across the blood-brain barrier (BBB) via a shared carrier-specific system that also transports phenylalanine and other dietary amino acids. The rate-limiting enzyme for synthesis of catecholamines is tyrosine hydroxylase (TH), which transforms L-tyrosine to L-dihydroxypenylalanine (L-DOPA, levodopa). This step is followed by decarboxylation of L-DOPA to DA via L-aromatic amino acid decarboxylase (L-AADC), which requires pyridoxal phosphate as a critical cofactor. In noradrenergic neurons, DA is converted to NE by action of dopamine-β-hydroxylase (DBH). In some neurons in the medulla, NE is transformed to epinephrine via the phenylethanolamine-N-methyltransferase (PNMT). In serotonergic neurons, the rate-limiting enzyme for 5-HT synthesis is tryptophan hydroxylase 2 (TPH2), which transforms L-tryptophan into 5-hydroxytryptophan (5-HTP), which is then decarboxylated by L-AADC to 5-HT. The initial steps of biosynthesis of DA, NE, and 5-HT critically depend on the availability of tetrahydrobiopterin (BH4), which

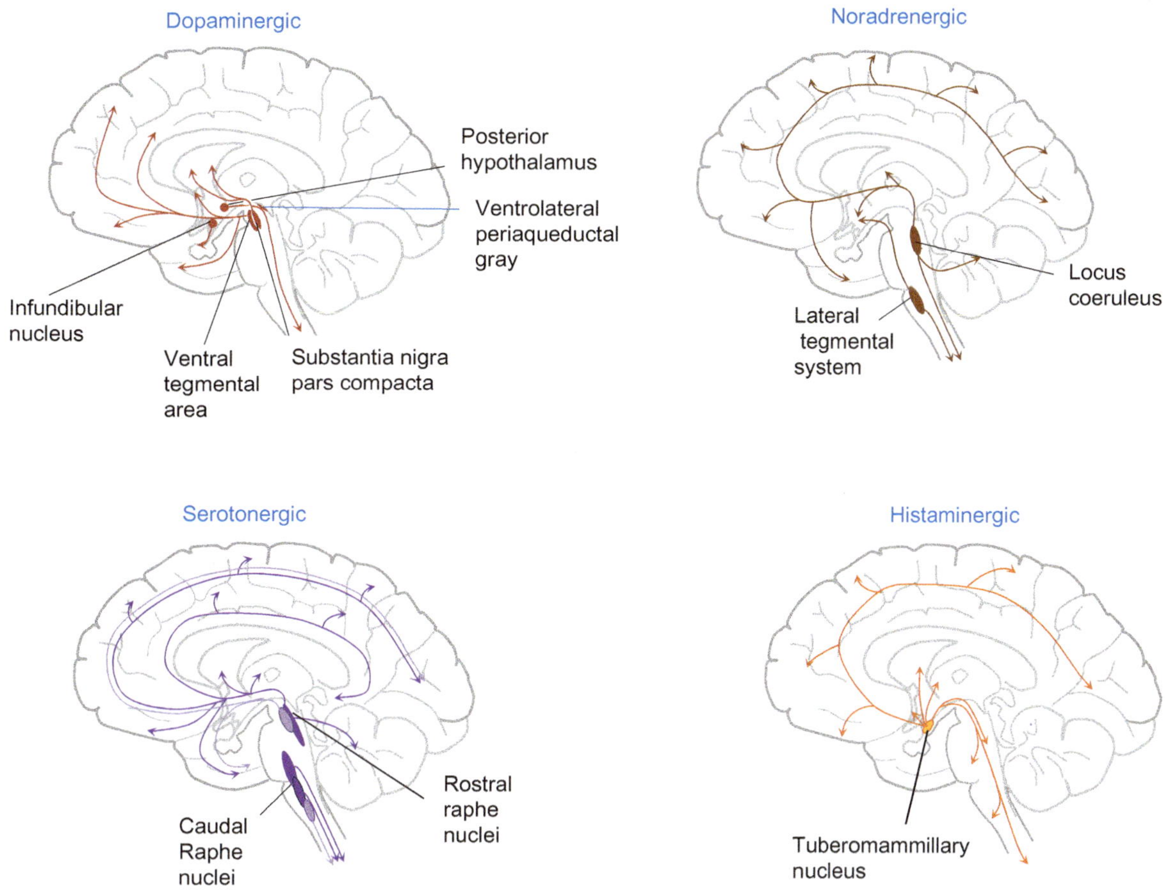

FIGURE 20.1 Distribution of central monoaminergic systems.
The central monoaminergic systems consist of neurons in restricted areas of the brainstem and hypothalamus that project to widespread areas and exert a global control of neuronal excitability that is fundamental for behavioral arousal, attention, motivation, stress responses. These monoaminergic systems include dopamine (DA)-synthesizing neurons of the substantia nigra pars compact (SNc) and ventral tegmental area (VTA); norepinephrine (NE)-synthesizing neurons of the locus coeruleus (LC) and NE- and epinephrine-synthesizing neurons in the ventrolateral medulla; serotonin (5-hydroxytryptamine, 5-HT)-synthesizing neurons the rostral and caudal raphe nuclei; and histamine (HA)-synthesizing neurons of the tuberomammillary nucleus (TMN) of the hypothalamus.

is an essential cofactor of TH, and TPH 2. BH4 is synthesized from guanosine triphosphate (GTP) in the three sequential steps. GTP cyclohydrolase I (GCH1, GCHY-I) mediates the first and rate-limiting step in BH4 synthesis. Histamine is synthesized from L-histidine by action of L-AADC.

Vesicular Storage and Release

Monoamines are incorporated into synaptic vesicles via members of the vesicular monoamine transporters (VMATs, *SLC18* family) family, which use the proton electrochemical gradient across the vesicular membrane maintained by the vesicular proton (H^+) ATPase.[2] The main transporter in the adult CNS is VMAT2, which can transport DA, NE, 5-HT, and HA. Monoamines are typically released from synaptic vesicles at synaptic terminals via Ca^{2+} mediated exocytosis. However, DA and 5-HT can also be released from dendrites by diffusion from the cytosol or reverse action of transporters located in the plasma membrane.

Reuptake

Monoamines undergo rapid reuptake at synapses via plasma membrane transporters that belong to the *SCL6* family and are expressed in the dendrites and axons of their respective monoaminergic neurons: the DA transporter (DAT), the NE transporter (NET), and the serotonin transporter (SERT), which are major determinants of monoaminergic synaptic signaling.[3] In addition to terminating the synaptic effects of monoamines, presynaptic reuptake is also critical to replenish the vesicular stores. The SCL6 transporters cotransport Na^+, Cl^-, K^+, and H^+ ions with the substrate molecule; Na^+ is transported along its electrochemical gradient, providing the driving force for the transport of the substrate. DAT, NET, and SERT segregate into lipid rafts in the presynaptic terminals and are confined to perisynaptic areas. Expression of these monoamine transporters is determined by the balance between insertion into the membrane via the secretory pathway and removal from the membrane

TABLE 20.1 *Common Features of Central Monoaminergic Neurons*

Distribution	Restricted areas of the brainstem or hypothalamus
Axonal projections	Widespread, releasing neurotransmitter both at synaptic and extrasynaptic sites (volume transmission)
Precursor	Essential dietary amino acids (L-tyrosine, L-tryptophan, L-histidine)
Biosynthetic pathway	Rate-limiting enzymes (hydroxylases or decarboxylases)
Vesicular storage	Vesicular monoamine transporter 2
Vesicular uptake	Presynaptic membrane transporters (except histamine)
Metabolism	Monoamine oxidases and methyltransferases
Receptor mechanisms	G protein-coupled receptors (except 5-HT3 receptor)
Firing pattern	Slow tonic activity during wakefulness regulated by inhibitory autoreceptors
State-dependent firing	Increased activity during active wakefulness, reduced firing in non-REM sleep, silent in REM sleep
Main synaptic inputs	Excitatory from the prefrontal cortex and orexin/hypocretin neurons; inhibitory from local neurons and ventrolateral preoptic nucleus
Functions	Arousal, attention, stress response, motivated behavior, inhibition of REM sleep, modulation of sensory, motor, and pain responses

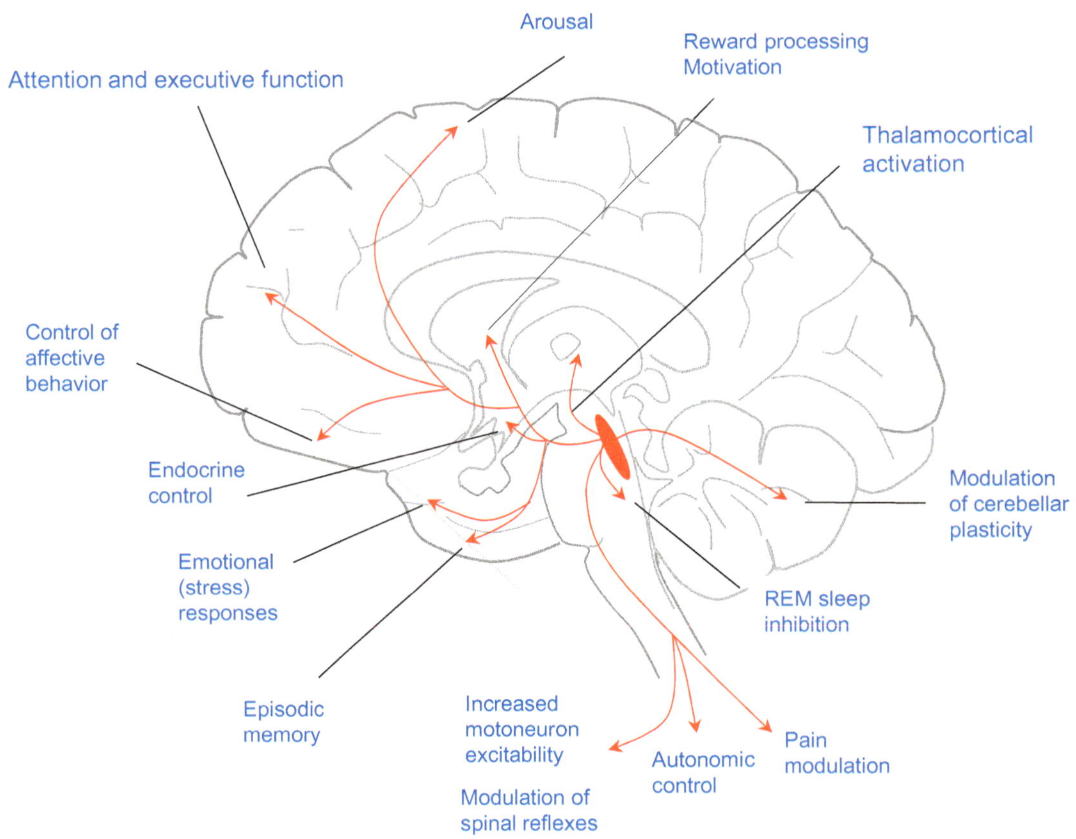

FIGURE 20.2 Major functions of the central monoaminergic systems.
Monoaminergic systems promote arousal and attention, modulate emotion and memory, and regulate excitability of segmental motor, nociceptive, and autonomic processes.

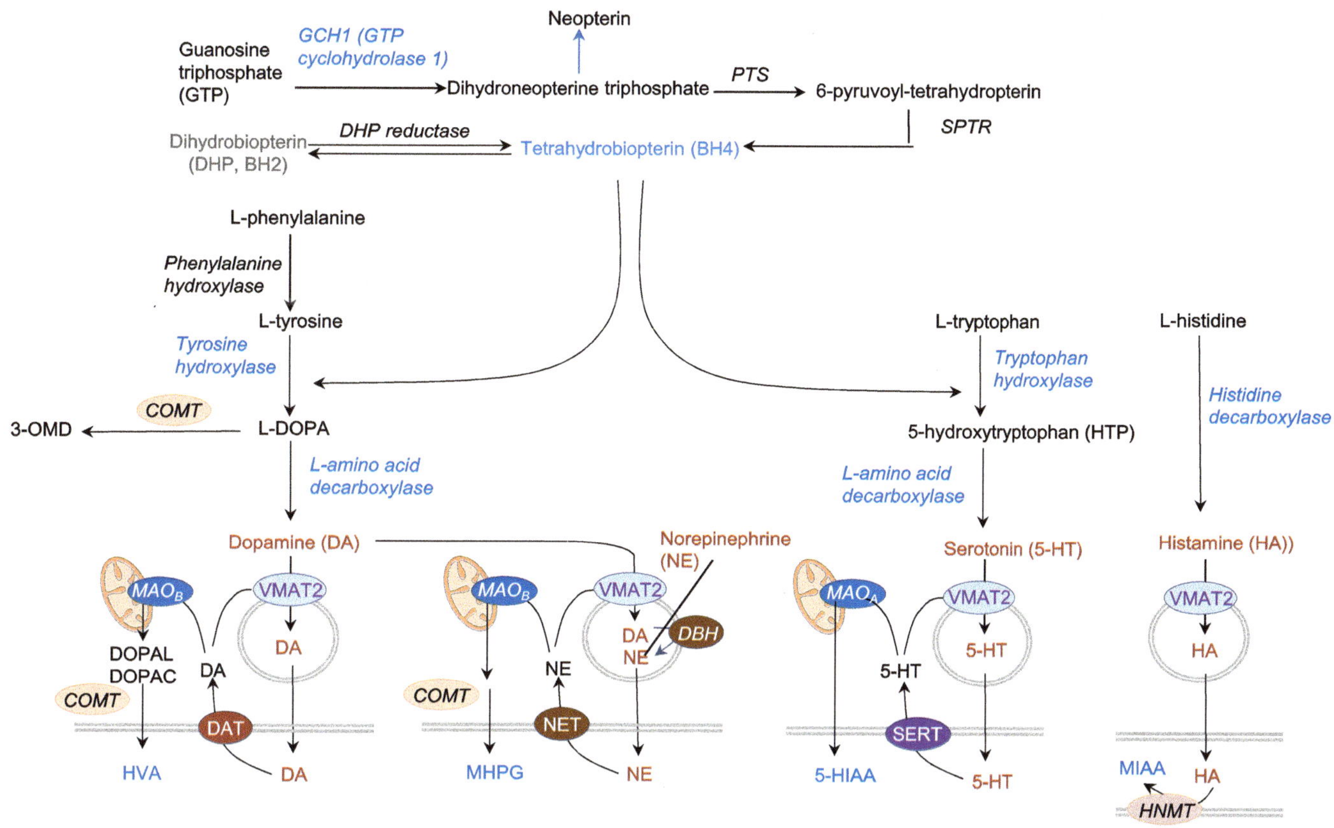

FIGURE 20.3 Major steps of monoamine neurotransmitter metabolism.
Monoamine neurotransmitters derive from L-tyrosine, L-tryptophan, and L-histidine provided from the diet. The rate-limiting enzyme for synthesis of dopamine (DA) and norepinephrine (NE) is tyrosine hydroxylase (TH), which transforms L-tyrosine to L-dihydroxypenylalanine (L-DOPA). L-DOPA is transformed to DA via L-aromatic amino acid decarboxylase (L-AADC). In noradrenergic neurons, DA is converted to NE by action of dopamine-β-hydroxylase (DBH). The rate-limiting enzyme for synthesis of serotonin (5-HT) is tryptophan hydroxylase 2 (TPH2), which transforms L-tryptophan into 5-hydroxytryptophan (5-HTP) which is then decarboxylated by L-AADC to 5-HT. The initial steps of biosynthesis of DA, NE, and 5-HT critically depend on the availability of tetrahydrobiopterin (BH4), which is an essential cofactor of TH and TPH 2. BH4 is synthesized from guanosine triphosphate (GTP) in the three sequential steps. GTP cyclohydrolase I mediates the first and rate-limiting step in BH4 synthesis. Histamine is synthesized from L-histidine by action of L-AADC. Monoamines are primarily incorporated into synaptic vesicles the vesicular monoamine transporter 2 (VMAT2) Monoamines undergo rapid reuptake at synapses via plasma membrane transporters: the DA transporter (DAT), the NE transporter (NET), and the serotonin transporter (SERT). Unlike other monoamines, HA does not undergo presynaptic reuptake. Catecholamines and serotonin are metabolized by monoamine oxidases (MAOs), which include MAO-A and MAO-B isoforms located in the outer mitochondrial membrane. Catecholamines are also metabolized by catechol-O-methyltransferase (COMT), which catalyzes the transfer of the methyl group of S-adenosyl methionine to L-DOPA and other compounds such as ascorbic acid and drugs such as α-methyldopa and carbidopa. Histamine undergoes metabolism by histamine-N-methyl transferase (HNMT) located in postsynaptic neurons. SEPTR, sepiapterin reductase; PTPS, 6-pyruvoyltetrahydropterin synthase.

by endocytosis; these processes are dynamically modulated by transporter glycosylation, phosphorylation, trafficking, and protein–protein interactions. Unlike other monoamines, HA does not undergo presynaptic reuptake.

Metabolism

Catecholamines and serotonin are metabolized by monoamine oxidases (MAOs), which include MAO_A and MAO_B isoforms. These enzymes are located in the outer mitochondrial membrane and catalyze oxidative deamination of the monoamines. MAO_A is highly expressed in noradrenergic neurons, and has high affinity for both NE and 5-HT. MAO_B is primarily located in serotonergic and histaminergic neurons and predominantly metabolizes DA. Catecholamines are also metabolized by catechol-O-methyltransferase (COMT), which includes a soluble and a membrane-bound

TABLE 20.2 *Presynaptic Events of Monoaminergic Neurotransmission*

Neurotransmitter	Dopamine	Norepinephrine	Serotonin	Histamine
Substrate	L-tyrosine	L-tyrosine	L-tryptophan	L-histidine
Rate-limiting enzyme	Tyrosine hydroxylase	Tyrosine hydroxylase	Tryptophan hydroxylase 2	Histidine decarboxylase
Further enzymatic steps	L-amino acid decarboxylase (L-AADC)	L-AADC Dopamine-β-hydroxylase	L-AADC	None
Vesicular storage	Vesicular monoamine transporter 2 (VMAT2)	VMAT2	VMAT2	VMAT2
Reuptake	Dopamine transporter (DAT)	Norepinephrine transporter (NET)	Serotonin transporter (SERT)	None
Metabolism	MAO_B COMT	MAO_A COMT	MAO_A	Histamine-N-methyltransferase MAO
Main product	Homovanillic acid (HVA)	Methyl-hydroxy-phenylglycol (MHPG)	5-hydroxy-indolacetic acid (5-HIAA)	N-methyl-imidazolacetic acid

COMT, catechol-O-methyltransferase; MAO, monoamine oxidase

isoform. Membrane bound COMT is the predominant form in the brain and is distributed in the endoplasmic reticulum (ER) of neurons and glial cells. COMT catalyzes the transfer of the methyl group of S-adenosyl methionine to the 3-hydroxyl group of L-DOPA, catecholamine metabolites generated by MAO, and other compounds such as ascorbic acid and drugs such as α-methyldopa and carbidopa. Histamine undergoes metabolism by histamine-N-methyl transferase (HNMT) located in postsynaptic neurons.

Receptor Mechanisms

Essentially all synaptic effects of monoamines are mediated by canonical signal pathways mediated by different subtypes of GPCRs (Table 20.3). Monoamine receptors coupled

TABLE 20.3 *Monoaminergic Signaling*

Neurotransmitter	$G\alpha_s$ / $G\alpha_{olf}$-coupled receptor Transduction pathway Adenylyl cyclase (AC)-cyclic AMP Protein kinase A (PKA)	$G\alpha_i$/ $G\alpha_o$-coupled receptor Transduction pathway Inhibition of AC GIRK activation Ca_v2 inhibition	$G\alpha_q$-coupled receptor Transduction pathway: Phospholipase C DAG/ IP_3 K^+ channel inhibition Intracellular Ca^{2+} Protein kinase C
Dopamine	Dopamine D1 (D5)	Dopamine D2* (D3, D4)	D1/D2 dimer
Norepinephrine	Beta (β1–3)	Alpha 2 (α2A, α2B)	Alpha 1 (α1A–C)
Serotonin**	5-HT4–7	5-HT1 ($5\text{-HT}1_A$, $5\text{-HT}1_{B/D}$, $5\text{-HT}1_F$)	5-HT2 (A–C)
Histamine	H2	H3	H1

* Also coupled to noncanonical signals via arrestin-mitogen-activated kinase pathways

** 5-HT3 receptor is a Ca^{2+} channel

DAG, diacylglycerol, GIRK, G protein-activated inward-rectifying K^+ channels; IP_3, inositol triphosphate; PLC, phospholipase C to G_s/G_{olf} signaling activate adenylyl cyclase, resulting in production of cyclic adenosine monophosphate (cAMP), which directly modulates ion channels and activates protein kinase A (PKA), triggering multiple downstream effects including facilitation of synaptic plasticity. Receptors coupled to $G_{i/o}$ signaling inhibit adenylyl cyclase, activate inward-rectifying K^+ channels ($K_{ir}3$, GIRK), and inhibit both postsynaptic Ca_v1 and presynaptic Ca_v2.channels. These mechanisms mediate presynaptic and postsynaptic inhibition. These receptors also function as somatodendritic inhibitory autoreceptors limiting the tonic firing of the corresponding monoaminergic cell. Monoamine receptors coupled to $G_{q/11}$ signaling activate phospholipase C, resulting in hydrolysis of membrane phosphatidylinositol (4,5) biphosphate resulting both in inhibition of K^+ channels and thus increased excitability, and production of inositol triphosphate (IP_3) and diacylglycerol (DAG). IP_3 triggers Ca^{2+} release from the ER, while DAG, together with Ca^{2+}, activates protein kinase C (PKC). Individual monoamines typically act via different subtypes of GPCRs and exert multiple effects that depend on receptor distribution and subtype. In addition, serotonin also acts via 5-HT3 receptors, which are ionotropic Ca^{2+} channels.

State-Dependent Activity

All monoaminergic neurons have a behavioral-state dependent patent of firing. They exhibit a slow tonic activity during quiet wakefulness, reduce their activity during drowsiness and NREM sleep, and are virtually silent during REM sleep. This tonic activity reflects the interplay between intrinsic ionic conductances, inhibitory somatodendritic autoreceptors, and local GABAergic inhibition by interneurons. Their changes of activity during the wake–sleep cycle is largely determined by the opposing effects of excitatory inputs from orexin (hypocretin) neurons in the posterior lateral hypothalamus that maintain the waking state and inhibitory GABAergic inputs from neurons in the ventrolateral and medial preoptic areas that induce sleep initiation. All monoaminergic groups increase their activity during active cortical states such as attention, exploration, and responses to stress. These responses are triggered either directly or indirectly by glutamatergic inputs from the prefrontal cortex (PFC).

DOPAMINERGIC SYSTEMS

Dopamine is an important modulator of neuronal activity and synaptic plasticity, particularly in the striatum and the cerebral cortex. It has a major role in reward-based motivated behavior, action selection, maintenance of effort, and attention to salient stimuli from the environment.

Anatomical Organization

The most important dopaminergic groups in the CNS are the midbrain neurons of the VTA (area A9), SNc (area A10), and the retrorubral field (Figure 20.4). Neurons in the VTA and SNc primarily target the striatum and the cerebral cortex with a partially segregated topography. The VTA projects primarily to the nucleus accumbens (NAc). The dorsal tier of the SNc primarily projects to most of the caudate nucleus; and the ventral tier of the SNC targets the putamen. These midbrain dopaminergic neurons also heavily innervate the prefrontal, motor, and posterior parietal areas and also provide inputs to the globus pallidus, subthalamic nucleus (STN), thalamus, and brainstem. There are two groups of dopaminergic neurons in the hypothalamus. Dopaminergic neurons in infundibular (arcuate) nucleus project to the anterior pituitary and tonically inhibit prolactin release. Dopaminergic neurons in the posterior lateral hypothalamus (A11) group, project to the brainstem and spinal cord. Dopamine is also present in neurons of the dorsal motor nucleus of the vagus, some amacrine cells of the retina, and some local neurons in the olfactory bulb.

Presynaptic Events of Dopaminergic Transmission

The rate-limiting step of DA biosynthesis is mediated by TH, which metabolizes L-tyrosine to L-DOPA, which is then converted to DA via the L-AADC (Figure 20.5). The expression and function of TH is highly regulated in an activity-dependent manner at the level of transcription, translation, and posttranslational modifications, particularly phosphorylation. The conversion of L-DOPA to DA via the L-AADC is important to prevent accumulation of L-DOPA. L-DOPA can be methylated by COMT to yield O-methyldopa in a reaction that reaction utilizes S-adenosyl methionine and may potentially lead to secondary 5-mehyl tetrahydrofolate deficiency. The incorporation of DA into synaptic vesicles via the VAMT2 is also a fundamental step that prevents excessive accumulation of cytosolic DA. Cytosolic DA could be target for oxidation by MAO_B, leading to DA depletion and production of toxic metabolites such as dihydroxyphenylacetaldehyde (DOPAL) that cause oxidative damage and may predispose to accumulation of α-synuclein. VMAT2 may also transport toxins such as the neurotoxin 1-methyl-4-phenyl-phenydium (MPP+) into synaptic vesicles. DAT mediated reuptake of DA from the synaptic space is critical for replenishment of synaptic vesicles. However, in certain conditions, DAT may act in a reverse direction and mediate nonvesicular release. This mechanism also allows DA release from dendrites. Dopamine uptake is followed by its metabolism by mitochondrial MAO_B and then cytosolic COMT; the main metabolite of DA is homovanillic acid (HVA).

Dopamine Receptors

Dopamine receptors are subdivided into D1-type and D2-type (Figure 20.5). The D1-type receptors include two subtypes, D1 (D1R) and D5 (D5R).[4] The most abundant is D1R; the D5R is primarily expressed in the striatum. D1-type receptors are coupled to $G\alpha_{olf}/G\alpha_s$ and thus to the

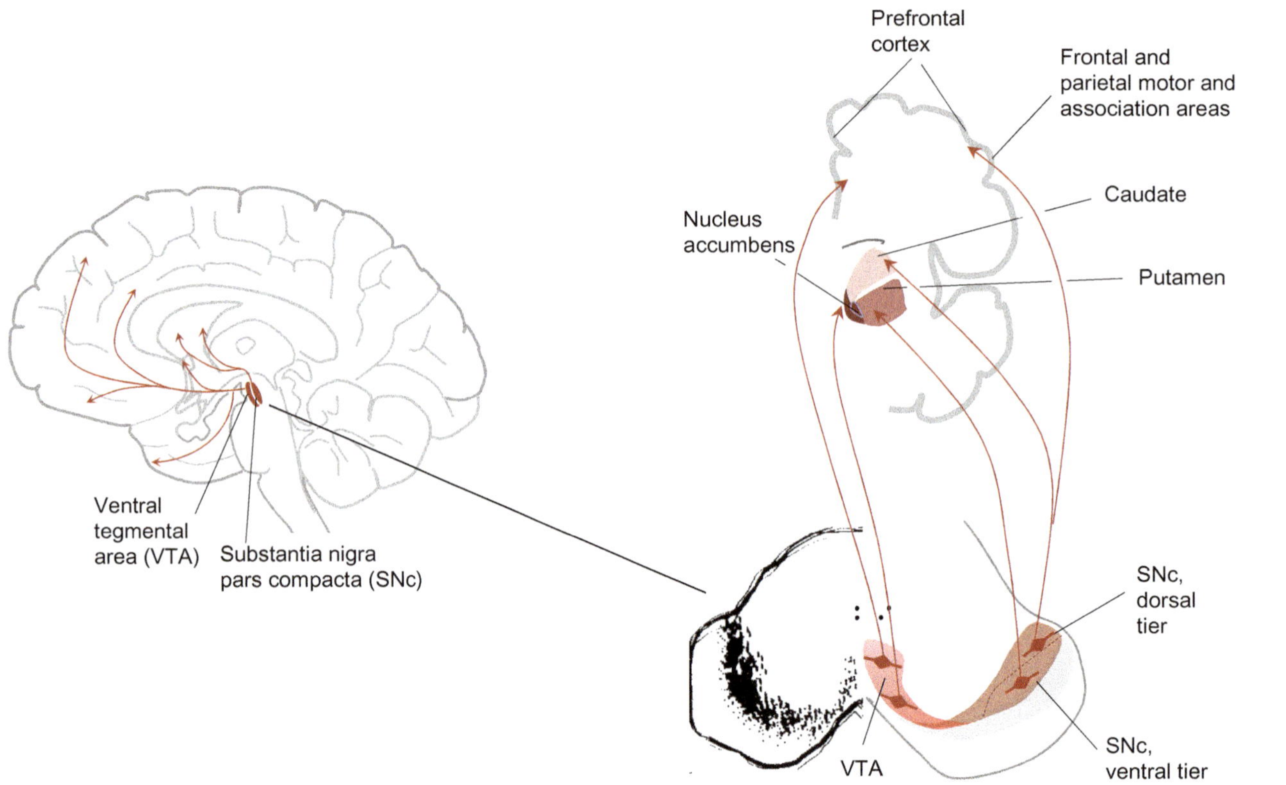

FIGURE 20.4 Organization of the midbrain dopaminergic system.
The most important dopaminergic system in the CNS includes neurons of the susbtantia nigra pars compacta (SNc, area A10), ventral tegmental area (VTA, area A9), and the retrorubral field. These neurons primarily target the striatum and the cerebral cortex with a partially segregated topography. The VTA projects primarily to the nucleus accumbens (NAc), ventral head of the caudate nucleus, and anterior putamen. The dorsal tier of the SNc primarily projects to most of the caudate nucleus; and the ventral tier of the SNC targets the posterior putamen. These midbrain dopaminergic neurons also heavily innervate the prefrontal, motor and posterior parietal areas and also provide inputs to the globus pallidus, subthalamic nucleus (STN) and brainstem (not shown).

adenylyl cyclase-cAMP-PKA pathway (Table 20.3). In many cases D1R activation increases neuronal excitability and promotes synaptic plasticity. For example, phosphorylation by PKA inhibits voltage-gated K^+ channels (K_v4) and Ca^{2+}-dependent K^+ channels (SK type), and increases Ca_v1 (L-type) Ca^{2+} channel currents, thus potentiating the effect of excitatory glutamatergic inputs. One important target of the D1R–cAMP–PKA pathway in the striatum is the phosphatase DARPP-32 (dopamine- and cyclic AMP regulated phosphoprotein of 32kD), which amplifies the PKA signal by inhibiting protein phosphatase 1. The D1R-triggered pathway is critical for synaptic plasticity, particularly N-methyl-D-aspartate receptor (NMDAR)-induced long-term potentiation (LTP). D1R signaling is turned off by phosphodiesterases that hydrolyze AMP.

D2-type receptors include three subtypes D2R, D3R, and D4R; the most abundant is the D2R; the D3R is also abundant in the ventral striatum. The D2Rs are coupled to $G_{i/o}$-triggered inhibitory signaling, including inhibition of adenylyl cyclase; activation of GIRKs and thus decreased neuronal excitability; and inhibition of presynaptic Ca_v2. channels and thus presynaptic inhibition of neurotransmitter release. Somatodendritic D2R and D3R function as inhibitory autoreceptors that restrain the tonic activity of dopaminergic neurons, whereas presynaptic inhibitory D2Rs inhibit release of DA, as well as that of other neurotransmitters. Signaling by D2Rs is turned off by regulator of G-proteinsignaling (RGS) proteins that activate GTPase activity of the $G\alpha_{i/o}$ subunit. Activation of D2Rs also triggers a noncanonical pathway that involves the β2-arrestin and activation of the protein phosphatase calcineurin, which leads to inhibition of both PKA and the growth factor signal activated kinase AKT and thus disinhibition of glycogen synthase kinase 3β (GSK-3β). By these mechanisms, D2R activation in general promotes long-term depression of glutamatergic synapses. Dopamine receptors may form complexes with each other and with other receptors, forming receptor mosaics in which allosteric interactions may lead to properties distinct from that of the individual receptors. For example, D1R/D2R heteromers are coupled to G_q

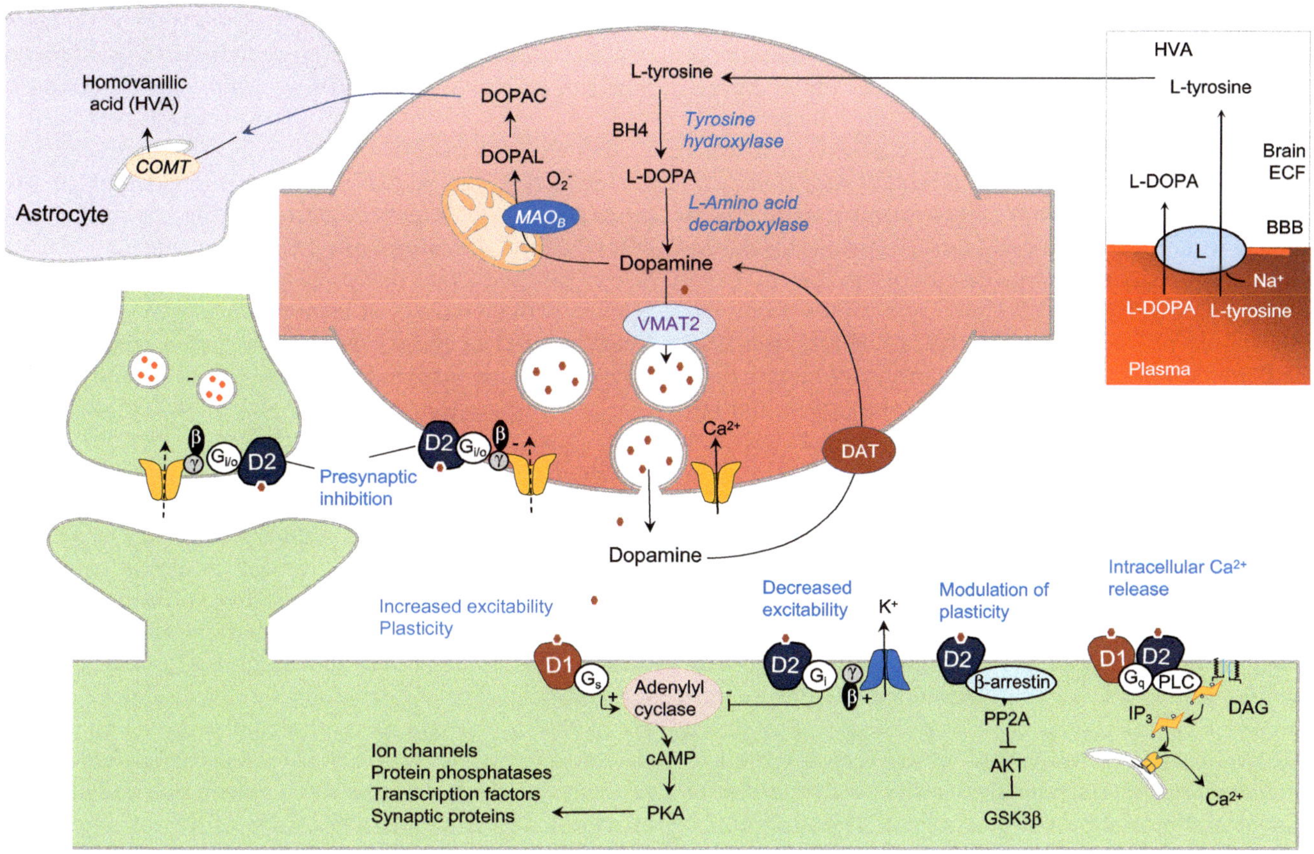

FIGURE 20.5 Dopaminergic neurotransmission.

The substrate for dopamine (DA) biosynthesis is L-tyrosine, which is transported across the blood-brain barrier (BBB) via the neutral amino acid transporter (L), which also transports L-dihydroxyphenylalanine (L-DOPA). The rate-limiting step for DA synthesis is mediated by tyrosine hydroxylase, which metabolizes L-tyrosine to L-DOPA, which is converted to DA via the L-amino acid decarboxylase. DA is incorporated in synaptic vesicles via the vesicular monoamine transporter 2 (VAMT2). Dopamine undergoes reuptake from the synaptic space via the dopamine transporter (DAT). This is followed by its metabolism by monoamine oxidase B (MAO_B) and then catechol-O-methyltransferase (COMT), yielding homovanillic acid (HVA). Dopamine acts via D1-type and D2-type receptors (D2Rs). The D1-type receptors (D1Rs) are coupled to $G\alpha_{olf}$ or $G\alpha_s$ and activate adenylyl cyclase and production of cyclic adenosine monophosphate (cAMP), which activates protein kinase A (PKA), which phosphorylates multiple targets, frequently increasing neuronal excitability and promoting synaptic plasticity. D2Rs are coupled to $G_{i/o}$ triggering inhibitory signaling, including inhibition of adenylyl cyclase and cAMP production, activation of inward-rectifying K^+ channels ($K_{ir}3$, GIRK) resulting in decreased neuronal excitability; and inhibition of presynaptic Ca_v2 channels and thus neurotransmitter release. Somatodendritic D2R and D3R function as inhibitory autoreceptors. In addition to $Gi_{/o}$, activation of D2Rs also triggers a noncanonical pathway that involves β2-arrestin and calcineurin, which leads to inhibition of signaling by PKA by the growth factor–activated kinase AKT, leading to disinhibition of glycogen synthase kinase 3β (GSK-3β). D1R/D2R heteromers couple to G_q and thus activate the phospholipase C transduction pathway linked to Ca^{2+} signaling.

and thus activate the transduction pathway linked to Ca^{2+} signaling. Dopamine receptors may also form heteromeric complexes with other receptors such as adenosine (A) receptors, forming A1R/D1R and $A2_A$R/D2R heteromers. These allosteric interactions lead to reduced dopamine receptor signaling. The D1R may form heteromers with the GluN2 subunit of NMDAR, promoting NMDAR signaling.

Physiology of Midbrain Dopaminergic Neurons

Midbrain dopaminergic neurons have two modes of discharge, tonic and burst firing. The tonic discharge reflects a pacemaker activity that primarily depends on hyperpolarization-activated cyclic nucleotide gated channels and, in the cases of neurons of the SNc, also by L-type ($Ca_v1.3$) channels. These channels also trigger dendritic Ca^{2+}

oscillations in mitochondria, which renders SNc neurons vulnerable to oxidative stress. A major influence on tonic pacemaker activity of midbrain dopaminergic neurons is feedback inhibition via D2 somatodendritic autoreceptors activated by DA released from dendrites of neighboring dopaminergic neurons. Burst firing of dopaminergic neurons reflects a rapid increase in intracellular Ca^{2+} triggered by L-glutamate acting via NMDARs. These glutamatergic inputs originate from the PFC and are conveyed primarily via the STN or the pedunculopontine/laterodorsal tegmental nuclear complex (PPT/LDT). Cholinergic inputs from the PPT/LDT acting via nicotinic acetylcholine receptors also contribute to burst firing of midbrain dopaminergic neurons. Bursting is suppressed by tonic GABAergic inhibition from local interneurons and by GABAergic inputs from the striatum and brainstem.

Dopamine Release as a Reward and Salience Signal

The tonic discharge of midbrain dopaminergic neurons maintains a steady baseline level of DA, which acts primarily via extrasynaptic D2Rs to maintain a low background inhibition critical for normal function circuits in the striatum and cerebral cortex. Burst or phasic firing produces rapid fluctuations or "transients" of extracellular DA levels that overwhelm DA reuptake via the DAT, resulting in spillover and activation of postsynaptic D1Rs and D2Rs. In contrast, pauses of midbrain DA neuron firing results in transient interruption of the D2R-mediated inhibition. Midbrain dopaminergic neurons are activated by alerting signals triggered by potentially relevant sensory cues. Most of these neurons further increase their activity in response to an unexpected reward or a cue signaling an upcoming reward whereas they become essentially silent in response to an aversive outcome or punishment. These neurons project primarily to the striatum and thus encode the motivational value of the stimulus for learning of reward-oriented behavior and action selection. A DA peak in the striatum activates D1Rs and promotes reward-based Pavlovian learning, goal-directed action selection, and habit formation, while via D2Rs it inhibits unwanted behaviors. In contrast, a fall in DA levels in response to an aversive outcome leads to suppression of the action that led to this outcome. A second population of midbrain dopaminergic neurons is activated both by rewarding and aversive outcomes. These neurons project primarily to the PFC and midcingulate cortex and code motivational salience of the stimulus to guide behavioral selection.[5] Dopamine signaling in the PFC is critical for attentional processing, including working memory.

NORADRENERGIC SYSTEMS

Norepinephrine is a major neurotransmitter in both the CNS and in the peripheral nervous system. In the CNS it has a major role in mechanisms of behavioral arousal, attention, stress response, and pain modulation. In the periphery, it mediates effect of the sympathetic nervous system in control of blood pressure and cardiac output, distribution of blood flow, response to exercise and stress, and other functions.

Anatomical Distribution

The major group of NE-synthesizing neurons in the brain is the LC (A6 group) located in the upper dorsolateral pontine tegmentum. The LC-NE neurons have extensively branched axons that project throughout the neuraxis (Figure 20.6). In humans, the most extensive noradrenergic innervation is in the somatosensory, motor, and association cortical areas including the PFC and lateral parietal cortex. Other targets include the amygdala, hippocampus, basal forebrain, thalamus, hypothalamus, superior colliculus, and cerebellum.[6] The LC sends descending projections that target preganglionic parasympathetic and sympathetic neurons, somatic cranial nerve and spinal motor nuclei, trigeminal nucleus, and dorsal horn of the spinal cord. The second major catecholaminergic system in the brain is the lateral tegmental system, which includes neurons that synthesize either NE (A1, A2, and A5 groups) or epinephrine (C1 and C2 groups). The rostral C1 and a caudal A1 groups are located in the ventrolateral medulla; the C2 and A2 in the dorsomedial medulla, and the A5 group in the pontine tegmentum. The lateral tegmental system primarily targets areas involved in homeostasis, such as the hypothalamus and brainstem and spinal autonomic nuclei, and has close anatomical and functional interactions with the LC system. In addition to its primary role as a central neurotransmitter, NE is the primary neurotransmitter of sympathetic ganglion neurons innervation all visceral targets.

Presynaptic Events in Noradrenergic Transmission

In noradrenergic neurons the initial steps of NE synthesis are identical to those of DA (Figure 20.7). In noradrenergic terminals, upon incorporation into synaptic vesicles by action of VMAT2, DA is converted into NE by action of dopamine-β-hydroxylase (DBH). This copper-dependent enzyme is located in the membrane of the storage vesicle and is coreleased with NE during exocytosis. The cytochrome b561 protein (CYB561) is a transmembrane electron carrier that maintains the redox state across the vesicular membrane and is required for proper DBH function. Ascorbic acid is critical in this redox reaction. Neurons of C1 and C2 groups that synthesize epinephrine-synthesizing neurons also contain phenyl ethanolamine-N-methyltransferase (PNMT), which transforms NE into epinephrine. Stress induces increased expression of the mRNAs encoding all enzymes synthesizing catecholamines. Like other monoamines, NE may be released both at typical synapses and at nonsynaptic release sites and act via volume transmission. The effects of NE are terminated by its uptake via the NET, which is regulated by phosphorylation triggered by neuronal activity. Like the DAT, the NET is competitively inhibited by cocaine and transports

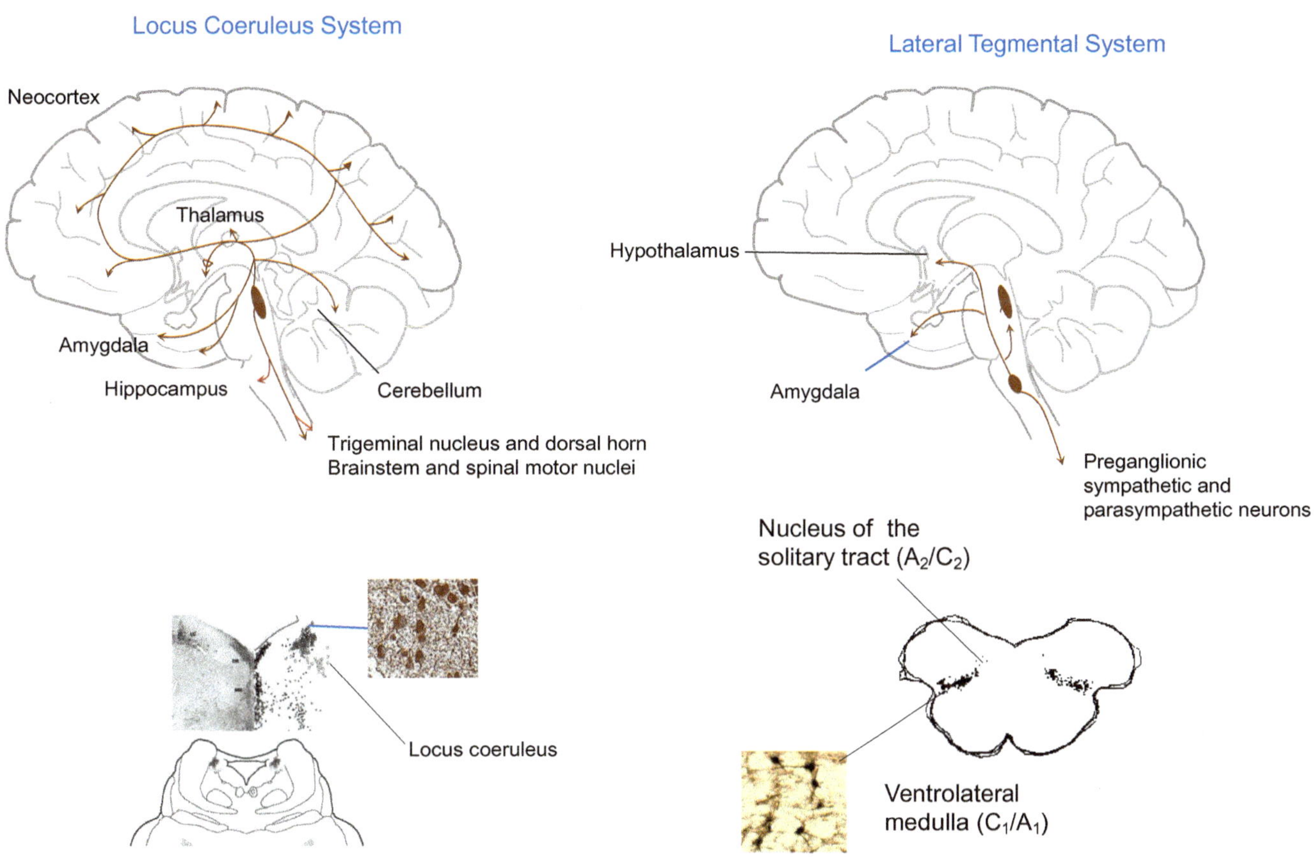

FIGURE 20.6 Major noradrenergic groups in the central nervous system.
The major group of norepinephrine (NE)-synthesizing neurons is the locus coeruleus (LC). The LC-NE neurons have extensively branched axons that project extensively to the somatosensory, motor and association cortical areas, hippocampus, amygdala, basal forebrain, thalamus, hypothalamus, superior colliculus, and cerebellum. The LC sends descending projections to brainstem and spinal autonomic, motor, and somatosensory nucle. The second major catecholaminergic system in brain is the lateral tegmental system. It includes different groups of neurons that synthesize either NE (A1, A2, and A5 groups) or epinephrine (C1 and C2 groups). The lateral tegmental system primarily targets areas involved in homeostasis, such as the hypothalamus and brainstem and spinal autonomic nuclei.

amphetamine. Amphetamine-like drugs, as well as tyramine, elicit a translocation of NE from the synaptic vesicles to the cytosol, triggering nonexocytotic release via a reversal of the transport mechanism. The NET is also the main transporter responsible for clearance of DA in the prefrontal cortex, as dopaminergic terminals in this region express low levels of DAT. Norepinephrine uptake is followed by its metabolism by mitochondrial MAO_A and then cytosolic COMT; the main metabolite of NE in the CNS is 3-methoxy-4-hydroxyphenylglycol (MHPG).

Adrenergic Receptors

The effects of NE are mediated by three families of GPCRs, also known as adrenoceptors (ARs): alpha 1 (α1), α2, and beta (β), each consisting of several subtypes (Figure 20.8). The α1ARs and βARs are present primarily at postsynaptic sites, whereas the α2ARs are present at both presynaptic and some postsynaptic sites. The α1ARs are coupled to G_q-and thus to the PLC signal transduction pathway, resulting in inhibition of K^+ channels and increased excitability, production of DAG and PKC activation, and IP_3-triggered Ca^{2+} release from the ER. The βARs (including β1 and β2 subtypes) are positively coupled to the adenylyl cyclase–cAMP–PKA cascade. The α2ARs are negatively coupled to adenylyl cyclase, activate K^+ currents thereby reducing neuronal excitability, and inhibit presynaptic Ca^{2+} channels reducing neurotransmitter release. Alpha 2 ARs act as inhibitory autoreceptors. Whereas in general α2ARs have an inhibitory function, they increase excitability of recurrent prefrontal cortical networks by inhibiting channels that dampen excitatory synaptic responses in in pyramidal neurons.[7]

Physiology of Locus Coeruleus Neurons

The LC-NE neurons fire in two distinct modes: tonic and phasic.[8] Their tonic regular baseline activity reflects the

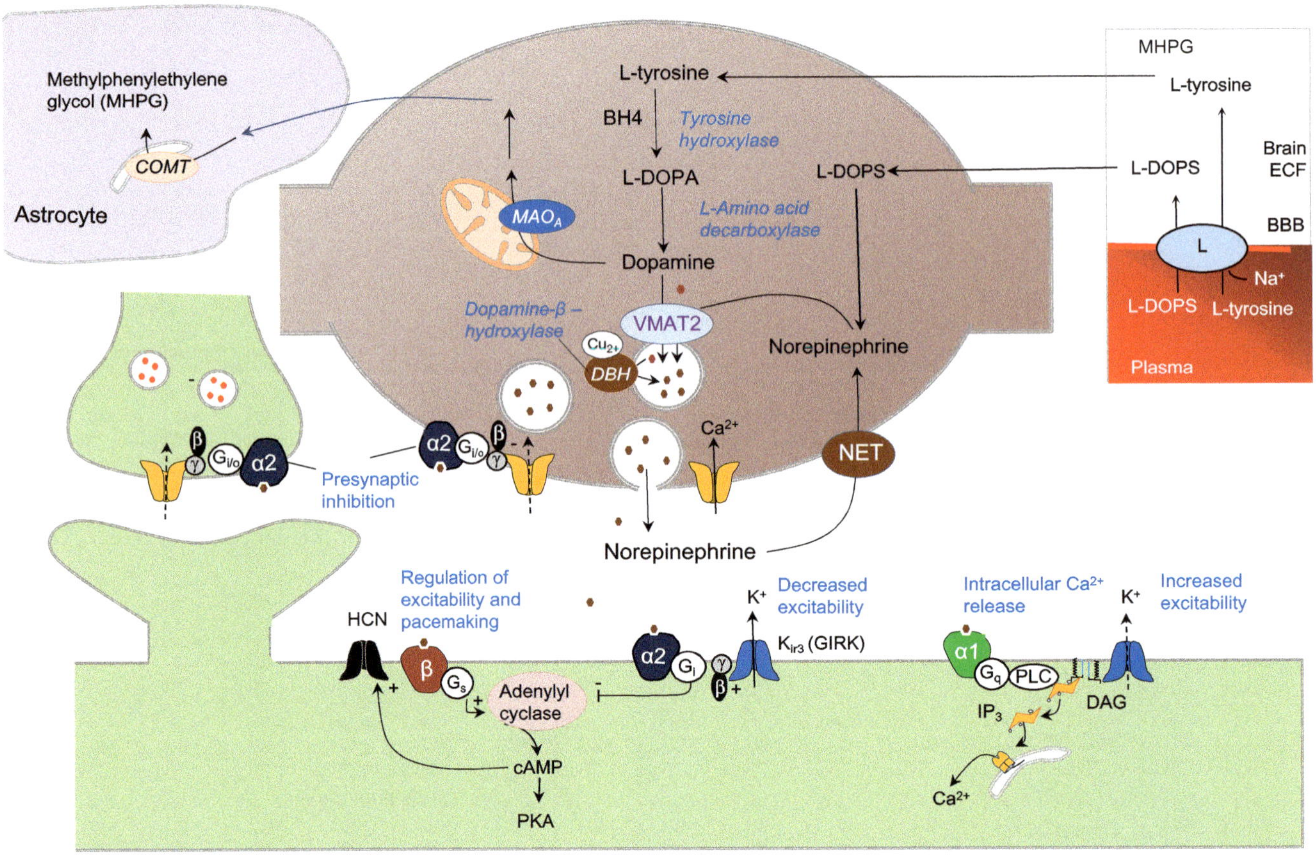

FIGURE 20.7 Noradrenergic neurotransmission.

The initial steps of norepinephrine (NE) are identical to those for dopamine (DA). The substrate is L-tyrosine, which is transported across the blood-brain barrier (BBB) via the neutral amino acid transporter (L), which also transports the synthetic precursors L-dihydroxyphenylalanine and L-dihydroxyphenylserine (L-DOPS). Tyrosine hydroxylase which metabolizes L-tyrosine to L-DOPA) which is converted to DA via the L-amino acid decarboxylase. DA is incorporated in synaptic vesicles via the vesicular monoamine transporter 2 (VAMT2). In noradrenergic terminals, upon incorporation into synaptic vesicles by action of VMAT2, DA is converted into NE by action of dopamine-β-hydroxylase (DBH). The effects of NE are terminated by its uptake via the norepinephrine transporter (NET). Reuptake is followed by its metabolism by mitochondrial monoamine oxidase A (MAO$_A$) and then cytosolic catechol-O-methyltransferase (COMT); the main metabolite of NE in the CNS is 3-methoxy-4-hydroxyphenylglycol (MHPG). The effects of NE are mediated by three families of adrenoceptors (ARs): alpha 1 (α1), α2, and beta (β). The α1ARs are coupled to G$_q$—and the phospholipase C (PLC) signal transduction pathway, resulting in inhibition of K$^+$ channels and increased excitability production of diacylglycerol (DAG) resulting in activation of protein kinase C (PKC) and IP$_3$- triggered Ca^{2+} release from the endoplasmic reticulum. The βARs are positively coupled to adenylyl cyclase increasing levels of cAMP, which affects synaptic excitability. The α2ARs are negatively coupled to adenylyl cyclase; they activate K$^+$ currents, thereby reducing neuronal excitability, and inhibit presynaptic Ca^{2+} channels (Ca$_v$2), thereby reducing neurotransmitter release. Alpha 2 ARs in somatodendritic and presynaptic axon domains of noradrenergic neurons act as inhibitory autoreceptors.

arousal state. They have slow tonic activity during unaroused states, moderate tonic activity during quiet wakefulness and engagement in a focused task, and high tonic activity while exploring a novel environment or in response to stress. During focused attention, LC neurons transiently interrupt their moderate tonic firing and respond with a phasic mode to task-relevant stimuli. This phasic discharge allows focused task performance by filtering irrelevant stimuli. Transitions between different tonic levels are enabled by cortical inputs from the orbitofrontal and anterior cingulate cortex. The transition between different firing states of LC-NE neurons is also regulated by local GABAergic neurons that receive strong input from the PFC and produce feedforward inhibition of LC-NE activity, thus controlling arousal level. Like other monoaminergic neurons, LC-NE neurons are essentially silent during REM sleep.

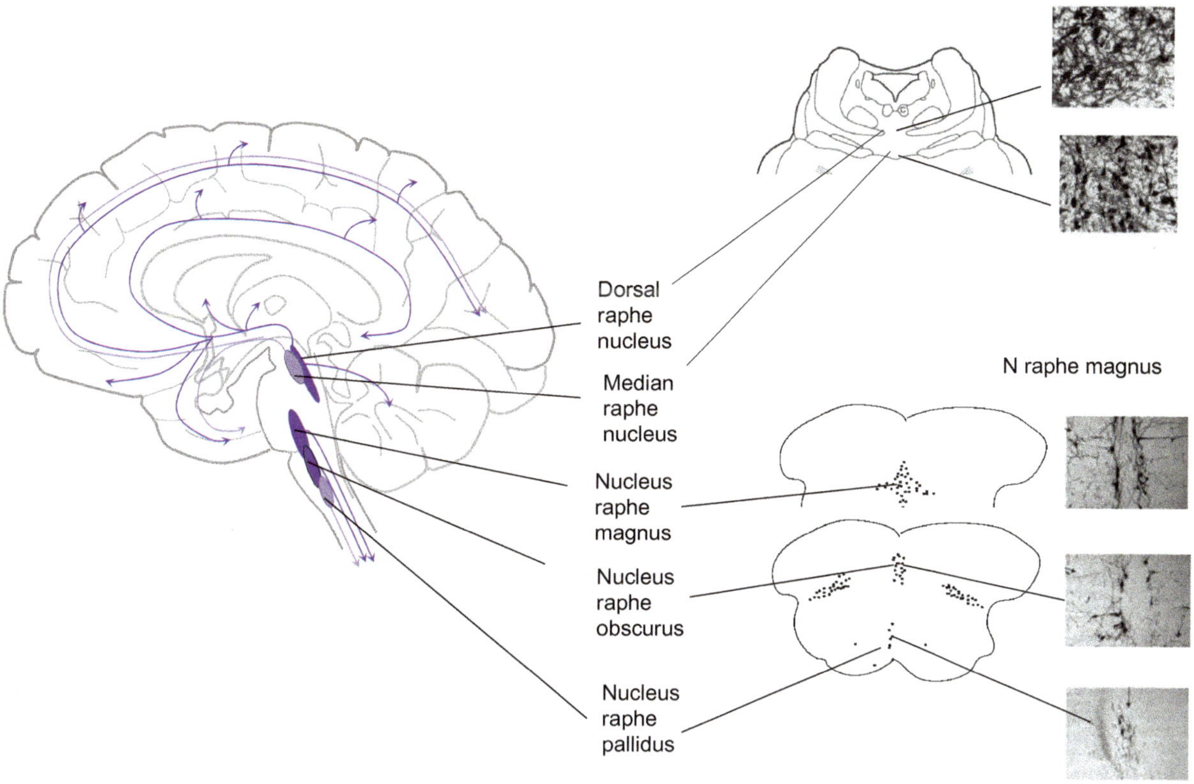

FIGURE 20.8 Distribution of serotonergic systems.
The raphe nuclei are broadly categorized into rostral and caudal groups, each subdivided into different nuclei. The rostral raphe nuclei include the dorsal raphe nucleus (DR), median raphe nucleus (MR), and the caudal linear nucleus. These nuclei send serotonergic projections via the median forebrain bundle to several targets in the forebrain, including the prefrontal cortex, amygdala, and hippocampal formation. The caudal raphe nuclei includes the nucleus raphe magnus (RMg), nucleus raphe pallidus (RPa), nucleus raphe obscurus (ROb), and nucleus paragigantocellularis located in the rostral ventrolateral medulla. These nuclei innervate sensory, motor, and autonomic nuclei of the brainstem and spinal cord.

Role of the Locus Coeruleus in Arousal, Attention and Stress Response

The LC-NE has a critical role in mechanisms of attention and working memory. Activation of α2ARs by a burst of firing of LC-NE arising from a moderate tonic firing promotes recurrent NMDAR-mediated excitation between pyramidal neurons in the lateral PFC; this is required by the maintenance of their activity during the delay period between the presentation of a stimulus and the appropriate response, which is the physiological basis of working memory.

The LC-NE system has a major role in behavioral and autonomic responses to stress. These neurons respond to inputs from the brainstem and orexin hypothalamic neurons during stress, promoting encoding of emotional memory via activation of β2AR receptors in the amygdala. During stress, high levels of NE resulting from high-frequency tonic firing also result in activation of both β2AR and α1ARs in the PFC, which reduces the efficacy of recurrent excitatory synapses thus impairing working memory and focused attention. The LC-NE system is also involved in homeostasis within the CNS. Norepinephrine released from extrasynaptic sites may diffuse in the extracellular fluid and astrocytes and microvessels via volume transmission. Activation of α1 and β2 receptors in astrocytes promotes Ca^{2+}signaling and activates glycogen metabolism and calcium signaling in astrocytes, leading to release of lactate. Via their effects of astrocytes, the LC-NE system participates in both neurovascular and neurometabolic coupling throughout the wake–sleep cycle.

Sympathetic Responses to Stress

The LC also participates in autonomic responses to stress via interactions with the premotor sympathoexcitatory C1 neurons of the rostral ventrolateral medulla. The C1 group constitutes a brain "alarm system" that triggers sympathoexcitatory cardiovascular responses via projections to spinal preganglionic sympathetic neurons.[9] The C1 neurons are also activated in response to internal stressors such as hypoxia or inflammation and promote arousal and ventilator responses via brainstem projections. In the periphery, NE is the primary neurotransmitter of the sympathetic nervous system. Its main effects include vasoconstriction mediated by α1ARs, cardiac stimulation via β1ARs, relaxation of vascular and visceral smooth muscle, and metabolic regulation via β2 and β3ARs.

SEROTONERGIC SYSTEMS

Serotonin has widespread actions in the CNS, yet its functional role remains poorly understood.[10] There is involvement of 5-HT in rewarding and aversive processing, hedonic experience, mood, and impulse control, but its precise contribution is controversial.

Anatomical Distribution

The serotonergic system operates as a conglomeration of subsystems (Figure 20.8). The raphe nuclei are broadly categorized into rostral and caudal groups, each subdivided into different nuclei. The rostral raphe nuclei are located in the upper pons and midbrain and include the dorsal raphe nucleus (DR), median raphe nucleus (MR), and the caudal linear nucleus. Individual serotonergic neurons of the DR and MR are highly branched and send input to multiple forebrain structures, but with target specificity. For example, neurons in the dorsolateral portion of the DR target the amygdala and interconnected areas, those in the ventromedial portion of the DR target the orbitofrontal cortex, and those in the caudal portion of the DR and in the MR target the hippocampus.[11] However, serotonergic neurons also provide collaterals to multiple targets, many of which are interconnected and have functional relationships with each other. Axon terminals containing 5-HT often form synaptic contacts with specific dendritic targets but may also signal through volume transmission. Serotonergic varicosities may occur in close proximity to presynaptic excitatory and inhibitory nerve terminals forming synaptic triads that may preferentially target excitatory or inhibitory neurons depending on the region.[12,13] The caudal raphe nuclei includes the nucleus raphe magnus (RMg), nucleus raphe pallidus (RPa), and nucleus raphe obscurus (ROb), which are located in the midline of the lower pons and medulla; serotonergic neurons are also present in the lateral paragigantocellular nucleus located in the rostral ventrolateral medulla. These nuclei innervate sensory, motor, and autonomic nuclei of the brainstem and spinal cord. Both the rostral and the caudal raphe send projections to other monoaminergic groups and the cerebellum.

Presynaptic Events in Serotonergic Transmission

The rate-limiting step of 5-HT biosynthesis is the hydroxylation of L-tryptophan by tryptophan hydroxylase 2 (TPH2) with formation of 5-hydroxytryptophan (5-HTP), which is converted to 5-HT via the nonspecific L-AADC (Figure 20.9). Serotonin is stored in synaptic vesicles by VMAT2; vesicles storing 5-HT differ from those storing catecholamine by their lack of ATP and the presence of a 5-HT-binding protein. Serotonin undergoes presynaptic reuptake by action via the SERT. Electroconvulsive therapy and chronic administration of MAO inhibitors increase 5-HT uptake, whereas chronic exposure to SERT inhibitors (selective serotonin reuptake inhibitors, SSRIs) decreases 5-HT uptake by inducing internalization and increased degradation of the transport protein. The anorexigenic agent fenfluramine and the drug of abuse 3, 4-methylenedioxymethamphetamine (ecstasy) inhibit the vesicular transport of 5-HT by competing for its substrate-binding site. This allows the accumulation of cytoplasmic 5-HT and triggers nonexocytotic release of 5-HT by a reversal transport mechanism. Upon reuptake, 5-HT is repackaged into vesicles or metabolized by MAO_A to its final metabolite 5-hydroxyindoleacetic acid (5-HIAA). Serotonergic cells contain predominantly MAO_B, for which 5-HT is not a preferred substrate. The role of MAO_B in these cells may be to prevent accumulation of DA or other substrates that could interfere with storage, release, or uptake of 5-HT. Concentrations of 5-HIAA in the CSF are an indirect index of central serotonergic neuron activity and 5-HT turnover.

Serotonin Receptors

There are many types of serotonergic receptors, each consisting of several receptor subtypes. They include 5-HT1, 5-HT2, 5-HT3, and 5-HT4 to 5-HT7 receptors. The 5-HT1 receptors (5-HT1Rs) are coupled to $G_{i/o}$ signaling, triggering inhibition of adenylyl cyclase, opening of inward-rectifying K^+ channels, and closure of presynaptic Ca^{2+} channels; these effects reduce both neuronal excitability and neurotransmitter release. 5-HT1_A receptors function as inhibitory somatodendritic autoreceptors that are activated by locally released 5-HT and inhibit the firing of the neighboring raphe neurons. The 5-HT1_A receptors also function as inhibitory somatodendritic receptors in other neurons, such as LC-NE neurons; this provides a basis for the anxiolytic effect of buspirone, a 5-HT1_A receptor agonist. The hallucinogenic agents mescaline, psilocybin, and lysergic acid diethylamide (LSD) are potent 5-HT1_A receptor agonists and thereby inhibit firing of raphe neurons. The $5HT1_{B/D}$ and 5-HT1_F receptors are primarily located on presynaptic terminals and function as inhibitory presynaptic receptors not only reducing release of serotonin (autoreceptors) but also that of acetylcholine, norepinephrine, and neuropeptides such as calcitonin gene-related peptide, which has relevance for treatment of acute migraine attacks.

The 5-HT2 receptor family includes several subtypes, including the 5-HT2_A, 5-HT2_B, and 5-HT2_C receptors. The 5HT2 receptors are mainly located postsynaptically and are coupled to G_q signaling pathways coupled to PLC; and thus elicit excitatory responses by decreasing K^+ conductances, increasing DAG production, and promoting IP_3-triggered Ca^{2+} release from the ER. The 5-HT2_A and 5-HT2_B receptors are widely distributed in several types of excitatory and inhibitory neurons; $5HT2_C$ receptors are expressed in a subpopulation of inhibitory cortical interneurons and

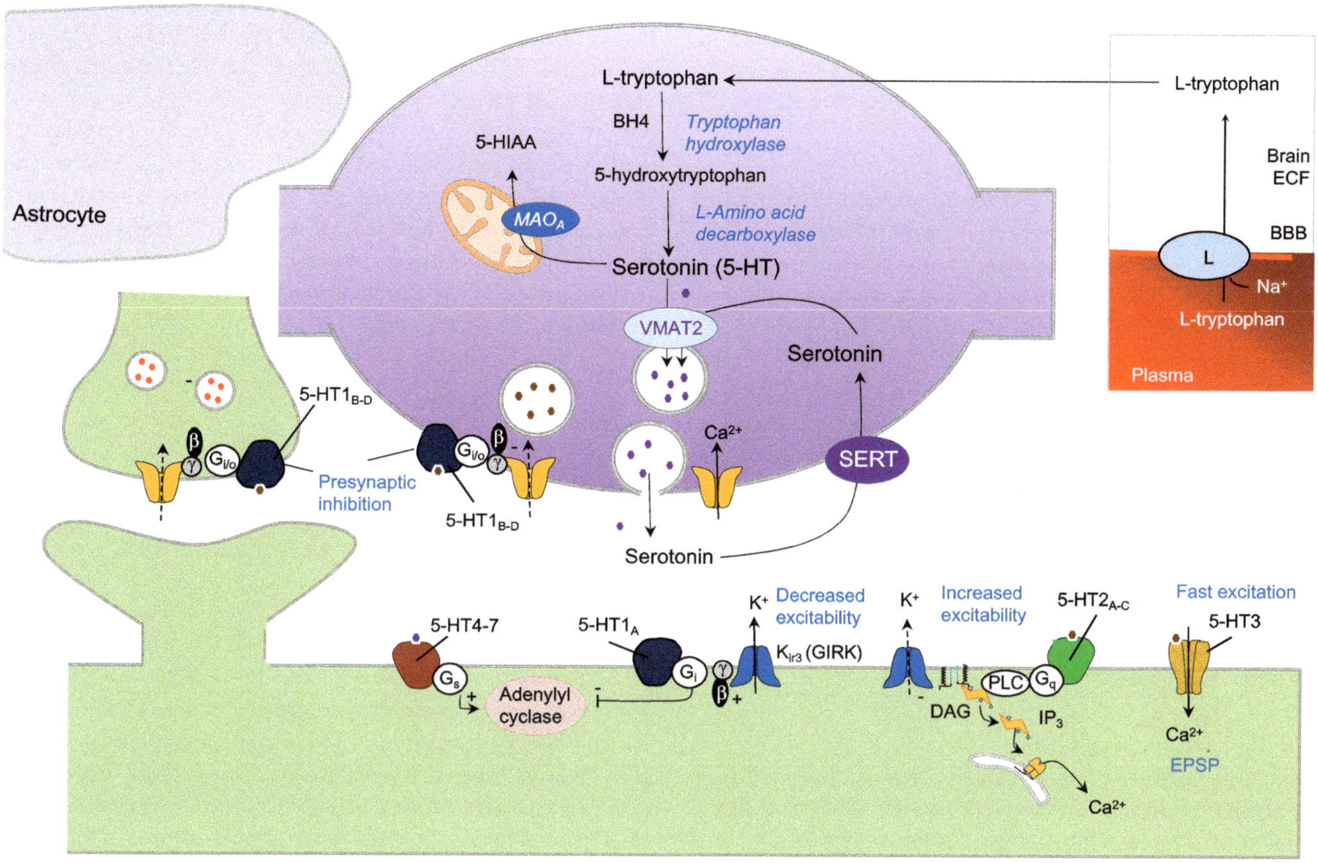

FIGURE 20.9 Serotonergic neurotransmission.

The substrate for serotonin (5-hydroxytyptamine, 5-HT) biosynthesis is L-tryptophan, which is transported across the blood-brain barrier (BBB) via the neutral amino acid transporter (L). The rate-limiting step of 5-HT biosynthesis is the hydroxylation of L-tryptophan by tryptophan hydroxylase 2 with formation of 5-hydroxytryptophan (5-HTP), which is converted to 5-HT via the nonspecific L-amino acid decarboxylase. Serotonin is stored in synaptic vesicles by the vesicular monoamine transporter 2 (VMAT2). Following release, serotonin undergoes presynaptic reuptake by action via the serotonin transporter (SERT) Upon reuptake, 5-HT is repackaged into vesicles or metabolized by MAO$_A$ to its final metabolite 5-hydroxyindoleacetic acid (5-HIAA). There are many types of serotonergic receptors, each consisting of several receptor subtypes. They include 5-HT1, 5-HT2, 5-HT3, and 5-HT4, to 5-HT7 receptors. The 5-HT1 receptors are coupled to $G_{i/o}$ signaling, triggering inhibition of adenylyl cyclase, opening of inward-rectifying K^+ channels, and closure of presynaptic Ca^{2+} channels. The 5-HT1$_A$ receptors are present in the soma and dendrites and function as inhibitory somatodendritic autoreceptors; 5HT$_{1B/D}$ receptors are primarily located on presynaptic terminals and function as inhibitory presynaptic autoreceptors reducing 5-HT release. They are also present in other presynaptic terminals such as cholinergic or noradrenergic terminals inhibiting neurotransmitter release. The 5-HT2 receptors are mainly located postsynaptically and are coupled to G_q-signaling pathways coupled to phospholipase C (PLC); their activation elicits excitatory responses by decreasing K^+ conductances, production of diacylglycerol (DAG) and stimulation of protein kinase C (PKC), and inositol triphosphate (IP$_3$)-triggered Ca^{2+} release from intracellular stores. The 5-HT3 receptors are cation channels that are highly permeable to Ca^{2+} and Na^+ and elicit fast postsynaptic or presynaptic depolarization. The 5-HT4 to 5-HT7 receptors are positively coupled to G_s and therefore stimulate the adenylyl cyclase–cAMP–PKA pathway.

constitutively active in the absence of agonist. The 5-HT3 receptors are cation channels that are highly permeable to Ca^{2+} and Na^+ and elicit fast postsynaptic or presynaptic depolarization. In the brain, these receptors are found postsynaptically in a subpopulation of GABAergic cortical and limbic neurons as well as in cholinergic and dopaminergic neurons. Activation of 5-HT3 receptors in dopaminergic neurons of the area postrema is one important trigger of vomiting and is inhibited by the potent antiemetic drugs ondansetron and granisetron. The 5-HT4, 5-HT6, and 5-HT7 receptors are positively coupled to G_s and therefore stimulate the adenylyl cyclase–cAMP–PKA pathway. The

5-HT4 receptors are highly concentrated in the striatum, substantia nigra, and hippocampus. In the enteric nervous system, serotonin acting via 5-HT3 and 5-HT4 receptors has an important role in gastrointestinal tract motility.

Physiology of Serotonergic Neurons

Serotonergic neurons constitute different subpopulations with respect not only to their targets but also to their electrophysiological characteristics and neurotransmission profile.[11] Some DR neurons rapidly respond to a variety of rewarding or aversive stimuli and to cues that predict these stimuli. Neurons of the ventromedial DR projecting to the PFC may be activated by reward and inhibited by punishment, whereas those in the dorsomedial DR projecting to the amygdala may be activated by both rewards and punishments. Cortical areas send excitatory projections that target the serotonergic neurons in the DR, whereas the central nucleus of the amygdala and hypothalamus send predominantly inhibitory GABAergic input that target local GABAergic interneurons. The interconnections are largely reciprocal, suggesting a role for feedback regulation of 5-HT projections by the target neurons.

Role of Serotonin in Control of Behavior

Specific subsets of serotonergic neurons have a differential role in distinct, wide-ranging behaviors and physiological processes. Serotonergic signals may produce both 5-HT2_A receptor-mediated excitation and 5-HT1_A receptor-mediated inhibition of principal cells or local GABAergic interneurons. In the cerebral cortex, serotonin elicits and 5-HT1_A receptor-mediated inhibition of principal cells; 5-HT3-mediated activation of a subset of GABAergic neurons targeting other GABAergic neurons, resulting in disinhibition of principal cells. Serotonergic neurons of the MR normally desynchronize hippocampal theta rhythms in the medial septum/diagonal band region. Optogenetic stimulation of serotonergic neurons in the dorsolateral portion of the DR that project to the amygdala produces anxiety-like behaviors; activation of serotonergic neurons in the ventromedial portion of the DR projecting to the orbitofrontal cortex decreases anxiety behavior. This indicates that the dorsolateral and the ventromedial DR systems functionally oppose one another.[11,14] Thus, globally targeting the serotonergic system using SSRI treatment is likely to activate antagonistic pathways.[14]

Role of Serotonin in Respiration, Thermoregulation, Motor Control, and Pain Modulation

Neurons of the caudal raphe are involved in central chemosensitivity, facilitation of respiratory reflexes, and control of body temperature. Subsets of neurons in the RMg respond to hypercapnia, and project to other chemosensitive respiratory areas of the brainstem. Neurons in the ROb and RPa heavily project to motor nuclei controlling airway and respiratory muscles. Descending projections from the RPa to the spinal cord also trigger thermogenic responses, including sympathetically mediated skin vasoconstriction, brown fat thermogenesis, and shivering. Serotonergic neurons in the ROb and RPa project to the ventral horn of the spinal cord targeting both motor neurons and interneurons.[15] Serotonin typically increases excitability of spinal motoneurons primarily via 5-HT2_A receptors. Serotonergic projections from the RMg and adjacent rostral ventromedial medulla to the dorsal horn are a fundamental component of the descending pain modulatory system that affects transmission of nociceptive inputs via presynaptic and postsynaptic mechanisms.

HISTAMINERGIC SYSTEM

The brain histaminergic system has an important role in maintenance of wakefulness. In addition, HA participates in suppression of REM sleep and control of circadian rhythms, feeding and endocrine function.[16]

Anatomical Organization

The tuberomammillary nucleus (TMN) is the sole source of histaminergic innervation of the CNS (Figure 20.10). The histaminergic TMN neurons include several cell clusters that have different physiological properties and are organized into distinct circuits.[17,18] Varicose axons of TMN neurons provide widespread input to all areas of the CNS, particularly the hypothalamus and cerebral cortex. Histaminergic pathways innervate the cholinergic and monoaminergic nuclei promoting wakefulness, as well as the basal forebrain, hippocampus, basal ganglia, cerebellum, and spinal cord. Microglia can also produce HA during inflammatory responses.

Presynaptic Events of Histaminergic Neurotransmission

Histamine is synthesized from L-histidine by action of the histidine-decarboxylase (HDC); this enzyme acts as an active homodimer and uses pyridoxal 5'-phosphate as a cofactor (Figure 20.11). Like other monoamines, HA is stored in synaptic vesicles via VMAT2 and released by exocytosis. However, unlike other monoamines, HA does not undergo presynaptic reuptake. Some HA may be taken up by the low-affinity organic cation transporter 3, which is expressed in astrocytes. Inactivation of HA in the extracellular space is achieved by the neuronal histamine N-methyltransferase (HNMT) with production of tele-methylhistamine, which undergoes oxidative deamination through a MAO_B to tele-methyl-imidazole acetic acid.

Histamine Receptors

The effects of histamine in the CNS are primarily mediated by H1, H2, and H3 receptors.[19] The H1 receptor (H1R) and H2 receptors (H2Rs) are located postsynaptically and, with few exceptions, mediate excitatory actions of HA. The H1R is coupled to $G_{q/11}$ proteins and triggers the PLC-DAG/

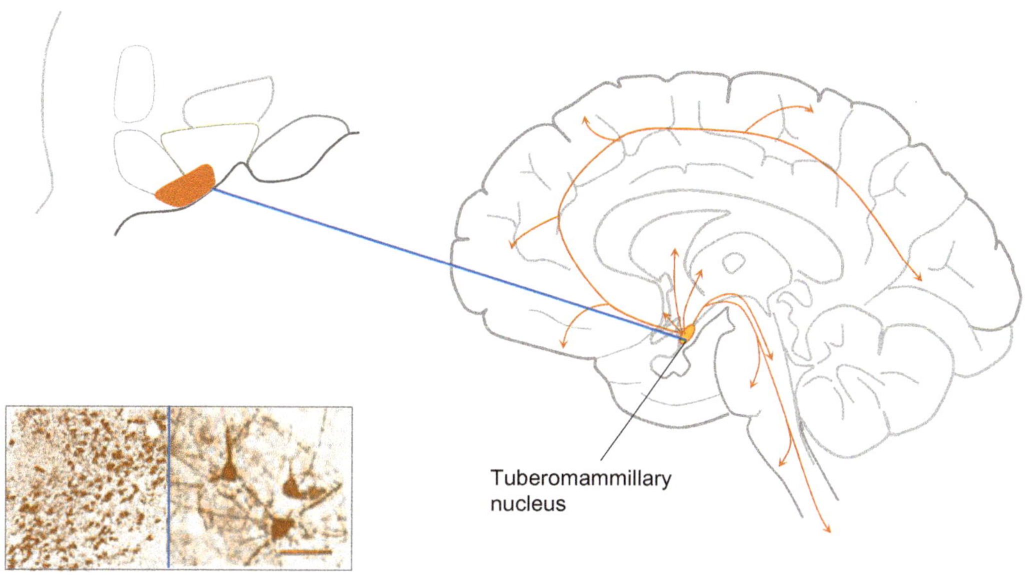

FIGURE 20.10 Anatomy of the histamine system.
The tuberomammillary nucleus (TMN) is the sole source of histaminergic innervation of the CNS. Varicose axons of TMN neurons provide widespread input to all areas of the CNS, particularly the hypothalamus, cerebral cortex as well as in the hippocampus, basal forebrain, basal ganglia, cerebellum, and spinal cord.

IP_3. H1Rs are widely distributed in the brain, particularly in the hypothalamus, monoaminergic and cholinergic brainstem nuclei, thalamus, and cortex. The H2R is coupled to G_s and activates the adenylyl cyclase–cAMP–PKA pathway. Phosphorylation by PKA inhibits Ca^{2+}-activated K^+ channels responsible for afterhyperpolarization and thus promotes repeated neuronal firing. The H3R is coupled to $G_i/_o$ signaling, inhibiting adenylyl cyclase and presynaptic Ca^{2+} channels responsible for neurotransmitter release. The H3R functions as a somatodendritic and presynaptic inhibitory autoreceptors in TMN neurons, inhibiting both firing of TMN neurons and HA release. H3Rs are also presynaptic inhibitory receptors in terminals releasing glutamate, GABA, acetylcholine, and other monoamines.

Physiology of Histaminergic Neurons

Histaminergic neurons in vitro have low frequency, rhythmic firing, broad action potentials, and a long latency to restart firing after sustained hyperpolarization, these properties largely reflect the effect of a prominent A-type K^+ potassium current. The TMN neurons fire fastest during wake, especially active wake state; they fire little during NREM sleep, and are essentially silent during REM sleep. Orexin neurons of the posterior lateral hypothalamus provide an important excitatory orexin 2 receptor mediated input to TMN neurons, maintaining the wake state. In the setting of a high histaminergic tone, HA can bind to H3R inhibitory somatodendritic autoreceptors in TMN neurons, reducing their pacemaker activity. Different TMN neuron subpopulations exhibit varied levels of baseline activity due to varied expression of inhibitory H3R autoreceptors and sensitivity to GABA, among other factors. For example, H3R antagonists increase HA release from terminals in the prefrontal cortex but not in the striatum. Histamine neurons respond to an increase in CO_2 and/or H^+ via both metabotropic glutamate receptors and acid-sensing ion channels. Activation of these neurons may affect central respiratory drive for example through activation of neurons in the nucleus of the solitary tract, which receives dense histaminergic innervation.

Function of Histamine in Wakefulness and Sleep

In the brain, HA participates in control of the circadian rhythm, maintenance of wakefulness, and inhibition of REM sleep.[16] There is a local circadian-like mechanism within the TMN that optimizes HA levels to maintain active wakefulness, with a peak of *Hdc* mRNA levels and HDC protein during the active period. Histamine maintains wakefulness via its effects on other wake-active groups of the brain stem and forebrain.[20] As the inhibitory H3R is expressed not only in TMN neurons but also presynaptically in terminals releasing glutamate, acetylcholine, DA, NE, or 5-HT, drugs that interfere with H3R signaling, such as pitolisant, can increase levels of many wake-promoting neurotransmitters. Since most H1Rs and H3Rs are constitutively active even in the absence of HA, sleep-promoting H1R antagonists such as diphenhydramine and wake-promoting H3R antagonists such as pitolisant are actually inverse agonists. In addition, HA projections excite local GABAergic neurons in the preoptic area, thereby inhibiting sleep-active GABAergic projection neurons in this

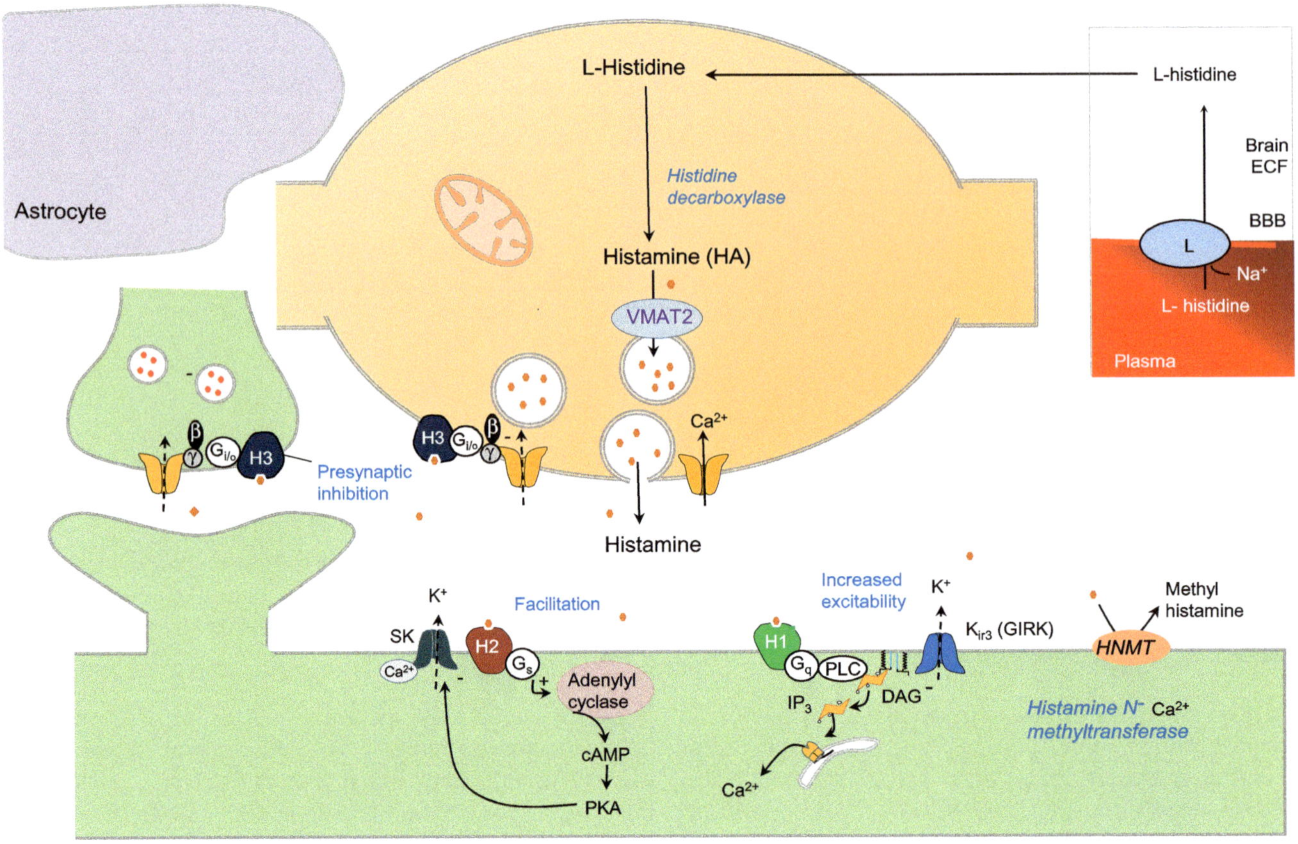

FIGURE 20.11 Histaminergic neurotransmission.
Histamine is synthesized from L-histidine by action of the histidine-decarboxylase. Like other monoamines, HA is stored in synaptic vesicles via the vesicular monoamine transporter 2 (VMAT-2), but unlike other monoamines, HA does not undergo presynaptic reuptake. Inactivation of HA in the extracellular space is achieved by the neuronal histamine N-methyltransferase (HNMT) with production of tele-methylhistamine, which undergoes oxidative deamination through a MAO_B to tele-methyl-imidazole acetic acid. The effects of histamine in the CNS are primarily mediated by H1, H2, and H3 receptors. The H1 receptor (H1R) and H2 receptors (H2Rs) are located postsynaptically and, with few exceptions, mediate excitatory actions. The H1R is coupled to $G_{q/11}$ proteins and triggers the phospholipase C (PLC)–diacylglycerol (DAG)–inositol triphosphate (IP_3) DAG/IP_3 pathway resulting in inhibition of Kir3 channels, activation of protein kinase C (PKC), and release of Ca^{2+} from intracellular stores. The H2R is coupled to G_s and activates the adenylyl cyclase–cAMP–PKA pathway. The H3R is coupled to $G_i/_o$ signaling, inhibiting adenylyl cyclase and presynaptic Ca^{2+} channels responsible for neurotransmitter release. The H3Rs thus function as somatodendritic and presynaptic inhibitory autoreceptors in TMN neurons. The H3Rs are also presynaptic inhibitory receptors in terminals releasing glutamate, GABA, acetylcholine, and other monoamines.

region. Knockout mice for HDC constitutively lacking HA or mice lacking H1Rs receptors have nearly normal amounts of wakefulness, indicating that other arousal systems can partially compensate for a chronic absence of HA. However the need of HA becomes evident when the mice are challenged to produce a high level of arousal. TMN neurons are capable of remarkable adaptation. Narcolepsy type 1 (NT1), which is characterized by a severe loss of orexin neurons, was found to be associated with increased number of HDC-immunoreactivity neurons in the TMN; this could reflect compensatory change in response to loss of orexin input.

Other Functions of Histaminergic Neurons

Histaminergic TMN neurons have also been implicated in control of cortical excitability, thermoregulation, stress response, control basal ganglia function, and feeding. Both H1Rs and H2Rs increase excitability of cortical interneurons; studies in several models of epilepsy indicate that H1Rs may a role in protection against seizures. Activation of H1R reduces food intake, whereas H3Rs promote food intake. H1R blockade has been implicated in the metabolic side effects, particularly weight gain, associated with chronic treatment with second-generation antipsychotics such as clozapine.[21] Histamine also regulates function in the striatum via through H1Rs, H2Rs, and H3Rs. Lack of HA synthesis due to *HDAC* mutations has been associated with Tourette syndrome.

PHARMACOLOGY OF MONOAMINERGIC TRANSMISSION

Monoaminergic transmission is an important target for treatment of neurological and psychiatric disorders. The major presynaptic targets include L-ADCC, VMATs, DAT, NET, and SERT, MAO_A, MAO_B, and COMT (Table 20.4). A large number of therapeutic drugs directly act via monoaminergic receptors (Table 20.5). Many drugs used to treat psychiatric disorders act via more than one mechanism. For example, new generation antipsychotic drugs used for schizophrenia and acute mania in bipolar disorders, such as clozapine, olanzapine, quetiapine, ziprasidone, and arsenapine block both 5-$HT2_A$ and D2 receptors. Aripiprazole has antagonist activity on 5-$HT2_A$ and is a weak agonist of D2 and 5-$HT1_A$ receptors. Overall, the antipsychotic effects of these drugs stems primarily from their activity as 5-$HT2_A$ and D2 receptors. Mirtazapine, which is used for treatment of depression is an antagonist of central presynaptic α2 inhibitory receptors thus enhancing central noradrenergic and serotonergic activity; it also has antagonist activity at central 5-HT2, 5-HT3, and H1 receptors and peripheral α1 and muscarinic receptors. Several antidepressant drugs that block 5-HT reuptake also have effects of 5-HT receptors. Many drugs inhibiting serotonin reuptake have additional mechanisms of action.

Trazodone, which is used for treatment of depression and insomnia, selectively inhibits 5-HT reuptake and acts as an antagonist at central 5-$HT2_A$ and 5-$HT2_C$ and peripheral α1 receptors. Vilazodone also inhibits 5-HT reuptake and

TABLE 20.4 *Presynaptic Pharmacological Targets of Monoaminergic Neurotransmission*

Target	Drugs (example)	Clinical use
L-AADC	Carbidopa	Parkinson disease (with levodopa) Action myoclonus (with 5-HTP) Autonomic spells (in HSAN3)
VMAT2	Tetrabenazine Valbenazine Deuterobenazine	Chorea Tardive dyskinesia
DAT	Bupropion	Depression Smoking cessation
NET	Atomoxetine	Depression Orthostatic hypotension
SERT (SSRI)	Fluoxetine, fluvoxamine, sertraline, paroxetine, citalopram, escitalopram	Depression Anxiety
SERT/NET (SNRI)	Tricycles (e.g., amitriptyline) Duloxetine Venlafaxine Desvenlafaxine Milnacipran	Depression Anxiety Pain Fibromyalgia
DAT/NET	Methylphenidate Dexamphetamine	Narcolepsy ADHD
MAO_A	Clorgyline Tranylcipromine	Depression
MAO_B	Selegiline Rasagiline Safinanide	Parkinson disease
COMT	Entacapone Opicapone	Parkinson disease (motor fluctuations)

L-ADDC, L amino acid decarboxylase; COMT, catechol-O-methyltransferase; DAT, dopamine transporter, MAO, monoamine oxidase; NET, norepinephrine transporter, SERT, serotonin transporter; VMAT2, vesicular monoamine transporter 2

TABLE 20.5 *Receptor Pharmacology in Neurologic and Psychiatric Disorders (examples)*

Neurotransmitter	Receptor Effect	Drug (example)	Therapeutic Use
Dopamine	D1R agonist	Levodopa Apomorphine	Parkinson disease
	D2R agonist	Levodopa, pramipexole, ropinirole, rotigotine	Parkinson disease Restless legs syndrome
	D2R antagonist	Haloperidol Clozapine Quetiapine Olanzapine Risperidone Ziprasidone	Hallucinations Bipolar disorder
Norepinephrine	α1AR agonist	Midodrine Droxidopa	Orthostatic hypotension
	α1AR antagonist	Prazosin	Nightmares
	α2AR agonist	Clonidine Guanfazine Tizanidine	ADHD Spasticity
	α2AR antagonist	Mirtazapine	Depression Sexual dysfunction?
	β2AR antagonist	Propranolol	Anxiety
Serotonin	$5HT1_A$R agonist	Buspirone	Anxiety
	$5HT1_{B/D}$ R agonist $5HT1_F$ R agonist	Triptans Lasmiditan	Migraine Cluster headache Migraine
	5-$HT2_A$R antagonist	Clozapine Quetiapine Olanzapine Risperidone Aripiprazole Ziprasidone Primavanserin*	Hallucinations Schizophrenia Bipolar disorder
	5-HT_3 antagonist	Ondasetron	Vomiting
Histamine	H1R antagonist	Diphenhydramine	Insomnia
	H3R antagonist	Pitolisant	Narcolepsy

* Lacks D2R blocking effects and is used for hallucinations in Parkinson disease

is a partial agonist of $5HT_{1A}$ receptors. Vortioxetine inhibits 5-HT reuptake, activates 5-$HT1_A$ receptors; is a partial agonist of 5-$HT1_B$ receptors; and an antagonist of 5-HT3, 5-$HT1_D$, and 5-HT7 receptors. A comprehensive review of this subject is beyond the scope of this chapter.

INHERITED MONOAMINE NEUROTRANSMITTER DISORDERS

Inherited disorders of neurotransmitters are rare metabolic diseases caused by impaired biosynthesis, breakdown or transport of neurotransmitters, or of lack of essential biosynthetic cofactors such as tetrahydrobiopterin (BH4) (Table 20.6). These disorders may result in a variety of clinical presentations ranging from late-onset movement disorders to early-onset lethal encephalopathies.[1,22,23] Primary monoamine neurotransmitter disorders can be clustered into (1) disorders of BH_4 synthesis or recycling, (2) primary enzyme defects in monoamine biosynthesis, (3) monoamine transporter defects, (4) monoamine catabolism disorders, and (5) chaperone-associated disorders.[23] Their clinical manifestations reflect deficits in dopaminergic, noradrenergic, and serotonergic neurotransmission.

TABLE 20.6 *Main Biochemical Features of Defects of Monoamine Metabolisms*

Defect	Neurotransmitter Affected	Neurochemical Profile in CSF	Other Neurochemical Markers
GCH1	DA>NE>5-HT BH4 cofactor	↓HVA, ↓5-HIAA ↓ biopterin	↑ plasma phenylalanine
Sepiapterin reductase	DA, NE, 5-HT BH4	↓HVA, ↓5-HIAA ↓ biopterin,	↑ plasma phenylalanine
PTPS	DA, NE, 5-HT BH4	↓HVA, ↓5-HIAA, ↓ biopterin,	↑ plasma phenylalanine
DHPR	DA, NE, 5-HTr ↓ folate	↓HVA, ↓5-HIAA, ↑ BH2	↑ plasma phenylalanine
TH	DA, NE	↓HVA, normal 5-HIAA ↓HVA/ 5-HIAA ratio	N/A
L-AADC	DA, NE, 5-HT	↓HVA, ↓5-HIAA ↑L-DOPA, ↑5-HTP ↑ 3-O-metyldopa	↑ plasma 3-MT (3-methoxytyrosine)-
DBH	NE	N/A	↓plasma NE, ↑plasma DA
VMAT2	DA, NE, 5-HT	↓HVA, ↓5-HIAA	*SLC18A2* mutation
DAT	DA	↑ HVA, normal 5-HIAA ↑ HVA/5-HIAA ratio	N/A
MAO_A, MAO_B		↓HVA, ↓5-HIAA, ↓MHPG	↑ Normetanephrine and 3-methoxytyramine in urine
DJ-1 chaperone	DA, NE, TH	↓HVA, ↓5-HIAA Normal biopterin	N/A

L-AADC, L-amino acid decarboxylase; DA, dopamine; DHPR, dihydropyridine reductase; 5-HT, HVA homovanillic acid; 5-hydroxytryptamine; 5-HIAA, 5-hydroxyindolaceti acid; MAO, monoamine oxidase; MHPG, methyl hydroxyphenylglycol; NE, norepinephrine; PTPS, 6-pyruvoyltetrahydropterin synthase; TH, tyrosine hydroxylase; VMAT, vesicular monoamine transporter 2.

Deficiency of DA is the most prominent contributor to the clinical phenotype, and the symptoms depend on the degree of DA deficit. They range from dopa-responsive dystonia (DRD) in children, to truncal hypotonia in infants with the progressive development of dystonia and parkinsonian features in the limbs, oculogyric crises, and occasionally dystonia-myoclonus or seizures. Norepinephrine deficits manifest with sympathetic dysfunction, including miosis, ptosis, nasal congestion, excessive salivation, excessive sweating, impaired thermoregulation, a predisposition to hypoglycemia, and in some cases orthostatic hypotension. Serotonin deficits may contribute to sleep disturbances and behavioral manifestations such as irritability. The diagnosis of genetic monoamine disorders is based on the history and examination, blood tests (plasma and dried blood spots), urine sampling, and CSF investigation. The deficit of individual neurotransmitters is determined by determination of CSF metabolites of DA (HVA), NE (MHPG), and serotonin (5-HIAA), as well as concentration of metabolites that accumulate due to interruption of a specific enzymatic step (Table 20.6).

Autosomal-Dominant GCH1 Deficiency as a Prototype of BH4 Deficiency

Autosomal-dominant GCH1 deficiency (Segawa disease, DYT5a, DYT/PARK-GCH1) is caused by autosomal-dominant *GCH1* mutations. Symptoms usually present within the first decade of life with dystonia starting in the lower extremities that asymmetrically progresses to the other limbs. Symptoms typically show a circadian fluctuation with worsening during the day and improvement after sleep. Parkinsonian symptoms can be present, especially later in the course. Sleep disturbance, anxiety, or depression are part of the phenotype. Levodopa/carbidopa supplementation drastically improves motor function, thereby having therapeutic and diagnostic value. Approximately 20% of patients develop levodopa-induced dyskinesia.

Primary Enzyme Defects in Monoamine Biosynthesis

Tyrosine hydroxylase deficiency (dopa-responsive dystonia, DYT5b, DYT/PARK-*TH*) is due to TH gene mutations resulting in isolated catecholamine deficiency. The clinical presentation includes dystonia, parkinsonism, ptosis, oculogyric crises, developmental delay, and autonomic dysfunction. Diagnosis is based on low CSF concentrations of HVA and 3MHPG, with a concurrent normal concentration of 5-HIAA and a low HVA/5-HIAA ratio. CSF HVA levels are helpful in determining L-dopa responsiveness. The treatment is levodopa-carbidopa; the patients are very sensitive and even low doses can produced dyskinesia or vomiting. Patients with poor response or fluctuations can benefit from MAO inhibitors such as selegiline or dopamine receptor agonists.

Aromatic L-amino acid decarboxylase deficiency results from mutations of the *ADDC* gene. The clinical phenotype reflects the combined absence or reduction of DA, NE, and 5-HT and thus resembles that of BH4 synthesis defects. Autonomic and behavioral dysregulation is more often seen in AADC deficiency than in other disorders. In the CSF, there is marked reduction in HVA and 5-HIAA combined with elevated levels of L-DOPA, 5-HT and 3-orthomethyldopa (3-OMD) a product of L-dopa methylation. Plasma levels of 3-methoxytyrosine (3-MT) are a viable biomarker for AADC deficiency. Treatment includes dopamine agonists and/or MAO inhibitors, and pyridoxal phosphate), the active form of pyridoxine, the cofactor of AADC.

Dopamine-β-hydroxylase deficiency due to *DBH* gene mutation is a very rare disease that results in increased levels of DA and impaired synthesis of NE. As a consequence, it manifests with severe orthostatic hypotension combined with ptosis, usually developing during late childhood. The phenotype includes hyperinsulinemia, increased glucose-triggered insulin secretion, and peripheral resistance toward insulin. Reduced or absent blood levels of NE and epinephrine simultaneously elevated DA levels are a biomarker of this disorder. Similar phenotypes have been described in members of families harboring mutations in the *CYB561* gene encoding CYB561, the vesicular electron carrier required for normal DBH function. The synthetic amino acid L-threo-dihydroxyphenylserine (L-threo-DOPS, droxidopa) is converted to NE by L-AADC and can maintain NE synthesis in patients with congenital DBH deficiency.

Monoamine Transporter Defects

Vesicular monoamine transporter 2 (VMAT2) deficiency due to *SLC18A2* gene mutations results in DA, NE, and 5-HT deficiency. It manifests with early childhood developmental delay, axial hypotonia, oculogyric crises, bulbar dysfunction, parkinsonian features, and dystonic attacks (reflecting DA deficiency); sweating, profuse nasal and oropharyngeal secretions, and postural hypotension (reflecting NE deficiency); and insomnia and depression (presumably due to 5-HT deficiency). Levodopa/carbidopa can worsen symptoms, pramipexole produces substantial symptom relief. Dopamine transporter (DAT) deficiency syndrome due *SLC6A3* mutations results in accumulation DA in the synaptic cleft and excessive activation of D2Rs. Activation of postsynaptic D2Rs lead to hyperkinesia and sleep disturbance; activation of presynaptic D2Rs probably decreases DA synthesis as a negative feedback-loop earlier or later in the course. Movement disorders develop during early childhood with axial hypotonia, chorea, dystonia, or dystonia-parkinsonism, and over time the hyperkinetic features shift toward parkinsonism. A later-onset subtype is characterized by juvenile-onset parkinsonism with dystonia. There is a combination of elevated HVA and normal 5-HTAA levels resulting in an increased HVA/5-HIAA ratio in the CSF. Treatment includes dopamine agonists showing high affinity to presynaptic autoreceptors, such as pramipexole, ropinirole, or rotigotine.

Disorders of Monoamine Metabolism

Monoamine oxidase deficiency is a rare X-linked condition due to mutations in the *MAOA* or *MAOB* genes on chromosome Xp11.23 Whereas isolated MAO_B deficiency is frequently asymptomatic, isolated MAO_A deficiency is associated with mental retardation and severe behavioral abnormalities including repeating aggressive and violent outbursts, and occasionally autonomic dysregulation with flushing and diarrhea have been reported. Combined MAO_A and MAO_B deficiency leads to mental retardation, sporadic episodes of hypotonia, stereotypical movements, and epilepsy. Biochemical features include increased levels of MAO_A substrates such as normetanephrine and 3-methoxytyramine in urine and reduced levels of products of MAO_A oxidation such as HVA, MHPG, and 5-HIAA in the CSF.

Chaperone-Associated Neurotransmitter Disorders

Biallelic mutations in the *DNAJC12*, encoding a heat shock co-chaperone of the HSP40 family that interacts with phenylalanine hydroxylase, TH, and TPH, produce hyperphenylalalinemia and deficiency of DA and 5-HT. There is a broad spectrum of symptoms including dystonia, speech delay, axial and limb hypertonia, parkinsonism, and psychiatric features. Another phenotype is that of slowly progressing parkinsonism and mild intellectual disability with disease onset in adolescence. CSF pattern shows decreased HVA and 5-HIAA concentrations with normal or elevated levels of biopterin.

KEY POINTS

- The central monoaminergic systems consist of neurons in restricted areas of the brainstem and hypothalamus that project to widespread areas of the CNS.
- Monoaminergic systems exert a global control of neuronal excitability and network activity which is fundamental for behavioral arousal, attention, motivation, and stress responses.
- These monoaminergic systems include dopamine (DA) neurons of the ventral tegmental area (VTA), substantia nigra pars compacta (SNc), and other groups; norepinephrine(NE) neurons of the locus coeruleus (LC) and ventrolateral medulla;

serotonin (5-HT) neurons the raphe nuclei; and histamine (HA) neurons of the tuberomammillary nucleus (TMN).

- Monoaminergic neurons have a slow, tonic activity during quiet wakefulness, increase their activity during tasks requiring attention and motivation, reduce their activity during non-rapid eye movement (NREM) sleep, and are virtually silent during REM sleep.
- Inputs from the prefrontal cortex (PFC) promote activity of monoaminergic groups promoting attention; excitatory inputs from orexin/hypocretin neurons to monoaminergic groups maintain wakefulness.
- Monoamine neurotransmitters are synthesized from essential amino acids by action of rate-limiting enzymes.
- The initial steps of biosynthesis of DA, NE, and 5-HT critically depend on the availability of tetrahydrobiopterin (BH4).
- The rate-limiting enzyme for synthesis of catecholamines is tyrosine hydroxylase (TH), leading to production of L-DOPA that is then decarboxylated to DA by L-amino acid decarboxylase (L-AADC).
- In noradrenergic neurons, DA is converted to NE by action of dopamine-β-hydroxylase (DBH).
- The rate-limiting enzyme of serotonin synthesis is tryptophan hydroxylase.
- The rate-limiting enzyme for histamine synthesis is histidine decarboxylase.
- Monoamines are incorporated into synaptic vesicles via a common vesicular monoamine transporter VMAT2.
- Monoamines undergo presynaptic reuptake via partially selective membrane transporters, including the DA transporter (DAT), NE transporter (NET), and serotonin transporter (SERT); histamine does not undergo reuptake.
- After uptake, DA, NE, and 5-HT undergo metabolism by monoamine oxidases (MAOs) and, in the case of catecholamines, also by the catechol-O-methyltransferase (COMT).
- Metabolites of monoamines can be detected in the CSF and serve as biomarkers of monoamine synthesis and turnover.
- Monoamines act both via synaptic and volume transmission mechanisms via several subtypes of G protein-coupled receptors (GPCRs), with the exception of the 5-HT3 receptor, which is a cation channel.
- Midbrain dopaminergic neurons of the VTA and SNc primarily target the striatum and the frontal cortex.
- The D1-type receptors (D1R) increase neuronal excitability and promote synaptic plasticity; D2-type (D2R) receptors mediate presynaptic and postsynaptic inhibition.
- The tonic discharge of midbrain dopaminergic neurons maintains a steady baseline level of DA, which acts primarily via extrasynaptic D2Rs to maintain a low background inhibition in the striatum, and PFC.
- Burst firing of midbrain dopaminergic neurons produces "transients" of extracellular DA levels that activates of postsynaptic D1Rs and D2Rs in the striatum, promoting reward-based action learning, goal-directed action selection, and habit formation.
- Dopamine transients in the PFC facilitate attentional processes such as working memory.
- The LC-NE-synthesizing neurons provide extensive innervation throughout the neuraxis.
- The lateral tegmental catecholaminergic targets the hypothalamus and autonomic nuclei.
- The effects of NE are mediated by α1, α2, and β receptors; postsynaptic α1 and β receptors mediate excitatory effects; α2 receptors mediate presynaptic inhibition and promote recurrent network activity in the PFC.
- The tonic activity of LC-NE neurons reflects the arousal state.
- During focused attention, LC neurons transiently interrupt their moderate tonic firing and respond with a phasic mode to task-relevant stimuli; this facilitates working memory and focused task performance by filtering of irrelevant stimuli.
- The LC-NE has a major role in response to stress via interaction with the amygdala, hypothalamus, brainstem, and spinal autonomic nuclei.
- The serotonergic neurons of the rostral raphe nuclei are subdivided into a rostral group—including the dorsal raphe (DR) and median raphe (MR) nuclei—that project to the forebrain and a caudal group—nucleus raphe magnus (RMg), raphe obscurus (ROb), and raphe pallidus-(RPa)—that project to the brainstem and spinal cord.
- Serotonin acts via a wide range of receptors, 5-HT1 receptors mediate postsynaptic and presynaptic inhibition; 5-HT2 receptors mediate postsynaptic excitation; 5-HT4-7 receptors have variable excitatory function; and 5-HT3 receptors are Ca^{2+} channels that elicit fast excitation.
- Rostral raphe neurons modulate reward, anxiety, and impulse control; those in the caudal raphe have a major role in descending modulation of pain and motor neuron excitability, activation of respiration, and thermoregulation.
- Histaminergic neurons of the TMN provide widespread projection through the CNS.
- The effects of histamine in the CNS are primarily mediated by H1 and H2 receptors, with primarily exert excitatory effects, and H3 receptors primarily mediate presynaptic inhibition.

- The central histaminergic system has a major role in maintenance of wakefulness and also participates in control of circadian rhythms, cortical excitability, feeding, and endocrine functions.
- Monoaminergic transmission is an important target for treatment of neurologic psychiatric disorders; the targets include L-ADCC, VMAT2, DAT, NET, SERT, MAO_A, MAO_B, COMT, and different subtypes of receptors.
- Inherited monoamine neurotransmitter disorders include disorders of BH_4 synthesis or recycling with (such as *GCH1s*), primary defects in monoamine biosynthesis (such as *TH, L-AADC* or *DBH* mutations), monoamine transporter defects (*VAMT2* mutations), monoamine catabolism disorders (*MAOA* or *MAOB* mutations), and chaperone-associated disorders (*DNAJC12* mutations).
- The clinical manifestations reflect deficit of dopamine, norepinephrine, and serotonin, either in isolation or combination and may result in a variety of clinical presentations ranging from late-onset movement disorders to early-onset lethal encephalopathies.
- Deficiency of DA is the most prominent contributor to the clinical phenotype, and manifests with dopa-responsive dystonia, progressive dystonia and parkinsonism, oculogyric crises, and occasionally dystonia-myoclonus or seizures.
- Norepinephrine deficits manifest with sympathetic dysfunction, including miosis, ptosis, nasal congestion, excessive salivation, excessive sweating, impaired thermoregulation, a predisposition to hypoglycemia, and in some cases orthostatic hypotension.
- Serotonin deficits may contribute to sleep disturbances and behavioral manifestations such as irritability.
- The deficit of individual neurotransmitters is determined by determination of CSF metabolites of DA (HVA), NE (MHPG), and serotonin (5-HIAA) as well as concentration of metabolites that accumulate due to interruption of a specific enzymatic step.

REFERENCES

1. Ng J, Papandreou A, Heales SJ, Kurian MA. Monoamine neurotransmitter disorders—clinical advances and future perspectives. Nat Rev Neurol 2015;11:567–584.
2. Mulvihill KG. Presynaptic regulation of dopamine release: Role of the DAT and VMAT2 transporters. Neurochem Int 2019;122:94–105.
3. Cheng MH, Bahar I. Monoamine transporters: structure, intrinsic dynamics and allosteric regulation. Nat Struct Mol Biol 2019;26:545–556.
4. Beaulieu JM, Espinoza S, Gainetdinov RR. Dopamine receptors—IUPHAR review 13. Br J Pharmacol 2015;172:1–23.
5. Schultz W. Updating dopamine reward signals. Curr Opin Neurobiol 2013;23:229–238.
6. Morrison JH, Foote SL. Noradrenergic and serotoninergic innervation of cortical, thalamic, and tectal visual structures in Old and New World monkeys. J Comp Neurol 1986;243:117–138.
7. Arnsten AF, Wang MJ, Paspalas CD. Neuromodulation of thought: flexibilities and vulnerabilities in prefrontal cortical network synapses. Neuron 2012;76:223–239.
8. Aston-Jones G, Waterhouse B. Locus coeruleus: from global projection system to adaptive regulation of behavior. Brain Res 2016;1645:75–78.
9. Stornetta RL, Guyenet PG. C1 neurons: a nodal point for stress? Exp Physiol 2018;103:332–336.
10. Fischer AG, Ullsperger M. An update on the role of serotonin and its interplay with dopamine for reward. Front Hum Neurosci 2017;11:484.
11. Ren J, Friedmann D, Xiong J, et al. Anatomically defined and functionally distinct dorsal raphe serotonin sub-systems. Cell 2018;175:472–487 e420.
12. Paul ED, Lowry CA. Functional topography of serotonergic systems supports the Deakin/Graeff hypothesis of anxiety and affective disorders. J Psychopharmacol 2013;27:1090–1106.
13. Okaty BW, Commons KG, Dymecki SM. Embracing diversity in the 5-HT neuronal system. Nat Rev Neurosci 2019;20:397–424.
14. Vahid-Ansari F, Zhang M, Zahrai A, Albert PR. Overcoming resistance to selective serotonin reuptake inhibitors: targeting serotonin, serotonin-1A receptors and adult neuroplasticity. Front Neurosci 2019;13:404.
15. Kawashima T. The role of the serotonergic system in motor control. Neurosci Res 2018;129:32–39.
16. Scammell TE, Jackson AC, Franks NP, Wisden W, Dauvilliers Y. Histamine: neural circuits and new medications. Sleep 2019;42:1–8.
17. Haas HL, Sergeeva OA, Selbach O. Histamine in the nervous system. Physiol Rev 2008;88:1183–1241.
18. Umehara H, Mizuguchi H, Fukui H. Identification of a histaminergic circuit in the caudal hypothalamus: an evidence for functional heterogeneity of histaminergic neurons. Neurochem Int 2012;61:942–947.
19. Panula P, Chazot PL, Cowart M, et al. International Union of Basic and Clinical Pharmacology. XCVIII. Histamine receptors. Pharmacol Rev 2015;67:601–655.
20. Parmentier R, Zhao Y, Perier M, et al. Role of histamine H1-receptor on behavioral states and wake maintenance during deficiency of a brain activating system: a study using a knockout mouse model. Neuropharmacology 2016;106:20–34.
21. Provensi G, Blandina P, Passani MB. The histaminergic system as a target for the prevention of obesity and metabolic syndrome. Neuropharmacology 2016;106:3–12.
22. Kurian MA, Gissen P, Smith M, Heales S, Jr., Clayton PT. The monoamine neurotransmitter disorders: an expanding range of neurological syndromes. Lancet Neurol 2011;10:721–733.
23. Brennenstuhl H, Jung-Klawitter S, Assmann B, Opladen T. Inherited disorders of neurotransmitters: classification and practical approaches for diagnosis and treatment. Neuropediatrics 2019;50:2–14.

Section III

Microenvironment and Mechanisms of Injury and Repair

21 Astrocytes and Astrocyte–Neuron Interactions

OVERVIEW

Astrocytes constitute a heterogeneous population that primarily includes protoplasmic and fibrous subtypes and express the intermediate filament glial fibrillary acid protein (GFAP). Astrocytes extend perisynaptic processes ensheathing synapses, endfoot processes that contact cerebral microvessels, perinodal processes around axons, and subpendymal processes that form the glia limitans. They are interconnected via gap junctions that provide for the formation of functional syncytia and are fundamental components of the neurovascular unit, including the blood-brain barrier (BBB) (Figure 21.1). Astrocytes express a large repertoire of ion channels, receptors, transporters, and other molecules, enabling them to sense a multitude of signals from neighboring synapses, other glial cells, vascular endothelium, and pericytes, and to participate in several homeostatic processes (Figure 21.2). Astrocytes have multiple fundamental functions in the CNS (Figure 21.3). They have major role in uptake and recycling of glutamate and GABA released at synaptic and extrasynaptic sites and provide metabolic support to active neurons by releasing lactate. They are also critical for buffering the increase in extracellular potassium (K^+) resulting from synaptic activity and they control water homeostasis in both the extracellular and intracellular compartments, including the myelin sheaths. Astrocytes sense neuronal activity, which triggers increases in intracellular calcium (Ca^{2+}), and they initiate both local transients and a propagating Ca^{2+} wave that propagates across the astrocyte network. In response to synaptic activity, astrocytes release chemical transmitters, referred to as gliotransmitters, such as glutamate, D-serine, and ATP (then converted to adenosine), which modulate transmission at neighboring synapses. Astrocytes also release signals such as lipid mediators, which have a critical role in coupling of synaptic activity with local blood flow. They also release extracellular matrix molecules and trophic factors that are important for synaptic development and plasticity, as well as multiple inflammatory mediators. Astrocytes are primarily affected in genetic disorders such as Alexander disease, hepatic encephalopathy, and autoimmune neuromyelitis optica spectrum disorders (NMOSD) and have a major role in epilepsy. They are critical elements of neuroinflammation in traumatic, vascular, inflammatory/demyelinating, and neurodegenerative disorders. Astrocyte senescence and age-associated adoption of a proinflammatory phenotype are important drivers of neurodegeneration. The aims of this chapter are to review (1) the functional heterogeneity and compartmentalization of astrocytes, (2) their role in regulation of extracellular ion and water homeostasis, (3) their fundamental function in control of neurotransmitter homeostasis and metabolic support, (4) calcium signaling and secretory functions of astrocytes, (5) their role in neurovascular coupling, (6) reciprocal neuron-astrocyte interactions regulating synaptic plasticity and network activity, and (7) representative examples of astrocytopathies.

HETEROGENEITY AND FUNCTIONAL COMPARTMENTALIZATION OF ASTROCYTES

Astrocytes constitute a heterogeneous population and differ in their morphology, developmental origin, gene-expression profiles, physiological properties, function, and response to injury and disease.[1,2] Astrocytes from different brain regions vary in their expression of membrane surface glycoproteins, ion channels, neurotransmitter receptors, transporters, and signaling molecules. Human astrocytes express specific genes that undergo transcriptome-wide transformations during development.[3] Astrocytes are classically subdivided into two main categories, protoplasmic

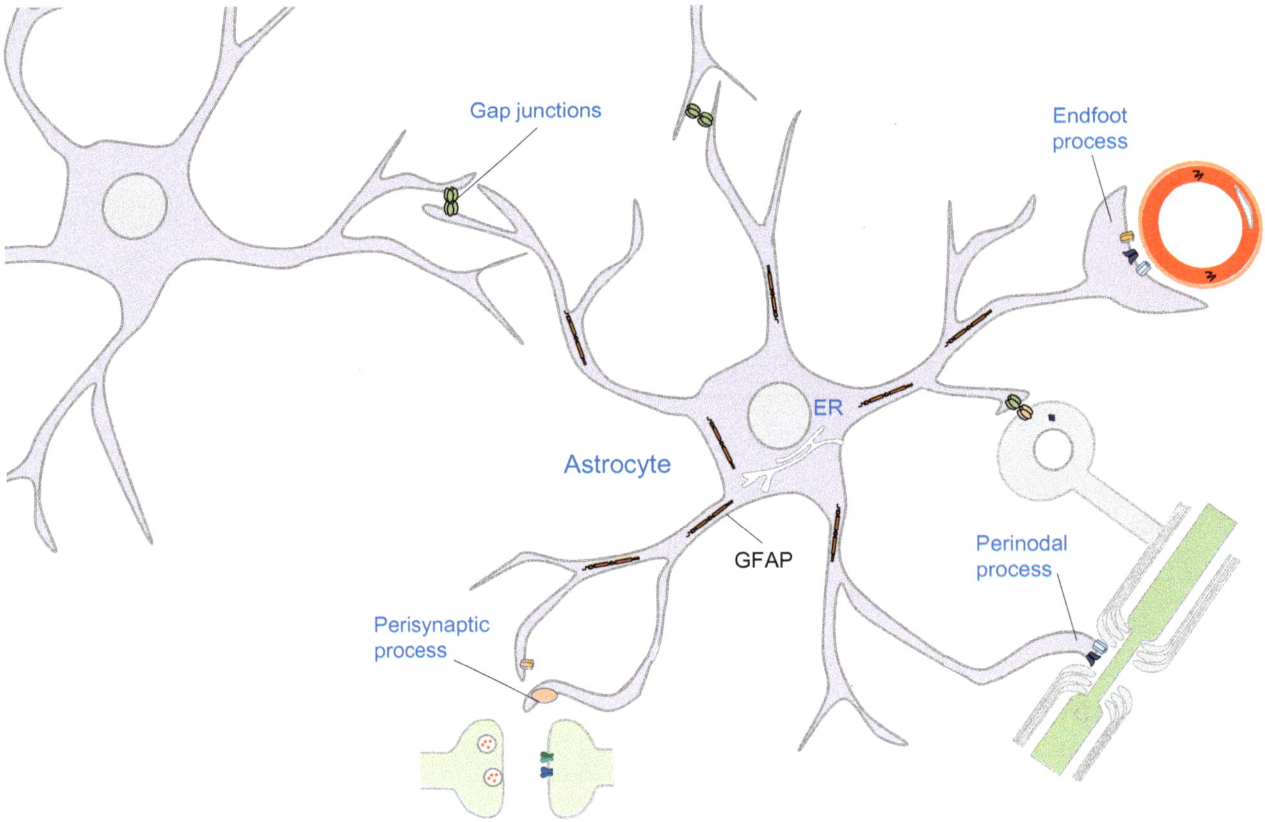

FIGURE 21.1 Functional compartments in astrocytes.
Astrocytes are characterized by the expression of the intermediate filament protein glial fibrillary acid protein (GFAP) and consist of several functional compartments with particular repertoires of ion channels and receptors. They extend perisynaptic processes ensheathing synapses endfoot processes that contact cerebral microvessels; perinodal processes around axons, and subependymal processes that form the glial limitans. They are interconnected via gap junctions that provide for the formation functional syncytia and are fundamental components of the neurovascular unit, including the blood-brain barrier (BBB). ER, endoplasmic reticulum.

and fibrous. Protoplasmic astrocytes represent the largest population of astrocytes in the gray matter, and are mainly found in the hippocampus and cerebral cortex. Their cell bodies are extremely ramified, which allows them to touch numerous synapses. In humans, cortical protoplasmic astrocytes are nearly three-fold larger in diameter, extend ten times more primary processes, and contact nearly 100-fold more synapses located in their territorial domains than their counterparts in rodents. Fibrous astrocytes are organized along white matter tracts; they are smaller and have fewer branching points than the protoplasmic astrocytes and can contact the nodes of Ranvier. The human brain also has exclusive subtypes of astrocytes, such as the interlaminar astrocytes located in the superficial cortical layers and sending long processes to deep layers, and varicose projection astrocytes located in deep cortical layers and sending very long varicose fibers in all directions in the cerebral cortex. There are other astrocyte-like cells that have important roles both during development and in the adult CNS. Radial glial cells are the main progenitor of neurons and glial cells during brain development and guide neuronal migration in the cerebral cortex. Bergmann glia are involved in granular cell migration and ensheath cerebellar synapses. Another example is Müller cells in the retina. Enteric glia constitute and heterogeneous cell populations that express genetic markers of either Schwann cells or astrocytes and are found within the enteric plexuses closely apposing and partially ensheathing ganglion neurons and form a dense diffuse network in the mucosae of the gut. Astrocytes are characterized by their expression of GFAP, which is responsible for their cytoskeletal architecture and mechanical strength.[4] However, GFAP is not broadly expressed by all astrocytes across brain areas and includes different isoforms that may be variably expressed in specific subsets of astrocytes.

In gray matter, astrocytes divide the parenchyma into relatively independent and nonoverlapping functional units known as neurovascular or astrogliovascular units. Astrocytes consist of different functional compartments with a unique repertoire of ion channels and transporters

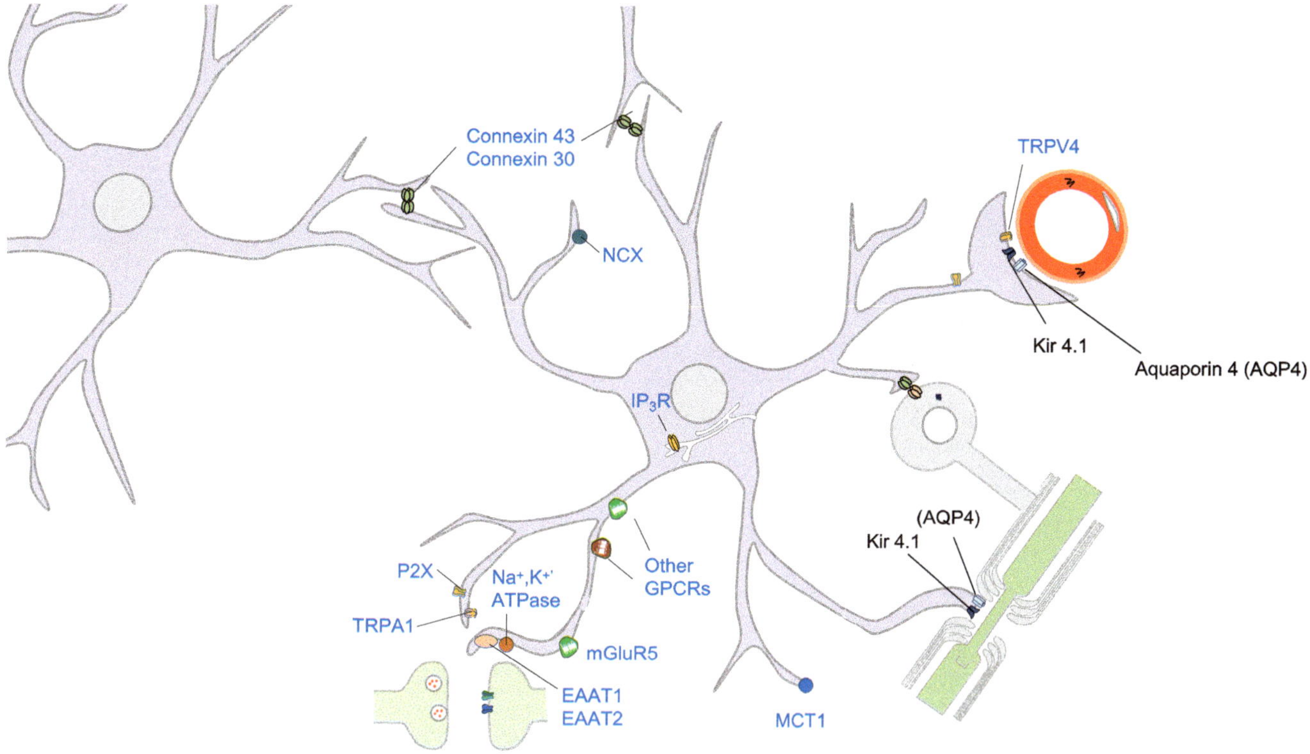

FIGURE 21.2 Compartmental distribution channels and receptors in astrocytes.
Astrocytes express a large repertoire of ion channels, receptors, transporters, and other molecules that have a preferential distribution in distinct compartments. The distal perisynaptic astrocytic processes are enriched with the excitatory amino acid transporters (EAATs) -1 and -2, which are critical for uptake of glutamate from synapses, and the transient receptor potential (TRP) ankyrin type 1 (TRPA1), which contributes to Ca^{2+} influx at distal astrocytic processes. In contrast, Ca^{2+} storage structures such as the endoplasmic reticulum (ER) are located far from the synapses and mediate the effects of a variety of guanine nucleotide (G) protein-coupled receptors (GPCRs), including metabotropic glutamate receptors (mGluRs), by releasing Ca^{2+} via inositol 3 phosphate receptors (IP_3Rs). Calcium signals also involve purinergic P2X and P2Y receptors, and activity of the Na^+/Ca^{2+} exchanger (NCX).

involved in maintenance of ion and water homeostasis (Table 21.1), metabolic support and recycling of neurotransmitters (Table 21.2), and receptors triggering Ca^{2+} signaling in astrocytes (Table 21.3).[5]

Perisynaptic Processes

The perisynaptic astrocytic processes interact with neurons via small, fiber-like structures referred to as leaflets or branchlets; the perisynaptic processes of a single protoplasmic astrocyte may cover up to 2 million synapses in human cerebral cortex,[6] These perisynaptic processes interact both structurally and functionally with the presynaptic and postsynaptic terminals, creating a tripartite synapse.[7,8] They embrace the synapse and create an "astroglial cradle" that confers isolation and spatial specificity to synaptic inputs by controlling local ion, neurotransmitter, and metabolic homeostasis.[9] The distal perisynaptic astrocytic processes are enriched by the excitatory amino acid transporters (EAAT) 1 and 2, which are critical for uptake of glutamate from synapses, and the transient receptor potential (TRP) ankyrin type 1 (TRPA1), which contributes to Ca^{2+} influx at distal astrocytic process. In contrast, Ca^{2+} storage structures such as the endoplasmic reticulum (ER) are located far from the synapses and mediate the effects of a variety of guanine nucleotide (G) protein-coupled receptors (GPCRs) expressed in astrocytes.

Astrocytic Endfeet

The endfeet of the astrocytes cover about 99% of the abluminal surface of blood vessels,[10] and together with vascular cells and neuronal terminals form the neurovascular unit.[11] At this level, astrocytes participate both in the structural and functional organization of the blood-brain barrier (BBB) and regulation of local cerebral blood flow (CBF) in response to neuronal activity.[12] The astrocytic endfoot processes are enriched by the inward-rectifying potassium channel 4.1 (Kir4.1), the water channel aquaporin 4 (AQP4), and the TRP vanilloid receptor type 4 (TRPV4).[5]

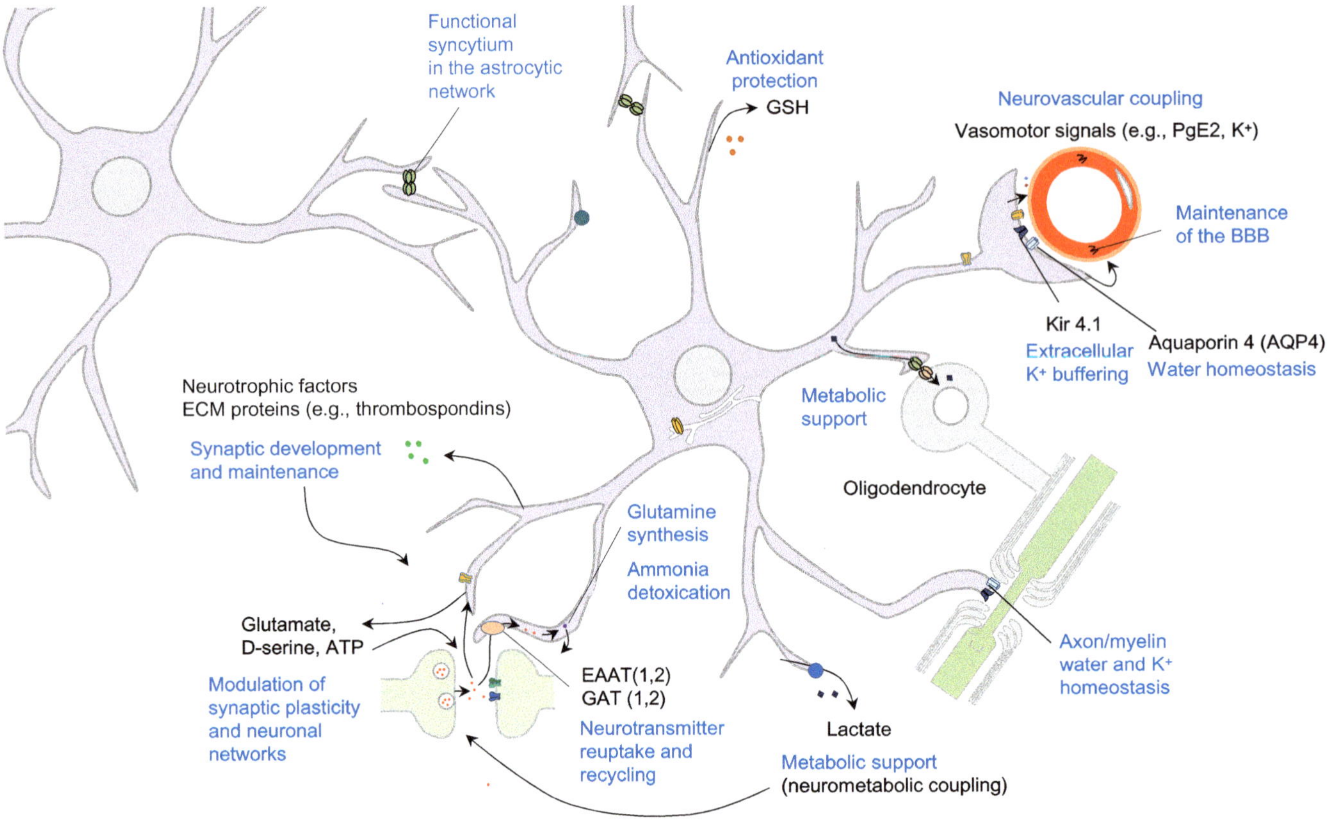

FIGURE 21.3 Main function of astrocytes.
Astrocytes have a major role in uptake of glutamate and GABA released at synaptic and extrasynaptic sites and synthesize glutamine as a substrate for resynthesis of these neurotransmitters. Astrocytes also provide metabolic support to active neurons as well as oligodendrocytes by releasing lactate, and are critical for buffering the increase in extracellular potassium (K^+) via inward-rectifying Kir4.1 and control water homeostasis via aquaporin 4 (AQP4) channels, both at the extracellular and intracellular compartments, including the myelin sheaths. Astrocytes release transmitters, referred to as gliotransmitters, such as glutamate, D-serine, and ATP (then converted to adenosine), which modulate transmission at neighboring synapses. They also release signals such as lipid mediators involved in coupling of synaptic activity with local cerebral blood flow (CBF). Astrocytes release trophic factors and extracellular matrix (ECM), proteins involved in formation and maintenance of synapses. EAAT, excitatory amino acid transporter; GAT, GABA transporter; GSH, glutathione; PgE2, prostglandin E2.

This differential localization reflects the presence of diffusion barriers between the astrocytic endfeet and the rest of the cell.[13]

Astrocytes also extend endfoot processes to the surface of the brain parenchyma. These processes and the associated basement membrane constitute the glial limitans that prevents the free access of immune cells to the CNS. Astrocytes in the CNS also extend processes that surround the nodes of Ranvier. These perinodal processes have a major role in the ion and water homeostasis in the axon and myelin sheath.

Gap Junction and Astrocyte Networks

In the adult brain, astrocytes are interconnected via gap junctions composed of connexins 43 and 30.[14,15] Gap junction channels are formed by the alignments of two connexin (Cx) hemichannels and provide for the formation of large syncytial networks composed of hundreds of astrocytes. Gap junctions allow localized signals to spread and amplify across broad regions via direct intercellular diffusion of ions (ionic coupling), and small molecules such as energy metabolites among interconnected astrocytes, as well as between astrocytes, oligodendrocytes, neurons, and blood vessels. Important functions attributed to astrocytic gap junction coupling include spatial buffering of K^+ and glutamate, regulation of cell volume, trafficking and delivery of energy metabolites from blood vessels to neurons and oligodendrocytes, and intercellular propagation of Ca^{2+} waves.[14,15] The permeability and selectivity of gap junction channels are regulated by a variety of signals. For example, the depolarizing actions of glutamate or K^+ may increase gap junction permeability via Ca^{2+} triggered phosphorylation of Cx43.[15]

TABLE 21.1 *Astrocytic Membrane Proteins Involved in CNS Ion and Water Homeostasis*

Protein	Function
Sodium (Na^+)/potassium (K^+) ATPase	Maintains transmembrane Na^+ gradient required to drive other transporters K^+ homeostasis Activation of glycolysis
Aquaporin 4	Water channel involved in volume regulation
Inward-rectifying K^+ channel (Kir) 4.1	K^+ homeostasis Volume regulation
Na^+/K^+/chloride (Cl^-) cotransporter 1 (KCC1)	K^+ homeostasis Maintenance of cell volume
Na^+/calcium (Ca^{2+}) exchanger (NCX)	Bidirectional regulation of Na^+ and Ca^{2+} influx or efflux
Na^+/bicarbonate cotransporter	Contributes to resting intercellular Na^+ levels Regulation of pH and volume
Na^+/proton (H^+) exchanger (NHE)	Pumps H^+ into cells Drives lactate efflux
Connexin 30 and 43 hemichannels	Gap junction formation Gliotransmitter release (hemichannels)

ASTROCYTES AND REGULATION OF ION AND WATER HOMEOSTASIS

Astrocytes express a variety of membrane transporters and channels that control ion and fluid homeostasis[16] (Figure 21.4) (Table 21.1).

Sodium and pH Homeostasis

Synaptic activity triggers Na^+ transients in astrocytes via influx through both Na^+ permeable channels and Na^+ transporters.[17–19] The main astroglial Na^+ transporter is the Na^+/ K^+ ATPase, consisting of α1 or α2 subunits containing isoforms and is the primary driver for secondary transport systems. Astrocytes can also transport Na^+ via the Na^+/bicarbonate cotransporter (NBC) and the Na^+/K^+/Cl^- chloride (Cl^-) cotransporter 1 (NKCC1), which are involved in regulation of intercellular pH and volume. Astrocytes express Na^+/Ca^{2+} exchangers (NCXs) that operate in both forward and reverse modes, according to transmembrane ion gradients and membrane potential.[20] Transmembrane Na^+ gradients have several fundamental roles in astrocytes. They drive glutamate, GABA, and glycine uptake via their respective transporters at synapses; promote Ca^{2+} signaling via reversal of the Na^+/Ca^{2+} exchanger; regulate K^+ homeostasis by driving uptake of extracellular K^+; participate in transport systems involved in pH homeostasis and cell volume; and initiate the astrocyte-to-neuron lactate shuttle via stimulation of glycolysis.[19,21,22] There are close

TABLE 21.2 *Astrocytic Membrane Proteins Involved in Neurotransmitter Homeostasis and Metabolic Support*

Protein	Function
Glucose transporter-1 (GLUT1)	Uptake of glucose from the blood stream
Monocarboxylic transporter 1	Lactate shuttle from the astrocyte to neurons
Excitatory amino-acid transporter (EAAT1 and EAAT2)	Sodium-dependent uptake of L-glutamate from the synaptic space
GABA transporters (GAT) 1 and 3	Sodium-dependent uptake of GABA from the synaptic space
Glycine transporter (GlyT) 1	Sodium-dependent uptake of glycine glutamate from the synaptic space
Glutamine transporter (SAT)	Glutamine export from the astrocytes to neurons

TABLE 21.3 *Astrocytic Receptor and Channels Involved Signaling Mechanisms*

Protein	Function
Purinergic P2X7 and P2Y1 receptors	Fast excitatory (P2X7) and modulatory (P2Y1) effects of ATP
Transient receptor potential (TRP) ankyrin 1 subtype (TRPA1)	Tonic Ca^{2+} influx at perisynaptic terminals
TRP vanilloid receptor 4 (TRPV4)	Mechanosensation at the astrocyte endfeet
Metabotropic glutamate receptor 5 (mGluR) 5	Inositol triphosphate receptor 2 (IP_3R_2)–mediated Ca^{2+} release from intracellular stores in response to excitatory synaptic activity
Noradrenergic α1 receptors	IP_3R_2-triggered intracellular Ca^{2+} release during arousal states
Cannabinoid CB1 receptor	Activated by endocannabinoids released from neurons; activate Ca^{2+}-triggered glutamate release from astrocytes
Bestrophin-1 (Best-1)	Glutamate and tonic GABA release
Two-pore domain weak inward-rectifying K channel-1 (TWIK-1)	Ammonia uptake
Mechanogated and arachidonic acid–activated TWIK-related channel 1 (TREK-1)	Fast glutamate release
Metabotropic glutamate receptor 3 (mGluR) 3	Activates TWIK-1 and Best-1

interactions among Ca^{2+} and Na^+ signaling and K^+ buffering in astrocytes regulating neuronal excitability. For example, intracellular Ca^{2+} increase due to release from intracellular stores in response to glutamate may promote Na^+ influx via the Na^+/Ca^{2+} exchanger; this may raise intracellular Na^+ sufficiently to activate the Na^+/K^+ ATPase, leading to a decrease of extracellular K^+ concentration and local hyperpolarization, reducing spontaneous excitatory synaptic activity. Aerobic glycolysis in neurons produces carbon dioxide (CO_2), which is converted to bicarbonate (HCO_3^-) and hydrogen (H^+) via the astrocytic carbonic anhydrase; HCO_3^- is exported out of the astrocyte via NBC.

Potassium Channels and Extracellular Potassium Buffering

Compared to neurons, astrocytes have a relative hyperpolarized resting membrane potential that reflects their high and selective permeability to K^+ due to the presence of Kir4.1 and two-pore forming K^+ channels. These channels and the low-resistance pathway formed by gap junctions allow the astrocyte network to provide for spatial K^+ buffering in response to synaptic activity. This spatial buffering primarily depends on the distribution and function of Kir4.1 channels and the water channel AQP4.[23] The Kir4.1 channel is encoded by the *KCNJ10* gene and expressed almost exclusively in astrocytes. This channel allows a bidirectional K^+ flux determined by the electrochemical gradient of K^+ and is thus ideally suited for regulation of K^+ homeostasis.[16] Gap junctions allow the cell-to-cell spread of K^+ toward the astrocyte endfeet, mediating the release of excess K^+ into the blood.

Aquaporin 4 Channels, Volume Regulation, and Glymphatic System

Aquaporin 4 includes two predominant isoforms, M1 and M23, which can form homo- or heterotetramers.[24] At the astrocyte endfeet, AQP4 interacts with the Kir4.1 channel via the dystrophin-associated protein complex and promotes K^+ clearance by allowing transmembrane flux of water and volume driven by osmotic imbalances created by K^+ redistribution.[25] Thus, AQP4 has a critical role in both volume and K^+ homeostasis.[26] Aquaporin 4 also interacts with TRPV4, a polymodal swelling-sensitive cation channel expressed in endfeet.[27] Water influx through AQP4 drives Ca^{2+} influx via TRPV4; reciprocally, Ca^{2+} regulates expression of AQP4 and Kir4.1, thus fine-tuning volume regulation in the astrocyte.[27] In addition to the perivascular endfoot processes, astrocytes express AQP4 in their subependymal, subventricular, and perinodal processes. The functional coupling of AQP4 with Kir4.1 channels in the perinodal process is important for regulation of ion and water environment in the axon and is also required for development and survival of oligodendrocytes. Contacts via gap junction between astrocyte and oligodendrocytes form a syncytium

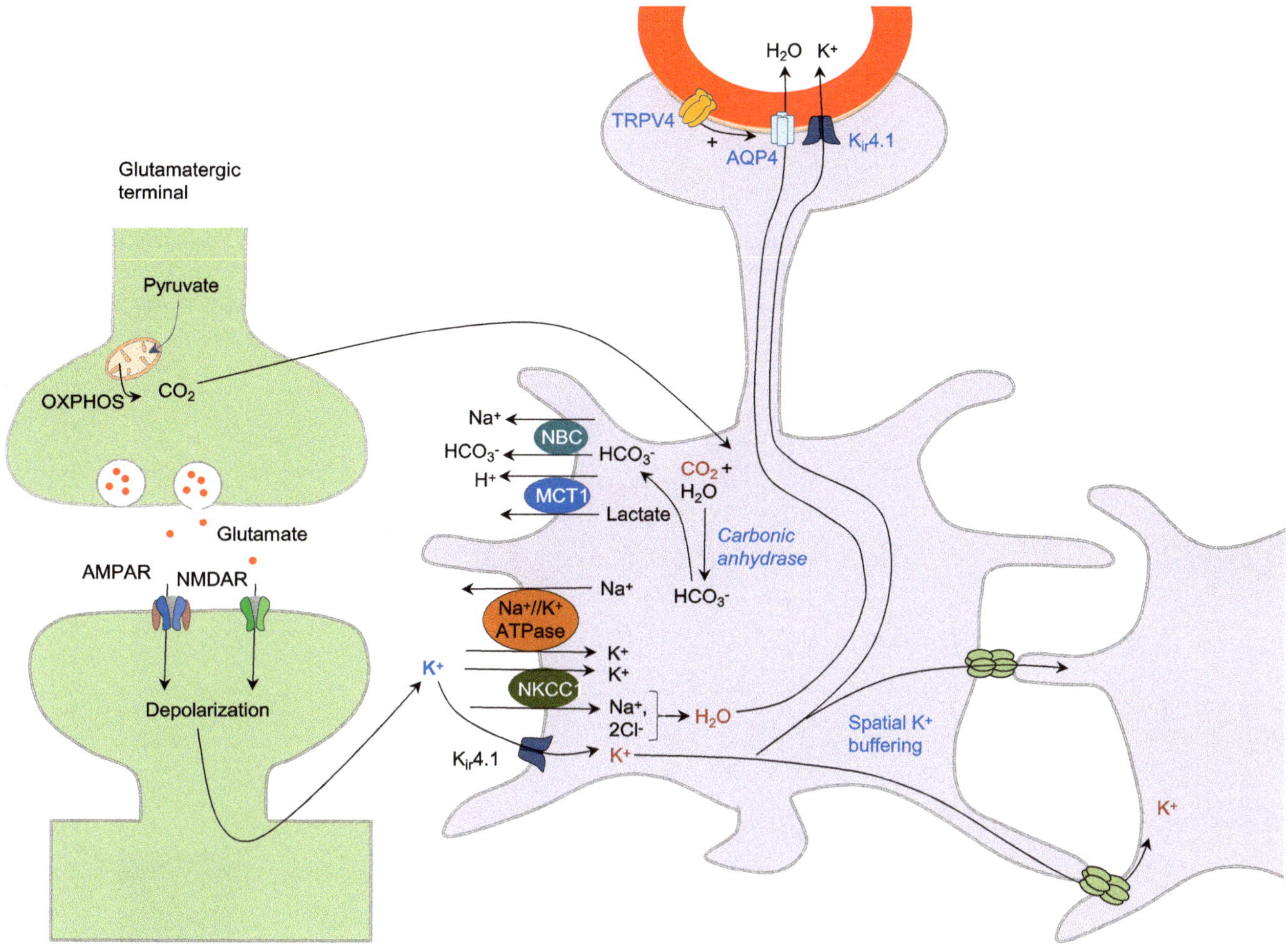

FIGURE 21.4 Astrocytic control of ion and fluid homeostasis.
Astrocytes express a variety of membrane transporters and channels that control ion and fluid homeostasis. Synaptic activity triggers sodium (Na^+) and calcium (Ca^{2+}) transients in astrocytes. The main astroglial Na^+ transporter is the Na^+/potassium (K^+) adenosine triphosphate (ATPase); astrocytes can also transport Na^+ via the Na^+/bicarbonate cotransporter (NBC) and the $Na^+/K^+/Cl^-$ cotransporter 1 (NKCC1). Aerobic glycolysis in neurons produces carbon dioxide (CO_2), which is converted to bicarbonate (HCO_3^-) and hydrogen (H^+) via the astrocytic carbonic anhydrase; HCO_3^- is exported out of the astrocyte via NBC. Buffering of extracellular potassium (K^+) following synaptic activity involves influx via inward-rectifying Kir4.1 channels, as well as NKCC1, its spatial distribution via gap junctions, and is elimination at the astrocytic endfeet coupled with water efflux via aquaporin 4 (AQP4) channels. Calcium influx via transient receptor potential vanilloid type 4 (TRPV4) channels regulates this process. Volume regulation in astrocytes also involves volume-regulated anion channels. MCT, monocarboxylic acid transporter; OXPHOS, oxidative phosphorylation.

that supports the unidirectional flow of cytosolic content from the astrocyte to the oligodendrocytes. This coupling also provides for potential spatial K^+ buffering to dissipate high K^+ concentration and is critical for volume regulation in the myelin sheath. Aquaporin 4 is proposed to be a major component of the glymphatic system.[28,29] This proposed tripartite system consists of a para-arterial CSF influx route, a transparenchymal pathway that depends on astroglial water transport via AQP4, and a paravenous interstitial route for clearance.[30] It has been proposed that the glymphatic system facilitates brain fluid clearance and waste removal during sleep. Both patients with idiopathic normal-pressure hydrocephalus and Alzheimer disease (AD) exhibit sleep disturbances, build-up of brain metabolic wastes and amyloid-beta (Aβ) plaques, perivascular reactive astrogliosis, and mislocalization of astrocyte AQP4. This implicates impaired glymphatic function in these disorders.[31] However, the role of astrocytes and AQP4 in this system has been questioned.[30,32] Volume regulation in astrocytes also involves volume-regulated ion channels permeable to Cl^-, bicarbonate, glutamate, glycine, and taurine.[33]

ROLE OF ASTROCYTES IN NEUROTRANSMITTER RECYCLING AND METABOLIC SUPPORT

Astrocytes have a major role in regulating neuronal synaptic levels of glutamate and GABA[34] and coupling of synaptic activity with energy metabolism[35] (Table 21.2).

Glutamine–Glutamate–GABA Shuttle and Control of Fast Neurotransmission

Astrocytes regulate fast synaptic transmission via a mechanism known as the glutamine–glutamate–GABA shuttle[34,36] (Figure 21.5). Glutamate uptake via the Na^+-dependent EAAT2 (expressed primarily in mature brain) and EAAT1 (in immature brain) is a fundamental mechanism for control of excitatory neurotransmission.[36,37] These transporters co-localize with and functionally couple to various intracellular Na^+-regulated and ATP-generating systems, including the Na^+/K^+ ATPase, the Na^+/Ca^{2+} exchanger, and glycogen-metabolizing and

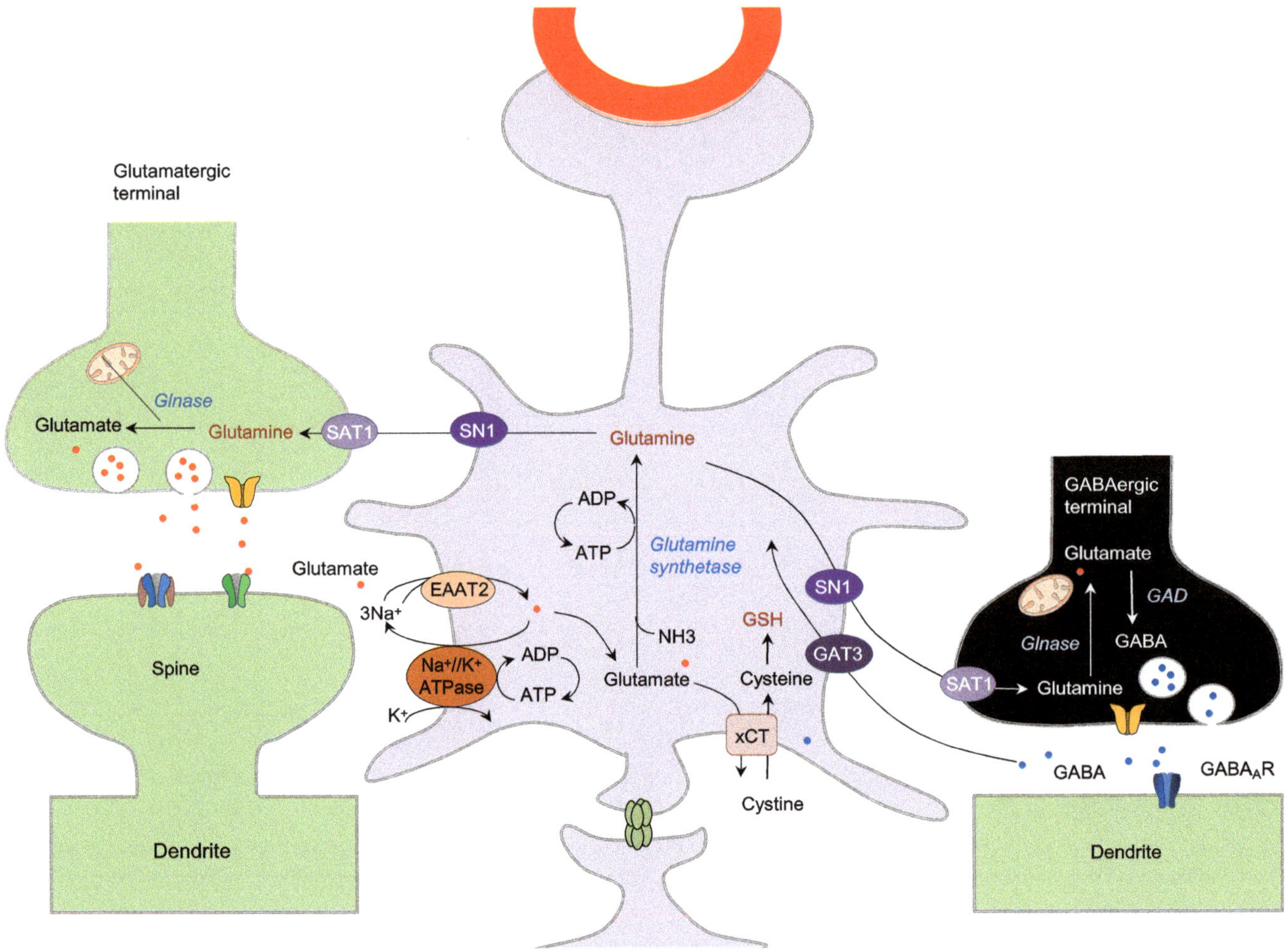

FIGURE 21.5 Role of astrocytes in neurotransmitter homeostasis.
Astrocytes regulate fast synaptic transmission via a mechanism known as the glutamine–glutamate–GABA shuttle. Synaptically released glutamate undergoes uptake via the Na^+-dependent astrocytic excitatory amino acid transporters (EAATs) particularly EAAT2, which co-localize the Na^+/ATPase. After uptake, glutamate is converted to glutamine via glutamine synthetase, which also buffers ammonia (NH_3) in the CNS. Astrocytes release glutamine into the extracellular space via the glutamine system N transporter (SN)1, whereas synaptic terminals import glutamine via the glutamine system A transporter (SAT)1. In synaptic terminals, glutamine serves as the substrate for synthesis of glutamate via the mitochondrial phosphate-activated glutaminase Glnase. This glutamate–glutamine shuttle thus recycles glutamate to both excitatory and inhibitory neurons. Astrocytes are involved in uptake of extrasynaptic GABA via the GABA transporter (GAT)3. Glutamate uptake provides a gradient for its export coupled to import of cystine by the cystine/glutamate antiporter XcT; which is critical for synthesis of the antioxidant glutathione (GSH). GAD, glutamic acid decarboxylase.

glycolytic enzymes, forming a supramolecular functional assembly termed a "glutamosome."[36] This functional coupling is bidirectional.[34] After uptake, glutamate is converted to glutamine via glutamine synthetase, which is expressed primarily, but not exclusively, in astrocytes.[38] Glutamine synthesis is a fundamental step in regulation of both intermediate metabolism and homeostasis of excitatory and inhibitory neurotransmitters[39] and is also the primary mechanism to buffer ammonia in the CNS. Astrocytes release glutamine into the extracellular space via the glutamine system N transporter (SN)1 whereas synaptic terminals import glutamine via the glutamine system A transporter (SAT)1. In synaptic terminals, glutamine serves as the substrate for synthesis of glutamate via the mitochondrial phosphate-activated glutaminase. This glutamate–glutamine shuttle thus recycles glutamate to both excitatory and inhibitory neurons. Most importantly, glutamine provides glutamate for synthesis of GABA in inhibitory neurons.[40–42]

Antioxidant Protection

One additional important consequence of glutamate uptake via EAATs is providing a gradient of glutamate for export coupled to import of cystine by the cystine/glutamate antiporter xCT (*SLC7A11*).[43] Within the cell, cystine is rapidly converted into cysteine, which is a fundamental substrate for the synthesis of glutathione (GSH). Astrocytes are the main source of this potent antioxidant in the CNS.[43] Cystine import by the xCT system is involved not only in GSH synthesis (and thus intracellular defenses against oxidative stress) but also in modification of the extracellular redox milieu and regulation of extracellular glutamate levels. Several neuroprotective stimuli promote xCT expression. These include nuclear factor-E2-related factor (NrF2), which is a master regulator of redox metabolism in response to oxidative stress and target of dimethyl fumarate; and activating transcription factor 4 (ATF4), which is a mediator of the unfolded protein response and a critical mediator of metabolic and oxidative homeostasis and cell survival.[44] Some drugs such as ceftriaxone (via NrF2), levetiracetam, and zonisamide also increase xCT expression. There is an important functional coupling between astrocyte uptake via EAAT and cystine import via xCT, which has major pathophysiological consequences. In many neurodegenerative disorders, epilepsy, and ischemia there is impaired EAAT activity and upregulation of xCT. Increased extracellular glutamate levels can compromise the proper functioning of system xCT, resulting in impaired cystine uptake, GSH depletion, and oxidative stress. In these disorders, xCT upregulation could potentially be protective. However, xCT upregulation might paradoxically contribute to injury by mediating nonsynaptic glutamate release, thereby promoting excitotoxic effects amplified by downregulation of EAATs, which usually balance system cXT–mediated glutamate release.[43]

Neuron–Astrocyte Metabolic Coupling (Lactate Shuttle)

Excitatory synaptic activity promotes glycolysis in astrocytes, leading to production and release of lactate as an energy substrate for active neurons (Figure 21.6). This is known as the astrocyte-neuron lactate shuttle.[35,45] Astrocytes take up glucose from the blood via the glucose transporter-1 (GLUT1) and synthesize glycogen, which serves as the substrate for glycolysis and production of lactate. The activity of both EAATs and glutamine synthetase consume ATP, leading to a decrease in the ATP/ADP ratio, which stimulates glycolysis in astrocytes.[19,22] Extracellular K^+ buffering indirectly triggers alkalinization of astrocytes, which also stimulates both glycogenolysis and glycolysis.[46] Lactate is shuttled from astrocytes to neurons via specific monocarboxylic acid transporters (MCTs), MCT1 and MCT4, and is used as substrate for energy metabolism in active neurons, In astrocytes, glycogen metabolism is regulated by several neurotransmitters; this contributes to variations in extracellular glucose and lactate across the sleep–wake cycle.[35] For example, norepinephrine, released from locus coeruleus afferents in the cerebral cortex during wakefulness and alerting reactions, activates Ca^{2+} transients[47] and promotes rapid glycogenolysis followed by glycogen resynthesis in astrocytes.

CALCIUM SIGNALS AND SECRETORY FUNCTION OF ASTROCYTES

Astrocytes show both spontaneous and synaptic activity–dependent increases in intracellular Ca^{2+} levels.[5,20,48,49] In response to these signals, astrocytes secrete a wide variety of molecules that contribute to the regulation of CNS development, synaptogenesis, synaptic plasticity, neuronal network synchronization, activity-dependent regulation of metabolism and blood flow, and both neuroprotective and deleterious responses in pathological conditions.[50,51]

Multiple Sources and Compartmentalization of Calcium Signals in Astrocytes

The astrocytic Ca^{2+} signaling is compartmentalized, with a gradient of intracellular Ca^{2+} increase from the distal processes to the soma, reflecting different receptor and transport mechanisms and intracellular Ca^{2+} sources. In distal processes, spontaneous Ca^{2+} signals occur at membrane microdomains, or "hot spots," primarily as a consequence of influx via a variety of channels (Table 21.3) (Figure 21.7). For example, at perisynaptic processes, spontaneous Ca^{2+} transients may reflect opening of TRPA1 channels and contribute secretory and transport functions in astrocytes, such as constitutive release of D-serine and expression of GABA transporters.[20] Glutamate can also trigger localized Ca^{2+} transients restricted to membrane hot spots near astrocytic branches, allowing astrocyte detection of local synaptic activity.[52] Astrocytes may integrate the activity

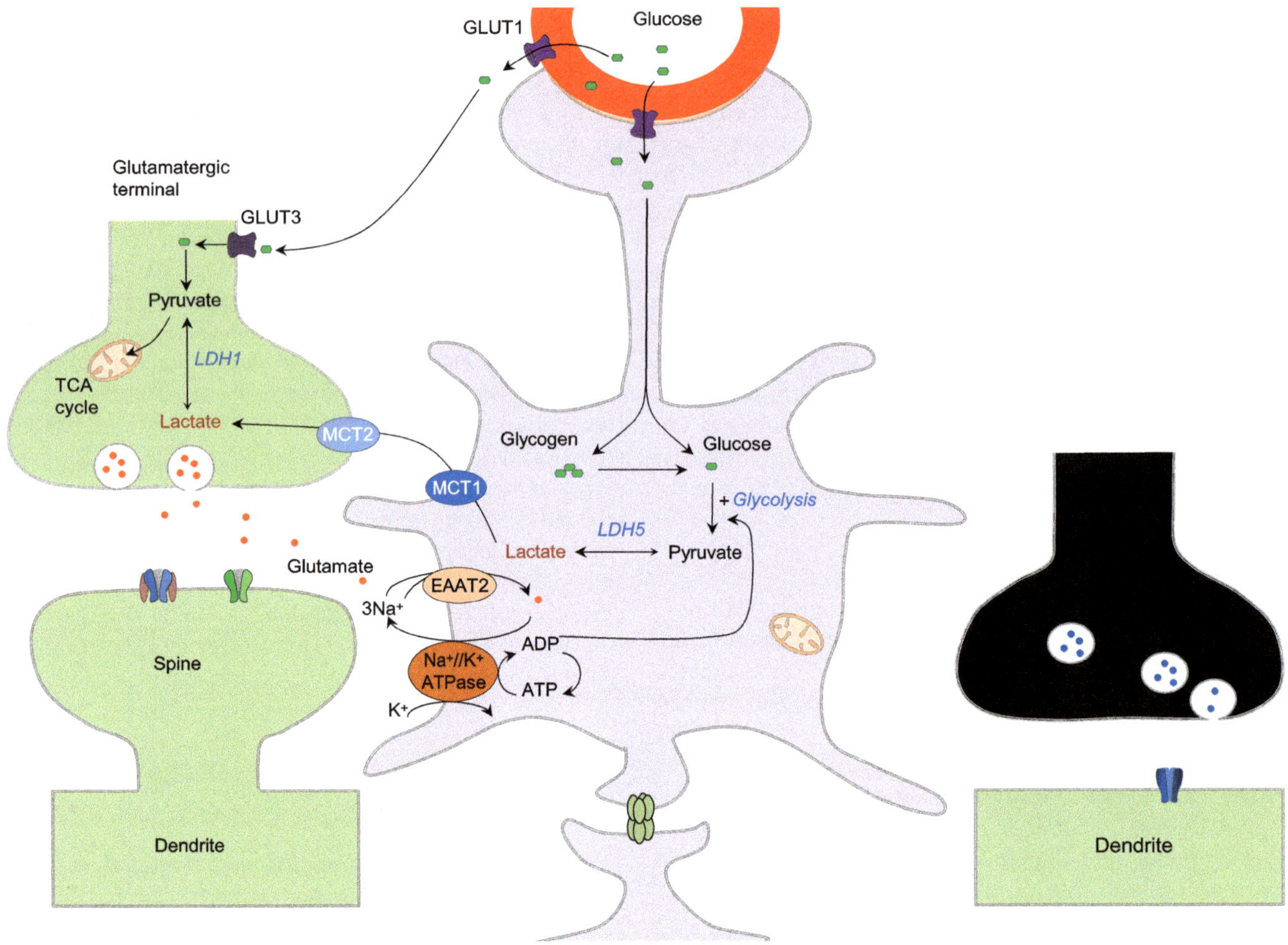

FIGURE 21.6 Astrocyte–neuron lactate shuttle.
Excitatory synaptic activity promotes glycolysis in astrocytes, leading to production and release of lactate as an energy substrate for active neurons. Astrocytes take up glucose from the blood via the glucose-transporter-1 (GLUT1) and synthesize glycogen, which serves as the substrate for glycolysis and production of lactate. The activity of both EAATs and glutamine synthetase consume ATP, leading to a decrease in the ATP/ADP ratio, which stimulates glycolysis in astrocytes. Glycolysis lead to the production of pyruvate, which is converted into lactate by lactate dehydrogenase (LDH)5. Lactate is shuttled from astrocytes to neurons via the monocarboxylic acid transporters (MCTs) MCT1 and MCT4 and is taken via MCT2 into neurons, where it is transformed by action of LDH1 back to pyruvate and is then metabolized in the mitochondria to fuel the tricarboxylic acid (TCA) cycle.

of individual synapses to generate a larger Ca^{2+} response.[53] Increase in intracellular Ca^{2+} at the level of the soma is primarily due to release from intracellular stores via inositol triphosphate type 2 (IP_3R_2) receptors, triggered by activation of a variety of GPCRs, including metabotropic glutamate receptor 5 (mGluR5), purinergic P2Y receptors, or adrenergic α1 receptors.[49,52]

Gliotransmitters and Other Signals Secreted by Astrocytes

Some signals released from astrocytes, such as L-glutamate, GABA, glycine, ATP, adenosine, D-serine, and neuropeptide Y, act on timescales of milliseconds to seconds and are directly involved in synaptic transmission and plasticity[50,51,53] (Figure 21.8) (Table 21.4). Others signals are released on timescales ranging from minutes to days and regulate energy metabolism, blood flow, synaptogenesis, and inflammation. They include lactate, GSH, neurosteroids, synaptogenic factors such as thrombospondins, trophic factors such as brain-derived neurotrophic factor (BDNF), mediators of inflammation such as cytokines and chemokines, and extracellular matrix proteins controlling repair, such as chondroitin sulfate proteoglycans (Table 21.5).

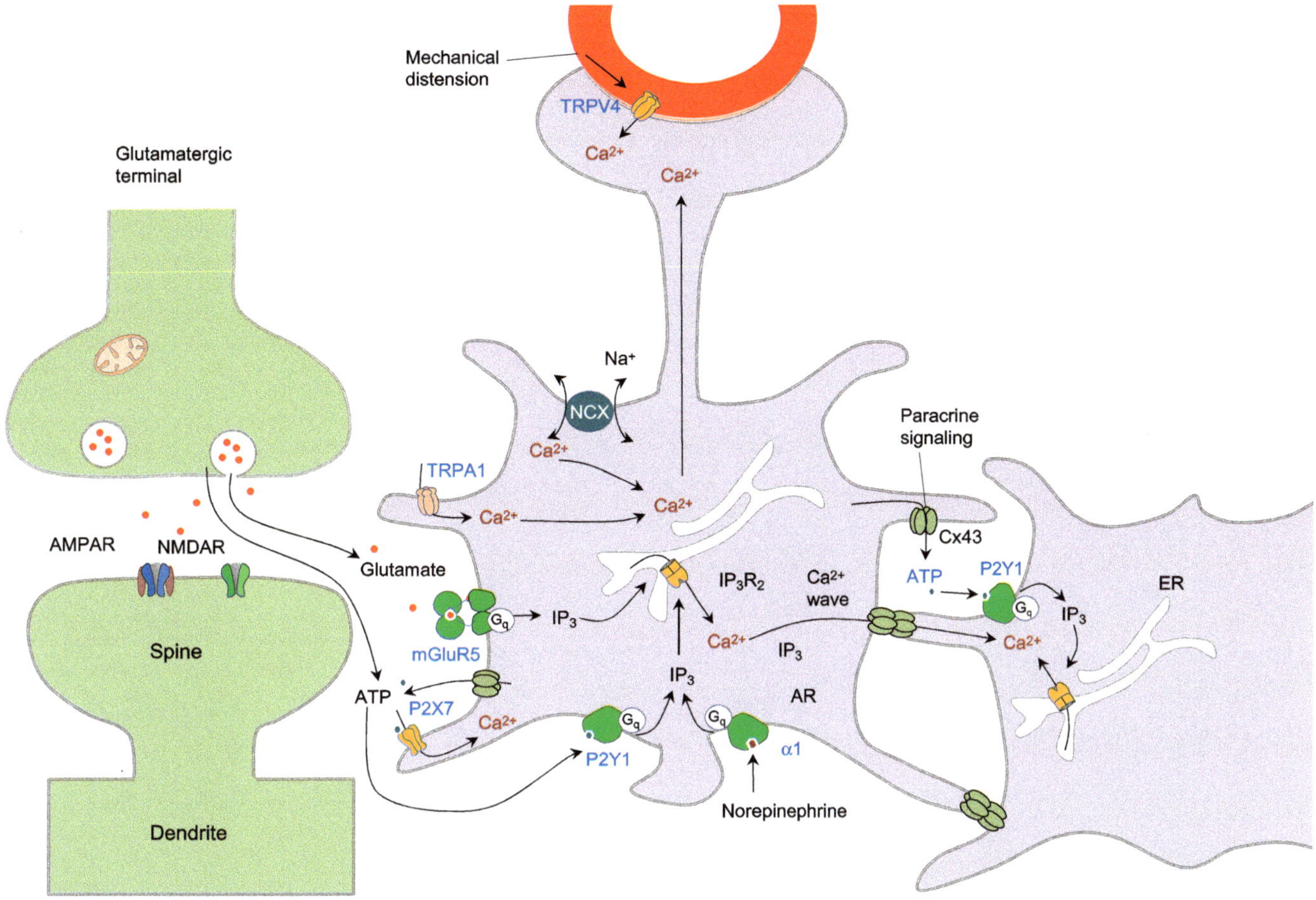

FIGURE 21.7 Calcium signaling in astrocytes.

There is a compartmentalization of calcium (Ca^{2+}) signaling in the astrocytes, with a gradient of intracellular Ca^{2+} increase from the distal processes to the soma. In the distal processes, spontaneous Ca^{2+} signals occur at membrane microdomains primarily as a consequence influx via a variety of channels, including transient receptor potential (TRP) ankyrin type 1 (TRPA1) channels in the perisynaptic processes and TRP vanilloid receptor type 4 (TRPV4) channels at the astrocytic endfeet, connexin hemichannels, and purinergic P2X7 receptors activated by adenosine triphosphate (ATP). Ca^{2+} influx also occurs via the sodium Na^+/Ca^{2+} exchanger (NCX). Synaptic activity triggers Ca^{2+} release from intercellular stores in the endoplasmic reticulum, via inositol triphosphate (IP_3) receptor type 2 (IP_3R_2) channels, in response to activation of guanine nucleotide $(G)_q$-coupled neurotransmitter receptors activating the phospholipase C (PLC) pathway. These include metabotropic glutamate receptor (mGluR) 5, purinergic P2Y1 receptors, alpha 1 adrenergic receptors (α1AR), and muscarinic cholinergic receptors (not-shown).

Connexin and Other Signaling Channels

Connexin hemichannels mediate direct exchange of signals between astrocytes and the extracellular space.[15] For example, Cx43 hemichannels allow tonic release of ATP, which mediates paracrine signals among astrocytes via purinergic P2X and P2Y receptors.[15] Two-pore K^+ channels not only contribute to the high resting (leak) K^+ permeability of astrocytes but also are activated in response to stimulation of metabotropic glutamate receptors (mGluRs) and regulate astrocyte signaling. For example, the weak inward-rectifying K channel (TWIK)-1 is a nonselective monovalent cation channel that allows ammonia uptake by astrocytes, which is critical for synthesis of glutamine. The mechano-gated and arachidonic acid–activated TWIK-related K^+ channel (TREK)-1 provides a mechanism for fast glutamate release by the astrocyte.[16] Bestrophin-1 is a Ca^{2+}-activated anion channel that is largely expressed in astrocytes, particularly in microdomains near synaptic junctions, and provides a pathway for both fast release of glutamate and tonic release of GABA.[54]

Mechanisms of Secretion by Astrocytes

Astrocytes secrete their multiple mediators through several mechanisms.[50] They include different forms of

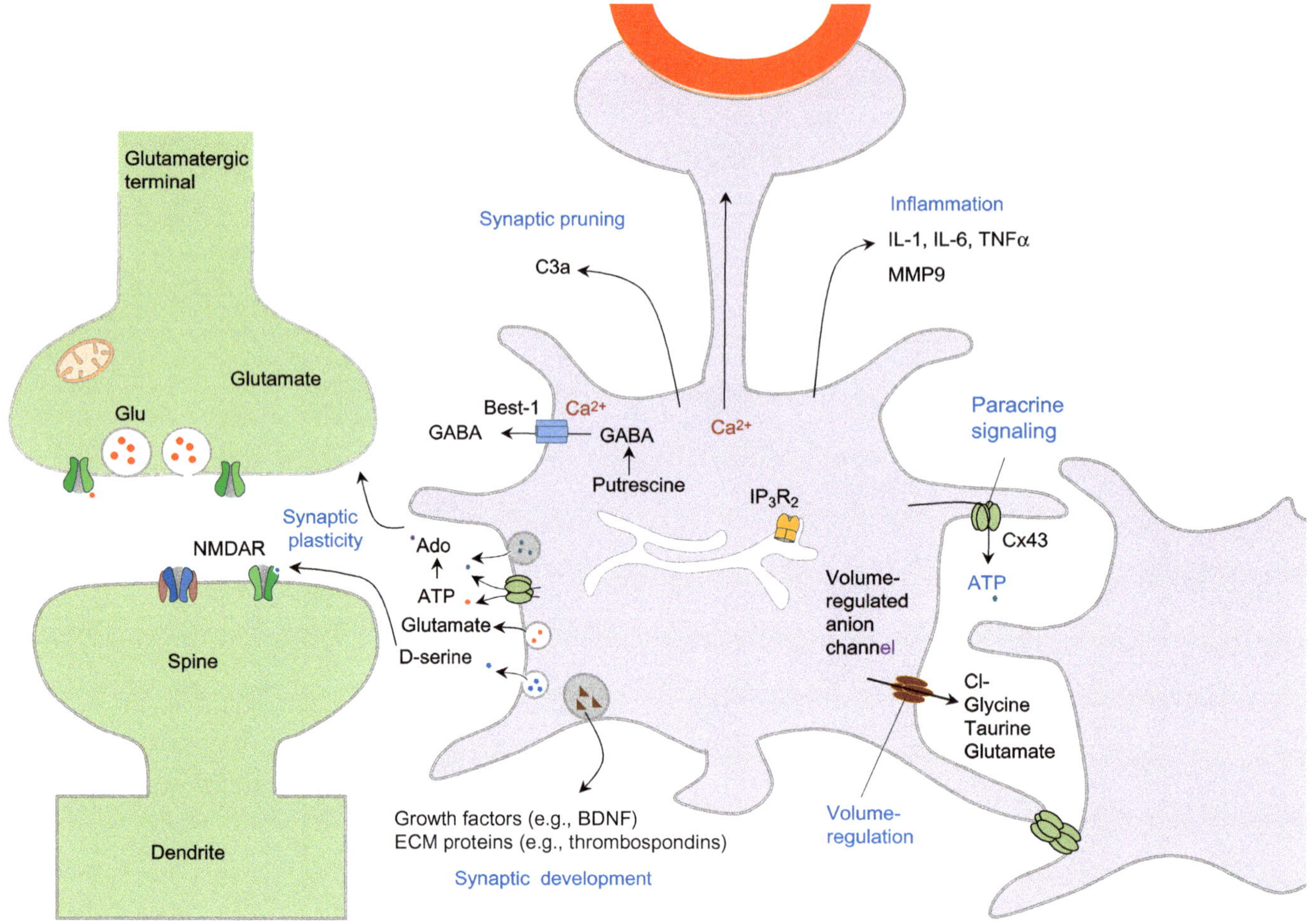

FIGURE 21.8 Secretory function of astrocytes and gliotransmission.
Astrocytes release a variety of gliotransmitters, including glutamate, γ-aminobutyric acid (GABA), D-serine, and ATP via several mechanisms, including Ca^{2+}-triggered exocytosis, connexin (Cx) 43 hemichannels, volume-operated ion channels, the mechano-gated and arachidonic acid–activated two-pore weak inward-rectifying K channel (TWIK)-related K^+ channel (TREK)-1, and bestrophin-1 (Best-1) channels; both TREK-1 and Best-1 are activated in response of mGluR3 activation. Gliotransmitters released at perisynaptic processes may affect synaptic transmission via several mechanisms, including activation of synaptic and extrasynaptic N-methyl-D-aspartate receptors (NMDARs) or $GABA_A$ receptors ($GABA_A$Rs), and via ATP conversion to adenosine (Ado), which regulates neurotransmitter release via adenosine receptors. C3a, complement component 3; IL, interleukin; MMP9, matrix metalloproteinase 9, TNF = tumor necrosis factor.

Ca^{2+}-triggered and vesicle-mediated exocytosis; diffusion through membrane ion channels; and extrusion via reverse operation of membrane transporters. Exocytosis may occur via synaptic-like microvesicles, as in the case of L-glutamate or D-serine; dense-core vesicles, as in the case of ATP and BDNF; secreting lysosomes, as in the case of proteolytic enzymes; or membrane-derived vesicles such as exosomes (e.g., protease receptor activator, microRNAs, and mitochondrial DNAs) and ectosomes (e.g., vascular endothelial growth factor, interleukin (IL) 1β, and matrix metalloproteinases).[50] Exocytosis may deliver membrane receptors, transporters, and channels to the astrocyte membrane; and, in pathological conditions, major histocompatibility complex-II molecules to reactive astrocyte membranes.[50] Astrocytes may release the same gliotransmitter via several mechanisms. For example, glutamate and ATP can be released via exocytosis, connexin hemichannels, bestrophin-1 channels, and P2X7 receptors. Glutamate, GABA, and glycine may also be released via the reversed operation of their transporters.[50] Volume-regulated anion channels permeable to Cl^- also release taurine, glutamate, and glycine to the extracellular space in response to cell swelling. The release of gliotransmitters to the extracellular space may be followed by their transport via the glymphatic system.[55]

TABLE 21.4 *Gliotransmitters Released from Astrocyte (examples)*

Signal	Release Mechanism	Effect
Glutamate	Exocytosis Connexin hemichannels P2X7 receptors Cysteine-glutamate antiporter Reverse action of EAATs	Presynaptic and postsynaptic modulation of synaptic transmission (ionotropic and metabotropic receptors) Network oscillations (extrasynaptic receptors)
ATP	Exocytosis Connexin hemichannels P2X7 receptors Lysosomes	Excitatory action via P2X receptors and modulatory actions via P2Y receptors Precursor of adenosine
D-serine	Exocytosis Volume-regulated channels Transporters	Substitutes for glycine at the NMDA receptor
Glutamine	Sodium-coupled neutral amino-acid transporters	Precursor of glutamate (and thereby GABA) Direct excitatory action
GABA	Bestrophin-1 channel Reverse action of GATs	Modulation of synaptic transmission and network oscillations ($GABA_A$ and $GABA_B$ receptors
Glycine	Reverse action of GlyT1	Inhibitory neurotransmitter NMDA receptor coagonist
Taurine	Volume-regulated channels Connexin 43 hemichannels	Agonist of glycine and $GABA_A$ receptors

Astrocytes and Neurovascular Coupling

There is a local increase of CBF triggered by synaptic activity, which is known as neurovascular coupling or functional hyperemia. This process involves signals from both neurons and astrocytes affecting vascular tone in capillaries by action on pericytes and in arterioles via effects on smooth muscle (Figure 21.9). For example, postsynaptic terminals release the potent vasodilator nitric oxide (NO) in response to activation of N-methyl-D-aspartate receptors (NMDARs) by glutamate. In response to synaptic activity, transient increases in intracellular Ca^{2+} levels in astrocytes also provide a major mechanism for neurovascular coupling (neuron-to-astrocyte-to vessel signaling) These activity-dependent Ca^{2+} transients in the astrocytic endfoot processes may be triggered by several signals, primarily ATP acting via P2X receptors. Resting Ca^{2+} levels in astrocytes provide for a tonic control of arteriolar diameter via continuous release of prostaglandin E2, producing steady-state vasodilation independent of synaptic activity.[56] Astrocytes may also function as sensors of cerebral hemodynamic influences (vessel-to-astrocyte-to neuron signaling).[12] For example, mechanosensitive TRPV4 channels expressed in astrocytic endfeet allow Ca^{2+} influx that activates phospholipase A2, leading to production of arachidonic acid and its metabolism by cyclooxygenase 2, with production of prostaglandin E_2, epoxyeicosatrienoic acid, or 20-hydroxyeicosatetraenoic acid, which regulate vascular tone.[57] Increases in intracellular Ca^{2+} in astrocyte endfeet can also activate large-conductance calcium-gated potassium channels (BK) and stimulate K^+ efflux onto vessels, resulting in vasodilation.[58,59]

ASTROCYTE–SYNAPSE INTERACTIONS

Astrocyte–synapse communication is a critical contributor to synaptic development, plasticity, and network oscillations (Figure 21.10). The synaptic role of astrocyte is both stimulus- and circuit-specific; the spatiotemporal diversity of astrocytic Ca^{2+} signals may allow astrocytes to encode and process different patterns of activation. Astrocytes contribute to synaptic transmission and plasticity both by undergoing plastic rearrangements of their contact with pre- and postsynaptic elements (morphological plasticity) and through bidirectional communication via regulatory signals.

Role of Astrocytes in Synaptic Development and Maintenance

Astrocytes have a key role in the formation and maturation of synapses, as well as maintenance, pruning, and remodeling of synapses, both during development and in

TABLE 21.5 *Metabolic and Trophic Molecules Released from Astrocytes (examples)*

Substance	Release Mechanism	Function
Lactate	Monocarboxylic transporter 1 Lactate channels	Energy substrate for active neurons and oligodendrocytes Synaptic effects
Glucose	Glucose transporters?	May contribute to neuronal metabolism and sustain glutamatergic transmission
Glutathione	ATP binding cassette subfamily member B1 transporter Connexin hemichannels	Buffering of reactive oxygen species
Ascorbate	Sodium-dependent ascorbate transporter	Buffering of reactive oxygen species
Eicosanoids (PgE2, ETE, HETE)	Direct release from membrane	Local regulation of cerebral blood flow Synaptic modulation Inflammatory responses
Atrial natriuretic peptide	Exocytosis	Local vasodilator
Thrombospondin-1	Unknown	Regulation of synaptogenesis
Glypican 4 and 6	Unknown	Formation of excitatory synapses
Cholesterol	Apolipoprotein E particles	Dendritic and synaptic differentiation
Thyroid hormone	L-type amino acid transporter	Astrocytes uptake T4 and converts T4 to T3 by deiodinase 2
Neurotrophins (NGF, BDNF)	Exocytosis	Regulation of neuronal survival, growth, differentiation, and synaptic plasticity
Transforming growth factor β	Unknown	Promotes synaptogenesis and myelinogenesis

BDNF, brain-derived neurotrophic factor; NGF, nerve growth factor

the adult CNS. Astrocytes guide neurite outgrowth, form barriers to neuronal connectivity, stimulate synaptogenesis, remove dendritic spines by pruning, and regulate structural dynamics of dendritic spines. Astrocyte-secreted signals regulate the formation of synaptic connections.[60] These signals include thrombospondin, hevin, and other ECM proteins that promote the formation of silent synapses. Glypican family proteoglycans promote the formation mature synapses. Secreted protein acidic and rich in cysteine (SPARC) and SPARC-like 1 (SPARCL1) produced by astrocytes oppositely control excitatory synaptogenesis; SPARCL1 directly promotes excitatory synapse formation, whereas SPARC antagonizes the synaptogenic actions of SPARCL1.[61] Chordin-like 1 is an astrocyte-secreted factor that induces the formation of mature glutamatergic synapses.[62] Chondroitin sulfate proteoglycans secreted by astrocytes contribute to the formation of perineuronal nets that stabilize synaptic structure and restrict synaptic plasticity.[63] Astrocyte-derived cholesterol is essential for neuronal dendritic elaboration and presynaptic function during development. Astrocytes, acting together with microglia, also participate in pruning of supernumerary excitatory synapses on dendritic spines. Astrocytes regulate synapse elimination during development by secreting transforming growth factor β (TGFβ), which induces components of the complement cascade in neurons (C1q),[64] and by direct phagocytosis of synapses.[65]

Activity-Dependent Structural Plasticity of Perisynaptic Processes

The perisynaptic astrocytic processes ensheath synaptic elements to variable extents, depending on the brain area and circuit. The extent to which such perisynaptic astrocytic processes structurally interact with synapses and regulate glutamatergic transmission is controlled by their actin-dependent motility and can change over time, in part as a function of neuronal activity. These structural rearrangements contribute to synaptic plasticity. For example, in

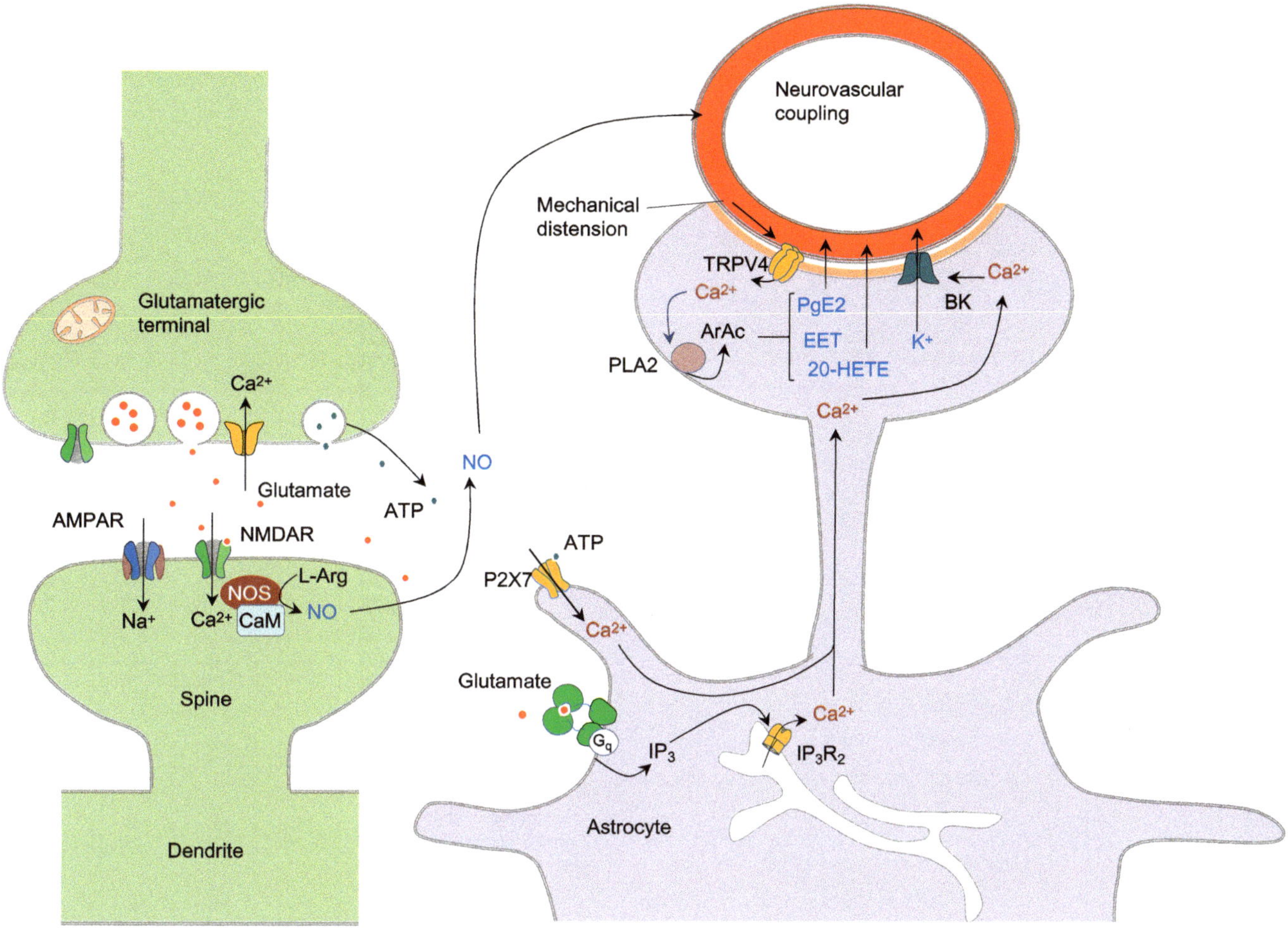

FIGURE 21.9 Neurovascular coupling.

Neurovascular coupling involves signals from both neurons and astrocytes. Postsynaptic terminals release the potent vasodilator nitric oxide (NO) in response to activation of N-methyl-D-aspartate receptors (NMDARs) by glutamate. In response to synaptic activity, transient increases in intracellular Ca^{2+} levels in astrocytes also provide a major mechanism for neurovascular coupling. These activity-dependent Ca^{2+} transients in the astrocytic endfoot processes may be triggered by several signals, primarily ATP acting via P2X receptors. Astrocytes may also function as sensors of cerebral hemodynamic influences (vessel-to-astrocyte-to neuron signaling). For example, mechanosensitive TRPV4 channels expressed in astrocytic endfeet allows Ca^{2+} influx that activates phospholipase A2, leading to production of arachidonic acid (ArAc) and its metabolism by cyclooxygenase 2 with generation of prostaglandin E_2 (PgE2), epoxyeicosatrienoic acid EET, or 20-hydroxyeicosatetraenoic 20-HETE regulating vascular tone. Increases in intracellular Ca^{2+} in astrocyte endfeet can also activate large-conductance calcium-gated potassium channels (BK) and stimulate K^+ efflux onto vessels, resulting in vasodilation.

the hippocampus, during induction of long-term potentiation (LTP) there is an increase in the number of astrocytic processes that approximate and tightly enwrap the most active enlarged dendritic spines. Activation of mGluR5 triggers Ca^{2+} increases that elicit transient motility of astrocytic perisynaptic processes and enhanced astrocytic coverage of the synapse.[66] Astrocytic and synaptic plastic changes occur coordinately and interdependently during synaptic remodeling. This rearrangement of the synaptic ensheathment modifies localization and efficacy of EAATs and gliotransmitter release, thereby contributing to changes in the synaptic gain.

Astrocyte–Synapse Signaling and Synaptic Plasticity

There is spatially and temporally complex bidirectional communication between astrocytes and synapses. Excitatory synaptic activity triggers Ca^{2+} transients in the perisynaptic astrocytic processes via several mechanisms, including activation of mGluR5 and P2X receptors; in response, astrocytes may release gliotransmitters such as glutamate, D-serine, and ATP, which exert complex pre- and postsynaptic effects.[53,49] Gliotransmitters may either increase or decrease excitatory or inhibitory

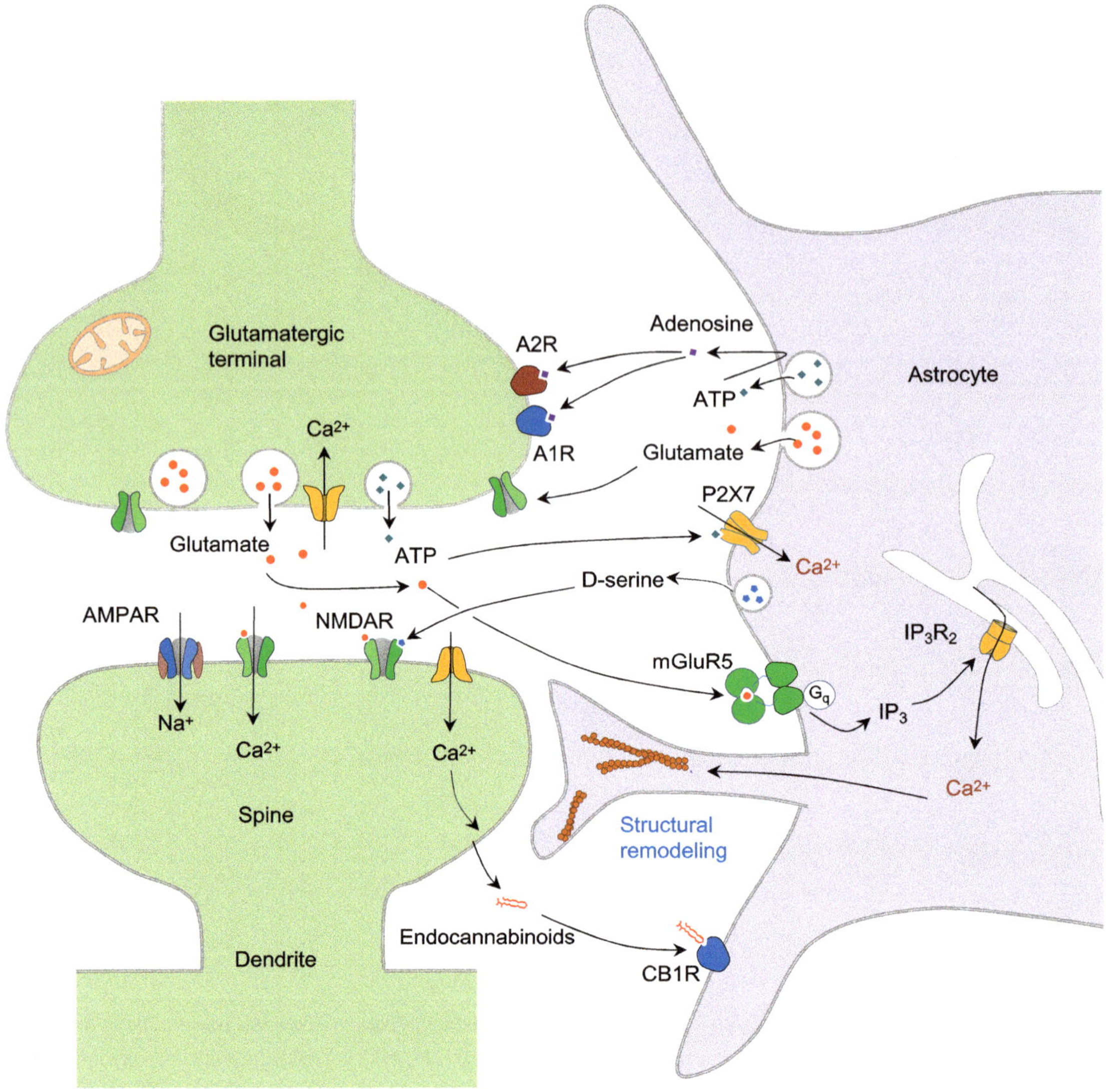

FIGURE 21.10 Astrocyte–synapse communication.
Reciprocal astrocyte–synapse communication is a critical contributor to synaptic development and plasticity. The extent to which perisynaptic astrocytic processes structurally interact with synapses and regulate glutamatergic transmission is controlled by their actin-dependent motility. Activation of mGluR5 triggers Ca^{2+} increases that elicit transient motility of astrocytic perisynaptic processes an enhanced astrocytic coverage of the synapse. Excitatory synaptic activity triggers Ca^{2+} transients in the perisynaptic astrocytic processes via activation of mGluR5 and P2X receptors; in response, astrocytes may release gliotransmitters such as glutamate, D-serine, and ATP. These gliotransmitters may either increase or decrease excitatory or inhibitory neurotransmission via a variety presynaptic or postsynaptic receptors. For example astrocytes release of D-serine, which increases the occupancy of the glycine co-agonist binding site of the NMDAR. Activity-dependent release of endocannabinoids from postsynaptic neurons stimulates both presynaptic and astrocytic cannabinoid-1 receptors (CB1Rs). Astrocytic glutamate modulates synaptic transmission and plasticity by activating pre- or postsynaptic NMDARs and, presynaptic mGluRs. A1R, adenosine 1 receptor; A2R, adenosine 2 receptor.

neurotransmission via a variety of presynaptic or postsynaptic receptors. The complexity of astrocyte-to-neuron signaling in part reflects the different properties of astrocytes and signaling mechanisms involved in different brain regions.[67] For example, classical NMDAR-dependent LTP at the CA1 area of the hippocampus requires transient astrocytic release of D-serine, which increases the occupancy of the glycine co-agonist binding site of the NMDAR and thus efficacy of glutamatergic transmission. Activity-dependent release of endocannabinoids from postsynaptic neurons stimulates both presynaptic and astrocytic cannabinoid-1 receptors (CB1Rs). Whereas activation of presynaptic CB1Rs exerts an inhibitory effect on neurotransmitter release, activation of astrocytic CB1Rs induces release of glutamate, D-serine, or both. Glutamate released from astrocytes modulates synaptic transmission and plasticity by activating pre- or postsynaptic NMDARs, presynaptic mGluRs, and dendritic (extrasynaptic) NMDARs. Depending on the circuit, the effect can be stimulatory or inhibitory. Activation of cholinergic, purinergic, and noradrenergic receptors on astrocytes also induces the release of fast-acting molecules that influence synaptic activity and plasticity via both pre- and postsynaptic mechanisms. For example, activation of nicotinic α7 receptors elicits release of D-serine; and activation of muscarinic receptors or purinergic P2Y1 receptors induces release of glutamate from astrocytes. Activation of β2 adrenoceptors by norepinephrine increases astrocytic glycogenolysis and production of lactate. In addition to entering neurons via MCT2 to function as a metabolic substrate, lactate also acts on putative membrane receptors inducing metabolic and/or signaling effects possibly involving control of NMDAR function. Lactate release from astrocytes is important for LTP in the CA3–CA1 synapses in the hippocampus, where lactate fosters memory consolidation via activation of protein synthesis.

Astrocytes' Sensing of Brain States and Modulation of Neuronal Ensembles

Astrocytes also participate in coordinated activity of ensembles of neurons and synaptic circuits. The excitability and responses of these neuronal networks to external stimuli are regulated by brain states such as arousal and attention. These behavioral states are generated by action of neuromodulators such as acetylcholine and monoamines, which produce spatially diffuse and slower effects in both neurons and astrocytic networks. Both the locus coeruleus–norepinephrine system and the basal forebrain cholinergic system have a critical role in arousal and attention and regulate synchronized brain-wide oscillations important for sensory processing and cognitive performance. These modulatory systems also activate astrocytes in the target areas, increasing the responsiveness of the astrocytic network to local cortical activity. For example, activation of astrocytic α1 adrenergic and nicotinic α7 receptors triggers the release of D-serine and ATP, which facilitate induction of LTP at excitatory synapses in the somatosensory cortex. At the cortical level, astrocytes contribute to the generation of slow-wave oscillations (<1 Hz), which occur prominently during non–rapid eye movement (NREM) sleep and have been associated with memory consolidation. Astrocytes also modulate oscillatory patterns in other frequency ranges, such as in the gamma range (25–80 Hz) required for local circuit synchronization. These effects of astrocytes reflect both inhibitory and stimulatory actions via coordinated control of pyramidal cells and GABAergic interneurons by gliotransmitters. For example, sustained interneuron firing in the hippocampus induces astrocyte $GABA_B$ signaling, which triggers gliotransmitter release and thereby indirectly controls the oscillatory activity of the neuronal network. Astrocytes may contribute to the coordinated activity across brain regions by multiple mechanisms.[68] For example, they can release glutamate simultaneously onto several neighboring neurons and coordinately activate extrasynaptic NMDARs. Astrocytes may also produce GABA via a putrescine degradation pathway and tonically release GABA via bestrophin-1 channels or reverse actions of the GABA transporters, leading to slow inhibitory currents mediated by extrasynaptic $GABA_A$ receptors. Astrocytes can extend their influence by forming astrocytic domains via gap-junction connectivity, coordinating activation and synchronizing bursting of the neuronal networks. Astrocytes may also regulate synaptic transmission indirectly via their effects on the axon. Calcium transients in periaxonal astrocytes associated with unmyelinated axons trigger glutamate and ATP release that depolarizes the axon; this produces broadening of the action potential and thereby increased Ca^{2+}-dependent synaptic transmission.[69] In myelinated axons, perinodal astrocytes surrounding the nodes of Ranvier modulate conduction velocity through regulation of extracellular K^+.[70]

Astrocytes can also contribute to modulation of memory function during the sleep–wake cycle. Sleep promotes memory consolidation particularly during early-night NREM phases characterized by cortical slow-wave oscillations. During prolonged wakefulness there is homeostatic increase in the need to sleep due to a progressive increase in adenosine, a sleep-inducing molecule, produced by astrocytes. Adenosine produced extracellularly from ATP released by astrocytes may contribute to slow inhibitory currents via adenosine A1 receptors.[68,71] In contrast, lactate produced by astrocytes in response to noradrenergic neurons of the locus coeruleus supports the activity of wake-promoting orexin neurons in the lateral hypothalamus.

PRIMARY ASTROCYTOPATHIES

Astroglial pathology includes astrocytopathies (or astrogliopathies) and reactive astrocytosis (or astrogliosis),[72] both of which alter the normal functions of astrocytes.[73,74]

Alexander Disease

Heterozygous gain-of-function mutations of the *GFAP* gene cause Alexander disease.[75–77] This disorder is a leukodystrophy with a variable, age-related phenotype. Alexander disease has been subdivided into two types: type I characterized by early onset, seizures, macrocephaly, motor delay, encephalopathy, failure to thrive, paroxysmal deterioration, and typical MRI features of leukodystrophy; and type II characterized by later onset, ocular movement abnormalities, bulbar symptoms (such as palatal myoclonus) autonomic dysfunction, and atypical MRI features including atrophy of the medulla and upper cervical spinal cord. The pathological hallmark is enlargement of the astrocytes, shortening of astrocytic processes, and accumulation of GFAP-containing aggregates (Rosenthal fibers), within their subpial, subependymal, and perivascular processes, particularly in the white matter and subpial portions of the CNS. Studies in experimental models indicate that GFAP accumulation in astrocytes leads to activation of cellular stress pathways; inhibition of proteasome activity and autophagy; and increased translation of GFAP mRNA. There is an early decrease in the Kir4.1 channel and the EAAT2 mRNA gene, leading to compromised ability to regulate extracellular K^+ and synaptic levels of glutamate; there is also loss of coupling via gap junctions and intramyelinic edema. Many of the morphological and functional changes in astrocytes in Alexander disease mimic those of reactive astrocytes in a variety of neurologic disorders. Astrocyte pathology elicits robust upregulation of chemokines and inflammatory cytokines and activation of microglia. Increased production of the CXCL10 chemokine by astrocytes is associated with demyelination, which in part may result from intramyelinic edema due to impaired astrocytic spatial buffering.

Neuromyelitis Optic Spectrum Disorders

Neuromyelitis optica (NMO) spectrum disorders (NMOSD) is an evolving group of relapsing CNS-inflammatory autoimmune demyelinating diseases associated with AQP4 antibodies. NMOSD is a relapsing disease, extending beyond the optic nerves and spinal cord to include brain (especially in children) and skeletal muscle. Some manifestations of NMOSD reflect involvement of AQP4-enriched regions in the CNS, including area postrema (causing intractable nausea and vomiting) and the hypothalamus (causing sleep disorders such as narcolepsy; impaired thermoregulation, and endocrine dysfunction such as syndrome of inappropriate secretion of antidiuretic hormone).[78] Binding of AQP4 antibodies triggers aggregation and internalization of the tetrameric AQP4 channel. This reduced expression in the astrocyte endfeet could result in myelin edema and depletion of EAAT2 from the plasma membrane, leading to extracellular glutamate accumulation and excitotoxic oligodendrocyte cell death.[79] Residual aggregates of AQP4 may activate locally available complement and produce the characteristic lesions of NMO.[78] Eculizumab, an antibody that targets the complement pathways, reduced the risk relapse in NMOSD patient compared to those who received placebo.[80] Inebilizumab, an anti-CD19 B cell-depleting antibody has potential application for patients with NMOSD.[81]

GFAP Astrocytopathy

Antibodies against GFAPα are associated with a distinct form of autoimmune meningoencephalitis,[82] GFAP astrocytopathy, which typically manifests with headache, meningeal signs, subacute encephalopathy, longitudinally extensive myelitis, optic papillitis tremor, and cerebellar ataxia. Typical MRI findings include perivascular radial enhancement extending out of the ventricles or in the cerebellum; leptomeningeal, serpentine, or subpial enhancement; and longitudinally extensive T2 hyperintensity with linear enhancement in the spinal cord and sometimes affecting the conus medullaris. Cerebrospinal fluid is inflammatory in more than 90% of patients. CSF GFAPα antibodies are highly specific. Neoplasia may occur in up to more than 35% of patients. One example is ovarian teratoma, with GFAPP coexisting with NMDAR and AQP4 autoimmunity. The disorder improves followed treatment with high-dose corticosteroids but has a tendency to relapse without long-term immunosuppression.[83]

Hyperammonemic States

The prototype metabolic astrocytopathy is hepatic encephalopathy. In this condition, excessive glutamine synthesis in ammonia-overloaded astrocytes contributes to astrocytic swelling and brain edema.[84] A large proportion of the newly formed glutamine enters mitochondria, leading to mitochondrial dysfunction. Ammonium may also produce dysregulation of astroglial Ca^{2+} signaling, in part due to upregulation of L-type channels[85] or activation of NMDARs.[86] Calcium-dependent glutamate release from astrocytes contributes to extracellular glutamate overload and excitotoxicity in this condition.[86,87] Ammonia also compromises astrocyte K^+ buffering, increasing extracellular K^+ concentration and neuronal excitability by reducing the efficacy of inhibitory GABAergic transmission.[88]

Familial Hemiplegic Migraine Type 2

Loss-of-function mutations in the α2 subunit of the Na^+/K^+ ATPase, which is primarily expressed in astrocytes, are linked to both familial and sporadic hemiplegic migraine type 2.[89,90] The decreased activity in the astrocytic Na^+/K^+ pump may be responsible for cortical spreading depression underlying the migraine aura; this may reflect impaired EAAT-mediated glutamate clearance from the synaptic cleft.[91] Mutations in the *SLC4A4* gene, encoding the electrogenic Na^+/bicarbonate cotransporter 1 have also been linked to familial hemiplegic migraine; this mutation impairs activity of this transporter in astrocytes, which potentially leads to dysregulation of synaptic pH.[92]

ROLE OF ASTROCYTES IN EPILEPSY

Impaired regulation of extracellular K^+ and synaptic homeostasis by astrocytes is a fundamental pathophysiological mechanism in epilepsy.[40–42,93] Several abnormalities occur during epileptogenesis, including structural and functional changes in receptors, ion channels, transporters, and enzymes regulating excitatory and inhibitory neurotransmission; gliosis; inflammation; impaired BBB function; aberrant dendritic and axonal plasticity; changes in neural circuits; reorganization of the ECM; and epigenetic reprogramming.[94–96] Studies on experimental models or in hippocampal tissue obtained during surgery in patients with medically refractory seizures showed several abnormalities in astroglial proteins. These include downregulation of both the Kir4.1 channel[97,98] and AQP4 expression[99] in astrocyte endfeet, which would affect astrocytic buffering of extracellular K^+, leading to neuronal depolarization and seizure propensity. In sclerotic hippocampus, there is substantial increase in glutamate concentrations and reduced expression of astrocytic glutamine synthetase, which reduces glutamate availability for GABA synthesis. Astrocytic dysfunction may also contribute to epileptogenesis in focal cortical dysplasia, which is associated with impaired AQP4 expression and gap junction connectivity in astrocytes.[42,100] In both sclerotic hippocampus and focal cortical dysplasia there is also downregulation of the K^+/Cl^- cotransporter 2 (KCC2) and upregulation of NKCC1, leading to abnormal regulation of transmembrane Cl^- gradients and efficacy of $GABA_A$ receptor-mediated inhibition.[101–103] Glioma cells share several characteristics of nonmalignant reactive astrocytes and are a common cause of seizures. Glioma cells have increased expression of the cystine/glutamate transporter system by which efflux of glutamate is coupled with influx of cystine for synthesis of GSH. In glioma cells, this transporter is a major mechanism of glutamate release, promoting excitatory drive, and thereby seizures. Abnormal peritumoral hyperexcitability may also reflect paradoxical excitatory rather than inhibitory responses to GABA, due to KCC2 downregulation and NKCC1 upregulation.[104] Impaired K^+ buffering in hyperammonemic states also increases NKCC1 activity reducing the efficacy of GABAergic inhibition.[88] Further supporting the relevance of impaired K^+ homeostasis in epileptogenesis, loss-of-function mutations of the *KCNJ10* gene encoding the Kir4.1 channel primarily expressed in astrocytes cause an autosomal recessive disorder characterized by seizures, sensorineural deafness, ataxia, mental retardation, and electrolyte abnormalities.[105,106]

INVOLVEMENT OF ASTROCYTES IN AGING AND NEURODEGENERATIVE DISORDERS

Phenotypic Heterogeneity of Reactive Astrocytes

Astrocytes acquire different reactive phenotypes in response to aging and numerous pathological stimuli, such as stroke, neurodegenerative disorders, tumors, trauma, and infection, and release several chemical signals in these conditions (Table 21.6). Astrocyte reactivity is characterized by changes in their gene expression profile and both morphological and functional changes that may vary from cellular hypertrophy or atrophy, to proliferation and scar formation. The type and extent of the astrocytic reaction is severely impacted by the size of the affected area, the nature of the insult and its severity, the intensity of BBB disruption, and the inflammatory response. Hallmarks of reactive astrocytes are overexpression of GFAP, which relates to the degree of hypertrophy of cell body and increase in the number of cellular processes; and other markers such as lipocalin-2 and the protease inhibitor serpin3. Aged astrocytes also upregulate expression of proteins of the complement system, such as components 3 (C3) and 4b (C4b), and decrease expression of enzymes involved in cholesterol synthesis. It has been proposed that, according to the type of insult, reactive astrocytes may adopt two phenotypes, a proinflammatory/cytotoxic A1 and an anti-inflammatory/neuroprotective A2 phenotype, related to similar phenotypes described in reactive microglia. In the setting of neuroinflammation, activated microglia induce a neurotoxic reactive astrocyte A1 phenotype by secreting interleukin (IL)-1a tumor necrosis factor (TNF)-α and complement component 1q (C1q). The A1 astrocytes lose normal functions and simultaneously gain new, harmful functions at the same time. For example, these reactive astrocytes lose their ability to induce synapse formation due to the increased expression of many classical complement cascade genes that are toxic to synapses. In contrast, other insults such as ischemia, can induce a

TABLE 21.6 *Inflammatory Mediators Released from Astrocytes (examples)*

Mediator	Mechanism of Release	Effect
Tumor necrosis factor-α	Exocytosis	Synaptic plasticity (scaling) Inflammatory response
Interleukins (IL-1, IL-6)	Unknown	Control of inflammatory response
Chemokines	Unknown	Activation of microglia and leukocytes by reactive astrocytes
C3a complement factor	Exocytosis	Synaptic maturation (pruning) Control of inflammatory response
Sphingosine-1 phosphate	ATP-binding cassette transporter A1	Regulation of cell proliferation and immune response

protective reactive astrocyte A2 phenotype, which may secrete neuroprotective molecules, such as thrombospondins neurotrophic factors, and promote CNS recovery and repair. However, as in the case of microglia, the dichotomy between "A1" and "A2" astrocytes is an oversimplification, as there is a spectrum astrocyte reactive states that blend elements of "A1" an "A2" astrocytes.[73,74]

Effects of Aging

Physiological aging is characterized by a chronic, low-grade brain and systemic inflammation, referred as "inflammaging." Astrocytes and microglia have a major role in controlling neuroinflammation and undergo age-related morphological, molecular, and functional changes that may result in pro- or anti-inflammatory phenotypes, depending on the pathological context.[107] Astrocytes undergo age-dependent hypertrophy, leading to increased surface and volume of somata and more complex astrocyte arborizations. These age-related changes are associated with increased expression of genes related to astrocyte reactivity, immune response, and synapse elimination.[108,109] These changes include upregulation of genes that have an important role in eliminating excess synapses during development, including the complement pathway and major histocompatibility complex MHC class I antigens, indicating that aging astrocytes provide an environment that is permissive for synapse elimination. Astrocytes in the aging brain undergo changes of reactive astrocytosis, including expression of GFAP and serine peptidase inhibitor (serpin) and upregulation of inflammatory cytokines.[104] Overall, these findings indicate that astrocytes in the aging brain alter their gene expression to produce an environment that will allow synapse elimination.[108] Astrocytes in regions more vulnerable to cognitive decline—the hippocampus and striatum—undergo more dramatic transcriptional changes compared to cortical astrocytes, with characteristic A1 reactive astrocyte genes that are induced in response to by interactions with microglia.[108,109] Aging astrocytes also show reduced expression of genes involved in the cholesterol synthesis pathway. In contrast, a majority of genes implicated in synaptogenesis in the developing brain appear to be unchanged in aging astrocytes.[108]

Astrocyte Contribution to Neurodegenerative Disorders

Neurodegeneration is a major age-related pathology. Both astrocytes and microglia have a key role in synaptic dysfunction, neuronal loss, and cognitive impairment associated with several neurodegenerative diseases, such AD, Parkinson disease (PD), Huntington disease (HD), and amyotrophic lateral sclerosis. A driver in these neurodegenerative disorders is cellular senescence, a cell fate that entails a permanent cell cycle arrest and pro-inflammatory senescence-associated secretory phenotype (SASP). The pathways for synaptic glutamate and potassium homeostasis pathway in astrocytes decline upon senescence, which may lead to excitotoxicity and neurodegeneration.[110]

For example, astrocytes may contribute to the several aspects of the pathogenesis of AD. In this disorder, there is a region-specific vulnerability to neurodegeneration and changes in morphology and gene expression in both astrocytes and microglia, consistent with neuroinflammation. Astrocytes may become either atrophic or hypertrophic, depending on the stage of the disease and proximity to amyloid plaque depositions. Atrophy occurs during early stages of AD pathology in non-plaque-associated astrocytes. A reduction in astrocyte territorial domains might result in diminished synaptic coverage and in impaired neurovascular coupling. These changes might underlie synaptic dysfunction and loss of metabolic support as well as impairment in synaptogenic and synaptic protective capacity at early disease stages. For example, Aβ oligomers rapidly interact with astrocytes, trigger astrocyte activation, and reduce the levels of TGF-β, which may result in impairment in the synaptogenic and neuroprotective potential of astrocytes. Astrocytic cytoskeletal abnormalities and degeneration with decreased size of both their perisynaptic and endfeet territory domains would likely contribute to the synaptic loss, vascular deficits, and impaired metabolism in AD.[72] During later stages of AD, astrocytes near plaques become highly hypertrophic and activated. Reactive astrocytes surround Aβ deposits and penetrate into amyloid plaques. In mouse models, neurons within the vicinity of Aβ deposition are often hyperexcitable, possibly due to an altered local microenvironment such as Aβ-mediated disruption of glutamate uptake, glutamate release, and GABAergic inhibition. Astrocytes in apposition to Aβ deposits are also hyperactive and display higher resting Ca^{2+} levels, more frequent and larger Ca^{2+} elevations and long-range coordinated Ca^{2+} waves, and increased gliotransmission. These astrocytes have increased expression of several receptors affecting the downstream signaling and synaptic function. They include α7 nicotinic, mGluR5, and P2Y1 receptors, leading to an abnormal astrocytic Ca^{2+} elevations and massive glutamate release. Astrocytes surrounding amyloid plaques also have enhanced synthesis and release of GABA, which increases tonic inhibition of dentate granule cells with a negative impact on memory processing.[111]

There is also astrocyte involvement in PD. In this disorder, protoplasmic astrocytes have α-synuclein-containing inclusions not only in areas containing neurons that develop Lewy bodies but also in the striatum, thalamus, and other brain regions. This suggests that astrocytes may internalize α-synuclein released by neurons or dysfunctional axon terminals. Astrocytes may also be able to transfer aggregated α-synuclein to neighboring astrocytes, via direct contact and tunneling nanotubes. Accumulation of α-synuclein induces upregulation of expression of pro-inflammatory genes and impairs the autophagosomal-lysosomal machinery in astrocytes. This results in ER swelling and mitochondrial damage, severe astrogliosis, downregulation of glutamate transporters, and disruption in the BBB. Alpha synuclein elicits these changes in vitro by promoting production of reactive oxygen species downstream of activation of Toll-like receptor 4 in glial cells. Studies in transgenic models show that astroglial dysfunction associated with mutated huntingtin accumulation is also a prominent feature in Huntington disease. There is decreased expression of EAAT2[112] and Kir4.1 channels[113] and reduced amplitude of spontaneous Ca^{2+} signals.[20]

Astrocytic Tauopathies

Astrocytic tau pathology with different morphologies is often found in association with abnormal neuronal tau accumulation in several tauopathies.[114] Studies in experimental models suggest that tau elicits cytoskeletal collapse in distal processes of astrocytes;[115,116] reduces EAAT2 expression;[117,118] and interferes with normal function of the BBB.[119]

Astrocytes may be primarily or secondarily affected in tauopathies.[120] Astrocytic plaques, tufted astrocytes, ramified astrocytes, and globular astroglial inclusions are seen predominantly in primary tauopathies such as progressive supranuclear palsy and corticobasal degeneration. Thorn-shaped astrocytes and granular/fuzzy astrocytes occur in aging-related tau astrogliopathy, which affects the white and gray matter in subpial, subependymal, and perivascular locations. Some of these findings overlap with the features of tau pathology seen in chronic traumatic encephalopathy. Astrocytic tau pathology in primary tauopathies can be observed in brain areas without neuronal tau deposition. The various morphologies of tau astrogliopathy might reflect a role in the propagation of pathological tau protein. Astrocyte tau pathology in the case of aging-related tau astrogliopathy may reflect a response to a repeated or prolonged pathogenic process such as BBB dysfunction or local mechanical impact.

KEY POINTS

- Astrocytes constitute a structural and functionally heterogeneous population and are critically involved in development, homeostasis, synaptic and neuronal network activity, and response to injury and repair in the CNS.
- Astrocytes are interconnected via gap junctions and extend perisynaptic processes, endfoot processes contacting microvessels, perinodal processes around axons, and subpendymal processes that form the glial limitans.
- The different compartments of the astrocytes contain a unique repertoire of ion channels, transporters, and receptors involved in maintenance of ion and water homeostasis, metabolic support, recycling of neurotransmitters, and Ca^{2+} signaling.
- Astrocytes have high and selective permeability to K^+ due to the presence of Kir4.1 and two-pore forming K^+ channels and have a major role in extracellular K^+ buffering following synaptic activity.
- Aquaporin 4 channels in the astrocytic endfeet interact with the Kir4.1 channel and are critical both for in volume and K^+ homeostasis.
- Aquaporin 4 is a component of the glymphatic system, which facilitates brain fluid clearance and Aβ removal during sleep.
- Astrocytes have a major role in regulating neuronal synaptic levels of glutamate and GABA via the glutamine–glutamate–GABA shuttle.
- Glutamate uptake via astrocytic excitatory amino acid transporters is a fundamental mechanism for control of excitatory neurotransmission and prevent glutamate toxicity.
- Astrocytes convert glutamate to glutamine via glutamine synthetase, which is fundamental for neurotransmitter homeostasis and ammonia buffering in the CNS.
- Glutamine is converted back to glutamate necessary for synthesis of GABA in inhibitory neurons.
- Astrocytes express the cystine/glutamate antiporter xCT, which provides the substrate for the glutathione the main source of antioxidant protection in the CNS.
- Excitatory synaptic activity promotes glycolysis in astrocytes, leading to production of lactate, which is shuttled from the astrocyte to the active neurons as metabolic substrate.
- Astrocytes show both spontaneous and synaptic activity-dependent compartmentalized increases in intracellular Ca^{2+} that propagate as waves within and between astrocytes.
- In response to Ca^{2+} signals, astrocytes release several gliotransmitters, such as L-glutamate, GABA, glycine, ATP, adenosine, and D-serine, which are involved in synaptic transmission and plasticity.
- Astrocytes also release molecules involved in regulation of energy metabolism, blood flow, synaptogenesis, and inflammation.
- In response to Ca^{2+} transients triggered by synaptic activity, astrocytic endfoot food processes release prostaglandin E and other vasoactive signals that mediate activity-dependent control of local blood flow.
- Astrocyte–synapse communication is critical contributor for synaptic development, plasticity, and network oscillations.
- Astrocytes have a key role in the formation and maturation of synapses, as well as maintenance, pruning, and remodeling of synapses.
- Astrocytes participate in the behavioral state–dependent coordinated activity of ensembles of neurons and synaptic circuits.

- Alexander disease is a primary astrocytopathy due to gain-of-function mutations of the *GFAP* gene and has a variable, age-related phenotype.
- Neuromyelitis optica spectrum disorders are a group of relapsing CNS-inflammatory autoimmune diseases associated with AQP4 antibodies.
- Antibodies against GFAPα are associated with a distinct form of autoimmune meningoencephalitis that may be paraneoplastic.
- Hepatic encephalopathy is a prototype metabolic astrocytopathy associated with excessive glutamine synthesis, astrocytic swelling, and mitochondrial dysfunction.
- Loss-of-function mutations in the α2 subunit of the Na^+/ K^+ ATPase, in astrocytes are linked to both familial and sporadic hemiplegic migraine type 2.
- Impaired regulation of extracellular K^+ and synaptic homeostasis by astrocytes is a fundamental pathophysiological mechanism in epilepsy.
- Astrocytes acquire different and overlapping reactive phenotypes in response to aging and numerous pathological stimuli.
- Age-dependent changes in astrocytes provide an environment for synapse elimination, neuroinflammation, and excitotoxicity.
- Glial senescence drives synaptic dysfunction and neuronal loss in neurodegenerative diseases.
- Astrocytic tau pathology with different morphologies is often found in association with abnormal neuronal tau accumulation in several tauopathies.

REFERENCES

1. Zhang Y, Barres BA. Astrocyte heterogeneity: an under-appreciated topic in neurobiology. Curr Opin Neurobiol 2010;20:588–594.
2. Tabata H. Diverse subtypes of astrocytes and their development during corticogenesis. Front Neurosci 2015;9:114–121.
3. Zhang Y, Sloan SA, Clarke LE, et al. Purification and characterization of progenitor and mature human astrocytes reveals transcriptional and functional differences with mouse. Neuron 2016;89:37–53.
4. Yang Z, Wang KK. Glial fibrillary acidic protein: from intermediate filament assembly and gliosis to neurobiomarker. Trends Neurosci 2015;38:364–374.
5. Rusakov DA, Bard L, Stewart MG, Henneberger C. Diversity of astroglial functions alludes to subcellular specialisation. Trends Neurosci 2014;37:228–242.
6. Oberheim NA, Wang X, Goldman S, Nedergaard M. Astrocytic complexity distinguishes the human brain. Trends Neurosci 2006;29:547–553.
7. Halassa MM, Fellin T, Haydon PG. The tripartite synapse: roles for gliotransmission in health and disease. Trends Mol Med 2007;13:54–63.
8. Perea G, Sur M, Araque A. Neuron-glia networks: integral gear of brain function. Front Cell Neurosci 2014;8:378.
9. Nedergaard M, Verkhratsky A. Artifact versus reality—how astrocytes contribute to synaptic events. Glia 2012;60:1013–1023.
10. McCaslin AF, Chen BR, Radosevich AJ, Cauli B, Hillman EM. In vivo 3D morphology of astrocyte-vasculature interactions in the somatosensory cortex: implications for neurovascular coupling. J Cereb Blood Flow Metab 2011;31:795–806.
11. Iadecola C, Nedergaard M. Glial regulation of the cerebral microvasculature. Nat Neurosci 2007;10:1369–1376.
12. Filosa JA, Morrison HW, Iddings JA, Du W, Kim KJ. Beyond neurovascular coupling, role of astrocytes in the regulation of vascular tone. Neuroscience 2015;323:96–109.
13. Nuriya M, Yasui M. Endfeet serve as diffusion-limited subcellular compartments in astrocytes. J Neurosci 2013;33:3692–3698.
14. Giaume C, Koulakoff A, Roux L, Holcman D, Rouach N. Astroglial networks: a step further in neuroglial and gliovascular interactions. Nat Rev Neurosci 2010;11:87–99.
15. Pannasch U, Rouach N. Emerging role for astroglial networks in information processing: from synapse to behavior. Trends Neurosci 2013;36:405–417.
16. Olsen ML, Khakh BS, Skatchkov SN, Zhou M, Lee CJ, Rouach N. New insights on astrocyte ion channels: critical for homeostasis and neuron-glia signaling. J Neurosci 2015;35:13827–13835.
17. Kirischuk S, Heja L, Kardos J, Billups B. Astrocyte sodium signaling and the regulation of neurotransmission. Glia 2015;64:1655–1666.
18. Rose CR, Chatton JY. Astrocyte sodium signaling and neuro-metabolic coupling in the brain. Neuroscience 2015;323:121–134.
19. Chatton JY, Magistretti PJ, Barros LF. Sodium signaling and astrocyte energy metabolism. Glia 2016;64:1667–1676.
20. Shigetomi E, Patel S, Khakh BS. Probing the complexities of astrocyte calcium signaling. Trends Cell Biol 2016;26:300–312.
21. Kirischuk S, Parpura V, Verkhratsky A. Sodium dynamics: another key to astroglial excitability? Trends Neurosci 2012;35:497–506.
22. Rose CR, Verkhratsky A. Principles of sodium homeostasis and sodium signalling in astroglia. Glia 2016;129:1045–1056.
23. Kofuji P, Newman EA. Potassium buffering in the central nervous system. Neuroscience 2004;129:1045–1056.
24. Mack AF, Wolburg H. A novel look at astrocytes: aquaporins, ionic homeostasis, and the role of the microenvironment for regeneration in the CNS. Neuroscientist 2013;19:195–207.
25. Soe R, Macaulay N, Klaerke DA. Modulation of Kir4.1 and Kir4.1–Kir5.1 channels by small changes in cell volume. Neurosci Lett 2009;457:80–84.
26. Nagelhus EA, Ottersen OP. Physiological roles of aquaporin-4 in brain. Physiol Rev 2013;93:1543–1562.
27. Jo AO, Ryskamp DA, Phuong TT, et al. TRPV4 and AQP4 channels synergistically regulate cell volume and calcium homeostasis in retinal Muller glia. J Neurosci 2015;35:13525–13537.
28. Plog BA, Nedergaard M. The glymphatic system in central nervous system health and disease: past, present, and future. Annu Rev Pathol 2018;13:379–394.
29. Rasmussen MK, Mestre H, Nedergaard M. The glymphatic pathway in neurological disorders. Lancet Neurol 2018;17:1016–1024.

30. Abbott NJ, Pizzo ME, Preston JE, Janigro D, Thorne RG. The role of brain barriers in fluid movement in the CNS: is there a '"glymphatic" system? Acta Neuropathol 2018;135:387–407.
31. Reeves BC, Karimy JK, Kundishora AJ, et al. Glymphatic system impairment in Alzheimer's disease and idiopathic normal pressure hydrocephalus. Trends Mol Med 2020;26:285–295.
32. Gakuba C, Gaberel T, Goursaud S, et al. General anesthesia inhibits the activity of the "glymphatic system." Theranostics 2018;8:710–722.
33. Pedersen SF, Okada Y, Nilius B. Biophysics and physiology of the volume-regulated anion channel (VRAC)/volume-sensitive outwardly rectifying anion channel (VSOR). Pflugers Arch 2016;468:371–383.
34. Robinson MB, Jackson JG. Astroglial glutamate transporters coordinate excitatory signaling and brain energetics. Neurochem Int 2016.
35. Petit JM, Magistretti PJ. Regulation of neuron-astrocyte metabolic coupling across the sleep-wake cycle. Neuroscience 2016;323:135–156.
36. Gegelashvili G, Bjerrum OJ. Glutamate transport system as a key constituent of glutamosome: Molecular pathology and pharmacological modulation in chronic pain. Neuropharmacology 2019;161:107623.
37. Jensen AA, Fahlke C, Bjorn-Yoshimoto WE, Bunch L. Excitatory amino acid transporters: recent insights into molecular mechanisms, novel modes of modulation and new therapeutic possibilities. Curr Opin Pharmacol 2015;20:116–123.
38. Schousboe A, Scafidi S, Bak LK, Waagepetersen HS, McKenna MC. Glutamate metabolism in the brain focusing on astrocytes. Adv Neurobiol 2014;11:13–30.
39. Rose CF, Verkhratsky A, Parpura V. Astrocyte glutamine synthetase: pivotal in health and disease. Biochem Soc Trans 2013;41:1518–1524.
40. Robel S, Sontheimer H. Glia as drivers of abnormal neuronal activity. Nat Neurosci 2015;19:28–33.
41. Coulter DA, Steinhauser C. Role of astrocytes in epilepsy. Cold Spring Harb Perspect Med 2015;5:a022434.
42. Steinhauser C, Grunnet M, Carmignoto G. Crucial role of astrocytes in temporal lobe epilepsy. Neuroscience 2015;323:157–169.
43. Lewerenz J, Hewett SJ, Huang Y, et al. The cystine/glutamate antiporter system x(c)(-) in health and disease: from molecular mechanisms to novel therapeutic opportunities. Antioxid Redox Signal 2013;18:522–555.
44. Fujii J, Homma T, Kobayashi S. Ferroptosis caused by cysteine insufficiency and oxidative insult. Free Radic Res 2019;Sep 23:1–12.
45. Pellerin L, Magistretti PJ. Glutamate uptake into astrocytes stimulates aerobic glycolysis: a mechanism coupling neuronal activity to glucose utilization. Proc Natl Acad Sci U S A 1994;91:10625–10629.
46. Bittner CX, Valdebenito R, Ruminot I, et al. Fast and reversible stimulation of astrocytic glycolysis by K+ and a delayed and persistent effect of glutamate. J Neurosci 2011;31:4709–4713.
47. Paukert M, Agarwal A, Cha J, Doze VA, Kang JU, Bergles DE. Norepinephrine controls astroglial responsiveness to local circuit activity. Neuron 2014;82:1263–1270.
48. Wu YW, Tang X, Arizono M, et al. Spatiotemporal calcium dynamics in single astrocytes and its modulation by neuronal activity. Cell Calcium 2014;55:119–129.
49. Bazargani N, Attwell D. Astrocyte calcium signaling: the third wave. Nat Neurosci 2016;19:182–189.
50. Verkhratsky A, Matteoli M, Parpura V, Mothet JP, Zorec R. Astrocytes as secretory cells of the central nervous system: idiosyncrasies of vesicular secretion. Embo J 2016;35:239–257.
51. Petrelli F, Bezzi P. Novel insights into gliotransmitters. Curr Opin Pharmacol 2016;26:138–145.
52. Panatier A, Vallee J, Haber M, Murai KK, Lacaille JC, Robitaille R. Astrocytes are endogenous regulators of basal transmission at central synapses. Cell 2011;146:785–798.
53. Araque A, Carmignoto G, Haydon PG, Oliet SH, Robitaille R, Volterra A. Gliotransmitters travel in time and space. Neuron 2014;81:728–739.
54. Park H, Oh SJ, Han KS, et al. Bestrophin-1 encodes for the Ca2+-activated anion channel in hippocampal astrocytes. J Neurosci 2009;29:13063–13073.
55. Jessen NA, Munk AS, Lundgaard I, Nedergaard M. The glymphatic system: a beginner's guide. Neurochem Res 2015;40:2583–2599.
56. Rosenegger DG, Tran CH, Wamsteeker Cusulin JI, Gordon GR. Tonic local brain blood flow control by astrocytes independent of phasic neurovascular coupling. J Neurosci 2015;35:13463–13474.
57. Shibasaki K, Ikenaka K, Tamalu F, Tominaga M, Ishizaki Y. A novel subtype of astrocytes expressing TRPV4 (transient receptor potential vanilloid 4) regulates neuronal excitability via release of gliotransmitters. J Biol Chem 2014;289:14470–14480.
58. Attwell D, Buchan AM, Charpak S, Lauritzen M, Macvicar BA, Newman EA. Glial and neuronal control of brain blood flow. Nature 2010;468:232–243.
59. Filosa JA, Iddings JA. Astrocyte regulation of cerebral vascular tone. Am J Physiol Heart Circ Physiol 2013;305:H609–619.
60. Allen NJ, Eroglu C. Cell biology of astrocyte-synapse interactions. Neuron 2017;96:697–708.
61. Blakely PK, Hussain S, Carlin LE, Irani DN. Astrocyte matricellular proteins that control excitatory synaptogenesis are regulated by inflammatory cytokines and correlate with paralysis severity during experimental autoimmune encephalomyelitis. Front Neurosci 2015;9:344.
62. Blanco-Suarez E, Liu TF, Kopelevich A, Allen NJ. Astrocyte-secreted chordin-like 1 drives synapse maturation and limits plasticity by increasing synaptic GluA2 AMPA receptors. Neuron 2018;100:1116–1132 e1113.
63. Dzyubenko E, Gottschling C, Faissner A. Neuron–glia interactions in neural plasticity: contributions of neural extracellular matrix and perineuronal nets. Neural Plast 2016;2016:5214961.
64. Bialas AR, Stevens B. TGF-beta signaling regulates neuronal C1q expression and developmental synaptic refinement. Nat Neurosci 2013;16:1773–1782.
65. Chung WS, Clarke LE, Wang GX, et al. Astrocytes mediate synapse elimination through MEGF10 and MERTK pathways. Nature 2013;504:394–400.
66. Aoyama K, Wang F, Matsumura N, et al. Increased neuronal glutathione and neuroprotection in GTRAP3–18-deficient mice. Neurobiol Dis 2012;45:973–982.

67. Fields RD, Woo DH, Basser PJ. Glial regulation of the neuronal connectome through local and long-distant communication. Neuron 2015;86:374–386.
68. Pal B. Astrocytic actions on extrasynaptic neuronal currents. Front Cell Neurosci 2015;9:474.
69. Sasaki T, Matsuki N, Ikegaya Y. Action-potential modulation during axonal conduction. Science 2011;331:599–601.
70. Bay V, Butt AM. Relationship between glial potassium regulation and axon excitability: a role for glial Kir4.1 channels. Glia 2012;60:651–660.
71. Lee HS, Ghetti A, Pinto-Duarte A, et al. Astrocytes contribute to gamma oscillations and recognition memory. Proc Natl Acad Sci U S A 2014;111:E3343–3352.
72. Pekny M, Pekna M, Messing A, et al. Astrocytes: a central element in neurological diseases. Acta Neuropathol 2016;131:323–345.
73. Sofroniew MV, Vinters HV. Astrocytes: biology and pathology. Acta Neuropathol 2010;119:7–35.
74. Sofroniew MV. Astrogliosis. Cold Spring Harb Perspect Biol 2014;7:a020420.
75. Olabarria M, Goldman JE. Disorders of astrocytes: Alexander disease as a model. Annu Rev Pathol 2017;12:131–152.
76. Prust M, Wang J, Morizono H, et al. GFAP mutations, age at onset, and clinical subtypes in Alexander disease. Neurology 2011;77:1287–1294.
77. Messing A. Alexander disease. Handb Clin Neurol 2018;148:693–700.
78. Pittock SJ, Lucchinetti CF. Neuromyelitis optica and the evolving spectrum of autoimmune aquaporin-4 channelopathies: a decade later. Ann N Y Acad Sci 2016;1366:20–39.
79. Hinson SR, Lennon VA, Pittock SJ. Autoimmune AQP4 channelopathies and neuromyelitis optica spectrum disorders. Handb Clin Neurol 2016;133:377–403.
80. Pittock SJ, Berthele A, Fujihara K, et al. Eculizumab in aquaporin-4-positive neuromyelitis optica spectrum disorder. N Engl J Med 2019;381:614–625.
81. Cree BAC, Bennett JL, Kim HJ, et al. Inebilizumab for the treatment of neuromyelitis optica spectrum disorder (N-MOmentum): a double-blind, randomised placebo-controlled phase 2/3 trial. Lancet 2019;394(10206):1352–1363.
82. Flanagan EP, Hinson SR, Lennon VA, et al. Glial fibrillary acidic protein immunoglobulin G as biomarker of autoimmune astrocytopathy: Analysis of 102 patients. Ann Neurol 2017;81:298–309.
83. Dubey D, Hinson SR, Jolliffe EA, et al. Autoimmune GFAP astrocytopathy: prospective evaluation of 90 patients in 1year. J Neuroimmunol 2018;321:157–163.
84. Zielinska M, Popek M, Albrecht J. Roles of changes in active glutamine transport in brain edema development during hepatic encephalopathy: an emerging concept. Neurochem Res 2014;39:599–604.
85. Wang F, Du T, Liang C, Verkhratsky A, Peng L. Ammonium increases Ca(2+) signalling and upregulates expression of Cav1.2 gene in astrocytes in primary cultures and in the in vivo brain. Acta Physiol (Oxf) 2015;214:261–274.
86. Haack N, Dublin P, Rose CR. Dysbalance of astrocyte calcium under hyperammonemic conditions. PLoS One 2014;9:e105832.
87. Montana V, Verkhratsky A, Parpura V. Pathological role for exocytotic glutamate release from astrocytes in hepatic encephalopathy. Curr Neuropharmacol 2014;12:324–333.
88. Rangroo Thrane V, Thrane AS, Wang F, et al. Ammonia triggers neuronal disinhibition and seizures by impairing astrocyte potassium buffering. Nat Med 2013;19:1643–1648.
89. Capendeguy O, Horisberger JD. Functional effects of Na+, K+-ATPase gene mutations linked to familial hemiplegic migraine. Neuromolecular Med 2004;6:105–116.
90. Weigand KM, Swarts HG, Russel FG, Koenderink JB. Biochemical characterization of sporadic/familial hemiplegic migraine mutations. Biochim Biophys Acta 2014;1838:1693–1700.
91. Leo L, Gherardini L, Barone V, et al. Increased susceptibility to cortical spreading depression in the mouse model of familial hemiplegic migraine type 2. PLoS Genet 2011;7:e1002129.
92. Suzuki M, Van Paesschen W, Stalmans I, et al. Defective membrane expression of the Na(+)-HCO(3)(-) cotransporter NBCe1 is associated with familial migraine. Proc Natl Acad Sci U S A 2010;107:15963–15968.
93. Patel DC, Tewari BP, Chaunsali L, Sontheimer H. Neuron–glia interactions in the pathophysiology of epilepsy. Nat Rev Neurosci 2019;20:282–297.
94. Goldberg EM, Coulter DA. Mechanisms of epileptogenesis: a convergence on neural circuit dysfunction. Nat Rev Neurosci 2013;14:337–349.
95. Kim SY, Porter BE, Friedman A, Kaufer D. A potential role for glia-derived extracellular matrix remodeling in postinjury epilepsy. J Neurosci Res 2016;94:794–803.
96. Hauser RM, Henshall DC, Lubin FD. The epigenetics of epilepsy and its progression. Neuroscientist 2018;24:186–200.
97. Das A, Wallace GCt, Holmes C, et al. Hippocampal tissue of patients with refractory temporal lobe epilepsy is associated with astrocyte activation, inflammation, and altered expression of channels and receptors. Neuroscience 2012;220:237–246.
98. Heuser K, Eid T, Lauritzen F, et al. Loss of perivascular Kir4.1 potassium channels in the sclerotic hippocampus of patients with mesial temporal lobe epilepsy. J Neuropathol Exp Neurol 2012;71:814–825.
99. Eid T, Lee TS, Thomas MJ, et al. Loss of perivascular aquaporin 4 may underlie deficient water and K+ homeostasis in the human epileptogenic hippocampus. Proc Natl Acad Sci U S A 2005;102:1193–1198.
100. Garbelli R, Frassoni C, Condorelli DF, et al. Expression of connexin 43 in the human epileptic and drug-resistant cerebral cortex. Neurology 2011;76:895–902.
101. Seifert G, Steinhauser C. Neuron-astrocyte signaling and epilepsy. Exp Neurol 2013;244:4–10.
102. Huberfeld G, Blauwblomme T, Miles R. Hippocampus and epilepsy: findings from human tissues. Rev Neurol (Paris) 2015;171:236–251.
103. Loscher W, Puskarjov M, Kaila K. Cation-chloride cotransporters NKCC1 and KCC2 as potential targets for novel antiepileptic and antiepileptogenic treatments. Neuropharmacology 2013;69:62–74.
104. Pallud J, Le Van Quyen M, Bielle F, et al. Cortical GABAergic excitation contributes to epileptic activities around human glioma. Sci Transl Med 2014;6:244ra289.
105. Bockenhauer D, Feather S, Stanescu HC, et al. Epilepsy, ataxia, sensorineural deafness, tubulopathy, and KCNJ10 mutations. N Engl J Med 2009;360:1960–1970.

106. Scholl UI, Choi M, Liu T, et al. Seizures, sensorineural deafness, ataxia, mental retardation, and electrolyte imbalance (SeSAME syndrome) caused by mutations in KCNJ10. Proc Natl Acad Sci U S A 2009;106:5842–5847.
107. Colombo E, Farina C. Astrocytes: key regulators of neuroinflammation. Trends Immunol 2016;37:608–620.
108. Boisvert MM, Erikson GA, Shokhirev MN, Allen NJ. The aging astrocyte transcriptome from multiple regions of the mouse brain. Cell Rep 2018;22:269–285.
109. Clarke LE, Liddelow SA, Chakraborty C, Munch AE, Heiman M, Barres BA. Normal aging induces A1-like astrocyte reactivity. Proc Natl Acad Sci U S A 2018;115:E1896–E1905.
110. Limbad C, Oron TR, Alimirah F, et al. Astrocyte senescence promotes glutamate toxicity in cortical neurons. PLoS One 2020;15:e0227887.
111. Jo S, Yarishkin O, Hwang YJ, et al. GABA from reactive astrocytes impairs memory in mouse models of Alzheimer's disease. Nat Med 2014;20:886–896.
112. Faideau M, Kim J, Cormier K, et al. In vivo expression of polyglutamine-expanded huntingtin by mouse striatal astrocytes impairs glutamate transport: a correlation with Huntington's disease subjects. Hum Mol Genet 2010;19:3053–3067.
113. Tong X, Ao Y, Faas GC, et al. Astrocyte Kir4.1 ion channel deficits contribute to neuronal dysfunction in Huntington's disease model mice. Nat Neurosci 2014;17:694–703.
114. Kahlson MA, Colodner KJ. Glial tau pathology in tauopathies: functional consequences. J Exp Neurosci 2015;9:43–50.
115. Yoshiyama Y, Zhang B, Bruce J, Trojanowski JQ, Lee VM. Reduction of detyrosinated microtubules and Golgi fragmentation are linked to tau-induced degeneration in astrocytes. J Neurosci 2003;23:10662–10671.
116. Forman MS, Lal D, Zhang B, et al. Transgenic mouse model of tau pathology in astrocytes leading to nervous system degeneration. J Neurosci 2005;25:3539–3550.
117. Dabir DV, Robinson MB, Swanson E, et al. Impaired glutamate transport in a mouse model of tau pathology in astrocytes. J Neurosci 2006;26:644–654.
118. Ferrer I, Legati A, Garcia-Monco JC, et al. Familial behavioral variant frontotemporal dementia associated with astrocyte-predominant tauopathy. J Neuropathol Exp Neurol 2015;74:370–379.
119. Blair LJ, Frauen HD, Zhang B, et al. Tau depletion prevents progressive blood-brain barrier damage in a mouse model of tauopathy. Acta Neuropathol Commun 2015;3:8.
120. Kovacs GG. Astroglia and tau: new perspectives. Front Aging Neurosci 2020;12:96.

22 Microglia and Neuroinflammation

OVERVIEW

Microglia are CNS-resident macrophages that represent approximately 10% of the total brain cell population. They have a critical role during development, synaptic homeostasis, and response to injury by functioning both as sensors and effector cells in the CNS (Figure 22.1). In the basal state microglia have a homeostatic function and actively survey their environment.[1] In response to challenges in CNS homeostasis, microglia cells become reactive and dynamically change their phenotype from a pro-inflammatory/cytotoxic phenotype to one that promotes tissue repair, depending on the type of stimulus and microenvironment.[2,3] Reactive gliosis is a prominent and common feature of CNS lesions and involves multiple cell types, including microglia, astrocytes, and neural/glial antigen 2 (NG2) expressing oligodendrocyte precursor cells (OPCs). Transcriptome and epigenome analysis and generation of glia-like cells from induced-pluripotent stem cells allow a large-scale analysis of phenotypic differentiation and subtypes of glial cells in humans.[4] Microglia and astrocytes not only initiate innate immune responses but also function as antigen-presenting cells that trigger adaptive immune responses. Immune cells rarely cross the unstimulated blood-brain barrier (BBB) but do so in the setting of neuroinflammation. Microglia and neuroinflammation have major roles in most neurologic disorders.[5] The main aims of this chapter are to review (1) the development of microglia, (2) the functions of the surveilling microglia, (3) the phenotypic heterogeneity of reactive microglia, (4) the components of gliosis, and (5) examples of disorders primarily or secondarily affecting microglia.

GENERAL FEATURES OF MICROGLIA

Origin, Development, and Lifespan

Microglia derive from erythromyeloid progenitors in the extraembryonic yolk sac, which spread via the bloodstream to the neuroepithelium and enter the brain via the ventricles, developing meninges, ventricular zone, and choroid plexus.[6] Under the influence of the CNS microenvironment, microglial precursors proliferate and mature from an amoeboid to a ramified phenotype and develop thin processes that form a regular nonoverlapping grid in the tridimensional space of the parenchyma.[7] Resident microglia predominate in the gray matter with the highest concentration in the substantia nigra, hippocampus, basal ganglia, and olfactory cortex. Microglia are capable of self-renewal, which maintains the microglial population throughout life.[7] Microglia establish a dense network with regional differences and slow overall turnover rates; microglial self-renewal under steady-state conditions constitutes a stochastic process.[8] The microglial landscape can be affected in several conditions, including seizures, acute injury, and sensory deprivation; the microglial P2Y12 receptors have a major role in regulating the microglial landscape through cellular translocation independent of proliferation, suggesting that microglia patrol the CNS through both process motility and soma translocation.[9]

In pathological conditions, this random proliferation shifts to a selected clonal expansion; in the resolution phase, excess disease-associated microglia are removed by cell egress and apoptosis to re-establish the stable microglial population.[8] In the absence of disruption of the BBB, circulating monocytes do not contribute to the population of microglia.[10] Transcriptome and epigenome analysis in mice indicate that microglia undergo four developmental phases, yolk sac, early microglia, pre-microglia, and adult microglia. Early microglia express genes related to cell cycle and proliferation; pre-microglia genes related to synaptic pruning; and late adult microglia genes related to immune surveillance.[4] Distinct microRNA expression patterns in microglia may have an important role in their phenotype and functions.

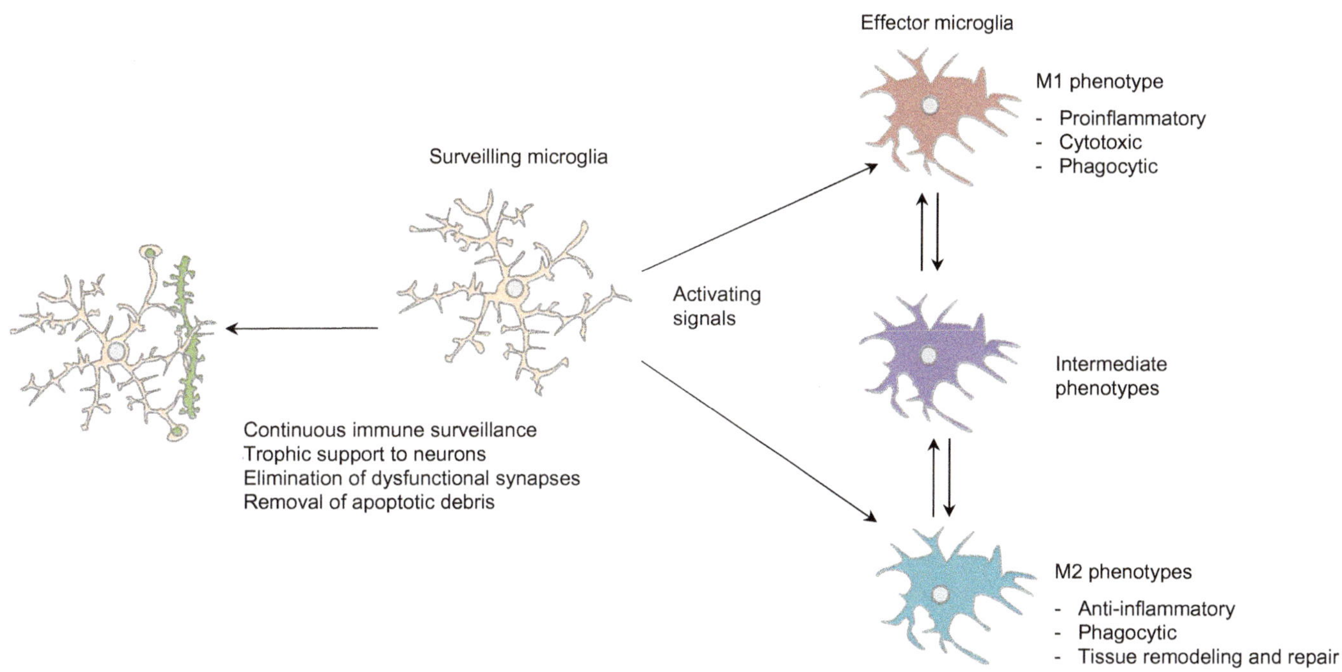

FIGURE 22.1 Overview of microglial functions.
Microglia includes surveilling and reactive (effector) phenotypes. Surveilling microglia have a homeostatic function and actively survey their environment and are involved in synaptic pruning and phagocytosis of cell debris. In response to challenges in CNS homeostasis, microglia cells become reactive and dynamically change their phenotype with a spectrum that ranges from a proinflammatoy/cytotoxic phenotype to one that promotes tissue repair depending on the type of stimulus and microenvironment.

Ion Channels and Receptors in Microglia

Microglia express a large number of membrane ion channels, receptors, transporters, adhesion molecules, and intracellular enzymes that control their surveillance and effector functions. The electrophysiology of microglia primarily depends on different types of potassium channels that are upregulated by stimuli that trigger glial activation. The voltage-gated proton channel Hv is highly expressed in microglia under physiological conditions and is coupled with NADPH oxidase to produce reactive oxygen species (ROS) during brain diseases.[11,12] Chloride channels and several transporters also control microglial activation and migration. Calcium signaling critically regulates microglial function and is triggered by calcium influx via ligand-gated channels, such as transient receptor potential (TRP) channels and purinergic P2X receptors, or by calcium release from the endoplasmic reticulum in response to activation of various G protein-coupled receptors. Microglia contain receptors for neurotransmitters, peptides, cytokines, chemokines, autacoids, complement proteins, and danger-associated molecular patterns (DAMPs), including toll-like receptors (TLRs); these receptors provide multiple converging signals that control the transition from surveillance to the different activated states. P2Y12 and β2 adrenergic receptors are highly expressed in resident microglia and importantly control microglia dynamics.[13–15] Overall, the signals to microglia have been subdivided into "off" and "on" receptor signals. "Off" signals have calming effects that prevent inappropriate activation of microglia (Table 22.1). "On" signals are novel signals that are recognized by the microglia and trigger their activation; many of such signals trigger innate immune responses (Table 22.2).

Receptors Regulating Microglial Development, Survival, and Function

One important receptor complex controlling microglial development, survival, and function is the triggering receptor expressed in myeloid cells 2 (TREM2). TREM2 is a transmembrane receptor that binds anionic ligands including bacterial lipopolysaccharides, phospholipids, apolipoprotein E (APOE), and amyloid β-beta (Aβ) oligomers. Interestingly, TREM2 variants are genetically linked to increased risk for Alzheimer disease (AD).[16,17] Ligand binding to TREM2 triggers downstream cascades via the DNAX activating protein of 12 kD (DAP12, also known as TYRO protein kinase-binding protein), which initiates a Syk tyrosine kinase signaling via extracellular signal regulated kinase, phosphatidylinositol 3-kinase, and intracellular calcium mobilization. The TREM2/DAP12 (TYRO) pathway promotes microglial proliferation and survival, increases motility and phagocytosis, and initiates inhibitory signals leading to suppression of TLR-induced inflammation. TREM2 has a major role in myelin degradation

TABLE 22.1 *Signals and Receptors Preventing Inappropriate Microglial Activation*

Signal	Microglial Receptor	Source of Interaction
CD200	CD200R	Neurons (contact)
Fractalkine (CX3CL1)	CX3CR1	Neurons (secreted)
Heat shock protein 60	TREM2	Apoptotic cells
CD47	SIRPα	Neurons
CD22	CD45	Synaptic terminals
Semaphorin 3A	Plexin A1 and neuropilin 1	Stressed neurons
IL-4, IL-10	IL-4 and IL-10 receptors	T_{H2} lymphocytes
Anandamide	Cannabinoid receptors (CB1R and CB2R)	Microglia (autocrine)
Specialized pro-resolving mediators (SPMs): lipoxins, resolvins, protectins, and maresins	SPMR	Microglia
Tryptophan	Aryl regulatory receptor (AHR)	Gut microbiota
Vasoactive intestinal polypeptide	VPAC	Neurons

SIRP, signal regulatory protein; TREM2, triggering receptor in myeloid cells-2; VPAC, vasoactive intestinal peptide (VIP) and pituitary adenylate cyclase-activating peptide (PACAP) receptors

and lipid metabolism both by acting as a lipid receptor that recognizes phagocytic cargo and by triggering downstream transduction pathways via phospholipase C γ2 (PLC γ2) required for the appropriate expression of genes involved in lipid metabolism.[18] TREM2-deficient microglia phagocytose myelin debris but fail to clear myelin cholesterol, resulting in cholesteryl ester accumulation.[19]

The second major pathway promoting microglia proliferation, survival, motility, and phagocytosis involves the colony stimulating factor 1 receptor (CSF1R), which is activated by CSF1 or interleukin (IL) 34. Signaling from CSF1R involves an effector tyrosine kinase that phosphorylates the intracellular motifs of DAP12, thereby providing for a cross-talk between CSF1 and TREM2 signaling.

TABLE 22.2 *Signals Triggering Microglial Activation (Examples)*

Signal	Microglial Receptor	Source of Interaction
ATP, ADP	P2X4, P2X7 P2Y6,P2Y12, P2Y13, P2Y14	Astrocytes Excessively active neurons Damaged axons
Complement C1q component	C3R	Aberrant or senescent synapses
Pathogen-activated molecular patterns	Toll-like receptor (TLR)-2 and TLR 4	Bacterial wall LPS Viral or bacterial DNA or RNA; HIV-1 protein gp120
Danger-associated molecular patterns	TLR4, TLR2, others	Heat shock proteins Misfolded proteins (e.g., Aβ) Tenascin, vesicans,
Advanced glycation end-products (AGE)	RAGE	Aβ, AGE
IFN-γ	Interferon (IFN)-γ receptor	T helper (Th) 1 lymphocyte
Tumor necrosis factor (TNF)-α	TNF receptor (TNFR1, TNFR2)	T helper (Th) 2 lymphocyte

Aβ, amyloid β; LPS, lipopolysaccharide; RAGE, receptor for advanced glycation end-products

SURVEILLANCE AND HOMEOSTATIC FUNCTION OF MICROGLIA

The "housekeeping" surveillance function of microglia is necessary to maintain CNS homeostasis. Resident microglial extend thin, rapidly motile processes that undergo rapid extension and retraction and actively survey a volume of parenchyma and, in normal conditions, target synaptic structures. Microglial processes make brief, repetitive contacts with synapses, remain in a close proximity to presynaptic boutons or postsynaptic spines, and then rapidly retract. These dynamic structural interactions between the microglial processes and dendritic spines respond to glutamatergic synaptic activity, particularly gradient concentrations of ATP and norepinephrine, acting via purinergic P2Y12 receptors and β2 adrenergic receptors in microglia.[3,14,15,20–22]

Markers of Surveilling Microglia

Transcriptome analysis indicates that surveilling microglia have a distinctive homeostatic gene signature that distinguish these cells from other CNS and myeloid cells.[4] Expression of these homeostatic genes depends on transforming growth factor β (TGF-β); they include those related to microglial ramification and motility (*P2RY12* encoding the P2Y12 receptors); synaptic remodeling (complement genes *C3* and *C1Q*); immune response (*HLA-DRA*); and microglial activation (*TREM2* and *APOE*). The expression profile of homeostatic gene transcription varies in different brain regions. In homeostatic conditions microglia perform continuous immune surveillance of the brain parenchyma, provide trophic support to neurons, eliminate dysfunctional synapses, and remove apoptotic debris; in the presence of immune stimulus they initiate an immune program. Recent studies in mice show that under basal network condition during wakefulness, noradrenergic tone suppresses surveillance processes by microglia via β2 receptor signaling; the relationship between neuronal network activity and microglia surveillance is not linear but rather follows an inverse U curve profile.[14,15]

Role of Microglia in Synaptic Pruning, Plasticity, and Homeostasis

During development and throughout adult life, microglia have important functions in refinement of synaptic circuits by synaptic pruning, phagocytosis of apoptotic cells, and promotion of programmed cell death. Microglia recognize aberrant synapses that need to be eliminated by pruning. One important tag for such synapses is complement protein C1q, which is recognized by complement receptor C3R expressed in microglia.[23,24] Astrocyte signals may contribute to the upregulation of complement and microglial activation preceding synapse elimination. Interactions of the microglia with synapses participate in not only brain development but also the control of synaptic plasticity in the adult brain. One example is synaptic scaling, which regulates the strength of excitatory synapses in response to changes in activity. Microglia clear apoptotic cells primarily in differentiating white matter tracts where OPCs undergo apoptosis. Several receptors and signaling pathways contribute to apoptotic cell clearance by microglia, depending on the environment context. Microglia also contribute to axonal guidance and neuronal support during development. In response to small disturbances in brain homeostasis, microglia may provide trophic support and reduce risk of excitotoxic damage to neurons. These neuroprotective effects may involve microglial production of growth factors such as glial derived neurotrophic factor, increased uptake of glutamate, and "synaptic stripping." Microglial processes intersperse between the pre- and the postsynaptic elements, engulfing the synapses and eliciting synapse elimination or inducing spine formation.[25,26]

Microglial Immune Checkpoints Mechanisms

Microglial cells receive constitutive signals from neurons that indicate a healthy state and impose a "calming" influence on microglia (Table 22.1). Because excessive microglial activation can produce damage to surrounding tissue, the transition from supporting homeostatic functions to immune activation is tightly regulated by a set of controlling mechanisms, referred to as microglial checkpoints.[27] Important checkpoints are interactions via direct contact with neighboring neurons (Figure 22.2). One example is the contact receptor–ligand interactions of neuronal CD200 and microglial CD200 receptor. Another example is fractalkine (CX3CL1), which is bound to the neuronal membrane and upon cleavage binds microglial CX3CR1 receptors. Another checkpoint is provided by soluble restraining factors, such as TGF-β, which is produced by astrocytes and abundantly expressed in the CNS in the steady state. TGF-β indirectly regulates synaptic pruning by microglia by controlling the expression of the complement factor C1q. The interactions between microglial signal regulatory protein (SIRP) α and postsynaptic CD47 may also protect maturing synapses from microglia-mediated clearance. Lipids mediators released from microglia, such as endocannabinoids, may also restrain proinflammatory responses by acting via cannabinoid 2 receptors (CB2Rs). Neurotransmitters such as GABA, acetylcholine, and norepinephrine, as well as neurotrophic factors such as nerve growth factor (NGF) and brain-derived neurotrophic factor (BDNF) also modulate microglia immunophenotype. Additional factors such as interleukin (IL)-4 and IL-13 may have neuroprotective effects by promoting microglial phagocytic activity and production of neurotrophic factors.[27]

MICROGLIAL ACTIVATION (EFFECTOR) STATES

Microglial activation encompasses a variety of morphological and functional responses of microglia toward different trigger signals (Table 22.3). Activated, or "effector"

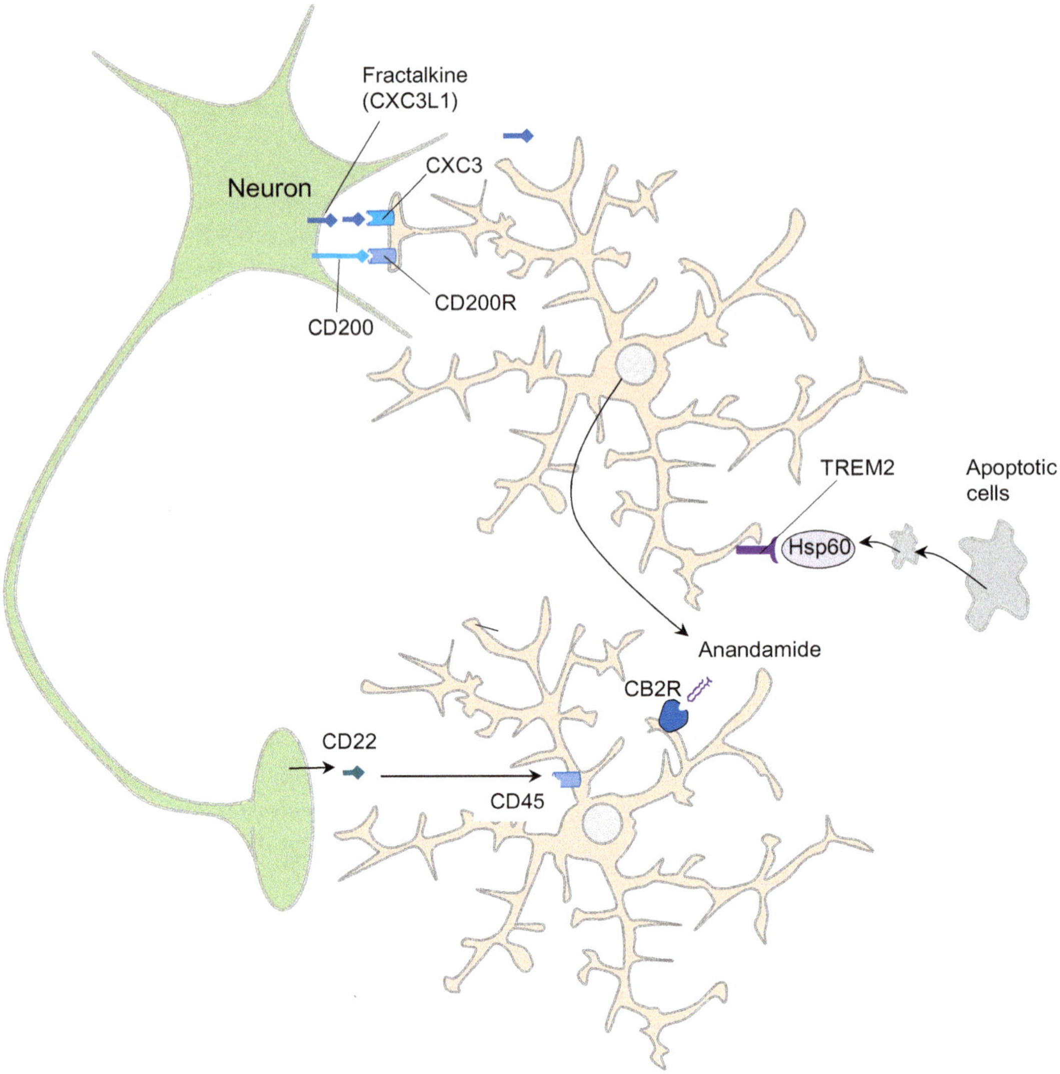

FIGURE 22.2 "Calming" signals for microglia.
Microglial cells receive constitutive signals from neurons that indicate a healthy state and impose a "calming" influence to these cells. Important checkpoints for microglial activation are interactions via direct contact with neighboring neurons. Typical examples are the contact receptor-ligand interactions of neuronal CD200 and microglial CD200 receptor (CD200R); and the interactions of fractalkine (CX3CL1). Lipids mediators released from microglia, such as endocannabinoids, may also restrain proinflammatory responses by acting via cannabinoid-2 receptors (CB2Rs). Apoptotic cells release heat shock protein 60 (Hsp60), which may interact with TREM2 (triggering receptor expressed in myeloid cells 2) promoting a repair function of microglia.

microglia are very plastic cells that can exist in multiple phenotypes and switch activity states in response to different chemical signals from various microenvironments (Figure 22.3). Effector microglia may adopt an amoeboid-like morphology that enables motility and phagocytic function during inflammation; rod-like, epithelioid, or multinucleated morphology in specific conditions; and hyperramified morphology in responses to stress or accelerated aging.[28,29]

"On" Signals Activating Microglia

One important "on" signal activating microglia is ATP, which is released from injured or activated neurons or astrocytes and acts as a paracrine signal that activates microglia via ionotropic P2X4 and P2X7 and metabotropic P2Y6 and P2Y12 receptors. Typical examples of signals activating microglia are DAMPs from pathogens such as bacterial wall lipopolysaccharides, viral envelopes, and bacterial or viral DNAs or RNAs; intracellular constituents released from necrotic cells; heat shock proteins; externalized phosphatidylserine on apoptotic cells; and misfolded proteins such Aβ and prion proteins. These signals activate microglial TLRs and other innate immune response receptors, such as receptors for advanced glycosylated end products (RAGE), and scavenger receptors. Complement proteins also activate

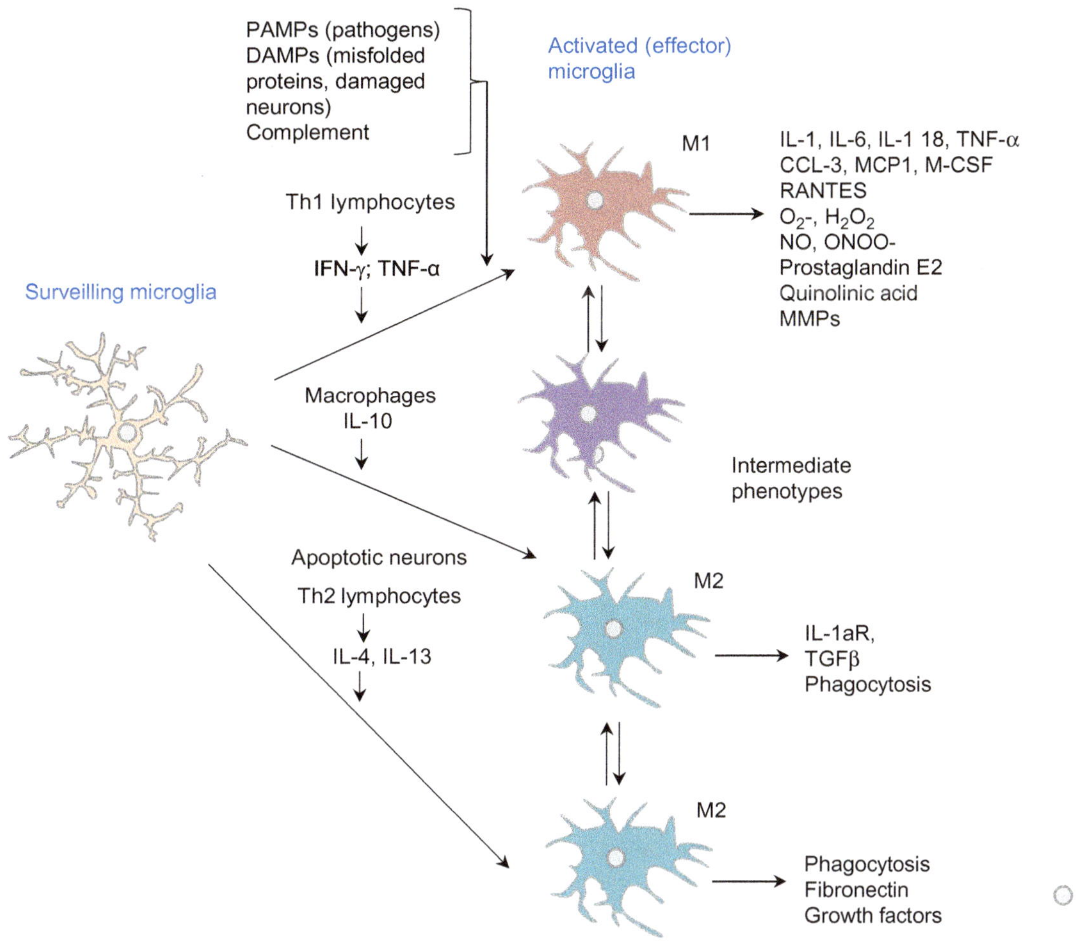

FIGURE 22.3 Activated states of microglia.

Activated macrophages, including microglia, have been classically subdivided into M1 and M2 phenotypes. The so-called M1 state is triggered by pathogen-associated molecular patterns (PAMPs) of damage-associated molecular patterns (DAMPs) that activate toll-like receptors (TLRs) or by interferon (IFN)-γ released from Th1 helper lymphocytes. M1 microglia release interleukin (IL)-1β, IL-6, IL-23, and tumor necrosis factor α (TNF-α); chemokines such as monocyte chemoattractant protein-1 (MCP-1); reactive oxygen species, nitric oxide, quinolinic acid, prostaglandin E_2, and matrix metalloproteinases (MMPs). In contrast, M2 microglia include different subtypes producing antiinflammatory cytokines such as IL-13, IL-14, IL-10, and transforming growth factor β(TGF-β); clear debris by phagocytosis; and promote tissue repair and tissue remodeling via extracellular matrix proteins. M2 microglia are induced by signals from apoptotic cells or by anti-inflammatory cytokines such as IL-4 and IL-13 released from Th2 helper cells. M1 and M2 patterns of activation represent a spectrum of response, and there are several intermediate states depending on the triggering stimulus. MCP-1, monocyte chemoattractant protein-1; M-CSF, macrophage colony stimulating factor; MIP, macrophage inflammatory protein; NGF, nerve growth factor; O_2^- (superoxide); NO, nitric oxide; $ONOO^-$, peroxynitrite; O_2^-, RANTES (regulated on activation, normal T cell expressed and secreted).

innate immune responses in microglia.[23] Another group of "on" signals are involved in adaptive immune responses and are mediated by cytokines released from different subsets of T-lymphocytes. Typical examples are pro-inflammatory cytokines, such as IL-1 and interferon-γ (IFN-γ). In general, "on" signals trigger proinflammatory cascades such as those mediated by p38 mitogen-activated protein kinase (p38MAPK) resulting in nuclear translocation of nuclear factor κB (NFκB) and subsequent transcriptional activation of various genes. Important target genes are those encoding cytokines, chemokines, cyclooxygenase 2, inducible nitric oxide (NO) synthase, nicotinamide adenine dinucleotide phosphate oxidase (NOX), major histocompatibility complex (MHC) receptors, and adhesion molecules.

Dynamic Phenotypic Heterogeneity of Activated Microglia

An early concept postulated a dichotomous categorization of activated macrophages, including microglia, into M1 and M2 phenotypes.[30] The classical M1 state (classical activation) can be triggered by ligands that activate TLRs during innate immune responses or by IFN-γ released from Th1 helper lymphocytes during adaptive immune responses. The M1 state consists of a phenotype associated with transcriptional activation mediated by NFκB, leading to production and release of pro-inflammatory cytokines and cytotoxic substance leading to an acute immune response. These include cytokines such as IL-1β, IL-6, IL-23, and TNF-α; chemokines such as monocyte chemoattractant protein-1 (MCP1); and cytotoxic substances such as reactive oxygen species, NO, quinolinic acid, prostaglandin E_2, and matrix metalloproteinases. In contrast, the M2 state (alternative activation) includes different subtypes determined by the microenvironment. These states are characterized by the production of anti-inflammatory cytokines such as IL-13, IL-14, IL-10, and TGF-β; facilitation of debris clearance by phagocytosis; promotion of tissue repair by releasing growth factors such as BDNF and glial-derived neurotrophic factor; and tissue remodeling via extracellular matrix proteins. M2 microglia are induced by signals from apoptotic cells that activate TREM2 or by anti-inflammatory cytokines such as IL-4 and IL-13 released from Th2 helper cells. It was classically assumed that microglia react to a stimulus with a M1 phenotype to address pathogens and damage, followed by transition to M2 state to promote tissue repair. However, transcriptome analysis disproves the existence of mutually exclusive M1–M2 polarization states.[4] Different stimuli trigger expression of a different transcription profile, including expression of M1 and M2 genes, indicating that the M1 and M2 patterns of activation represent a spectrum of response and there are several intermediate states of microglial activation depending on the triggering stimulus. Therefore, the extrapolation of the M1 and M2 phenotypes described in macrophages to define microglia phenotypes is an oversimplification that may be misleading.[31]

Effects of Aging on Microglia

Microglia undergo changes in morphology and function with normal aging.[32,33] They acquire a reactive state characterized by decreased size, number, and branching of the individual ramifications and dystrophic changes such as increased tortuosity, cytoplasmic beading, and fragmentation of microglial processes. Human transcriptome studies show increased expression of genes associated with actin dynamics (disassembly), which is consistent with evidence that microglial senescence results in decreased motility and rate of migration to focal tissue injury. The effects of aging in microglia may result in both loss of neuroprotective function and gain of pro-inflammatory function. In addition to morphological features of an activated state, senescent microglia also show upregulation of expression of MHC II, and activation of inflammasome-related signaling, including increased production of IL-1β and other pro-inflammatory cytokines. Upregulation of expression of TLR4 and other pattern recognition receptors and decreased CXC3L-CX3CR1 signaling may also occur in aged microglia. Reduced activity of the TREM2-DAP12 may reduce their phagocytic ability and increase production of inflammatory cytokines. This altered inflammatory response in immunosenescent microglia may predispose the brain to neurodegenerative conditions such as Alzheimer disease and Parkinson disease.[5]

REACTIVE GLIOSIS

Cells that are dying, or damaged but recoverable express or release many types of molecules, including neurotransmitters, chemokines, cytokines, neuroimmune regulators, and DAMPs that stimulate reactive gliosis, debris clearance, and specific immune responses.

Signals for Reactive Gliosis

According to cell type or injury severity there is release of different combinations of these molecules, which trigger different responses. For example, mild cellular insults can increase extracellular levels of ATP or glutamate that attract microglial processes or elicit calcium responses in astrocytes and microglia without triggering full-blown inflammation. Within the astrocytic syncytium, connexin-dependent release of ATP in response to increased intracellular calcium contributes to increase extracellular ATP levels and thus amplifies this danger signal. More severe cell damage or cell death results in release of intracellular DAMPs and "alarmins," such as heat shock proteins (e.g., Hsp60 and αB-crystallin), the S100 family of calcium-binding proteins, Aβ peptide, DNA, and RNA. All these molecules serve as "danger" signals to alert the innate immune system to areas of tissue injury and promote clearance of altered cells and cell debris. Similar responses are triggered by "non-self" signals including pathogen-associated molecular patterns (PAMPs). Both endogenous and exogenous alarm signals activate pattern-recognition receptors, such as TLRs and RAGEs. Healthy neurons and glia, either in normal conditions or near the area of CNS insults express neuroimmune regulatory molecules and self-defense proteins that signal "healthy self"; these signals include both secreted and membrane-bound molecules and serve to prevent phagocytosis of viable cells and confine potential noxious neuroinflammatory signaling. For example, sialic acid in the membrane of healthy cells interacts with sialic acid receptors on innate immune cells and functions as a "don't eat me" signal. As mentioned previously, the CD200 cytokine secreted by neurons, astrocytes, and oligodendrocytes binds to its C200R in microglia reducing microglial activation and phagocytosis. Fractalkine (CXC3L1) is another important constitutive signal from neurons that maintains microglia in a quiescent, surveillance (homeostatic) state and prevents microglial activation.

Heterogeneity of Reactive Astrocytes

Like microglia, astrocytes respond to signals from active synapses and regulate growth and differentiation of synapses and functional organization of the axons during development. As discussed in the previous chapter, in the adult CNS astrocytes provide metabolic support to neurons; regulate local cerebral blood flow, water and ion metabolism, and synaptic levels of neurotransmitters; modulate activity at individual synapses and neuronal networks; provide antioxidant protection to both neurons and oligodendrocytes; and interact with oligodendrocytes and axons to maintain myelin sheath and axon integrity. Reactive gliosis is triggered and regulated by a multitude of molecular signals.[34] They include danger signals released from pathogens or damaged or dead neurons and glial cells; cytokines, chemokines, ATP, and other molecular signals released from reactive microglia, other astrocytes, oligodendrocytes, endothelial cells, and pericytes; and similar signals from infiltrating leukocytes that gain access to the CNS via a leaky BBB. The coordinated interactions among these different cell types and signals allow for the fine-tuned regulation and resolution of the inflammatory response. In response to these signals, reactive glia alter their gene expression, morphology, and function in a selective and specific way, which depends both on the type and severity of the insult and the combination of signals that they receive. Reactive astrocytes, like microglia, are highly diverse and encompass a broad spectrum that includes pro-inflammatory/neurotoxic, phagocytic (scavenging), neuroprotective, and repair-promoting phenotypes (Figure 22.4).[34,35]

Astrogliosis is aimed functionally at increasing neuroprotection and trophic support of stressed neurons; isolation of the damage area from the rest of the CNS; repair of the damaged BBB; and, in some cases, remodeling of brain circuits in areas surrounding the lesioned region.[34] Features of reactive astrocytes include hypertrophy of the astrocyte process and upregulation of expression of glial fibrillary acid protein (GFAP). Transcriptome studies show that in addition of *GFAP* other genes are upregulated in reactive astrocytes. This reactive profile led to the identification of at least two different types of reactive astrocytes, referred to as "A1" and "A2" to parallel the M1 and M2 nomenclature applied to macrophages.

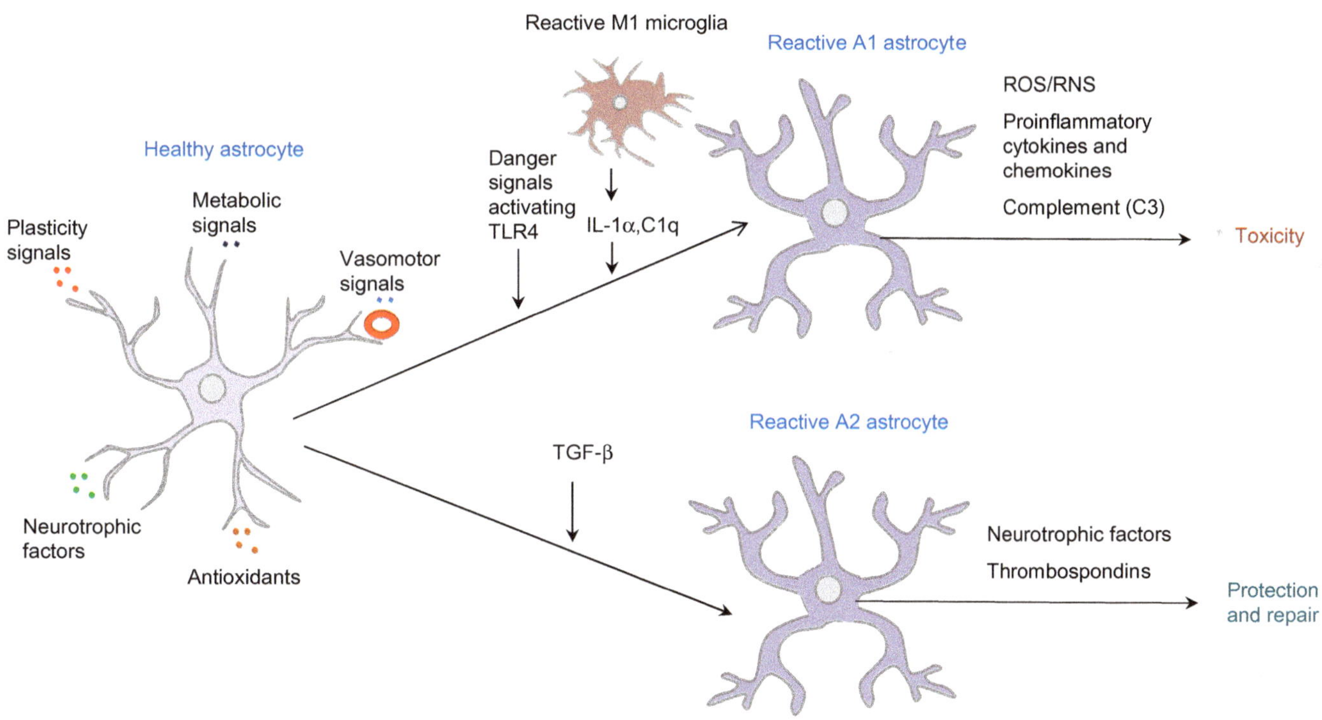

FIGURE 22.4 Patterns of astrocytic activation during inflammation.
Reactive astrocytes are highly diverse and encompass a broad spectrum that includes proinflammatory/neurotoxic, phagocytic (scavenging), neuroprotective, and repair-promoting phenotypes. A1 astrocytes are activated by signals from reactive M1 microglia such as interleukin (IL)-1α, tumor necrosis factor (TNF)-α, and C1q, in response to toll-like receptor (TLR4) oligodendrocyte death. A2 astrocytes upregulate neurotrophic factors that promote neuronal survival. As in the case of microglia, there are several intermedia states between the A1 and A2 phenotypes. RNS, reactive nitrogen species; ROS, reactive oxygen species.

The A1 astrocytes are activated by signals from reactive M1 microglia, such as IL1α, TNFα, and the complement component subunit C1q in the setting of inflammation or exposure to TLR4 receptor agonists. A1 astrocytes upregulate genes encoding C3 and other components of the complement cascade that are destructive to synapses, and secrete neurotoxins that promote neuronal and oligodendrocyte death. In contrast, reactive A2 astrocytes are activated in the setting of ischemia, upregulate expression of neurotrophic factors that promote neuronal survival, and secrete thrombospondins that promote synaptic repair. However, as in the case of microglia, A1 and A2 astrocytes represent the extremes of a phenotypic continuum that is determined by the type of insult and type and timing of the resulting environmental signals.[34] Unlike other cells such as microglia and infiltrated leukocytes involved in neuroinflammation, astrocytes do not migrate toward the site of injury. Rather, they stay within their domains; some become functionally polarized or can proliferate associated with blood vessels.

Glial Scar

Upon damage to the CNS, microglia, newly proliferated astrocytes and NG2 cells form a compact border, or glial scar, around the area of tissue damage, or lesion core.[35] The glial scar clearly demarcates the lesion and separates it from the rest of the CNS. The lesion core, also known as fibrotic or mesenchymal scar, contains perivascular-derived fibroblasts, pericytes, phagocytic macrophages, and ependymal cells and is rich in extracellular matrix proteins that inhibit axonal growth and remyelination. For example, reactive astrocytes secrete chondroitin sulfate proteoglycans that form barriers to axon growth. However, studies in animal models indicate that at least some astrocytes promote axonal growth by eliminating myelin debris and may support both tissue survival and repair. Oligodendrocyte progenitor NG2 cells constitute a large percentage of cells forming the glial scar. Like astrocytes, NG2 cells proliferate and undergo hypertrophy and increased expression of NG2 proteoglycans. Several developmental signals, such as platelet-derived growth factor, promote the differentiation of NG2 glia into oligodendrocytes and are upregulated in the glial scar. However, many NG2 glia do not differentiate to myelinating oligodendrocytes; some may generate astrocytes or Schwann cells according to the site of injury. NG2-derived Schwann cells may contribute to remyelination in the injured spinal cord but not in other CNS areas.

ADAPTIVE IMMUNITY IN THE CNS

In contrast to the ventricular and subarachnoid spaces, which allow entry and exit of peripheral immune cells and provide limited drainage of parenchymal antigens, the CNS parenchyma is protected from the immune system.

Barriers for Entrance of Immune Cells into the Brain Parenchyma

The major barriers to the entry of immune cells into the CNS are the vascular endothelium forming the BBB, the choroid plexus epithelium, and the glial limitans surrounding blood vessels at the surface of the parenchyma. Immune cells may enter the CSF via the choroid plexus or by extravasation through the walls of subarachnoid veins. The arachnoid consists of a layer of cells connected by tight junctions that forms a blood-CSF barrier between the dura and the subarachnoid space. Whereas the pia covering the brain is permeable to solutes and immune cells, the surface of the parenchyma is covered by the glia limitans formed by compacted astrocytic processes and an overlying basement membrane. The BBB encompasses a barrier for solutes formed by tight junctions between endothelial cells and a barrier in the postcapillary venules that regulates the entrance of immune cells. To reach the brain parenchyma from the blood, T cells have to penetrate first the vascular endothelium and then the glia limitans. Whereas solutes and immune cells can pass from the blood to the stroma of the choroid plexus, the choroid epithelium contains gap junctions forming a blood CSF barrier that regulates the composition of the CSF and the passage of immune cells.

Features of the BBB Relevant to Neuroinflammation

The BBB is a fundamental functional feature of the neurovascular unit, which includes the microvascular endothelial cells, pericytes, astrocytes, neuronal processes, and microglia. A unique feature of neurovascular endothelial cells is the low expression of leukocyte adhesion molecules, which prevents immune cells from crossing the BBB in basal, unstimulated conditions. The endothelial basement membrane is permissive for T cell infiltration in inflammatory conditions. Once extravasated, T cells are trapped in the perivascular space due to the presence of the parenchymal basement membrane formed by the glia limitans, which prevents transmigration of immune cells into the CNS. Entrance of T cells into the parenchyma requires their reactivation by local antigen-presenting perivascular macrophages that reside in the perivascular space around postcapillary venules. Neuroinflammation in the CNS parenchyma is initiated by events in the periphery and subarachnoid space. Activated memory T cells can directly pass into the CSF through meningeal vessels or the choroid plexus. BBB breakdown may result from mechanical shear injury of microvessels, resulting in a massive, non-selective passage of blood- and brain-derived inflammatory components. Inflammatory factors released from cells of the neurovascular unit, including pro-inflammatory cytokines, reactive oxygen species, MMPs, and vascular endothelial growth factor (VEGF), can induce an activated phenotype in the endothelium and mediate alteration of the architecture of tight junctions. Reactive oxygen species elicit oxidation of junctional proteins, upregulation of inflammatory mediators, and activation of MMPs, particularly MMP-9, which can directly degrade components of the basement membranes. During inflammation endothelial activation leads to increased vascular permeability due to partial loss of junctional integrity, upregulation of cell adhesion molecules to recruit immune cells from the periphery, and release of cytokines and chemokines that further support infiltration of peripheral immune cells. Upregulation of cell adhesion molecules such as intercellular adhesion molecule-1 (ICAM-1) promotes leukocyte trafficking via a multistep process including rolling, activation of integrins such as α4β1 integrin leading to arrest and firm adhesion, crawling, and diapedesis. Once leukocytes have overcome the endothelial, basement membrane, and pericyte layer, they accumulate at perivenular spaces forming inflammatory perivascular cuffs. Activation of MMPs is then required for leukocytes to further traverse the parenchymal basement membrane and layer of astrocyte endfeet to reach the neural tissue.

Role of the Choroid Plexus

In addition to the BBB, there are alternative routes for entrance of immune cells and cytokines to the CNS, including the circumventricular organs, which have capillaries that lack BBB-type tight junctions. Immunoglobulins (mainly IgG and IgM) can penetrate at a low rate through the blood-CSF barrier at the level of the choroid plexus and are present as polyclonal populations in healthy persons. The choroid plexus macrophages and dendritic cells are located primarily in the stroma and may serve as a port for macrophages/leukocytes to enter the CSF and then the ventricular surface. Epithelial choroid cells express adhesion molecules and chemokines that facilitate the transepithelial passage of macrophages and leukocytes into the CSF. Infiltrating immune cells first migrate from the blood across the fenestrated endothelium into the stromal surface, move along the basolateral surface of the choroid epithelium and gain access across the epithelium to the CSF. Epiplexus Kolmer cells are macrophages that migrate from the circulation to the choroid stroma and then to the apical surface of the choroid epithelium, where they may function as antigen-presenting cells to lymphocytes.

INFLAMMATION AS A COMMON DISEASE MECHANISM IN NEUROLOGIC DISORDERS

Acute Focal Disorders

Acute brain injury from trauma or stroke leads to rapid degeneration of neurons and their process, resulting in release of DAMPS that activate innate immune responses in microglia via TLRs, RAGE, and ATP receptors. Microglia in the core of an acute lesion and in the surrounding penumbra rapidly respond by adopting an M1 phenotype with upregulation of IL-1, IL-16, TNF-α, NO, quinolinic acid and other cytotoxic molecules that contribute to neuronal death this; innate inflammatory response may exacerbate lesion size following acute focal injury, but is limited in time. In addition, microglia can form a protective barrier around the injury site via their unique P2Y12 receptors.[13] There is also microglial activation along the degenerating fibers undergoing Wallerian degeneration, which is followed by removal of degenerating axons and myelin by microglia and macrophages. However, these cells are relatively ineffective in removal of myelin or axonal debris and may persist for several years at the site of injury.

Acute CNS injury results in global immune activation throughout the body, mostly within the cervical lymph nodes, meningeal spaces including the CSF, and the site of injury. This adaptive response is preceded by an innate immune response, as damaged tissue promptly releases alarmins, such as ATP and particularly IL-33, which rapidly activate glia and recruit granulocytes and monocytes to the site of injury.

Inflammatory and Immune Disorders

In the case of infection, innate immunity leads to pathogen-specific adaptive immune responses that, in turn, further regulate the innate immune response, skewing the microglia phenotype from a pathogen-fighting to a tissue-building phenotype once the infection has cleared. The adaptive response then regulates itself by suppressing effector T cells and retaining a small number of memory clones that can be rapidly reactivated in response to the same infection. The regulation of T-cell responses is critical to prevent potentially self-reactive T cells from attacking the brain.

The CNS damage in multiple sclerosis (MS) results from immune attack by T- and B cells and macrophages leading to damage of the BBB, myelin, axons, and neurons. In this disorder, proinflammatory B cells have a major role in presentation of antigens to T-helper cells, secretion of cytokines, and antibody production. Microglia have a key role in the initiation and perpetuation of both demyelination and remyelination in MS due to their ability to present antigens, release neurotoxic molecules and pro-inflammatory or anti-inflammatory cytokines, clear myelin debris and apoptotic cells, recruit endogenous OPCs, and deliver trophic factors that support remyelination. Active microglia are present in the areas of active demyelination, the white matter beyond the plaque, and the gray matter. Whereas inflammatory microglial mediators such as TNF-α and NO trigger axonal injury in demyelinating disease, microglia also release mediators that promote remyelination. Phagocytosis during demyelination is associated with upregulation of TREM2 and other phagocytic receptors; TNF-α and growth factors such as insulin-like growth factor 1 are also upregulated during demyelination and promote remyelination. In the mouse model experimental autoimmune encephalomyelitis (EAE), resident microglia and infiltrating monocytes play differential roles: monocyte-derived macrophages associate with nodes of Ranvier and initiate demyelination, whereas microglia appear to clear debris.[36]

Autoimmune Encephalitis

Autoreactive B cells can drive autoimmunity through production of antibodies, immune complex formation, presentation of autoantigen to T cells, and production of cytokines. Autoantibodies against neural self-antigens may arise spontaneously, in response to an underlying malignancy, or as consequence of viral or bacterial infections. Antibody-mediated encephalitis may manifest with changes in memory, cognition and behavior, psychosis, seizures, abnormal movements, disturbance in arousal and sleep, and autonomic disturbances.[37] Autoimmune encephalitis associated with autoantibodies directed against membrane antigens such as ion channels or neurotransmitter receptors manifests with loss-of-function of the target membrane proteins. The pathogenic effects of antibodies include blocking receptor function, cross-linking internalization of receptors, and interference with intercellular protein–protein interactions. Autoimmune response may be initiated by antigens released by tumors, viral destruction (e.g., in herpes simplex type 1 [HSV1] encephalitis), or immune checkpoint inhibitors. In these disorders, memory B cells reach the brain, where they undergo restimulation, antigen-driven maturation, clonal expansion, and differentiation into antibody-producing plasma cells. The intrathecal synthesis of antibodies is reflected by the presence of oligoclonal bands in the CSF, with little evidence of BBB dysfunction and low or undetectable levels of serum antibodies. These autoimmune encephalitides respond to immunomodulatory therapy, including rituximab, a monoclonal antibody that targets the CD20 antigen in autoreactive B cells. Autoimmune encephalitides due to antibodies against intracellular antigens are typically paraneoplastic and have poor response to immunotherapy. These paraneoplastic antibodies are directed against nucleocytoplasmic onconeural antigens such as mRNA-splicing factors. Peptides derived from these antigens are by MCH class I expressing cells cytokine environment and recognized by cytotoxic CD8+ T cells; tissue-specific CD8+ cells may then be activated as a consequence of molecular mimicry or viral infection of the target tissue.

Innate immune responses and neuroinflammation have a contributory role in autoimmune encephalitis. Infiltrating monocytes and microglial proliferation at the site of pathology could contribute to the pathogenesis of the disease with resultant BBB, disruption and subsequent activation of adaptive immune response. Both innate and adaptive immune cells can produce pro-inflammatory molecules, which can perpetuate ongoing neuroinflammation and drive manifestations such as ongoing seizure activity and ultimately neurodegenerative changes.[38] For example, HSV-1 encephalitis produces a pro-inflammatory CNS environment, leading to activation of microglia and production of pro-inflammatory cytokines, such as TNF-α, IL-1β, IL-6, and CCL2, which could drive upregulation and infiltration of innate cells such as monocytes into the CNS. This results in BBB dysfunction and then recruitment of B cells to produce antibodies. Imaging studies also demonstrated the importance of neuroinflammation and altered BBB permeability in autoimmune encephalitis. Arterial spin labeling MRI of patients with N-methyl-D-aspartate receptor (NMDAR) encephalitis show early increased BBB permeability prior to parenchymal neuroinflammation. Fluorodeoxyglucose (FDG)-PET neuroimaging in various subtypes of autoimmune encephalitis show areas of both hypometabolism and hypermetabolism, which could reflect seizure activity, neuroinflammation, or early increase in BBB permeability. Neuroinflammation may contribute to ongoing seizure activity in autoimmune encephalitis, by the combination of ongoing release of mediators and alterations in neuronal excitability due to antibody effects on receptors. Microglial activation and proliferation may also contribute to long-term cognitive changes seen in patients with autoimmune encephalitis. Antibody-mediated encephalitis can also be associated with antibodies against glial antigens, such as astrocytic aquaporin 4 (AQP4) in neuromyelitis optica spectrum disorders or myelin-oligodendrocyte glycoprotein (MOG). For example, astrocyte–microglia interaction drives evolving neuromyelitis optica lesions.[39]

Neurodegenerative Disorders

Microglia-mediated neuroinflammation is an important feature of neurodegenerative disorders. The primary mechanism is expansion of resident microglia; increased number of perivascular and other CNS macrophages derived from circulating monocytes is a major contributor in conditions associated with BBB disruption. The persistent activation of microglia in these disorders may reflect an innate immune response to the accumulation of misfolded proteins, neuronal degeneration, or both. Endogenous stimuli including aggregated Aβ, α-synuclein, or tau oligomers may persistently activate microglial pro-inflammatory responses and finally lead to irreversible neuron loss. Transcriptome analysis in experimental models indicates that in all these disorders gene expression is characterized by downregulation of homeostatic signature genes and upregulation of genes associated with inflammation, phagocytosis, and lipid metabolism. Microglia may have either a protective or a neurotoxic effect depending on their predominant phenotype, determined by environmental signals in a time-dependent manner. For example, *APOE*, *TREM2*, and *HLA-DR* are highly expressed in microglia surrounding dense-core plaques in early stages of AD. Missense *TREM2* variants are a risk factor for late-onset AD.[16,17] These mutations lead to loss of TREM2 function by reducing lipid–ligand affinity and subsequent signaling. Variants of *PLCG2* encoding phospholipase C γ2, which cleaves membrane phospholipids downstream of TREM2 and TLR signaling to induce inflammatory response are also risk factors of late-onset AD.[40] In the absence of TREM2, microglia may lose their ability to process lipids through the TREM2–PLCγ2 signaling pathway,

TABLE 22.3 *Features of Microglial Phenotypes*

Phenotype	M1	M2	M2
Function	Pro-inflammatory Killing of pathogens Cytotoxicity Phagocytosis	Anti-inflammatory Phagocytosis	Tissue repair ECM remodeling Phagocytosis
Stimulus	PAMPs, DAMPS Misfolded proteins Complement IFN-γ, TNF-α	IL-10	IL-4, IL-13
Source of stimulus	Pathogens Damaged neurons Th1 lymphocytes	Macrophages	Apoptotic neurons Th2 lymphocytes
Receptors	TLRs, TNFR, IFNR MHC1, MHC-II,	CCL17, CCL22, CD163	TREM2 Mannose receptor
Products	IL-1, IL-18; IL-6 TNF-α CCL3 (MIP-1α) MCP-1, MCSF RANTES ROS (O_2^-, H_2O_2) RNS (NO, $ONOO^-$) Prostaglandin E2 Quinolinic acid MMPs	IL-10 receptor IL-1R antagonist (IL-1Ra) TGF-β Anandamide	ECM components Fibronectin Growth factors (BDNF, GDNF, NGF, IGF)

BDNF, brain-derived neurotrophic factor; GDNF, glial-derived neurotrophic factor); H_2O_2, hydrogen peroxide; IGF, insulin-like growth factor; IFN-γ, interferon-γ; IL, interleukin; MCP-1, monocyte chemoattractant protein-1; M-CSF, macrophage colony stimulating factor; MIP, macrophage inflammatory protein; NGF, nerve growth factor; O_2^- (superoxide); MHC, major histocompatibility complex; MMP, matrix metalloprotease; NO, nitric oxide; NOO^-, peroxynitrite; O_2^-, RANTES (regulated on activation, normal T cell expressed and secreted superoxide); RNS, reactive nitrogen species; ROS, reactive oxygen species; TGF-β, transforming growth factor β; TNF-α, tumor necrosis factor α; TREM2, triggering receptor expressed in myeloid cells 2.

which leads to increased lipid burden in these cells resulting in amplified TLR–PLCγ2 signaling downstream of TLR activation, promoting detrimental inflammatory responses.[18] In addition, some *TREM2* variants have also been described in families with behavioral-variant frontotemporal dementia with atypical features, including seizures and corpus callosum atrophy. TREM2 has been suggested as part of a functional network involved in other neurodegenerative diseases including PD and other synucleinopathies, amyotrophic lateral sclerosis, tauopathies, and Creutzfeldt-Jakob disease.

INVOLVEMENT OF MICROGLIA IN SELECTIVE NEUROLOGIC DISORDERS

Primary Microgliopathies and Leukoencephalopathy

Primary microglial disorders result from loss-of-function mutations affecting TREM-DAP12 or CSF1-CSF1 receptor signaling. Mutations of the *TREM2* or *DAP12 (TYROBP)* genes produce polycystic lipomembranous dysplasia with sclerosing leukoencephalopathy (Nasu-Hakola disease). This is an autosomal recessive disorder that manifests with multiple bone cysts (due to impairment of osteoclasts) and early-onset progressive dementia associated with white matter lesions presumably related to abnormal microglial activation. Mutations of the *CSF1R* gene cause adult-onset leukoencephalopathy with axonal spheroids and pigmented glia (ALSP).[41] This is an autosomal dominant disorder that manifests with relatively rapidly progressive cognitive and psychiatric symptoms (resembling frontotemporal dementia), parkinsonism (sometimes resembling corticobasal syndrome), and spasticity with bilateral involvement of the corticospinal tract extending from the subcortical white matter to the spinal cord. Typical MRI findings in ALSP include increased T2 signal in the anterior white matter, small cysts, thinning of the corpus callosum and small symmetric calcifications adjacent to the anterior horns and parietal subcortical white matter. Neuropathologically, ALPS is characterized by the presence of activated and pigmented microglia and dystrophic axons with thin and knot-like spheroids. Similar findings have been described in leukoencephalopathy associated with mutations of the *AARS2* gene encoding alanyl-transfer RNA synthetase 2.

Role of Microglia in Seizures

Studies in experimental models and observations in brain tissue of patients with epilepsy indicate robust microglial activation in the setting of seizures.[42,43] Microglial activation may occur rapidly in response to excessive neuronal activity, as shown in the CA3 region of the hippocampus. These studies show that in the acute phase microglia respond to ATP released from hyperactive neurons by a P2Y12 receptor-mediated extension of microglial processes that target these hyperactive neurons, thereby attenuating seizure severity and having a neuroprotective role. In the subacute phase, fractalkine released from neurons activates microglia, likely causing neuronal degeneration. In the chronic phase microglia may be able to recognize DNA from degenerating neurons via TLR9 receptors, which initiates signaling that prevents aberrant neurogenesis following induction of seizures.[43]

Role of Microglia in Pain

Microglia in the spinal cord are strongly activated after peripheral nerve injury.[44] While C-fiber activation is sufficient to elicit spinal microglial reactivity, stimulation of large A-fibers is also important to maintain microglial activation. Multiple signaling molecules released from damaged primary afferents play a major role in the induction and development of spinal microgliosis. They include CSF1; chemokines such as CCL2 acting via microglial CCR2 receptors; MMP9, which induces cleavage and activation of IL-1β; caspase6, which triggers TNF release from microglia; and neuregulin-1. Following nerve injury, there is upregulation of purinergic receptors, including P2X4, P2X7, P2Y12, and P2Y13 in microglia, which promotes microglial activation in response to ATP released from damaged afferents and contribute to the development of mechanical allodynia. Peripheral nerve injury also results in upregulation of the CX3CR1 chemokine receptor; expression of cathepsin S, which cleaves and activates fractalkine (CXCL1); and upregulation of complement components C1q, C3, and C4 in spinal microglia. Microglial activation is reflected by upregulation of p38 MAPK and other phosphorylation cascades.[44]

KEY POINTS

- Microglia maintain cellular, synaptic, and myelin homeostasis during development and normal function and response to injury.
- Microglia are capable of self-renewal, which maintains the microglial population throughout life.
- Microglia development is controlled by the triggering receptor expressed in myeloid cells 2 (TREM2) and is activated by the colony stimulating factor 1 receptor (CSF1R).
- The "housekeeping" surveillance function of microglia is necessary to maintain CNS homeostasis including synaptic pruning and clearance of debris.
- Activated ("reactive" or "effector") microglia constitute a heterogeneous population that dynamically changes in phenotype depending on the type of stimulus and microenvironment.
- Reactive gliosis is an heterogeneous reaction that includes microglia, astrocytes and NG2 cells an varies according to the type and timing of the triggering insult.
- Entrance of T cells into the parenchyma requires their reactivation by local antigen-presenting perivascular macrophages.
- Acute CNS injury results in an innate immune response followed by an adaptive immune activation.
- Innate immune responses and neuroinflammation have a contributory role in autoimmune encephalitis.
- Microglia-mediated neuroinflammation is an important feature of neurodegenerative disorders.
- *TREM2* variants may be risk factors for Alzheimer disease.
- Mutations of the *CSF1R* gene cause adult-onset leukoencephalopathy with axonal spheroids and pigmented glia.
- There is robust microglial activation in the setting of seizures.
- Microglia in the spinal cord are strongly activated after peripheral nerve injury.

REFERENCES

1. Eyo UB, Wu LJ. Microglia: lifelong patrolling immune cells of the brain. Prog Neurobiol 2019;179:101614.
2. Hanisch UK, Kettenmann H. Microglia: active sensor and versatile effector cells in the normal and pathologic brain. Nat Neurosci 2007;10:1387–1394.
3. Wake H, Moorhouse AJ, Miyamoto A, Nabekura J. Microglia: actively surveying and shaping neuronal circuit structure and function. Trends Neurosci 2013;36:209–217.
4. Wes PD, Holtman IR, Boddeke EW, Moller T, Eggen BJ. Next generation transcriptomics and genomics elucidate biological complexity of microglia in health and disease. Glia 2016;64:197–213.
5. Bohlen CJ, Friedman BA, Dejanovic B, Sheng M. Microglia in brain development, homeostasis, and neurodegeneration. Annu Rev Genet 2019;53:263–288.
6. Gomez Perdiguero E, Schulz C, Geissmann F. Development and homeostasis of "resident" myeloid cells: the case of the microglia. Glia 2013;61:112–120.
7. Tay TL, Hagemeyer N, Prinz M. The force awakens: insights into the origin and formation of microglia. Curr Opin Neurobiol 2016;39:30–37.

8. Tay TL, Mai D, Dautzenberg J, et al. A new fate mapping system reveals context-dependent random or clonal expansion of microglia. Nat Neurosci 2017;20:793–803.
9. Eyo UB, Mo M, Yi MH, et al. P2Y12R-dependent translocation mechanisms gate the changing microglial landscape. Cell Rep 2018;23:959–966.
10. Ransohoff RM, Cardona AE. The myeloid cells of the central nervous system parenchyma. Nature 2010;468:253–262.
11. Wu LJ, Wu G, Akhavan Sharif MR, et al. The voltage-gated proton channel Hvl enhances brain damage from ischemic stroke. Nat Neurosci 2012;15:565–573.
12. Wu LJ. Voltage-gated proton channel HV1 in microglia. Neuroscientist 2014;20:599–609.
13. Haynes SE, Hollopeter G, Yang G, et al. The P2Y12 receptor regulates microglial activation by extracellular nucleotides. Nat Neurosci 2006;9:1512–1519.
14. Liu YU, Ying Y, Li Y, et al. Neuronal network activity controls microglial process surveillance in awake mice via norepinephrine signaling. Nat Neurosci 2019;22:1771–1781.
15. Stowell RD, Sipe GO, Dawes RP, et al. Noradrenergic signaling in the wakeful state inhibits microglial surveillance and synaptic plasticity in the mouse visual cortex. Nat Neurosci 2019;22:1782–1792.
16. Guerreiro R, Wojtas A, Bras J, et al. TREM2 variants in Alzheimer's disease. N Engl J Med 2013;368:117–127.
17. Jonsson T, Stefansson H, Steinberg S, et al. Variant of TREM2 associated with the risk of Alzheimer's disease. N Engl J Med 2013;368:107–116.
18. Andreone BJ, Przybyla L, Llapashtica C, et al. Alzheimer's-associated PLCgamma2 is a signaling node required for both TREM2 function and the inflammatory response in human microglia. Nat Neurosci 2020;23:927–938.
19. Nugent AA, Lin K, van Lengerich B, et al. TREM2 regulates microglial cholesterol metabolism upon chronic phagocytic challenge. Neuron 2020;105:837–854 e839.
20. Tremblay ME. The role of microglia at synapses in the healthy CNS: novel insights from recent imaging studies. Neuron Glia Biol 2011;7:67–76.
21. Nimmerjahn A, Kirchhoff F, Helmchen F. Resting microglial cells are highly dynamic surveillants of brain parenchyma in vivo. Science 2005;308:1314–1318.
22. Fontainhas AM, Wang M, Liang KJ, et al. Microglial morphology and dynamic behavior is regulated by ionotropic glutamatergic and GABAergic neurotransmission. PLoS One 2011;6:e15973.
23. Zabel MK, Kirsch WM. From development to dysfunction: microglia and the complement cascade in CNS homeostasis. Ageing Res Rev 2013;12:749–756.
24. Hammond TR, Robinton D, Stevens B. Microglia and the brain: complementary partners in development and disease. Annu Rev Cell Dev Biol 2018;34:523–544.
25. Parkhurst CN, Yang G, Ninan I, et al. Microglia promote learning-dependent synapse formation through brain-derived neurotrophic factor. Cell 2013;155:1596–1609.
26. Miyamoto A, Wake H, Ishikawa AW, et al. Microglia contact induces synapse formation in developing somatosensory cortex. Nat Commun 2016;7:12540.
27. Deczkowska A, Amit I, Schwartz M. Microglial immune checkpoint mechanisms. Nat Neurosci 2018;21:779–786.
28. Boche D, Perry VH, Nicoll JA. Review: activation patterns of microglia and their identification in the human brain. Neuropathol Appl Neurobiol 2013;39:3–18.
29. Hanisch UK. Proteins in microglial activation—inputs and outputs by subsets. Curr Protein Pept Sci 2013;14:3–15.
30. Mosser DM, Edwards JP. Exploring the full spectrum of macrophage activation. Nat Rev Immunol 2008;8:958–969.
31. Ransohoff RM. A polarizing question: do M1 and M2 microglia exist? Nat Neurosci 2016;19:987–991.
32. Mecca C, Giambanco I, Donato R, Arcuri C. Microglia and aging: the role of the TREM2-DAP12 and CX3CL1-CX3CR1 axes. Int J Mol Sci 2018;19.
33. Spittau B. Aging microglia-phenotypes, functions and implications for age-related neurodegenerative diseases. Front Aging Neurosci 2017;9:194.
34. Pekny M, Pekna M, Messing A, et al. Astrocytes: a central element in neurological diseases. Acta Neuropathol 2016;131:323–345.
35. Adams KL, Gallo V. The diversity and disparity of the glial scar. Nat Neurosci 2018;21:9–15.
36. Yamasaki R, Lu H, Butovsky O, et al. Differential roles of microglia and monocytes in the inflamed central nervous system. J Exp Med 2014;211:1533–1549.
37. Dalmau J, Graus F. Antibody-mediated encephalitis. N Engl J Med 2018;378:840–851.
38. Wesselingh R, Butzkueven H, Buzzard K, Tarlinton D, O'Brien TJ, Monif M. Innate immunity in the central nervous system: a missing piece of the autoimmune encephalitis puzzle? Front Immunol 2019;10:2066.
39. Chen T, Lennon VA, Liu YU, et al. Astrocyte-microglia interaction drives evolving neuromyelitis optica lesion. J Clin Invest 2020;130:4025–4038.
40. Sims R, van der Lee SJ, Naj AC, et al. Rare coding variants in PLCG2, ABI3, and TREM2 implicate microglial-mediated innate immunity in Alzheimer's disease. Nat Genet 2017;49:1373–1384.
41. Miura T, Mezaki N, Konno T, et al. Identification and functional characterization of novel mutations including frameshift mutation in exon 4 of CSF1R in patients with adult-onset leukoencephalopathy with axonal spheroids and pigmented glia. J Neurol 2018;265:2415–2424.
42. Patel DC, Tewari BP, Chaunsali L, Sontheimer H. Neuron-glia interactions in the pathophysiology of epilepsy. Nat Rev Neurosci 2019;20:282–297.
43. Eyo UB, Murugan M, Wu LJ. Microglia-neuron communication in epilepsy. Glia 2017;65:5–18.
44. Chen G, Zhang YQ, Qadri YJ, Serhan CN, Ji RR. Microglia in pain: detrimental and protective roles in pathogenesis and resolution of pain. Neuron 2018;100:1292–1311.

23 Microenvironment in the Central Nervous System

OVERVIEW

The structural and functional integrity of the CNS, including cell survival, signaling, plasticity, and response to injury, requires a highly controlled microenvironment. Fundamental mechanisms include the coupling between cerebral blood flow (CBF) and neuronal activity; regulation of permeability of and transport across the blood-brain barrier (BBB); and dynamic interchange between the cerebrospinal fluid (CSF) and the brain interstitial fluid (ISF) compartments. The control of local CBF and BBB function requires the coordinated activity of the components of a neurovascular unit, which includes perivascular neuronal processes, astrocytic endfoot processes, brain endothelial cells, pericytes, and vascular smooth muscle cells. The choroid plexus–CSF system and its interactions with the ISF allow transport of trophic and signaling molecules and detoxification of xenobiotics. The endothelium of the BBB, the choroid plexus epithelium, and the ependymal glia limitans formed by astrocytes limit the access of inflammatory cells into the CNS parenchyma in normal conditions. Disturbances of local CBF regulation, BBB permeability, and CSF production and dynamics are fundamental disease mechanisms in many neurologic disorders. The aims of this chapters are to review: (1) the components of the neurovascular unit and their function; (2) the mechanisms of regulation of local CBF; (3) the structure and function of the BBB; (4) the production, composition, and dynamics of the CSF; (5) the fluid interchange between the CSF and in brain interstitial fluid; and (6) some clinical examples of disturbances of these functions.

NEUROVASCULAR UNIT

The neurovascular unit consists of processes of excitatory and inhibitory neurons, astrocytes, and microglia surrounding and interacting with vascular pericytes, vascular smooth muscle, and endothelial cells[1,2] (Figure 23.1). The neurovascular unit is functionally heterogeneous throughout the brain. The arteries that penetrate the brain from the subarachnoid space consist of endothelial cells, a basement membrane, and smooth muscle cells, surrounded by a perivascular space, pia mater, and end-foot processes of astrocytes. As vessels continue deeper into the brain, they lose their smooth muscle cell and pia mater coverage, gaining pericytes between the capillary endothelial cells and the astrocytic endfeet.

Interactions within the neurovascular unit enables the tight coupling of neuronal activity with local CBF (known as neurovascular coupling or functional hyperemia) and substrate availability for energy metabolism (neurometabolic coupling); regulation of the formation, permeability, and transport function of the BBB; trophic interactions among its different components (neurotrophic coupling); angiogenesis and vascular remodeling; and neuroimmune responses.[3–11] All components of the neurovascular unit secrete multiple chemical signals and express a variety of receptors that allow for complex paracrine interactions.

Cellular Components

The brain endothelial cells are the core unit of the BBB.[9] They are joined by tight junctions and adherens junctions, which provide a physical barrier that impedes paracellular diffusion of ions, macromolecules, and other polar solutes. In addition to a physical barrier, brain vascular endothelial cells form a selective transport interface between the blood and the brain. In the human brain, capillaries contribute to 85% of the vessel length and provide ~12 m^2 of the endothelial surface area available for transport exchanges. Pericytes extend thin processes around and along the outer wall of precapillary arterioles, capillaries, and postcapillary venules and are separated from endothelial cells by a basement membrane.[11,12] Pericytes are multifunctional cells that have an important role in regulation of CBF and maintenance of

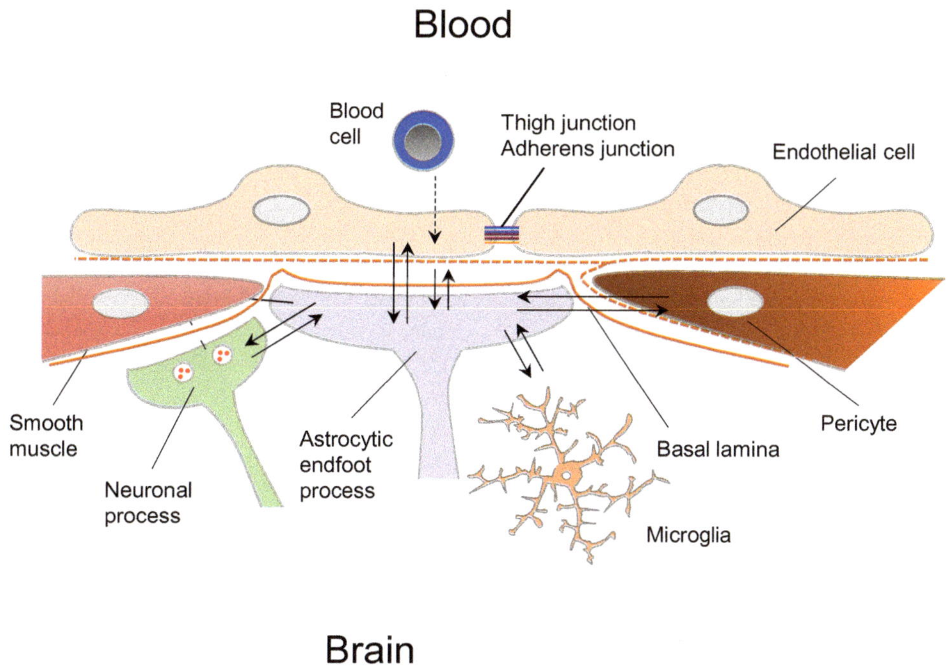

FIGURE 23.1 Neurovascular unit.

The neurovascular unit consists of processes of excitatory or inhibitory neurons, astrocytes, and microglia surrounding and interacting with vascular cells including pericytes, vascular smooth muscle, and endothelial cells. Interactions within the neurovascular unit enables the tight regulation of blood flow through the brain vasculature, vascular permeability, and neuroimmune responses.

the BBB, control of vascular development and angiogenesis, and neuroinflammatory processes.[10–12] They communicate both with each other via peg-and-socket contacts and with cerebral endothelial cells through gap junctions. This allows the propagation of signals up or down the capillary.[6,11,13] Astrocytes occupy a strategic position between capillaries and neurons and are a pivotal component of the neurovascular unit. They respond dynamically to synaptic activity and are a critical link in the mechanisms of neurovascular coupling and neurometabolic coupling. Their endfoot processes provide ~99% of the coverage of the abluminal surface of cerebral blood vessels, creating gliovascular units.[3,4] These processes express the water channel aquaporin 4 (AQP4) and the inward-rectifying potassium channel Kir4.1, which contribute to the coupling of local regulation of blood flow and activity-dependent water and potassium homeostasis.[14,15] The presence of AQP4 may allow the astrocytes to participate in ISF clearance via the so-called-glymphatic system.[16,17] Astrocytic perivascular endfoot processes also secrete growth factors that induce tight junction formation and upregulate transport system proteins in vascular endothelial cells. Astrocytes and endothelial cells also interact with microglia and perivascular macrophages, affecting BBB permeability during inflammation.[18]

In the brain, neuronal processes are in physical contact with the vasculature, and release mediators that elicit local increase in CBF in response to metabolic demand resulting from synaptic activity.

Basement Membrane

Secreted proteins make up a specialized extracellular matrix (ECM) that forms the basement membrane (or basal lamina) around blood vessels. A basement membrane is present both between endothelial cell and pericytes and between astrocytes and pericytes. As the coverage of the vasculature by pericytes is discontinuous, in areas of discontinuity astrocytes and endothelial cells share a single basement membrane. The protein composition of the ECM in the basement membrane surrounding brain vasculature differs from that present in the periphery. Within the brain the protein composition of the basement membrane also varies between large and small vessels.[19] Key proteins of the basement membranes include ECM collagens (particularly collagen type IV), fibrillins, laminins, vitronectin, and fibronectin; proteins that bind to ECM such as lectins and semaphorins; enzymes responsible for matrix degradation and processing, including matrix metalloproteases (MMPs); and soluble factors such as growth factors and cytokines.[19]

REGULATION OF CEREBRAL BLOOD FLOW

The human brain has both a limited capacity for substrate storage and a high metabolic rate, making the precise regulation of CBF critical for the maintenance of constant nutrient and O_2 supply. While the brain represents ~2%

of body weight, it receives up to 15%–20% of total cardiac output. The elevated metabolic requirements of the brain, which relies to an important extent on oxidative metabolism, necessitate a great proportion of cardiac output. The cerebral cortex is supplied by a two-dimensional network of pial arterioles that feed a three-dimensional network of subsurface microvessels located in close proximity to neurons and glia. The penetrating arterioles that connect the pial network to the subsurface network are bottlenecks to blood flow. Collateral flow is insufficient to compensate for the occlusion of a penetrating arteriole.[20]

Cerebral Autoregulation

Cerebral autoregulation ensures constant cerebral blood flow over a wide range of systemic arterial blood pressure.[21,22] The classic description of cerebral autoregulation is that CBF is maintained at a constant level across a wide range of mean arterial blood pressure between 60 and 150 mmHg. The relationship between average CBF and average perfusion pressure is known as static cerebral autoregulation. However, studies using transcranial Doppler ultrasonography allowing relatively high fidelity recordings of CBF velocity (and by assumption CBF) showed that CBF is very dynamic at rest, and could change markedly in response to dynamic changes in blood pressure. This provides for the concept of dynamic cerebral autoregulation.[21] Static versus dynamic cerebral autoregulation is an experimental, not a physiological, distinction. There are several limitations of the experimental approaches to assessing cerebral autoregulation in humans.[23] Static cerebral autoregulation is typically described as operating over several minutes to hours and represents the steady-state relationship between mean arterial pressure and CBF. In contrast, dynamic cerebral autoregulation commonly refers to the cerebral pressure–flow relationship as observed during transient changes in mean arterial pressure as occurs for example, with changes in posture, and takes place over a period of seconds. Short-term (dynamic) and long-term (static) regulation of CBF could represent the same mechanism, although they may dissociate, for example, in some pathological conditions. A classical study showed that in response to transient hypotension flow velocity in the middle cerebral artery recovers more rapidly than blood pressure.[24] There are several hypothesis about the mechanisms underlying cerebral autoregulation.[25] Findings from studies in healthy humans indicate the potential contribution of endothelial-related regulation via nitric oxide (NO), neurogenic regulation through sympathetic activity, and intrinsic myogenic control. However, the role of NO in human cerebral autoregulation appears negligible. The brain circulation is richly supplied by perivascular adrenergic nerves, and smooth muscle cells in the arterioles have alpha- and beta-adrenergic receptors.[26,27] Transcranial Doppler (TCD) measures support a modest role of autonomic nerves in regulating dynamic cerebral autoregulation. Some, but not all, studies suggest that the posterior circulation seems to have a less effective dynamic cerebral autoregulation, characterized by transfer function analysis, compared to the anterior circulation. The myogenic hypothesis proposes that stretching of vascular smooth muscles activates stretch-sensitive nonselective cation channels, resulting in the influx of Ca^{2+} through voltage-gated Ca^{2+} (L-type) channels, and consequently smooth muscle contraction. A study using pharmacological blockade of alpha-adrenergic-, muscarinic-, and calcium channel-mediated mechanisms suggest that myogenic effects occur outside the active region of autoregulation, whereas neurogenic influences are largely responsible for cerebral blood flow control within it.[28] Dynamic cerebral autoregulation may be more able to compensate for transient hypertension than for hypotension. These asymmetric pressure–flow relationships may reflect an adaptation for protecting the cerebral circulation against arterial pressure surges. For example during exercise, despite progressive elevations in systolic blood pressure during exercise, CBF only increases by 15%–25% up to 70% of maximal oxygen uptake. Animal data indicate that cerebral sympathetic nerves are activated during acute hypertension, but not hypotension. However, human pial arteries are sparsely innervated and are insensitive to topical norepinephrine. Both chronic hypertension and hypotension are generally associated with paradoxical reductions in CBF. With chronic hypertension, long-term structural changes in small cerebral vessels, brain atrophy, and altered BBB permeability are likely the result of reductions in CBF. With chronic hypertension, the static autoregulatory curve shifts rightward, which may place patients at risk of impaired ability to tolerate hypotension. Long-term treatment of hypertension may partially reverse this rightward shift. With chronic hypotension the related brain cerebral hypoperfusion has been shown to cause cognitive deficits in attention and memory. Particularly in the elderly, cerebral autoregulation does not necessarily protect the brain from chronic low blood pressure and low cardiac output, and can result in CBF insufficiency.[29]

Effects of Blood Gases

Products of cerebral tissue metabolism and chemical stimuli, such as arterial carbon dioxide tension ($PaCO_2$) are among the key factors that influence the diameter of the cerebral vessels. In awake and healthy humans, $PaCO_2$ is the most potent regulator of CBF, and even small fluctuations can result in large changes in CBF. Elevations in $PaCO_2$ cause a reduction in cerebrovascular resistance and a consequent increase in CBF, while reductions in PaCO2 cause an increase in cerebrovascular resistance and a decrease in CBF. The magnitude of this response is referred to as cerebrovascular CO_2 reactivity. As changes in $PaCO_2$ do not typically occur in isolation, the integrative influence of physiological factors such as intracranial pressure, arterial oxygen content, cerebral perfusion pressure, and sympathetic nervous activity must be considered.[30] Alterations in $PaCO_2$ induce changes in blood vessel diameter not only in small pial vessels but also in large vessels such as the middle cerebral artery.[31] One of the putative mechanisms for hypercapnia-induced vasodilation is via vasodilator prostaglandins, such as prostaglandin E2 (PGE2). One study showed that the internal carotid artery dilates in response to hypercapnia and modestly constricts in response to hypocapnia; this response is markedly blunted by indomethacin but no other nonsteroidal anti-inflammatory agents, indicating an effect independent of cyclooxygenase inhibition.[32] Hypoxia also increases CBF and one of the potential signals is adenosine. However, a study using the adenosine receptor blocker theophylline showed that adenosine is not obligatory for CBF regulation in response to hypoxia.[33]

Neurovascular Coupling

Neurovascular coupling, or functional hyperemia, is the spatial and temporal coupling of increased CBF based on the energy demands in response to neural activity. Functional hyperemia is primarily driven by excitatory synaptic activity and involves signals from both neurons and astrocytes to smooth muscle in arterioles and pericytes surrounding capillaries. These signals include NO, prostanoids such as PGE2, extracellular K^+, hydrogen (H^+) ions, and adenosine.[3–8] Functional hyperemia provides the basis for blood-oxygen-level-dependent (BOLD) signals on functional MRI. The relative role of synaptic and spiking activity in driving hemodynamic signals is controversial. Studies using two-photon microscopy to measure sensory-evoked responses of individual blood vessels while imaging synaptic and spiking activity in the surrounding tissue with fluorescent glutamate and calcium sensors showed that local neural and hemodynamic signals may be partly decoupled.[20,34] In vivo, when sensory input increases blood flow, capillaries dilate before arterioles and are estimated to produce 84% of the blood flow increase. Dilation of capillaries critically depends on pericyte relaxation driven by astrocyte mediators, whereas arteriolar dilation directly depends on signals from local neurons and interneurons. This indicates that different signaling cascades regulate cerebral blood flow at the capillary and arteriole levels.[35] The pial arteries on the surface of the cerebral cortex offer the greatest cerebrovascular resistance and are the main site of control of regional CBF. Downstream vasodilator signals from the intraparenchymal capillaries and arterioles at the site of neuronal activity may be transmitted to pial arteries via a mechanism of intramural vascular signaling, resulting from increased velocity and shear stress in upstream branches. The relative contributions of neurons and astrocytes and neurons to vasomotor responses vary as a function of brain region and local anatomy. However, the vasoactive mediators released from both cell populations act together either synergistically or antagonistically to precisely regulate CBF within their microdomains.

The primary basis of functional hyperemia is excitatory synaptic activity resulting in release of L-glutamate from excitatory synapses. Glutamate drives local vasodilation both via production of NO in target cells and activation of astrocytes to release PGE2 and other vasodilator prostanoids. Activation of N-methyl-D-aspartate receptors (NMDARs) elicits Ca^{2+} influx and calmodulin kinase II (CaMKII)-triggered activation of neuronal NO synthase, resulting in NO release.[3,35] Nitric oxide induces vasodilation through activation of cytosolic guanylyl cyclase and generation of cyclic guanosine monophosphate (cGMP) in arteriolar smooth muscle cells.[3–8] Neuronal activity also triggers an increase in intracellular Ca^{2+} in perisynaptic astrocytes both via activation of metabotropic glutamate receptors leading to Ca^{2+} release from the endoplasmic reticulum stores and via release of ATP that activates Ca^{2+} influx via P2X receptors. The Ca^{2+} signal reaches the astrocytic endfeet and activates phospholipase A_2 (PLA_2), leading to production of arachidonic acid, which is then metabolized by cyclooxygenase-2 to PGE2 and via epoxygenase to the vasodilator epoxyeicosatrienoic acid (EET) and the vasoconstrictor 20-hydroxy-epoxyeicosatrienoic acid (HETE). The main astrocyte-derived mediator triggering vasodilation is PGE2, which acts vie EP4 receptors in pericytes, causing capillary vasodilation. This vasodilator effect requires NO release from neurons to suppress the synthesis of HETE. Increases in intracellular Ca^{2+} in astrocyte endfeet also trigger K^+ efflux via large-conductance calcium-gated potassium channels (BK); increase in perivascular K^+ concentration leads to vasodilation via activation of inward-rectifying K^+ channels producing hyperpolarization and reduced Ca^{2+} signaling of perivascular contractile cells.[3,36] Whereas modest increase in astrocytic Ca^{2+} elicits vasodilation, large increases may trigger vasoconstriction. For example, astrocytes contribute to pressure-induced increases in vascular tone via release 20-HETE, triggered by mechanical activation of transient receptor potential channel of the vanilloid family 4 (TRPV4) in astrocytics endfoot processes.

Pericytes contain contractile proteins including smooth muscle actin, tropomyosin, and myosin; respond to signals from neighboring astrocytes and endothelial cells; and contribute to neurovascular coupling.[12,37,38] Ischemia and other causes of oxidative stress result in capillary constriction by pericytes, which may contribute to the long-lasting blood flow decrease and neuronal damage after stroke.[37,38] The vascular endothelium may have a key role in the long-range propagation of vasodilation during functional hyperemia.[39] Capillary endothelial cells may directly sense neuronal activity and respond to extracellular K^+, which activates inward-rectifying K^+ channels and produces a rapidly propagated retrograde membrane hyperpolarization that is communicated as a vasodilator signal from the endothelium to upstream arterioles.[40] Since capillaries are embedded in the O_2-consuming neuropil, activity-dependent dips in O_2 tension drive capillary hyperemia. Red blood cells act as O_2 sensors that autonomously regulate their own deformability and thereby flow velocity through capillaries in response to physiological decreases in O_2 tension.

Neuronal Networks and Behavioral State-Dependent CBF Regulation

Neuromodulatory signals from forebrain cholinergic neurons and brainstem monoaminergic neurons, including the locus-coeruleus-norepinephrine system, elicit a behavioral state-dependent control of CBF in cortical networks. These neuromodulatory signals produce these effects by acting on pyramidal neurons, local GABAergic neurons, and astrocytes. GABAergic interneurons within local cortical circuits express vasoactive polypeptides such as vasoactive intestinal polypeptide (VIP) and neuropeptide Y and have processes that terminate onto both the cerebral microvessels and astrocytes, contributing to the local regulation of CBF.[2] Experimental studies show that in response to sensory activation, acetylcholine potentiates sensory-evoked hemodynamic responses by recruiting both pyramidal neurons and GABA/VIP-containing interneurons, whereas concurrent increase of norepinephrine levels reduce the spread of the sensory-evoked hemodynamic response in the cortex.[2]

BLOOD-BRAIN BARRIER

The BBB is the key interface for molecular exchange between the blood and the brain interstitial fluid. It restricts ionic and fluid movements between the blood and the brain, supplies the brain with essential nutrients, and mediates efflux of waste and other potential toxic products.[9,41,42] The endothelial cells that form the BBB are characterized both by the presence of tight junctions and by the polarized expression of membrane of ion channels, transporters, receptors, and metabolite-degrading enzymes. The BBB is also critical in long-range crosstalk between the periphery and CNS via microRNA (miRNA)-containing exosomes.

Tight Junctions

The tight junctions are primarily formed by claudins and occludin. These are integral membrane proteins that are located close to the apical endothelial membrane and form dimers with their counterparts on adjacent endothelial cells (Figure 23.2). Tight junction proteins are connected via scaffolding zonula occludens (ZO) proteins to the actin and vinculin-based cytoskeletal filaments via the dystrophin complex. Adherens junction proteins, vascular endothelial cadherin, and platelet endothelial cell adhesion molecule-1 form homophilic endothelial-to-endothelial contacts. Gap junction proteins, including connexin-37 (Cx37), Cx40, and Cx43, form hemichannels between endothelial cells, enabling endothelial intercellular communications maintaining tight junction integrity.

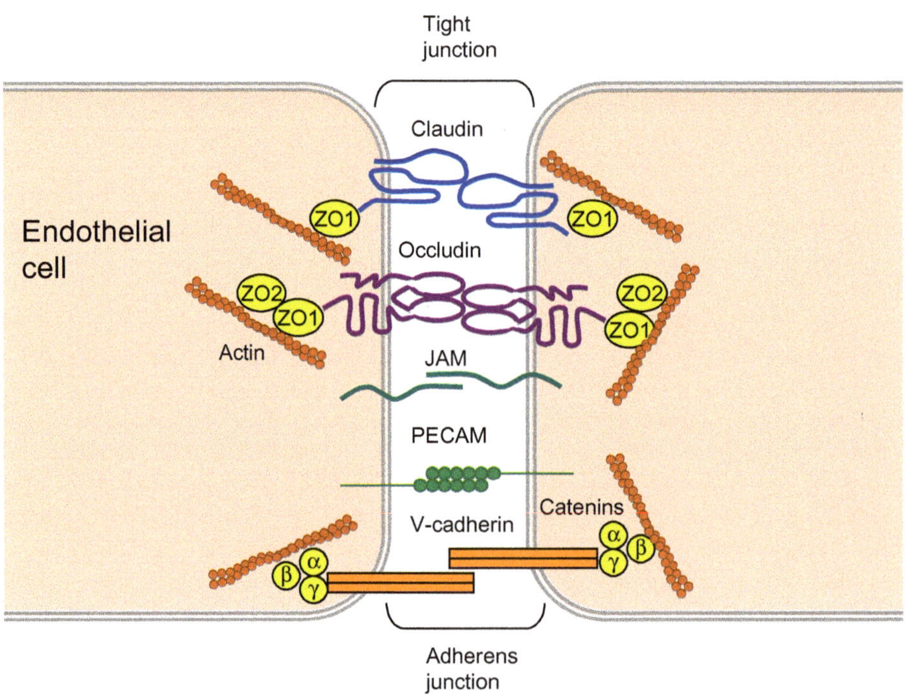

FIGURE 23.2 Blood-brain barrier.
The brain endothelial cells are the core unit of the blood-brain barrier (BBB). Adjacent brain endothelial cells are joined by tight junctions and adherens junctions. The tight junction proteins claudins and occludin are connected via zonula occludens (ZOs) proteins to the cytoskeleton. Gap-junction proteins, including connexin-37 (Cx37), Cx40, and Cx43, form hemichannels between endothelial cells. JAM, junctional adhesion molecule; PECAM, platelet endothelial cell adhesion molecule.

Formation, Maturation, and Maintenance of the BBB

Both cerebral angiogenesis and BBB formation require precise cues from various growth factors, guidance molecules, and other molecules such as microRNAs, as well as tightly tuned intracellular signaling pathways and gene expression. These signals originate from endothelial cells, pericytes, astrocytes, and the ECM. Endothelial cells and pericytes communicate by juxtacrine and paracrine signaling.[12] Endothelial cells secrete growth factors such as angiopoietin 1, transforming growth factor beta (TGF-β) and platelet-derived growth factor (PDGF) BB to direct pericytes to migrate to new vessels in order to stabilize the vascular wall. Pericytes share a common basement membrane with brain capillary endothelial cells and have a critical role in angiogenesis and BBB maintenance.[10,11]

Pericytes control the cell cycle of endothelial cells, secrete angiogenic-promoting factors such as vascular endothelial growth factor (VEGF) and Notch homolog protein (NOTCH) 3 to activate angiogenesis, and directly contribute to the formation of the basement membrane by secreting ECM proteins such as laminin and vimentin.[43] Pericytes can also modulate and maintain the BBB through the release of signaling factors to determine the number of endothelial cell tight junctions and direct the polarization of the end-foot processes of astrocytes. Pericytes also have stem cell potential; they are similar to mesenchymal stem cells and can differentiate into multiple cell types, including angioblasts, neural progenitors, vascular cells, and microglia. WNT signaling is crucial for both angiogenesisi and BBB genesis. Several WNT ligands secreted in the local environment including those derived from astrocytes induce gene expression promoting differentiation of endothelial cells.

Astrocytes join the neurovascular unit during the maturation stage and provide additional support to the BBB, through the formation of perivascular astrocytic endfeet around capillaries and the glial limitans that ensheathes the penetrating arterioles. Astrocytes also strengthen the basement membrane by producing laminins, and release signals such as retinoic acid, sonic hedgehog, TGFβ, glial-derived neurotrophic factor, and angiopoietin 1, which regulate gene expression in endothelial cells and enhance formation of intercellular junctions. Astrocytes alsosecreteapolipoprotein E which bind to the low-density lipoprotein receptor-related protein 1 receptor (LRP1) on pericytes, thus promoting astrocyte–pericyte interactions.

Neuronal activity also contributes to BBB maintenance For example, exposure to light increases transcription of BBB-related genes in the visual cortex. Molecules expressed in the basement membrane have signaling functions and mediate interactions within the neurovascular unit. For example, astrocytes and endothelial cells associate with the ECM and basal lamina via integrins and dystroglycans. Integrins are receptors that bind to laminins, and fibronectin links the ECM to the cytoskeleton; dystroglycans also bind to laminins, agrin, and perlecan to provide additional links of the ECM to the cytoskeleton. Astrocytic endfeet are strongly linked to the basal side of the endothelial cells by numerous integrin–dystroglycan complexes. Integrins in the endothelial basal cell membrane interact with extracellular laminin and fibronectin, connecting collagen IV and proteoglycans in the extracellular space to dystroglycans inserted in the underlying astrocytic endfeet membrane.[44] The basal lamina also determines the functional polarity of the astrocytes. For example, agrin, a proteoglycan of the basal lamina induces segregation of AQP4 and Kir4.1 to the perivascular astrocytic endfeet via signaling mechanism that involves the α-dystroglycan-syntrophin complex.

Regulation of BBB Permeability and Transport Function

The BBB is a highly metabolic structure that contains several specialized transport systems at both its luminal (blood-facing) and abluminal (brain-facing) sides. Transporters at the luminal side allow entry of specific nutrients, such as glucose, amino acids, nucleosides, neurotransmitter transports, and some peptides such as transferrin, whereas transporters at the abluminal side eliminate potentially toxic molecules, such as excitatory neurotransmitters, metabolic waste products, and amyloid β peptide (Aβ). Thus, normal BBB function is critical to maintain the composition of the extracellular and intracellular compartments in the CNS. Reciprocal interactions among astrocytes, endothelial cells, pericytes, and ECM proteins via a large number of paracrine signals maintain the integrity of the BBB.[9,41] Regulation of tight junction proteins involves several signaling pathways mediated by intracellular Ca^{2+}, cyclic adenosine monophosphate, protein kinases, and Rho guanosine triphosphatases; these signals affect transcription factors and cytoskeletal proteins. For example, increased intracellular Ca^{2+} activates protein kinase C, which phosphorylates occludin and disrupts the tight junctions. Several regulatory mechanisms influence expression of transporters and carriers in endothelial cells. For example, hypoxia-inducible factor-1, ATP, and other signals from astrocytes promote glucose transporter 1 (GLUT1) expression aimed to supply more glucose in the setting of increased synaptic activity. Similarly, PGE2 and inflammatory cytokines regulate P-glycoprotein expression and activity. The BBB may also become permeable to specific molecules, such as insulin-like growth factor 1 (IGF1) in response to neural activity. In epilepsy, which is associated with increased glutamatergic activity there is opening of BBB although the mechanism involved is still undetermined.

Solute Transport Systems at the BBB

With the exception of gases (e.g., oxygen and CO_2) and small lipophilic molecules such as ammonia, ethanol, or benzodiazepines, which freely diffuse across the endothelium, molecular exchanges between blood-and-brain and brain-and-blood are regulated by endothelial transport systems as well as by pericyte transporters. Substrate-specific endothelial solute carrier transporters encoded by *SLC* genes enable solutes such as carbohydrates, amino acids, monocarboxylic acids, hormones, fatty acids, nucleotides, inorganic ions, amines, choline, and vitamins to cross the BBB (Table 23.1) (Figure 23.3). One important example is the GLUT1 uniporter, which is expressed in endothelial cells, can be accessed from both the luminal and abluminal endothelial membrane, and transports glucose down its concentration gradient. GLUT1 deficiency due to loss-of-function *SLC2A1* gene mutations manifests with a widely variable phenotype associated with an inappropriate low CSF glucose concentration (typically <40 mg/d).[45] All essential amino acids that are substrates for monoamine neurotransmitter synthesis are transported across the BBB via the large neutral amino acid transporter (LNAA, LAT1/LAT2, *SCL7A5*).[46] This transporter also transports levodopa, which competes with other neutral amino acids for its access from the blood to the brain; this provides the rationale for a protein-restricted diet and taking levodopa on an empty stomach to increase its CNS availability in patients with Parkinson disease (PD).[47] The expression of LAT1 was reduced in a mouse model of PD.[48] Glutamine has higher levels in the brain ISF than in the blood; it is transported into the endothelium via sodium-coupled transporters, then hydrolyzed in the endothelium to glutamate via glutaminase, and finally removed into circulation. There are several transporters that exchange glutamine for other amino acids at the BBB. Glutamine exchangers have a role in conditions of extreme ISF glutamine loads (glutaminosis) where excessive glutamine efflux across the BBB enhances influx of tryptophan, which overloads the brains with neuroactive products such as serotonin, kynurenic acid, and quinolinic acid.[49] Transporters of excitatory amino acids, glycine, taurine, and GABA mediate high-affinity, sodium-dependent transport from the brain to the endothelium.

TABLE 23.1 *Solute Carriers at the Blood-Brain Barrier (Examples)*

Transporter	Function/Comments
Glucose transporter-1 (GLUT1)	Transports glucose and other hexoses from blood to brain
Sodium/myo-inositol transporter (SMIT)	Transports of myo-inositol by facilitated diffusion into the brain
Large amino acid transporters (LAT 1,2)	Transport of tryptophan and tyrosine into the brain
Cationic amino acid transporters (CAT1-3)	Transport of lysine and arginine
Sodium-coupled neutral amino acid transporters (SNAT 1,2,3,5)	Transport of glutamine out of the brain
Sodium-dependent excitatory amino acid transporters (EAATs 1,2,3)	Transport of glutamate and aspartate out of the brain
Sodium-dependent amino acid transporters ASCT1/2 and GLYT1	Transport alanine, serine and cysteine, and glycine out of the brain
Monocarboxylic acid transporter-1 (MCT1)	Transports lactate and ketone bodies from the blood to the brain
Fatty acid transporter protein (FATP1-4)	Transports fatty acids from blood to brain
Organic cation/carnitine transporter-2 (OCTN2)	Transports carnitine from blood to brain
Plasma membrane monoamine transporter (PMAT)	Transport serotonin and dopamine from brain to endothelium to blood
Choline transporter-like protein1 (CTL1)	Bidirectional transport of choline
Concentrative nucleoside transporter-2 (CNT2) and equilibrative nucleoside transporter-1 and 2 (ENT1/2)	Sodium-independent transport of nucleotides and nucleobases
Organic anion transporter-3 (OAT3) and organic anion transporting polypeptides (OATP 1A4 and 2b1)	Bidirectional transport of organic anions
Thyroid hormone transporters MCT8 (for T3) and organic transport polypeptide 1c1 (OATP1C1, for T4)	Transports thyroid hormones from blood to brain
Sodium-dependent vitamin transporter (SVT1)	Transports multivitamins from blood-to-brain

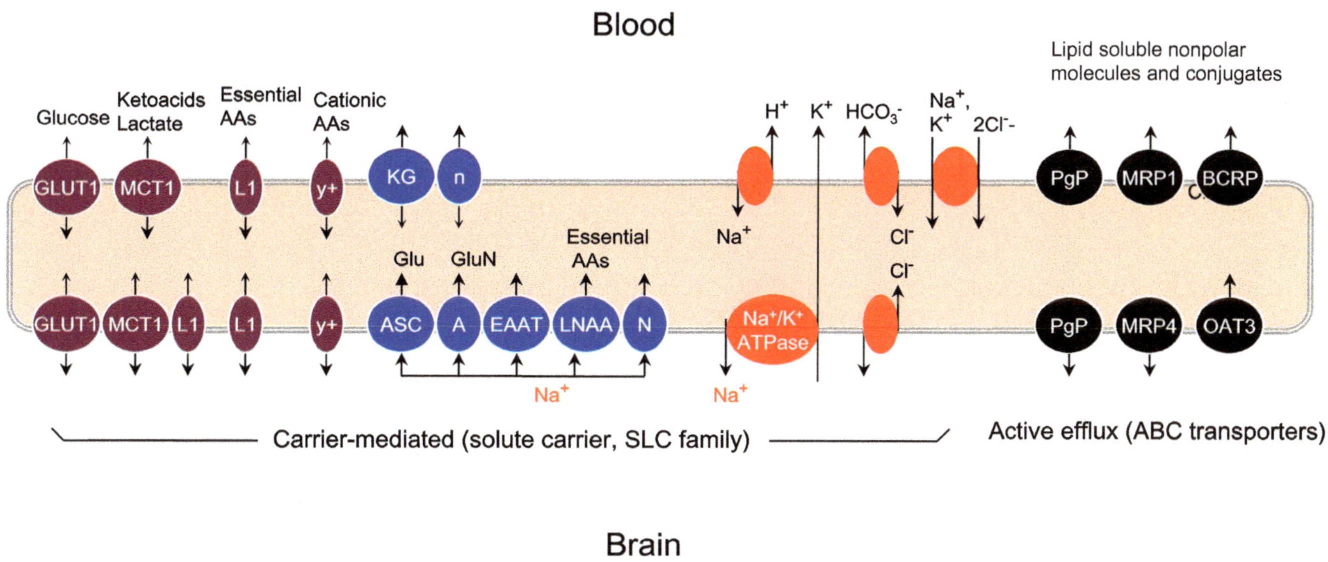

FIGURE 23.3 Solute transport across the BBB.
Substrate-specific endothelial solute carrier transporters encoded by *SLC* genes enable solutes such as carbohydrates, amino acids, monocarboxylic acids, hormones, fatty acids, nucleotides, inorganic ions, amines, choline, and vitamins to cross the BBB. They include the GLUT1 uniporter, transporters for myo-inositol, essential amino acids, excitatory amino acid transporters (EAATs), transporters for neutral amino acids, and monocarboxylate transporter-1 (MCT1) for lactate. The abluminal sodium pump (Na^+/K^+ ATPase) is a key regulator of sodium (Na^+) influx into the brain and potassium (K^+) efflux from the brain. Other transporters and ion channels have a major role in maintaining endothelial cell volume and pH or participate in mechanisms of CBF regulation. Endothelial cells of the BBB express ATP-binding cassette (ABC) transporters. They include ABCB1 (also known as P-glycoprotein, P-gp), ABCA2, breast cancer resistance protein (BCRP), and multidrug resistance-associated proteins (MRPs).

Lactate released from skeletal muscles during exercise and ketone bodies derived from liver from metabolism of fatty acids are transported from blood into the brain across the BBB by the monocarboxylate transporter-1 (MCT1) and then utilized as alternative energy metabolites by the brain.

Endothelial Ion Transport

The BBB has a major role in controlling concentration of ions in the CNS. The abluminal Na^+/K^+-ATPase is a key regulator of sodium (Na^+) influx into the brain and potassium (K+) efflux from the brain. This keeps high concentrations of Na^+ and low levels of K^+ in brain interstitial fluid, which is critical both for regulating neuronal excitability and for maintaining the Na^+ concentration gradient to drive Na^+-dependent transport across the BBB. Other transporters and ion channels have a major role in maintaining endothelial cell volume and pH or participate in mechanisms of CBF regulation. The ion transporters expressed in brain endothelium are also expressed in the choroid plexus epithelium, but with an opposite polarity in distribution. For example, the Na^+/K^+ ATPase is located in the apical (luminal) membrane, where it constitutes the primary driver for CSF secretion.

Endothelial Active Efflux and Enzymatic Barrier

Endothelial cells of the BBB express ATP-binding cassette (ABC) transporters primarily at their luminal side; these transporters utilize ATP as an energy source and function to prevent brain accumulation of drugs, xenobiotics, drug conjugates, and nucleosides via active efflux from endothelium to blood. They include ABCB1 (also known as P-glycoprotein or multidrug resistance protein 1) and multidrug resistance-associated proteins (MRPs). Genetic polymorphisms of *ABCB1* gene have been proposed to affect the bioavailability of antiepileptic drugs.[50] The endothelial cells forming the BBB also express enzymes that metabolize endogenous and exogenous molecules, including neurotransmitters. Examples of this enzymatic barrier include monoamine oxidase, γ-glutamyl transpeptidase, and angiotensin-converting enzyme 2 (ACE2). In experimental models, ACE2 deficiency impaired endothelial function in cerebral arteries and augmented endothelial dysfunction during aging.[51] Of note, ACE2 is a receptor for SARS-Covid-2.[52]

Endothelial Receptor-Mediated Transport

Some proteins and peptides use receptor-mediated transport to traverse the BBB and enter into or exit the brain (Figure 23.4). For example, transferrin receptor, insulin receptor, and leptin receptor mediate blood-to-brain transport of their respective ligands. The arginine-vasopressin V1 receptor mediates bidirectional transport of this peptide across the endothelium. Given its potential pathophysiological and therapeutic implications for Alzheimer

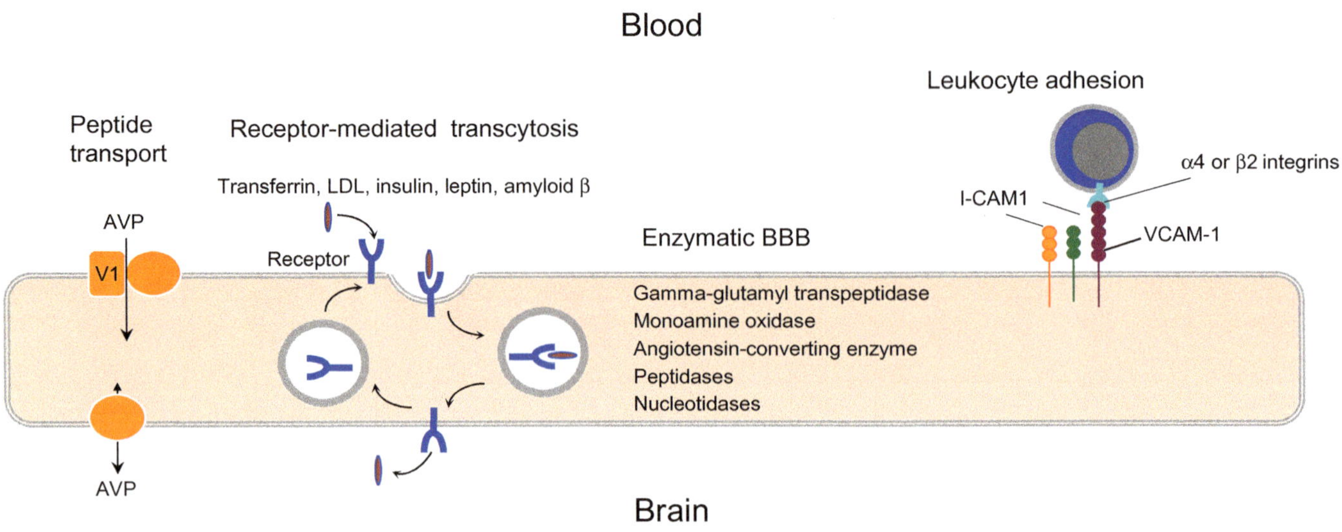

FIGURE 23.4 Other mechanisms regulating passage across the BBB.
Some proteins and peptides use receptor-mediated transport to traverse the BBB and enter into the brain. For example, transferrin receptor, insulin receptor, and leptin receptor mediate blood-to-brain transport of their respective ligands. The arginine-vasopressin V1 receptor mediates bidirectional transport of this peptide across the endothelium. Lipoprotein receptors (LPR1 and LPR2) colocalize mainly on the abluminal side of the endothelium and are important for clearance of amyloid β (Aβ) peptides from the brain to the blood. The endothelial cells forming the BBB also express enzymes that metabolize endogenous and exogenous molecule, including neurotransmitters. Leukocyte migration across the BBB is determined by interactions between endothelial cell adhesion molecules such as vascular cell adhesion molecule 1 (VCAM-1) and integrins expressed in the leukocytes, particularly α4/β2 integrin.

disease (AD), the mechanisms of transport of amyloid β (Aβ) across the BBB have been extensively investigated.[53] Both, the ABCB1 and the receptor low-density lipoprotein receptor-related protein 1 (LRP1) have an important roles Aβ efflux from brain. Both proteins are functionally linked, mediating a concerted Aβ transcytosis through endothelial cells. The phosphatidylinositol-binding clathrin assembly protein (PICALM) is associated with both ABCB1 and LRP1, representing a functional link and guiding both proteins through the brain endothelium.[54] Of note, PICALM polymorphisms may be a risk factor for late-onset AD.[55,56] However, LRP1 has a dual role in the metabolism of the amyloid precursor protein (APP) as it also enhances Aβ generation via APP internalization[57] LRP2 (megalin) is a member of the low-density lipoprotein receptor binds APOJ (also known as clusterin) and also mediates $A\beta_{42}$ transport from brain to blood. In contrast to lipoprotein receptors, the receptor for advanced glycation endproducts (RAGE) is expressed mainly at the luminal membrane of the BBB and, under pathological conditions, mediates reentry or influx of circulating Aβ across the BBB into the brain.[58] Pericytes express multiple transporters, receptors, and ion channels. For example, they express carbohydrate transporters such as insulin-regulated glucose transporter GLUT4, the sodium/myo-inositol cotransporter, the high-affinity excitatory amino acid transporter (EAAT), GABA transporters, and others. Pericytes clear Aβ 42 aggregates via LRP1 interactions with ApoE3, but not ApoE4.[59]

Passage of Immune Cells Across the BBB

The BBB also has a critical role in mediating the bidirectional crosstalk between the immune cells and endothelium, which is an essential element of normal immune surveillance and under inflammatory conditions. Circulating monocytes are able to penetrate the intact BBB by a process of diapedesis through the cytoplasm of the endothelial cells. Leukocyte migrations across the BBB are determined by interactions between endothelial cell adhesion molecules such as vascular cell adhesion molecule 1 (VCAM-1) and integrins expressed in the leukocytes, particularly α4/β2 integrin.

CHOROID PLEXUS AND CSF PRODUCTION

The choroid plexus consists of a monolayer of cuboidal epithelial cells that contacts the ventricular surface and surrounds a stromal core of connective tissue and fenestrated capillaries (Figure 23.5). Choroid epithelial cells have an apical brush border containing microvilli and scarce cilia and are joined by tight junctions forming a brain-CSF barrier that is much more permeable than the BBB. Choroid microvilli largely increase (~10-fold) the apical surface of the epithelium, and are enriched with the machinery required for CSF production. There is an age-dependent reduction in size of microvilli that relates to reduced ability for CSF production. The choroidal plexus stroma has

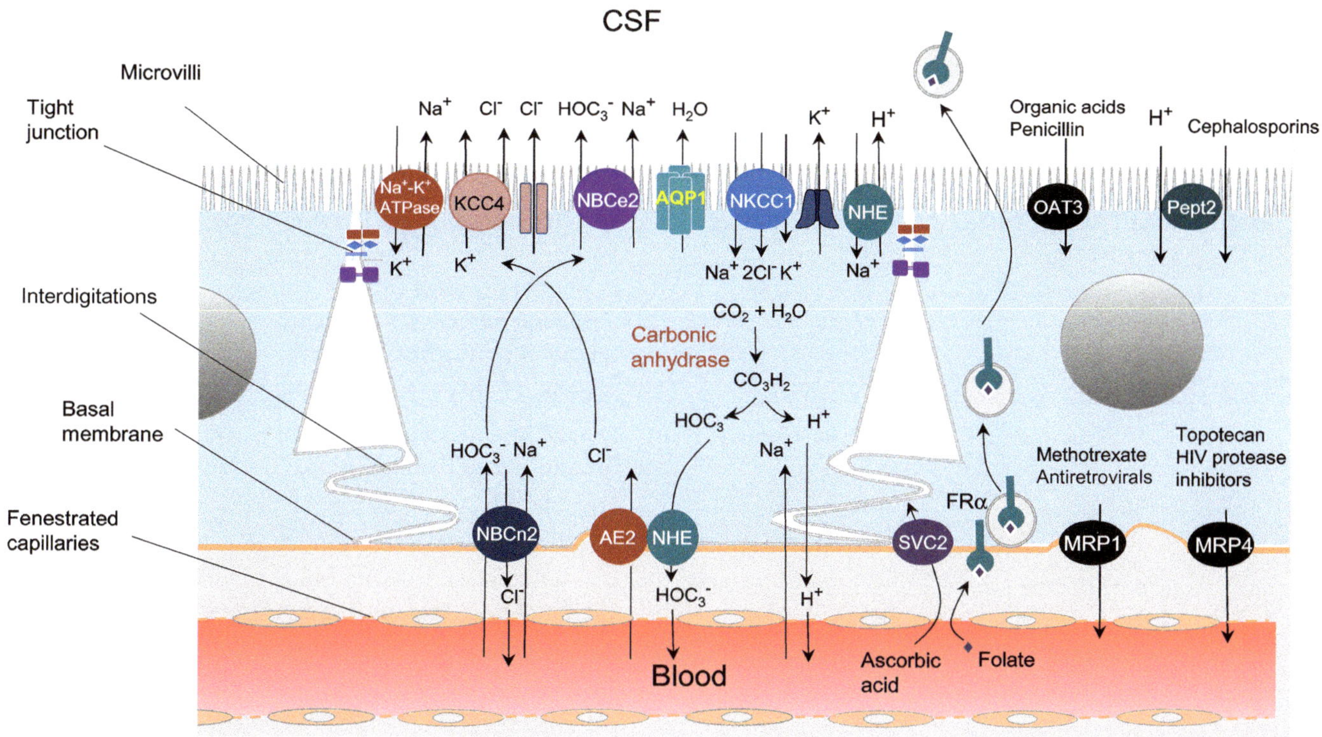

FIGURE 23.5 Structure and functions of the choroid plexus.
The choroid plexus consists of a monolayer of cuboidal epithelial cells that contact the ventricular surface and surround a stromal core of connective tissue and fenestrated capillaries. Choroid epithelial cells have an apical brush border containing microvilli and scarce cilia, establish endfeet at a basalmembrane opposite to the ventricular surface, have complex interdigitations between their lateral walls, and are joined by tight junctions forming a brain-CSF barrier. The main determinants of CSF secretion are the active secretion of Na^+ via the Na^+/K^+ ATPase located in the apical membrane, the secretion of chloride (Cl^-) via an anion-permeable channel and Cl^-/K^+ cotransporter, the transport of bicarbonate (HCO_3^-) ions synthesized by action of carbonic anhydrase, and the passive osmotically driven water efflux via aquaporin 1 (AQP1) channels. The supply of Cl^- for CSF production primarily depends on its interchange for HCO_3^- at the basolateral membrane. The choroid plexus transports nutrients, metabolic precursors, and trophic factors. These include the sodium-dependent vitamin C transporter-2 (SVC2) and folate receptor α (FRα) which transports the active metabolite of folic acid from the bloodstream to the CSF. Choroid epithelial cells also express efflux transporters, such as multidrug resistance proteins (MRP1)1 and 4, organic acid transporter-3 (OA3), and peptide transporter 2 (Pept2), that transport penicillin G, cephalotin, sulfonamides, and other substrates.

fenestrated blood vessels with high permeability to small molecules and water. Both blood flow and CSF production by the choroid epithelium are regulated by sympathetic and parasympathetic fibers.

Mechanisms of CSF Secretion

Approximately 80% of CSF is secreted by the choroid plexus; the remaining 20% originates from the brain ISF. The rate of CSF secretion is approximately 0.4 ml per minute per gram of tissue, so that about 500–600 ml are produced in 24 hours. The total CSF volume in human CNS is about 140–150 ml, indicating the CSF is replaced three to four times a day. Maximal CSF production occurs during the middle of the sleep cycle and the minimum occurs in the afternoon. The choroid plexus epithelial cells express a wide range of ion pumps and transporters that contribute, to various degrees, to CSF secretion (Figure 23.5, Table 23.2). The main determinants of CSF secretion are the active secretion of Na^+ via the Na^+/K^+ ATPase located in the apical (luminal) membrane, the secretion of chloride (Cl^-) via an anion permeable channel and $Cl\text{-}/K^+$ cotransporter, the transport of bicarbonate (HCO_3^-) ions synthesized by action of carbonic anhydrase, and the osmotically driven water efflux via apical AQP1 channels. The supply of Cl^- for CSF production primarily depends on its interchange for HCO_3^- at the basolateral membrane. Inhibition of carbonic anhydrase by acetazolamide reduces CSF production by 50%–100%; topiramate also inhibits this enzyme. Furosemide inhibits the Na^+/K^+ ATPase, and amiloride inhibits the Na^+/H^+ exchanger, but their clinical effect in conditions such as idiopathic intracranial hypertension is minimal. In contrast, caffeine increases expression of the

TABLE 23.2 *Molecules Involved in CSF Secretion*

Pump/Channel/Transporter	Location	Functional Significance
Na^+/K^+ ATPase	Luminal (apical)	Extrudes Na^+ to the ventricular space Establishes and maintains the Na+ and K+ gradients that drive other transporters
Inward-rectifying Cl^- and HCO_3^- channels	Luminal (apical)	Secretes Cl^- and HCO_3^- into the ventricles
K^+-Cl^- cotransporter (KCC)		Facilitates outward transport of ions driven by transmembrane K^+ gradients Inhibited by furosemide
Na^+-HCO_3^- cotransporter (NBCe2)	Luminal	Regulates CSF pH by extruding HCO_3-
Na^+-HCO_3^- cotransporter (NBCn2)	Basolateral	Contributes to accumulation of Na^+ and HCO_3^- in the choroid epithelial cell
Epithelial Na^+ channel (ENAC)	Basolateral	Possible entry pathway for Na^+ at the basolateral membrane.
Na^+-K^+-$2Cl^-$ cotransporter (NKCC1)	Luminal (apical)	Still uncertain role in ion influx or efflux. Inhibited by bumetanide and furosemide
Na^+/H^+ exchanger (NHE1)	Luminal	Electroneutral H^+ extruder into the CSF driven by the inward Na+ gradient
	Basolateral	pH sensitive Na^+ uptake in basolateral membrane
Cl^-/HCO_3^- exchanger (AE2)	Basolateral	Mediates uptake of Cl- and extrusion of HCO_3^- Main mechanism of Cl^- entry in the choroid epithelium to sustain CSF secretion
Aquaporin 1(AQP1)	Luminal	Passive water transport across the epithelium driven by osmotic gradient

Na^+/K^+ ATPase, leading to increased CSF production. Both secretion and composition of the CSF are regulated by autonomic and humoral signals.

Transport Mechanisms in the Choroid Plexus

The choroid plexus transports nutrients, metabolic precursors, and trophic factors (Table 23.3). These signal molecules are either directly synthesized by choroid plexus epithelial cells or transported from the blood. The choroid plexus epithelium secretes transthyretin (TTR), which transports thyroxine to the CSF, expresses transporters for ascorbic acid, and transports 5-methyltetrahydrofolate (5-MTHF) via a receptor mechanism that includes folate receptor-α (FRα) present in the basolateral membrane and mediates 5-MTHF endocytosis followed by exosome delivery into the CSF. Cerebral folate deficiency due to mutations of the *FOLR-1* gene encoding the folate receptor-α in the choroid plexus epithelium is a neuropsychiatric condition associated with progressive movement disorders, psychomotor decline, and epilepsy, with reduced CSF levels of 5-methyl-tetrahdrofolate (MTHF) but normal folate status outside the CNS.

Choroid plexus efflux transporters have a major role in clearance of metabolites, drugs, and toxins and thus maintenance of CNS homeostasis. For example, the apical membrane expresses high levels of organic acid transporter-3, which transports penicillin G, cephalotin, sulfonamides, and other substrates. The ABC class transporters transport substrates such as include HIV-1 protease inhibitors from the choroid epithelial cells to the brain ISF. The choroid plexus epithelium is involved in receptor-mediated endocytosis of peptides. It participates in CSF-mediated Aβ clearance, direct Aβ absorption, and production of Aβ chaperones and proteases.

Immune Function

The choroid plexus also harbors different types of immune cells and is a gateway for immune cell entry into the CNS. Macrophages and dendritic cells are located primarily in the choroid plexus stroma. Infiltrating immune cells first migrate from the blood across the fenestrated endothelium into the stromal surface, move along the basolateral surface of the choroid epithelium and gain access across the epithelium to the CSF.

Choroid epithelial cells express adhesion molecules and chemokines that facilitate the transepithelial passage of macrophages and leukocytes into the CSF. Epiplexus

TABLE 23.3 *Choroid Plexus Transporters*

Transporter	Substrates (example)	Implications
Transthyretin (TTR)	Thyroxine (T4) Retinol-binding protein Amyloid β (Aβ)	Main determinant of the T4 pool in the cerebral extracellular May contribute to Aβ clearance
Sodium-dependent vitamin C transporter (*SCL23*A1)	Ascorbic acid	Essential for maintenance of ascorbic acid levels in the brain
Folate receptor-α (FRα)	Folate	Mediates 5-MTHF endocytosis in the basolateral membrane followed by exosome delivery into the CSF
Reduced folate carrier 1	Folate	Present in the apical membrane, and together with FRα regulates folate levels
Peptide transporter-2 (PEPT-2)	Aminolevulinic acid Cephalexin, cefadroxil	Limits bioavailability in the CSF
Organic anion transporter-3 (OAT3)	Penicillin G, Cephalotin, Cimetidine Riboflavin	Limits bioavailability in the CSF
Multidrug resistance-related protein 1 (MRP1)	Etoposide Topotecan HIV-1 protease inhibitors	May limit availability in the CSF
MRP4	Cyclic nucleotides Eicosanoids Methotrexate Topotecan Nucleoside analogue antivirals (e.g., adefovir, tenofovir) Cephalosporins Furosemide	May limit availability in the CSF
Low-density lipoprotein receptor-related protein-2 (LRP2, megalin)	Leptin Amyloid β peptide (Aβ)	Mediates entry of leptin into the brain Participates in clearance of amyloid β

Kolmer cells are macrophages that migrate from the circulation to the stroma and the choroid plexus epithelium into the apical surface, where they remain attached to epithelial cells via intercellular cell adhesion molecule. Both choroid plexus epithelial cells and Kolmer cells can serve as antigen presenting cells to lymphocytes.

FLUID DYNAMICS IN THE CNS

Brain fluids are tightly regulated to provide stable environments for neuronal function and signaling, minimize neurotoxicity, and removal of neuronal and astroglial waste products.[42]

CSF Circulation and Drainage

The CSF produced continuously in the choroid plexus passes through the ventricles to the subarachnoid space. In the ventricle, the CSF is in contact with the ependymal epithelium, which constitutes a leaky barrier; in the subarachnoid space the CSF is separated from the brain parenchyma by the pia mater. There is a second-to-second pulsatile movement of CSF through the ventricular system; CSF flows approximately 8 mm/s toward the posterior brain during systole and then gently back at 5 mm/s to the anterior brain during diastole. Respiratory motion results in cyclical movement of CSF at the foramen magnum over and above the fluctuation due to cardiac pulsation; inspiration increases flow of CSF into the ventricular system, and expiration has the opposite effect. Although the net direction of CSF flow is toward the posterior brain, plasticity would act to mix CSF contents between ventricles and promote the sink action of CSF. Superimposed on these acute pulses is a circadian rhythm. From the subarachnoid space CSF primarily drains into the sagittal and transverse venous sinuses via arachnoid granulations. However the dural venous sinuses also have many arachnoid villi, which are smaller than granulations and can mediate drainage of CSF. A small fraction of CSF may return to the blood stream via the perineural sheet of cranial nerves and lymphatics in nasal sinus tissue that underlies the cribriform plate.

Exchange Between the CSF and ISF: Glymphatic System

The brain ISF fills the narrow extracellular space between neurons and glia and primarily originates as a secretion across the brain capillary endothelium via ion channels and transporters that are expressed at the BBB. Whereas the ISF has the same composition as the CSF, the abundant ECM may affect CSF/interstitial fluid transport and exchange by impacting diffusion of certain ions and other molecules.[42] Elegant studies led to the proposal of the presence of a tripartite paravascular pathway, named glymphatic system, for fluid passage between the CSF and brain interstitium.[14,15,17] In this proposal, the glymphatic pathway involves three serial steps: initial convective flow of subarachnoid CSF into the brain along periarterial spaces; astrocytic AQP4-facilitated water and solute flow from the periarterial space through the brain extracellular space ("transparenchymal" convection) resulting in transport of interstitial fluid toward venules or veins; and clearance out of the brain along perivenous spaces.[14,15,17] Consistent with this hypothesis, AQP4 is particularly enriched in the brain at CSF interfaces, with polarized expression in astrocytes at glia limitans facing the pial surface, perivascular endfeet between the parenchymal blood vessels and the neuropil, and ependymal cells facing the surface of the ventricle. Several experimental studies show that AQP4 has a critical role in the transport of water between brain compartments as well as the formation and resolution of brain edema. Reduced AQP4 expression may promote accumulation of Aβ accumulation in experimental models of AD.[14,15,17] However, the role of the glymphatic mechanism and astrocytic AQP4 for convective or bulk flow of interstitial fluid has been more recently questioned,[42] as some studies indicate that local transport of small and large molecules through the brain extracellular space is predominantly by diffusion.

Perivascular Space and Role of Arterial Pulsations

The perivascular space visible in the brain parenchyma on MRI surrounds arterioles and runs perpendicular to the brain's surface.[60] Perforating arterioles are surrounded by pia mater at the surface and within the brain; at the capillaries, the pial membrane is replaced by a basal lamina that is surrounded by astrocytic endfeet. Perforating arterioles that enter the basal ganglia are covered by two layers of leptomeninges along the arteriole length, and the perivascular spaces between these layers communicate with the subarachnoid space at the base of the brain. Whether the perivascular space surrounding arterioles that enter the convexity cortex communicate with the subarachnoid space or only with the subpial space is currently under debate. In the rigid skull, limited tissue compliance promotes propagation of arterial pressure pulsation throughout the brain, leading to pulsatile flow in the microvasculature, which may help move fluid and waste through the brain. Arterial pulsation may lead to fast para-arterial solute transport through the combined effect of local mixing and diffusion in the para-arterial space;[61] and large molecule solutes would be more easily cleared from the brain interstitial by diffusion than by bulk flow.[42,62] During acute blood pressure elevation, which increases arteriole stiffness, the pulsations in distal vessels increase in amplitude, resulting in jerky movement which may result in intermittent reversal of the flow, reduction in net flow in the perivascular spaces, and failure to clear debris. In MRI studies, an increase in intracranial vascular pulsatility was associated with a reduction in the pulsatile flow of volume of CSF and increased visibility of basal ganglia perivascular spaces, suggesting fluid stagnation and less effective flushing of perivascular spaces. Sleep and wakefulness may affect the extracellular space volume and thus clearance, with increased volume and clearance during the sleep state.[63] During wakefulness, 85% of Aβ is reportedly removed via transport across the BBB and just 15% via passive ISF bulk. During sleep, total Aβ clearance is increased ~2.2-fold; 60% occurs via BBB transport, and 40% occurs via ISF flow.[12] Disruption of slow-wave sleep led to higher CSF levels of Aβ the following day, and worse sleep efficiency in the week preceding a lumbar puncture was associated with increased CSF levels of tau.

Drainage Pathways for the CSF and ISF: Brain Lymphatic System

Meningeal lymphatics drain alongside the major dural venous sinuses via cranial perineuronal channels to cervical lymph nodes and are thought to be major drainage routes for CSF and ISF. The vessels of this lymphatic system express all molecular markers of lymphatic endothelial cells and carry both fluid and immune cells from the CSF to the deep cervical lymph node. Nasal lymphatics drain from the frontal subarachnoid space, through the cribriform plate via the nasal mucosa and to the cervical lymph nodes. This lymphatic system may represent a second step in the drainage of the interstitial fluid into the periphery, following its drainage into the CSF via the glymphatic system.

DISORDERS OF THE NEUROVASCULAR UNIT AND BLOOD-BRAIN BARRIER

Disturbances of the cerebral microcirculation and BBB are major pathophysiological mechanisms in a wide range of neurologic disorders, including traumatic brain injury, stroke, epilepsy, inflammatory disorders, neurodegenerative disorders, neoplasm, and some genetic and metabolic disorders. These disorders are associated, either primarily or in various combinations, with impaired neurovascular coupling, disruption of the BBB, altered expression and function of membrane transporters or enzymes in endothelial cells, pericyte damage; astrocyte dysfunction, microglial activation, passage of inflammatory cells from the blood the CNS, and in some cases aberrant angiogenesis. Only some examples will be discussed here.

Impaired Neurovascular Coupling

Alterations of neurovascular coupling occurs in several neurologic disorders, including stroke, AD, and small vessel disease. Studies in experimental models of ischemic stroke show impaired hemodynamic responses to sensory stimuli in the perilesional tissue weeks following a microinfarct, despite recovery of neuronal activity, indicating neurovascular uncoupling.[64,65] One important mechanism of impaired reactive hyperemia is oxidative stress. Excessive production of superoxide ion leads to its reaction with NO to produce peroxinitrite; the decrease in free NO may affect its ability to promote vasodilation and to prevent the vasoconstrictor effects of HETE and other compounds.

Blood-Brain Barrier Disruption, Astrocytic Dysfunction, and Cerebral Edema

Cerebral edema is the accumulation of excess fluid in the brain, either in the extracellular compartment (vasogenic edema) or intracellular compartments (cytotoxic edema). However, these two types of fluid accumulation rarely occur independently from each other. Vasogenic edema results from breakdown of the BBB in many disorders associated with downregulation of tight junctions and degradation of basement membrane proteins. These changes commonly reflect the downstream effects of signals triggered by cytokines, chemokines, and other substances released during inflammation, including matrix metalloproteinases such as MMP-9 and VEGF. These signals commonly interact and potentiate their disruptive effects on the BBB via engagement of astrocytes and microglia. One important consequence of BBB dysfunction is transendothelial migration of inflammatory cells. In response to proinflammatory cytokines, brain endothelial cells upregulate their expression of chemokines and cell adhesion molecules such as VCAM-1 at their luminal surface. Endothelial chemokines bind to their specific receptors on the leucocyte, triggering the activation of $\alpha 4/\beta 2$ integrins, which mediate leukocyte adhesion via interactions with VCAM-1 and other endothelial cell adhesion molecules. Pericytes also have properties of immune-regulating cells, responding to and expressing many inflammatory molecules, presenting antigens, and displaying phagocytic ability.[66]

Leukocyte-derived chemokines, acting on receptors on the endothelium, trigger cytoskeletal reorganization, which promotes further transmigration of leukocytes across the BBB. Finally, opening of tight junctions as a result of the actions of cytokines and MMP-9 further allows leukocyte migration via a paracellular route. For example, CD20+ B lymphocytes can permeate the BBB and have a major role in several disorders including multiple sclerosis, AQP4 IgG induced neuromyelitis spectrum disorder, and autoimmune encephalitis.

Vasogenic edema leads to secondary impairment in capillary blood flow and astrocyte dysfunction. Disruption of the basement membrane results in loss of agrin from the abluminal surface of the brain endothelial cells adjacent to astrocytic endfeet; this may contribute to redistribution of AQP4 and Kir4.1 channels, leading to impaired K^+ homeostasis and secondarily to cytotoxic edema. In some conditions, such as early stages of ischemia or hepatic encephalopathy, the BBB may stay intact but there is a disturbance of cellular metabolism that impairs ion transport in glial cell membranes, leading to cellular retention of sodium and water and cell swelling (cytotoxic edema). Cytotoxic edema may be associated with a reduced extracellular space volume, further hindering diffusional transport of edema fluid. This is potentiated by upregulation of AQP4 in astrocytes, as occurs in the setting of ischemia, inflammation, or neoplasm. Bulk flow pathways, including white matter tracts and perivascular spaces, are important for resolution of edema. Aquaporin water channels may also play a role in this process.[67]

Neoplastic Disease

In both glioma and brain metastasis, neoplastic cells can first survive within the perivascular space of the neurovascular unit and later remodel, destroy, and produce new vasculature with aberrant components and function.[68] Glioma cells can migrate within perivascular spaces and come into direct contact with the basement membrane and its signaling molecules, and then migrate through the brain extracellular space using the blood vessels or axons as their guide via interactions with the ECM mediated by integrins and other cell adhesion molecules. Gliomas may secrete their own promigratory ECM proteins, including hyaluronic acid, brevican, tenascin-C, and thrombospondin as well as basement membrane fibronectin, which increase glioma cell motility and support their invasiveness. Glioma cell migration requires not only adhesion of the leading edge of the migrating cell and anchoring to the ECM, but also detachment of the trailing end, which depends on proteases such as MMP-9. These proteases degrade the basement membrane and activate protease secretion by endothelial cells, astrocytes, and microglia. Displacement of normal astrocytic end-feet promotes vascular "leakiness" through downregulation of tight junction protein expression and disrupted regulation of vascular tone. Malignant glioma cells also upregulate expression of heparan sulfate proteoglycans that act as coreceptor that facilitates signaling by growth factors such as PDGF and VEGF, which promote cell proliferation and angiogenesis. Many tumor types rely on angiogenesis for growth, for which pericytes are critical. Imatinib, which blocks the phosphorylation of PDGFR-β in pericytes, prevents pericyte proliferation, thus reducing tumor growth.

MICROVASCULAR AND BLOOD-BRAIN BARRIER DYSFUNCTION IN DEMENTIA

Neurovascular Unit Abnormalities in Alzheimer Disease

Dysfunction of the neurovascular unit and BBB are early events in AD.[5,6,9,11] Soluble Aβ oligomers induce vascular oxidative stress by increasing production of reactive oxygen species in astrocytes and microglia. Superoxide ions react with NO and impair NO-mediated vasodilatation both directly and by inhibiting synthesis of vasodilator prostaglandins, which is essential for neurovascular coupling. Pericytes are also affected in AD, as they endocytose perivascular debris and participate in clearance of Aβ. Accumulation of Aβ causes pericyte degeneration that may contribute to neurovascular dysfunction.[69] Pericyte death leads to reduced CBF and loss of BBB integrity, which may in turn accelerate neuronal degeneration and Aβ plaque buildup. Soluble PDGFR-β is a CSF biomarker of pericyte injury during early cognitive impairment and correlates with BBB disruption independent of Aβ and tau.[70] Together, these alterations contribute to the chronic cerebral hypoperfusion observed in AD. One important pathogenic mechanism in AD is impaired Aβ clearance from the brain due to dysfunction of LRP1 receptor-mediated transcytosis across the BBB. As mentioned previously, polymorphisms associated with downregulation of PICALM, which guides transendothelial trafficking, have been linked to risk for development of late-onset AD.[9] In contrast, there is upregulation of RAGE receptors, which mediate reentry of circulating Aβ across the BBB into the brain. According to one hypothesis, APP and its Aβ cleavage products accumulate in swollen axons due failure of axonal transport; Aβ may then be extruded through the axonal membranes into the brain ISF, taken up by nearby neurons and astrocytes via (LRP1) and finally degraded.[71,72] Changes in astrocytes in AD have been linked with the development of perivascular Aβ deposits. Impaired Aβ clearance via the glymphatic system is an additional proposed pathogenic mechanisms in AD.[15–17] There are also morphological and functional alterations of the choroid plexus with aging and AD. There is also reduced expression of choroid plexus epithelium proteins that bind Aβ and contribute to its clearance, such as TTR and apolipoprotein J. Reduced expression of AQP1 can also lead to increased Aβ burden by reduced production of CSF and thereby the sink action for brain Aβ clearance.

Small Vessel Disease

Increased visibility of perivascular spaces on MRI in humans is a marker of impaired flushing of brain ISF. It occurs in association with several vascular risk factors, inflammation, and BBB leakage, in conjunction with other features of small vessel disease. CNS small vessel disease is the attributable cause of 25% of strokes and it contributes to 45% of dementia cases.[73] MRI biomarkers include recent small subcortical infarct, white matter hyperintensity, lacunes, cerebral microbleeds, enlarged perivascular spaces, and cerebral atrophy. The most important modifiable risk factor for CNS small vessel disease is hypertension. In small vessel disease, alterations of the vessel wall with thickened arteriolar basement membrane increased tortuosity and reduced number of capillaries contribute to impaired neurovascular coupling. Cerebral amyloid angiopathy (CAA) is due to Aβ deposition in small to medium cortical and leptomeningeal vessels with greater concentrations in the perivascular basement membrane surrounding the smooth muscle cells in the tunica media. An important component of CAA pathogenesis may be failure of perivascular drainage of Aβ from the brain parenchymal arteriolar adventitia, as a typical example of the so-called protein elimination failure angiopathies.[74,75] Sequelae of CAA include loss of vessel compliance; decreased cerebral vascular reactivity; increased susceptibility to cortical cerebral microbleeds, convexal subarachnoid hemorrhage, and cortical superficial siderosis; white matter disease (posterior predominance); altered structural network connectivity; and cortical atrophy. CAA commonly presents with transient focal neurologic episodes, also known as amyloid spells, which typically include recurrent stereotyped focal weakness or numbness (or both). Some evidence suggests that these spells may be caused by cortical spreading depression from acute blood resulting from cortical subarachnoid hemorrhage. There is a distinction between capillary CAA, which is associated with AD and strongly with the ApoE epsilon 4 allele, and arteriolar and capillary CAA, which is more often associated with microinfarcts and larger hematomas. CAA-related vasculopathic changes and fragility associated with ApoE epsilon 2 allele might have a role in the pathophysiology and severity of cortical superficial siderosis.[76]

Genetic Cerebral Vasculopathies

There are several genetic disorders resulting in altered development or maintenance of cerebral vasculature.[75,77,78] Autosomal dominant familial forms of CAA are fairly rare and localized to distinct geographic regions. One example is hereditary cerebral hemorrhage with amyloidosis of the

Dutch type (HCHWA-D), resulting from an *APP* mutation and characterized by abundant amyloid deposition in blood vessels. Cerebral autosomal dominant arteriopathy with subcortical infarcts and leukoencephalopathy (CADASIL) associated with *NOTCH3* mutations is the most common genetic cause of stroke and vascular dementia in adults.[79] *NOTCH3* encodes a transmembrane receptor that regulates development of vascular smooth muscle cells and pericytes; mutations alter the number of cystine residues in the its extracellular domain, leading to accumulation of Notch 3. Notch 3 binds to the tissue inhibitor of metalloproteinase 3 and vitronectin, forming extracellular granular osmiophilic material, leading to degeneration of vascular smooth muscle.[60] Cerebral autosomal recessive arteriopathy with subcortical infarcts and leukoencephalopathy (CARASIL) is due to mutations of the *HTRAS* gene encoding a serine peptidase that is highly expressed in vascular smooth muscle cells and has a key role in regulating TGFβ signaling during vessel development. Cathepsin A-related arteriopathy with strokes and leukoencephalopathy (CARASAL) is due to mutations of the *CTSAS* gene encoding cathepsin A. Cathepsin-A degrades endothelin-1, which is a potent vasoconstrictor expressed in astrocytes and may contribute to vasoconstriction and hypoxia and inhibition of oligodendrocyte precursor cell.[80] Mutations of the *COL4A1* and *COL4A2* genes encoding the basement membrane collagen proteins COL4A1 and COL4A2 lead to cerebral small vessel disease associated with lacunar ischemic strokes, intracerebral hemorrhages, and white matter hyperintensities. Mutations of the *CCM* and *PDCD10* genes produce cerebral cavernous malformations by affecting proteins that are critical for maintaining for endothelial differentiation, leading to formation of enlarged and irregular small vessels, including thin-walled and leaky capillaries. Loss-of-function mutations in endothelial *PDGFB* or pericyte *PDGFRB* genes cause primary familial brain calcification also known as idiopathic basal ganglia calcification or Fahr disease.

KEY POINTS

- The structural and functional integrity of the CNS requires a highly controlled microenvironment through the coupling between cerebral blood flow (CBF) and neuronal activity; regulation of transport across the blood-brain barrier (BBB), and dynamic interchange between the cerebrospinal fluid (CSF) and the brain interstitial fluid (ISF).
- The neurovascular unit consists of processes of excitatory or inhibitory neurons, astrocytes, and microglia, and their interactions with pericytes, vascular smooth muscle, and endothelial cells.
- All components of the neurovascular unit interact with each other and contribute to local regulation of CBF, development and maintenance of the BBB, and neuroinflammation.
- The brain endothelial cells are the core unit of the BBB; they are joined by tight junctions and adherens junctions that provide the physical barrier to diffusion of ions, macromolecules, and other polar solutes.
- Pericytes are multifunctional cells with contractile properties and have a major role in local CBF regulation, maintenance of the BBB, control of vascular development and angiogenesis, and neuroinflammation.
- Astrocytes extend endfoot processes that occupy a strategic position between capillaries and are critical for neurovascular coupling, water and potassium homeostasis, and dynamics of ISF via the so-called glymphatic system.
- Microglia and perivascular macrophages have a major role in the neurovascular unit, primarily by affecting BBB permeability during inflammation.
- Neuronal processes contact the vasculature, and release mediators that elicit local increase in CBF in response to metabolic demand resulting from synaptic activity.
- Secreted proteins make up a specialized extracellular matrix (ECM) that forms the basement membrane (basal lamina) between endothelial cell and pericytes and between astrocytes and pericytes.
- Cerebral blood flow is controlled by three major processes, cerebral autoregulation, responses to systemic carbon dioxide, and neurovascular coupling or functional hyperemia.
- Neurovascular coupling is primarily driven by excitatory synaptic activity and involves neurochemical and metabolic signals from neurons and associated astrocytes.
- Pericytes contribute to neurovascular coupling by actively relaxing or contracting in response to localized changes in neuronal activity.
- Ascending inputs from cholinergic and monoaminergic modulatory systems act via cortical interneurons and astrocytes for coupling of cortical behavioral states with blood flow.
- The BBB restricts ionic and fluid movements between the blood and the brain, supplies the brain with essential nutrients, and mediates efflux of waste and potential toxic products.
- The formation of tight junctions depends on claudins and occludins.
- Cerebral angiogenesis and BBB formation require precise cues from various growth factors, guidance molecules, and other signals released from endothelial cells, pericytes, and astrocytes.
- The interactions between astrocytes, endothelial cells, and pericytes occur in part through associations with the ECM and basal lamina.

- There is a polarized expression of membrane of ion channels, transporters, receptors, and metabolite-degrading enzymes in endothelial cells.
- Some proteins and peptides, such as transferrin, leptin, and amyloid β (Aβ), use receptor-mediated transport to traverse the BBB.
- Endothelial cells of the BBB express ATP-binding cassette (ABC) transporters and prevent brain accumulation of drugs, xenobiotics, and other substances.
- The BBB has a critical role in mediating the bidirectional crosstalk between the immune cells and endothelium.
- The choroid plexus epithelium is the main source of CSF production and forms a brain-CSF barrier.
- The choroid plexus secretes transthyretin, ascorbic acid, active folic acid metabolites, trophic factors, and other molecules that reach many brain areas via the CSF.
- Choroid plexus cells also express efflux transporters that have a major role in clearance of metabolites, drugs, and toxins.
- The dynamic interchange between the brain ISF and the CSF is integral to brain homeostasis.
- The glymphatic pathway involves initial convective flow of CSF into the brain along periarterial spaces; astrocytic AQP4-facilitated water and solute flow and clearance out of the brain along perivenous spaces.
- Arterial pulsation is a major driver for solute transport through the combined effect of local mixing and diffusion in the perivascular space around arterioles.
- Sleep and wakefulness may affect the extracellular space volume and thus clearance, with increased volume and clearance during the sleep state.
- Drainage of CSF and ISF occurs within dural lymphatic vessels to the cervical lymph nodes.
- Impaired neurovascular coupling occurs in several neurologic disorders, including stroke, small vessel disease, and Alzheimer disease (AD).
- Vasogenic edema results from breakdown of the BBB in disorders associated with downregulation of tight junctions and degradation of the basement membrane.
- Cytotoxic edema may be associated with a reduced extracellular space volume, potentiated by upregulation of AQP4 in astrocytes.
- Dysfunction of the neurovascular unit and BBB are early events in AD.
- Soluble Aβ oligomers induce vascular oxidative stress and impair neurovascular coupling.
- Accumulation of Aβ causes pericyte degeneration.
- One important pathogenic mechanism in AD is impaired Aβ clearance from the brain due to dysfunction of LRP1 receptor-mediated transcytosis.
- Cerebral amyloid angiopathy and CADASIL are important causes of small vessel disease.

REFERENCES

1. McConnell HL, Kersch CN, Woltjer RL, Neuwelt EA. The translational significance of the neurovascular unit. J Biol Chem 2017;292:762–770.
2. Lecrux C, Hamel E. Neuronal networks and mediators of cortical neurovascular coupling responses in normal and altered brain states. Philos Trans R Soc Lond B Biol Sci 2016;371.
3. Attwell D, Buchan AM, Charpak S, Lauritzen M, Macvicar BA, Newman EA. Glial and neuronal control of brain blood flow. Nature 2010;468:232–243.
4. Filosa JA, Morrison HW, Iddings JA, Du W, Kim KJ. Beyond neurovascular coupling, role of astrocytes in the regulation of vascular tone. Neuroscience 2016;323:96–109.
5. Iadecola C. The neurovascular unit coming of age: a journey through neurovascular coupling in health and disease. Neuron 2017;96:17–42.
6. Kisler K, Nelson AR, Montagne A, Zlokovic BV. Cerebral blood flow regulation and neurovascular dysfunction in Alzheimer disease. Nat Rev Neurosci 2017;18:419–434.
7. Cauli B, Hamel E. Brain perfusion and astrocytes. Trends Neurosci 2018;41:409–413.
8. Lecrux C, Bourourou M, Hamel E. How reliable is cerebral blood flow to map changes in neuronal activity? Auton Neurosci 2019;217:71–79.
9. Sweeney MD, Zhao Z, Montagne A, Nelson AR, Zlokovic BV. Blood-brain barrier: from physiology to disease and back. Physiol Rev 2019;99:21–78.
10. Brown LS, Foster CG, Courtney JM, King NE, Howells DW, Sutherland BA. Pericytes and neurovascular function in the healthy and diseased brain. Front Cell Neurosci 2019;13:282.
11. Hirunpattarasilp C, Attwell D, Freitas F. The role of pericytes in brain disorders: from the periphery to the brain. J Neurochem 2019;150:648–665.
12. Sweeney MD, Ayyadurai S, Zlokovic BV. Pericytes of the neurovascular unit: key functions and signaling pathways. Nat Neurosci 2016;19:771–783.
13. Wei HS, Kang H, Rasheed ID, et al. Erythrocytes are oxygen-sensing regulators of the cerebral microcirculation. Neuron 2016;91:851–862.
14. Iliff JJ, Lee H, Yu M, et al. Brain-wide pathway for waste clearance captured by contrast-enhanced MRI. J Clin Invest 2013;123:1299–1309.
15. Plog BA, Nedergaard M. The glymphatic system in central nervous system health and disease: past, present, and future. Annu Rev Pathol 2018;13:379–394.
16. Iliff J, Simon M. Crosstalk proposal: the glymphatic system supports convective exchange of cerebrospinal fluid and brain interstitial fluid that is mediated by perivascular aquaporin-4. J Physiol 2019;597:4417–4419.
17. Rasmussen MK, Mestre H, Nedergaard M. The glymphatic pathway in neurological disorders. Lancet Neurol 2018;17:1016–1024.
18. Thurgur H, Pinteaux E. Microglia in the neurovascular unit: blood-brain barrier-microglia interactions after central nervous system disorders. Neuroscience 2019;405:55–67.

19. Joutel A, Haddad I, Ratelade J, Nelson MT. Perturbations of the cerebrovascular matrisome: a convergent mechanism in small vessel disease of the brain? J Cereb Blood Flow Metab 2016;36:143–157.
20. O'Herron P, Chhatbar PY, Levy M, et al. Neural correlates of single-vessel haemodynamic responses in vivo. Nature 2016;534:378–382.
21. Tzeng YC, Ainslie PN. Blood pressure regulation IX: cerebral autoregulation under blood pressure challenges. Eur J Appl Physiol 2014;114:545–559.
22. Ainslie PN, Brassard P. Why is the neural control of cerebral autoregulation so controversial? F1000Prime Rep 2014;6:14.
23. Tan CO, Taylor JA. Integrative physiological and computational approaches to understand autonomic control of cerebral autoregulation. Exp Physiol 2014;99:3–15.
24. Aaslid R, Lindegaard KF, Sorteberg W, Nornes H. Cerebral autoregulation dynamics in humans. Stroke 1989;20:45–52.
25. Peterson EC, Wang Z, Britz G. Regulation of cerebral blood flow. Int J Vasc Med 2011;2011:823525.
26. Edvinsson L, Hardebo JE, Owman C. Influence of the cerebrovascular sympathetic innervation on regional flow, autoregulation, and blood-brain barrier function. Ciba Found Symp 1978;56:69–95.
27. Sandor P. Nervous control of the cerebrovascular system: doubts and facts. Neurochem Int 1999;35:237–259.
28. Hamner JW, Tan CO. Relative contributions of sympathetic, cholinergic, and myogenic mechanisms to cerebral autoregulation. Stroke 2014;45:1771–1777.
29. Kennelly S, Collins O. Walking the cognitive "minefield" between high and low blood pressure. J Alzheimers Dis 2012;32:609–621.
30. Hoiland RL, Fisher JA, Ainslie PN. Regulation of the cerebral circulation by arterial carbon dioxide. Compr Physiol 2019;9:1101–1154.
31. Verbree J, Bronzwaer AS, Ghariq E, et al. Assessment of middle cerebral artery diameter during hypocapnia and hypercapnia in humans using ultra-high-field MRI. J Appl Physiol (1985) 2014;117:1084–1089.
32. Hoiland RL, Tymko MM, Bain AR, Wildfong KW, Monteleone B, Ainslie PN. Carbon dioxide-mediated vasomotion of extra-cranial cerebral arteries in humans: a role for prostaglandins? J Physiol 2016;594:3463–3481.
33. Hoiland RL, Bain AR, Tymko MM, et al. Adenosine receptor-dependent signaling is not obligatory for normobaric and hypobaric hypoxia-induced cerebral vasodilation in humans. J Appl Physiol (1985) 2017;122:795–808.
34. Denfield GH, Fahey PG, Reimer J, Tolias AS. Investigating the limits of neurovascular coupling. Neuron 2016;91:954–956.
35. Mishra A, Reynolds JP, Chen Y, Gourine AV, Rusakov DA, Attwell D. Astrocytes mediate neurovascular signaling to capillary pericytes but not to arterioles. Nat Neurosci 2016;19:1619–1627.
36. Filosa JA, Iddings JA. Astrocyte regulation of cerebral vascular tone. Am J Physiol Heart Circ Physiol 2013;305:H609–619.
37. Hall CN, Reynell C, Gesslein B, et al. Capillary pericytes regulate cerebral blood flow in health and disease. Nature 2014;508:55–60.
38. Hamilton NB, Attwell D, Hall CN. Pericyte-mediated regulation of capillary diameter: a component of neurovascular coupling in health and disease. Front Neuroenergetics 2010;2:5.
39. Chen BR, Kozberg MG, Bouchard MB, Shaik MA, Hillman EM. A critical role for the vascular endothelium in functional neurovascular coupling in the brain. J Am Heart Assoc 2014;3:e000787.
40. Longden TA, Dabertrand F, Koide M, et al. Capillary K+-sensing initiates retrograde hyperpolarization to increase local cerebral blood flow. Nat Neurosci 2017;20:717–726.
41. Liebner S, Dijkhuizen RM, Reiss Y, Plate KH, Agalliu D, Constantin G. Functional morphology of the blood-brain barrier in health and disease. Acta Neuropathol 2018;135:311–336.
42. Abbott NJ, Pizzo ME, Preston JE, Janigro D, Thorne RG. The role of brain barriers in fluid movement in the CNS: is there a 'glymphatic' system? Acta Neuropathol 2018;135:387–407.
43. Ribatti D, Nico B, Crivellato E. The role of pericytes in angiogenesis. Int J Dev Biol 2011;55:261–268.
44. Engelhardt B, Carare RO, Bechmann I, Flugel A, Laman JD, Weller RO. Vascular, glial, and lymphatic immune gateways of the central nervous system. Acta Neuropathol 2016;132:317–338.
45. Klepper J, Akman C, Armeno M, et al. Glut1 Deficiency Syndrome (Glut1DS): State of the art in 2020 and recommendations of the international Glut1DS study group. Epilepsia Open 2020;5:354–365.
46. Karkkainen J, Gynther M, Kokkola T, et al. Structural properties for selective and efficient l-type amino acid transporter 1 (LAT1) mediated cellular uptake. Int J Pharm 2018;544:91–99.
47. Wang L, Xiong N, Huang J, et al. Protein-restricted diets for ameliorating motor fluctuations in Parkinson's disease. Front Aging Neurosci 2017;9:206.
48. Ohtsuki S, Yamaguchi H, Kang YS, Hori S, Terasaki T. Reduction of L-type amino acid transporter 1 mRNA expression in brain capillaries in a mouse model of Parkinson's disease. Biol Pharm Bull 2010;33:1250–1252.
49. Albrecht J, Zielinska M. Exchange-mode glutamine transport across CNS cell membranes. Neuropharmacology 2019;161:107560.
50. Orlandi A, Paolino MC, Striano P, Parisi P. Clinical reappraisal of the influence of drug-transporter polymorphisms in epilepsy. Expert Opin Drug Metab Toxicol 2018;14:505–512.
51. Pena Silva RA, Chu Y, Miller JD, et al. Impact of ACE2 deficiency and oxidative stress on cerebrovascular function with aging. Stroke 2012;43:3358–3363.
52. Roman GC, Spencer PS, Reis J, et al. The neurology of COVID-19 revisited: a proposal from the Environmental Neurology Specialty Group of the World Federation of Neurology to implement international neurological registries. J Neurol Sci 2020;414:116884.
53. Sharma HS, Castellani RJ, Smith MA, Sharma A. The blood-brain barrier in Alzheimer's disease: novel therapeutic targets and nanodrug delivery. Int Rev Neurobiol 2012;102:47–90.
54. Storck SE, Hartz AMS, Bernard J, et al. The concerted amyloid-beta clearance of LRP1 and ABCB1/P-gp across the blood-brain barrier is linked by PICALM. Brain Behav Immun 2018;73:21–33.
55. Juul Rasmussen I, Tybjaerg-Hansen A, Rasmussen KL, Nordestgaard BG, Frikke-Schmidt R. Blood-brain barrier transcytosis genes, risk of dementia and stroke: a prospective cohort study of 74,754 individuals. Eur J Epidemiol 2019;34:579–590.

56. Kim JH. Genetics of Alzheimer's disease. Dement Neurocogn Disord 2018;17:131–136.
57. Van Gool B, Storck SE, Reekmans SM, et al. LRP1 has a predominant role in production over clearance of abeta in a mouse model of Alzheimer's disease. Mol Neurobiol 2019;56:7234–7245.
58. Cai Z, Qiao PF, Wan CQ, Cai M, Zhou NK, Li Q. Role of blood-brain barrier in Alzheimer's disease. J Alzheimers Dis 2018;63:1223–1234.
59. Ma Q, Zhao Z, Sagare AP, et al. Blood-brain barrier-associated pericytes internalize and clear aggregated amyloid-beta42 by LRP1-dependent apolipoprotein E isoform-specific mechanism. Mol Neurodegener 2018;13:57.
60. Wardlaw JM, Benveniste H, Nedergaard M, et al. Perivascular spaces in the brain: anatomy, physiology and pathology. Nat Rev Neurol 2020;16:137–153.
61. Asgari M, de Zelicourt D, Kurtcuoglu V. Glymphatic solute transport does not require bulk flow. Sci Rep 2016;6:38635.
62. Holter KE, Kehlet B, Devor A, et al. Interstitial solute transport in 3D reconstructed neuropil occurs by diffusion rather than bulk flow. Proc Natl Acad Sci U S A 2017;114:9894–9899.
63. Xie L, Kang H, Xu Q, et al. Sleep drives metabolite clearance from the adult brain. Science 2013;342:373–377.
64. Sutherland BA, Fordsmann JC, Martin C, et al. Multi-modal assessment of neurovascular coupling during cerebral ischaemia and reperfusion using remote middle cerebral artery occlusion. J Cereb Blood Flow Metab 2017;37:2494–2508.
65. Summers PM, Hartmann DA, Hui ES, et al. Functional deficits induced by cortical microinfarcts. J Cereb Blood Flow Metab 2017;37:3599–3614.
66. Rustenhoven J, Jansson D, Smyth LC, Dragunow M. Brain pericytes as mediators of neuroinflammation. Trends Pharmacol Sci 2017;38:291–304.
67. Clement T, Rodriguez-Grande B, Badaut J. Aquaporins in brain edema. J Neurosci Res 2020;98:9–18.
68. Charles N, Holland EC. The perivascular niche microenvironment in brain tumor progression. Cell Cycle 2010;9:3012–3021.
69. Kisler K, Nelson AR, Rege SV, et al. Pericyte degeneration leads to neurovascular uncoupling and limits oxygen supply to brain. Nat Neurosci 2017;20:406–416.
70. Nation DA, Sweeney MD, Montagne A, et al. Blood-brain barrier breakdown is an early biomarker of human cognitive dysfunction. Nat Med 2019;25:270–276.
71. Kanekiyo T, Cirrito JR, Liu CC, et al. Neuronal clearance of amyloid-beta by endocytic receptor LRP1. J Neurosci 2013;33:19276–19283.
72. Liu CC, Hu J, Zhao N, et al. Astrocytic LRP1 mediates brain abeta clearance and impacts amyloid deposition. J Neurosci 2017;37:4023–4031.
73. Cannistraro RJ, Badi M, Eidelman BH, Dickson DW, Middlebrooks EH, Meschia JF. CNS small vessel disease: a clinical review. Neurology 2019;92:1146–1156.
74. Carare RO, Hawkes CA, Jeffrey M, Kalaria RN, Weller RO. Review: cerebral amyloid angiopathy, prion angiopathy, CADASIL and the spectrum of protein elimination failure angiopathies (PEFA) in neurodegenerative disease with a focus on therapy. Neuropathol Appl Neurobiol 2013;39:593–611.
75. Vinters HV, Zarow C, Borys E, et al. Review: Vascular dementia: clinicopathologic and genetic considerations. Neuropathol Appl Neurobiol 2018;44:247–266.
76. Charidimou A, Zonneveld HI, Shams S, et al. APOE and cortical superficial siderosis in CAA: meta-analysis and potential mechanisms. Neurology 2019;93:e358–e371.
77. Mancuso M, Arnold M, Bersano A, et al. Monogenic cerebral small-vessel diseases: diagnosis and therapy. Consensus recommendations of the European Academy of Neurology. Eur J Neurol 2020;27:909–927.
78. Fazekas F, Enzinger C, Schmidt R, et al. Brain magnetic resonance imaging findings fail to suspect Fabry disease in young patients with an acute cerebrovascular event. Stroke 2015;46:1548–1553.
79. Wang MM. Cadasil. Handb Clin Neurol 2018;148:733–743.
80. Bugiani M, Kevelam SH, Bakels HS, et al. Cathepsin A-related arteriopathy with strokes and leukoencephalopathy (CARASAL). Neurology 2016;87:1777–1786.

Section IV

Neuronal Interactions in Cortical and Subcortical Circuits

24 Neocortical Organization and Circuits

OVERVIEW

Over the past several years, information gathered using multimodal magnetic resonance imaging (MRI) supported by the Human Connectome Project (HCP) has led to a multimodal parcellation of the cerebral cortex that allowed the delineation of 180 areas per hemisphere.[1,2] In all cortical areas, the two major cell types are excitatory principal cells, which with few exceptions have pyramidal morphology and harbor dendritic spines; and different subtypes of GABAergic interneurons that target different portions of the principal cells and differ in their neurochemical composition and firing patters. Principal cells and interneurons participate in canonical microcircuits that constitute the basic operational units of the cerebral cortex. Information processing in cortical networks critically depends on the precise synchronization of neuronal ensembles, both within local networks and across relatively long distances between separate brain regions.[3] Cortical neurons process information on a background of spontaneous, ongoing activity with distinct spatiotemporal profiles defining different cortical states. According to current models, background information also provides a "predictive" code about the expected sensory consequences of an external stimulus. Disturbances within excitatory and/or inhibitory circuits in the neocortex both at a single neuron and circuit level lead to cognitive impairment, seizures, or both. The main aims of this chapter are to review: (1) general principles of cortical connectivity, (2) the types of excitatory neurons in the cerebral cortex, (3) the functional heterogeneity of GABAergic interneurons, (4) canonical circuits between and within cortical columns, (5) mechanisms and functional relevance of cortical network oscillation, (6) some of the principles of cortical states and large-scale network organization, and (7) cortical mechanisms underlying seizures. This chapter is focused on neocortical circuits. Circuits within the hippocampus and amygdala are discussed in the next chapter.

CYTOARCHITECTONICS AND CONNECTIVITY OF THE NEOCORTEX

The two histological types of human cortical areas are the isocortex (or neocortex) and allocortex, which show a stepwise transition of cytoarchitecture (distribution of neuronal cell bodies) and myeloarchitecture (myelin fiber content). The allocortical areas include the hippocampal formation (archicortex) and olfactory cortex (paleocortex), which are the first steps in the architectonic differentiation toward progressively more differentiated cortices, ending in the typical six-layered (layers 1-6, L1-L6) isocortex or neocortex. This differentiation occurs via two parallel streams. The so-celled hippocampocentric stream gives rise to areas in the medial and dorsolateral portion of the cerebral hemispheres; the so-called olfactocentric stream gives rise to areas in the inferior and ventrolateral portions of the hemispheres. Areas of intermediate differentiation between the allocortex and the neocortex are known as "paralimbic" and are interconnected both with the limbic cortex and with association areas of the neocortex.[4]

Cytoarchitectonics, Mapping, and Gradients of the Neocortex

The six-layered architecture of the neocortex exhibits spatially ordered gradual changes of laminar differentiation (cortical gradients) both in terms of cytoarchitectonic organization (Brodmann areas, BA)[4,5] and differences in the density of myelinated fibers in the different cortical layers.[6] The gradual cytoarchitectonic changes include the emergence of the granular layer (layer 4), and successive increase of neuronal density of upper (supragranular) layers 2 and 3, compared with lower (infragranular) layers 5 and 6. Hence, the cerebral cortex forms a gradient spanning from less to more differentiated cortical areas.[4,7] At one end of the spectrum, primary sensory areas, somatosensory, visual, and auditory, are characterized by their prominent layer 4 containing spiny stellate cells and constitute the granular cortical areas. At the other end, the frontal motor cortex lacks a granular layer (agranular cortex) and is characterized by the presence of large pyramidal neurons in deep layer 5. There is systematic structural variation in the cortex, extending from the simplest limbic cortices to eulaminate areas and this is reflected by the strength and topography of connections between nearby or distant cortices and subcortical structures. Cortical area topography is in part determined by a conserved genetic program involving different morphogens and transcription factors but also has high degree of plasticity.[8] Areas at the similar position within this hierarchical gradient are functionally interconnected with each other.[7] The primary sensory areas receive their primary input from modality-specific, first-order relay nuclei of the thalamus and are distinguished by their high degree of myelination and high expression of receptors for neuromodulatory neurotransmitters. Primary sensory areas project to their respective higher-order unimodal sensory areas (secondary and tertiary areas), which in turn project to multimodal association areas located in the posterior parietal, lateral temporal, and prefrontal cortex (PFC)[4] (Figure 24.1).

A cortical area is defined not only on the bases of its microstructure and functional properties but also according to its connectivity, both anatomical and functional. Functional connectivity has been extensively studied using resting-state functional MRI (fMRI), based on synchronous fluctuations in low frequency blood-oxygen-level-dependent (BOLD) signal between different brain regions.[2,9–12] In general, but not always, functional connectivity reflects structural connectivity. Information gathered from data provided by the HCP combining different MRI modalities to assess cortical thickness, myelin content, and cortical folding pattern; diffusion tensor imaging to assess fiber tracts; and resting-state and task- fMRI to assess functional connectivity has allowed the multimodal parcellation of the cerebral cortex.[1] Whereas the classical cytoarchitectonic map of Brodmann divided the cortex into 43 areas based on the distribution of cell bodies,[5] this multimodal approach has led to identification of 180 distinct areas per cerebral hemisphere.[1]

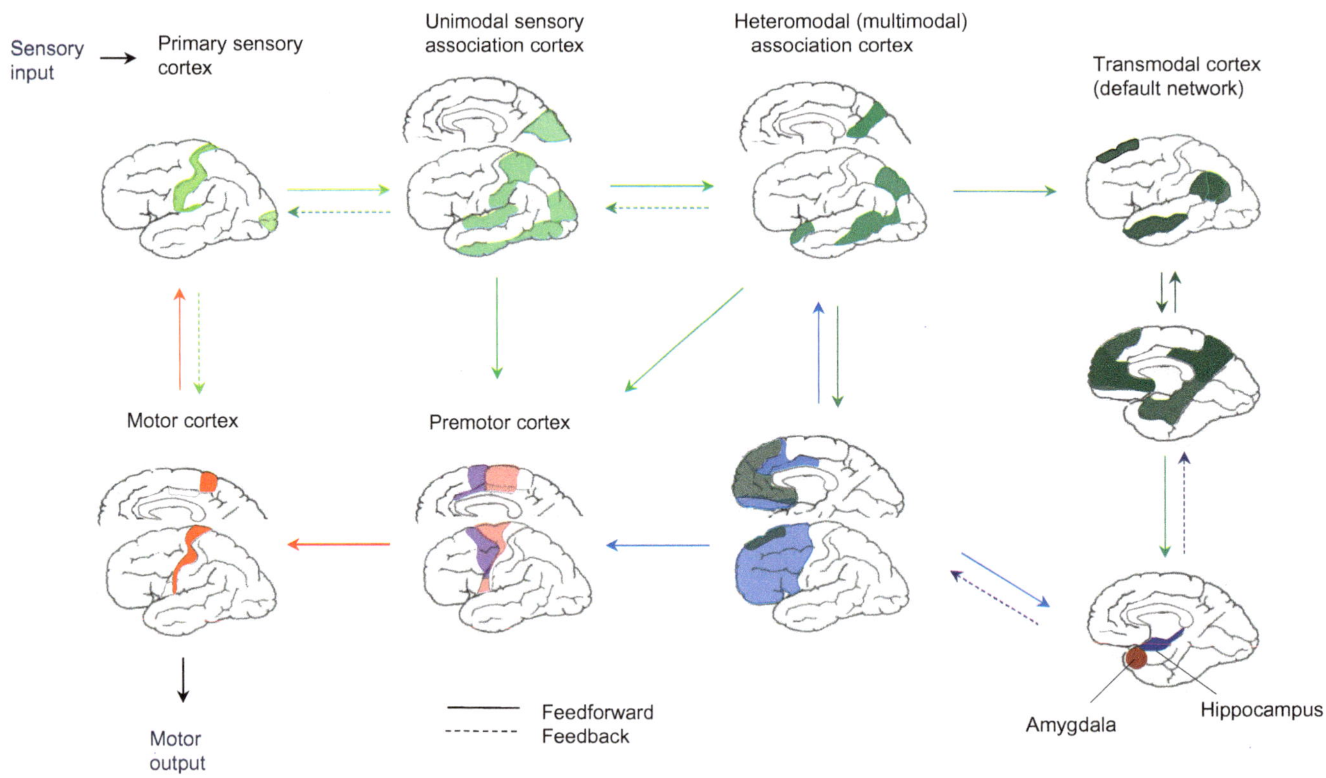

FIGURE 24.1 Overview of connectivity in the cerebral cortex.
There is as serial processing of information in the cerebral cortex from primary sensory, to unimodal sensory, to heteromodal areas. There is a strong interaction between the posterior and prefrontal heteromodal areas. The prefrontal cortex controls motor outputs via premotor areas that project to the primary motor cortex. The heteromodal areas are interconnected with paralimbic areas that channel the information to the hippocampus and amygdala. Many of the connections are reciprocal, consistent with feedforward and feedback interactions.

A key feature of cortical organization is the spatial arrangement of areas along a global gradient between sensorimotor and transmodal regions.[4, 13] This sensorimotor-to-transmodal cortical gradient reflects the microstructural changes resulting from the temporal sequence of neurogenesis. Human structural MRI studies show that primary sensorimotor areas have high myelin content and cortical thickness, which systematically decrease toward transmodal areas in the parietal, temporal, and particularly the PFC.[1,14] Functional MRI studies show a gradient of strength of connectivity from the different primary sensorimotor areas that converges in multimodal integration areas such as the anterior cingulate cortex and the temporooccipital junction, and finally reach transmodal regions of the medial prefrontal, posterior cingulate, and temporal cortex.[15] There is also a gradient of gene expression patterns between primary sensory and motor cortex on one end of the spectrum to transmodal temporal and frontal areas on the other.[16] Distant cortical regions can have similar gene expression patterns if they share long-range connections, particularly between their supragranular layers.[17] There is also a functional integration ranging from unimodal to transmodal areas. For example, in the case of processing of speech, there is a smooth transition from concrete perceptual and quantitative descriptions in sensorimotor areas to abstract category representations related to emotional and social processing in transmodal regions.[18] There is also a hierarchy of temporal integration of information. For example, primary sensory areas track fast changes in a scene in the order of milliseconds to seconds, whereas transmodal association areas that encode complex concepts and situations integrate information across seconds, minutes or longer.[19] All this evidence has led to the proposal of an "intrinsic coordinate system" along the sensorimotor-to-transmodal axis aligning functionally equivalent areas based on both their connectivity and functional gradients.[13]

Feedforward and Feedback Connectivity

One organizing principle of cortical connectivity is that of "cortical hierarchy" based on the presence of feedforward, feedback, and lateral connections.[7] Feedforward connections originate from a cortical area with more elaborate laminar structure than the destination cortical area; for example the primary visual cortex (V1) provides feedforward projection to the higher order visual association area V2. According to the classical view, feedforward connections originate from supragranular layers (particularly layer 3) of lower cortical areas and target layer 4 in higher cortical areas. Feedback connections occur in opposite direction from the higher-order (less laminated) to lower-order cortical areas. These feedback connections originate largely from infragranular layers (particularly layer 5) of higher cortex and terminate outside of layer 4 in lower-level cortex, primary on layer 1, containing the apical dendrites of pyramidal neurons as well as local interneurons.[20] At each cortical area the long-range connections originate from projection neurons with the largest soma size.[21]

The PFC provides a prototypical example of laminar-specific connectivity. High-order prefrontal areas are heavily interconnected with high-order association areas of the parietal cortex. In contrast, paralimbic prefrontal areas such as the anterior cingulate cortex and posterior orbitofrontal cortex, have unique reciprocal connections with the hippocampus, amygdala, and hypothalamus.[7] The large pyramidal neurons of the CA1 region of the hippocampus send feedback projections to CA1 to layer 1 of the neocortex.[22]

Parallel Processing of Cortical Information: Dorsal and Ventral Streams

From the primary sensory cortical areas, information is subsequently processed first at unimodal (sensory modality-specific) cortical association and then heteromodal (multimodal) cortical areas via two distinct streams (Figure 24.2). The dorsal stream consists of pathways that convey information to the posterior parietal cortex. These pathways are involved in processing of spatial information, including representation of space in egocentric (body-centered) coordinates for control of movements and in allocentric (landmark-centered) coordinates to allow navigation.[23] The ventral stream consists of pathways that convey information to the lateral temporal cortex. These pathways allow identification of objects and faces for semantic knowledge and emotional responses.[24] In addition to this hierarchical and parallel feedforward system, higher-order parietal and temporal sensory areas, together with the PFC, provide feedback modulatory inputs to areas involved in early sensory processing. This constitutes the basis of attention, which selects relevant sensory stimuli at the expense of others. Both the dorsal and ventral streams converge in the hippocampal formation, which integrates spatial (place) and feature information to encode episodic memory. Inputs from the dorsal stream to the dorsolateral PFC and from the ventral stream to the ventrolateral and ventromedial PFC provide for high-order executive functions, including decision-making, behavioral planning and adaptation, and control of emotion and social interactions. These pathways and functions are further discussed in other chapters of this book.

EXCITATORY CIRCUITS IN THE NEOCORTEX

Excitatory cells constitute ~80% or more of cortical neurons. Most of them are pyramidal cells, which have a long apical dendrite that arborizes in tufts in layer 1 as well as extensive basal dendrites, both containing dendritic spines. Pyramidal cells originate from precursors in the subventricular zone of the developing brain, which reach the cortex via several waves of radial migration along radial glial processes, and organize into the different layers in

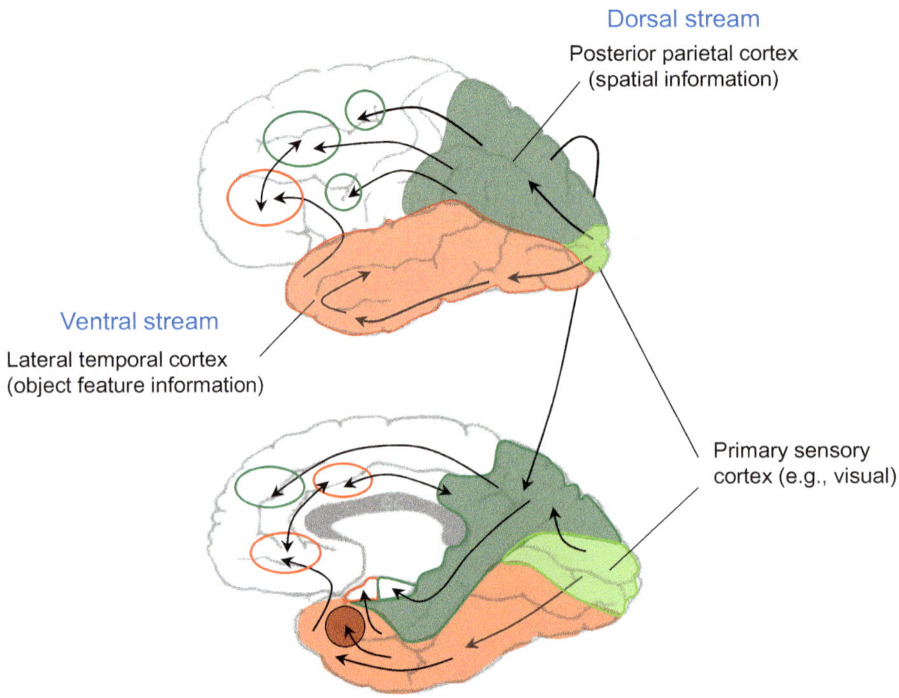

FIGURE 24.2 Dorsal and ventral streams of cortical processing.
Primary sensory cortical information is subsequently processed first at unimodal (sensory modality-specific) cortical association and then heteromodal (multimodal) cortical areas via two distinct processing streams. The dorsal stream conveys information to the posterior parietal cortex and is involved in processing of spatial information. The ventral stream involves connections to the lateral temporal cortex and is involved identification of objects and faces for semantic knowledge and emotional responses.

such a way that newly generated neurons occupy the most superficial layers.[8,25]

Physiology of Pyramidal Neurons

The apical and basal dendrites of pyramidal cells consist of several semi-independent functional compartments, each with a characteristic distribution of ion channels and receptors and receiving different types of inputs (Figure 24.3). The intrinsic electrophysiological properties of these cells depend on the expression of fast inactivating sodium (Na^{+}) currents responsible for the spike of action potential, persistent Na^{+} currents responsible for plateau potentials, several types of voltage-gated calcium (Ca^{2+}) conductances in the soma and dendrites that contribute to a Ca^{2+} spike, and several potassium (K^{+}) conductances that control excitability and shape the firing pattern of pyramidal cells. The distal portions of the dendrites also contain hyperpolarization-activated, cyclic nucleotide-gated (HCN) channels that locally regulate excitability and responses to synaptic inputs. Most cortical pyramidal cells show a regular spiking pattern of firing, which reflects the presence Ca^{2+}-activated K^{+} currents (particularly SK currents) that mediate spike frequency adaptation. Some pyramidal cells may also have intrinsic bursting firing patterns involving T-type Ca^{2+} channels. The activity of the pyramidal cells is shaped by several influences. They include excitatory glutamatergic inputs from both corticocortical and thalamocortical projections targeting the dendritic spines, GABAergic inhibition by different types of local interneurons targeting distinct portions of the pyramidal cell, and modulatory cholinergic and monoaminergic inputs from the brainstem and basal forebrain. Glutamatergic excitation is primarily mediated by α-amino-3-hydroxy-5-methyl-4 isoxazole propionic acid receptors (AMPARs), which generate local excitatory postsynaptic potentials that spread along dendritic branches and summate at a branching point. Dendritic spines also express N-methyl-D-aspartate receptors (NMDARs) that are involved in synaptic plasticity. The probability of excitatory postsynaptic potentials to reach the axonal initial segment depends on the generation of local voltage-gated Na^{+} and Ca^{2+}spikes as well NMDAR-mediated spikes that serve as a boost that allows depolarization from the distal dendrites to reach the soma.[26] Whether this activity reaches the soma depends on modulatory gating by both excitatory glutamatergic corticocortical or thalamocortical inputs and inhibitory GABAergic inputs along the apical dendritic shaft. Local GABA release at distal dendrites and dendritic branches can decrease the probability of postsynaptic potentials to reach the soma; these local GABAergic influences also

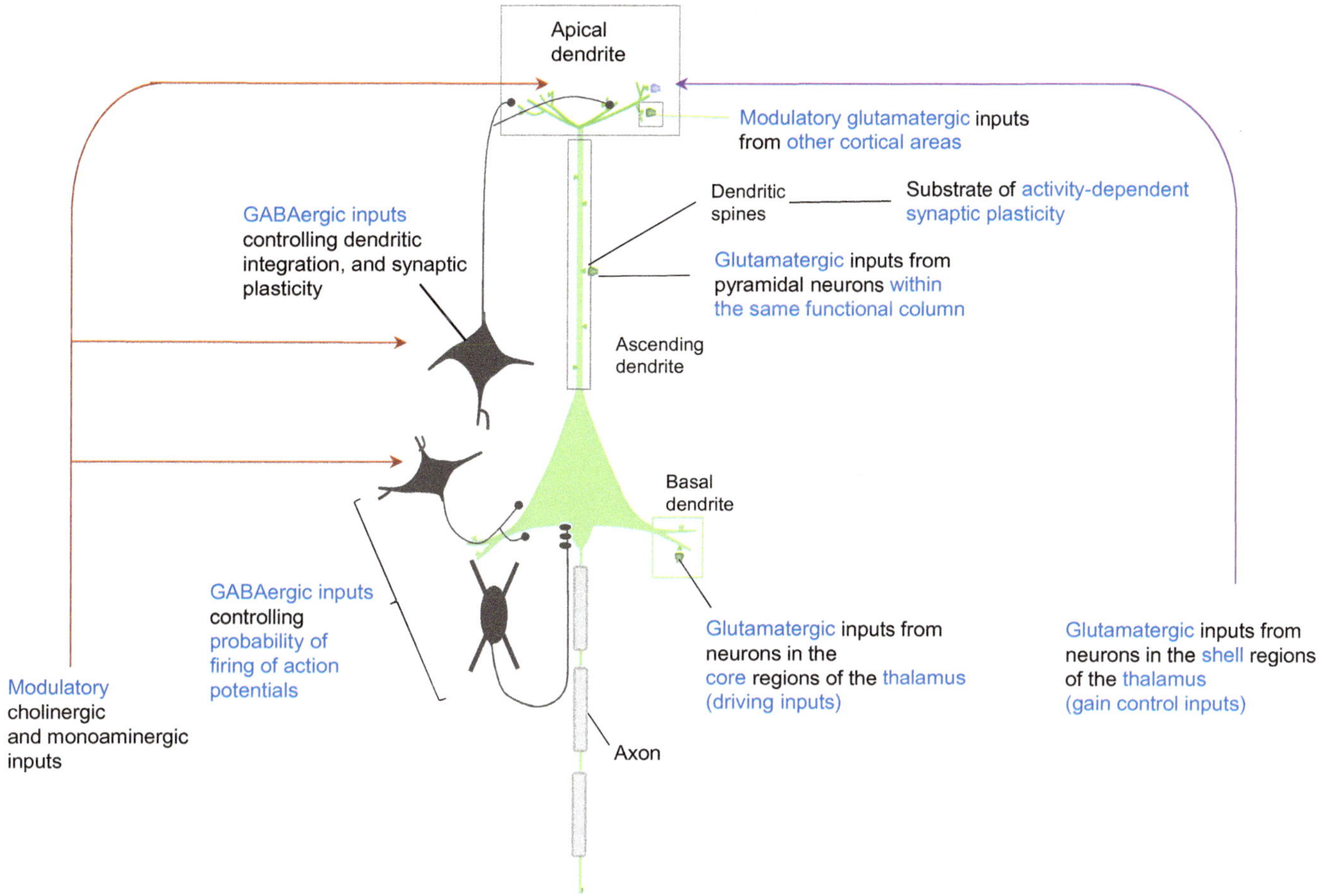

FIGURE 24.3 Functional compartmentalization of pyramidal neurons.

The apical dendrite and basal dendrites of pyramidal cells consist of several semi-independent functional compartments, each with a characteristic distribution of ion channels and receptors and receiving different types of inputs. The activity of the pyramidal cells is shaped by excitatory glutamatergic inputs from other pyramidal neurons and thalamocortical projections; GABAergic inhibition by local interneurons, and modulatory cholinergic and monoaminergic inputs from the brainstem and basal forebrain. Dendritic spines receive most of the excitatory synapses. Local GABA release at distal dendrites and dendritic branches can decrease the probability of postsynaptic potentials to reach the soma, control the efficacy and integration of glutamatergic inputs from different sources, and reduce Ca^{2+}-dependent synaptic potentiation. The soma and basal dendrite areas receive feedforward excitatory glutamatergic inputs as well as robust GABAergic inhibition providing for the global integration and modulation of neuronal output.

control the efficacy of integration of glutamatergic inputs from different sources and reduce Ca^{2+}-dependent synaptic potentiation. After summation of currents spreading from the apical and basal dendrites to the soma, electrical activity is integrated at the level of the axon hillock and initial segment, which determines the probability to trigger an action potential (spike). Backpropagation of the action potential from the axon initial segment to the soma and dendrites increases this probability and is opposed by the several K^+ conductances in the somatodendritic compartment. The soma and basal dendrites receive feedforward excitatory glutamatergic inputs as well as robust GABAergic inhibition, which provides for the global integration and modulation of neuronal output. Inhibition at the level of the soma, proximal dendrites, and axon initial segment globally modulates the output of the pyramidal cell and strongly influences spike timing and thus the firing synchrony of populations of neurons.

Neocortical Excitatory Microcircuits

Pyramidal cells are subdivided into three classes, intratelencephalic (IT), pyramidal tract (PT), and corticothalamic (CT)[27] (Figure 24.4). Intrinsic connections constitute approximately 95% of cortical connectivity and are mediated by different subclasses of IT neurons (Figure 24.5). Intratelencephalic neurons are found in layers 2–6, and project only within the telencephalon. One special type are layer 4 ITs, which have pyramidal or spiny stellate morphology and are particularly abundant in primary sensory areas. Layer 4 is the first station for

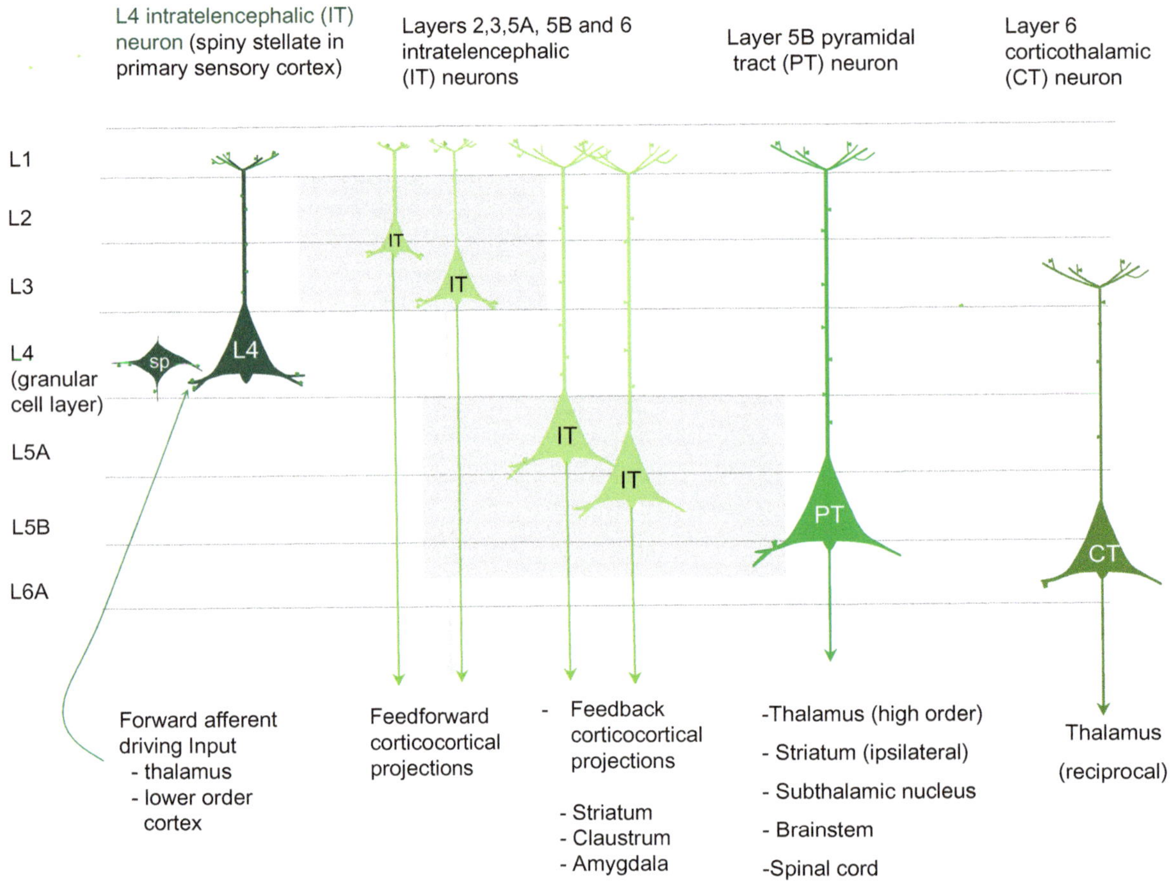

FIGURE 24.4 Subtypes of cortical pyramidal cells.
Pyramidal cells are subdivided into three classes, intratelencephalic (IT), pyramidal tract (PT), and corticothalamic (CT), each consisting of multiple subclasses. Layer 4 ITs are the primary recipient of feedforward inputs from the thalamus or other cortical areas. The majority of IT neurons are located in supragranula in layer 5B and project to multiple subcortical regions as well as association nuclei of thalamus, striatum, subthalamic nucleus, tectum, brainstem, and spinal cord; PT also have axonal branches in the ipsilateral cortex, striatum, and thalamus. The CT neurons that are located in layer 6 project primarily to ipsilateral thalamus.

extrinsic forward excitatory (drive) inputs to the cortex. In primary sensory cortex, the driving projections to L4 IT neurons originate from core-type thalamocortical neurons located in first-order thalamic relay nuclei receiving modality-specific sensory information. Layer 4 neurons in higher-order sensory areas receive long-range inputs from thalamic association nuclei as well as corticocortical feedforward inputs from lower-order areas. Layer 4 IT neurons project heavily to IT neurons in layers 2/3 and layers 5/6, which constitute the second stage of the local excitatory circuit. Neurons of superficial layers 2/3 project forward to the next cortical area, forming a disynaptic route between thalamus and secondary cortical areas. Information from layers 2/3 is then sent to layers 5 and layers 6, which send intrinsic feedback projections back to layer 4. The layer 5 IT cells also send long-range feedback projections to superficial layers of earlier cortical areas. The large PT neurons of layer 5B represent the third and final stage of the local excitatory circuit. They receive extensive inputs from IT neurons of multiple layers, strong direct thalamocortical inputs from thalamic association nuclei, and both feedforward and feedback corticocortical inputs. Whereas PT neurons in any particular neocortical area often project to a characteristic target, their axons tend to branch to innervate the thalamus, striatum, subthalamic nucleus, brainstem, and spinal cord. Therefore PT neurons function as downstream elements in the local circuit broadcasting the results of cortical computations to distant subcortical structures.[27] The CT neurons of layer 6 receive little thalamic and local input but instead receive input primarily from high-order cortical areas. These CT neurons project back to the thalamic relay nucleus that provides the thalamocortical input to the corresponding portion of the cortex, and thus participate in excitatory thalamocortical loops specialized for integrating long-range signals to modulate thalamocortical activity. All classes of excitatory cortical neurons form recurrent connections with local neurons of the same class.

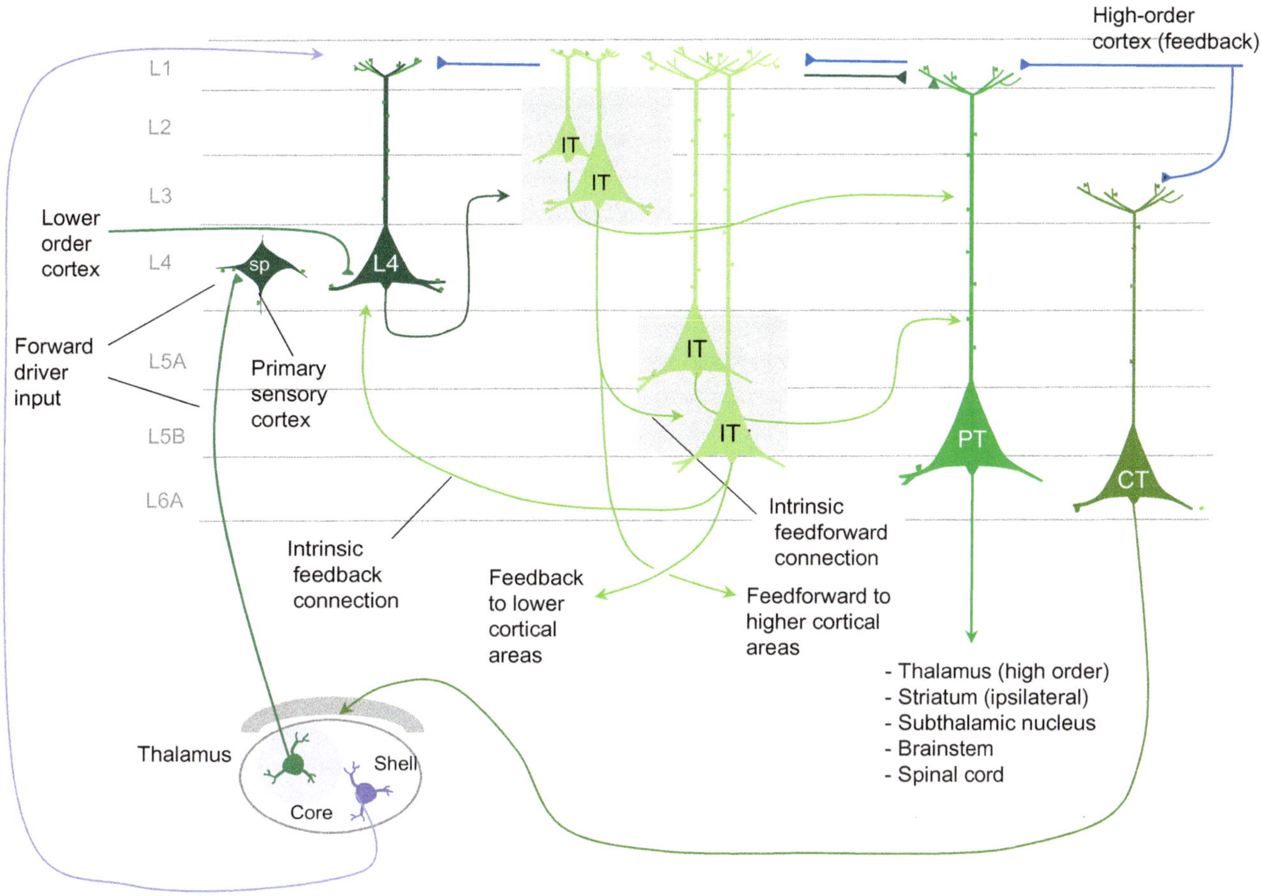

FIGURE 24.5 Information flow in local excitatory cortical circuits.
Layer 4 intratelencephalic (IT) neurons are the first station for extrinsic forward excitatory (drive) inputs to the cortex, In primary sensory cortex, layer 4 IT neurons receive driving inputs from core-type thalamocortical neurons located in first-order thalamic relay nuclei. Layer 4 IT neurons in higher-order sensory areas receive long-range inputs from thalamic association nuclei sources as well as corticocortical feedforward inputs from lower-order areas. Layer 4 IT neurons project heavily to IT neurons in layers 2/3 and to layers 5/6, which constitute the second stage of the local excitatory circuit. Neurons of superficial layers L2/3 project forward to the next cortical area, forming a disynaptic route between thalamus and secondary cortical areas. Information from L2/3 is then sent to L5 and L6, which sends (intrinsic) feedback projections back to L4. The L5 IT cells originate feedback connections to earlier cortical areas. The large pyramidal tract (PT) neurons of layer 5B receive extensive inputs from IT neurons of multiple layers, strong direct thalamocortical inputs from thalamic association nuclei, and both feedforward and feedback corticocortical inputs and function act as downstream elements in the local circuit projecting to distant subcortical structures. The corticothalamic (CT) neurons of layer 6 receive input primarily from high-order cortical areas and project back to the thalamic relay nucleus, which provides the thalamocortical input to the corresponding portion of the cortex.

Cortical Columns

The functional unit of the neocortex cortex is the cortical column (Figure 24.6),[28] which can vary over three orders of magnitude between minicolumns, columns, and hypercolumns. The minicolumn extends vertically across layers 2–6 and includes principal cells and interneurons that are heavily connected in the vertical direction. Several hundreds of minicolumns are bound together to form functional columns. Columns are the elementary functional unit of the neocortex; they vary from 300 to 600 μm in dimension and each consists of 10^3–10^4 neurons. A cortical column is classically defined as a vertical alignment of cells containing neurons with similar receptive field properties, such as orientation preference and ocular dominance in V1[29] or touch in somatosensory cortex.[28] The properties of every cortical column are shaped by the spatial and temporal integration of excitatory thalamocortical and corticocortical inputs and inhibitory GABAergic local circuit neurons. These properties are transitory and are determined by the fraction of the synaptic inputs that the column receives at a given time. Excitatory and inhibitory interactions between cortical columns preferentially connect neurons situated

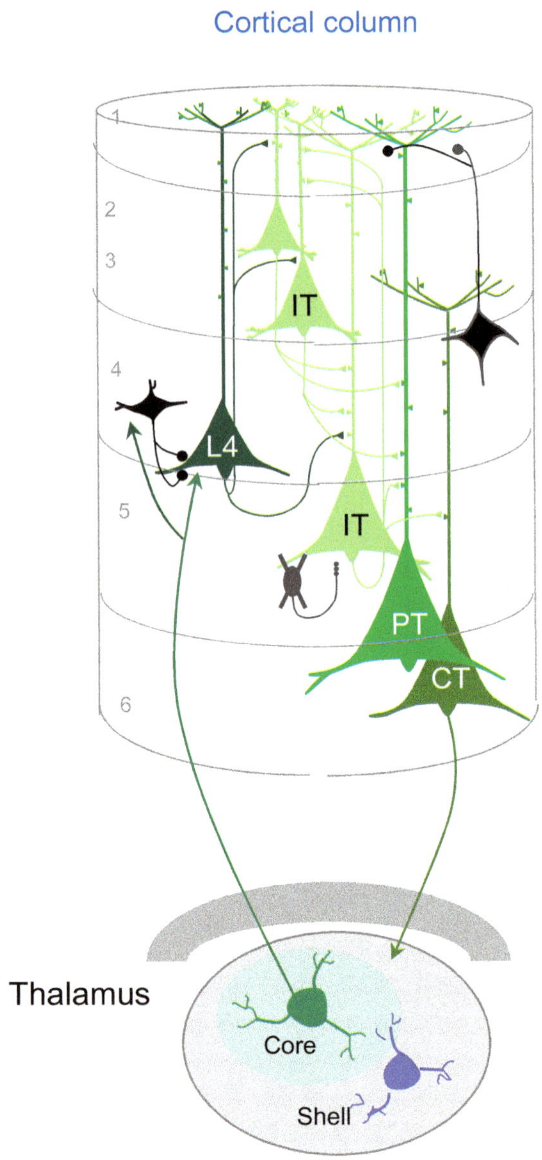

FIGURE 24.6 Cortical column.
Columns are the elementary functional unit of the neocortex; they vary from 300 to 600 μm in dimension and each consists of 10^3–10^4 neurons. A cortical column was classically defined as a vertical alignment of cells containing neurons with similar receptive field properties. The properties of every cortical column are shaped by the spatial and temporal integration of excitatory thalamocortical and corticocortical inputs and inhibitory GABAergic local circuit neurons. Columnar identity is maintained dynamically by per columnar (lateral) inhibition mediated by GABAergic interneurons. CT, corticothalamic neurons; IT, intratelencephalic neurons; PT, pyramidal tract neuron.

in close proximity to one another and thus link neurons with similar receptive-field properties. Columnar identity is maintained dynamically by per columnar (lateral) inhibition mediated by GABAergic interneurons.

INHIBITORY CORTICAL CIRCUITS

Information processing in the cerebral cortex depends on a large diversity of GABAergic interneurons, which constitute 25%–30% of all cortical neurons in primates.[27] These neurons form a highly heterogeneous group, which in part reflects their different developmental origins; some groups originate from the median ganglionic eminence and others from the lateral ganglionic eminence and other sources. GABAergic neuron precursors reach the cerebral cortex primarily via tangential migration. Cortical inhibitory interneurons are interconnected by gap junctions, primarily among interneurons of the same class. This connectivity results in the generation of interneuron networks that fire synchronously.

Heterogeneity of Cortical Inhibitory Neurons

Cortical interneurons are classified according to their expression of neurochemical markers, electrophysiological properties, targets, and functions[27,30,31] (Figure 24.7). There are multiple groups of cortical GABAergic interneurons. A simplified classification subdivides them into those expressing the calcium-binding protein parvalbumin (PV), those expressing somatostatin (SOM), and those expressing the ionotropic serotonin 5HT3a receptor (5HT3aR). However these groups are highly diverse.[32] The PV interneurons are fast-spiking and include basket cells and axon-axonic chandelier neurons. Basket cells form perisomatic synapses on both pyramidal cells and other interneurons; chandelier neurons form candlestick-like synaptic terminal arrays that specifically target the axon initial segment of pyramidal cells. The fast-spiking of these PV neurons depends on the expression and kinetics of their fast $Na_v1.1$ and $K_v3.3$ channels, and ensures that they produce a fast, reliable, strong, and temporally precise inhibition on their target cells. By producing hyperpolarizing and/or shunting inhibition close to the site of action potential generation, both types of PV GABAergic neurons influence the output of their target neurons. In the neocortex, GABAergic synapses of chandelier cells may elicit depolarization due to a higher intracellular Cl^- concentration at the axon initial segment; whether these synapses are excitatory or inhibitory may depend on the excitatory state of the postsynaptic cell. The prototype SOM expressing GABAergic interneurons are Martinotti cells, which are present in layers 2/3 and 5/6 and form axonal plexuses in layer 1, targeting the tuft dendrites and dendritic spines of pyramidal cells. SOM interneurons are activated by axon collaterals of pyramidal cells and thus have a major role in feedback inhibition in the cerebral cortex. SOM neurons have a low-threshold spiking pattern and receive weak excitatory synaptic input but are strongly facilitated during repetitive stimulation. The 5-HT3aR-expressing GABAergic interneurons constitute a heterogeneous group. They include vasoactive intestinal polypeptide (VIP)-expressing neurons,

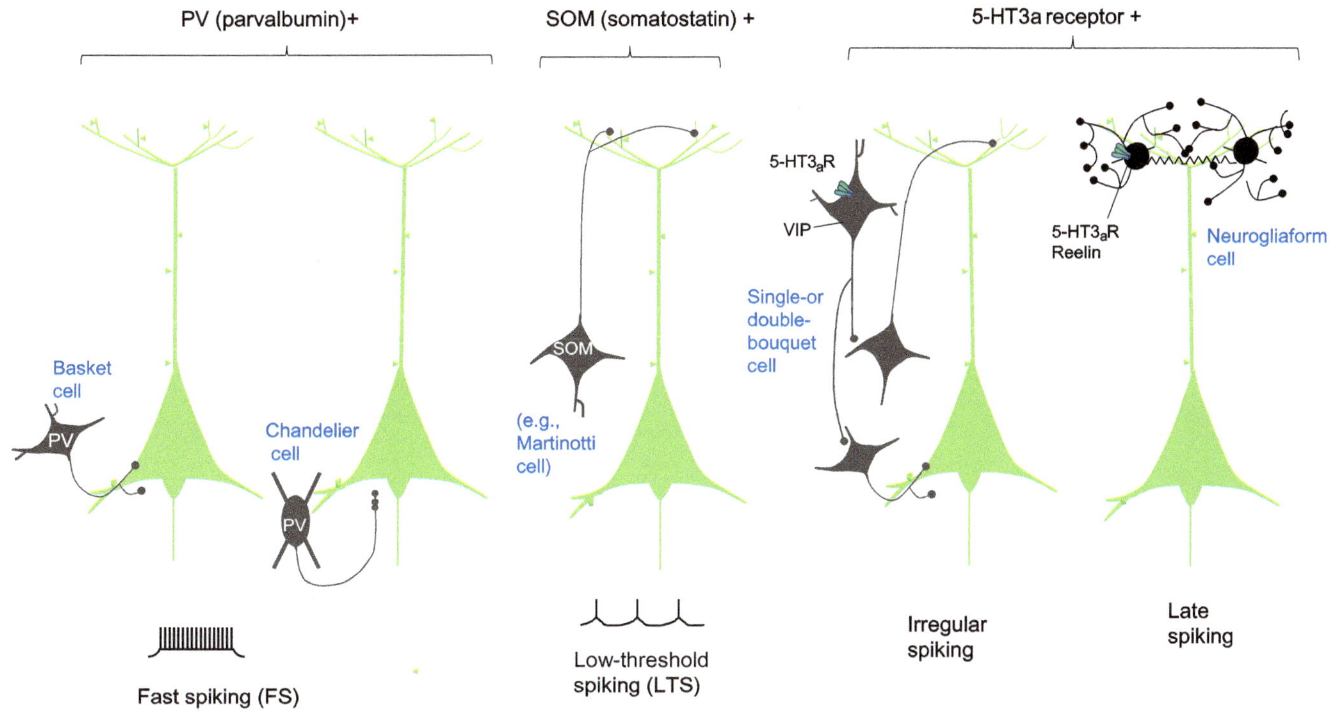

FIGURE 24.7 Main classes of cortical inhibitory neurons.
There are three main groups of cortical GABAergic interneurons: those expressing the calcium-binding protein parvalbumin (PV), those expressing somatostatin (SOM), and those expressing the ionotropic serotonin 5-HT3a receptor (5-HT3aR). The PV interneurons are fast-spiking neurons and include basket cells and axon-axonic chandelier neurons. The prototype SOM neurons are Martinotti cells, which are present in layers 2/3 and 5/6 and form axonal plexuses in layer 1 targeting the tuft dendrites and dendritic spines of pyramidal cells. The 5-HT3aR-expressing interneurons constitute a heterogeneous group. They include vasoactive intestinal polypeptide (VIP)-expressing neurons; cholecystokinin (CCK)-expressing basket cells (not shown), and neurogliaform cells. The VIP interneurons are present mainly in layers 2/3 and have vertically oriented, bipolar-like dendrites. VIP neurons primarily target other inhibitory interneurons, particularly SOM but also PV neurons. Neurogliaform cells have small, round soma from which multiple, very short dendrites spread radially in all directions and a wider, spherical, very dense axonal plexus composed of fine branches with widespread connections with neighboring neurons.

cholecystokinin (CCK) expressing basket cells, and neurogliaform cells. The VIP interneurons are present mainly in layers 2/3 and their majority have vertically oriented, bipolar-like dendrites and an axon that targets other inhibitory interneurons. The dendrites of VIP neurons cross several layers in either direction, can sample inputs restricted to one column, and can be targeted by many intracortical and subcortical projections. The axons of layer 2/3 VIP interneurons are also directed vertically, in a narrow columnar fashion often reaching layer 4 and layers 5/6. Neocortical and hippocampal CCK basket cells expressing 5-HT3Ra also express CB1 cannabinoid receptors and provide perisomatic inhibition to principal cells. Activation of the CB1 receptors by endocannabinoids generated in postsynaptic cells inhibits GABA release from CCK basket cells and suppresses this inhibition. Neurogliaform cells are located in layer 1 and have small, round soma from which multiple, very short dendrites spread radially in all directions and a wider, spherical, very dense axonal plexus composed of fine branches with widespread connections with neighboring neurons. Layer 1 contains several types of neurogliaform and other types of interneurons that express neuron-derived neurotrophic factor (NDNF), α7 nicotinic receptors, reelin, neuropeptide Y, and nitric oxide synthase.

Canonical Inhibitory Circuits in the Cerebral Cortex

The main inhibitory circuit motifs in the neocortex are feedforward inhibition, feedback inhibition, and disinhibition. Feedforward inhibition in the neocortex is largely mediated by PV fast spiking basket cells (Figure 24.8). These cells are recruited by thalamocortical afferents in layer 4 of primary sensory cortices. As the synaptic effects of thalamic afferents are faster and greater on PV interneurons than on pyramidal neurons, thalamocortical inputs elicit a strong, disynaptic feedforward inhibition of the principal cells that lags with a very short delay behind the monosynaptic thalamocortical excitation. This creates a limited

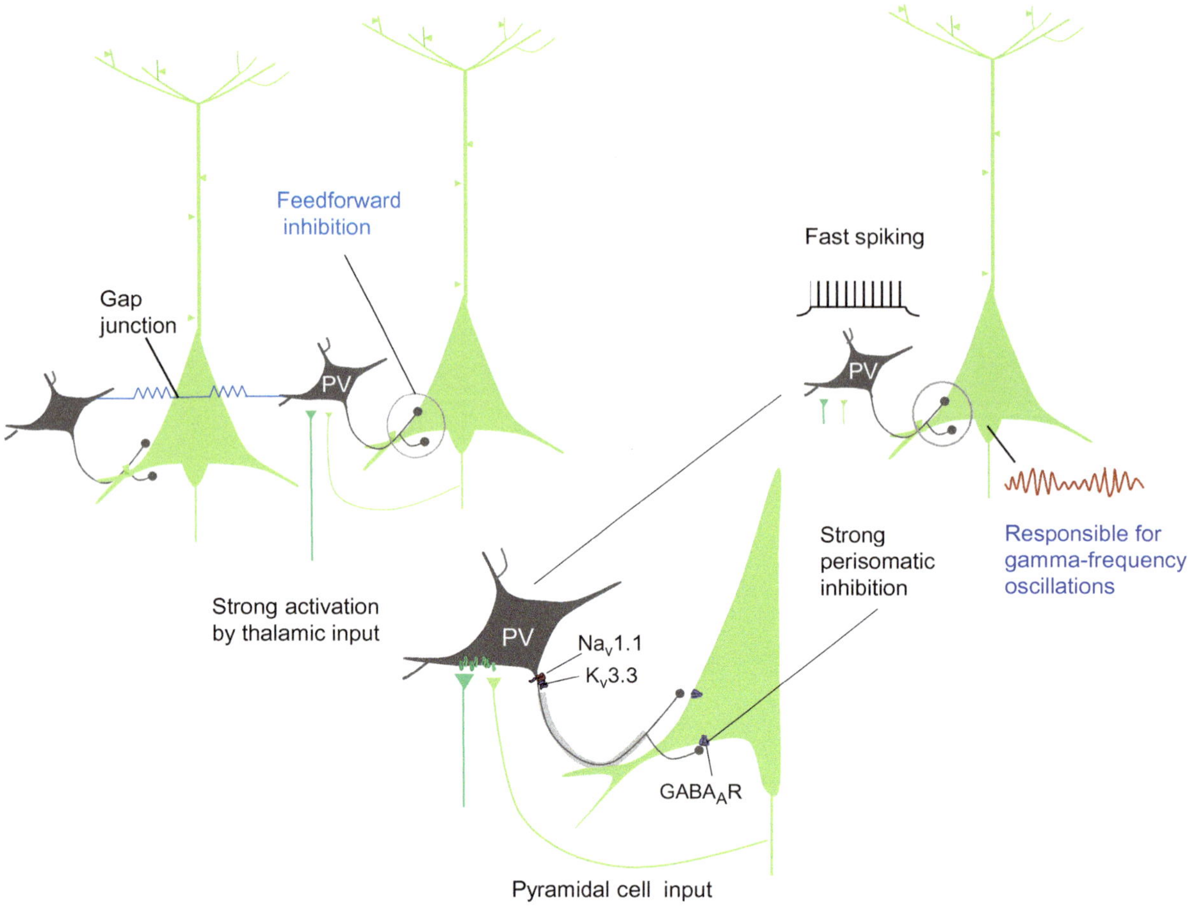

FIGURE 24.8 Roles of parvalbumin neurons in the neocortex.
Fast-spiking parvalbumin (PV) basket cells mediate feedforward in the neocortex. They are recruited by thalamocortical afferents and produce disynaptic feedforward inhibition of the principal cells. This creates a limited temporal window of opportunity for the principal cells to summate afferent inputs and to fire in response to sensory signals. Basket cells also receive inputs from their target pyramidal cells and are thus important for oscillatory activity in local cortical networks. Although PV basket interneurons interconnect with other PV interneurons, their strong connectivity to principal cells can result in synchronizing a highly interconnected population on the short time scale.

temporal window of opportunity for the principal cells to summate afferent inputs and to fire in response to sensory signals. Basket cells are also recruited by inputs from their target pyramidal cells, and their fast-spiking activity and strong inhibitory effects on pyramidal cells provide the basis for circuit oscillation at gamma frequency. The gamma cycle reflects the alternation of periods of strong inhibition, during which pyramidal neurons are less receptive to synaptic inputs, with short periods with weak inhibition, during which pyramidal neurons can fire an action potential. Although PV basket interneurons interconnect with other PV interneurons, their strong connectivity to principal cells can result in synchronizing a highly interconnected population on a short timescale. This feedforward inhibitory circuit is suppressed via presynaptic muscarinic M2 cholinergic and $GABA_B$ receptors on GABAergic terminals of PV basket cells.

The second major circuit motif is feedback (recurrent) inhibition, in which the source of excitation of the interneurons are axon collaterals from local principal cells (Figure 24.9). This inhibitory feedback reduces or prevents further discharges of the excitatory cell and controls the excitatory-inhibitory balance of local populations of principal cells. Interneurons can inhibit not only the principal cell from which it received excitation but also others that are part of either local or neighboring populations; this phenomenon is referred to as lateral inhibition. Feedback inhibitory circuits in the neocortex may involve either PV or SOM interneurons. Whereas the response of PV interneurons to repetitive inputs is initially high and rapidly decreases, SOM interneurons are recruited more slowly but undergo synaptic facilitation and excitatory postsynaptic potential summation. Thus, these interneurons function as detectors of the most active excitatory cells in the local network

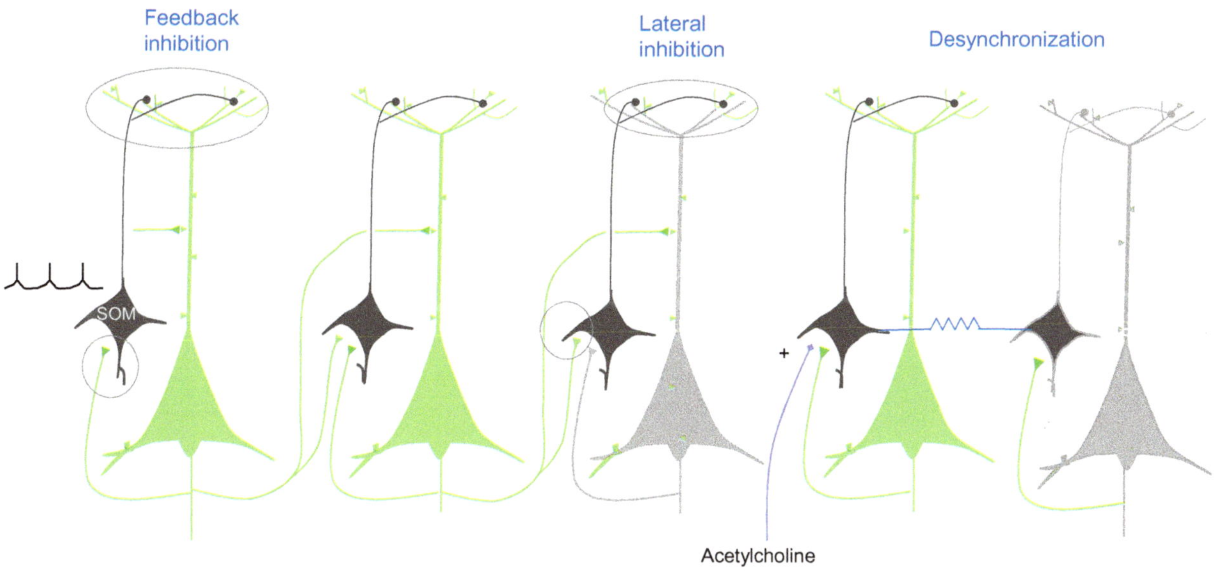

FIGURE 24.9 Neocortical somatostatin neurons and feedback inhibition.
Somatostatin (SOM) neurons receive input from collateral highly active pyramidal cells and project to their apical dendrites, exerting powerful feedback inhibition and also inhibit neighboring populations (lateral inhibition). These neurons are activated by acetylcholine and may be involved in mechanisms of cortical desynchronization.

and prevent synchronized activity of pools of pyramidal neurons. SOM interneurons also receive robust cholinergic input that depolarizes these neurons largely via M1 muscarinic receptors. These cholinergic inputs promote feedback inhibition via SOM interneurons and thus desynchronize background cortical activity.

The third major inhibitory circuit motif is disinhibition, which is mediated by VIP interneurons in layers 2/3 that target SOM and to a lesser extent PV interneurons (Figure 24.10). As VIP neurons are excited by corticocortical feedback projections from higher-order cortices, they have a major role in mediating attentional modulation of excitability of pyramidal neurons by reducing their inhibition by SOM or PV interneurons. The VIP neurons are also strongly depolarized by serotonin via 5HT3Rs and by acetylcholine via nicotinic receptors and thus also mediate attentional effects of these ascending neuromodulatory systems.

In some cases, feedback connections can inhibit sensory processing via inputs to neurogliaform cells in layer 1, which are interconnected with each other via electrical connections and provide strong monosynaptic inhibition to layer 2/3 pyramidal cells. Neurogliaform neurons participate in mechanisms of volume transmission and elicit slow, long-lasting inhibition on pyramidal cells and other interneurons through a combined activation of extrasynaptic $GABA_B$ and δ-subunit-containing $GABA_A$ receptors. Layer 1 contains the apical dendritic tufts of pyramidal cells and receives converging top-down projections from other cortical areas, higher-order thalamus and basal forebrain. When action potentials backpropagating from the soma into the apical dendrites coincide with dendritic excitatory inputs, they facilitate the generation of dendritic Ca^{2+} spikes thus enhancing probability of action potential generation. This may constitute a coincidence detector mechanism for top-down and bottom-up inputs on pyramidal cells. GABAergic inputs from SOM positive Martinotti cells and layer 1 interneurons shape local dendritic integration in pyramidal cells and thus control circuit plasticity and learning. Reduction in SOM interneuron signaling promotes learning by enabling top-down inputs to elicit plastic changes on apical pyramidal cell dendrites. Layer 1 interneurons receive strong excitatory long-range top-down projections from other cortical areas, high-order thalamic nuclei, and basal forebrain. These interneurons not only elicit long-lasting inhibition of apical dendrites of pyramidal cells but also engage a disinhibitory circuit by inhibiting PV expressing GABAergic interneurons in other layers. Thus the balanced influences of SOM interneurons and lamina 1 inhibitory neurons may differentially shape associative learning in the cortex.

Long-Range Projecting GABAergic Interneurons

Whereas the majority of cortical GABAergic neurons target nearby cells and control the local network activity, some cortical GABAergic neurons also project to other brain areas. Within the neocortex, these long-range GABAergic projections connect different areas both within same or in the contralateral hemisphere.[33] A potential function of these projections is to synchronize rhythmic activity between distant neocortical areas and to participate in interhemispheric inhibition via the corpus callosum. For example, a group of PV GABAergic neurons

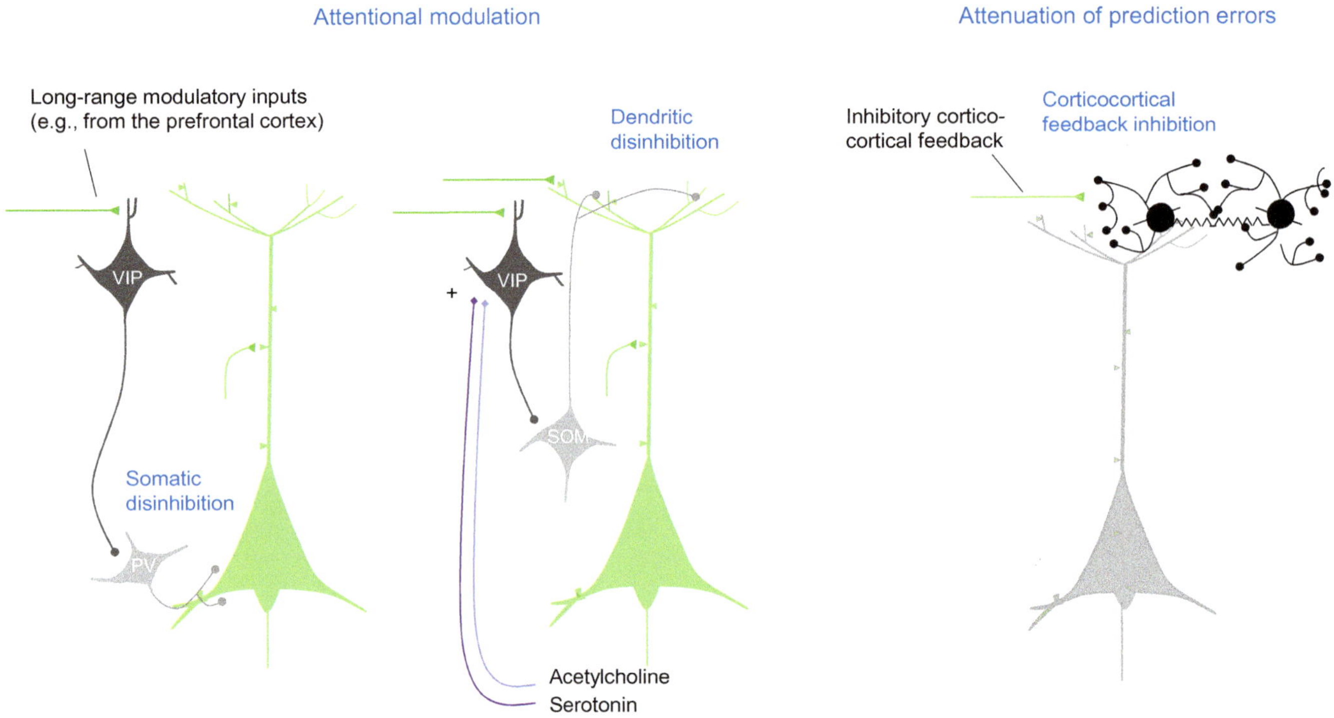

FIGURE 24.10 Disinhibitory circuits in the neocortex.
Disinhibition in the neocortex is mediated by vasoactive intestinal polypeptide (VIP) interneurons in layers 2/3 that target somatostatin (SOM) and to a lesser extent parvalbumin (PV) inhibitory neurons. These VIP neurons are excited by corticocortical feedback projections from higher order cortices, by cholinergic inputs acting via nicotinic and M1 muscarinic receptors, and via serotonergic inputs via 5-HT3aRs.

provide callosal inhibitory projections from the visual, and motor cortices to their corresponding cortex in the contralateral hemisphere.[34] Long-range GABAergic cells also interconnect cortical with subcortical areas. For example, GABAergic neurons of the frontal cortex project to striatum and globus pallidus.[35]

CORTICAL OSCILLATIONS

Information processing in neuronal networks is critically dependent on the precise synchronization of ensembles of neurons. This synchronous activity is reflected by neuronal oscillations, which produce extracellular local field potentials that can be recorded with microelectrodes, electroencephalogram (EEG), and magnetoencephalogram (MEG). The EEG oscillations include slow (<1 Hz), delta (~1–4 Hz), theta (~4–8 Hz), alpha and mu (~8–13 Hz), beta (~13–30 Hz), gamma (>30–80 Hz), ripple (>80–200 Hz), fast ripple (>200–600 Hz), and sigma (≥600 Hz).[36,37]

Role of Interneurons

Interneurons play a key role in coordinating activity both within local networks and across the relatively long distances that separate different brain regions. Networks of interneurons are the backbone of many brain oscillators as they provide rhythm-based timing to principal cells in the brain.[38] Most oscillations are called "relaxation" or pulse type; spikes of principal cells are typically concentrated within a narrow window of opportunity during the phase when inhibitory neurons are less active. By this mechanism, interneurons coordinate activity both within local networks and across different brain regions.[39] A fundamental function of inhibitory interneurons is to allow the dynamic organization of principal cells into functional ensembles. Because of inhibitory connections, competing cell assemblies can be functionally isolated, such that excitatory pathways can be rerouted though the coordinated interneuron groups. Thus specific firing patterns of principal cells in a network will depend largely on the temporal and spatial distribution of inhibition. In response to the same input, the same network can potentially produce several different output patterns at different times, depending on the distribution of inhibition.[38]

Slow Oscillations

Slow and delta oscillations represent the dominant network activity in neocortical areas during non-rapid eye movement (NREM) sleep. During the slow oscillation, cortical neurons display synchronous bursts of depolarization (UP states) separated by periods of relative quiescence (DOWN states) and oscillate between these two states. (Figure 24.11). These UP- and DOWN-states reflect spontaneous synaptic events sustained through a balance of recurrent fast ionotropic excitatory neurotransmission in principal cells and its termination by strong inhibitory inputs via both $GABA_A$ and $GABA_B$ receptors. Basal forebrain cholinergic neurons reduce the power of neocortical slow oscillations by promoting activity of SOM interneurons, preventing synchronization of populations of pyramidal neurons. Whereas slow oscillations can be generated within the cortex alone, pacemaking activity of the thalamus also has an important role during deep NREM sleep.

Theta Oscillations

Theta oscillations typically occur in hippocampal circuits but are also present in the neocortex. The hippocampal theta oscillations occur during voluntary movements and REM sleep, where the oscillation modulates the timing of action potentials. Both excitatory pyramidal cells and GABAergic interneurons contribute to generating theta oscillations. Theta oscillations have a critical role in coordinating the activity of the PFC and hippocampus during memory encoding and retrieval, as described in the next chapter.

Alpha Oscillations

The alpha rhythm is typically 9.5–12.5 Hz and its frequency varies among individuals. It is more pronounced in the parietooccipital region, especially during the alert relaxed state, but is present across the cortex, including the

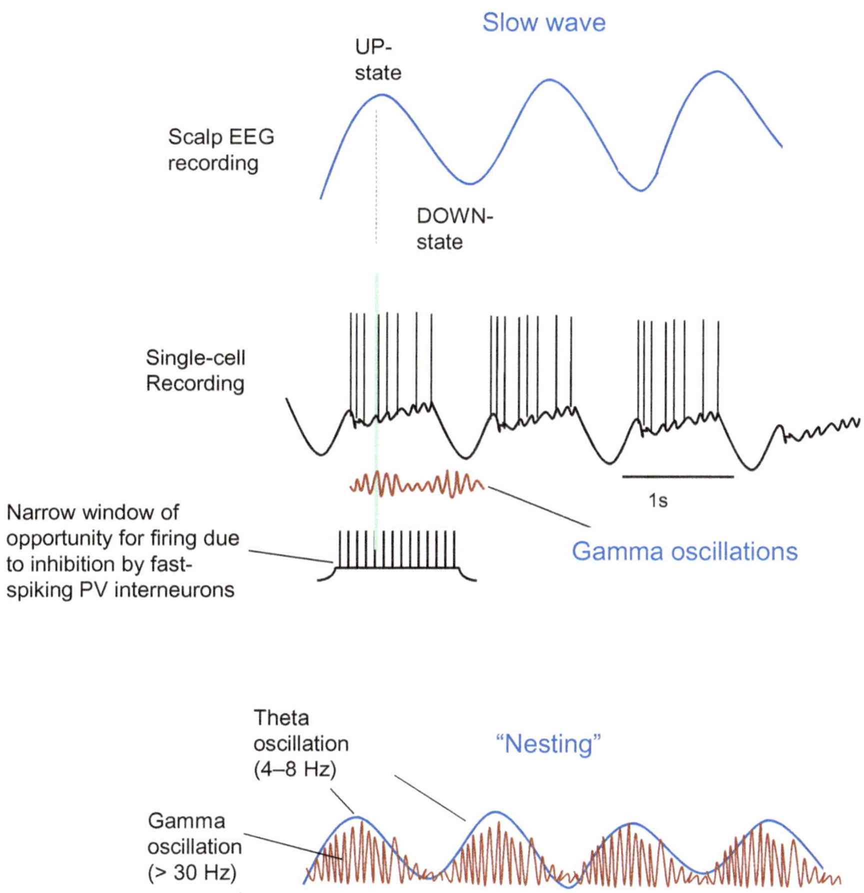

FIGURE 24.11 Slow and gamma cortical oscillations.
Slow oscillations and delta activity represent the dominant network activity during non-rapid eye movement sleep in neocortical areas. During the slow oscillation, cortical neurons display synchronous bursts of depolarization (UP states) separated by periods of relative quiescence (DOWN states). The basis for the gamma-rhythm is the strong feedforward inhibition of pyramidal cells by fast-spiking parvalbumin (PV) basket cells. This inhibition provides a narrow window for spike generation in principal cells in response to incoming inputs. Slow oscillation can affect the faster oscillations; this is reflected by cross-frequency phase-amplitude coupling, or "nesting," so that the phase of the slow oscillations modulates the power of the faster ones.

sensorimotor cortex (where it is called mu rhythm), auditory cortex, and association cortex. Alpha oscillations have an important effect on neural excitability; when the alpha power increases in a given region, neuronal activity decreases at the peak of the alpha oscillation cycle (pulsed inhibition). The alpha rhythm is related to tonic alertness, sustained self-initiated attention, or preparedness to process information and to respond. Thalamocortical interactions, primarily via the pulvinar, may be pivotal in originating cortical alpha oscillations and translating control signals from parietal and prefrontal regions to other cortical areas. During selective attention, alpha oscillation power decreases and cortical excitability increases over the area processing the attended information.

Beta Oscillations

Oscillations at the beta frequency (~13–30 Hz) are prominent in the cortical sensorimotor areas. They reflect periodic and synchronous activity in essentially all elements of the sensorimotor control system. Beta oscillations are prominent during postural holds when muscles are tonically active or during anticipation of somatosensory stimulation in preparation for movement. They disappear during movement. Beta oscillations also have a major role in communication between the PFC and other cortical areas, both directly and via the thalamus.

Gamma Oscillations

Gamma band oscillations (~30–100 Hz) synchronized among spatially distributed cortical areas are thought to represent the neuronal correlate of the perceptual binding between stimulus features. Gamma oscillations are associated with numerous cognitive processes and are present in all neocortical areas, hippocampus, and amygdala. The gamma power closely relates to the BOLD signal in fMRI. The basis for the gamma rhythm is the strong feedforward inhibition of pyramidal cells by fast-spiking PV basket cells. This inhibition provides a narrow window for spike generation in principal cells in response to incoming inputs (Figure 24.11). The gamma cycle reflects the alternation of periods with strong inhibition, when neurons are less responsive to synaptic inputs, with short periods with weak inhibition, during which pyramidal neurons have a stronger response. For effective communication between brain regions, these time periods need to be aligned such that synaptic inputs consistently arrive during periods when postsynaptic neurons are not inhibited. This is in part determined by the rapid communication between PV neurons via gap junctions.

High-Frequency Oscillations

High-frequency oscillations (HFOs) are defined as transient, sinusoid-like events that contain spectral power between 80 and 600 Hz. In the normal brain, local inhibitory cells, primarily fast-spiking basket cells in the neocortex and the CA1 region of the hippocampus, have a prominent role in physiological HFOs via synchronous $GABA_A$ receptor-mediated inhibition of principal cells. The tightly orchestrated pattern of firing between interneurons and principal cells during normal HFOs has been implicated with encoding information, sensorimotor integration, and, in the hippocampus, memory consolidation during NREM sleep.

Laminar Organization of Cortical Oscillations

Whereas superficial and deep layers are anatomically interconnected, they constitute functionally distinct processing streams. For example, in visual cortical areas different connectivity pathways seem to exert their influence via specific frequency bands. Connections originating in supragranular layers 2/3 influence other cortical areas mostly via gamma frequency band oscillations, whereas connections originating infragranular layers 5/6 exert their influence via low frequencies, predominantly in the beta frequency band. Such a tight connectional–functional association was also empirically demonstrated for the visual system of the human cortex.[40] Since feedforward connections originate predominately from superficial layers and feedback connections from deep layers, these differences suggest that feedforward connections use relatively high frequencies, compared to feedback connections.[41]

Grouping and Routing of Neocortical Processing by Inhibition-Based Oscillations

The system of cortical rhythms is hierarchical both in space and time, largely due to anatomical wiring of networks and the limited speed of axon conduction. High-frequency oscillations involve interconnected neurons within local circuits. Synchronization in the gamma band provides for local functional network ensembles of pyramidal cells. In contrast, slow oscillations allow long-range communication between interacting distant cortical areas. As a result, when multiple rhythms are present simultaneously, the slow oscillation can affect the faster oscillations. This interaction is reflected by cross-frequency coupling, so that the phase of the slow oscillations in the theta- or alpha range rhythm modulates the power of the faster ones, for example in the gamma range (Figure 24.11). This cross-frequency phase-amplitude coupling or "nesting" is critical for neuronal interactions both within and between networks. For example, gamma oscillations are often nested within theta oscillations in prefrontal and hippocampal circuits; variation of amplitude of the gamma oscillation in phase with the theta rhythm is important for encoding and retrieval of episodic memory.

CORTICAL STATES

The brain is constantly active, even in the absence of any external sensory input or motor activity. Cortical neurons process information on a background of spontaneous, ongoing activity that has distinct spatiotemporal profiles that define different cortical states. These cortical states provide for a dynamic control of information processing by affecting the balance of activity between specific subtypes of neurons, synchronization between nearby neurons, and functional coupling between distant cortical areas.[42]

Active Versus Inactive Cortical States

Cortical activity changes during different levels of waking and across the wake–sleep cycle. Small-amplitude high-frequency fluctuations of the EEG occur during wakefulness and are followed by a progressive transition to higher-amplitude and slower fluctuations, with are slowest during deep NREM sleep. Based on classical EEG studies, wakefulness is often described as a state of global neocortical desynchronization, dominated by low-voltage, high-frequency (>20 Hz) activity, whereas NREM sleep is described as a state of global synchronization dominated by high-voltage, low-frequency (<10 Hz) activity. However, during different levels of waking, cortical activities, particularly in the gamma frequency range, can be highly synchronous both within and across cortical areas. Thus, the active cortical state has been more recently defined as the cortical activity characterized by a low ratio between low frequency (1–10 Hz) and high frequency (20–100 Hz) oscillations.[42] Studies in mice show that during quiet wakefulness the cortex fluctuates between an activated and a deactivated state in relation to behavioral context, attentional level, or general motor activity. In the wake state, there are rapid changes in spontaneous cortical activity from high-amplitude, low-frequency fluctuations predominantly in layer 2/3 during quite wakefulness to faster and smaller amplitude fluctuations when animals are active.[42] Fast-spiking PV interneurons fire at high frequency during quiet wakefulness and reduce their activity during active wakefulness, whereas VIP interneurons increase their firing during active wakefulness, promoting disinhibition and facilitating cortical information processing.

State-Dependent Synchrony of Brain Activity and Encoding Information

Cortical activation or deactivation can occur locally but is highly correlated in functionally linked cortical regions. Whereas local synchronization between small neuronal populations may allow the formation of functional neuronal ensembles coding for similar aspects of a stimulus, local desynchronization may enhance the information content of neuronal population activity by reducing the signal-to-noise ratio. On the other hand, long-range synchronization between brain regions may allow functional coupling between of areas co-engaged in a given cognitive task. Neuronal synchrony is highly dynamic and is strongly affected by brain states. During quiet wakefulness, the slow, high-amplitude fluctuations of nearby excitatory neurons are highly synchronous, both within the same cortical layer and across layers. This low-frequency activity is also synchronized across more distant cortical areas. During active waking there is a decrease in both local neuronal synchrony and power in the low-frequency band; however this is associated with an increased coherence in the low-frequency band between cortical areas. This contrasts with NREM sleep, where low-frequency activity increases locally but its coherence between cortical areas strongly decreases, which is consistent with a decrease in cortical functional connectivity.[42]

Sensory processing highly depends on attentional, behavioral, and motivational states as well as context and past experience. Behavioral context and learning defines and enhances the processing of relevant sensory stimuli. The strongest effect of cortical activation in sensory areas is to reduce background fluctuations in membrane potential that may interfere with activity driven by sensory stimuli. As a consequence, cortical activation often results in an increased reliability of the sensory evoked neuronal responses by increasing the signal-to-noise ratio. Thus, task performance is higher with high than with low level of arousal.

Thalamic and Extrathalamic Modulation of Cortical States

Whereas corticocortical connectivity is critical for the generation of slow spontaneous cortical activity during sleep, direct inputs from other cortical areas or subcortical structures markedly contribute to the generation and modulation of cortical activities during the waking state. These influences include glutamatergic inputs from the thalamus, top-down glutamatergic inputs from other cortical areas, cholinergic inputs from the basal forebrain, and monoaminergic inputs from the brainstem. For example, tonic release of acetylcholine determines the degree of cortical activity, whereas peaks of acetylcholine, norepinephrine, and dopamine signal salient events of the environment that engage attention and improve both sensory processing and performance of a task. These modulatory influences are further discussed in chapter 28.

EMERGING PROPERTIES OF THE NEOCORTEX

Predictive Coding

The predictive code model poses that the brain actively constructs perception using past experience.[43,44] A central aspect of this model is that the brain predicts upcoming sensory experience to reduce or "explain away" activity in lower-level areas receiving the actual sensory input. Predictive coding involves the filtering of sensory inputs to reduce the mismatch between predicted (internal) and externally induced sensations. According to this model, top-down predictions based on previous experience are compared with bottom-up incoming sensory information to form a prediction error.[43,44] At each level of processing, the discrepancy between the predictions received from higher-level brain areas and the actual sensory input conveyed by lower-level areas represents a prediction error signal that generates a response. Consistent with this model, human imaging studies show smaller responses in early sensory cortical areas to predictable compared to unpredictable or deviant stimuli. In a familiar environment, even minor deviations from perceptual predictions may generate a sensory response. Predictions are sent as feedback signals in the hierarchy, whereas prediction errors are sent in a feedforward direction. The prediction errors are used to update the higher-level representations that provided the top-down predictions; and these optimized predictions then reduce prediction error at lower levels. These prediction error signals are thus used to update representations to ensure better estimates for future experience. In this scheme, feedback connections should have an inhibitory influence on earlier areas to suppress feedforward driving inputs. This may reflect direction of information flow along gradients of laminar differentiation from limbic to neocortical areas.[45] For example, in addition to its critical role in episodic memory, the hippocampus may also be involved in online prediction, anticipating upcoming sensory information using recent sensory inputs together with internally generated stored information.[46] Whereas during episodic recall the hippocampus may exert an excitatory influence on the neocortex to reinstate activity patterns across cortical circuits, the hippocampus can also provide sensory predictions to "explain away" prediction errors via inhibitory hippocampal-neocortical interactions.[46] Feedback inhibitory predictions can coexist with feedforward top-down attentional enhancement of processing of new sensory information. Attention enhances neural activity and effectively opposes the inhibitory effect of prediction by enhancing the precision of neocortical representation. In predictive coding, attention would increase the gain of neuronal populations encoding a novel stimulus and thus prediction error. Thus the cortical microcircuitry provides the basis for predictive coding as the interface between feedforward (prediction error) and feedback (prediction) interaction.[44]

Large-Scale Networks

Functional neuroimaging and recordings of cortical activity show that complex behaviors, such as attention, language, and inner thought processing emerge from distributed functional networks involving several cortical regions[8,9,11,47] (Figure 24.12). Multiple functionally distinct but anatomically overlapping components of different brain networks may exist within the same cortical region. Examples of these large-scale cortical networks include attention networks, control networks, and the default mode network.

There are two attention networks involved in deployment of attention and reorientation to unexpected events.[48,49] A dorsal attention network is involved in goal-oriented attention and includes areas in superior parietal lobule, lateral PFC along the precentral sulcus, and the frontal eye field. The ventral attention network registers salient events in the environment; this network includes areas at the temporoparietal junction and the ventral lateral frontal cortex, and is lateralized to the right hemisphere. The frontoparietal control network is critical for the ability to coordinate behavior in a rapid, accurate, and flexible goal-driven manner. This network includes regions of the lateral PFC, intraparietal sulcus, and ventral inferior temporal lobe and flexibly interacts with other networks.[50] The salience network responds to homeostatically relevant stimuli and outcomes and has its hub in the anterior cingulate cortex and ventral anterior insular (frontoinsular) cortex.[51] These areas contain large layer 5 projection neurons, called von Economo neurons, that provide input to brainstem autonomic nuclei; the salience network responds to bodily sensations and controls output to visceral organs. The cingulo-opercular task-control network, including the dorsal anterior insula and anterior midcingulate cortex appears to be critical for task set initiation and maintenance, perhaps by providing the sustained vigilance or "tonic alertness."[52] The default mode network, unlike the other networks, is active at resting state and becomes inactivated during tasks that involve attention to the external environment. It has been proposed that the default mode network comprises multiple subsystems, each contributing to self-generated thought processes.[53] A core group of regions in this network, including the areas of the medial prefrontal and posterior cingulate cortex represents information that is personally relevant; a medial temporal subsystem involving the hippocampus and parahippocampal regions allows construction of coherent mental scenes to reflect about the past and project the future; and a dorsal medial subsystem including the dorsomedial PFC allows inferring about the mental state of the self and others.[54] The functions of these large-scale networks are further discussed in another chapters of this book. A recent study revealed a core of 10 widely distributed "multiple-demand" parcels per hemisphere that are activated during many tasks and are functionally interconnected.[55] These areas are located along the lateral frontal surface above the anterior insula and dorsal part of the lateral frontal surface; in the dorsomedial frontal surface; within and surrounding the intraparietal sulcus; the dorsomedial parietal cortex; and the posterior temporal cortex.[55]

Neural Correlates of Consciousness

Consciousness has been described as the subjective experience of "what it is like" to perceive a scene, recognize a face, or reflect on the experience itself.[56] The neural correlates of consciousness have been defined as the minimum neural mechanisms sufficient for any one specific conscious percept.[56–58] Based on evidence provided by lesion, stimulation, and recording studies, it has been proposed that these

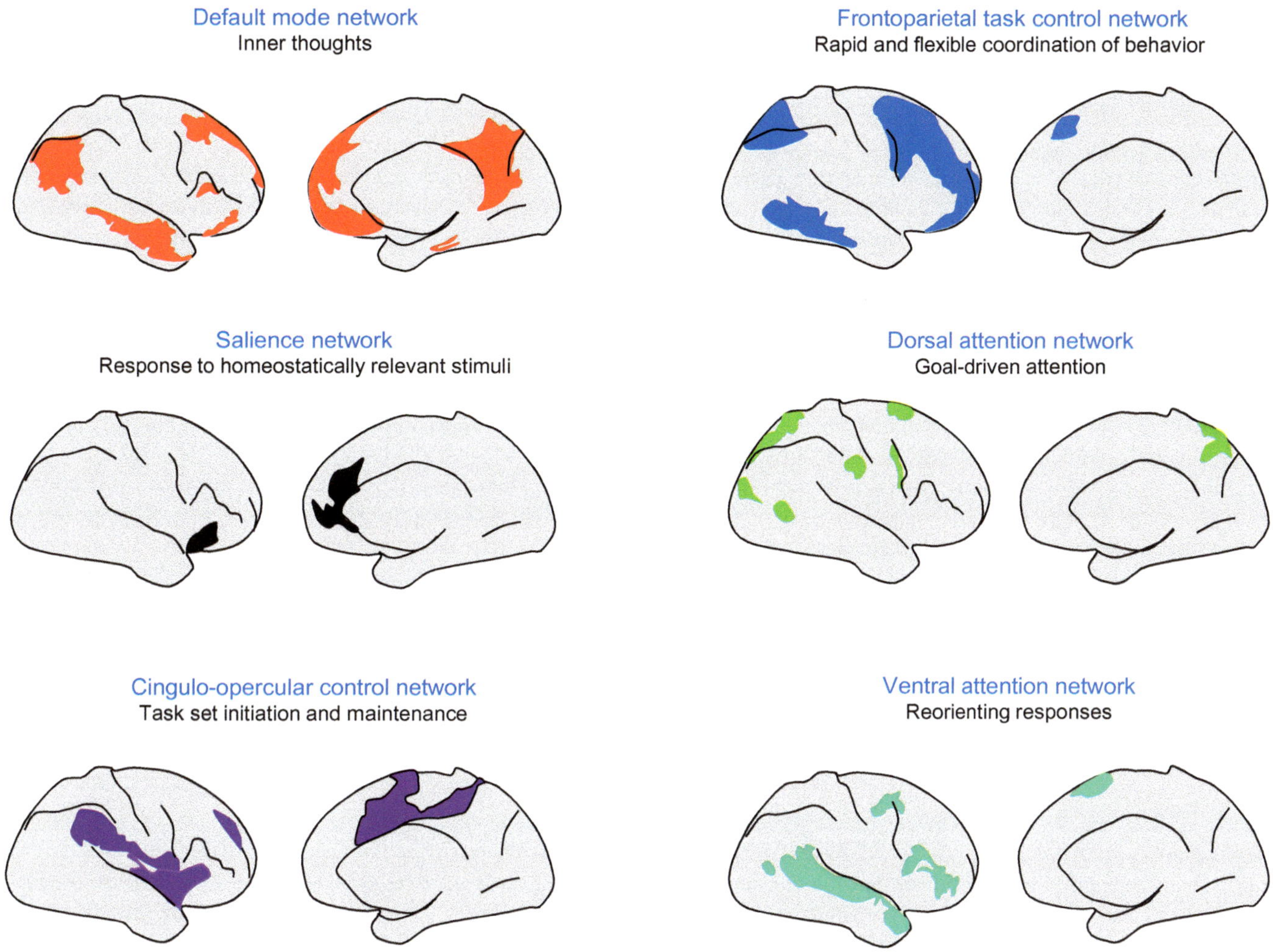

FIGURE 24.12 Schematic representation of the large-scale networks in the cerebral cortex.
Functional neuroimaging and recordings of cortical activity show that complex behaviors, such as attention, language, and inner thought processing emerge from distributed functional networks involving several cortical regions. A dorsal attention network is involved in goal-oriented attention and includes areas in superior parietal lobule, lateral prefrontal cortex (PFC)along the precentral sulcus, and the frontal eye field. The ventral attention network registers salient events in the environment and includes areas at the temporoparietal junction and the ventral lateral frontal cortex and is lateralized to the right hemisphere. The frontoparietal control network is critical for the ability to coordinate behavior in a rapid, accurate, and flexible goal-driven manner and includes regions of the lateral PFC, intraparietal sulcus, and ventral inferior temporal lobe. The cingulo-opercular task-control network, including the dorsal anterior insula and anterior midcingulate cortex, appears to be critical for task set initiation and maintenance. The salience network responds to homeostatically relevant stimuli and outcomes and has its hub in the anterior cingulate cortex and ventral anterior insula. The default mode network comprises multiple subsystems, each contributing to self-generated thought processes.

neural correlates are primarily localized to a posterior cortical "hot zone" that includes parietotemporooccipital regions.[57] This model is largely based on observations that large bilateral prefrontal lesions do not affect subjective perception. In this view, content-specific neural correlates of consciousness directly contribute to phenomenal distinctions such as visual features, face, or places; the full neural correlate of consciousness would consist of the combination of all these content-specific neural correlates. In this model, areas in the PFC would be primarily involved in monitoring and reporting the conscious experience, but the PFC activity per se does not reflect specific perceptual content; PFC activation during perceptual awareness would be driven by the need to monitor and report the subjective experience rather than subjective experience per se. However, an alternative view is that PFC should not be dismissed as a substrate of conscious perception.[58] Thus, the relative role of the "anterior" (prefrontal") versus the "posterior" (parietotemporooccipital) cortex in conscious perceptual experience is still a matter of controversy.

CORTICAL NETWORK PATHOPHYSIOLOGY IN EPILEPSY

Seizures result from an imbalance between excitation and inhibition in a discrete cortical area, or seizure onset focus, resulting in aberrant activity in a distributed network and subsequent recruitment of adjacent cortex. Epileptogenesis creates a persistent increased probability of spontaneous seizures. In chronic epilepsy the timing of seizures is unpredictable and seizures typically represent less than 1% of the total brain activity except in the most severe epileptic encephalopathies.[59]

Mechanisms Increasing Neuronal Excitability

Some genetic epilepsies are due to mutations affecting inhibitory or excitatory conductances, as occurs in channelopathies or synaptopathies. Representative examples are mutations affecting voltage-gated Na^+ or K^+ channels or subunits of $GABA_A$ or NMDA receptors. Many mutations producing epilepsy affect proteins involved in exocytosis or transduction of synaptic signals. This supports the idea that functional shifts in the balance between inhibition and excitation due to abnormal synaptic plasticity could transform normal levels of network activity into ictal activity.[59] One prominent mechanism of activity-dependent disinhibition involves dysregulation of ionic concentrations. Seizure activity results in increases in extracellular K^+ that overwhelms the activity of the Na^+/K^+ ATPase, elicits membrane depolarization, and compromises the cotransport of other ions. Large influxes of Ca^{2+} through voltage- and ligand-gated channels may lead to reductions in extracellular Ca^{2+} and neurotransmitter release. Prolonged activation of inhibitory $GABA_A$Rs can degrade inhibition due to changes in the reversal potential of Cl^- by overwhelming the transport capacity of the cation-chloride cotransporter KCC2. In these circumstances the $GABA_A$R conductance becomes depolarizing and thus excitatory. Astrocyte dysfunction also has a major role in ictogenesis by impairing their ability to buffer extracellular K^+, synthesize glutamine as the source of glutamate for GABA synthesis in inhibitory neurons, and uptake glutamate from the synaptic cleft.[61]

Microcircuit Interactions and Seizures

Several cortical microcircuits may contribute to initiation of seizures.[60] Impaired feedforward inhibition by PV interneurons may be a major mechanism of ictogenesis. For example, loss-of-function *SCN1A* mutations impairing $Na_v1.1$ channels in the axon initial segment in these cells may underlie epilepsy in Dravet syndrome. Studies using optical and electrophysiological methods in experimental models, as well as intra-operative intracranial recordings in patients with epilepsy, show that the earliest synaptic abnormality preceding seizure onset is the presence of multiphasic, repetitive, and potent inhibitory signals that are initially associated with normal (nonictal) background network activity. This is followed by a sudden collapse of inhibition resulting in predominance of strong excitatory signals that produce step-like waves of local excitation at the network level. This cycle then repeats to propagate seizure activity to the next microcircuit. The SOM neurons involved in feedback inhibition of pyramidal cell dendrites are progressively recruited by simultaneous repetitive activity in multiple pyramidal cells and could be important for dampening activity and locally suppressing seizures in the microcircuit. Chandelier cells targeting the axon initial segment of pyramidal neurons may also be recruited by epileptic activity and serve as a microcircuit emergency brake. In contrast, disinhibitory circuits mediated by VIP interneurons may contribute to ictogenesis by suppressing the inhibitory activity of the other types of GABAergic interneurons. The final type of circuit involved in most epilepsies is local recurrent excitation, which is a common motif in cortical networks as ~80% of neurons and synapses are excitatory. A typical example is recurrent excitation in the dentate gyrus shown in temporal lobe epilepsy (TLE) models; recurrent excitatory connections also occur in the neocortex in the setting of injury or cortical dysplasia. Activity can be propagated between microcircuits through efferent projections to circuit elements outside of the microcircuit.

Electrophysiological Patterns and Epilepsy Networks

Interictal, preictal, and seizure discharges produce different patterns on surface and stereo EEG and microelectrode recordings. Electroencephalographic recordings in patients with epilepsy typically show interictal spikes and sharp waves.[61] In focal epilepsies, the interictal spikes are usually closely related to the epileptogenic zone or "primary irritative zone" but may also occur in regions remote from the epileptogenic zone, referred to as "secondary irritative zone." High local synchrony may be a marker of epileptogenic cortex. Invasive studies using wide bandwidth recording and small-diameter electrodes show typical patterns of pathological HFOs (80–600 Hz), as well as electrographic seizure-like events referred to as microseizures and focal microperiodic epileptiform discharges, which may could be potential biomarkers of epileptogenicity.[62] Microseizures are interictal local field potential events whose spatial extent is restricted to approximately the width of a neocortical column and are not contiguous but rather surrounded by microdomains generating normal-appearing interictal physiology. Microseizures or microperiodic epileptiform discharges lead directly into clinical seizures as much as 20% of the time.[62] One study showed a trend to reduction of functional connectivity assessed by fMRI but increased functional connectivity assessed by surface EEG in the epileptogenic zone compared to noninvolved regions; this discrepancy was attributed to altered neurovascular coupling.[63] Simultaneous intracortical EEG and fMRI recordings showed that the zones initiating the interictal spikes and seizures have increased homogeneity in self-sustaining pathological oscillatory states.[64]

Several patterns of seizure onset may be observed during surface EEG recording. A common pattern is a low-voltage fast discharge that may be preceded by preictal spikes, train of spikes, or slow-wave complexes. Low-voltage fast discharge may range from beta/low gamma (15–30 Hz) in mesial temporal seizures to gamma range (30–100 Hz) in neocortical seizures. Seizures in humans are associated with abnormal synchronization of distant brain areas as indicated by functional connectivity measures. Whereas seizure onset is often marked by a decrease of synchrony among recorded brain structures, increased network synchrony occurs during seizure spread and termination. Ictal clinical symptoms could be related to the abnormal activation of physiologic neural networks by epileptic rhythm or by the disruption of normal brain control mechanisms.

The information gathered from multiscale and multimodal studies of epilepsy has stimulated the development of computational modeling ranging from single neuron to network, to whole-brain activity. At the neuronal (microscale) level, synchronization among firing patterns of pyramidal cells can explain the switch between epileptic spikes and HFOs; whereas at the microcircuit (mesoscale) level, transitions of dynamics toward seizures could be explained by a gradual decrease of dendritic inhibition. In all models, epilepsy is considered a dynamic brain disease. On the basis of key concepts from mathematical theory of dynamical systems, seizures are thought to be enabled by loss of balance between order and disorder in the epileptic brain. In this context, a seizure represents a self-initiated and self-terminated event that emerges as a result of a bistability property of the brain, which allows spontaneous switching from seemingly normal physiological dynamics to periods of pathological activity. This switching might be induced not only by altered properties of neurons or groups of neurons but also by changes in the gross connections of the neuronal network.

DEMENTIA

The disruption of brain networks is characteristic of neurodegenerative dementias. For example, one study in patients with frontotemporal dementia (FTD) showed attenuation of beta desynchronization during tests of behavioral motor inhibition such as the Go-No Go trials.[65] This study also showed loss of connectivity of the inferior frontal gyrus particularly in the gamma band, loss theta-to-alpha coupling with other cortical areas; and enhanced gamma band connectivity between the presupplementary and primary motor cortical areas.[65] These findings could be linked to increased impulsivity in this disorder.[65] Gamma oscillations are impaired in the entorhinal-hippocampal circuit in patients with Alzheimer disease.[66] In animal models, accumulation of amyloid β (Aβ) peptides alters the excitatory/inhibitory balance, causing hyperactivity in cortical and hippocampal neurons, a breakdown of slow-wave oscillation, and network hypersynchrony.[67] A magnetoencephalography study on patients amnestic Alzheimer disease, posterior cortical atrophy, and different forms of frontotemporal lobar degeneration showed consistent large-scale changes in brain networks, with reductions in local efficiency of functional connectivity compared to controls; the frequency range of altered connectivity was consistent across clinical syndromes and separated the disorders from each other and from controls.[68]

PSYCHIATRIC DISORDERS

Several psychiatric disorders have been associated with impairment of neural oscillations.[69] In particular, patients with schizophrenia have reduced neural oscillations during sensory and cognitive processing. In this disorder, auditory hallucinations are considered the consequence of aberrant hyperactivity of the left temporoparietal junction and hypoactivity of the left dorsolateral PFC. This abnormal activity is associated with loss of functional connectivity between these two regions and reduced resting-state alpha oscillations. There is also a reduction in gamma band oscillations during execution of executive tasks in this disorder. Administration of ketamine, which blocks NMDARs, reproduces the positive symptoms of schizophrenia, such as hallucinations. NMDAR blockade increases local gamma oscillations but impairs long-range gamma band synchrony, thus reducing coordination of large-scale networks by altering corticocortical interactions preferentially in superficial cortical layers 2/3. Prolonged NMDA-receptor hypofunction is associated with reduced GABAergic neurotransmission, as there is also loss of PV interneurons in the PFC. This is consistent with evidence of impaired GABAergic inhibition in schizophrenia.[70] Abnormal oscillatory activity can be affected by transcranial magnetic stimulation in this disorder.[71] Aberrant neural synchrony also occurs in autism spectrum disorders.[72–74] In these conditions, there is reduction of high-frequency oscillation entrainment during sensory processing, particularly in frontoparietal networks. As in the cases of schizophrenia, in autism there is reduced long-range coherence in the low alpha band, with a shift toward increased local connectivity. The alterations of gamma-band oscillations suggest that changes in the excitatory/inhibitory balance is a feature of both schizophrenia and autism spectrum disorders. Studies in mouse models show that mutations of the *MeCP2* gene, which are linked to Rett syndrome, autism, and childhood-onset schizophrenia, are associated with impaired GABAergic signaling in forebrain neurons and reduction in amplitude and phase locking of event-related oscillations at both low and high frequencies.[75]

KEY POINTS

- Structural and functional MRI information obtained under the Human Connectome Project (HCP) has allowed the parcellation of the cerebral cortex into 180 areas per hemisphere.
- There is a global organization of cortical areas along a gradient based on cytoarchitecture, myeloarchitecture, connectivity, and function.
- The hierarchical cortical processing involves feedforward connections from earlier areas to higher areas of processing and feedback modulatory projections form higher areas to earlier areas.
- The dorsal stream of sensory processing conveys sensory information to the posterior parietal cortex for spatial information.
- The ventral stream of sensory processing conveys information to the lateral temporal cortex for object recognition and semantic knowledge.
- Higher-order cortical areas, provide feedback modulatory inputs to areas involved in early sensory processing.
- In all cortical areas, the two major cell types are excitatory principal (mostly pyramidal) cells and different subtypes of GABAergic interneurons.
- The activity of pyramidal cell is shaped by inputs from the thalamus, corticocortical connections, local circuits mediated by GABAergic neurons, and modulatory cholinergic and monoaminergic projections.
- Cortical pyramidal cells include intratelencephalic (IT), pyramidal tract (PT), and corticothalamic (CT) cells.
- Layer 4 IT neurons are the primary recipient of feedforward inputs from the thalamus or other cortical areas.
- Most IT neurons are located in supragranular layers 2/3and infragranular layers 5/6 and participate in intracortical excitatory circuits both locally, and at a distance.
- The large pyramidal tract (PT) neurons located in layer 5 project to multiple subcortical regions.
- The CT neurons of layer 6 project back to the thalamic relay nucleus.
- The functional unit of the neocortex cortex is the cortical column.
- Cortical GABAergic interneurons include several populations that are distinguished by their neurochemical signature and firing pattern, and target different domains of the pyramidal cells.
- Parvalbumin-expressing, fast-spiking GABAergic basket cells mediate feedforward inhibition.
- Somatostatin-expressing GABAergic neurons participate in feedback and lateral inhibitory circuits.
- Vasoactive intestinal polypeptide GABAergic mediating disinhibitory circuits.
- Information processing in cortical networks critically depends on the precise synchronization of neuronal ensembles, both within local networks and across relatively long distances.
- During quiet wakefulness the cortex fluctuates between an activated and a deactivated state in relation to behavioral context.
- The brain actively constructs action and perception using past experience; predictive coding filters sensory inputs to reduce the mismatch between predicted (internal) and externally induced sensations.
- Complex behaviors, such as attention, language, and inner thought processes, emerge from distributed functional networks involving several cortical regions.
- Large-scale cortical networks include the dorsal attention and ventral attention networks; the salience network; the cingulo-opercular task-control network; the frontoparietal control network; and the default mode network.
- Disturbances within excitatory and/or inhibitory circuits in the neocortex lead to seizures and cognitive dysfunction.
- Seizures result from an imbalance between excitation and inhibition in a discrete cortical area, resulting in aberrant activity in a distributed network and subsequent recruitment of adjacent cortex.
- Alterations in cortical dynamics may contribute to cognitive and behavioral manifestations of dementia and psychiatric disorders.

REFERENCES

1. Glasser MF, Coalson TS, Robinson EC, et al. A multi-modal parcellation of human cerebral cortex. Nature 2016;536:171–178.
2. Eickhoff SB, Yeo BTT, Genon S. Imaging-based parcellations of the human brain. Nat Rev Neurosci 2018;19:672–686.
3. Singer W. Neuronal oscillations: unavoidable and useful? Eur J Neurosci 2018;48:2389–2398.
4. Mesulam MM. From sensation to cognition. Brain 1998;121 (Pt 6):1013–1052.
5. Zilles K, Amunts K. Centenary of Brodmann's map: conception and fate. Nat Rev Neurosci 2010;11:139–145.
6. Nieuwenhuys R, Broere CA. A map of the human neocortex showing the estimated overall myelin content of the individual architectonic areas based on the studies of Adolf Hopf. Brain Struct Funct 2017;222:465–480.
7. Barbas H. General cortical and special prefrontal connections: principles from structure to function. Annu Rev Neurosci 2015;38:269–289.
8. Alfano A, Studer M. Neocortical arealization: evolution, mechanisms, and open questions. Dev Neurobiol 2013;73:411–447.

9. Yeo BT, Krienen FM, Sepulcre J, et al. The organization of the human cerebral cortex estimated by intrinsic functional connectivity. J Neurophysiol 2011;106:1125–1165.
10. Power JD, Cohen AL, Nelson SM, et al. Functional network organization of the human brain. Neuron 2011;72:665–678.
11. Jones DT, Vemuri P, Murphy MC, et al. Non-stationarity in the "resting brain's" modular architecture. PLoS One 2012;7:e39731.
12. Destrieux C, Fischl B, Dale A, Halgren E. Automatic parcellation of human cortical gyri and sulci using standard anatomical nomenclature. Neuroimage 2010;53:1–15.
13. Huntenburg JM, Bazin PL, Margulies DS. Large-scale gradients in human cortical organization. Trends Cogn Sci 2018;22:21–31.
14. Burt JB, Demirtas M, Eckner WJ, et al. Hierarchy of transcriptomic specialization across human cortex captured by structural neuroimaging topography. Nat Neurosci 2018;21:1251–1259.
15. Taylor P, Hobbs JN, Burroni J, Siegelmann HT. The global landscape of cognition: hierarchical aggregation as an organizational principle of human cortical networks and functions. Sci Rep 2015;5:18112.
16. Hawrylycz MJ, Lein ES, Guillozet-Bongaarts AL, et al. An anatomically comprehensive atlas of the adult human brain transcriptome. Nature 2012;489:391–399.
17. Krienen FM, Yeo BT, Ge T, Buckner RL, Sherwood CC. Transcriptional profiles of supragranular-enriched genes associate with corticocortical network architecture in the human brain. Proc Natl Acad Sci U S A 2016;113:E469–E478.
18. Huth AG, de Heer WA, Griffiths TL, Theunissen FE, Gallant JL. Natural speech reveals the semantic maps that tile human cerebral cortex. Nature 2016;532:453–458.
19. Murray JD, Bernacchia A, Freedman DJ, et al. A hierarchy of intrinsic timescales across primate cortex. Nat Neurosci 2014;17:1661–1663.
20. Felleman DJ, Van Essen DC. Distributed hierarchical processing in the primate cerebral cortex. Cereb Cortex 1991;1:1–47.
21. Goulas A, Zilles K, Hilgetag CC. Cortical gradients and laminar projections in mammals. Trends Neurosci 2018;41:775–788.
22. Ferreira-Fernandes E, Pinto-Correia B, Quintino C, Remondes M. A gradient of hippocampal inputs to the medial mesocortex. Cell Rep 2019;29:3266–3279 e3263.
23. Kravitz DJ, Saleem KS, Baker CI, Mishkin M. A new neural framework for visuospatial processing. Nat Rev Neurosci 2011;12:217–230.
24. Kravitz DJ, Saleem KS, Baker CI, Ungerleider LG, Mishkin M. The ventral visual pathway: an expanded neural framework for the processing of object quality. Trends Cogn Sci 2013;17:26–49.
25. Borrell V. Recent advances in understanding neocortical development. F1000Res 2019;8.
26. Stuart GJ, Spruston N. Dendritic integration: 60 years of progress. Nat Neurosci 2015;18:1713–1721.
27. Harris KD, Shepherd GM. The neocortical circuit: themes and variations. Nat Neurosci 2015;18:170–181.
28. Mountcastle VB. The columnar organization of the neocortex. Brain 1997;120 (Pt 4):701–722.
29. Hubel DH, Wiesel TN. Laminar and columnar distribution of geniculo-cortical fibers in the macaque monkey. J Comp Neurol 1972;146:421–450.
30. DeFelipe J, Lopez-Cruz PL, Benavides-Piccione R, et al. New insights into the classification and nomenclature of cortical GABAergic interneurons. Nat Rev Neurosci 2013;14:202–216.
31. Tremblay R, Lee S, Rudy B. GABAergic interneurons in the neocortex: from cellular properties to circuits. Neuron 2016;91:260–292.
32. Mihaljevic B, Benavides-Piccione R, Guerra L, DeFelipe J, Larranaga P, Bielza C. Classifying GABAergic interneurons with semi-supervised projected model-based clustering. Artif Intell Med 2015;65:49–59.
33. Caputi A, Melzer S, Michael M, Monyer H. The long and short of GABAergic neurons. Curr Opin Neurobiol 2013;23:179–186.
34. Rock C, Zurita H, Lebby S, Wilson CJ, Apicella AJ. Cortical circuits of callosal GABAergic Neurons. Cereb Cortex 2018;28:1154–1167.
35. Tomioka R, Sakimura K, Yanagawa Y. Corticofugal GABAergic projection neurons in the mouse frontal cortex. Front Neuroanat 2015;9:133.
36. Worrell GA, Jerbi K, Kobayashi K, Lina JM, Zelmann R, Le Van Quyen M. Recording and analysis techniques for high-frequency oscillations. Prog Neurobiol 2012;98:265–278.
37. Herrmann CS, Struber D, Helfrich RF, Engel AK. EEG oscillations: from correlation to causality. Int J Psychophysiol 2016;103:12–21.
38. Buzsaki G. Neural syntax: cell assemblies, synapsembles, and readers. Neuron 2010;68:362–385.
39. Roux L, Buzsaki G. Tasks for inhibitory interneurons in intact brain circuits. Neuropharmacology 2015;88:10–23.
40. Michalareas G, Vezoli J, van Pelt S, Schoffelen JM, Kennedy H, Fries P. Alpha-beta and gamma rhythms subserve feedback and feedforward influences among human visual cortical areas. Neuron 2016;89:384–397.
41. Bosman CA, Schoffelen JM, Brunet N, et al. Attentional stimulus selection through selective synchronization between monkey visual areas. Neuron 2012;75:875–888.
42. Poulet JFA, Crochet S. The cortical states of wakefulness. Front Syst Neurosci 2018;12:64.
43. Adams RA, Shipp S, Friston KJ. Predictions not commands: active inference in the motor system. Brain Struct Funct 2013;218:611–643.
44. Bastos AM, Usrey WM, Adams RA, Mangun GR, Fries P, Friston KJ. Canonical microcircuits for predictive coding. Neuron 2012;76:695–711.
45. Chanes L, Barrett LF. Redefining the role of limbic areas in cortical processing. Trends Cogn Sci 2016;20:96–106.
46. Barron HC, Auksztulewicz R, Friston K. Prediction and memory: a predictive coding account. Prog Neurobiol 2020;192:101821.
47. Damoiseaux JS, Rombouts SA, Barkhof F, et al. Consistent resting-state networks across healthy subjects. Proc Natl Acad Sci U S A 2006;103:13848–13853.
48. Corbetta M, Shulman GL. Control of goal-directed and stimulus-driven attention in the brain. Nat Rev Neurosci 2002;3:201–215.
49. Vossel S, Geng JJ, Fink GR. Dorsal and ventral attention systems: distinct neural circuits but collaborative roles. Neuroscientist 2014;20:150–159.
50. Marek S, Dosenbach NUF. The frontoparietal network: function, electrophysiology, and importance of individual precision mapping. Dialogues Clin Neurosci 2018;20:133–140.

51. Seeley WW. The salience network: a neural system for perceiving and responding to homeostatic demands. J Neurosci 2019;39:9878–9882.
52. Dosenbach NU, Visscher KM, Palmer ED, et al. A core system for the implementation of task sets. Neuron 2006;50:799–812.
53. Greicius MD, Krasnow B, Reiss AL, Menon V. Functional connectivity in the resting brain: a network analysis of the default mode hypothesis. Proc Natl Acad Sci U S A 2003;100:253–258.
54. Andrews-Hanna JR, Smallwood J, Spreng RN. The default network and self-generated thought: component processes, dynamic control, and clinical relevance. Ann N Y Acad Sci 2014;1316:29–52.
55. Assem M, Glasser MF, Van Essen DC, Duncan J. A domain-general cognitive core defined in multimodally parcellated human cortex. Cereb Cortex 2020;30:4361–4380.
56. Tononi G, Boly M, Massimini M, Koch C. Integrated information theory: from consciousness to its physical substrate. Nat Rev Neurosci 2016;17:450–461.
57. Koch C, Massimini M, Boly M, Tononi G. Neural correlates of consciousness: progress and problems. Nat Rev Neurosci 2016;17:307–321.
58. Boly M, Massimini M, Tsuchiya N, Postle BR, Koch C, Tononi G. Are the neural correlates of consciousness in the front or in the back of the cerebral cortex? clinical and neuroimaging evidence. J Neurosci 2017;37:9603–9613.
59. Staley K. Molecular mechanisms of epilepsy. Nat Neurosci 2015;18:367–372.
60. Paz JT, Huguenard JR. Microcircuits and their interactions in epilepsy: is the focus out of focus? Nat Neurosci 2015;18:351–359.
61. Bartolomei F, Lagarde S, Wendling F, et al. Defining epileptogenic networks: contribution of SEEG and signal analysis. Epilepsia 2017;58:1131–1147.
62. Staba RJ, Stead M, Worrell GA. Electrophysiological biomarkers of epilepsy. Neurotherapeutics 2014;11:334–346.
63. Bettus G, Ranjeva JP, Wendling F, et al. Interictal functional connectivity of human epileptic networks assessed by intracerebral EEG and BOLD signal fluctuations. PLoS One 2011;6:e20071.
64. Ridley B, Wirsich J, Bettus G, et al. Simultaneous intracranial EEG-fMRI shows inter-modality correlation in time-resolved connectivity within normal areas but not within epileptic regions. Brain Topogr 2017;30:639–655.
65. Hughes LE, Rittman T, Robbins TW, Rowe JB. Reorganization of cortical oscillatory dynamics underlying disinhibition in frontotemporal dementia. Brain 2018;141:2486–2499.
66. Nakazono T, Jun H, Blurton-Jones M, Green KN, Igarashi KM. Gamma oscillations in the entorhinal-hippocampal circuit underlying memory and dementia. Neurosci Res 2018;129:40–46.
67. Busche MA, Konnerth A. Impairments of neural circuit function in Alzheimer's disease. Philos Trans R Soc Lond B Biol Sci 2016;371.
68. Sami S, Williams N, Hughes LE, et al. Neurophysiological signatures of Alzheimer's disease and frontotemporal lobar degeneration:pathology versus phenotype. Brain 2018;141:2500–2510.
69. Uhlhaas PJ, Singer W. Neuronal dynamics and neuropsychiatric disorders: toward a translational paradigm for dysfunctional large-scale networks. Neuron 2012;75:963–980.
70. Shaw AD, Knight L, Freeman TCA, et al. Oscillatory, computational, and behavioral evidence for impaired GABAergic inhibition in schizophrenia. Schizophr Bull 2020;46:345–353.
71. Vittala A, Murphy N, Maheshwari A, Krishnan V. Understanding cortical dysfunction in schizophrenia with TMS/EEG. Front Neurosci 2020;14:554.
72. An KM, Ikeda T, Yoshimura Y, et al. Altered gamma oscillations during motor control in children with autism spectrum disorder. J Neurosci 2018;38:7878–7886.
73. Seymour RA, Rippon G, Gooding-Williams G, Schoffelen JM, Kessler K. Dysregulated oscillatory connectivity in the visual system in autism spectrum disorder. Brain 2019;142:3294–3305.
74. Casanova MF, Sokhadze EM, Casanova EL, et al. Translational neuroscience in autism: from neuropathology to transcranial magnetic stimulation therapies. Psychiatr Clin North Am 2020;43:229–248.
75. Ho EC, Eubanks JH, Zhang L, Skinner FK. Network models predict that reduced excitatory fluctuations can give rise to hippocampal network hyper-excitability in MeCP2-null mice. PLoS One 2014;9:e91148.

25 Hippocampal and Amygdala Circuits

OVERVIEW

The term "limbic" used by Broca referred to structures that are at the border or edge of the hemispheres and led to the development of the concept of a limbic system.[1] Anatomical and functional evidence indicates that this system is not a unique entity but rather includes three components.[2] An "anterior" limbic system includes the amygdala, orbitofrontal cortex, insula, and anterior cingulate cortex. These structures are involved in processing emotion and reward value via their connections with areas of the ventral stream that provide information about stimulus features ("what" pathway). A "posterior limbic" circuit includes the hippocampus and the perirhinal, parahippocampal, and posterior cingulate cortices. These structures are involved in object–spatial associations via connections with the dorsal stream that provides information about space, action, and "where" events occur. The hippocampus is a key structure in episodic memory as it receives inputs both from the dorsal and the ventral processing stream. A third "limbic" system, which involves the midcingulate cortex, associates value-based information conveyed via the anterior cingulate cortex with action outcome information conveyed via the posterior cingulate cortex and sends inputs to premotor cortical areas to control further actions. The amygdala and hippocampus are thus core elements of different subsystems that interact to integrate emotion, value, and outcomes to control behavior[3–5] (Figure 25.1). Despite their different yet overlapping functions, the hippocampus and amygdala share several features, including their relatively simple cellular organization, their operations mediated by serial excitatory connections between principal neurons and strongly regulated by local GABAergic interneurons; robust mechanisms of coincidence detection leading to synaptic plasticity, and feedforward and feedback interneuron circuits promoting the formation of cell ensembles.[6–19] These medial temporal lobe structures also share vulnerability in a wide range of neurologic disorders, including limbic encephalitis, medial temporal lobe seizures, and neurodegenerative disorders associated with dementia. The aims of this chapter are to briefly review: (1) the organization of the intrinsic circuits of the hippocampus, (2) the role of the hippocampus in encoding of episodic memory and navigation, (3) the organization of the intrinsic circuits of the amygdala, (4) the role of the amygdala in formation and extinction of conditioned responses, and (5) examples of disruption of these circuits in neurologic disorders.

HIPPOCAMPAL CIRCUITS

The hippocampus includes several subdivisions: dentate gyrus; CA3, CA2, and CA1 fields; and subiculum (Figure 25.2). All the subfields of the hippocampal formation contain excitatory neurons that are connected via largely unidirectional pathways.[20]

Extrinsic Hippocampal Connections

The entorhinal cortex serves as the gateway for access of neocortical information to the hippocampus. Association areas send projections to the perirhinal and parahippocampal cortices, which in turn project to the entorhinal cortex.[10] These connections are topographically and functionally segregated (Figure 25.3).[21–23] The perirhinal cortex conveys inputs to the lateral entorhinal cortex, whereas the parahippocampal cortex provides input to the medial entorhinal cortex. Inputs from the perirhinal cortex provide information from the ventral stream of sensory involved in object recognition and discrimination ("what/content" pathway). This perirhinal-lateral entorhinal pathway primarily targets the anterior hippocampus. Neurons in this anterior circuit, referred to as anterior temporal circuit, participate in object feature and emotional processing for recognition memory. Inputs from the parahippocampal

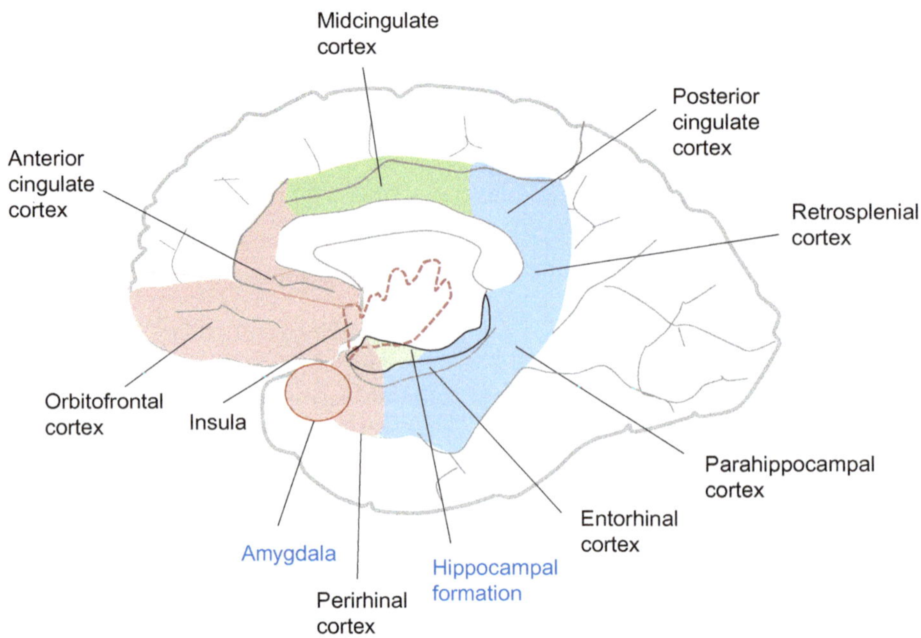

FIGURE 25.1 Anterior and posterior limbic circuit.
The hippocampus, together with the amygdala, is a core area of the so-called limbic system. Based on connectivity patterns and functions, this system contains a posterior limbic circuit centered in the hippocampus and involved in episodic and visuospatial memory and an anterior limbic circuit centered in the amygdala and involved in emotional and social processing.

cortex provide information from the dorsal stream of sensory processing in the posterior parietal cortex, involved in encoding of visuospatial coding ("where/context" pathway). This parahippocampal-medial entorhinal cortex targets the posterior hippocampus. Neurons in this posteromedial circuit encode highly specific locations and time signals and participate in spatiotemporal organization of the event memories and navigation. Inputs from the lateral and medial entorhinal cortex converge in the dentate gyrus, and reach different portions of CA3, CA1 and subiculum.

Information processed in the hippocampus is fed back via CA1 to the entorhinal cortex, which in turn projects back via the perirhinal and parahippocampal areas to the neocortex. These feedback projections are functionally segregated and respect the topographic organization of the inputs to the hippocampus. The subcortical outputs of the hippocampus originate from CA1 and subicular cortex and are conveyed via the fornix to the septal area, anterior nucleus of the thalamus, mammillary bodies, and nucleus reuniens.

Intrinsic Excitatory Hippocampal Circuit

The entorhinal cortex projects to the different components of the intrinsic hippocampal circuit via two separate excitatory pathways (Figure 25.4). Pyramidal neurons of layer 2 of the entorhinal cortex send excitatory inputs to the dentate gyrus via the perforant pathway. The dentate gyrus contains granule cells that convey these inputs via mossy fibers to pyramidal cells of CA3 and CA2. Granule cells also provide excitatory inputs to mossy neurons in the hilus of the dentate gyrus, which interconnect different territories of the dentate gyrus via projections along the longitudinal extent of the hippocampus. Pyramidal neurons within CA2 and CA3 are interconnected via recurrent autoexcitatory collaterals and provide excitatory inputs to CA1 via the Schaffer collaterals. This constitutes the classical trisynaptic entorhinal–dentate gyrus–CA3–CA1 pathway. Hippocampal area CA2 has several features that distinguish it from CA1 and CA3, including a unique gene expression profile, failure to display long-term potentiation, and relative resistance to cell death.[24] There is a second parallel pathway from the entorhinal cortex to the hippocampal circuit. This pathway originates from pyramidal and stellate cells of layer 3 in the entorhinal cortex, which project directly to CA1 and subiculum; this is known as temporo-ammonic pathway. Information processed in the hippocampus is fed back via CA1 and subiculum to layers 5 and 6 of the entorhinal cortex, which in turn projects back via the perirhinal and parahippocampal areas to the neocortex. The CA1 neurons integrate novel information originating from the entorhinal cortex with stored information provided by CA3 (or CA2) via the Schaffer collaterals and thereby detect mismatches between new and old information. The CA1 neurons also send direct top-down projections to neocortical areas, including the perirhinal cortex (a component of the ventral stream) and the retrosplenial cortex (a component of the dorsal stream).

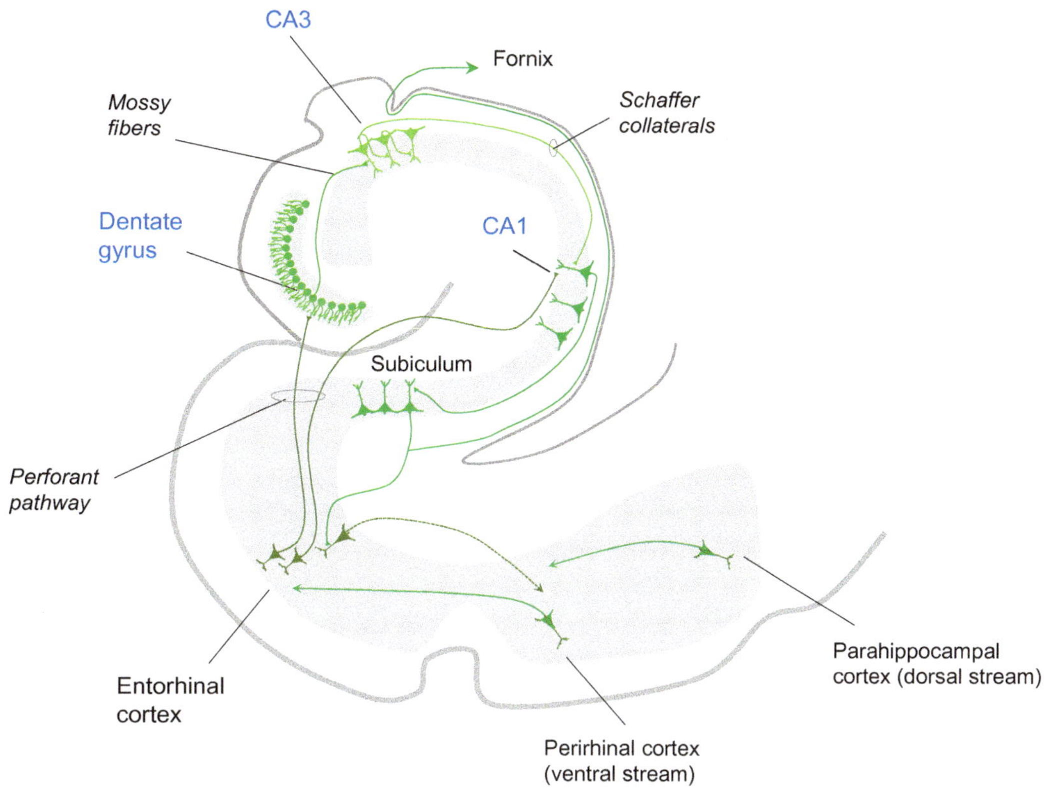

FIGURE 25.2 Components of the hippocampal circuits.
The hippocampus includes several subdivisions: dentate gyrus, CA3, CA2, and CA1 fields, and subiculum. All these subfields of the hippocampal formation consist of excitatory projection neurons that are connected by largely unidirectional pathways. The entorhinal cortex serves as a gateway for neocortical information to the hippocampus. Neocortical association areas send projections to the parahippocampal region, which includes the perirhinal and parahippocampal cortices; these areas project to the entorhinal cortex, which channels this information to the hippocampus.

Inhibitory Circuits in the Hippocampal Formation

The hippocampus contain several types of GABAergic cell types, many of which are neurochemically and functionally similar to those in the neocortex[25] (Figure 25.5). They include parvalbumin- and cholecystokinin-expressing basket cells targeting the perisomatic territories, somatostatin cells targeting the distal segments of the dendrites, and axo-axonic cells targeting the axon initial segments. These neurons provide for feedforward and feedback inhibition in hippocampal circuits. In the dentate gyrus, basket cells receive inputs from the entorhinal cortex and mediate powerful feedforward inhibition of granule cells. These basket cells are also activated by granule cells both directly and via disynaptic excitation via mossy neurons. In the CA1 and CA3 fields, fast-spiking parvalbumin-expressing and regular-spiking cholecystokinin-expressing basket cells target the perisomatic territories of pyramidal neurons and contribute to feedback circuits. Although both types of basket cells innervate overlapping territories of target pyramidal neurons, they have different properties. Fast-spiking basket cells respond rapidly and reliably to glutamatergic excitation and generate fast and precise inhibitory postsynaptic currents; regular-spiking cholecystokinin basket cells integrate excitatory afferent activity and generate endocannabinoid-sensitive inhibitory postsynaptic potentials. The somatostatin interneurons provide feedback inhibition via projections to the apical dendrites of pyramidal cells. In CA1 most of GABAergic interneurons are also innervated Schaffer collateral axons from CA3 pyramidal neurons and are involved in feedforward circuits.

In addition to local GABAergic interneurons, there are also bidirectional long-range GABAergic projections connecting the hippocampus with the medial entorhinal cortex or medial septum; many of these GABAergic projection cells express somatostatin and contribute to dendritic inhibition of pyramidal cells and also target other GABAergic neurons.

OSCILLATORY ACTIVITY IN HIPPOCAMPAL CIRCUITS

Hippocampal circuits exhibit synchronized theta and gamma oscillations during active states and typically

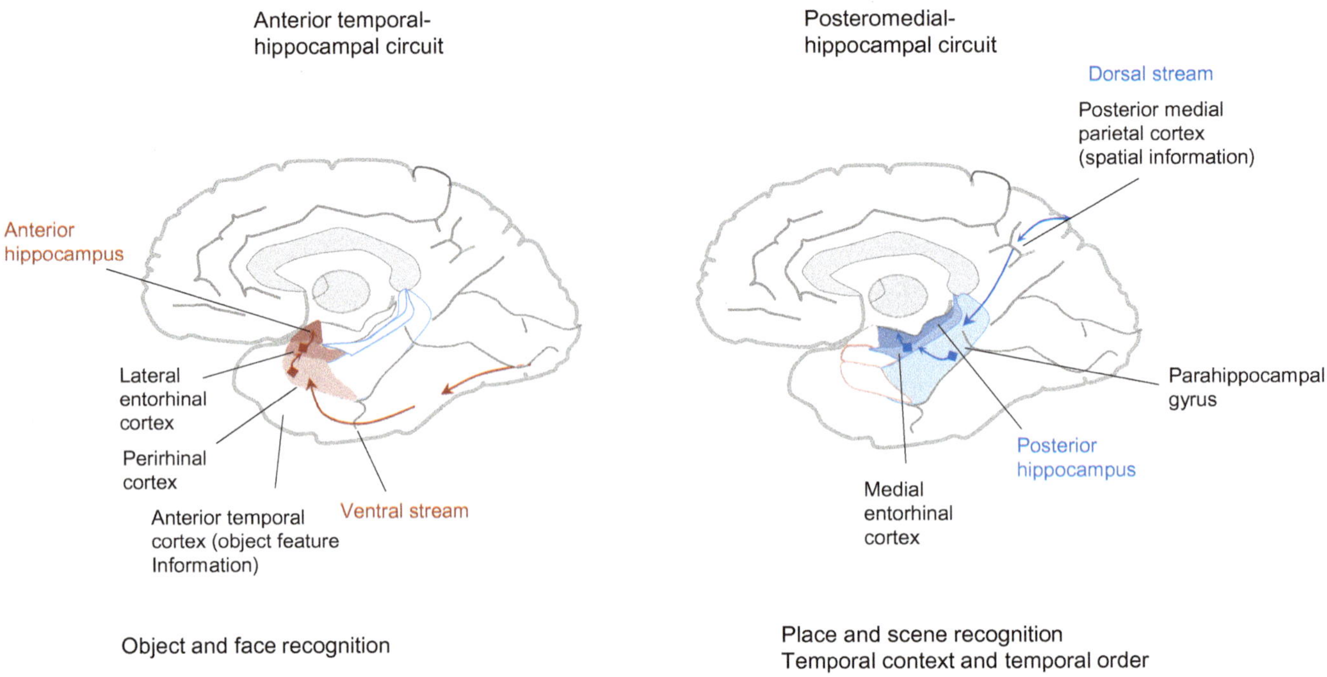

FIGURE 25.3 Extrinsic hippocampal connections.
Cortical association areas send projections to the perirhinal and parahippocampal cortices, which in turn project to the entorhinal cortex that provides the gateway to the hippocampal circuits. The lateral entorhinal cortex receives inputs from the perirhinal cortex, which conveys sensory information from the ventral pathway required from object recognition and discrimination. This perirhinal-lateral entorhinal pathway primarily targets the anterior hippocampus. The medial entorhinal cortex receives inputs from the parahippocampal cortex, which conveys spatial and temporal information, required for encoding of contextual information and navigation. This pathway primarily targets the posterior hippocampus.

generate sharp wave-ripple activity primarily during non-rapid eye movement (NREM) sleep.[26]

Theta Oscillations

Theta oscillations provide for timing of coordinated activity within and across brain regions during successful encoding and retrieval of memory. They are most regular and have the highest amplitude in CA1 but can also be generated in CA3 and in the subiculum and can "reverse propagate" through CA1 to entrain the CA3 network. In humans, hippocampal theta oscillations at 7–9 Hz occur during real-world navigation; slower 3–4 Hz theta oscillations are recorded during navigation in a virtual reality environment. The hippocampal theta rhythm depends on inputs from cholinergic and GABAergic projection neurons in the medial septum and diagonal band, which exhibit a pacemaker activity at theta frequency.[27] In the hippocampus, acetylcholine (ACh) produces excitation of both pyramidal cells and GABAergic interneurons, whereas GABAergic projections from the medial septum inhibit the GABAergic interneurons (Figure 25.6). The timing of pyramidal cell firing relative to the phase of the theta rhythm is required for successful memory encoding. The theta rhythm is in part triggered by inputs from the ascending reticular formation, including the oral pontine reticular nucleus, via a synapse on the supramammillary nucleus of the posterior hypothalamus. Theta activity is then transmitted throughout the hippocampal system.

Gamma Oscillations

Gamma activity represents local spiking in hippocampal networks and promotes binding of separate details of events. Gamma oscillations in CA1 include fast gamma (~90 Hz), driven by the medial entorhinal cortex and promoting formation of new memories, and slow gamma (~40 Hz), driven by CA3 and promoting retrieval in familiar contexts (Figure 25.7). Direct hippocampal recording in patients evaluated for epilepsy surgery show that gamma power synchronization and its coherence between the hippocampus and entorhinal cortex increase during successful memory encoding. Gamma activity in CA3 and CA1 occurs at different phases of the theta cycle in CA. Fast gamma oscillations driven by novel information via the entorhinal cortex occur at the peak of the theta wave; slow gamma oscillations driven by stored representations from CA3 occur during the theta wave trough. This gamma/theta coupling is important for representation and off-line maintenance of signals triggered by events and sequences of events, assessment of novelty, and induction of plasticity during encoding, consolidation, and retrieval of stored memories.

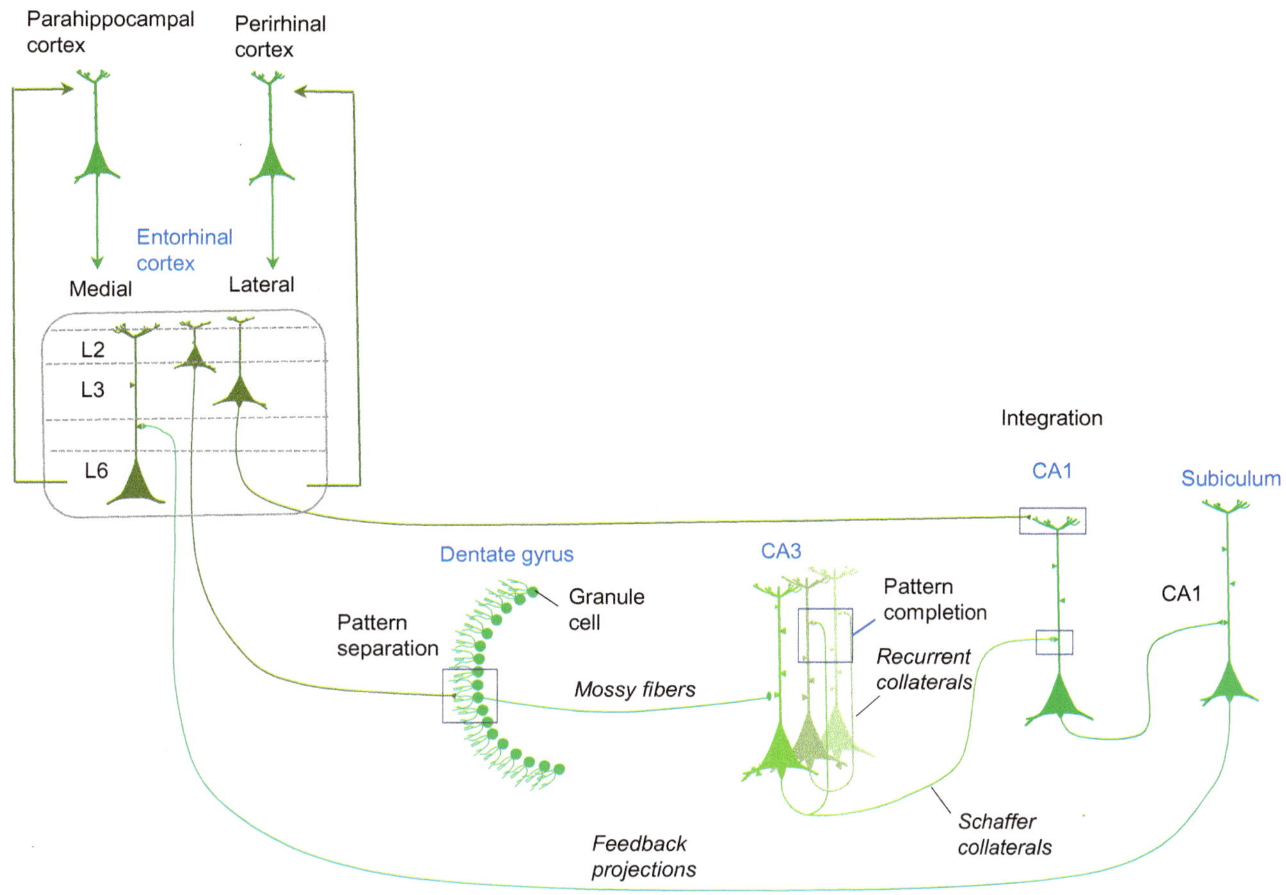

FIGURE 25.4 Intrinsic circuit of the hippocampus.
The entorhinal cortex projects to the different components of the intrinsic hippocampal circuit via two separate excitatory pathways that participate in different processing of information. Pyramidal neurons of layer 2 of the entorhinal cortex send excitatory inputs to the dentate gyrus via the perforant pathway. The dentate gyrus contains granule cells that convey these inputs via mossy fibers to pyramidal cells of CA3 and CA2. Granule cells also provide excitatory inputs to mossy neurons in the hilus of the dentate gyrus; which interconnect different territories of the dentate gyrus via projections along the longitudinal extent of the hippocampus. Pyramidal neurons within CA2 and CA3 are interconnected via recurrent autoexcitatory collaterals and provide excitatory inputs to CA1 via the Schaffer collaterals. A second parallel pathway from pyramidal and stellate cells of layer 3 of the entorhinal cortex that project directly to CA1 and the subiculum; this is known as temporo-ammonic pathway. Information processed in the hippocampus is fed back via CA1 and subiculum to layers 5 and 6 of the entorhinal cortex, which in turn projects back via the perirhinal and parahippocampal areas to the neocortex.

Sharp Wave-Ripple Oscillations

Hippocampal sharp wave-ripples are irregular, synchronous bursts consisting of slow sharp waves (0.1–3 Hz) and associated ripples (~200 Hz) that occur primarily in NREM sleep. Sharp wave-ripples are thought to be involved in memory consolidation by representing reactivation of memories encoded during wakefulness.[12] Sharp waves are initiated by a population burst of reciprocally interconnected CA3 pyramidal cells and trigger a subsequent burst in CA1 resulting in local ripples. GABAergic neurons, including basket parvalbumin cells and most long-range projecting GABAergic cells, are consistently activated during sharp wave-ripple, which contributes to entrain the excitability of the dendritic and somatic domains of CA1 pyramidal cells to ripple frequencies.

FUNCTIONAL SEGREGATION IN HIPPOCAMPAL CIRCUITS FOR EPISODIC MEMORY

The different stations within the intrinsic hippocampal circuits participate in different aspects of memory encoding, based on novelty and behavioral relevance.

Pattern Separation in the Dentate Gyrus

Pattern separation refers to the encoding of distinct nonoverlapping representations from similar overlapping inputs. This operation enables processing of similar experiences as distinct memories, even though the general context may be the same. By minimizing the overlap between the representations of two similar events at the time of

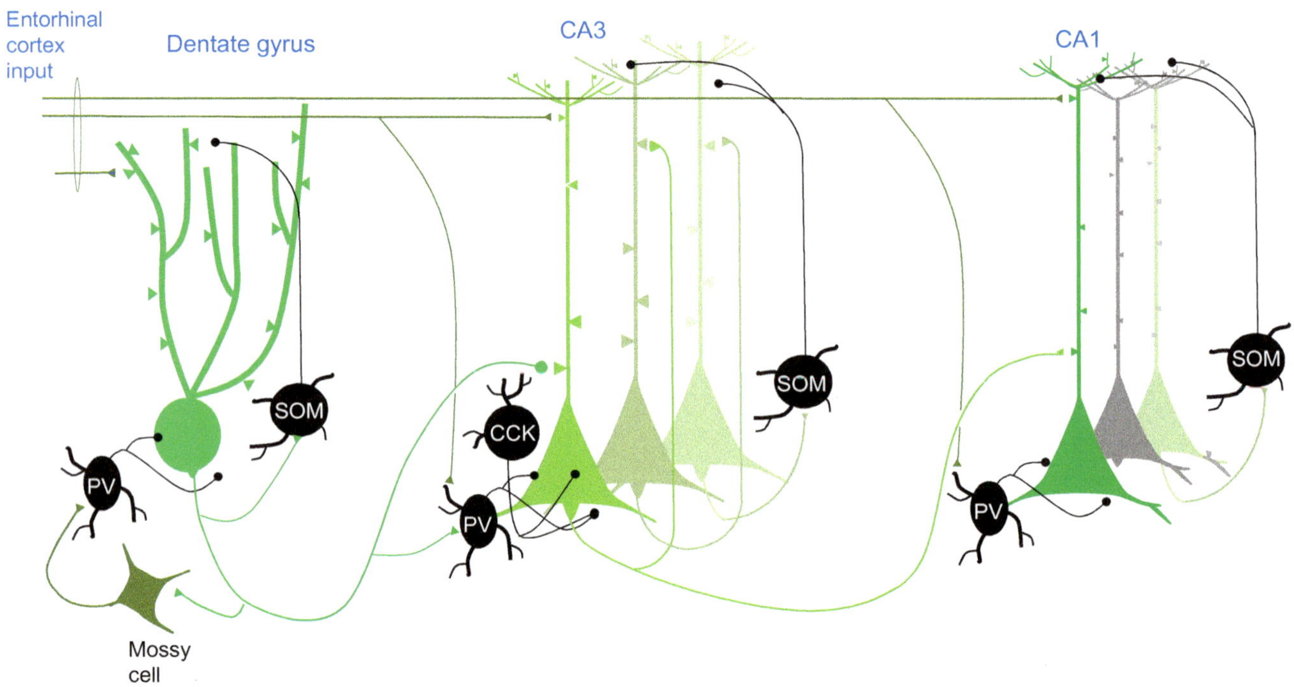

FIGURE 25.5 Intrinsic inhibitory circuits in the hippocampus.
The hippocampus contain several types of GABAergic cell types, many of which are neurochemically and functionally similar to those in the neocortex. They include parvalbumin (PV)- and cholecystokinin (CCK)-expressing basket cells targeting the perisomatic territories, somatostatin (SOM) cells targeting the distal segments of the dendrites, and axo-axonic cells targeting the axon initial segments. In the dentate gyrus basket cells receive inputs from the entorhinal cortex and mediate powerful feedforward inhibition of granule cells. These basket cells are also activated by granule cells both directly and via disynaptic excitation via mossy neurons. In the CA1 and CA3 fields, fast-spiking PV and regular-spiking CCK basket cells targeting the perisomatic territories of pyramidal neurons, contribute to feedback circuits.

encoding (learning) pattern separation decreases interference between different memories during the retrieval process. Studies in experimental animals, as well as functional magnetic regional imaging (fMRI) and effects of lesions in humans, show that the dentate gyrus is selectively involved in pattern separation.[28,29] The role of the dentate gyrus in this process reflects its pattern of connectivity. Dentate granule cells largely outnumber the cells of both entorhinal cortex and CA3, and therefore receive highly divergent excitatory input and provide divergent output to CA3. Mossy fiber terminals from dentate granule cells provide a very strong synaptic contact to the soma and proximal dendrites of the CA3 pyramidal neurons so that inputs from a single dentate granule cells are able to trigger an action potential in CA3 pyramidal cells. Another mechanism potentially contributing to pattern separation is adult neurogenesis in the subgranular zone of the dentate gyrus.[29] Neurons born in the subgranular zone integrate into the local networks and differentiate into excitatory granule cells in the dentate gyrus. Compared to mature cells, immature dentate granule cells are more excitable in response to glutamate, are less sensitive to GABAergic inhibition, and have increased potential for synaptic plasticity. These features make them more likely to be engaged in information processing and undergo use-dependent plasticity triggered by new information, while mature dentate granule cells preserve the information that is already represented. Recent evidence indicates that pattern separation also occurs in proximal fields of CA3.

Pattern Completion in CA3

Pattern completion is the ability to lump together similar or related experiences or events. It provides a specific mechanism for memory retrieval and allows the recall of a complete representation even in the presence of a partial input. Pattern completion involves primarily the distal CA3 field and depends on autoassociative connections that functionally couple coactive CA3 pyramidal cells at the time of encoding. By this mechanism, activation of a sufficient subset of CA3 neurons would propagate to all members of the cell ensemble, allowing the complete reinstantation of the learned episode. Since the hippocampus stores memories via these associative networks within CA3, it is necessary that this region receives highly separated inputs from the granule cells of the dentate gyrus to prevent interference among similar, but distinct memories.

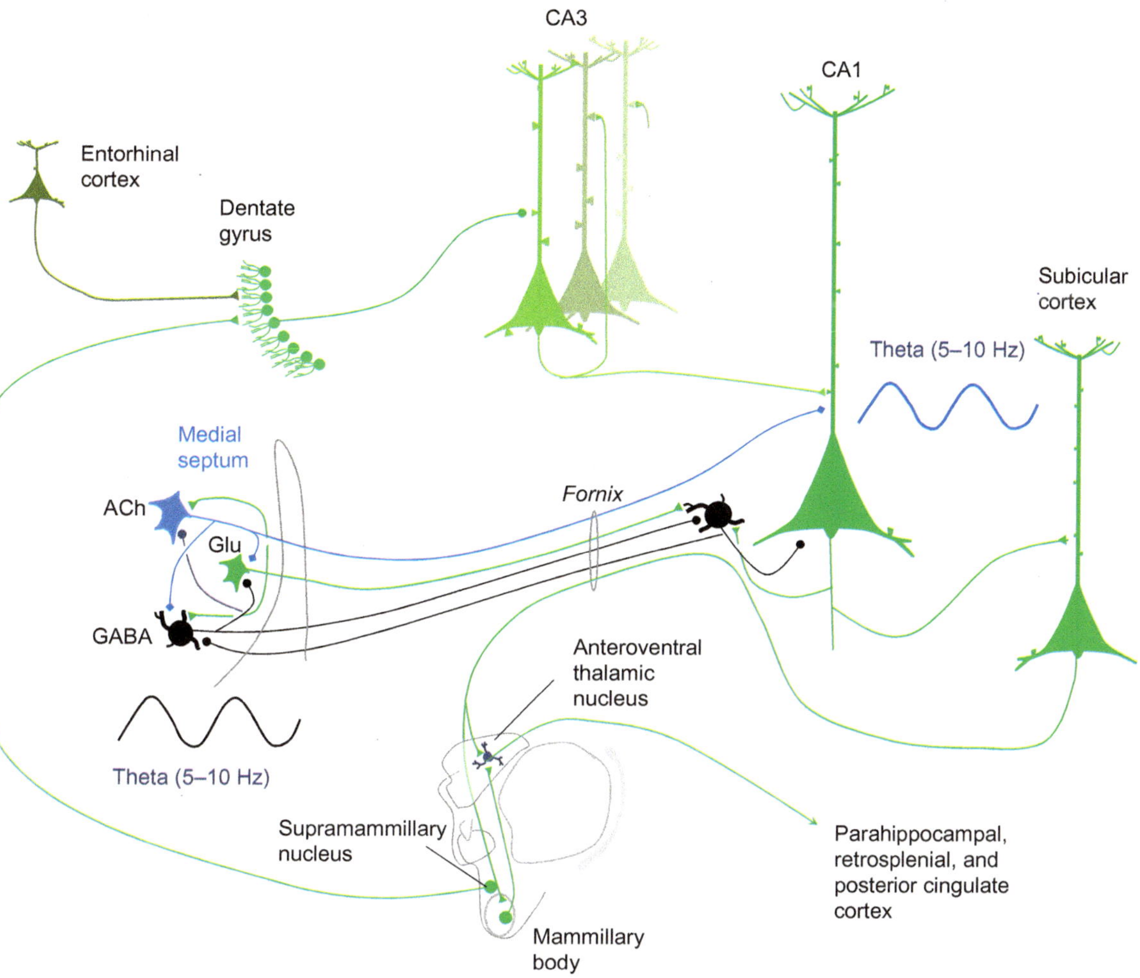

FIGURE 25.6 Generation of the theta rhythm in hippocampal circuits.
The hippocampal theta rhythm depends on inputs from cholinergic and GABAergic projection neurons in the medial septum and diagonal band, which exhibit a pacemaker activity at theta frequency. Acetylcholine produces excitation of both pyramidal cells and GABAergic interneurons, whereas projections from medial septum GABAergic neurons inhibit the GABAergic interneurons. The theta rhythm is in part triggered by inputs from the ascending reticular formation, including the oral pontine reticular nucleus, via a synapse on the supramammillary nucleus of the posterior hypothalamus and is transmitted through the hippocampal system, including the anterior nucleus of the thalamus and medial mammillary nucleus via projections from the subiculum via the fornix.

Signal Integration at CA1

CA1 pyramidal neurons receive direct inputs from both the entorhinal cortex and CA3 (or CA2). Inputs from the entorhinal cortex terminate in the distal dendrites and signal new information. In contrast, inputs from CA3 Schaffer collaterals terminate in the ascending dendrite and signal information stored in the autoassociative CA3 networks (Figure 25.7). Thus, CA1 neurons integrate novel information originating from the entorhinal cortex with stored information provided by CA3.[30] Via this mechanism CA1 integrates and detects mismatches between new and old information and may be able to switch between encoding and retrieval modes based on comparison of novel versus already stored information.[11,31] Invasive electrophysiological recordings and noninvasive functional brain imaging in humans have provided evidence for the rapid formation of hippocampal representations and the ability of the hippocampus to both pattern-separate and pattern-complete input from the neocortex. The hippocampus represents associations between multimodal stimuli, while simultaneously acting as a hub within an extended cortical network during memory retrieval.

MODULATORY INFLUENCES ON THE HIPPOCAMPUS

Cholinergic and Dopaminergic Modulation of Hippocampal Function

Acetylcholine (ACh) released from afferents originating in the medial septum and diagonal band can directly affect several elements of the hippocampus including

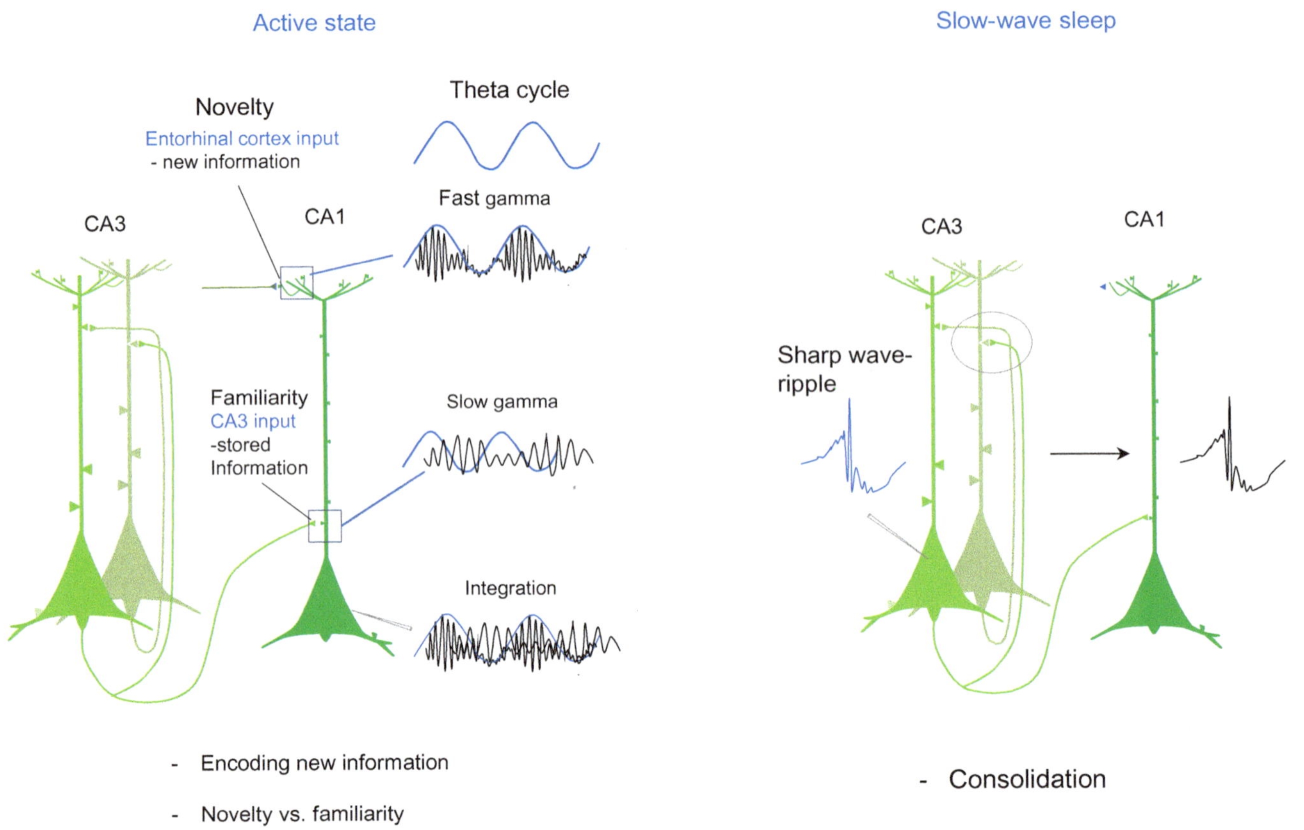

FIGURE 25.7 Gamma and sharp wave-ripple oscillations in the hippocampus.
Gamma activity represents local spiking in hippocampal networks and promotes binding of separate details of events by facilitating learning-related synaptic changes. Gamma oscillations in CA1 include fast gamma (~90 Hz) driven by the medial entorhinal cortex and slow gamma (~40 Hz) driven by CA3. Fast gamma rhythm promotes the transmission of current sensory information to the hippocampus during new memory. Slow gamma activity in CA1 is with inputs from CA3 and may promote memory retrieval by facilitating CA3 inputs to CA1 in familiar environments. Gamma activity in CA3 and CA1 occurs at different phases of the theta cycle. In CA1, fast gamma oscillations occur at the peak of the theta wave; slow gamma oscillations driven by stored representations arising from CA3 occur during the theta wave trough. Hippocampal sharp wave-ripples are irregular, synchronous bursts that occur as slow sharp waves (0.1–3 Hz) and associated ripples (~200 Hz) that occur primarily in non-rapid eye movement (NREM) sleep and are thought to be involved in memory consolidation. Sharp waves are initiated by a population burst of reciprocally interconnected CA3 pyramidal cells and trigger a subsequent burst in CA1 resulting in local ripples.

glutamatergic and GABAergic neurons, presynaptic terminals, postsynaptic receptors, and astrocytes.[32] Acetylcholine is released in response to novel signals and may modulate the shift of hippocampal operation between a storage and a retrieval state[33] (Figure 25.8). During active waking, the hippocampus exhibits prominent theta rhythm oscillations associated with high levels of ACh. Novel patterns presented to neurons in the dentate gyrus lead to brief periods of depressed firing in the hippocampal circuitry; as the hippocampus has an inhibitory influence on the medial septum, pauses in hippocampal activity lead to increased firing of medial septum cholinergic neurons. The resulting increase in ACh release in the hippocampus produces network dynamics that favor learning of new information over retrieval of old information.[32] Acetylcholine reduces recurrent activity in CA3 by activating dendrite projecting GABAergic neurons and also reduces glutamate release from Schaffer collaterals via presynaptic M2 receptors. ACh also elicits an M3 muscarinic receptor-mediated activation of inhibitory interneurons, leading to activation of $GABA_B$ receptors and decreased responsiveness of CA1 cells to Schaffer collateral inputs. Acetylcholine may thus impose rhythmic inhibition of CA1 pyramidal neurons at theta frequencies, reducing their output while facilitating synaptic integration within CA1 pyramidal cell dendrites by increasing their excitability via M1 receptors. In contrast, during NREM sleep, the reduced level of ACh in the hippocampus promotes recurrent autoexcitation in CA3, manifested as sharp wave-ripples, and therefore storage of information learned during wakefulness. At this sleep stage, intrahippocampal CA3–CA1 interactions via Schaffer collater also dominate the hippocampal CA1

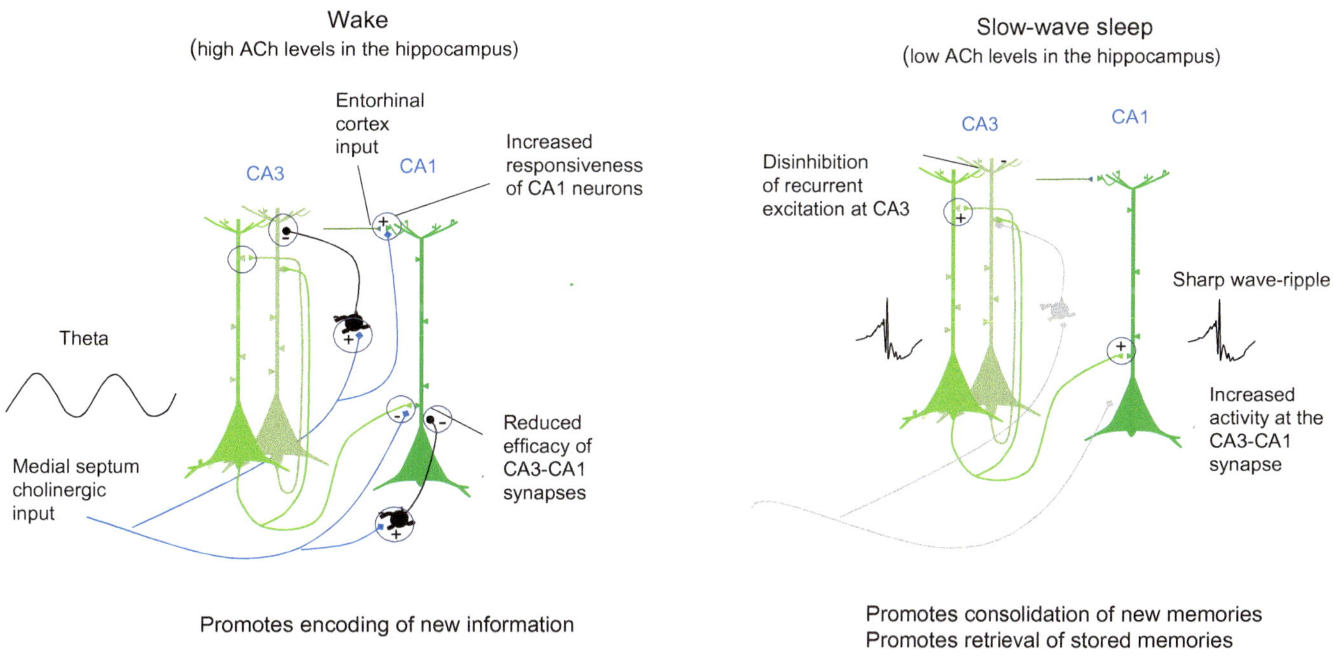

FIGURE 25.8 Effects of acetylcholine on hippocampal circuits.
Acetylcholine is released in response to novel signals and may modulate the shift of hippocampal operation between a storage and a retrieval state. During active waking, the hippocampus exhibits prominent theta-rhythm oscillations associated with high levels of ACh. During alert states, higher ACh concentrations would favor processing of novel inputs from the entorhinal cortex, thus permitting the transient formation of episodic memories in CA1. Acetylcholine reduces recurrent activity in CA3 by activating dendrite projecting GABAergic neurons and also reduces glutamate release from Schaffer collaterals. During NREM sleep, the reduced level of ACh promotes recurrent autoexcitation in CA3, manifested as sharp wave-ripples, and therefore storage of information learned during wakefulness. Lower ACh concentrations would permit intrahippocampal CA3–CA1 interactions via Schaffer collaterals to dominate hippocampal CA1 output and memory retrieval.

output, promoting memory retrieval. During REM sleep, increased ACh levels may promote long-term potentiation (LTP) at the CA3–CA1 synapses.

Dopaminergic inputs provide novelty (salience) and reward components to information being processed by the hippocampus, and thereby promote encoding of episodic memory. The anterior hippocampus may detect newly arrived information that is not already stored in its long-term memory, and provide a novelty signal to the ventral tegmental area via a pathway that includes the subiculum, nucleus accumbens, and ventral pallidum. This signal would contribute to novelty-dependent firing of ventral tegmental area neurons and dopamine release in the hippocampus. Dopaminergic inputs to the hippocampus and the PFC may have an important role in regulating their interaction during memory encoding and retrieval.

Plasticity of Hippocampal Circuits

Hippocampal representations undergo a continuous process of strengthening, weakening, and modification. Memories are formed in the hippocampus by creating ensembles of strongly coupled neurons that encode a specific event or episode.[18] This involves long-term synaptic plasticity, either long-term potentiation (LTP) or long-term depression (LTD) of glutamatergic synapses. In the hippocampus, LTP involves activation of synaptic N-methyl-D-aspartate receptors (NMDARs) allowing influx of calcium (Ca^{2+}), activation of Ca^{2+}/calmodulin kinase II and phosphorylation of the GluA1 subunit of α-amino-3 hydroxy-5-methyl-isoxazoleproprionic acid receptors (AMPARs), increasing their trafficking to the synapse. In contrast, LTD can be induced by extrasynaptic NMDARs or type 5 metabotropic glutamate receptors and results in internalization of AMPARs.[34] Several neuromodulators, including ACh, dopamine, norepinephrine, and serotonin, are released to focus attention on events in which the predicted outcome does not match the expected reality. Through a variety of presynaptic and postsynaptic receptor mechanisms on both principal cells and GABAergic interneurons, all these neuromodulators facilitate the induction and/or expression of long-term synaptic plasticity within the hippocampus, and therefore may function as a filter that ensures that only the most salient events are memorized. For example, activation of D1 receptors promotes LTP of both dentate gyrus and CA1 synapses, thereby increasing the probability of formation of reward-associated memories. This process may be needed to update memory representations to make better future predictions and reduce uncertainty.

Diencephalic Inputs to the Hippocampus

The intrinsic circuits of the hippocampus receive two major external inputs from the diencephalon, one from the supramammillary nucleus of the posterior hypothalamus and the second from the nucleus reuniens of the midline thalamus.[35] These two afferent systems project to separate, nonoverlapping, regions of the hippocampus. Inputs from the supramammillary nucleus distribute to the dentate gyrus and to CA3/CA2 and amplify signals from the entorhinal cortex to the dental gyrus. The supramammillary nucleus is a major part of an ascending brainstem system generating the theta rhythm in the hippocampus. Inputs from the nucleus reuniens target CA1 and subiculum and amplify signals from CA3 (and entorhinal cortex) to CA1. The nucleus reuniens also routes reciprocal information between the prefrontal cortex (PFC) and hippocampus.

HIPPOCAMPAL NAVIGATION SYSTEM AND FORMATION OF EVENT ENGRAMS

The hippocampus has a critical role in navigation by providing a representation of space.[36] Space may also represent a frame to organize all experiences within episodic memories, what is referred to as "cognitive map."[37] Temporally organized activity of hippocampal neurons helps organize these memories both in space and time by formation of "event engrams."[4]

Place Cells, Grid Cells, and Spatial Coding for Navigation

Seminal studies from O'Keefe and coworkers in rodents showed that the CA3 and CA1 regions contains a special type of cells, called place cells, that selectively fire when the animal is in a specific location of space.[37] This activity provides a mechanism by which space (allocentric frame of reference) generates an internal cognitive map for integration of all the features that constitute a given experience or episode.[38] The hippocampal system also uses a path integration reference frame for spatial coding and navigation.[8,9] The entorhinal cortex and subiculum contain different types of cells that encode self-motion and environment cues. These include grid cells, border cells, head direction cells, and speed cells. Grid cells in the medial entorhinal cortex fire in multiple locations of the environment to form a hexagonal grid-like pattern and provide direct input to place cells in CA1. Border cells fire exclusively along geometric borders of the environment and relate the firing of place and grid cells to the fixed features of the environment. Head-direction cells signal the orientation of the subject's head in the horizontal plane and integrate direction and velocity signals into a coherent two-dimensional space. In humans, functional MRI studies during imagined navigation tasks and presurgical intracranial recordings on patients with epilepsy show map-like spatial codes in the hippocampus and grid-like codes in the entorhinal cortex.[11,39]

Formation of Event Engrams for Episodic Memory

The hippocampus is a convergence zone that rapidly forms associations between stimuli represented in distinct neocortical regions. Neocortical representations of the elements of an episodic event, such as locations and people, form links within individual neurons in the hippocampus. These include not only place cells that encode the spatial location of the individual at the time of the event but also "concept"' cells that encode object information during the event. Concept cells can respond to the identity of a person in a stimulus-invariant manner; for example, one neuron can respond to both the written name and a photo of the same person. Hippocampal place cells and concept cells may act as the building blocks of episodic memory as they can rapidly form direct associations when firing together during a given experience, thereby forming event engrams. Individual neurons that initially fire selectively in response to viewing a person or a landmark, may also respond after exposure to a composite image (i.e., an image of both the person and landmark) such that they subsequently fire to either image in isolation. At retrieval, when the location is cued, all associated elements are retrieved via the process of pattern completion, supported by the recurrent connections of subfield CA3. Subsequently, the retrieved elements are reinstated in the neocortex, allowing for the experience of recollection under the executive control from the PFC.[40] Hippocampal networks also map temporally organized experiences. Space and time are integrated in the representation of memories through overlapping and interacting systems that converge on the hippocampal region.[4] Whereas spatial and temporal aspects of memory are processed somewhat differently in hippocampal subregions, they become fully integrated within CA1 networks as independent representations of space and time.

Hippocampal–Prefrontal Interactions

The hippocampus participates in important reciprocal network interactions with PFC.[41–43] Whereas the hippocampus establishes the relationships between events and their context for encoding, storage, and retrieval of new episodic memories, the PFC has an integral role in long-term memory and executive control of retrieval. The PFC contributes to episodic memory by top-down control of memory processing. These two cortical areas are strongly interconnected via direct and indirect pathways. There is a direct projection from CA1 and proximal subiculum to the medial PFC; a direct bidirectional connection between the medial PFC and the perirhinal and lateral entorhinal cortex; and bidirectional connections between the medial PFC and hippocampus via nucleus reuniens. These connections promote transfer of theta oscillations between the hippocampus and the PFC during memory encoding and retrieval. Hippocampal theta precedes medial PFC theta during contextual learning, whereas medial PFC theta precedes hippocampal theta during retrieval.[44,45] The nucleus reuniens may function to coordinate these interactions by resynchronizing and reversing the direction of information flow between these two cortical areas.[46] A second pathway for theta synchronization between the hippocampus and the medial PFC is via the anteromedial subdivision of the anterior nucleus of the thalamus, which receives inputs from CA1 and subiculum and projects to the medial PFC. The hippocampal–prefrontal interactions also occur via other network oscillatory patterns, including sharp wave-ripples and gamma oscillations. Slow gamma oscillations in the medial PFC are strongly linked to attentional processing, rule representation, and flexible rule switching and are coupled to hippocampal theta oscillations. The parahippocampal, perirhinal, and entorhinal cortices project via the mediodorsal nucleus of the thalamus to the PFC. In this system, beta band synchronization between the medial temporal lobe and the PFC may promote recognition memory and cue-based recollection. The medial PFC may also have a role in directing neocortical learning independent of the hippocampus during the shift from medial temporal lobe to neocortical representations during consolidation. The main functions of the medial PFC would be to detect the congruency of new information with existing information in the neocortex.[47]

CIRCUITS OF THE AMYGDALA

The amygdala provides automatic tagging of positive or negative valence of environmental stimuli and their intensity and therefore encodes their relevance. A major role of the amygdala is associative learning, or Pavlovian conditioning. The amygdala is characterized by its very strong internuclear and intranuclear connectivity and by its extensive cortical and subcortical connections. Formation of new emotional memories as well as extinction of previous emotional memories involve complex excitatory and inhibitory circuits within the amygdala.

Nuclear Organization

The amygdala is a nuclear complex subdivided into three main regions: a basolateral nuclear group including the lateral nucleus (LA) and the basal complex (BA) encompassing the basolateral and basomedial nucleus; a superficial cortical laminated region; and a centromedial group including the central and the medial nucleus (Figure 25.9). The central nucleus includes a centromedial (CeM) and centrolateral (CL) divisions. The basolateral complex and the laminated region have a structure similar to the cerebral cortex; about 80% of neurons are pyramidal neurons and about 20% GABAergic interneurons. The centromedial group consists primarily of GABAergic neurons; the CeL nucleus has been considered a homolog to the striatum and the CeM a homolog to the ventral pallidum. In addition, there are also two clusters of GABAergic neurons, a lateral intercalate cluster at the external capsule, which borders the amygdala laterally, and the medial intercalate cluster at the intermediate capsule, located in between the basolateral and the centromedial groups. The cortical laminated region and the medial nucleus of the amygdala are largely involved in olfactory processing and will not be further discussed in this chapter.

Extrinsic Connections

The amygdala has strong connections with cortical and subcortical areas involved in innate survival responses, reward processing, behavioral arousal, attention, adjudication of value for decision-making, motivation, social cognition, and episodic memory (Figure 25.10).

The LA is the primary recipient of sensory inputs that originate from the neocortex and the thalamus.[3,48] Cortical sensory inputs originate primarily from high-order visual and auditory temporal areas and from the insula conveying somatosensory information. The LA provides input to the other nuclei of the amygdala. There are also connections of the LA with the entorhinal cortex, hippocampal formation, temporal association cortex, and insula. The basolateral nuclear complex is strongly innervated by basal forebrain cholinergic and midbrain dopaminergic inputs and has strong direct and indirect connections with the orbitofrontal, medial prefrontal, and anterior cingulate cortices as well as the entorhinal and perirhinal cortex. Via these projections, the basolateral nucleus has an important role in attention and consolidation of emotional memory. The basomedial nucleus has high expression of estrogen receptors and provides the major output of the amygdala to the hippocampal, entorhinal, and perirhinal cortex, as well as to the orbitofrontal and medial prefrontal cortices. The superficial cortical laminated region is surrounded by the piriform (olfactory) and entorhinal cortex and receives inputs from the olfactory bulb and thus constitutes the "olfactory amygdala." The CeM provides the main output of the amygdala to the hypothalamus and brainstem to generate innate survival responses, and arousal.[49] The medial nucleus is involved in food intake, sexual behavior, and aggressive and defensive behaviors.

Intrinsic Circuits

The LA sends excitatory inputs to all nuclei of the amygdala, primarily the basolateral and the basomedial nuclei, and all three nuclei provide excitatory input to the CeM (Figure 25.11). The convergence of cortical and subcortical input onto single pyramidal cells on the LA provides the basis for associative learning or Pavlovian conditioning. The unidirectional intrinsic excitatory flow of information from the LA to the basolateral and basomedial nuclei and then to the CeM is strongly controlled by a different groups of GABAergic neurons.[6,7] Local inhibitory neurons control the probability of associative learning at the level of the LA

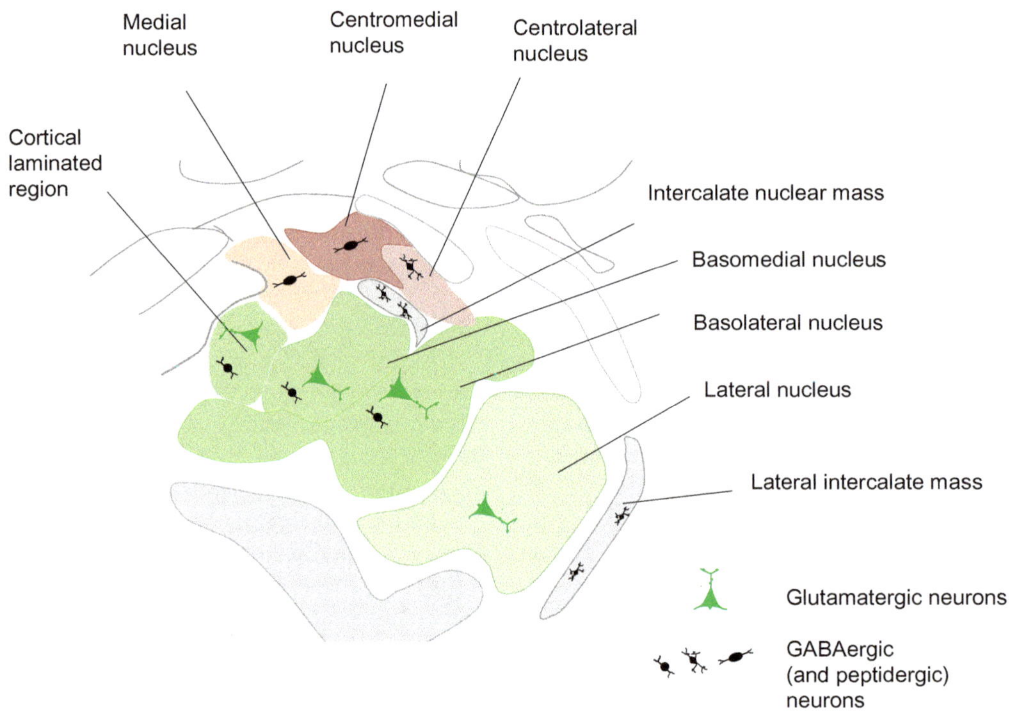

FIGURE 25.9 Nuclear organization of the amygdala.
The amygdala is a nuclear complex subdivided into a basolateral nuclear group, a centromedial group, intercalate masses, and a superficial cortical laminated region. The basolateral complex and the laminated region have a structure similar to the cerebral cortex; about 80% of neurons are pyramidal neurons and about 20% GABAergic interneurons. The centromedial group has a structure resembling the striatum, and consisting primarily of GABAergic neurons. Similarly, GABAergic neurons form two major clusters, a lateral intercalate cluster at the external capsule, which borders the amygdala laterally, and the medial intercalate cluster at the intermediate capsule, located in between the basolateral and the centromedial groups.

and transfer of information by the basolateral and basomedial nuclei. Fast-spiking parvalbumin GABAergic interneurons targeting the soma and proximal dendrites receive strong inputs from the principal cells and are thus involved in feedback inhibition, whereas somatostatin neurons targeting the distal dendrites receive strong cortical input, and are mainly involved in feedforward inhibition of pyramidal cells in the LA. Transfer of information from the LA via the basolateral and basomedial nuclei to the CeM is flexibly gated via local inhibitory and disinhibitory circuits. In addition to direct excitatory projections to the CeM, pyramidal neurons of the basolateral and basomedial nuclei also project to GABAergic neurons of the CeL. Studies in mice show that the CeL contains at least two subpopulations of inhibitory neurons. One population expresses oxytocin receptors and protein kinase Cδ and tonically inhibits CeM cells. A second population expresses somatostatin and inhibits the oxytocin receptor-expressing CeL neurons, thereby disinhibiting the CeM neurons. In addition, axons of pyramidal neurons of LA and basolateral and basomedial nuclei synapse with GABAergic neurons of the medial intercalated cell mass that targets either the CeL or the CeM. Via these projections, the basolateral amygdala influences the CeM in two ways, via direct glutamatergic excitation and indirectly, via feedforward inhibition through the intercalated cell mass (Figure 25.11). The medial intercalated GABAergic cell clusters also receive excitatory inputs from the medial PFC, including the anterior cingulate gyrus, and mediate the inhibitory effect the PFC on transfer of emotional information to the CeM. Intercalated GABAergic neurons located in the external capsule also receive cortical input and, via their projections to the BA allow for a flexible regulation of cortical influences over the basolateral amygdala.[6,7]

CIRCUITS FOR ACQUISITION, EXPRESSION, AND EXTINCTION OF CONDITIONED RESPONSES

The amygdala has a key role in acquisition of associative learning and automatically attributes emotional value, either negative or positive, to sensory stimuli. The classical paradigm of associative learning is Pavlovian fear conditioning.[48] After a single exposure to a neutral or conditioned stimulus (CS) with a noxious or unconditioned stimulus (US) that generates an emotional reaction (such as

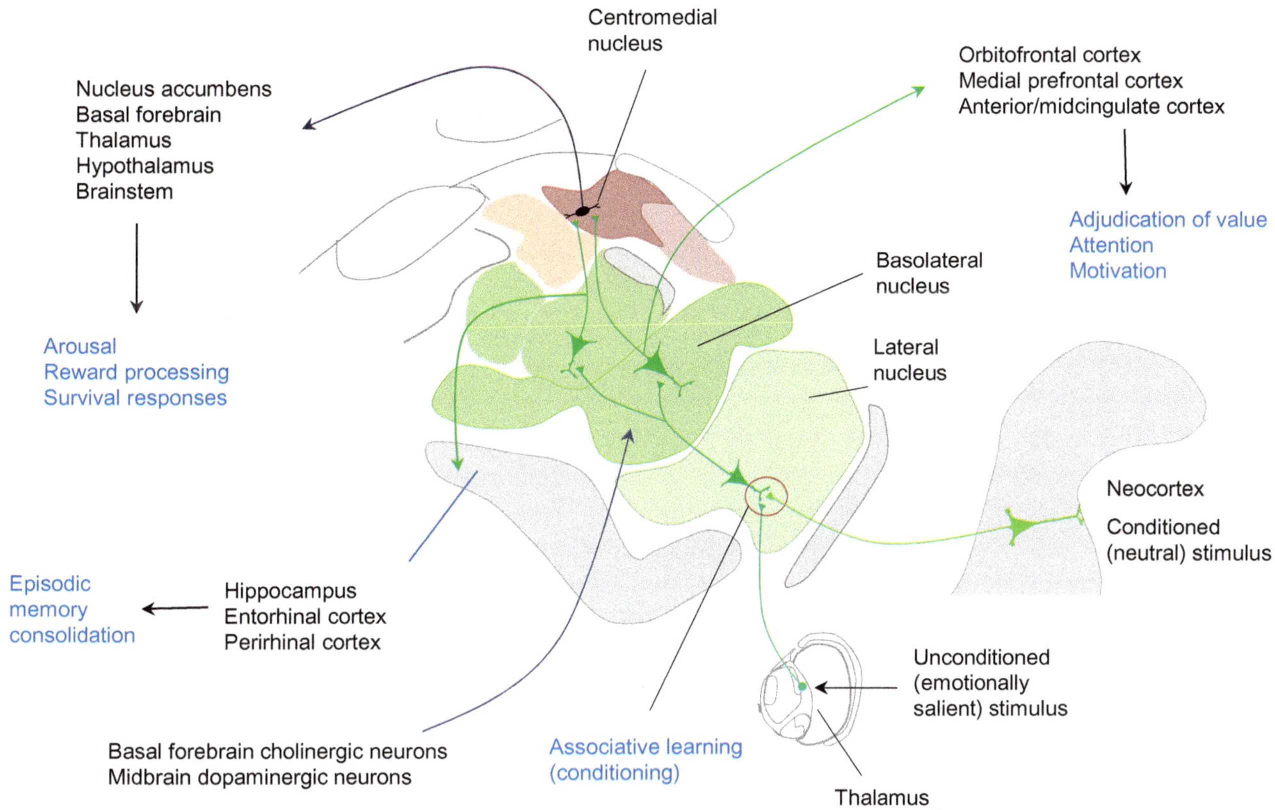

FIGURE 25.10 Intrinsic excitatory and extrinsic connections of the amygdala.
The lateral nucleus of the amygdala (LA) is the primary recipient of sensory inputs that originate from the neocortex and the thalamus. The convergence of cortical and subcortical input onto single pyramidal cells of the lateral amygdala provides the basis for associative learning or Pavlovian conditioning. The LA then conveys this information to the basolateral and basomedial nuclei, which then project to the centromedial nucleus (CeM). Both the basolateral and the basomedial nuclei provide projection to the orbitofrontal, medial prefrontal, and anterior cingulate cortices, as well as the hippocampal, entorhinal, and perirhinal cortices. The CeM provides the output of the amygdala to the basal forebrain, thalamus, hypothalamus, and brainstem.

sympathetic activation) a link is formed between the CS and the US, so that thereafter, exposure to the CS alone is able to induce the complete emotional response. Fear conditioning is a rapidly acquired and long-lasting form of memory.

Acquisition of Fear Conditioning as Prototype of Associative Learning

The LA is the critical site of synaptic plasticity for the acquisition of Pavlovian fear. Inputs from cortical neurons processing CS (such as innocuous auditory or visual stimulus) and thalamic neurons receiving US (such as pain) can converge onto single LA neurons. The convergence of these two glutamatergic inputs onto single LA neurons results NMDAR-mediated LTP of the synapses conveying CS via a mechanism similar to that occurring in the hippocampus. Whereas CS inputs are relatively weak prior to conditioning, the potentiation of CS synapses as a result of pairing with the US would allow CS alone to activate LA neurons and elicit the emotional response. Consolidation of fear memory requires activation of intracellular phosphorylation cascades, new gene transcription and local translation of synaptic proteins. Inhibitory circuits mediated by GABAergic neurons in the LA have a key role in regulating associative conditioning. These GABAergic neurons are important targets of neuromodulators. For example, dopamine and norepinephrine suppress feedforward inhibition onto principal LA neurons through inhibition of somatostatin interneurons, thereby promoting acquisition of emotional response; in contrast, serotonin excites inhibitory interneurons and constrains plasticity in the LA.

Circuits for Fear Extinction

Fear extinction is the process of learning that stimuli previously associated with adverse outcome no longer represent a threat. Fear extinction occurs upon repeat presentation of the CS alone, leading to a gradual reduction of the conditioned fear response. Extinction does not erase the previous CS-US associations or underlying fear memory but rather depends on the formation of a new inhibitory memory that competes with the previous fear memory.

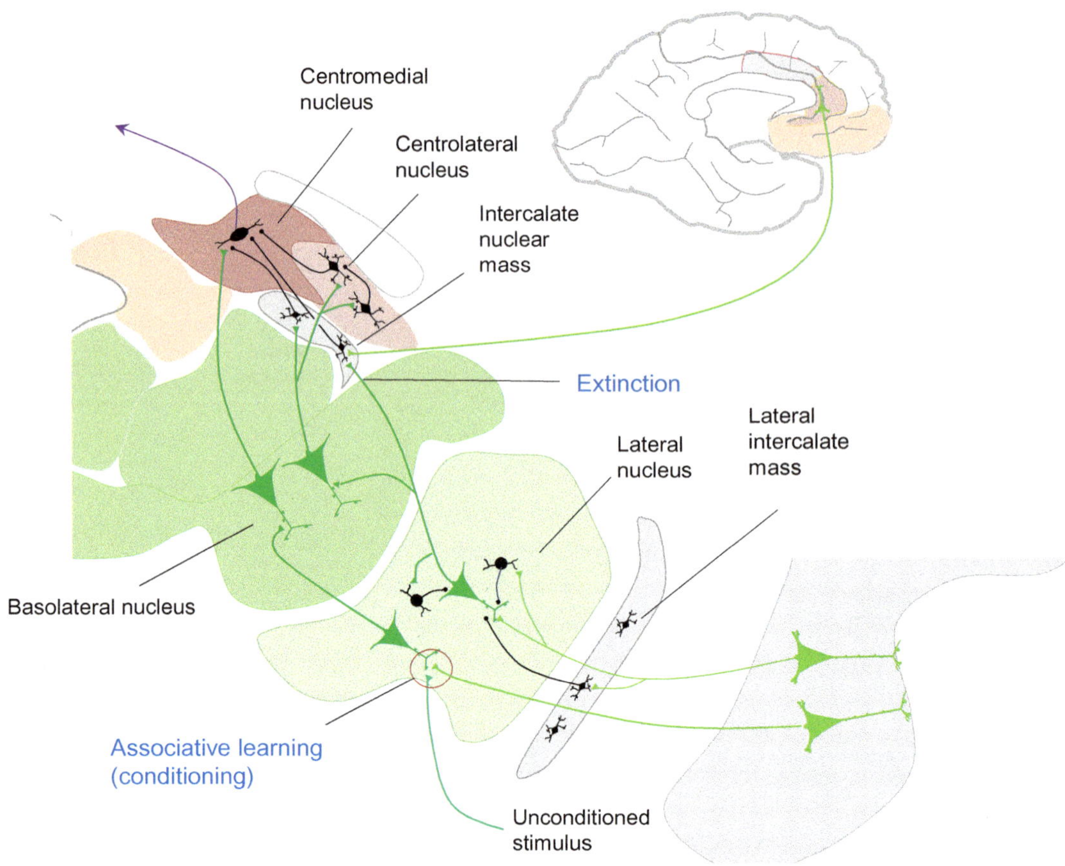

FIGURE 25.11 Intrinsic circuit of the amygdala regulating conditioned learning and gear extinction.
The unidirectional intrinsic excitatory flow of information from the lateral amygdala (LA) to the basolateral and basomedial nuclei and then to the centromedial nucleus (CeM) is strongly controlled by different groups of GABAergic neurons. Parvalbumin (PV) interneurons in the LA receive strong inputs from the principal cells and are thus involved in feedback inhibition, whereas somatostatin (SOM) neurons receive strong cortical input affecting conditioning. Transfer of excitatory information from the LA via the basal nuclei to the CeM is flexibly gated via local inhibitory and disinhibitory circuits mediated by GABAergic neurons in the intercalated cell mass, and centrolateral nucleus (CeL) The medial intercalated GABAergic cell clusters also receive excitatory inputs from the medial prefrontal cortex including the orbitofrontal cortex anterior cingulate gyrus, and mediate the inhibitory effect the PFC on transfer of excitatory information to the CeM.

Fear extinction is mediated by a distributed network that includes the amygdala, medial PFC, and hippocampus.[14,15] At the level of the amygdala, extinction largely involves local inhibitory circuits that cause a shift in the networks responsible for transferring CS information from the LA and involves different subtypes of BA cells. These cells may respond either during fear conditioning or extinction and the rapid switching of activity between these two types of BA neurons suggests the coexistence of different circuits involving differential recruitment of particular subpopulations of GABAergic interneurons (Figure 25.11). Extinction training is also associated with increased levels of endocannabinoids, which acting via presynaptic CB1 receptors reduce release of GABA from a population of inhibitory interneurons that target the extinction cells. Another inhibitory circuit involves medial intercalated GABAergic neurons that prevent the activation of CeM cells by BA neurons. These intercalated GABAergic neurons receive excitatory inputs from an area of the medial PFC corresponding to the subgenual anterior cingulate in humans.

Engrams and Network Oscillations in the Amygdala

Synaptic plasticity in the basolateral amygdala allows subsets of neurons to be recruited during learning and reactivated during memory retrieval, thereby forming cell engrams.[6] Acquisition of an emotional memory forms an engram of activated neurons in the basolateral amygdala by inducing LTP at pathways relaying associative cues to pyramidal cells in the LA. Both the induction of LTP and the selection of the engram are critically dependent on the excitability of these neurons, which is controlled by several factors including intrinsic cell membrane properties, strength of local excitatory connections, activity of GABAergic interneurons, and release of neuromodulators. Retrieval of emotional memories occurs, at least in part, via reactivation of the engram formed during acquisition and stabilized during consolidation. These processes depend on protein synthesis for LTP and oscillatory mechanisms occurring during sleep. Synchronous oscillations in the theta and gamma bands between the basolateral amygdala, CA1 field of the hippocampus, and PFC occur during consolidation and retrieval of emotional memories. The extinction of fear memories involves changes in plasticity at multiple pathways and remodeling of interneuron-pyramidal neuron connections. At the network level, extinction reduces CA1-basolateral amygdala theta synchrony, but increases the theta oscillation drive from the mPFC to the basolateral amygdala.

Modulation of Emotional Memory Acquisition and Consolidation by Stress

Stress strongly affects emotional learning by activating locus coeruleus neurons, resulting in release of norepinephrine from their projections to the amygdala.[17] Stress also activates neurons of the paraventricular nucleus of the hypothalamus that secrete and release corticotrophin-releasing factor, leading to activation of the adrenocortical axis and release of glucocorticoids. Acute stress promotes fear memory consolidation via activation of local glucocorticoid receptors and norepinephrine release in the basolateral amygdala. This results in activation of β-adrenoceptors and increased trafficking and synaptic stabilization of glutamate receptors in principal cells of the basolateral amygdala. Norepinephrine and dopamine also inhibit GABAergic neurons that produce feedforward inhibition of pyramidal cells. Serotonergic axons from a group of neurons in the dorsal raphe nuclei innervate both the principal neurons and interneurons predominantly the BA, and to a lesser extent the LA and CeM. Presentation of both CS and US, inescapable stress, and fear memory retrieval are associated with increased serotonin release in the basolateral amygdala. Serotonin may modulate acquisition of conditioned fear through complex effects on principal neurons and interneurons via different receptor subtypes.[16]

CLINICAL CORRELATIONS

Classical disorders affecting the hippocampus, amygdala, or both include mesial temporal sclerosis, limbic encephalitis, and neurodegenerative disorders. Involvement of hippocampal or amygdala circuits underlie impaired episodic memory, behavioral and emotional dysregulation, and seizures in these conditions. The amygdala and hippocampus have also been implicated in psychiatric disorders such as anxiety, depression, and schizophrenia. A discussion of these disorders is beyond the scope of this chapter. Only the putative circuit pathophysiology will be briefly discussed here.

Cognitive Disorders

Patients with lesions to the hippocampus have marked deficits in episodic and spatial memory. Selective hippocampal damage disrupts performance in memory tasks that require multimodal associations and relational representations. One hypothesized mechanism for disorders that affect episodic memory, such as amnestic type Alzheimer disease (AD), is imbalance within the excitatory/inhibitory networks in the hippocampus. Studies in mouse models of AD showed that amyloid β (Aβ) affects such balance, leading to hyperactivity in hippocampal neurons, a breakdown of slow-wave oscillations, disruption of gamma oscillations, and network hypersynchrony; these changes precede amyloid plaque formation.[50] Optogenetic excitation of medial septum or hippocampal fast-spiking parvalbumin interneurons at slow gamma frequency[51] or transcranial magnetic stimulation of the hippocampus,[52] attenuated Aβ production and improved memory performance in these models. Deep brain stimulation targeting different components of the hippocampal systems, including the hippocampus and entorhinal cortex, is being explored as an approach to improve memory performance in patients with AD or epilepsy.[53]

Mesial Temporal Lobe Seizures

The hippocampus has the lowest seizure threshold in the brain, which reflects its basic circuit involving serial excitatory synapses and positive feedback loops. Several features of the CA3 region make it especially prone to generate and sustain seizure activity. Pyramidal CA3 neurons tend to fire in bursts, receive a powerful excitation by mossy fiber projections from dentate granule cells, and give rise to highly collateralized axons that distribute widely within the hippocampus to contact many CA3 and CA1 neurons. Recurrent excitatory connections among CA3 pyramidal cells can generate synchronous firing and bursts of population spikes. Under normal conditions, the strong inhibitory activity of GABAergic interneurons prevents the expression of this latent hyperexcitability. The GABAergic basket cells of the dentate gyrus receive direct excitatory inputs from the granule cells and provide feedback inhibition to these neurons. Basket cells also receive indirect disynaptic excitation via mossy neurons located in the hilus of the dentate gyrus. Several cellular and circuit abnormalities in the dentate gyrus predispose to epileptogenesis. These include vulnerability of mossy cells leading to loss of glutamatergic mossy fiber input to basket cells ("dormant cell hypothesis"), collateral sprouting of dentate granule cell axons, ectopic localization of newborn dentate granule cells in the hilus, and abnormal development of basal dendrites in these newborn cells.[54,55] Recurrent excitation is an important circuit motif in the dentate gyrus that may contribute to epileptogenesis. This involves increased collateral inputs to granule cells from aberrant sprouting of their axons, from hilar excitatory neurons, and from CA3 neurons. In experimental models, kainic acid induces both acute seizures and temporal lobe epilepsy through GluK1- and GuK2-containing receptors expressed in inhibitory neurons or CA3 cells.[56] Mossy fiber sprouting targeting granule cells recruits kainic acid receptors;[56] these receptors are also expressed in the astrocytes in the hippocampus of patients with medial temporal lobe seizures.[57] Microglia regulate both adult neurogenesis in the hippocampus and seizure susceptibility by eliminating viable newborn cells in the adult dentate gyrus after status epilepticus, maintaining homeostasis of the dentate circuitry.[58]

High-frequency oscillations (HFOs) at a frequency 80 and 600 Hz occur spontaneously in the hippocampal formation during interictal episodes, primarily during slow-wave sleep or waking quiescence, and to a lesser extent during the onset of some seizures.[59] In the normal brain, local inhibitory cells, primarily basket cells in CA1, have a prominent role in physiological HFOs. The tightly orchestrated pattern of firing between these interneurons and principal cells during normal HFOs has been implicated with encoding information and memory consolidation.[60] In contrast, in the epileptic hippocampal formation, fast ripple-frequency HFOs reflect brief bursts of population spikes generated from a cluster of pathologically interconnected neurons. These bursts also occur in the dentate gyrus, an area that does not generate such events in normal conditions. Pathological HFOs reflect both increased principal cell spike firing and reduced interneuron firing and coincide and with spontaneous population spikes. In mesial temporal lobe epilepsy due to hippocampal sclerosis, hippocampal atrophy and neuronal loss correlate with both disruption of normal ripple-frequency HFOs and generation of pathological fast ripple-frequency HFOs. Depth electrode recordings from the dentate gyrus of rats with experimental TLE showed two typical seizure onset patterns, low-voltage fast and hypersynchronous patterns.[61] The low-voltage fast pattern reflects initial synchronous excessive inhibitory parvalbumin interneuron discharge that leads to activation of $GABA_A$Rs in both in pyramidal cells and in interneurons. This is followed by an increase in extracellular K^+, reduced inhibitory postsynaptic potentials, network hyperexcitability, and spiking of principal cells. Ripples (80–200 Hz) predominate during low-voltage fast seizures, and synchronized activity generated by principal cells is entrained by synchronously active interneuron networks. The hypersynchronous seizure onset pattern is characterized by focal periodic spiking at frequency of ~1 Hz and reflects excessive and coordinated discharge of pyramidal cells and connected interneurons. This leads both to excessive activation of $GABA_A$Rs and progressive accumulation of extracellular K^+, followed by progressive weakening of inhibition at pyramidal cell dendrites, recurrent principal cell discharge, and eventually to a hypersynchronous seizure onset. Fast ripples (250–500 Hz) are thought to reflect the hypersynchronous firing of principal glutamatergic neurons during hypersynchronous onset seizures. Long-term intracranial-depth recordings obtained during presurgical stereo-EEG monitoring have revealed that low voltage–fast seizure onset is the most common pattern of ictal discharge initiation and occurs both in focal neocortical focal and in mesial TLE. In contrast, the hypersynchronous-onset pattern is observed only in mesial TLE with hippocampal sclerosis. A number of studies in patients have detected HFOs or an increase in HFO power during or preceding ictal onset by several minutes to seconds. Intracranial EEG monitoring showed that engagement in spatial and episodic memory tasks promotes temporal lobe spikes in patient with temporal lobe seizures.[62]

KEY POINTS

- The hippocampus and the amygdala are core areas of the so-called limbic system.
- The posterior limbic circuit centered in the hippocampus is involved in episodic memory and navigation.
- The hippocampal formation includes the dentate gyrus; CA3, CA2, and CA1 fields; and subiculum.
- The entorhinal cortex serves is the gateway for access of neocortical information to the hippocampus
- The entorhinal cortex projects to the intrinsic hippocampal circuit via two separate excitatory pathways, a trisynaptic pathway sequentially involving the dentate gyrus, CA3, and CA1 and a direct projection from the entorhinal cortex the CA1 and subiculum.
- The hippocampus contain several types of GABAergic cell types, which provide feedforward and feedback inhibition within hippocampal circuits.
- Hippocampal circuits exhibit synchronized theta and gamma oscillations during active states and generate sharp wave-ripple activity primarily during non–rapid eye movement (NREM) sleep.
- Theta oscillations provide for coordinated activity within and across brain regions during successful encoding and retrieval of memory.
- The hippocampal theta rhythm depends on inputs from cholinergic and GABAergic projection neurons in the medial septum.
- Gamma activity represents local spiking in hippocampal networks and promotes binding of separate details of events.
- Hippocampal sharp wave-ripples are thought to be involved in memory consolidation.
- The dentate gyrus is involved in pattern separation, which minimizes the overlap between the representations of two similar events.
- Adult neurogenesis in the subgranular zone of the dentate gyrus may contribute to pattern separation.
- Pattern completion allows the recall of a complete representation even in the presence of a partial input and depends on autoassociative connections within CA3.
- CA1 neurons integrate novel information originating from the entorhinal cortex with stored information provided by CA3.

- Acetylcholine (ACh) is released in the hippocampus during theta oscillations during wakefulness and promotes encoding of new information.
- During NREM sleep, reduced ACh levels promote recurrent autoexcitation in CA3, leading to consolidation and storage of information.
- Dopaminergic inputs provide novelty (salience) and reward components to the hippocampus, and thereby promote encoding of episodic memory.
- Hippocampal representations undergo a continual process of strengthening, weakening, and modification via synaptic plasticity.
- The hippocampus has a critical role in navigation by providing a representation of space, which provides a frame to organize all experiences within episodic memories.
- Neocortical representations of the elements of an episodic event form links with individual neurons in the hippocampus referred to as "concept cells."
- The prefrontal cortex contributes to episodic memory by top-down control of memory processing and retrieval.
- The amygdala provides automatic tagging of positive or negative valence to environmental stimuli and has a major role in associative learning, emotional memory, and social cognition.
- The lateral nucleus of the amygdala (LA) receives convergent inputs from the neocortex and thalamus and is the site of associative learning, or Pavolvian conditioning.
- The basal nucleus (BA) receives inputs from the LA and is strongly interconnected with areas involved in attention and consolidation of emotional memory.
- Both the LA and BA project to the centromedial nucleus (CeM), which triggers emotional responses via its inputs to the hypothalamus and brainstem.
- Formation of new emotional memories and extinction of previous emotional memories involve complex excitatory and inhibitory intrinsic circuits in the amygdala.
- Synaptic plasticity in the basolateral amygdala allows subsets of neurons to be recruited during learning and reactivated during retrieval of emotional memories.
- Stress strongly affects emotional learning by activating locus coeruleus neurons resulting in release of norepinephrine from their projections to the amygdala.
- Memory deficits in amnestic type Alzheimer disease may reflect excitatory/inhibitory imbalance and disruptions of gamma oscillations.
- Deep brain stimulation targeting the hippocampus and entorhinal cortex is may improve memory performance in patients with AD or epilepsy.
- Several cellular and circuit abnormalities in the dentate gyrus predispose to epileptogenesis.
- In patients with medial temporal lobe seizures, high-frequency oscillations (HFOs) occur spontaneously in the hippocampal formation during interictal episodes.

REFERENCES

1. Pessoa L, Hof PR. From Paul Broca's great limbic lobe to the limbic system. J Comp Neurol 2015;523:2495–2500.
2. Rolls ET. The cingulate cortex and limbic systems for action, emotion, and memory. Handb Clin Neurol 2019;166:23–37.
3. Rolls ET. Limbic systems for emotion and for memory, but no single limbic system. Cortex 2015;62:119–157.
4. Eichenbaum H. On the integration of space, time, and memory. Neuron 2017;95:1007–1018.
5. Lisman J, Buzsaki G, Eichenbaum H, Nadel L, Ranganath C, Redish AD. Viewpoints: how the hippocampus contributes to memory, navigation and cognition. Nat Neurosci 2017;20:1434–1447.
6. Bocchio M, Nabavi S, Capogna M. Synaptic plasticity, engrams, and network oscillations in amygdala circuits for storage and retrieval of emotional memories. Neuron 2017;94:731–743.
7. Duvarci S, Pare D. Amygdala microcircuits controlling learned fear. Neuron 2014;82:966–980.
8. Moser EI, Moser MB, McNaughton BL. Spatial representation in the hippocampal formation: a history. Nat Neurosci 2017;20:1448–1464.
9. Sanders H, Renno-Costa C, Idiart M, Lisman J. Grid cells and place cells: an integrated view of their navigational and memory function. Trends Neurosci 2015;38:763–775.
10. van Strien NM, Cappaert NL, Witter MP. The anatomy of memory: an interactive overview of the parahippocampal-hippocampal network. Nat Rev Neurosci 2009;10:272–282.
11. Sasaki T, Leutgeb S, Leutgeb JK. Spatial and memory circuits in the medial entorhinal cortex. Curr Opin Neurobiol 2015;32:16–23.
12. Sasaki T, Piatti VC, Hwaun E, et al. Dentate network activity is necessary for spatial working memory by supporting CA3 sharp-wave ripple generation and prospective firing of CA3 neurons. Nat Neurosci 2018;21:258–269.
13. Johnson EL, Knight RT. Intracranial recordings and human memory. Curr Opin Neurobiol 2015;31:18–25.
14. Maren S. Seeking a spotless mind: extinction, deconsolidation, and erasure of fear memory. Neuron 2011;70:830–845.
15. Gilmartin MR, Balderston NL, Helmstetter FJ. Prefrontal cortical regulation of fear learning. Trends Neurosci 2014;37:455–464.
16. Bocchio M, McHugh SB, Bannerman DM, Sharp T, Capogna M. Serotonin, amygdala and fear: assembling the puzzle. Front Neural Circuits 2016;10:24.
17. Aubry AV, Serrano PA, Burghardt NS. Molecular mechanisms of stress-induced increases in fear memory consolidation within the amygdala. Front Behav Neurosci 2016;10:191.
18. Horner AJ, Doeller CF. Plasticity of hippocampal memories in humans. Curr Opin Neurobiol 2017;43:102–109.
19. Palacios-Filardo J, Mellor JR. Neuromodulation of hippocampal long-term synaptic plasticity. Curr Opin Neurobiol 2019;54:37–43.
20. Dickerson BC, Eichenbaum H. The episodic memory system: neurocircuitry and disorders. Neuropsychopharmacology 2010;35:86–104.

21. Strange BA, Witter MP, Lein ES, Moser EI. Functional organization of the hippocampal longitudinal axis. Nat Rev Neurosci 2014;15:655–669.
22. Ritchey M, Libby LA, Ranganath C. Cortico-hippocampal systems involved in memory and cognition: the PMAT framework. Prog Brain Res 2015;219:45–64.
23. Ranganath C, Ritchey M. Two cortical systems for memory-guided behaviour. Nat Rev Neurosci 2012;13:713–726.
24. Dudek SM, Alexander GM, Farris S. Rediscovering area CA2: unique properties and functions. Nat Rev Neurosci 2016;17:89–102.
25. English DF, McKenzie S, Evans T, Kim K, Yoon E, Buzsaki G. Pyramidal cell-interneuron circuit architecture and dynamics in hippocampal networks. Neuron 2017;96:505–520 e507.
26. Hanslmayr S, Staresina BP, Bowman H. Oscillations and episodic memory: addressing the synchronization/desynchronization conundrum. Trends Neurosci 2016;39:16–25.
27. Dannenberg H, Pabst M, Braganza O, et al. Synergy of direct and indirect cholinergic septo-hippocampal pathways coordinates firing in hippocampal networks. J Neurosci 2015;35:8394–8410.
28. Bakker A, Kirwan CB, Miller M, Stark CE. Pattern separation in the human hippocampal CA3 and dentate gyrus. Science 2008;319:1640–1642.
29. Aimone JB, Deng W, Gage FH. Resolving new memories: a critical look at the dentate gyrus, adult neurogenesis, and pattern separation. Neuron 2011;70:589–596.
30. Duncan K, Ketz N, Inati SJ, Davachi L. Evidence for area CA1 as a match/mismatch detector: a high-resolution fMRI study of the human hippocampus. Hippocampus 2012;22:389–398.
31. Butler JL, Paulsen O. The hippocampal cacophony: multiple layers of communication. Neuron 2014;84:251–253.
32. McQuiston AR. Acetylcholine release and inhibitory interneuron activity in hippocampal CA1. Front Synaptic Neurosci 2014;6:20.
33. Hasselmo ME. The role of acetylcholine in learning and memory. Curr Opin Neurobiol 2006;16:710–715.
34. Nicoll RA. A brief history of long-term potentiation. Neuron 2017;93:281–290.
35. Vertes RP. Major diencephalic inputs to the hippocampus: supramammillary nucleus and nucleus reuniens. Circuitry and function. Prog Brain Res 2015;219:121–144.
36. Moser EI, Kropff E, Moser MB. Place cells, grid cells, and the brain's spatial representation system. Annu Rev Neurosci 2008;31:69–89.
37. O'Keefe J. Place units in the hippocampus of the freely moving rat. Exp Neurol 1976;51:78–109.
38. Epstein RA, Patai EZ, Julian JB, Spiers HJ. The cognitive map in humans: spatial navigation and beyond. Nat Neurosci 2017;20:1504–1513.
39. Jacobs J, Weidemann CT, Miller JF, et al. Direct recordings of grid-like neuronal activity in human spatial navigation. Nat Neurosci 2013;16:1188–1190.
40. Bulkin DA, Law LM, Smith DM. Placing memories in context: hippocampal representations promote retrieval of appropriate memories. Hippocampus 2016;26:958–971.
41. Anderson MC, Bunce JG, Barbas H. Prefrontal-hippocampal pathways underlying inhibitory control over memory. Neurobiol Learn Mem 2016;134 Pt A:145–161.
42. Eichenbaum H. Prefrontal-hippocampal interactions in episodic memory. Nat Rev Neurosci 2017;18:547–558.
43. Benchenane K, Peyrache A, Khamassi M, et al. Coherent theta oscillations and reorganization of spike timing in the hippocampal- prefrontal network upon learning. Neuron 2010;66:921–936.
44. Backus AR, Schoffelen JM, Szebenyi S, Hanslmayr S, Doeller CF. Hippocampal-prefrontal theta oscillations support memory integration. Curr Biol 2016;26:450–457.
45. Colgin LL. Oscillations and hippocampal-prefrontal synchrony. Curr Opin Neurobiol 2011;21:467–474.
46. Ketz NA, Jensen O, O'Reilly RC. Thalamic pathways underlying prefrontal cortex-medial temporal lobe oscillatory interactions. Trends Neurosci 2015;38:3–12.
47. van Kesteren MT, Ruiter DJ, Fernandez G, Henson RN. How schema and novelty augment memory formation. Trends Neurosci 2012;35:211–219.
48. LeDoux J. The amygdala. Current biology: CB 2007;17:R868–874.
49. Murray EA. The amygdala, reward and emotion. Trends Cogn Sci 2007;11:489–497.
50. Busche MA, Konnerth A. Impairments of neural circuit function in Alzheimer's disease. Philos Trans R Soc Lond B Biol Sci 2016;371.
51. Etter G, van der Veldt S, Manseau F, Zarrinkoub I, Trillaud-Doppia E, Williams S. Optogenetic gamma stimulation rescues memory impairments in an Alzheimer's disease mouse model. Nat Commun 2019;10:5322.
52. Zhen J, Qian Y, Weng X, et al. Gamma rhythm low field magnetic stimulation alleviates neuropathologic changes and rescues memory and cognitive impairments in a mouse model of Alzheimer's disease. Alzheimers Dement (N Y) 2017;3:487–497.
53. Mankin EA, Fried I. Modulation of human memory by deep brain stimulation of the entorhinal-hippocampal circuitry. Neuron 2020;106:218–235.
54. Chen L, Wang Y, Chen Z. Adult neurogenesis in epileptogenesis: An update for preclinical finding and potential clinical translation. Curr Neuropharmacol 2020;18:464–484.
55. Cavarsan CF, Malheiros J, Hamani C, Najm I, Covolan L. Is mossy fiber sprouting a potential therapeutic target for epilepsy? Front Neurol 2018;9:1023.
56. Falcon-Moya R, Sihra TS, Rodriguez-Moreno A. Kainate receptors: role in epilepsy. Front Mol Neurosci 2018;11:217.
57. Kitaura H, Shirozu H, Masuda H, Fukuda M, Fujii Y, Kakita A. Pathophysiological characteristics associated with epileptogenesis in human hippocampal sclerosis. EBioMedicine 2018;29:38–46.
58. Luo C, Ikegaya Y, Koyama R. Microglia and neurogenesis in the epileptic dentate gyrus. Neurogenesis (Austin) 2016;3:e1235525.
59. Stead M, Bower M, Brinkmann BH, et al. Microseizures and the spatiotemporal scales of human partial epilepsy. Brain 2010;133:2789–2797.
60. Worrell GA, Jerbi K, Kobayashi K, Lina JM, Zelmann R, Le Van Quyen M. Recording and analysis techniques for high-frequency oscillations. Prog Neurobiol 2012;98:265–278.
61. Avoli M, de Curtis M, Gnatkovsky V, et al. Specific imbalance of excitatory/inhibitory signaling establishes seizure onset pattern in temporal lobe epilepsy. J Neurophysiol 2016;115:3229–3237.
62. Vivekananda U, Bush D, Bisby JA, et al. Spatial and episodic memory tasks promote temporal lobe interictal spikes. Ann Neurol 2019;86:304–309.

26 Thalamus and Thalamocortical Interactions

OVERVIEW

The thalamus has a critical role in regulation of cortical activity. It is crucial for relay of sensory information to the cortex, selective attention, cortical arousal, motor control, gating sensory input to the cerebral cortex, and generation of sleep spindles during non–rapid eye movement (NREM) sleep. The thalamus includes two major components, the dorsal thalamus (thalamus proper, hereafter referred to as thalamus) and the thalamic reticular nucleus (TRN). The thalamus consists of different types of nuclei containing glutamatergic thalamocortical (TC) projection neurons that project to the cerebral cortex (Figure 26.1).[1] First-order relay nuclei receive modality-specific input from sensory pathways and project to the respective primary cortical sensory area. Higher-order relay nuclei receive their main input from layer 5 of the neocortex and participate in cortico-thalamo-cortical circuits that have a major role in attention and other high-level cognitive functions.[2]

The motor thalamus receives inputs from the cerebellum and basal ganglia and projects to the motor cortex. Intralaminar nuclei receive inputs from the brainstem reticular formation and other sources, send diffuse projections to the cerebral cortex promoting cortical arousal, and provide a powerful input to the striatum. Midline thalamic nuclei participate in mechanisms of arousal and memory. Unlike all other thalamic nuclei, the TRN contains GABAergic neurons that project to all other thalamic nuclei but not to the cortex both. The TRN functions as a gate for transfer of information between the rest of the thalamus and the cerebral cortex both during sleep and during attentional selection. The reciprocal interactions between TRN and TC neurons provide the basis for spindle oscillations during NREM sleep.

The relay of information from the thalamus to the cerebral cortex is also strongly modulated by reciprocal projections from corticothalamic (CT) neurons; modulatory inputs from cholinergic and monoaminergic neurons of the brainstem; and GABAergic projections from the pontine reticular formation, globus pallidus, and other extrathalamic sources. Disruptions in thalamocortical communication resulting from focal thalamic lesions,[3] or abnormal oscillatory activity in thalamocortical circuits, or "thalamocortical dysrhythmia,"[4] result in profound disturbances in attention, sleep-wake regulation, sensory processing, and motor control. For example hypersynchronous thalamocortical discharges are associated with transient behavioral arrest during typical absence seizures. Impaired awareness in temporal lobe seizures may also reflect thalamic involvement. The main aims of this chapter are to review: (1) the functional organization of thalamic nuclei, (2) the organization of the TRN, (3) the firing patterns of thalamic neurons, (4) the thalamocortical activity during NREM sleep, (5) the role of the thalamus in arousal and attention mechanisms, and (6) the involvement of the thalamus in seizures and other neurologic disorders.

ANATOMICAL AND FUNCTIONAL ORGANIZATION OF THE DORSAL THALAMUS (THALAMUS PROPER)

The integration of cytoarchitecture, myeloarchitecture, connectivity, and neuroimaging data has led to an updated parcellation and nomenclature of the human thalamus.[1]

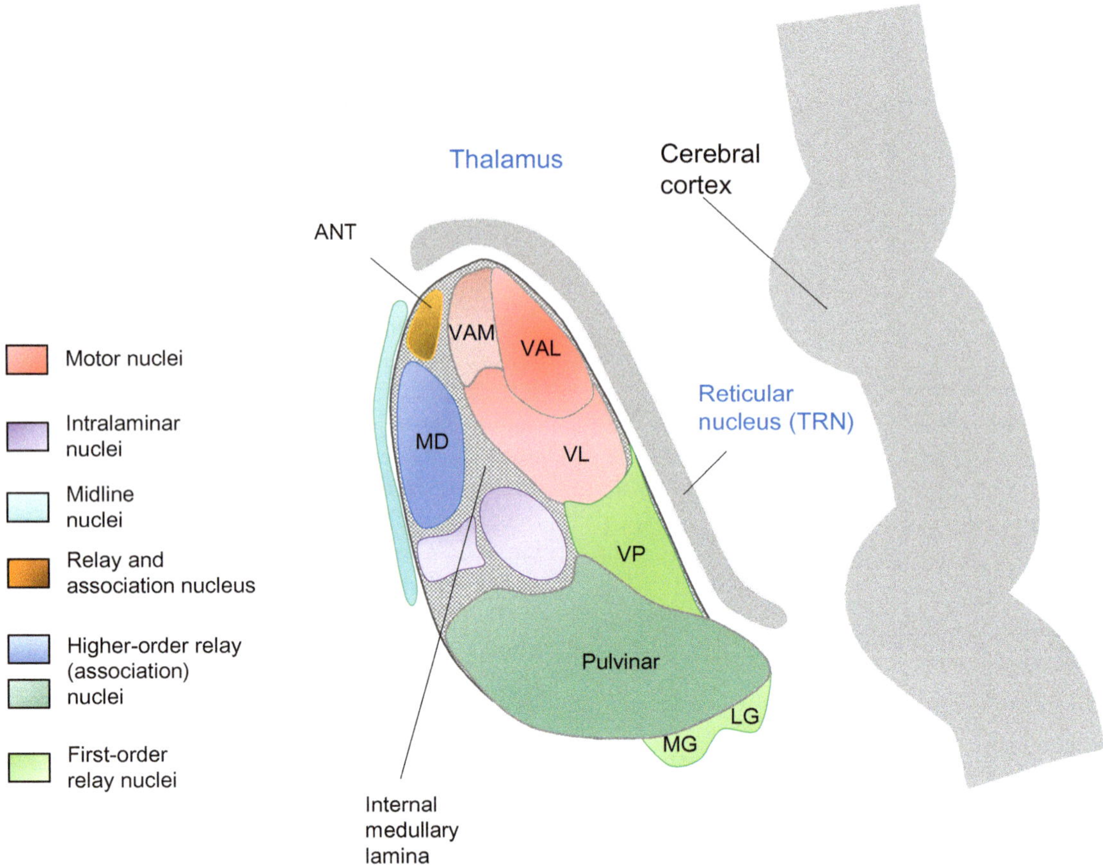

FIGURE 26.1 Components of the thalamus.
The thalamus includes two major components, the dorsal thalamus (thalamus proper, hereafter referred to as thalamus), which contains thalamocortical projection neurons, and the thalamic reticular nucleus (TRN). The superior region of the thalamus includes the anterior nucleus (ANT). The medial region includes the mediodorsal nucleus (MD). The lateral region includes the ventral anterior nucleus (VA), including medial (VAM) and lateral (VAL) portions; the ventrolateral nucleus (VL); and the ventroposterior nuclear complex (VP). The intralaminar nuclei are divided into an anterior, central, and posterior groups. The periventricular formation includes the midline nuclei; the posterior region consists of the pulvinar; and the geniculate region includes the medial geniculate nucleus (MG) and lateral geniculate nucleus (LG). First-order relay nuclei receive modality-specific driver input from subcortical afferent sources and project to the modality-specific primary sensory area of the cerebral cortex. Higher-order relay nuclei receive their main input from the neocortex and participate in cortico-thalamo-cortical circuits. Intralaminar nuclei have diffuse projections to cortex and also target the striatum. The motor thalamus receives and conveys inputs from deep cerebellar nuclei and basal ganglia to the motor cortex. Nuclei in the periventricular region participate in mechanisms of arousal and memory. The TRN contains GABAergic neurons that project to all other thalamic nuclei.

Anatomical Subdivisions

The internal medullary lamina contains the intralaminar nuclei and divides the thalamus into medial, lateral, and anterior nuclear regions. The anterodorsal region of the thalamus consists primarily of the anterior nuclear complex (ANT). The medial region consists of the mediodorsal nucleus (MD). The region between the ependyma of the third ventricle and the MD comprises a sheet of small neurons that are a component of the periventricular ventricular gray and small clusters of neurons known as midline nuclei and subdivided into a dorsal and a ventral group. The lateral region of the thalamus contains nuclei that are characterized both by their source of afferent inputs and their cortical targets. They include the motor thalamus, which receives inputs from the basal ganglia, cerebellum, and vestibular nuclei, and the sensory thalamus, which receives somatosensory and visceral input. The nomenclature of these nuclei varies according to different authors. According one nomenclature, these nuclei can be subdivided into a ventral anterior (VA), ventrolateral (VL), and ventroposterior nuclear complex (VP). The VA is subdivided into a medial region receiving inputs from the substantia nigra pars reticulata (SNr) and a lateral region receiving inputs from the globus pallidus pars interna (GPi). The VL is subdivided into an anterior region (VLa) and a posterior region (VLp, also referred to as ventral intermedius) receiving input from the cerebellum. The VP complex receives somatosensory and visceral inputs via the medial lemniscus, spinothalamic tract, or trigeminothalamic tract. The VP is subdivided into a lateral ventroposterior nucleus (ventral posterolateral nucleus, VPL), medial ventroposterior nucleus (ventral posteromedial nucleus, VPM), superior ventroposterior nucleus (VPS), ventral posterior inferior nucleus (VPI), and the medial ventroposterior nucleus, parvocellular part (ventral posteromedial nucleus, parvocellular part, VPMpc). The metathalamus includes the lateral geniculate and the medial geniculate bodies. The lateral geniculate body is composed primarily of the lateral geniculate nucleus (LGN or, more precisely, dorsal LGN), which receives input from the retina. The medial geniculate body is divided into a lateral or principal portion and a medial division, which receives auditory inputs via the inferior colliculus. The posterior region of the thalamus consists of the pulvinar. The pulvinar nuclei include the medial, lateral, anterior, and inferior nuclei and the lateral posterior nucleus.

Driver Versus Modulatory Inputs to the Thalamus

Thalamic nuclei receive two general types of afferents, referred to as drivers and modulators.[2] Driver afferents target the proximal dendrites and reliably evoke spikes in thalamic cells, triggering faithful transmission of information to the cerebral cortex. Driver afferents are glutamatergic and elicit fast excitation via ionotropic receptors. In contrast, modulatory afferents target primarily the distal dendrites and control excitability of thalamic neurons, thereby fine-tuning the message relayed by thalamic cells. These modulatory inputs include glutamatergic afferents from the cortex and cholinergic and monoaminergic inputs from the brainstem and affect thalamic cell excitability via metabotropic receptors. On the basis of the source of driver input, to TC neurons, thalamic nuclei are subdivided in two groups, first-order and higher-order relay nuclei.[2]

First-Order Relay Nuclei

First-order relay nuclei receive modality-specific driver input from subcortical sources and project to the corresponding primary sensory area of the cerebral cortex (Figure 26.2). These nuclei include the different components of the VP, which relays somatosensory and visceral input to the primary sensory cortex; the LGN, which relays inputs from retinal ganglion cells to the primary visual cortex (V1); and the ventral portion of the MGN, which relays auditory inputs to the primary auditory cortex. Projection TC neurons in these nuclei target layer 4 of the corresponding primary sensory cortex. Within each major sensory modality, there are submodality-specific channels that target different cortical columns. These pathways are further discussed in chapter 29.

Higher-Order Relay Nuclei

Higher-order nuclei receive driver input primarily from layer 5 of the neocortex. These nuclei participate in cortico-thalamic-cortical circuits (also referred to transthalamic circuits) that modulate or gate the transfer of information between cortical areas, in parallel to their direct corticocortical connections. The main higher-order thalamic nuclei are the pulvinar and the MD (Figure 26.3). The pulvinar has a critical role in visual processing and attention via its widespread reciprocal connectivity with cortical visual areas. It consists of inferior, lateral, and medial divisions that receive direct inputs from the retina or primary visual cortex and convey these inputs to visual cortical association areas. The MD is characterized by its strong interconnectivity with the prefrontal cortex (PFC) and has a major role in attention, recognition memory, and emotion. The MD consists of three major subdivisions; the medial subdivision interacts with the orbitofrontal cortex, medial PFC and anterior cingulate cortex; the lateral subdivision with the lateral PFC; and the paralaminar subdivision with the frontal eye fields. Higher order thalamic nuclei employ more complex and heterogeneous circuitry than do first order nuclei. Many neurons across the pulvinar and MD receive convergent inputs from multiple cortical areas. In addition to their prominent driver input from layer 5, a subset of thalamic cells in these nuclei receive a driver input from the superior colliculus, which is involved in attention and orienting responses.

Anterior Nucleus

The ANT includes the principal anteroventral the anteromedial, and anterodorsal nuclei. The inputs to the ANT originate in the subicular cortex of the hippocampal formation via the fornix, either directly or with a relay in the mammillary bodies. The anteroventral nucleus receives inputs from the medial mammillary nucleus, has extensive interactions with the retrosplenial cortex and has a major role in relaying the theta rhythm during encoding of episodic memory. The anteromedial subnucleus has extensive reciprocal connections with the anterior cingulate and medial PFC and participates in emotional processing. The anterodorsal nucleus receives inputs from the lateral mammillary nucleus, is interconnected with the retrosplenial cortex and has major role in spatial navigation.[5] These functions are further discussed in chapter 40.

Midline Nuclei

The midline nuclei are divided into a ventral and a dorsal group. The ventral group includes the nucleus reuniens, which has reciprocal connections with both the hippocampus (CA1 region and subiculum) and the PFC and

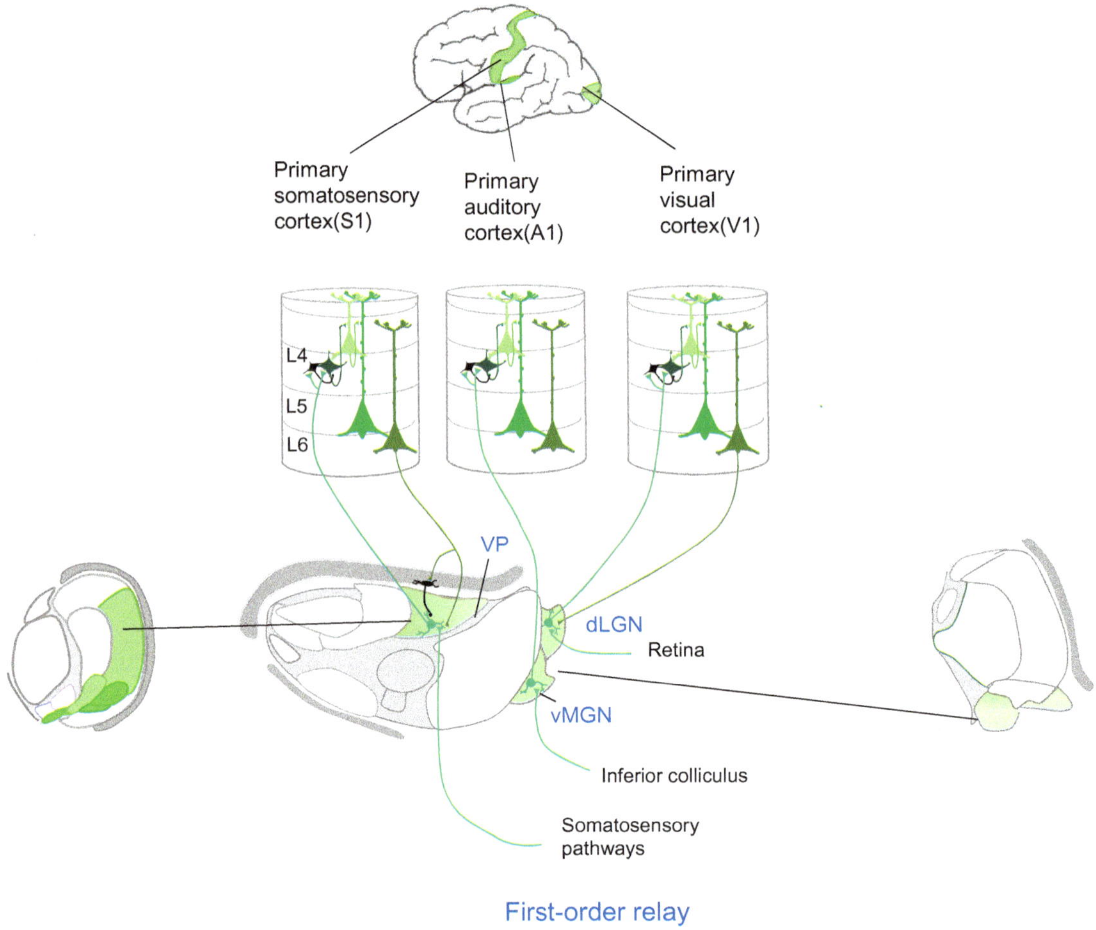

FIGURE 26.2 First-order relay nuclei.
First-order relay nuclei receive modality-specific driver input from subcortical sources and project to the corresponding primary sensory area of the cerebral cortex. They include subdivisions of the ventroposterior complex (VP), which relay somatosensory inputs to the somatosensory cortex; the dorsal lateral geniculate nucleus (dLGN), which relays retinal inputs to the primary visual cortex; and the ventral portion of the medial geniculate nucleus (vMGN), which receives inputs from inferior colliculus and projects to the primary auditory cortex.

constitutes the principal route for transferring information between these two structures, which is required for executive control of episodic memory. The dorsal group includes the paraventricular nucleus, which targets the anterior cingulate cortex, insula, amygdala, nucleus accumbens, and hypothalamus and receives inputs from the medial PFC, insula, hypothalamus, and brainstem. Via these connections, the paraventricular nucleus participates in responses associated with emotion and to stress responses.[6]

Intralaminar Nuclei

The intralaminar nuclei are embedded in the internal medullary lamina and are characterized both by their diffuse projections to the cerebral cortex and their dense projections to the striatum.[1,7] They are subdivided into an anterior, central, and posterior groups. The anterior group includes central medial and the central lateral nucleus (CL); the central group includes the centromedian (CMn), parafascicular (PF), and subparafascicular nucleus; and the posterior nuclear complex includes the posterior nucleus and the suprageniculate nucleus. The CL receives inputs from the frontal and parietal cortex, cerebellum, brainstem, and spinal cord and sends projections back to the frontal and parietal cortex and the striatum. The CL conveys inputs from the cerebellum to the striatum. The CMn/PF complex provides the most substantial projection to the striatum. The posterior nucleus conveys multimodal sensory inputs to the cerebral cortex. Through their diffuse cortical projections, the intralaminar nuclei have a major role in cortical activation.

Motor Nuclei of the Thalamus

The thalamus contains two regions that receive inputs from the cerebellum and basal ganglia. The ventrolateral

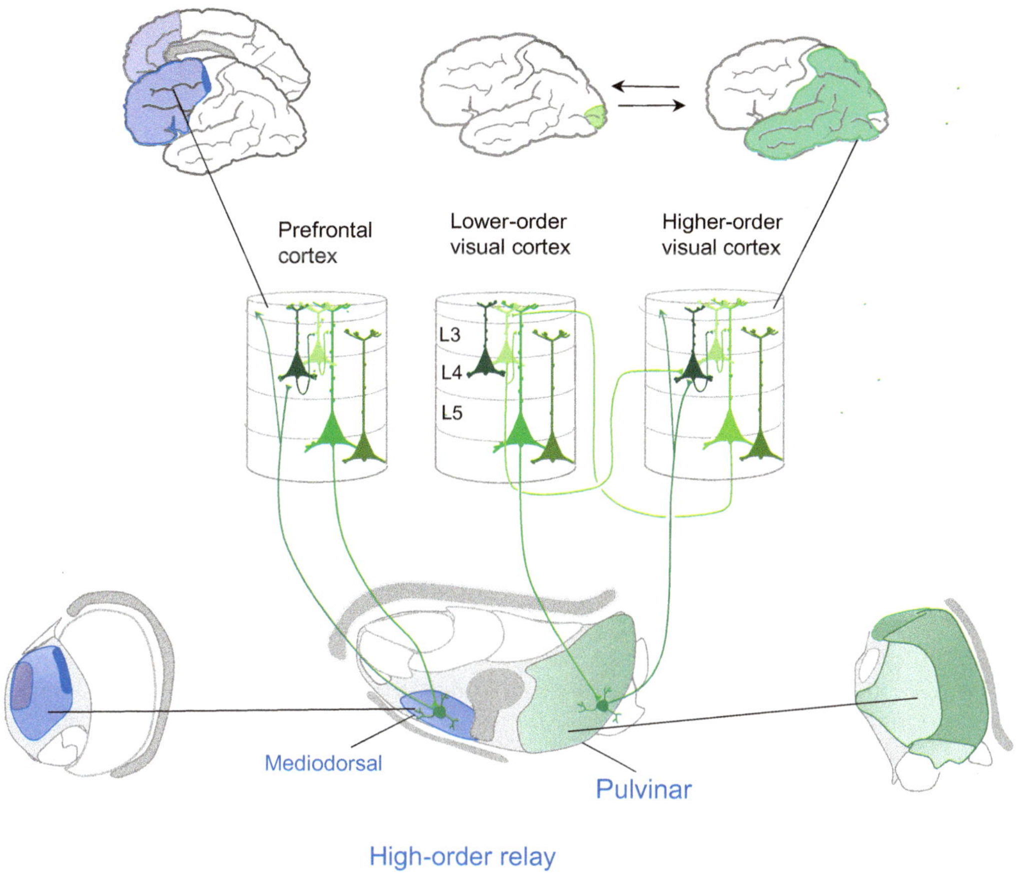

FIGURE 26.3 Higher-order relay nuclei.
Higher-order nuclei participate in cortico-thalamic-cortical circuits that are often parallel to direct cortico-cortical connections. The prototype higher-order thalamic nuclei are the pulvinar and the mediodorsal nuclei. The pulvinar is primarily associated with visual processing. The mediodorsal is characterized by its strong interconnectivity with the prefrontal cortex.

region, classically referred to the "motor thalamus," consists of the VA and VL and can be subdivided, from anterior to posterior, into a nigral, pallidal, and cerebellar territory. The nigral territory receives inputs from the SNr and projects to the PFC and frontal eye fields. The pallidal territory receives input from the GPi and projects to the supplementary motor area and premotor cortex. The cerebellar territory involves the VL, particularly its posterior portion (VLp or ventral intermedius), receives input from the deep cerebellar nuclei and projects mainly to the primary motor and lateral premotor areas. The functions of these nuclei are discussed in chapters 33 and 34. A second thalamic territory receives sparse convergent input from both the basal ganglia and cerebellum, and includes the lateral parts of MD, parts of CL and CMn/Pf, the VA-VL border, and the ventromedial nucleus. There is a fundamental difference between the influences of the cerebellum and basal ganglia on the thalamus. The cerebellar inputs are driving glutamatergic inputs; in contrast, the output from the GPi and SNr provide tonic GABAergic inhibition.[8]

Innervation of Motor Areas by Branching of Thalamic Driver Inputs

Driver inputs to first- and higher-order thalamic relay nuclei typically consist of branching axons that also innervate brainstem motor centers. For example, first-order axons from retinal ganglion cells projecting to the LGN branch to also innervate the superior colliculus; axons from the medial lemniscus projecting to the VP branch to innervate motor nuclei of the brainstem reticular formation; and axons from the cerebellar nuclei projecting to the VL branch to innervate the red nucleus. Furthermore, cortical axons from layer 5 neurons that provide driver inputs to high-order thalamic relay nuclei also branch to motor areas of the brainstem. For example, cortical projections from the visual cortex to the pulvinar branch to innervate the superior colliculus; and pyramidal tract neurons from motor cortex branch extensively to innervate the VL, brainstem, and spinal cord. This suggests that the thalamus participates in motor control by providing efference copies to motor nuclei.[2]

RECIPROCAL THALAMO-CORTICO-THALAMIC INTERACTIONS

The projections from TC neurons to the cortex have been subdivided into distinct patterns, referred to as "core"-type and "matrix"-type projections. Reciprocally, corticothalamic (CT) neurons in layer 6 of the targeted cortical area send reciprocal inputs to both core- and matrix -type TC neurons (Figure 26.4).

Core-Type Inputs

Core-type TC relay neurons are located mainly in the first-order sensory relay nuclei and provide driving input to layer 4 of their corresponding primary sensory cortices. This thalamic core input not only targets layer 4 intratelencephalic (IT) neurons that convey sensory information to other cortical layers but also strongly activates fast-spiking parvalbumin (PV) GABAergic basket interneurons targeting the soma and proximal dendrites of the same layer 4 IT neurons. Thus, local processing of core thalamocortical inputs by layer 4 IT neurons depends on the precise timing of direct excitation and feedforward inhibition via GABAergic interneurons triggered by the same thalamocortical core afferent. This creates a narrow window of opportunity for cortical neurons to fire an accurately timed spike and to respond selectively to specific stimuli.

Layer 4 neurons in higher-order sensory areas receive long-range core-type inputs from different thalamic sources as well as corticocortical feedforward inputs from lower-order areas.

Matrix-Type Inputs

Matrix-type TC neurons send projections to lamina 1, targeting the apical dendrites of pyramidal cells in widely distributed cortical columns. Matrix-type projection neurons are located in several thalamic regions, including high-order relay nuclei, regions surrounding the core neurons, and in the intralaminar thalamic nuclei. For example axons from the pulvinar may project either diffusely to superficial layer 1 and function as modulators or terminate in a denser and localized fashion in layers 3 and 4 and function as drivers. The TC neurons in the intralaminar nuclei, particularly the CL, send diffuse projections to layer 1, as well as layer 5 and 6 mostly in motor and frontal cortex. These matrix-type projections are important to increase the responsiveness of pyramidal neurons to core-type inputs. For example, the coincidence of matrix-type excitatory input targeting the apical dendrites in layer 1 with inputs from core TC input targeting the soma or proximal dendrites in layer 4 increases the probability of the pyramidal cell to fire an action potential in response to an incoming driver input.

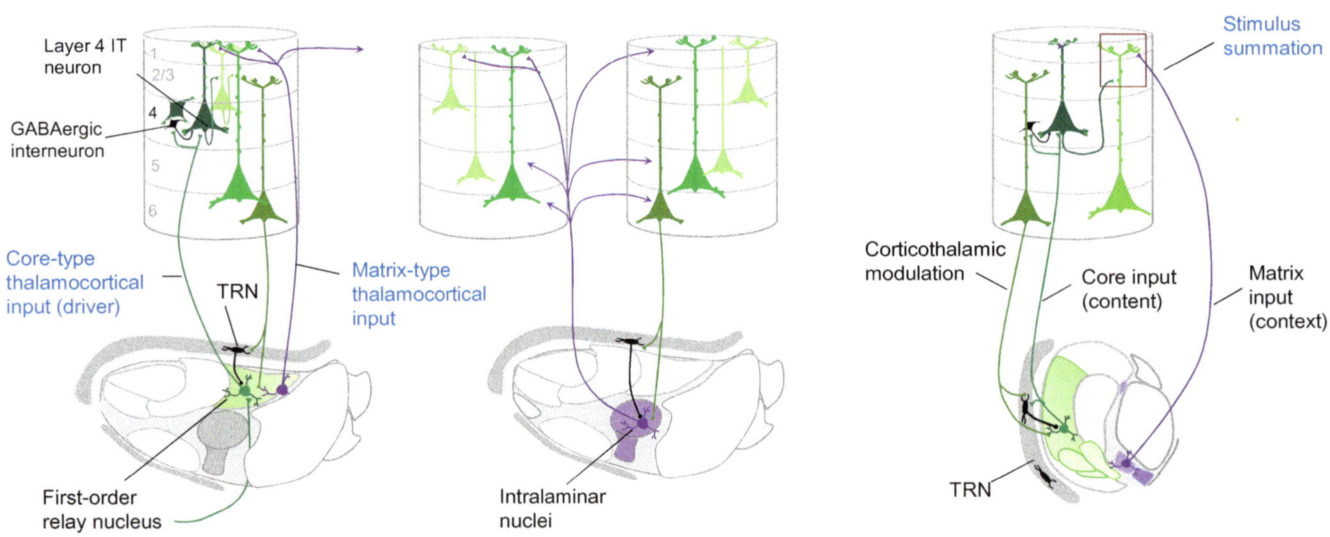

FIGURE 26.4 Reciprocal thalamocortical and corticothalamic interactions.
The projections from thalamocortical neurons to the cortex have been subdivided into distinct patterns, originating from different types of relay cells and referred to as "core" type and "matrix" type projections. Core-type thalamocortical relay neurons are located mainly in the primary (first-order) relay nuclei and project in a topographic manner to primary sensory cortices, projecting to layer 4, targeting both intratelencephalic (IT) neurons specific for each sensory modality and parvalbumin (PV) GABAergic basket interneurons. Matrix-type relay neurons are located predominantly in higher-order thalamic nuclei and project to layer 1. For example, neurons in the intralaminar nuclei, particularly the central lateral (CL), send diffuse projections to layer 1, as well as layer 5 and 6 mainly in the motor and frontal cortex, providing influence on widespread cortical areas. Corticothalamic (CT) neurons in layer 6 of the targeted cortical area send reciprocal inputs to both core and shell type thalamocortical neurons as well as neurons of the thalamic reticular nucleus (TRN) targeting these thalamic neurons.

Cortical Modulatory Inputs to the Thalamus

About 30%–50% of the pyramidal cells in layer 6 are corticothalamic (CT) neurons, which send topographically precise and specific modulatory glutamatergic projections to the thalamic nuclei selective for each sensory modality.[9] Layer 6 CT neurons receive input from all cortical layers and thus integrate processed cortical information with the direct input from the thalamus. Modulatory projections from layer 6 CT neurons target the most distal portion of the dendrites of both TC and TRN neurons and act via group I metabotropic receptors (particularly mGluR1) to elicit both direct excitation of TC neurons and disynaptic inhibition via TRN neurons. Corticothalamic modulatory inputs are critical for sensory processing in relay nuclei. Higher order nuclei receive layer 6 CT inputs from multiple cortical areas. There may also be contribution from the contralateral hemisphere to these corticothalamic projections.

THALAMIC RETICULAR NUCLEUS

In addition to TC projection neurons, which represent the majority of thalamic neurons, each thalamic nucleus also contain GABAergic interneurons that participate in local sensory processing. However, the TRN is the main source of GABAergic influence to the thalamus. The TRN forms a thin layer of tissue surrounding the thalamus and separating it from the cortex, and is thus a unique position to function as a gateway for thalamocortical information (Figure 26.5).

Organization and Connectivity

The TRN contains at least two different subtypes of GABAergic neurons targeting the TC cells in the relay nuclei.[10,11] Parvalbumin positive neurons target the first-order sensory nuclei and are primarily responsible for generation of sleep spindles. A given PV neuron of the TRN receives excitatory inputs both from its targeted TC neuron and from CT neurons of the topographically aligned deep layer 6 of the cortex. In sensory nuclei, this organization allows the PV neurons of the TRN to provide sensory modality-specific inhibition that reflects both "bottom-up" inputs coming through the thalamus and "top-down" feedback from cortex. A second group of TRN neurons expresses somatostatin (SOM). These TRN neurons receive inputs not only from the cortex but also from subcortical areas such as the amygdala, and mainly participate in circuits

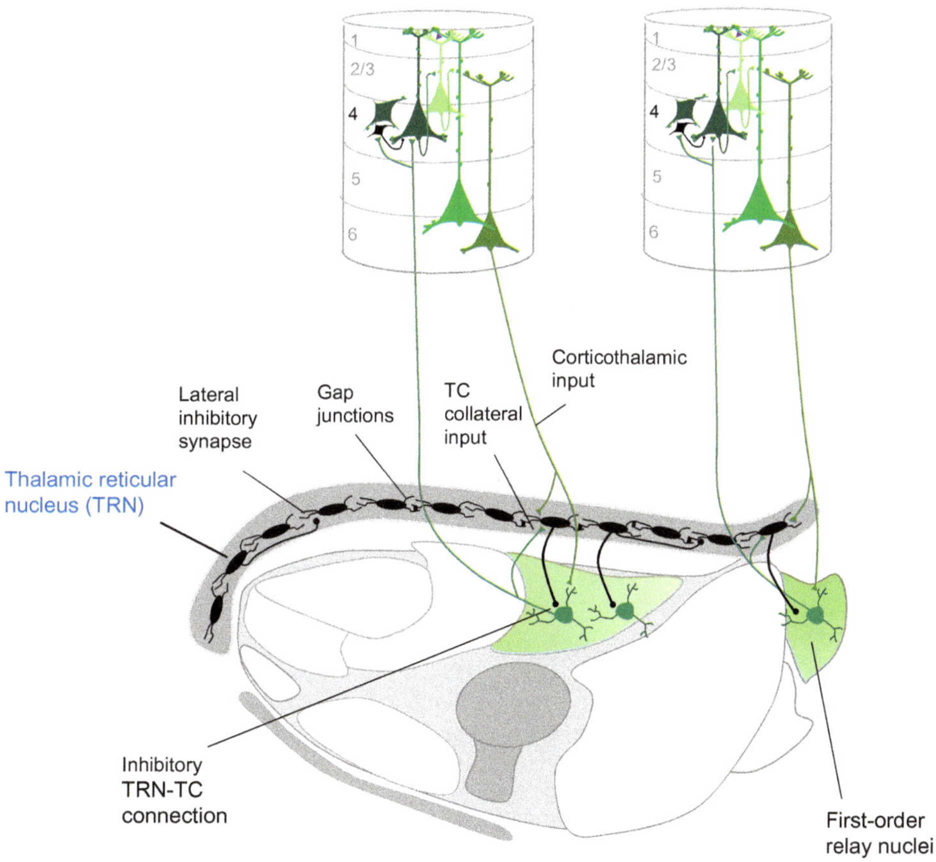

FIGURE 26.5 The thalamic reticular nucleus (TRN) is the main source of GABAergic influence on thalamocortical (TC) neurons. The TRN contains at least two different subtypes of GABAergic neurons projecting to the TC cells in the relay nuclei. A given TRN neuron receives excitatory inputs both from its targeted TC neuron and from the topographically aligned deep layer 6 of the cortex. The TRN neurons establish mutual connections both via gap junctions and via dendrodendritic and axo-axonic GABAergic synapses.

involving the intralaminar and association nuclei.[10] Via these projections SOM neurons may be preferentially involved in bottom-up limbic modulation of cortical circuits involving the PFC. In addition to their extrinsic connections, TRN neurons establish mutual connections both via gap junctions and via dendrodendritic and axo-axonic GABAergic synapses. The electrical coupling of TRN by gap junctions may enable coordinated firing and display activity-dependent plasticity; most of gap junction-coupled TRN cells project to a single nucleus. The interconnections between TRN neurons through GABAergic synapses may establish mutual inhibitory networks via $GABA_A$ receptors; these inhibitory connections may be important to prevent hypersynchronization within the TRN. Astrocytes in the TRN may release an endogenous benzodiazepine site ligand, producing a constitutive positive allosteric modulation of $GABA_A$ receptors ($GABA_ARs$) that suppresses synchrony in the TRN network.[12]

Effects of TRN Input on TC Neurons

At the TRN-TC synapse, GABA activates three different types of receptors (Figure 26.6). Postsynaptic $GABA_ARs$ containing α1β2γ2 subunits drive fast, phasic inhibition in TC neurons. The lack of a complete glia sheet around TRN terminals promotes GABA spillover and therefore the availability of GABA to activate extrasynaptic $GABA_ARs$ (containing α4β2δ subunits) and $GABA_B$ receptors ($GABA_BRs$). The uptake of GABA by the astrocytic GABA transporters GAT-1 and GAT-3 tightly regulates the activation of these extrasynaptic receptors at the TRN-TC synapse. Activation of extrasynaptic $GABA_A$ and particularly $GABA_B$ receptors results in large and prolonged inhibitory postsynaptic currents. As GAT-1 is localized closer to synapses, GAT-3 has a major role in limiting GABA spillover at sites located far from the synapses and required for sustained $GABA_B$-mediated inhibition (Figure 26.6).

FIRING MODES OF THALAMIC NEURONS AND THALAMIC OSCILLATIONS

The pattern of firing of TC and TRN neurons and thalamocortical oscillations have a major role in determining the cortical state and thus information processing.

Tonic- Versus Burst-Firing Modes

Both TC and TRN neurons display two types of firing mode: tonic and bursting (Figure 26.6). Tonic firing is mediated by sodium (Na^+) spike trains that allow TC cells to respond in a linear fashion to their inputs and reliably transmit information to the cortex. Tonic firing typically occurs during wakefulness and rapid eye movement (REM) sleep. Bursting is mediated by large-amplitude low-threshold calcium (Ca^{2+}) spikes (LTS) crowned by high-frequency Na^+ spikes. The LTS are generated by Ca_v3 (T-type) channels that are recruited at hyperpolarized membrane potentials. Thalamocortical neurons express $Ca_v3.1$ channels, whereas TRN neurons express Ca_v 3.3 channels. The majority of these T-channels are located in the soma, and their recruitment and spatial distribution leads to transient increases in intracellular Ca^{2+} throughout the somatodendritic tree. This results in activation of small-conductance calcium-dependent potassium channels (SK) and thus a prominent afterhyperpolarization following each LTS. In TC neurons a modest hyperpolarization to just 5–10 mV below normal resting potential (about -60mV) results in a switch from tonic- to burst-firing mode. This level of hyperpolarization de-inactivates Ca_v3 channels so that depolarizing stimuli elicit a LTS lasting 20–70 milliseconds, supporting a burst of action potentials.

Role of TRN–TC Interactions in Setting the Firing Patterns in the Thalamus

The intrinsic properties and synaptic actions of TRN neurons contribute to the time course of inhibition of TC neurons and thus to their gradual shift from tonic to burst mode. During tonic spike firing, GABA released from TRN neurons activates synaptic $GABA_ARs$ producing fast, phasic inhibition in TC neurons. During burst firing, GABA released from terminals of TRN neurons spills over and activates extrasynaptic $GABA_ARs$ and $GABA_BRs$ in TC neurons, resulting in large and prolonged inhibitory postsynaptic currents that promote de-inactivation of T-type channels, leading to reverberating TC–TRN–TC oscillations. Burst firing occurs typically during "inactive" states such as NREM sleep. However, compared to tonic firing, burst firing provides higher reliability of signal transmission, as it is less sensitive to noise and more effective to trigger responses in some neocortical neurons, thereby providing an "alert" signal in response to a novel, unexpected stimulus.

Pacemaker Activity of Thalamic Neurons

Whereas modest hyperpolarization to just 5–10 mV below normal resting potential allows the TC neurons to switch from a tonic- to burst-firing mode in response to GABAergic input from the TRN, further membrane potential hyperpolarization to ~ -80 mV leads to autonomous rhythm generation characterized by periodic LTS at frequencies of 1–2 Hz. This intrinsic (pacemaker) oscillation results from the interaction between the low-threshold currents mediated by Ca_v3 channels and a cation current mediated by hyperpolarization-activated, cyclic nucleotide-gated (HCN) channels followed by activation of Ca^{2+}-activated K^+ channels.

EXTRATHALAMIC INPUTS REGULATING THALAMIC ACTIVITY

The firing of TC neurons is controlled not only by their reciprocal interactions with the TRN and descending

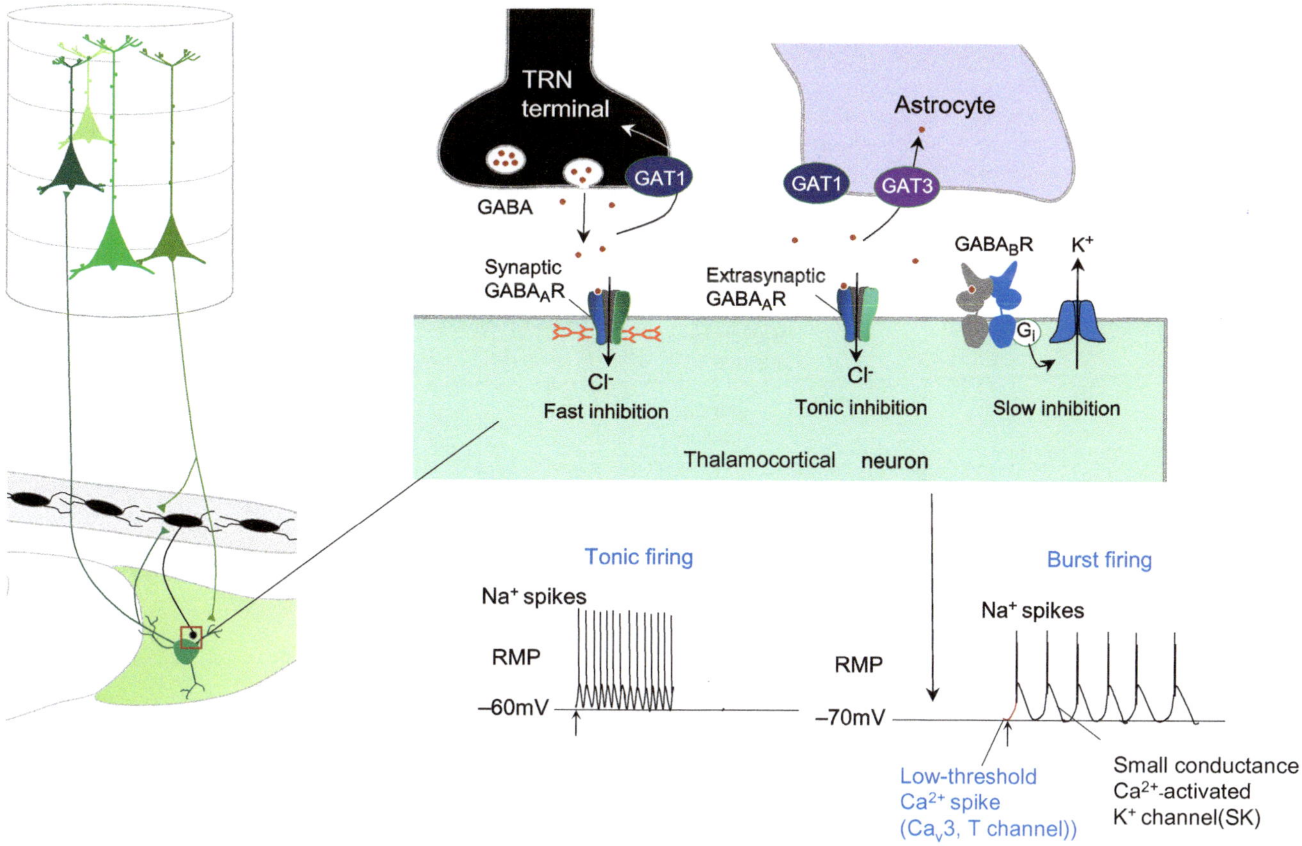

FIGURE 26.6 Effects of thalamic reticular inputs on thalamocortical neurons.

At the TRN-TC synapse, GABA can activate three different types of receptors, including synaptic GABA$_A$ receptors (GABA$_A$Rs) containing α1β2γ2 subunits driving fast, phasic inhibition in TC neurons; GABA that escapes uptake from astrocytes activates extrasynaptic GABA$_A$Rs (containing α4β2δ subunits); and GABA$_B$Rs receptors located up to tens of microns away from TRN synapses. Activation of extrasynaptic GABA$_A$ and particularly GABA$_B$ receptors results in large and prolonged inhibitory postsynaptic currents. Thalamic neurons display two types of firing mode: tonic and bursting. Tonic spiking consists of trains of sodium (Na^+) spikes and typically occurs during wakefulness and rapid eye movement (REM) sleep. A burst is a large-amplitude low-threshold calcium (Ca^{2+}) spike (LTS) crowned by high-frequency Na^+ spikes. The LTS are generated by Ca$_v$3 (T-type) channels that are recruited at hyperpolarized membrane potentials. The transient increases in intracellular Ca^{2+} results in activation of small-conductance calcium-dependent potassium channels (SKs) and thus a prominent afterhyperpolarization following each LTS, limiting the bursts to a precise duration. In TC neurons a modest hyperpolarization to just 5–10 mV below normal resting potential (about -60mV) results in a switch from tonic to burst-firing mode. During burst firing, GABA released from terminals of TRN neurons spills over and activates extrasynaptic GABA$_A$Rs and more distant GABA$_B$ receptors in TC neurons, resulting in large and prolonged inhibitory postsynaptic currents that promote de-inactivation of T-type channels in these cells, leading to reverberating TC-TRN-TC oscillations.

modulatory inputs from the CT neurons of layer 6 of the cerebral cortex but also by inputs originating from cholinergic and monoaminergic groups and extrathalamic GABAergic neurons (Figure 26.7).

Effect of Cholinergic and Monoaminergic Neuromodulatory Systems

The thalamus receives modulatory cholinergic and monoaminergic inputs from several sources.[9] These projections are particularly dense in the midline and intralaminar thalamic nuclei. Cholinergic inputs originate primarily from the pedunculopontine tegmental and laterodorsal tegmental nuclei. Acetylcholine excites TC neurons via both nicotinic and M1 muscarinic receptors and hyperpolarizes TRN neurons via M2 receptors. Monoaminergic inputs originate from noradrenergic neurons of the locus coeruleus, serotonergic neurons of the dorsal raphe, dopaminergic neurons of the ventral tegmental area, and

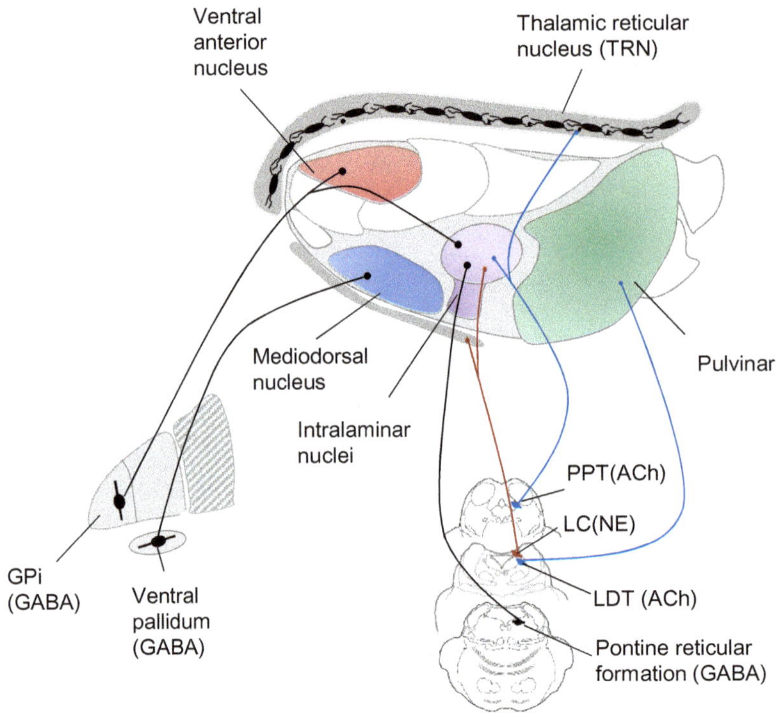

FIGURE 26.7 Extrathalamic inputs regulating thalamic activity.
Activity in thalamic nuclei is affected by local inhibitory interneurons and, particularly, by strong influence from extrathalamic GABAergic inputs. Furthermore, the activity of both the TC and TRN neurons is modulated in a behavioral state-dependent manner by inputs from cholinergic and monoaminergic cell groups. Extrathalamic GABAergic inputs originate from the output nuclei of the basal ganglia including the globus pallidus pars interna (GPi), substantia nigra pars reticulata (SNr) and ventral pallidum; and pontine reticular formation as well as zona incerta and anterior pretectal nucleus (not shown). Modulatory cholinergic inputs from the pedunculopontine nucleus (PPT) and laterodorsal tegmental nucleus (LDT) and monoaminergic systems such as the locus coeruleus (LC) are particularly dense in the midline and intralaminar thalamic nuclei. ACh, acetylcholine; NE, norepinephrine.

histaminergic neurons of the tuberomammillary nucleus. As in other areas, monoamines exert complex effects both on TC and TRN neurons via a variety of presynaptic and postsynaptic receptors. The modulation of excitability of TC and TRN neurons by cholinergic and monoaminergic inputs affects the firing patterns in the thalamus and strongly influence the cortical states. During NREM sleep, reduced of cholinergic-mediated depolarization of TC neurons promotes the deactivation of T-channels and thus the probability of TC neurons to switch from the tonic to burst firing in response to GABAergic inputs from the TRN.

Extrathalamic GABAergic Inputs

Extrathalamic GABAergic inputs originate from the output nuclei of the basal ganglia (GPi, SNr, and ventral pallidum), zona incerta, anterior pretectal nucleus, and pontine reticular formation.[11] One common feature among all extrathalamic GABAergic systems is their lack of projections to primary sensory relay nuclei. Instead, the GPi and SNr innervate motor territories; the ventral pallidum innervates the MD; the zona incerta and anterior pretectal nucleus innervate higher order sensory nuclei such as the posterior nucleus; and the pontine reticular formation innervates the midline and intralaminar nuclei. Extrathalamic GABAergic afferents exert a strong influence on TC neurons given their large terminals with many boutons that converge on a proximal dendrite of the TC neurons. Unlike the TRN, the extrathalamic GABAergic nuclei do not receive feedback from the thalamus and do not exert global inhibitory influence to synchronize thalamic activity. Rather, their global effects reflect inhibition of thalamic nuclei that have widespread cortical projections. For example, selective stimulation of GABAergic pontine reticular formation afferents to the intralaminar thalamus elicits cortical slow oscillations and interruption of ongoing behavior. Whereas neurons of the TRN receive input from CT neurons of layer 6, extrathalamic inhibitory nuclei receive inputs from layer 5. This layer 5 input provides for the emergence of an inhibitory loop cortico–extrathalamic–TC loop parallel to the cortico–TRN–TC loops triggered by CT inputs from layer 6.[11]

THALAMIC ACTIVITY DURING SLEEP

From the state of relaxed, inattentive wakefulness through the deepest stages of NREM (N) sleep, the EEG pattern progressively increases in amplitude and decreases in frequency from alpha waves (8–13 Hz) during relaxed wakefulness, to theta waves (4–7 Hz) in stage N1; sleep spindles (7–15 Hz) in stage N2; and delta waves (0.5–4 Hz) and slow waves (<1 Hz) in stage N3. These transitions in part reflect the progressive decrease of activity of wake-active cholinergic and monoaminergic neurons in the forebrain and brainstem. Intracellular recordings on TC and TRN neurons indicate that a common feature of these low-vigilance states is the rhythmic occurrence of action potential bursts driven by voltage-dependent Ca^{2+} spikes[13–15] (Figure 26.8). During sleep spindles, delta sleep and slow-wave sleep, these bursts have high frequency (100–500 Hz) and are driven by LTS mediated by T-type (Ca_v3) channels following short periods of membrane hyperpolarization. The membrane potential strongly influences whether a TC neuron will entrain spindle, delta, or slow oscillations.

Spindle Oscillations

Spindles consist of 7–15 Hz oscillations lasting between 1 and 3 seconds and separated by a refractory period of 5–20 seconds. The amplitude of spindle oscillations first waxes and wanes and later drops out as the spindle progresses. Spindles are generated by the PV positive GABAergic neurons in the TRN that primarily target first-order sensory relay nuclei. The strong recurrent connectivity between TC and TRN neurons enables thalamic spindle oscillations. During a spindle oscillation, groups of synchronized TRN neurons transiently inhibit TC cells via $GABA_A$ and $GABA_B$ receptors; upon release from inhibition, TC neurons fire rebound bursts that re-excite TRN neurons, initiating another TRN burst and the next. The neocortical feedback to TRN and TC neurons contributes to the properties of sleep spindles. There are two spindle-range oscillations in humans. Spindles in centrotemporal areas are faster than those in the frontal cortex and propagate in a posterior-to-anterior direction. In contrast, the cortical slow oscillations, which may be the trigger for global spindle initiation, travel in an anterior-to-posterior direction. Optogenetic studies in mice show that TRN neurons projecting to sensory relay nuclei are highly engaged in spindle activity whereas TRN neurons projecting to limbic thalamic nuclei such as the ANT do not engage in spindles but instead show reduced spiking during sleep.[10] This indicates that during sleep TRN-mediated inhibition is higher for sensory thalamic nuclei processing outside information and lower for memory-associated thalamic processing. This would presumably allow the replay of memory traces and enhance offline consolidation of information encoded in the hippocampus during wakefulness.

Delta Oscillations and Slow Waves

Delta and slow oscillations in TC and TRN neurons can occur via cell-intrinsic pacemaker mechanisms in the absence of neocortical inputs. During a transition into slow-wave sleep, progressive reduction in activity of neuromodulators leads to further hyperpolarization across the thalamus, biasing thalamic oscillations from spindles to delta and then slow oscillations (Figure 26.8). Thalamocortical neurons are capable of firing periodic bursts of action potentials at 1–2 Hz that, when synchronized, generate delta oscillations. These oscillations depend on the dynamic interaction between T-channels and HCN channels in TC neurons and Ca^{2+}-activated K^+ channels in TRN neurons. However, both the neocortex and the thalamus participate in producing delta and slow rhythms on the EEG. During sleep, the cortex generates a 0.3–1 Hz rhythm, termed the slow oscillation, which consists of alternating periods of high activity ("UP" states) and silence ("DOWN" states). During the "UP" state corticothalamic output drives widespread and coordinated TRN-mediated hyperpolarization across the TC population resulting in phase-locked rebound bursting, which once entrained initiates clocklike thalamic delta oscillations that are propagated back to the cortex. Whereas slow oscillations in the neocortical networks are primarily generated by interactions between excitation and inhibition, slow oscillations in TC and TRN neurons are generated by cell-intrinsic mechanisms. Tonic TRN firing may evoke targeted TC hyperpolarization and thus a spatially restricted version of global sleep-related delta or slow oscillations even during wakefulness. In humans, slow-wave power is amplified and slow activity during NREM sleep becomes more localized in task-related regions after learning. This allows offline processing and enhancement of hippocampal encoded memories and promotes their consolidation during sleep.

Thalamic Oscillations and Thalamic Plasticity

In addition to its critical role in generation of state-dependent oscillations during low-vigilance states, the increase in somatodendritic Ca^{2+} elicited during the LTS strongly affects thalamic synaptic plasticity.[14] The strength of the TRN-TC GABAergic synapse varies according to the frequency of LTS and thus the stage of NREM sleep. For example when LTS occur at slow oscillation frequency (< 1 Hz) they promote a Ca^{2+} influx via postsynaptic L-type channels; this triggers a retrograde signal mediated by nitric oxide and resulting in long-term potentiation of

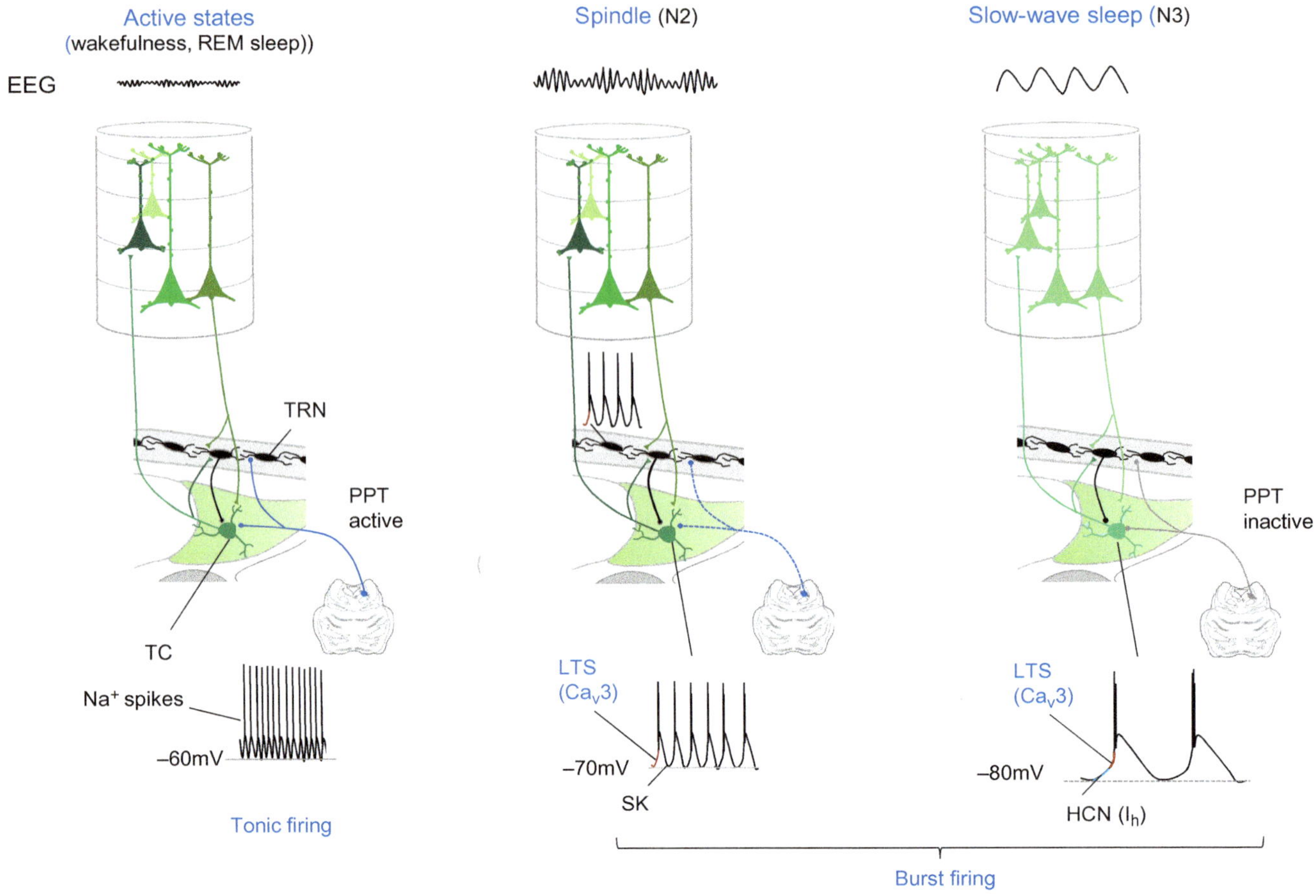

FIGURE 26.8 Firing patterns of the thalamus during sleep.
A common feature of low-vigilance states is the rhythmic occurrence of action potential bursts driven by voltage-dependent Ca^{2+} spikes in the thalamus. During sleep spindles and slow-wave sleep, these bursts are driven by low-threshold spikes (LTS) mediated by T-type (Ca_v3) channels following short periods of membrane hyperpolarization. The membrane potential strongly influences whether a TC neuron will entrain spindle, delta, or slow oscillations. Spindles are generated by GABAergic neurons in the TRN that primarily target first-order sensory relay nuclei. The strong recurrent connectivity between TC and TRN neurons enables thalamic spindle oscillations. Delta oscillations in TC and TRN neurons can occur in the absence of neocortical inputs via cell-intrinsic (pacemaker) mechanisms. Thalamocortical neurons are intrinsic pacemakers capable of firing periodic bursts of action potentials at 1–2 Hz that, when synchronized, generate delta oscillations. These oscillations depend on the dynamic interaction between T-channels and HCN channels in TC neurons and Ca^{2+}-activated K^+ channels in TRN neurons. PPT, pedunculopontine tegmental nucleus.

the GABAergic synapses from TRN on TC neurons. In contrast, when LTS occur at delta frequency, they trigger Ca^{2+}-dependent activation of calcineurin and long-term depression of the TRN-TC inhibitory synapse. The excitatory synapses onto TC and TRN also undergo LTS-dependent long-term potentiation or depression via activation of N-methyl-D-aspartate receptors. Thalamic activity may participate in homeostatic modifications of synaptic strength that occurs during sleep.[16] This involves downscaling of strength at particular synapses while preserving or increasing strength at synapses that have been strongly activated by novel features during the preceding period of wakefulness.

THALAMUS AND CORTICAL AROUSAL

Consciousness has two major components: wakefulness (i.e., the level of consciousness) and awareness of the environment and of self (i.e., the content of consciousness). Cortical arousal involves complex interactions among the brainstem, hypothalamus, basal forebrain, and thalamus. Fluctuations in the arousal state and vigilance are reflected both by changes in the EEG and functional connectivity in human fMRI.[17] In general, EEG indicators of cortical arousal and vigilance show an inverse correlation with the cortical fMRI signal. In contrast, states of low arousal are associated with increases in global fMRI signal at the cortical level and reduction in fMRI signal in arousal-promoting reagions including the midline thalamus and basal forebrain. The role of the thalamus in maintaining arousal is still incompletely defined. Classically the thalamus has been considered a critical relay for inputs to the brainstem reticular activating system to maintain the waken state. However, recent experimental studies emphasize the role of extrathalamic pathways in this function.

Thalamic Regions Implicated in Cortical Activation

The intralaminar nuclei, particularly the CL, have long been implicated in arousal, given their extensive projections that activate widespread regions of cortex. The CL receives direct excitatory inputs from brainstem glutamatergic, cholinergic, and monoaminergic arousal systems and sends diffuse cortical projections, thereby promoting overall excitability of the cortex during states of alertness. In contrast, GABAergic input from the pontine reticular formation to the CL may result in global cortical inactivation. In rodents, high-frequency optogenetic stimulation of the centromedial thalamus elicited cortical EEG desynchronization and behavioral arousal via glutamatergic mechanisms, whereas low-frequency stimulation elicited slow-wave and spindle-like oscillations, absence seizure-like spike-and-wave discharges, and behavioral quiescence through GABAergic inputs to the thalamus.[18] Selective activation of tonic neuronal firing in the centromedial thalamus preceded cortical UP states and transitions between NREM sleep and wakefulness, whereas burst activation elicited a state resembling sleep.[19] Glutamatergic neurons of the paraventricular thalamus may also have a critical role in maintaining wakefulness.[20] Whereas all the studies support a primary role of the thalamus in cortical arousal, another study in mice showed that extensive thalamic lesions had little effect on EEG activity, cortical activation, or wakefulness.[21] Rather, this study showed that the critical areas required for maintenance of wakefulness included the parabrachial nucleus and precoeruleus region via a relay to the basal forebrain and then to the cerebral cortex.[21]

THALAMUS, ATTENTION, AND MEMORY

Attentional operations include the ability to select relevant environmental stimuli from among less relevant ones (enhancing feature detection); to transition the focus of attention from one feature to another according to the environmental context (attentional switching or reorienting response); and to maintain "on-line" and manipulate the selected information in the absence of stimuli in order to guide behavior (working memory). These processes are under the control of interconnected frontoparietal networks. The thalamus has a critical role in attentional processing by controlling functional connectivity both within and across these cortical regions and is an integrative hub for functional brain networks.[22,23] The three major thalamic nuclei involved in these functions are the pulvinar, the MD, and the TRN.

Pulvinar and Functional Connectivity Among Visual Areas

The pulvinar has a critical role in visual processing and attention via its widespread reciprocal connectivity with multiple cortical visual areas. The inferior and lateral divisions of the pulvinar contain retinotopic maps receiving inputs from early visual cortex. The inferior pulvinar also receives direct input from the retina and superior colliculus and projects to dorsal visual stream areas processing object motion. The lateral pulvinar receives projections from V1 and early visual association areas of the ventral stream representing object features and projects to these areas. Pulvinar microcircuits and their outputs regulate cortico-cortical information flow by modifying the synaptic efficacy and functional connectivity within and across visual cortical regions. The pulvinar controls the interactions between primary visual and extrastriate visual areas during sustained visuospatial attention through coordinated spiking across pulvinar neurons, particularly in the alpha frequency band (~10 Hz). Alpha oscillations reflect the precise temporal parsing of cortical activity via phasic inhibition of layer 5 projection neurons in the posterior parietal cortex. This alpha-band synchronization may act to gate or suppress the processing of incoming sensory information at early stages in the visual cortex. During low arousal states cortical alpha oscillations drive the synchronized activity between the posterior parietal cortex and the pulvinar. During higher arousal states, the pulvinar drives the posterior parietal cortex in the theta frequency band during visual processing, particularly during active sampling of the external environment via saccades. The pulvinar is an integration zone for the interaction between visual networks (comprising primary visual and visual association areas), and the dorsal attention network, which comprises the posterior parietal cortex and the frontal eye fields.[24] Projections from the frontal eye fields and intraparietal sulcus indirectly innervate the pulvinar via the superior colliculus, forming cortico–colliculo–pulvino–cortical loops. This suggests that the pulvinar may coordinate attentional functions via integration of the visual and dorsal attention networks.

Mediodorsal Nucleus and Modulation of Prefrontal Cortical Function

Individual MD neurons can target multiple regions of the PFC and, like the case of the pulvinar, the same neuron can innervate one region with modulatory terminals and another region with driving terminals. These MD projections promote relevant recurrent synaptic interactions in the PFC, which maintain representations of task rules, for example those required for sensory selection. Via these mechanisms, the different MD subdivisions participate in multiple cognitive processes, including attention, working memory, familiarity-based recognition and retrieval, and emotional processing.[25] The medial portion of the MD is a component of a perirhinal-prefrontal system involved in familiarity-based recognition and retrieval processing[26] and also has a central role in emotional processing by interconnecting the amygdala and the posterior orbitofrontal cortex.[27] The lateral division of the MD receives converging inputs from the dorsolateral PFC and the superior colliculus, processes visuospatial information, and has a major role in working memory. The dorsal thalamus, including the MD, together with the caudate nucleus, are major cognitive integration zones and sites of convergences among different cortical cognitive networks, including the default, ventral attention, salience, and frontoparietal control networks.[24] Both subcortical areas are interconnected with core cortical components of these networks, including the ventromedial PFC (default network), ventrolateral PFC (ventral attention network), anterior cingulate cortex (salience network), and dorsal PFC (frontoparietal control network). Of note, another large-scale cortical network, the cingulo-opercular network, is integrated with cortical motor networks at the level of the VL (ventral intermedius) nucleus, which functions as a motor integration zone, suggesting a role of cingulo-opercular network in top-down control of motor functions via the thalamus.[24]

Thalamic Reticular Nucleus and Gating of Incoming Sensory Information

The TRN helps direct attention during behavioral tasks by becoming engaged in relevant thalamic inhibition. For example, neurons of the visual TRN sending inhibitory projections to the LGN decrease their firing in anticipation to presentation of a stimulus during a visual detection task. However, when behavior requires the selective gating of visual or auditory information, the activity of the corresponding TRN neurons may either decrease or increase, according to the sensory modality that is favored over the other. This differential TRN activity is important for distractor suppression and optimal task performance according to the target selected. Recent studies in mice indicate that in response to top-down corticothalamic input, SOM-positive TRN neurons enhance feature detection while decreasing attentional switching between features.[28] The PFC may also filter sensory inputs, augmenting relevant signals and suppressing noise through modality-specific TRN subnetworks via the basal ganglia.[29] The amygdala, via inputs of the TRN, may also promote emotional bias.[30]

Thalamic Oscillations and Cortical Interactions for Memory Processing

Oscillatory dynamics in several brain regions are associated with different aspects of memory encoding and retrieval via different thalamic-based circuits.[31] One model proposes that the thalamus participates in two different diencephalic circuits, a recollection-based and a recognition-based circuit. According to this model, the recollection-based circuit involves the ANT and its interactions with the hippocampus and mammillary nuclei; and the familiarity-based recognition circuit involves the MD and its interaction with the perirhinal and entorhinal cortex, PFC, and amygdala.[32] Another model proposes that the thalamus participates in oscillatory interactions within three different circuits. The circuit involving the ANT, hippocampus, and medial septum would maintain theta oscillations critical in encoding and retrieval of episodic memory. A circuit including the MD connecting the entorhinal, parahippocampal, and perirhinal cortex to the medial, orbital, and lateral PFC via synchronized beta oscillations may be involved in familiarity-based recognition memory. A third circuit involving the pulvinar and its interconnections with both parietal and visual cortex and the medial, orbital, and lateral PFC via alpha oscillation may be important for bottom-up memory control by inhibiting incoming sensory information during memory processing.[31]

INVOLVEMENT OF THE THALAMUS IN DISORDERS OF CONSCIOUSNESS

Depressed Vigilance or Coma

Lesions affecting the central thalamus can produce coma and vegetative state.[33] Coma may result from disruption of white matter pathways connecting brainstem arousal nuclei to the basal forebrain and thalamic intralaminar and reticular nuclei, for example in the case of traumatic brain injury.[34] In one study, strokes involving the paramedian posterior thalamus near the CMn/PF nuclei, posterior hypothalamus, and midbrain tegmentum were associated with impaired arousal; however, all patients with stupor or coma had lesions extending into the midbrain and/or pontine tegmentum, whereas purely thalamic lesions did not severely impair arousal.[35] This finding supports the concept that arousal primarily depends on extrathalamic pathways.[21] Consistent with this view, lesions involving a small region in the rostral dorsolateral pontine tegmentum corresponding to the parabrachial area were found to be typically associated with coma.[36] This region is functionally connected to the ventral anterior insula and pregenual anterior cingulate cortex, which are part of the salience cortical network regions and may become disconnected from the brainstem in disorders of consciousness.[36]

Disorders of the Sleep–Wake Cycle

Despite its still debated role in maintaining the state of arousal, the thalamus has a fundamental role in regulation of the sleep–wake cycle.[37] This is reflected by the sleep disturbances resulting from disorders such as stroke[3] or fatal familial insomnia.[38] Fatal familial insomnia is a prion disorder associated with pathological involvement of the anteroventral subnucleus of the ANT and the MD[38] and selective hypometabolism in the thalamus.[39] Fatal familial insomnia, like delirium tremens associated with alcohol withdrawal, and Morvan syndrome associated with contactin-associated related protein 2 (CASPR2) autoantibodies, produces a syndrome referred to as "agrypnia excitata." This refers to a profound loss of slow-wave sleep with reduction of sleep spindles and K complexes, associated with REM sleep behavior disorder.[40]

INVOLVEMENT OF THE THALAMUS IN ABSENCE AND TEMPORAL LOBE SEIZURES

Absence Seizures

The thalamocortical network is capable of generating high-amplitude generalized 3 Hz spike-wave (SW) discharges lasting 2–30 s that are characteristic of typical absence seizures. During this condition, TRN and TC neurons are simultaneously excited by synchronous, transient cortical input. As the cortical excitatory effect on the TRN overrides that on the TC neurons, the latter become hyperpolarized and produce a rebound LTS that propagates back to the TRN and to the cortex, triggering the next cycle of the oscillation. Studies in behaving animals show that synchronous bidirectional cortico-thalamo-cortical communication during absence seizures requires T-channel activation in TRN neurons.[41] The TRN bursts triggered by corticothalamic input elicit tonic feedforward inhibition and markedly reduced ictal firing of TC neurons throughout most of the spike-wave cycle, which may be responsible for loss of awareness. The slow wave reflects reciprocal excitation of TC and cortical neurons as well as excitation of TRN neurons by the corticothalamic input.[41] The precise timing of excitation may depend on both intracortical rhythmogenic mechanisms and corticothalamic interactions. Ethosuximide, a drug selectively used for treatment of absence seizures, modestly reduces T-currents in both TRN and TC neurons and increases the threshold for burst firing across the thalamus. Absence seizures tend to begin in frontal cortical areas; activity rapidly generalizes throughout the cortex in less than one second—within 1–2 cycles of spike-and-wave discharge.[42] In absence epilepsy, focal subnetworks, particularly those involving higher-order intralaminar and midline thalamic nuclei, may be particularly susceptible to hypersynchronization and global propagation of oscillations and thus able to evoke an absence-like state. Absence seizures are associated with widespread decrease in fMRI signal in the cortex and focal increases in the median portion of the thalamus.

Mutations affecting the control of thalamic oscillations may increase the probability of synchronization and allow a latent focal cortical network to generate SW discharges typical of absence seizures.[43] One such mechanism is activation of T-currents in TRN neurons. *CACNA1H* gene mutations affecting the $Ca_v3.2$ channels in these neurons have been associated with generalized epilepsy, as well as focal or multifocal epilepsy.[44] The susceptibility to hypersynchronization in the thalamus causing absence seizures is also affected by local GABAergic circuits. Gain-of-function of extrasynaptic $GABA_A$ receptors may also explain the electrical silence, marked decrease of tonic firing, and paucity of rebound bursts in TC neurons during the SW discharge. Variants of the *SLC6A1* gene encoding the GABA transporter GAT-1 expressed in presynaptic terminals are linked to a wide spectrum of epilepsy phenotypes, including myoclonic-atonic epilepsy, absence, myoclonic, and atonic seizures associated with intellectual disability.[45] Whereas excessive GABAergic inhibition at the TRN-TC synapse may predispose to SW discharge, GABAergic inhibition within the TRN may prevent hypersynchronization.[46] This inhibition is mediated by β3 receptor subunit containing $GABA_A$ receptors. Mutations of the *GABRB3* gene encoding this subunit are associated with childhood absence epilepsy and early onset epileptic encephalopathy that may respond to clonazepam.[47]

Temporal Lobe Seizures with Impaired Awareness

Experimental studies suggest that focal temporal lobe seizures depress subcortical arousal systems[46] and affect thalamocortical activity producing a pattern resembling slow-wave sleep, which may relate to impaired awareness.[48,49] For example, experimental temporal lobe seizures are associated with reduced activity of ascending cholinergic systems;[50] a switch from a tonic to a burst firing in the CL; a trend toward increased activity in the ANT reflecting polyspike seizure discharges seen in the hippocampus; and increased spindle activity in the first-order relay nuclei such as the VPM.[48,49] Reduced tonic and increased burst-firing in the CL as well as spindle activity in the VPM resemble the NREM sleep state, depressing thalamocortical relay of information and consistent with reduction of ascending cholinergic input to these areas.[50] The ANT, as part of the so-called extended hippocampal system, may be involved in maintenance and propagation of focal limbic seizures. Morphometric MRI studies show that patients with temporal lobe seizures and mesial temporal sclerosis have bilateral volume loss in the ANT that correlates with CA1 volume loss and thinning of the mesial temporal cortex. Microelectrode recordings in awake patients with severe epilepsy showed that the majority of ANT neurons had a bursting pattern of activity. Studies with simultaneous EEG recordings and functional MRI in patients with idiopathic generalized epilepsy showed abnormal activity in CMn/PF preceding that of the ANT, suggesting that the CMn/PF may be involved in epileptic discharge initiation or early propagation, while the ANT may have a role in its maintenance.[49,50]

INVOLVEMENT OF THE THALAMUS IN OTHER NEUROLOGIC DISORDERS

Focal Syndromes

The thalamus receives supply from four arteries, tuberothalamic (from the posterior communicating artery), paramedian (from the P1 segment of the posterior cerebral artery), inferolateral (from the P2 segment), and posterior choroidal (from the P2 segment). Vascular lesions manifest with different combinations of symptoms that vary according of the arterial territory[3] (Table 26.1). Some strategically located thalamic lesions produce cognitive and behavioral manifestations that mimic those resulting from lesions affecting their cortical targets.[51] Tuberothalamic territory strokes involve the ANT, which receives inputs from the hippocampal formation and mamillothalamic tract and projects to anterior orbital and medial PFC, anterior cingulate gyrus, and parahippocampal gyrus. Most patients with anterior infarcts show a unique behavioral pattern including disorganized speech with superposition of unrelated information ("palipsychism, from *palin* –again and *psyche*–soul) and perseveration (anterior behavioral syndrome), apathy, and anterograde amnesia with better performance in recognition tasks. Interruption of inputs from the ANT to the medial PFC may also explain the confabulations that are common in both anterior thalamic and medial PFC lesions. The episodic memory deficit that characterizes Korsakoff syndrome reflects involvement of the medial mammillary nucleus and ANT, as well as the MD. Vascular thalamic amnesia manifests primarily with declarative anterograde memory, with less consistent deficit in retrograde declarative memory. Paramedian territory strokes affecting the medial portion of the MD lesions affect familiarity-based memory for novel faces; lateral MD lesions impair recognition accuracy and cued recall. These lesions may also result in confabulation, temporal disorientation, and impaired social skills and personality resembling the manifestations of PFC disorders. Pulvinar lesions, particularly on the right side, resulting from posterior choroidal artery stroke produce a thalamic neglect syndrome resembling cortical neglect resulting from posterior parietal cortex lesions. These patients have deficits in encoding spatial information in the contralateral visual field, localizing stimuli on the affected visual field, binding visual features based on spatial information and filtering distracting information. Bithalamic lesions can occur with strokes due to occlusion of a single paramedian artery (of Percheron); venous infarction, Creutzfeld-Jakob disease, Wernicke encephalopathy, viral encephalitis (particularly due to flaviviruses and more recently SARS-Cov2), or autoimmune encephalitis. These lesions may manifest with confusional state, memory impairment, speech difficulties, day-night reversal of sleep pattern; sleep-wake reversal, and frontal lobe signs.

Thalamic Deep Brain Stimulation

The thalamus is a therapeutic target for deep brain stimulation (DBS) for several neurologic disorders, including tremor, seizures, tics, and neuropathic pain as well as psychiatric disorders such as depression.[52] For example, the VL (Vim) nucleus is a major target for treatment of tremor

TABLE 26.1 *Vascular Syndromes of the Thalamus*

Vascular Territory (% of Cases)	Nuclei Affected	Clinical Manifestations
Tuberothalamic (15%)	Anterior Anterior pole of mediodorsal Ventral anterior Rostral ventral lateral Reticular	Palipsychism Perseveration Apathy Anterograde amnesia Confabulation
Paramedian (35%)	Mediodorsal Intralaminar Midline	Decreased alertness Vertical gaze palsy Personality changes Disinhibited behavior Apathy Impaired familiarity-based Recognition memory and clued recall Aphasia Temporal disorientation
Inferolateral (45%)	Ventral posterior complex Ventral lateral	Hemisensory loss Thalamic pain Hemiataxia Lateropulsion Executive dysfunction
Posterior choroidal 8%)	Lateral geniculate Pulvinar	Homonymous sectoranopsia Spatial neglect

using DBS, radiofrequency or radiosurgery thalamotomy, and, more recently, focused ultrasound.[53] Effective DBS therapy for tremor critically requires optimal targeting to modulate the tremor network, which is more precise after determining thalamic connectivity mapped onto somatotopic maps of both motor cortex and cerebellum.[54] Studies also show a substantial improvement in seizure control upon DBS of the ANT in patients with medically intractable seizures.[55,56] Stimulation of the CMn nucleus appears to be more suitable for the control of absence and generalized seizures, especially in patients with Lennox-Gastaut syndrome.[57] In isolated cases, DBS of the anterior intralaminar thalamic nuclei increased arousal from a minimally conscious state, improved thalamocortical functional connectivity, and increased EEG activation.[58,59] Pallidothalamic oscillations may be implicated in the pathophysiology of Tourette syndrome.[60] A recent study showed that high-frequency DBS in the CMn/PF may suppress striatal output and reduce tic production; suppression of the motor and insula networks correlate with motor tic reduction, whereas suppression of frontal and parietal networks correlate with vocal tic reduction.[61]

KEY POINTS

- The thalamus has a critical role in relay of sensory information to the cortex, selective attention, cortical arousal, motor control, and generation of sleep spindles during non-REM (NREM) sleep.
- The thalamus includes several nuclei that contain glutamatergic thalamocortical (TC) projection neurons and the thalamic reticular nucleus (TRN), which contains GABAergic neurons that project to the other thalamic nuclei but not to the cortex.
- First-order relay nuclei receive modality-specific input from sensory afferent pathways and project to the modality-specific primary cortical sensory areas.
- Higher-order relay nuclei receive their main input from layer 5 of the neocortex and participate in cortico-thalamo-cortical circuits involved in attention and other high-level cognitive functions.
- The prototype higher-order thalamic nuclei are the pulvinar, which primarily interacts with visual association areas, and the mediodorsal nucleus, which interacts with the prefrontal cortex.
- The anterior nucleus participates in hippocampal circuits involved in episodic memory and spatial navigation.
- Intralaminar nuclei have diffuse projections to the cerebral cortex promoting cortical arousal and also project a powerful input to the striatum.
- The motor thalamus receives inputs from the deep cerebellar nuclei and output nuclei of the basal ganglia and projects to the motor cortex.
- Core-type TC relay neurons provide driving input to layer 4 of the target cortical areas, whereas matrix-type neurons send diffuse projections to layer 1, influencing widespread cortical areas.
- Corticothalamic (CT) neurons in layer 6 mediate reciprocal interactions between the cerebral cortex and both TC and TRN neurons and have a major modulatory role on thalamic function.
- The TRN functions as a gateway for thalamocortical information both during NREM sleep and during selective attention.
- The majority of TRN neurons are responsible for generation of sleep spindles.
- The TRN neurons establish mutual inhibitory connections, which are important to prevent hypersynchronization within the TRN.
- At the TRN-TC synapse, GABA activates synaptic $GABA_{A,}$ and extrasynaptic $GABA_A$ and $GABA_B$ receptors that shape the strength and frequency of oscillations in the TRN-TC circuit.
- Modulatory cholinergic and monoaminergic inputs promote arousal by preventing burst activity at the TRN-TC circuits.
- Extrathalamic GABAergic inputs strongly affect thalamic output to widespread cortical areas.
- The EEG transitions from light to deep NREM sleep reflect progressive decreased input from wake-active neurons and rhythmic occurrence of action potential bursts dependent on T-channel-mediated Ca^{2+} spikes in the setting of progressive hyperpolarization of TC neurons.
- The pulvinar has a critical role in visual processing and attention via its widespread reciprocal connectivity with multiple cortical visual areas.
- The MD promotes recurrent synaptic interactions in the PFC during attention, working memory, familiarity-based recognition and retrieval, and emotional processing.
- The TRN helps direct attention during behavioral tasks by engaging in relevant thalamic inhibition.
- The ANT has a critical role in episodic memory encoding and navigation.
- Lesions affecting the central thalamus can produce coma and vegetative state.
- Development of stupor or coma requires involvement of the parabrachial nucleus and surrounding areas.
- The thalamus is affected in sleep disorders such as fatal familial insomnia.
- Abnormal thalamic activity underlies disorders of awareness such as typical absence and temporal lobe seizures.
- Synchronization of spike-and-wave discharge during typical absence seizures involves activation of T-channels in TRN neurons, reduced ictal firing of TC neurons, and hypersynchronization of TRN circuits.

- Temporal lobe seizures with impaired awareness are associated with reduced activity of ascending cholinergic systems, tonic burst firing in the CL, increased activity in the ANT, and spindle activity in the first-order somatosensory relay nucleus resembling NREM sleep.
- Focal lesions affecting associative thalamic nuclei produce behavioral syndromes that mimic those produced by lesions affecting their targeted cortical regions.
- The ventral lateral VL (ventral intermedius) nucleus is a major target for treatment of tremor.
- DBS of the anterior thalamic nucleus may benefit patients with medically intractable seizures, whereas DBS of the intralaminar nuclei may benefit generalized seizures.
- Thalamic DBS may relieve symptoms in Tourette syndrome and, in isolated cases, promote cortical arousal in patients with minimally conscious state.

REFERENCES

1. Mai JK, Majtanik M. Toward a common terminology for the thalamus. Front Neuroanat 2018;12:114.
2. Sherman SM. Thalamus plays a central role in ongoing cortical functioning. Nat Neurosci 2016;19:533–541.
3. Schmahmann JD. Vascular syndromes of the thalamus. Stroke 2003;34:2264–2278.
4. Llinas RR, Ribary U, Jeanmonod D, Kronberg E, Mitra PP. Thalamocortical dysrhythmia: a neurological and neuropsychiatric syndrome characterized by magnetoencephalography. Proc Natl Acad Sci U S A 1999;96:15222–15227.
5. Jankowski MM, Ronnqvist KC, Tsanov M, et al. The anterior thalamus provides a subcortical circuit supporting memory and spatial navigation. Front Syst Neurosci 2013;7:45.
6. Vertes RP, Linley SB, Hoover WB. Limbic circuitry of the midline thalamus. Neurosci Biobehav Rev 2015;54:89–107.
7. Saalmann YB. Intralaminar and medial thalamic influence on cortical synchrony, information transmission and cognition. Front Syst Neurosci 2014;8:83.
8. Hintzen A, Pelzer EA, Tittgemeyer M. Thalamic interactions of cerebellum and basal ganglia. Brain Struct Funct 2018;223:569–587.
9. Varela C. Thalamic neuromodulation and its implications for executive networks. Front Neural Circuits 2014;8:69.
10. Clemente-Perez A, Makinson SR, Higashikubo B, et al. Distinct thalamic reticular cell types differentially modulate normal and pathological cortical rhythms. Cell Rep 2017;19:2130–2142.
11. Halassa MM, Acsady L. Thalamic inhibition: diverse sources, diverse scales. Trends Neurosci 2016;39:680–693.
12. Christian CA, Huguenard JR. Astrocytes potentiate GABAergic transmission in the thalamic reticular nucleus via endozepine signaling. Proc Natl Acad Sci U S A 2013;110:20278–20283.
13. Fogerson PM, Huguenard JR. Tapping the brakes: cellular and synaptic mechanisms that regulate thalamic oscillations. Neuron 2016;92:687–704.
14. Crunelli V, Lorincz ML, Connelly WM, et al. Dual function of thalamic low-vigilance state oscillations: rhythm-regulation and plasticity. Nat Rev Neurosci 2018;19:107–118.
15. Mak-McCully RA, Rolland M, Sargsyan A, et al. Coordination of cortical and thalamic activity during non-REM sleep in humans. Nature Communications 2017;8:15499.
16. de Vivo L, Bellesi M, Marshall W, et al. Ultrastructural evidence for synaptic scaling across the wake/sleep cycle. Science 2017;355:507–510.
17. Calabro RS, Cacciola A, Bramanti P, Milardi D. Neural correlates of consciousness: what we know and what we have to learn! Neurol Sci 2015;36:505–513.
18. Liu J, Lee HJ, Weitz AJ, et al. Frequency-selective control of cortical and subcortical networks by central thalamus. Elife 2015;4:e09215.
19. Gent TC, Bandarabadi M, Herrera CG, Adamantidis AR. Thalamic dual control of sleep and wakefulness. Nat Neurosci 2018;21:974–984.
20. Ren S, Wang Y, Yue F, et al. The paraventricular thalamus is a critical thalamic area for wakefulness. Science 2018;362:429–434.
21. Fuller PM, Sherman D, Pedersen NP, Saper CB, Lu J. Reassessment of the structural basis of the ascending arousal system. J Comp Neurol 2011;519:933–956.
22. Halassa MM, Kastner S. Thalamic functions in distributed cognitive control. Nat Neurosci 2017;20:1669–1679.
23. Hwang K, Bertolero MA, Liu WB, D'Esposito M. The human thalamus is an integrative hub for functional brain networks. J Neurosci 2017;37:5594–5607.
24. Greene DJ, Marek S, Gordon EM, et al. Integrative and network-specific connectivity of the basal ganglia and thalamus defined in individuals. Neuron 2020;105:742–758 e746.
25. Golden EC, Graff-Radford J, Jones DT, Benarroch EE. Mediodorsal nucleus and its multiple cognitive functions. Neurology 2016;87:2161–2168.
26. Pergola G, Ranft A, Mathias K, Suchan B. The role of the thalamic nuclei in recognition memory accompanied by recall during encoding and retrieval: an fMRI study. Neuroimage 2013;74:195–208.
27. Timbie C, Barbas H. Pathways for emotions: specializations in the amygdalar, mediodorsal thalamic, and posterior orbitofrontal network. J Neurosci 2015;35:11976–11987.
28. Makinson CD, Huguenard JR. Attentional flexibility in the thalamus: now we're getting SOMwhere. Nat Neurosci 2015;18:2–4.
29. Nakajima M, Schmitt LI, Halassa MM. Prefrontal cortex regulates sensory filtering through a basal ganglia-to-thalamus pathway. Neuron 2019;103:445–458 e410.
30. John YJ, Zikopoulos B, Bullock D, Barbas H. The emotional gatekeeper: a computational model of attentional selection and suppression through the pathway from the amygdala to the inhibitory thalamic reticular nucleus. PLoS Comput Biol 2016;12:e1004722.
31. Ketz NA, Jensen O, O'Reilly RC. Thalamic pathways underlying prefrontal cortex-medial temporal lobe oscillatory interactions. Trends Neurosci 2015;38:3–12.
32. Aggleton JP, Dumont JR, Warburton EC. Unraveling the contributions of the diencephalon to recognition memory: a review. Learn Mem 2011;18:384–400.

33. Honig A, Eliahou R, Eichel R, Shemesh AA, Ben-Hur T, Auriel E. Acute bithalamic infarct manifesting as sleep-like coma: a diagnostic challenge. J Clin Neurosci 2016;34:81–85.
34. Edlow BL, Haynes RL, Takahashi E, et al. Disconnection of the ascending arousal system in traumatic coma. J Neuropathol Exp Neurol 2013;72:505–523.
35. Hindman J, Bowren MD, Bruss J, Wright B, Geerling JC, Boes AD. Thalamic strokes that severely impair arousal extend into the brainstem. Ann Neurol 2018;84:926–930.
36. Fischer DB, Boes AD, Demertzi A, et al. A human brain network derived from coma-causing brainstem lesions. Neurology 2016;87:2427–2434.
37. Gent TC, Bassetti C, Adamantidis AR. Sleep-wake control and the thalamus. Curr Opin Neurobiol 2018;52:188–197.
38. Lugaresi E, Tobler I, Gambetti P, Montagna P. The pathophysiology of fatal familial insomnia. Brain Pathol 1998;8:521–526.
39. Prieto E, Dominguez-Prado I, Riverol M, et al. Metabolic patterns in prion diseases: an FDG PET voxel-based analysis. Eur J Nucl Med Mol Imaging 2015;42:1522–1529.
40. Montagna P, Lugaresi E. Agrypnia excitata: a generalized overactivity syndrome and a useful concept in the neurophysiopathology of sleep. Clin Neurophysiol 2002;113:552–560.
41. McCafferty C, David F, Venzi M, et al. Cortical drive and thalamic feed-forward inhibition control thalamic output synchrony during absence seizures. Nat Neurosci 2018;21:744–756.
42. Miao A, Wang Y, Xiang J, et al. Ictal source locations and cortico-thalamic connectivity in childhood absence epilepsy: associations with treatment response. Brain Topogr 2019;32:178–191.
43. Depaulis A, Charpier S. Pathophysiology of absence epilepsy: insights from genetic models. Neurosci Lett 2018;667:53–65.
44. Chourasia N, Osso-Rivera H, Ghosh A, Von Allmen G, Koenig MK. Expanding the phenotypic spectrum of CACNA1H mutations. Pediatr Neurol 2019;93:50–55.
45. Johannesen KM, Gardella E, Linnankivi T, et al. Defining the phenotypic spectrum of SLC6A1 mutations. Epilepsia 2018;59:389–402.
46. Sohal VS, Huntsman MM, Huguenard JR. Reciprocal inhibitory connections regulate the spatiotemporal properties of intrathalamic oscillations. J Neurosci 2000;20:1735–1745.
47. Zhang Y, Lian Y, Xie N. Early onset epileptic encephalopathy with a novel GABRB3 mutation treated effectively with clonazepam: a case report. Medicine (Baltimore) 2017;96:e9273.
48. Furman M, Zhan Q, McCafferty C, et al. Optogenetic stimulation of cholinergic brainstem neurons during focal limbic seizures: Effects on cortical physiology. Epilepsia 2015;56:e198–202.
49. Feng L, Motelow JE, Ma C, et al. Seizures and sleep in the thalamus: focal limbic seizures show divergent activity patterns in different thalamic nuclei. J Neurosci 2017;37:11441–11454.
50. Motelow JE, Li W, Zhan Q, et al. Decreased subcortical cholinergic arousal in focal seizures. Neuron 2015;85:561–572.
51. Carrera E, Bogousslavsky J. The thalamus and behavior: effects of anatomically distinct strokes. Neurology 2006;66:1817–1823.
52. Lee DJ, Lozano CS, Dallapiazza RF, Lozano AM. Current and future directions of deep brain stimulation for neurological and psychiatric disorders. J Neurosurg 2019;131:333–342.
53. Dallapiazza RF, Lee DJ, De Vloo P, et al. Outcomes from stereotactic surgery for essential tremor. J Neurol Neurosurg Psychiatry 2019;90:474–482.
54. Al-Fatly B, Ewert S, Kubler D, Kroneberg D, Horn A, Kuhn AA. Connectivity profile of thalamic deep brain stimulation to effectively treat essential tremor. Brain 2019;142:3086–3098.
55. Salanova V, Witt T, Worth R, et al. Long-term efficacy and safety of thalamic stimulation for drug-resistant partial epilepsy. Neurology 2015;84:1017–1025.
56. Zangiabadi N, Ladino LD, Sina F, Orozco-Hernandez JP, Carter A, Tellez-Zenteno JF. Deep brain stimulation and drug-resistant epilepsy: a review of the literature. Front Neurol 2019;10:601.
57. Velasco AL, Velasco F, Jimenez F, et al. Neuromodulation of the centromedian thalamic nuclei in the treatment of generalized seizures and the improvement of the quality of life in patients with Lennox-Gastaut syndrome. Epilepsia 2006;47:1203–1212.
58. Schiff ND. Central thalamic deep brain stimulation to support anterior forebrain mesocircuit function in the severely injured brain. J Neural Transm (Vienna) 2016;123:797–806.
59. Magrassi L, Maggioni G, Pistarini C, et al. Results of a prospective study (CATS) on the effects of thalamic stimulation in minimally conscious and vegetative state patients. J Neurosurg 2016;125:972–981.
60. Neumann WJ, Huebl J, Brucke C, et al. Pallidal and thalamic neural oscillatory patterns in Tourette's syndrome. Ann Neurol 2018;84:505–514.
61. Jo HJ, McCairn KW, Gibson WS, et al. Global network modulation during thalamic stimulation for Tourette syndrome. Neuroimage Clin 2018;18:502–509.

27 Sleep–Wake Cycle and Circadian Rhythms

OVERVIEW

Wake and sleep states are defined by changes in behavior associated with concomitant changes in electrocortical activity reflected in the electroencephalogram (EEG) and changes in motor and autonomic functions (Figure 27.1). The control of the wake–sleep cycle primarily depends on glutamatergic and GABAergic neurons distributed in the basal forebrain, hypothalamus, thalamus, and brainstem. The activity of these neurons is modulated in a state-dependent manner by cholinergic, monoaminergic, and peptidergic inputs.[1,2] The two primary triggers of sleep are homeostatic sleep "pressure" produced by periods of wakefulness or sleep deprivation, and circadian influences from the suprachiasmatic nucleus (SCN). Sleep promotes memory consolidation and clearance of brain metabolites and interacts with other homeostatic mechanisms, such as thermoregulation. Sleep disturbances are a major manifestation of neurologic disorders, including neurodegenerative, autoimmune, and focal brainstem or hypothalamic disorders. The aims of this chapter are to review: (1) areas involved in maintenance of wakefulness; (2) mechanisms that trigger onset of sleep; (3) the control of REM sleep and its associated phenomena; (4) the roles of the SCN in circadian rhythms; (5) the relationship between sleep and memory, and its age-dependent changes; and (6) primary disorders of sleep regulation.

PHENOMENOLOGY OF SLEEP

During wakefulness the EEG shows low-amplitude, fast frequencies, and the EMG shows variable amounts of muscle activity. Brain activity during sleep is characterized by circuit-specific oscillations, including spindles, theta waves, and slow waves, which are nested in thalamocortical or hippocampal networks.[3]

Non–rapid eye movement (NREM) sleep is associated with EEG patterns that define three stages; stage 1 (N1) at the beginning of sleep; stage 2 (N2) characterized by sleep spindles; and deep or stage 3 sleep (N3) characterized by low-frequency (0.5–2 Hz) delta waves. Sleep spindles during stage N2 are generated by interactions between the reticular nucleus (TRN) of the thalamus and thalamocortical neurons. Slow waves and delta waves in stage N3 reflect both UP and DOWN states in cortical neurons and pacemaker-activity of thalamic neurons. NREM sleep is associated with reductions of muscle tone. REM sleep is associated with low-amplitude mixed frequency in the EEG and absent muscle tone; tonic REM is interrupted by phasic phenomena characterized by brief irregular distal muscle twitches, rapid eye movements, and arousal reflected by increases in EEG frequency and muscle tone. There are also state-related changes in sympathetic and parasympathetic activity, baroreflex sensitivity, respiratory rhythm, chemosensitivity, and airway tone during sleep.[4] Whereas wakefulness and NREM sleep are often considered discrete states, arousal levels vary within these states. For example, levels of arousal vary during wakefulness and may sometimes correlate with pupil diameter. Levels of wakefulness fluctuate during the day, with a "physiological dip" in alertness in the early afternoon that correlates with a tendency for napping. Further, there is a "second wind" of alertness in the early evening, which interferes with falling asleep between 4 and 6 pm. NREM sleep is punctuated by spontaneous or stimulus-induced microarousals detected by spontaneous increase in EEG frequencies, K complexes, or delta bursts. Whereas REM sleep resembles wakefulness on the basis of the EEG, it differs from the waking state in several important aspects. Differences between

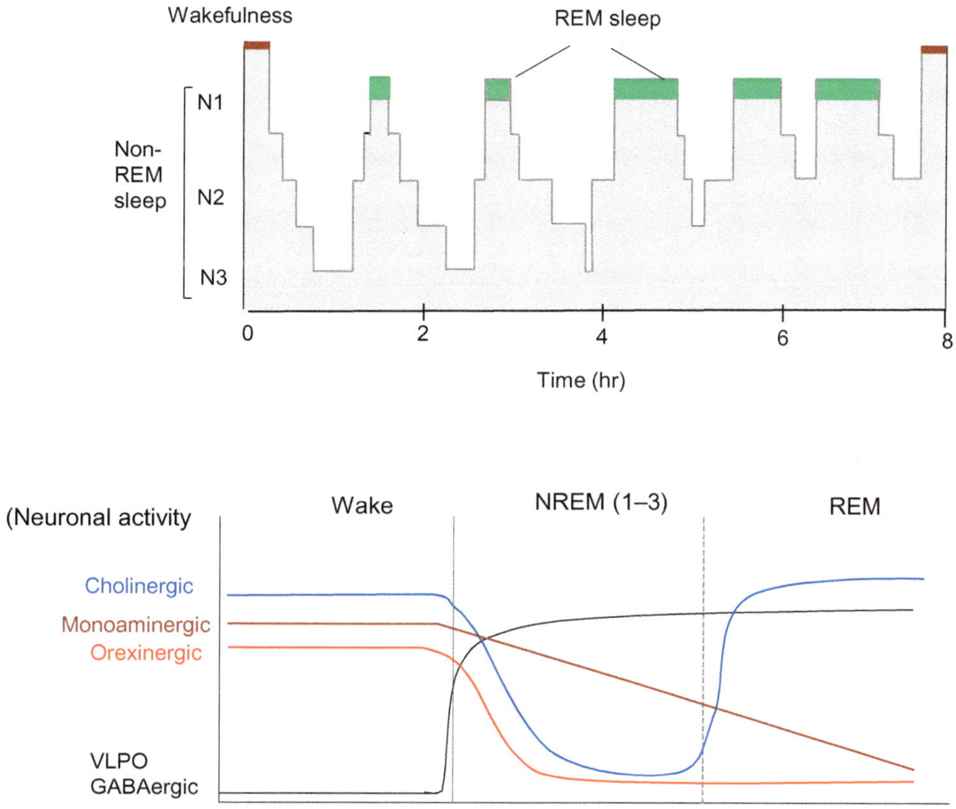

FIGURE 27.1 Architecture and neurochemical changes during sleep.
Wake and sleep states are defined by changes in behavior and electrophysiological associated with concomitant changes in electrocortical activity reflected in the electroencephalogram (EEG) and changes in motor and autonomic functions. VLPO, ventrolateral preoptic area.

REM dreaming and waking cognition are at least partly reflected in regional patterns of cerebral blood flow and glucose metabolism. For example, limbic and paralimbic areas (amygdala, hippocampus and anterior cingulate cortex) are more activated during REM sleep than during wakefulness, which may explain the emotional aspects of dreaming. Increased activity of posterior temporo-occipital cortices during REM sleep is consistent with the visual nature of dreams. In contrast, REM sleep is characterized by relative quiescence of frontoparietal associative networks, which could contribute to the lack of insight and control that is typical of dreaming.[5] Cerebral blood flow is higher during REM sleep than in NREM sleep. Dreaming may be reported in at least 50% of NREM sleep awakenings; compared with REM sleep dreams, NREM sleep experiences are shorter, less vivid, less bizarre, and less emotional and more related to current concerns.

The cerebellum also shows changes of activity during sleep. The functional connectivity between the cerebellum and the cerebral cortex is generally decreased during N3 stage; cerebellar activity is increased in REM compared to NREM sleep.[6]

MAINTENANCE OF WAKEFULNESS

Several neurochemical systems promote arousal and fast cortical activity typical of wakefulness. Brainstem wake-promoting pathways ascend through the paramedian region of the midbrain and then split into a dorsal pathway that innervates the thalamus and a large ventral pathway that innervates the hypothalamus, basal forebrain, and cortex. The dorsal pathway enables thalamic processing necessary for the content of consciousness. Patients with lesions limited to the thalamus are usually in an awake but unresponsive vegetative state. The ventral pathway via the hypothalamus and forebrain is essential for the behavioral state of wakefulness. Patients with injury affecting this pathway have difficulty staying awake.

Brainstem Arousal Nuclei

The brainstem contains several groups of glutamatergic, cholinergic, and monoaminergic neurons that change their firing pattern during the wake–sleep cycle (Figure 27.2). These neurons are active during wakefulness and decrease their firing before onset of NREM sleep. This activity reflects

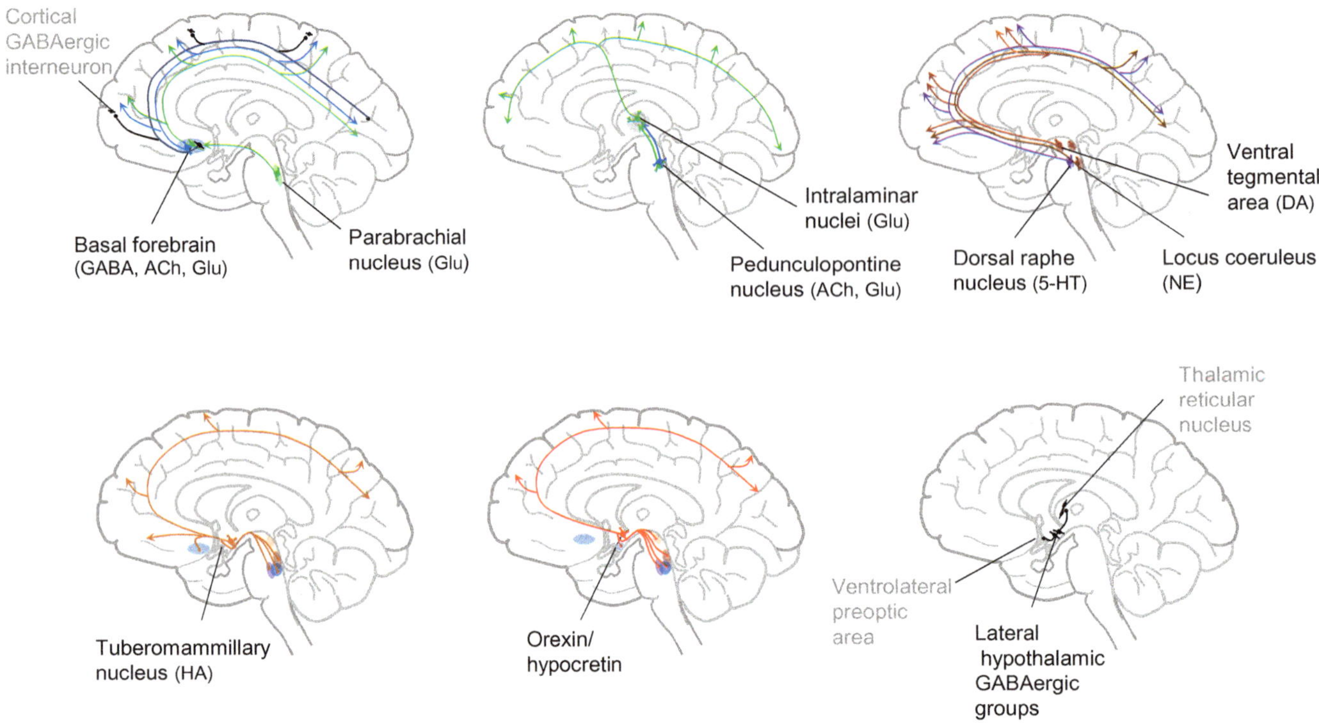

FIGURE 27.2 Areas involved in maintenance of wakefulness.
The brainstem contains several groups of glutamatergic, cholinergic, and monoaminergic neurons that change their firing pattern during the wake-sleep cycle. They include neurons in the basal forebrain releasing acetylcholine (ACh), GABA, or glutamate (Glu). Neurons in the parabrachial nucleus releasing Glu activate the basal forebrain and may be critical for maintenance of wakefulness. The pedunculopontine tegmental nucleus sends cholinergic projections of the intralaminar thalamic nuclei that activate the cortex via widespread glutamatergic projections. Monoaminergic arousal-promoting neurons including noradrenergic (NE) neurons of the locus coeruleus, serotonergic (5-HT) neurons of the dorsal raphe, and dopaminergic (DA) neurons of the ventral tegmental area (VTA). The posterior lateral hypothalamus contains histaminergic (HA) neurons of the tuberomammillary nucleus; orexin/hypocretin neurons that promote arousal both directly and via other arousal nuclei; and GABAergic neurons that inhibit several sleep-promoting regions.

the antagonistic influence of excitatory inputs from orexin (ORX, also known as hypocretin) neurons in the posterior lateral hypothalamus maintaining wakefulness and inhibitory inputs from GABAergic neurons in the preoptic region triggering NREM sleep.[1,2,7]

The parabrachial nucleus (PB) in the dorsolateral pons contains glutamatergic neurons that project to the forebrain and have a major role in arousal.[8] Neurons in the medial PB heavily innervate the basal forebrain, which in turn provides arousal signals to the cerebral cortex. Brainstem lesions affecting the PB region and surrounding areas are associated with coma in humans.[9] Glutamatergic neurons of the external lateral PB that also express calcitonin gene-related peptide are activated by hypercapnia and mediate hypercapnia arousal,[10,11] which has important implications for sleep apnea.

The pedunculopontine tegmental nucleus (PPN/PPT) contains cholinergic, glutamatergic, and GABAergic neurons that provide input to the thalamus, targeting primarily intralaminar nuclei that project diffusely to the cortex. Both cholinergic and glutamatergic PPN/PPT inputs to the thalamus promote thalamocortical activation, manifested by cortical gamma oscillations and EEG desynchronization. Cholinergic inputs promote tonic firing in thalamocortical neurons via nicotinic and M1 muscarinic receptors and inhibit neurons in the TRN via M2 receptors. The response of cholinergic PPN neurons to sensory stimulation is only transient whereas glutamatergic PPN neurons maintain a high discharge their more substantial role in maintaining cortical activation.[12,13]

Monoaminergic arousal-promoting neurons include noradrenergic (NE) neurons of the locus coeruleus (LC), serotonergic neurons of the dorsal raphe (DR), and dopaminergic neurons of the ventral tegmental area (VTA). These neurons promote arousal via several mechanisms. For example, the LC-NE system promotes arousal via α2 receptor-mediated inhibition of sleep-active neurons in the preoptic area, α1- and β-receptor-mediated activation of local GABAergic neurons in this region, α1 receptor mediated activation of cholinergic neurons of the basal forebrain, and α1 and β adrenergic receptors in the thalamus, hypothalamus, and cerebral cortex. Clonidine, which activates inhibitory α2 autoreceptors in LC neurons, reduces LC firing and has sedating effects. A recent study in humans with a loss-of-function mutation of the gene encoding β1 receptors that resulted in reduced need to sleep led to identification of wake-active neurons in the dorsal pons that express this receptor and were affected by the mutation.[14] Dopaminergic neurons of the VTA may promote wakefulness especially under conditions of high motivation. Drugs that increase dopamine signaling, such as amphetamines and modafinil, strongly promote wakefulness.

Basal Forebrain

The basal forebrain contains cholinergic, glutamatergic, and GABAergic neurons that innervate the cerebral cortex and target both pyramidal neurons and interneurons. These different groups of basal forebrain neurons make different contributions in promoting cortical activation.[15] Cholinergic neurons mainly promote fast cortical EEG activity without substantially affecting sleep/wake states. Parvalbumin-expressing fast-spiking GABAergic basal forebrain neurons target and inhibit local inhibitory interneurons in the cerebral cortex, thereby promoting both fast EEG activity and wakefulness. In contrast, somatostatin-expressing GABAergic neurons in the basal forebrain increase NREM sleep by inhibiting local wake-promoting cholinergic, GABAergic, and glutamatergic projection neurons.[15]

Hypothalamic Arousal Systems

The posterior lateral hypothalamus contains several groups of neurons that are critical for maintenance of the awake state (Figure 27.3). Injury to this region often causes severe sleepiness. At least three neuronal groups in the posterior lateral hypothalamus have an important role in maintenance of wakefulness: histaminergic neurons of the tuberomammillary nucleus (TMN); ORX (hypocretin) neurons; and GABAergic neurons. Histamine promotes wakefulness by several mechanisms.[16] Via H1 receptors, it activates the cerebral cortex, thalamus, and several wake-promoting brainstem neurons and also activates GABAergic inhibitory neurons in the sleep-promoting preoptic area. The relevance of H1 receptors in promoting wakefulness explains the sleep-promoting effects of H1 receptor antagonists such as diphenhydramine and doxepin.[17] In contrast, presynaptic H3 receptors inhibit the release of

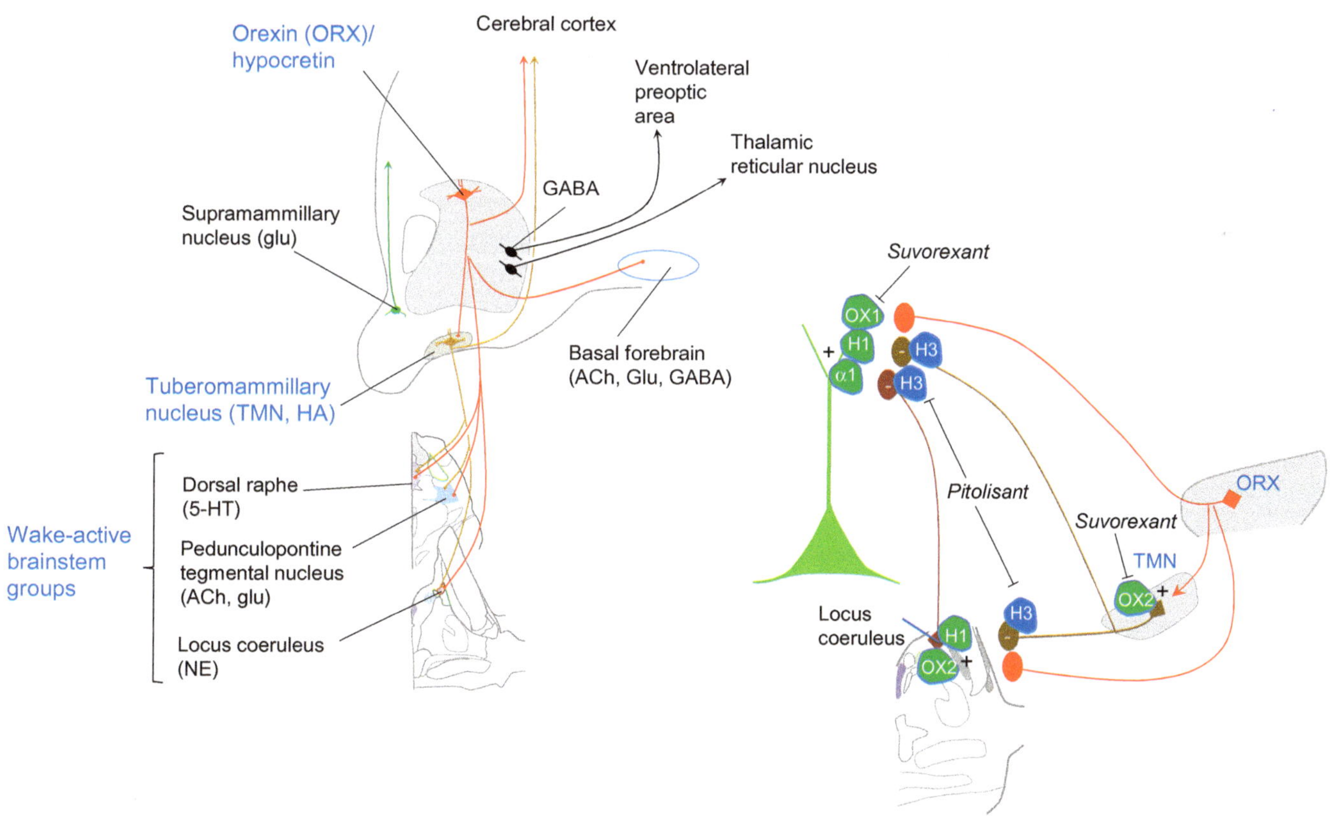

FIGURE 27.3 Orexin system and its effectors.
Orexin/hypocretin neurons are active during wakefulness, particularly during active wakefulness in response to stress, homeostatic challenges, and reward. They fire less during quiet wakefulness and very little during NREM or REM sleep. Orexin neurons heavily innervate and activate several regions that promote arousal, including the basal forebrain and brainstem cholinergic and monoaminergic nuclei. These effects are mediated by orexin 1 (OX1R, orexin A) and orexin2 (OX2R, orexin B) receptors.

histamine and other wake-promoting neurotransmitters. Pitolisant is a histamine H3 receptor antagonist/inverse agonist that triggers a long-lasting activation of histaminergic neurons and has been approved for treatment of narcolepsy.

Orexin/hypocretin neurons are scattered across the lateral hypothalamus and include two separate groups, one located around the fornix and the other in the lateral hypothalamic area. These neurons are active during wakefulness, particularly during active wakefulness in response to stress, homeostatic challenges, and reward. They fire less during quiet wakefulness and very little during NREM or REM sleep. Orexin neurons heavily innervate and activate several regions that promote arousal, including the basal forebrain and brainstem cholinergic and monoaminergic nuclei (Figure 27.3). These effects are mediated by orexin 1 (OX1R, orexin A) and orexin 2 (OX2R, orexin B) receptors. Via this mechanism, ORX stabilizes wakefulness and orchestrates REM sleep physiology.[18] Orexin neurons also release glutamate locally, triggering a local feedforward autoexcitatory circuit that maintains ORX neuron activity.[19] They may also co-release dynorphin, which inhibits local GABAergic neurons via κ-opioid receptors. These local circuits allow maintenance of extracellular ORX levels promoting prolonged maintenance of wakefulness. Suvorexant blocks both OX1 and OX2 receptors and is approved for treatment of insomnia.[17] In addition to their role in maintenance of wakefulness, ORX neurons participate in mechanisms of reward and motivation via projections to the VTA, and promote autonomic and respiratory responses during active behavioral states and stress via projections to the hypothalamus and brainstem.[20] Reciprocally, ORX neurons receive inputs from brain regions that regulate sleep–wake states, circadian rhythms, reward processing, fear and anxiety, autonomic activity, and visceral sensation. For example, ORX neurons are activated by arousal promoting glutamatergic inputs from the PB.[21]

There are two populations of GABAergic neurons in the posterior lateral hypothalamus that promote wakefulness by inhibiting neuronal group that promote NREM sleep.[22] One population innervates the TRN; the second innervates the sleep-promoting brain in the preoptic area. The supramammillary nucleus in the posterior hypothalamus contains a group of glutamatergic neurons that produce sustained behavioral and EEG arousal as well as theta and gamma frequency EEG activity.[23]

TRANSITION FROM WAKEFULNESS TO NREM SLEEP

The transition from wakefulness to NREM sleep is regulated by two main influences: previous duration of wakefulness (homeostatic mechanism or sleep pressure) and circadian rhythms. Thermoregulation also affects this transition. There is a functional overlap among these three sleep-promoting mechanisms. Neurons that promote the transition from wakefulness to NREM sleep are primarily distributed in the preoptic area of the hypothalamus.

Preoptic and Other Sleep-Promoting Areas

The ventrolateral preoptic area (VLPO) and median preoptic nucleus (MnPO) contain GABAergic neurons that are essential for promoting the transition from wakefulness to NREM sleep (Figure 27.4). VLPO neurons also produce the neuropeptide galanin. Both the VLPO and MnPO send inhibitory inputs to all arousal-promoting neuronal groups of the hypothalamus, basal forebrain, and brainstem. Reciprocally, arousal promoting nuclei provide inhibitory projection to the VLPO, either directly or via local GABAergic neurons. One model proposes that the mutual inhibition between the VLPO and wake-promoting areas generates patterns of activity akin to an electrical flip-flop switch.[1] This dynamic interaction should enable rapid transitions between states and the generation of full sleep and awake states with little time spent in intermediate drowsy states.

The VLPO and MnPO are not the only sleep-promoting areas. The basal forebrain contains GABAergic neurons that produce somatostatin and increase NREM sleep via local inhibition of wake-active basal forebrain neurons.[15] There is a cluster of NREM sleep-active GABA/glycinergic neurons in a region located just dorsal and lateral to the facial nerve in the rostral medulla and referred to as the parafacial zone in rodents; these neurons directly inhibit glutamatergic PB neurons that project to the basal forebrain and promote wakefulness.[24] There is also a subpopulation cortical GABAergic interneurons that express nitric oxide synthase, are active during NREM sleep, and may respond to homeostatic sleep drive by synchronizing slow cortical rhythms via long-range, intracortical projections. GABAergic neurons of the TRN are active during NREM sleep, are fundamental for sleep spindles in N2 stage, and contribute to slow oscillations during N3 stage.

Homeostatic Mechanism of Sleep Induction

Prolonged periods of wakefulness are followed by long periods of deep NREM sleep as revealed by a rebound of slow-wave sleep activity. This homeostatic response is likely mediated by sleep-promoting substances (somnogens) that accumulate during wakefulness and act as paracrine mediators to promote sleep. They include adenosine, prostaglandin D2, and cytokines such as interleukin-1 and tumor necrosis factor-α. The best-characterized somnogen is adenosine. Levels of adenosine increase in the setting of ATP depletion, thus representing a state of relative energy deficiency. Astrocytes and microglia may influence sleep pressure, duration, and intensity.[25] Astrocytes have multiple roles in sleep. One such role is to modulate the process of sleep

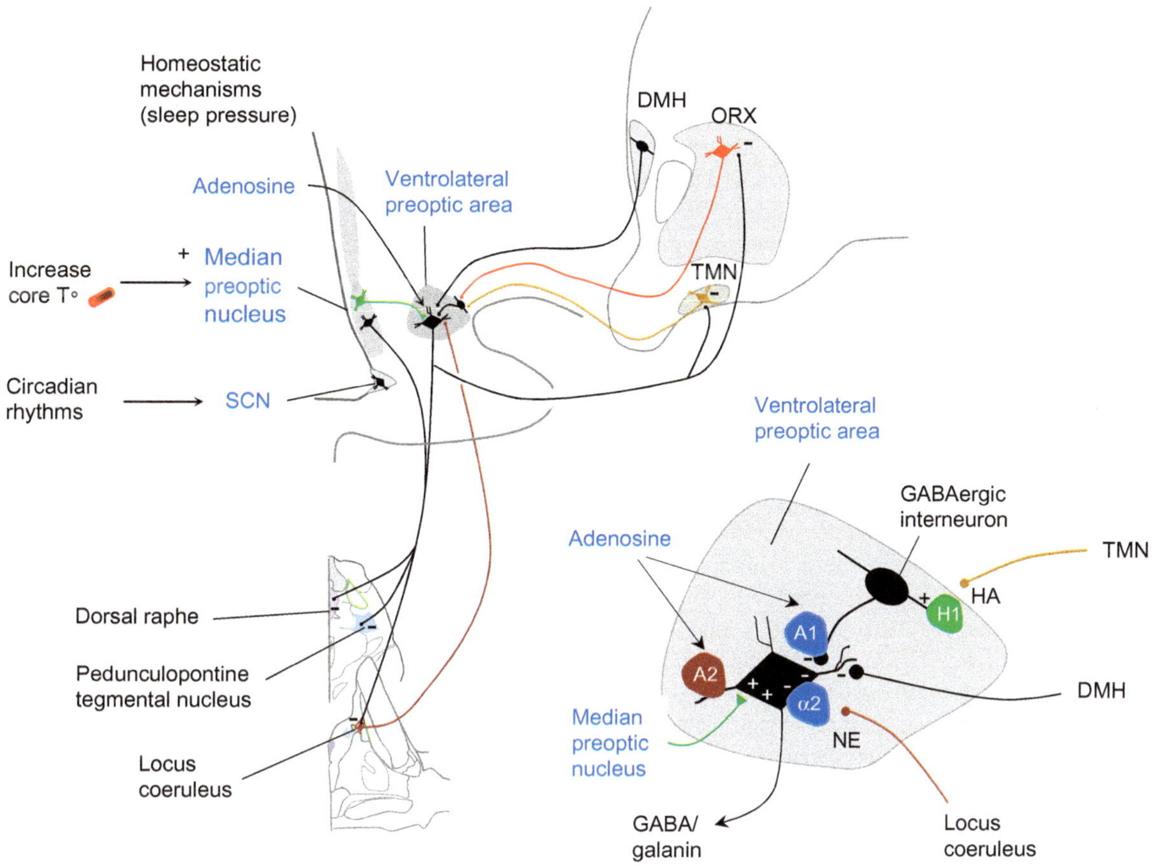

FIGURE 27.4 Sleep-promoting areas and their regulation.

The transition from wakefulness to NREM sleep is regulated by previous duration of wakefulness (homeostatic mechanism or sleep pressure) in part via signals such as adenosine and circadian rhythms controlled by the suprachiasmatic nucleus (SCN); as well as increase in body temperature (T°). The neurons that promote the transition from wakefulness to NREM sleep are located in the ventrolateral preoptic area (VLPO) and median preoptic nucleus, which contain GABAergic neurons that send inhibitory inputs to all arousal-promoting neuronal groups of the hypothalamus, basal forebrain, and brainstem. Reciprocally, arousal promoting nuclei, including the tuberomammillary nucleus (TMN), locus coeruleus, orexin (ORX) groups, and dorsomedial nucleus of the hypothalamus (DMH), provide inhibitory projections to the VLPO, either directly or via local GABAergic neurons.

homeostasis through the release of adenosine.[25,26] Adenosine promotes sleep via A1 receptors (A1Rs) and $A2_A$ receptors ($A2_A$Rs). The A1Rs mediate presynaptic and postsynaptic inhibition of wake-active neurons in the hypothalamus, basal forebrain, and brainstem; activation of A1Rs also inhibits local GABAergic neurons in the VLPO, thereby disinhibiting sleep-active VLPO neurons. Positron emission tomography studies in humans show increased A1R expression during sleep deprivation and normalization after recovery of sleep.[27] Activation of A2Rs promotes both NREM and REM sleep by increasing VLPO neuron activity. Caffeine antagonizes both A1Rs and A2Rs. Studies in knockout mice indicate that its wake-promoting effects are mediated by $A2_A$R blockade. It has been proposed that activation of $A2_A$Rs promotes sleep by suppressing arousal, whereas A1Rs mediate the homeostatic response to sleep deprivation.[28]

Suprachiasmatic Nucleus and Circadian Regulation of Sleep

Circadian rhythms dominate all physiological and metabolic functions, primarily via the sleep–wake cycle.[29] The principal circadian pacemaker is the SCN, which consists of GABAergic neurons that exert their effects on biological rhythms via projections to other hypothalamic nuclei. Via indirect projections, the SCN inhibits the sleep-promoting neurons in the VLPO and MnPO. The circadian clock integrates external and internal timing cues. This requires entrainment—the synchronization of the autonomous oscillator with an external timing cue, or *zeitgeber*. The most potent circadian *zeitgeber* is light, which activates the SCN via the retinohypothalamic tract. The circadian clock thus promotes wakefulness during the day even as homeostatic sleep drive builds. This wake-promoting influence turns off just before habitual bedtime. The functions of the SCN are discussed later in this chapter.

Thermoregulatory Influences on Sleep Onset

The circadian clock regulates timing and quality of sleep both directly and via its effects on thermoregulation.[29,30] There is a circadian rhythm in core body temperature of around one degree, with higher values at daytime and lower values during nighttime. Sleep onset is fundamentally connected with thermoregulation and occurs simultaneously with a reduction in core temperature.[30] Sleep promotes body cooling. Direct skin warming can shorten sleep-latency and promote NREM sleep. In humans, immersion in warm water between 1 and 8 h before but not immediately before going to bed promotes sleep this is known as the "warm bath effect." The interactions between changes in body temperature and sleep onset involves a microcircuitry in the preoptic area. Warm-sensitive neurons in the MnPO facilitate induction of NREM sleep both via direct inhibitory GABAergic projections to wake-active brainstem neurons and via excitatory glutamatergic/nitroxidergic projections to sleep-active VLPO neurons. There is a strong link between circadian cycle of core temperature and the onset of the first NREM sleep episode. If sleep onset is postponed by sleep deprivation, then the circadian temperature rhythm is disrupted.[30]

Role of the Basal Ganglia

There is increasing evidence that the basal ganglia control wakefulness and sleep.[31] Dopaminergic inputs from the VTA to the nucleus accumbens (NAc) promote wakefulness during motivational states. The shell of the NAc contains a group of GABAergic neurons that promote sleep via projections the ventral pallidum, lateral hypothalamus, VTA, and PB.[28] These NAc neurons are inhibited by dopaminergic inputs from the VTA via D2 receptors and activated by adenosine via A2Rs. In the absence of motivating stimuli, wakefulness is depressed via activation $A2_A$Rs in the NAc.[32] The NAc also contains a second population of neurons that express D1 receptors, are activated by dopamine, and promote wakefulness. These neurons project to the midbrain and lateral hypothalamus, and might disinhibit midbrain dopamine neurons and lateral hypothalamus orexin neurons via their inhibitory effects on local GABAergic neurons.[33] Recent evidence also supports a role of the external globus pallidus (GPe) on sleep control. The GPe contains GABAergic neurons that target the TRN, and both local GABAergic and projection neurons of the PFC. The GPe is a target of $A2_A$R-expressing GABAergic neurons in the striatum, which promote sleep via their inhibitory effect on the GPe.[34] A recent report showed that deep brain stimulation of the GPe improved objective and subjective sleep quality indices in a patient with severe insomnia.[35]

REGULATION OF REM SLEEP

The initiation and phenomenology of REM sleep depends on neurons in the dorsal pons, and is affected by several influences from the brainstem and hypothalamus (Figure 27.5).

Pontine REM-on Generator

Onset of REM sleep depends on a pontine region referred to as subcoeruleus nucleus (in primates, including humans) or sublaterodorsal nucleus (in rodents).[36,37] Neurons in this region fire tonically throughout REM sleep (REM-on neurons), and their activation rapidly produces low-voltage EEG, prominent EEG theta activity, and muscle atonia. Glutamatergic REM-on subcoeruleus neurons project to the gigantocellular reticular nucleus in the medulla, which sends an inhibitory GABA/glycinergic projection to spinal motor neurons; this pathway is responsible for muscle atonia during REM sleep. There may also be a glutamatergic projection that excites spinal glycine and/or GABAergic interneurons, indirectly inhibiting the motor neurons. Other neurons in the subcoeruleus nucleus promote rapid eye movements and EEG desynchronization via projections to adjacent nuclei in the pons and lower midbrain. Lesions that extend into adjacent regions can reduce the total amount of REM sleep.

REM Sleep-Suppressing (REM-off) Pontine Neurons

Several neuronal populations in the pons are thought to suppress REM sleep. There is a population of GABAergic REM sleep-suppressing neurons located in the ventrolateral periaqueductal gray matter (vlPAG) and the lateral pontine tegmentum. These neurons are silent during REM sleep and active during wakefulness and NREM sleep and send an inhibitory GABAergic projection to the REM-on subcoeruleus neurons. Reciprocally, during REM sleep, the vlPAG/lateral pontine tegmentum REM-off neurons are held in check by projections from REM-sleep active GABAergic neurons of the subcoeruleus nucleus. This mutually inhibitory circuit regulates REM sleep.[36,37]

Brainstem Modulation of REM Sleep

The neurons involved in the REM-on/REM-off switch receive modulatory inputs from the hypothalamus and brainstem. Cholinergic neurons of the PPT/LDT are positive modulators of the REM-on subcoeruleus neurons and increase their firing prior to REM sleep onset. In contrast, noradrenergic neurons of the LC and serotonergic neurons in the DR are REM-off neurons that inhibit the subcoeruleus REM-on nucleus and become nearly silent during REM sleep. Antidepressants that increase monoamine levels often suppress REM sleep. There is a group of neurons located in the dorsal and lateral paragigantocellular nuclei of the medulla that promote REM sleep by sending inhibitory

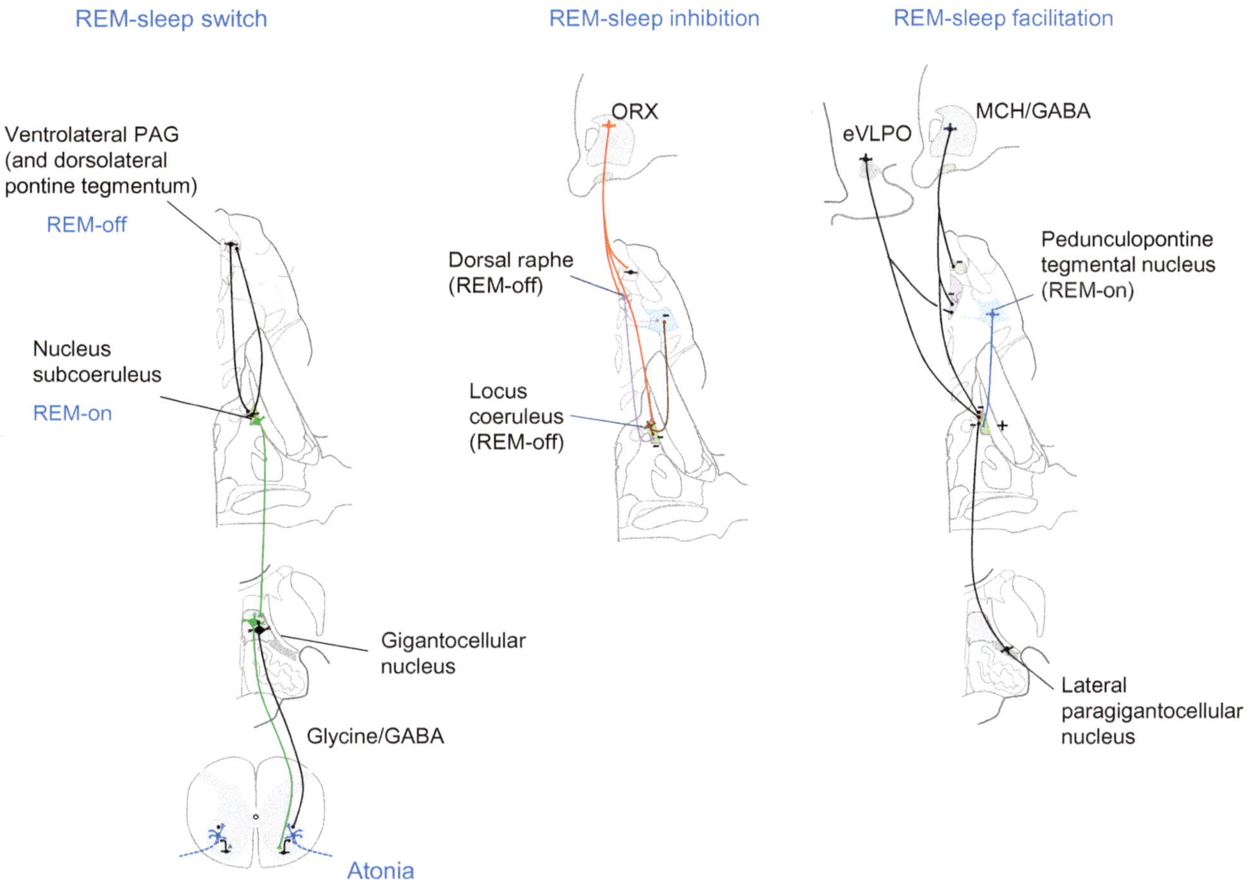

FIGURE 27.5 Regulation of REM sleep.

Onset of REM sleep depends on a pontine region referred to as subcoeruleus nucleus (in primates, including humans) or sublaterodorsal nucleus. Glutamatergic REM-on subcoeruleus neurons project to the gigantocellular reticular nucleus in the medulla, which sends an inhibitory GABA/glycinergic projection to spinal motor neurons; this pathway is responsible for muscle atonia during REM sleep. A population of GABAergic REM sleep-suppressing neurons located in the ventrolateral periaqueductal gray matter (vlPAG) and the lateral pontine tegmentum send an inhibitory GABAergic projection to the REM-on subcoeruleus neurons. Reciprocally, during REM sleep, the vlPAG/lateral pontine tegmentum REM-off neurons are held in check by projections from REM-sleep active GABAergic neurons of the subcoeruleus nucleus. The neurons involved in the REM-on/REM-off switch receive modulatory inputs from the hypothalamus and brainstem. Cholinergic neurons of the pedunculopontine and laterodorsal tegmental nuclei are positive modulators of the REM-on subcoeruleus neurons, whereas noradrenergic neurons of the locus coeruleus (LC) and serotonergic neurons in the dorsal raphe (DR) are REM-off neurons that inhibit the subcoeruleus REM-on nucleus. There is a group of neurons located in the dorsal and lateral paragigantocellular nuclei of the medulla that promote REM sleep by sending inhibitory GABAergic projections to REM sleep-off neurons. Orexin (ORX) neurons inhibit REM sleep via their input to REM sleep-suppressing regions such as the LC, DR, and vlPAG/lateral pontine tegmentum. In contrast, neurons producing melanin-concentrating hormone (MCH) promote REM sleep by inhibiting the REM-off groups, either directly or via co-release of GABA. One group of neurons in the extended ventrolateral preoptic area (eVLPO) send inhibitory GABA/galanin projections to REM-off neurons and also promote REM sleep.

GABAergic projections to REM sleep-suppressing neurons of the LC, DR, and vlPAG/lateral poutine tegmentum.[38]

Hypothalamic Modulation of REM Sleep

There are several hypothalamic groups that modulate REM sleep. ORX neurons inhibit REM sleep via their input to REM sleep-suppressing regions such as the LC, DR, and vlPAG/lateral pontine tegmentum. In contrast, neurons scattered across the lateral and posterior hypothalamus and producing melanin-concentrating hormone (MCH)[39] are strongly activated during REM sleep. These neurons are intermingled with ORX neurons and widely project to the brainstem, where they inhibit the REM-off groups, either directly via MCH-1 receptors or via co-release of GABA. Furthermore, glutamate released from these MCH neurons may directly activate pontine REM sleep-promoting neurons. In addition, MCH neurons send GABAergic inhibitory inputs to TMN histamine neurons, thereby reducing wakefulness. The firing pattern of MCH neurons is reciprocal to that of the ORX neurons; MCH neurons discharge maximally during REM sleep when complete muscle atonia occurs, whereas the ORX neurons are silent during REM sleep but fire maximally during active wakefulness when muscle tone is high. These two groups of neurons innervate each other, potentially exerting mutually inhibitory effects. One group of neurons located just dorsal and medial to the VLPO, in a region referred to as the extended VLPO, sends inhibitory GABA/galanin projections to REM-off neurons in the LC, DR, and vlPAG/lateral pontine tegmentum and also promotes REM sleep.

During REM sleep there is activation of the anterior cingulate, retrosplenial, medial entorhinal, and dentate gyrus, whereas other cortical areas are inactivated. The tonic activation of these limbic areas may reflect projections from glutamatergic neurons in the claustrum and GABA/glutamatergic neurons in the supramammillary nucleus driven by GABAergic neurons in the medial septum involved in generation of the theta rhythm.[5]

CIRCADIAN RHYTHMS

Circadian rhythms are driven by cellular "clocks" that are distributed throughout the body and prepare the body to perform functions appropriate for the anticipated day or anticipated night. The defining property of circadian clocks is that their intrinsic oscillation persists "free-running" with a period of approximately (*circa-*) one day (*diem*) when deprived of environmental cues. Circadian rhythms result from programs of negative feedback oscillations of transcription and translation that direct tissue-specific patterns of gene expression.

Molecular Clock Mechanisms

The cellular basis of circadian timekeeping in the SCN and other tissue is a cell-autonomous clock consisting of interlocking transcriptional–translational feedback loops that drive spontaneous oscillations of gene and protein expression[40–44] (Figure 27.6). These self-sustaining loops begin at circadian dawn (circadian time 0) with the formation of a heterodimer of the transcription factors CLOCK and BMAL1. These heterodimers bind to E-boxes in DNA sequences, driving the expression of an estimated 10%–15% of all genes in all tissues. Among them are the genes encoding the repressor factors (PER) and cryptochrome (CRY). At the end of the circadian day (circadian time 12) large PER-CRY multimeric complexes that have translocated into the nucleus repress their own transcription and that of CLOCK/BMAL1 activated genes. During the course of the ensuing circadian night (circadian time 12–24/0) the *PER* and *CRY* mRNA levels fall and PER and CRY undergo posttranslational modifications and then proteasomal degradation, ultimately allowing the start of a new circadian cycle. In addition to this central circuit, there is an additional regulatory loop that involves the nuclear retinoic acid receptor-related orphan receptors RORα and REV-ERB that regulate *BMAL1* transcription. A variety of signaling pathways influence core clock regulators by inducing several posttranslational modifications that ultimately lead to changes in clock control. They include acetylation, phosphorylation, and sumoylation. One important example is posttranslational phosphorylation of PER, which affects its nuclear localization. PER phosphorylation is regulated by the balanced activity of casein kinase 1 and protein phosphatase 1. Changes in phosphorylation of PER resulting from missense mutation at a putative phosphorylation site in PER2 cause familial advanced sleep phase syndrome, which is characterized by a lifelong pattern of sleep onset in the early evening and offset in the early morning.[45,46] Several other mutations have been linked to this disorder.[47]

The control of circadian gene expression by the clock is associated with chromatin remodeling. Among chromatin remodelers, the nicotine adenine dinucleotide (NAD)-dependent sirtuin 1 (SIRT1) deacetylase provides a molecular link between metabolism, epigenetics, and the circadian clock. By this mechanism, circadian oscillations in kinase pathways, energy metabolism (AMP/ATP ratio), and redox state (NAD/NADH ratio) link global control of cellular physiology and metabolism to the molecular clock. For example, CLOCK–BMAL1 complexes control the expression of nicotinamide phosphoribosyl transferase (NAMPT), which is the rate-limiting enzyme of NAD biosynthesis. Thus, NAMPT oscillations control circadian fluctuations in NAD levels, which in turn modulate SIRT1 activity and signaling. High levels of NAD+ activate SIRT1 which interacts directly with CLOCK–BMAL1 to deacetylate BMAL1 and inhibit CLOCK-driven transcription.

Properties of SCN Neurons

The SCN is composed of approximately 10,000 interconnected neurons in humans. All SCN neurons are GABAergic, and are subdivided into two functionally distinct and interconnected regions: the ventral core and the dorsal shell (Figure 27.7). Neurons in the core also contain vasoactive intestinal polypeptide (VIP) and are the recipients of retinal inputs via the retinohypothalamic tract (RHT). Neurons in the shell also express arginine vasopressin (AVP) and other neuropeptides; they receive input from the core region, provide feedback to the core, and send direct outputs to other brain areas. A key feature of SCN neurons is their spontaneous firing cycle, which oscillates between <1 Hz and >10 Hz and encodes the solar time. The ability of SCN neurons to sustain autonomous circadian oscillations reflects their

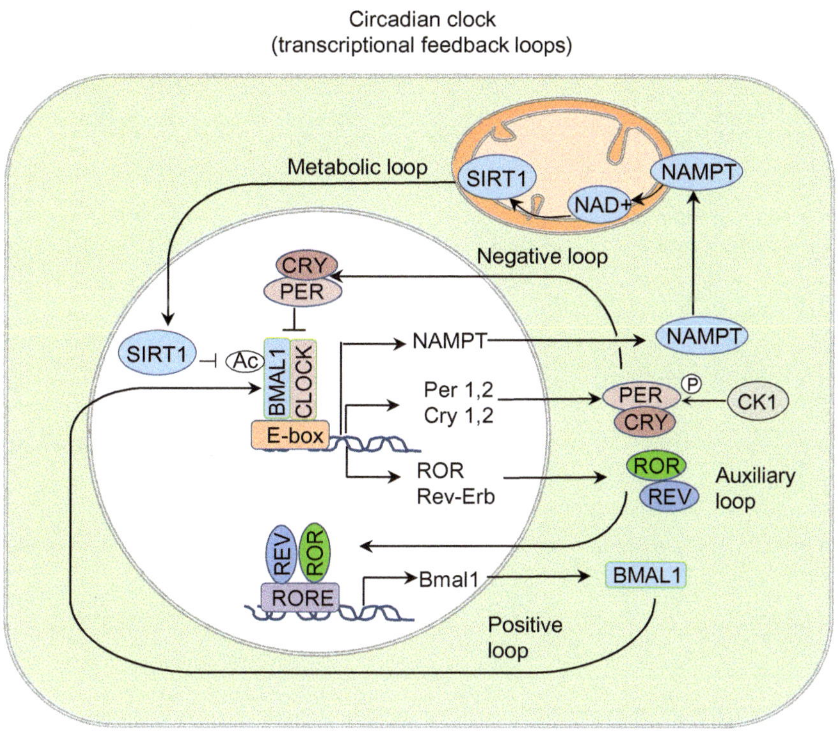

FIGURE 27.6 Molecular circadian clocks.

The cellular basis of circadian timekeeping is in a cell-autonomous clock consisting of interlocking transcriptional–translational feedback loops. These self-sustaining loops begin at circadian dawn with the formation of a heterodimer of the transcription factors CLOCK and BMAL1. These heterodimers bind to E-boxes in DNA sequences encoding repressors period (PER) and cryptochrome (CRY). At the end of the circadian day (circadian time 12) large PER-CRY multimeric complexes that have translocated into the nucleus repress their own transcription and that of CLOCK/BMAL1-activated genes. There is an additional regulatory loop that involves the nuclear retinoic acid receptor-related orphan receptors RORα and REV-ERB that regulate *BMAL1* transcription. One important mechanism that regulates the feedback loops is posttranslational phosphorylation of PER controlled by the balanced activity of casein kinase 1 (CK1). The control of circadian gene expression by the clock is associated with chromatin remodeling. The nicotine adenine dinucleotide (NAD)–dependent sirtuin 1 (SIRT1) deacetylase participates in this processs. CLOCK–BMAL1 complexes control the expression of nicotinamide phosphoribosyl transferase (NAMPT), which is the rate-limiting enzyme of NAD+ biosynthesis.

powerful intercellular coupling conferred by electrophysiological and synaptic activity.[48] Individual SCN neurons exhibit spontaneous rhythms in membrane potential and firing rate that peaks in the middle of day; the resting membrane potential spontaneously switches between daytime depolarization (about -45 mV) and nocturnal hyperpolarization (about -55mV). The circadian regulation of the membrane potential in SCN neurons reflects an alternating state determined by the complementary circadian changes in depolarizing sodium and calcium conductances and hyperpolarizing potassium conductances (i.e., the "bicycle" model). The linkage between balanced daily programs of ionic conductances and molecular oscillations in the SCN probably involves second-messenger signals such as circadian oscillations of cyclic AMP (cAMP) and intracellular calcium, which peak in the middle of circadian day and correlate with the daily peak of membrane depolarization and neuronal firing rate.

Retinohypothalamic Tract and Light Entrainment of the Circadian Rhythm

The major source of light information to the SCN is the RHT, which primarily originates in intrinsically photosensitive melanopsin-synthesizing retinal ganglion cells. These cells are most sensitive to relatively short wavelengths, paralleling the particularly strong effect of blue light in entrainment. In response to light, melanopsin causes depolarization of these cells, resulting in the release of glutamate and pituitary adenylyl-cyclase-activating peptide from RHT terminals in the ventral core of the SCN. Glutamate activates these core neurons, which then propagate this activity to the surrounding shell in a paracrine fashion via VIP and GABA. Light-induced increase in SCN firing causes a phase shift in the transcriptional–translational feedback loop, which likely involves circadian oscillations of cAMP and intracellular calcium. Given that the *PER* genes contain calcium/cAMP-response elements in their

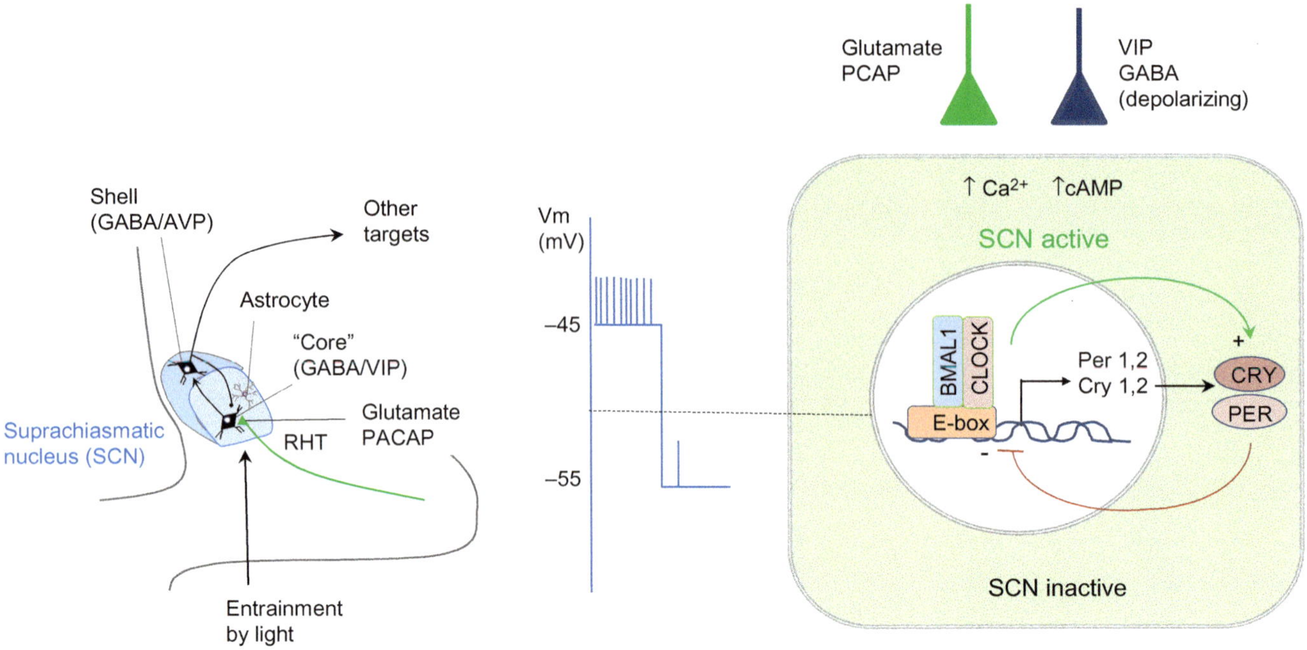

FIGURE 27.7 Physiology of the suprachiasmatic nucleus (SCN).
The SCN includes a core that contains GABA/vasoactive intestinal polypeptide (VIP) neurons that receive retinal inputs via the retinohypothalamic tract (RHT) and a shell that contains GABA/arginine vasopressin (AVP) neurons that receive input from the core region, provide feedback to the core, and send direct outputs to other brain areas. SCN neurons have a spontaneous firing cycle. Individual SCN neurons exhibit spontaneous rhythms in membrane potential and firing rate that peaks in the middle of day; the resting membrane potential spontaneously switches between daytime depolarization (about -45 mV) and nocturnal hyperpolarization (about -55mV). The linkage between balanced daily programs of ionic conductances and molecular oscillations in the SCN probably involves second-messenger signals such as circadian oscillations of cyclic AMP (cAMP) and intracellular calcium (Ca^{2+}), which peak in the middle of circadian day and correlate with the daily peak of membrane depolarization and neuronal firing rate. The major source of light information to the SCN is the RHT, which primarily originates in intrinsically photosensitive melanopsin-synthesizing retinal ganglion cells that release of glutamate and pituitary adenylyl-cyclase activating peptide (PACAP) from RHT terminals.

promoters, these cytosolic oscillations can influence core clock gene expression. Other robust afferent projections are the geniculohypothalamic tract originating from the thalamic intergeniculate leaflet, serotonergic input from the median raphe, and histaminergic input from the TMN.[49]

Intrinsic Circuitry of the SCN

The overall function of SCN circuits depends on VIP signaling via VIP receptor 2 located in shell neurons. GABA may operate synergistically with VIP to maintain a phase-divergent state, opposing synchrony via $GABA_A$ receptors. Intracellular chloride concentration may regionally track the photoperiod; high intracellular chloride during long photoperiods may switch $GABA_A$ receptor signaling from inhibitory to excitatory. $GABA_B$ receptor signaling can contribute to phase-shift of electrical rhythms. By controlling the relative phase of different SCN subregions, the combined effects of signaling by glutamate (RHT), VIP (core to shell), and GABA (reciprocal connections) may ultimately maintain and sculpt the emergent properties of the SCN circuit.

The SCN is also densely populated by astrocytes, which potentially influence the SCN by at least two mechanisms. Circadian changes in astrocyte morphology alter the access of signals between neurons and may regulate the activity of RHT synapses in the SCN core. Astrocytes show strong intracellular calcium oscillations that are antiphasic to neuronal oscillations, peaking during the circadian night, when neurons are inactive. This nocturnal increase of activity in astrocytes in the circadian night may regulate extracellular glutamate levels via uptake by the astrocytic excitatory amino acid transporters. The SCN may also be sensitive to astrocytic uptake of GABA via GABA transporters. The nocturnal increase in intracellular calcium in astrocytes may trigger their release of glutamate as a gliotransmitter. Glutamate released by astrocytes during the night acts via presynaptic N-methyl-D-aspartate receptors in GABAergic neurons, promoting GABA release in the SCN shell. Astrocytes also supply lactate as a metabolic substrate to neurons. Glucose consumption in the SCN is rhythmic, and brain lactate concentrations show daily variations that peak during the active phase, possibly suggesting the existence of a rhythmic neurometabolic coupling mechanism among astrocytes and neurons throughout the SCN. Dopamine may regulate SCN function via D1 receptors, which are expressed in most VIP-expressing and approximately 60% of AVP neurons. Reciprocally, the circadian pacemaker strongly regulates dopamine signaling.

Efferent Connections of the Suprachiasmatic Nucleus

The SCN sends GABAergic projections throughout the CNS, mainly targeting other hypothalamic nuclei, primarily indirectly via the subparaventricular zone located just above the SCN[50] (Figure 27.8). The subparaventricular zone contains GABAergic neurons and consists of different portions that receive distinct inputs from the SCN, project to different targets, and have different functions in circadian regulation.[50] The ventromedial subparaventricular zone is involved in regulation of sleep–wake rhythms and provides heavy inputs to areas involved in control of arousal and sleep. The SCN promotes wakefulness through an indirect pathway via the supraventricular zone, resulting in increased activity in the dorsomedial nucleus of the hypothalamus (DMH).[29] Glutamatergic neurons of the DMH

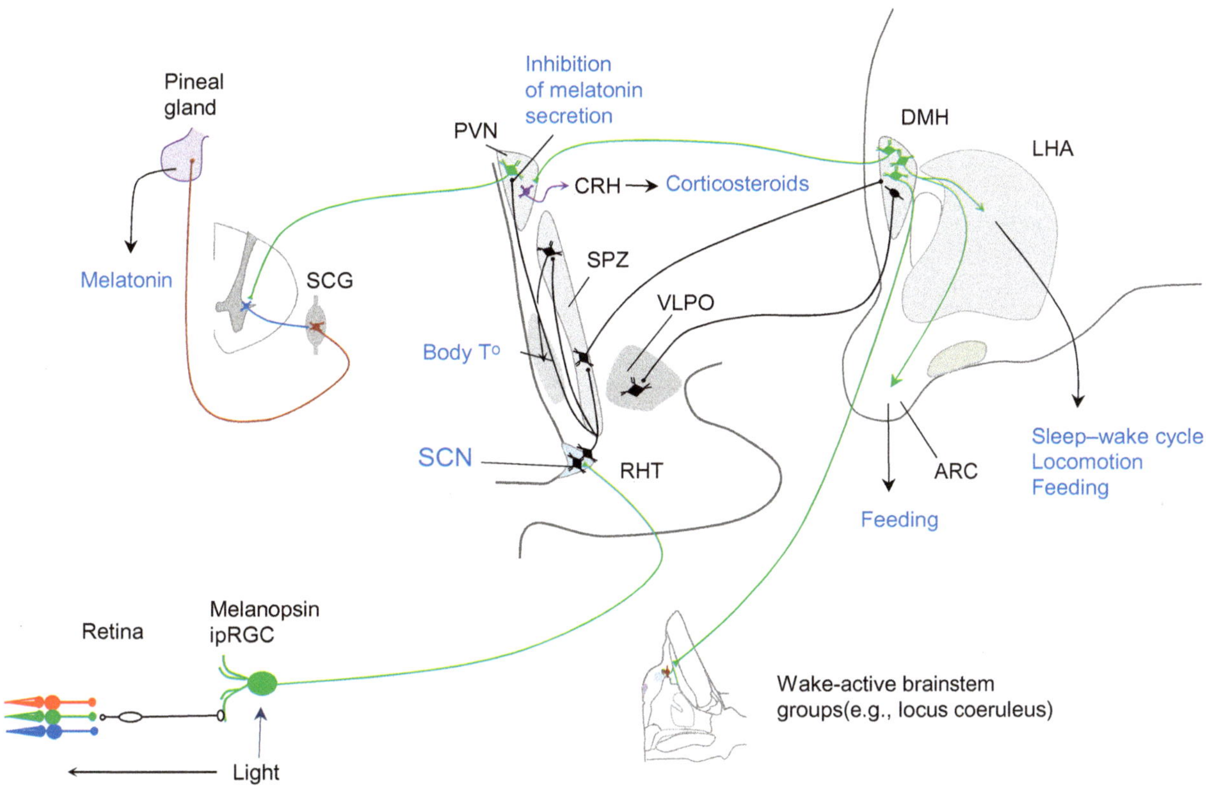

FIGURE 27.8 Extrinsic connections and effects of the suprachiasmatic nucleus (SCN).
The SCN entrainment by light depends on intrinsically photosensitive melanopsin-synthesizing retinal ganglion (ipRGC) that project via the retinohypothalamic tract (RHT). The SCN sends GABAergic projections throughout the CNS, mainly targeting other hypothalamic nuclei, primarily indirectly via the subparaventricular zone (SPZ),which contains GABAergic neurons that project to different targets. The SCN promotes wakefulness through an indirect pathway via the SPZ resulting in increased activity in the dorsomedial nucleus of the hypothalamus (DMH); glutamatergic neurons of the DMH innervate wake-promoting brain regions in the brainstem and lateral hypothalamic area (LHA), whereas GABAergic DMH neurons inhibit sleep-promoting regions including the ventrolateral preoptic area (VLPO). Signals from the SPZ also regulate the circadian rhythms of feeding. In part via the arcuate (ARC), infundibular nucleus. Melatonin is released from the pineal gland during the dark period. The pineal gland receives noradrenergic innervation from the superior cervical ganglion (SCG); this sympathoexcitatory pathway is initiated by projections from the paraventricular nucleus of the hypothalamus (PVN) to neurons of the intermediolateral cell column of the spinal cord targeting the superior cervical ganglion. During the daytime, GABAergic inputs from the SCN to the PVN inhibit this sympathoexcitatory pathway. Inputs from the SCN to the PVN may also provide circadian regulation of release of corticotrophin-releasing hormone (CRH).

innervate wake-promoting brain regions, including the ORX group, the TMN, and cholinergic and monoaminergic brainstem areas. In addition, GABAergic DMH neurons innervate sleep-promoting regions including the VLPO and MnPO. Direct inhibitory projections from the SCN to the VLPO and MnPO may also contribute to circadian control of sleep onset.[50] Signals from the subparaventricular zone also regulate the circadian rhythms of heart rate, blood pressure, body temperature, locomotor activity, and feeding. The dorsomedial portion of the subparaventricular zone primarily regulates endocrine rhythms; the dorsolateral portion may have a major role in modulating energy hemostasis and aggressive and reproductive behavior.[49]

Role of Melatonin

One important physiological timing cue to the SCN is melatonin, which is released from the pineal gland during the dark period. The pineal gland receives noradrenergic innervation from the superior cervical ganglion, which activates a cascade of circadian events that leads to the nightly formation of melatonin from serotonin.[51] This sympathoexcitatory pathway is initiated by projections from the paraventricular nucleus of the hypothalamus (PVN) to neurons of the intermediolateral cell column of the spinal cord targeting the superior cervical ganglion. During the daytime, GABAergic inputs from the SCN to the PVN inhibit this sympathoexcitatory pathway to the pineal gland, suppressing melatonin secretion. Melatonin elicits circadian phase-shifting effects on SCN firing that inversely mirror those of light, suggesting its role as an internal timing signal. Melatonin acts through two types of receptors, type 1 (MT1R) and type 2 (MT2R).[52] These receptors trigger downstream inhibitory signals and mediate a feedback mechanism by which melatonin controls the SCN activity.[52,53] The MT1R is mostly involved in regulation of circadian rhythms, whereas the MT2R is mostly involved in sleep induction.[54] The nonselective MT1/MT2 receptor agonist ramelteon is used for treatment of insomnia.[17] Tasimelteon has been approved for the treatment of non-24-h sleep–wake rhythm disorder in blind people due to its efficacy in resynchronizing to the 24-h sleep–wake rhythm. Agomelatine acts as both a nonselective MT1R/MT2R agonist and a 5-HT2C receptor antagonist.

Mutations of the *RAI1* gene encoding retinoic acid-induced gene-1, which regulates several processes including circadian rhythms, cause Smith-Magenis syndrome, a genetic disorder characterized by distinctive physical features, developmental delay, cognitive impairment, and a typical behavioral phenotype. A distinctive feature of this disorder is inversion of the circadian rhythm of melatonin secretion, associated with impaired sleep maintenance with a phase advance and intense sleepiness around noon. The inversion of circadian melatonin secretion could be linked to alterations in light signal transduction, global misalignment of the circadian system, or a specific impairment in the melatonin secretion pathway.[55]

Circadian Rhythms and Cognitive Performance

Circadian rhythms can be observed in the performance of most tasks and activities such as sensory, motor, reaction time, time estimation, memory tasks, verbal tasks, arithmetic calculations, and simulated driving tasks. Performance increases during the day and decreases during the night. One of the basic cognitive functions affected by circadian rhythms is attention, which reaches its lowest levels during nighttime and early morning hours, and increases around noon and even further during afternoon and evening hours. Several factors modulate the temporal course of cognitive performance: chronotype, age, sleep deprivation, and drugs. Polymorphisms in clock genes that are associated with abnormal circadian disorders also produce more subtle nonpathological phenotypes like chronotypes. For example, a *PER3* polymorphism (rs228697) was significantly associated with diurnal preference phenotype.[56]

Age also modulates the time course of cognitive rhythms; adolescents tend to delay while aged people tend to advance their sleep–wake cycle. The greater the sleep deprivation the greater the deterioration in executive function throughout the day, with a greater decrease in the morning, the post-lunch dip, and in the first hours of the night. Some drugs such as caffeine can modulate the temporal course of circadian rhythms in cognitive performance.

SLEEP AND MEMORY

Sleep is necessary for many aspect of declarative memory including primarily consolidation of episode memory but also other aspects of memory. There are two main proposals regarding the role of sleep memory consolidation. One is that of "active" system consolidation through global and synchronized information exchange between the hippocampus and the neocortex.[57,58] The second is that of local synaptic cortical homeostasis by a mechanism of "down selection," in the setting of global reduction (depotentiation) of synaptic activity, with preservation of representations in only those synapses that have been most strongly activated during wakefulness.[59] These two mechanisms may not be mutually exclusive but rather occur at different stages of NREM sleep.[59–61]

Sleep Replay as an Active Mechanism for Memory Consolidation

Neocortical slow oscillations during NREM sleep are distributed throughout large areas of the neocortex and are temporally connected to sharp wave-ripple complexes, which are distributed throughout the hippocampus. This reflects a bidirectional interplay of neocortical and hippocampal activity. Correlative patterns of hippocampal and neocortical activities that occur during learning are spontaneously reactivated during sharp wave-ripples. This phenomenon is known as "replay" and is thought to have a major role in active memory consolidation during NREM sleep. The bidirectional link would promote exchange of information between the initial stage of memory acquisition (hippocampus) and the final memory store that is activated during the time of acquisition (neocortex). Neocortical slow oscillations also generate sleep spindle oscillations in the thalamus.[62] Cortical waves impose periodically recurrent excitation upon TRN neurons and thus entrain intrathalamic spindles. Fast spindles (~13–15 Hz) occur in parietal and central cortical regions, primarily at the depolarized (UP state) of slow cortical oscillations. In contrast, slow spindles (7–8 Hz) occur over the frontal cortex riding over the hyperpolarized (DOWN) state. Sleep spindles occur more frequently after learning, and have been associated with synaptic plasticity and improved retention. They may promote memory formation by "phase-locking" rhythmic neocortical, thalamic, and hippocampal activities. The power of hippocampal sharp wave–ripples increases just before the peaks of spindle activity. Ripples are nested into succeeding troughs of spindles, generating spindle-ripple events. Typically fast spindles precede the slow spindles in the EEG. It has been proposed that fast spindles are involved in hippocampal-neocortical transfer of memory-related information and at a second stage slow spindles recruit frontal areas for memory storage.[63]

Cortical Synaptic Homeostasis During Deep NREM Sleep

Delta waves may support the homeostatic process that dominates during deep NREM sleep.[59,64] According to the "down-selection" hypothesis, synapses that have been potentiated during wakefulness are downscaled (depotentiated) during sleep.[59] Downscaling would improve memory retention by silencing weak synaptic connections while sparing stronger ones, thereby increasing the signal-to-noise ratio and freeing the space for new learning.[59] Delta waves during deep NREM sleep occur in the setting of reduced level of excitatory neuromodulators such as NE and thus create optimal conditions for synaptic depotentiation. Periodic slow oscillations, as occur during deep NREM sleep, trigger synaptic depression. Downscaling at this stage may occur at the level of single cells or synapses. Most delta waves are local and are regulated in relationship to previous experience. This is consistent with the breakdown of cortico-cortical connectivity and more local network clustering during slow-wave sleep. Whereas during light NREM sleep global, transient fluctuations of activity and replay of memory traces via hippocampal-neocortical connections may be important for active system consolidation, after this process takes place more local slow oscillations at hyperpolarization levels favoring synaptic depression may produce downscaling and improve the signal-to-noise ratio of the surviving memories.[64]

Sleep deprivation impairs memory consolidation by interfering with these processes. The role of REM sleep in memory function is less well understood. However, recent studies show that neural activity during REM sleep is also critical for normal memory consolidation.[65] Activity of GABAergic neurons in the medial septum associated with theta oscillation is involved in spatial and contextual memory consolidation during REM sleep. Theta activity may also have a role in synaptic downscaling at this stage. The global process of downscaling may occur together with upscaling via interplay between ripple-associated and theta-associated replay activity across the sleep–wake cycle.

ASTROCYTES AND BRAIN HOMEOSTASIS DURING SLEEP

Studies using microdyalis and amperometry in behaving mice have provided important information about the changes in brain homeostasis during sleep.[66] Brain energy expenditure in NREM sleep only decreases to 85% of the waking value. REM sleep is as expensive as wakefulness, and the suspension of thermoregulation during REM sleep increases brain metabolic heat production and temperature. State transitions from wakefulness to sleep are associated with changes in brain energy metabolism governed by oxygen consumption and state-dependent metabolic shift, with sleep being more oxidative than wakefulness. The transition from wakefulness to sleep is also accompanied by a marked expansion of extracellular space, as well as rapid and sustained decrease in extracellular K^+ and increase in extracellular Ca^{2+} and Mg^{2+}. These changes in large part reflect an important role of astrocytes during sleep in addition to homeostatic sleep induction via release of adenosine.[26]

Functional Changes in Astrocytes from Wakefulness to Sleep

Cognitive processing requires coordinated activity of synaptic ensembles and astrocytes during both wakefulness and sleep.[66] During wakefulness the LC-NE system acting via β2 adrenergic receptors increases both glucose utilization and lactate production in astrocytes. Lactate promotes memory processing by potentiating neuronal NMDAR signaling necessary for long-term potentiation and by triggering expression of genes involved in synaptic plasticity; lactate can also regulate NE availability by stimulating its release from LC axonal varicosities. Arousal upregulates genes related to extracellular matrix and cytoskeleton involved in the elongation of peripheral astrocytic processes, bringing them closer to the synaptic cleft. Astrocytes also release adenosine, which may affect memory consolidation via A2Rs in inhibitory neurons and presynaptic A1Rs in glutamatergic afferents. During wakefulness, NE inhibits astrocytic Na^+/K^+ ATPase; this results in increased extracellular K^+, which promotes swelling in response to synaptic activity. The sleep state is associated with profound changes in astrocyte physiology that reflect cessation of LC-NE activity.[66] The reduced LC-NE activity prevents production of lactate by astrocytes and contributes to a shift of brain metabolism to a predominant oxidative state. The reduced LC activity also results in transient disinhibition of the astrocytic Na^+/K^+ ATPase, thus promoting removal of extracellular K^+ and increase in extracellular volume. The reduction of extracellular K^+ and lactate during sleep may also reflect their clearance via the lymphatic system. The decrease in interstitial K^+ concentration is consistent with widespread neuronal hyperpolarization and consequent reduction in neuronal firing rates that occurs during NREM sleep. Reduced synaptic coverage by astrocytes during sleep results in decreased glutamate reuptake and consequent increase in glutamate dwell time and spillover, with profound consequences on neuronal synchronization and synaptic plasticity.[65]

Clearance Function of Sleep

Sleep facilitates the efflux of lactate, glutamate, K^+, and potentially toxic products such as amyloid β (Aβ)from perivascular and nonperivascular spaces into the vascular component. Sleep stimulates the clearance of these and other substances through the glymphatic system.

This proposed tripartite pathway allows the convective flow of CSF into the brain along arterial perivascular spaces, then into the interstitium facilitated by aquaporin 4 water channels in astrocytes, and then into the venous perivascular and perineuronal spaces, ultimately clearing solutes from the neuropil into meningeal and cervical lymphatic drainage vessels. The volume of extracellular space increases during NREM sleep, promoting clearance of Aβ and other toxic products via this tripartite system. Glymphatic function robustly increases during sleep, eliminating various metabolic byproducts from the extracellular space that accumulate during wakefulness.[67–69] There are also circadian changes in the permeability of the blood–brain barrier (BBB), which is higher at night. Studies in *Drosophila* show that this permeability rhythm is driven by circadian regulation of efflux and depends on a molecular clock in the perineural glia.[70]

SLEEP AND AGING

Normal aging is associated with a reduced ability to initiate and maintain sleep. Deficits in sleep physiology, including NREM sleep and its associated neural oscillations, are especially prominent in later life.

Changes in Sleep Architecture and Brain Oscillations

Both sleep architecture and oscillations change during progression into older age.[59,70] Changes in sleep architecture include advanced sleep timing (i.e., earlier bedtimes and rise times); longer sleep-onset latency; shorter overall sleep duration; increased sleep fragmentation; more fragile sleep; reduced amount of deep-stage NREM (N3) sleep; increased time spent in lighter NREM (N1 and N2) stages; shorter and fewer NREM-REM sleep cycles; and increased time spent awake throughout the night.[71] Age-related reductions in REM sleep are subtler and only emerge into the eighth decade and beyond or as a symptom of degenerative dementias. Men experience far greater relative disruption and impairment in NREM sleep than women later in life; this may reflect significantly greater relative loss of VIP neurons within the SCN and galanin-expressing neurons in the VLPO.

There are also substantial changes in the electrical oscillations occurring at the different sleep stages. The most prominent are changes in slow waves and sleep spindles during NREM sleep. The maximal age-related decrements in absolute slow wave activity occur over the PFC and in the first NREM sleep cycles. There is also slowing in average frequency of slow waves across most cortical areas. In older adults, the homeostatic buildup of sleep pressure is slower and weaker and the dissipation of homeostatic sleep drive is also shallower across a night of sleep relative to younger adults. Whereas older adults have higher levels of adenosine accumulation with increasing time awake compared to younger adults, there is reduced sensitivity to adenosine due to reduction in adenosine A1Rs with aging. The amplitude and frequency range of sleep spindles is also reduced with aging; maximal impairments in spindle density and amplitude occur over frontal lobe regions, whereas reductions in spindle duration are maximal over posterior head regions.

These age-related changes in sleep structure and sleep stages have been linked to instability in sleep–wake maintenance systems.[70] There is an age-dependent reduction in the number of GABA/galanin cells in the VLPO and ORX neurons and reduced α2 adrenoceptor responsivity within the LC. Reduced sleep time at night in older adults is associated with thinning of gray matter within regions in the prefrontal, superior temporal and insular cortices; this is one factor underlying impairments in NREM sleep slow-wave oscillations.[71]

Sleep, Aging, and Memory Impairment

Age-related cognitive decline is associated with impaired ability to form new hippocampal-dependent memories. In older adults, there is an association between poor and shorter sleep and the extent of impairment on numerous cognitive tests, including those requiring verbal memory encoding. The magnitude of impairment in fast-frequency spindle density predicts the failure of the hippocampus to engage in episodic associative memory encoding the following day. Age-related impairment in NREM slow-wave activity in the PFC predicts worse overnight hippocampal–neocortical memory transformation, which is associated with accelerated forgetting. Age-related disruption of fast-frequency sleep spindles over the PFC attenuates hippocampal encoding activity. In young adults, low-frequency transcranial direct-current stimulation at <1 Hz during slow-wave sleep increases slow oscillation power and almost doubles overnight memory retention. In older adults, enhancing the slow oscillation using this approach during an afternoon nap leads to a memory enhancement.

Impaired Circadian Rhythms with Aging

Several, but not all, studies have reported decline in melatonin levels with aging. Older individuals show lower-amplitude body temperature rhythms, with the minimum of the endogenous phase occurring nearly two hours earlier than in younger individuals. The number of VIP- and AVP-expressing cells in the SCN decreases with age. Studies in vitro show that SCN neurons lose phase coherence with age; this leads to desynchronization and a reduction in the amplitude of neuronal activity. In older adults, less-robust circadian rhythms and more fragmented patterns of activity are risk factors for the development of dementia.

SLEEP AND CIRCADIAN RHYTHMS IN NEURODEGENERATIVE DEMENTIAS

Sleep disruption is especially pervasive in neurodegenerative dementias, such as Alzheimer disease (AD) and Parkinson disease (PD).[72] Measures of poor sleep correlate with cortical Aβ and cerebrospinal fluid measures of Aβ42 and phosphorylated tau. Accumulation of tau-associated neurofibrillary tangles within the medial temporal lobe is relevant given the role of the hippocampus in generating sharp wave-ripples supporting memory consolidation. Patients with mild cognitive impairment (MCI) and AD have significantly fewer posterior fast sleep spindles relative to healthy older adults. In AD, accumulation of neurofibrillary tangles within the preoptic area correlates with the severity of sleep fragmentation.

Sleep Disturbances and Impaired Aβ Clearance

The link between degenerative dementia and sleep disruption is bidirectional. The levels of Aβ levels increase with time spent awake, and NREM sleep is thought to promote the clearance of Aβ. One proposed link between sleep disturbances and dementia risk is reduced Aβ clearance via the glymphatic system. In transgenic mouse models of AD, impaired glymphatic function in AQP4-knockouts resulted in marked reduction in the clearance and increased brain levels of Aβ compared with those in transgenic mice expressing AQP4. Studies in mice also showed that glymphatic clearance of $A\beta_{1\text{-}40}$ increased during sleep compared with the awake states; sleep deprivation caused a marked reduction in the clearance of various CSF metabolites.

Circadian Rhythm Dysfunction in Neurodegenerative Disorders

Disrupted circadian rhythms occur in AD, PD, depression, and autism.[72,73] Single-nucleotide polymorphisms in *CLOCK*, *BMAL1*, and *PER1* have been associated with increased risk of AD and PD. Compared with healthy aged people, individuals with AD or PD show considerably lower melatonin rhythm amplitudes. Some studies indicate that morning light therapy may improve circadian rhythms and cognitive and behavioral functions particularly in the early stages of AD; in severe cases of dementia light therapy reduces agitation. Sundowning syndrome is prevalent in people with dementia and is characterized by increases in aggression, restlessness, delirium, and agitation specifically in the late afternoon or early evening. Lack of appropriate light–dark cues, reductions in REM sleep, and a deterioration of the SCN pacemaker activity and its outputs may all contribute to this syndrome. Aggression may be modulated by the circadian system. Studies in mice show that rhythms in the propensity of aggressive behaviors are modulated via a polysynaptic circuit from VIP neurons in the SCN to GABAergic neurons of the subparaventricular zone, which in turn innervate the ventromedial hypothalamus, an area known to regulate aggression. Circadian rhythm disruption also occurs in depression.

NARCOLEPSY

Narcolepsy is the most common cause of excessive diurnal sleepiness (EDS) and is caused by the selective loss of ORX-producing neurons.[74,75] Narcolepsy type 1 is the classic phenotype and is associated with cataplexy and low or undetectable ORX levels in the CSF. Narcolepsy type 1 is an autoimmune disease mediated by T cells.[74] Narcolepsy type 2 has less severe symptoms, is not associated with cataplexy, and 90% of patients have normal CSF ORX levels. In rare cases, narcolepsy results from brain injuries or immune attack affecting ORX neurons or their projections, for example in the setting of neuromyelitis optic spectrum disorders (NMOSD) associated with AQP4 autoantibodies[76] and paraneoplastic disorders associated with testicular carcinoma and anti-Ma antibodies.[77]

Loss of ORX neurons underlies the two major pathophysiological manifestations of narcolepsy: poor maintenance of wakefulness and poor regulation of REM sleep.[78] Most patients with narcolepsy have poor quality sleep but most feel well rested in the morning or after a nap. Orexin neuron loss destabilizes arousal circuits by reducing excitatory drive to the wake-promoting neurons in the TMN, LC, and other brainstem groups.[79] Patients with narcolepsy also exhibit dysregulation of REM sleep; this manifests with poor circadian timing, rapid transitions into REM sleep, and disruption of REM sleep physiology, including REM sleep behavior disorder (RBD) or sleep paralysis. In normal conditions, REM sleep exhibits a strong circadian rhythm and is suppressed during the active period via signals initiated by the SCN and conveyed via the DMH to ORX neurons. A major manifestation of narcolepsy type 1 is cataplexy.[80] Cataplexy is the sudden loss of muscle tone triggered by strong, generally positive emotions, such as when laughing. Cataplexy shares physiological bases with atonia during REM sleep, including loss of muscle stretch reflexes and H-reflexes on EMG. Functional MRI studies show that areas that are active during REM sleep-induced atonia are also active during cataplexy. Cataplexy thus reflects excessive activity of the pathway from REM-on neurons in the subcoeruleus region to GABA/glycinergic neurons of the gigantocellular medullary reticular nucleus projecting the ventral horn. In normal conditions, inputs from ORX neurons to pontine REM-off neurons ensure a strong suppression of REM sleep phenomena during wakefulness. In contrast, neurons of the centromedial nucleus of the amygdala (CeM) activated by emotional stimuli send strong inhibitory projections to these REM-off neurons. Studies in knockout mice show that serotonergic neurons of the DR mediate the effects of ORX in preventing cataplexy by inhibiting the CeM.[18] Strong positive emotions normally engage the medial PFC, which excites both CeM and ORX neurons. Normally the excitatory effects of ORX neurons offset the inhibitory effects of the CeM on the REM-off pontine neurons. In narcolepsy with cataplexy lack of ORX activity allows strong emotions to unmask the inhibitory effect of the CeM on REM-off neurons, resulting in disinhibition of the subcoeruleus REM-on neurons and loss of muscle tone. Furthermore, lack of ORX reduces the inhibitory serotonergic DR inputs to the CeM.[18]

Narcolepsy type 1 can be caused by an autoimmune process, as evidenced during the H1N1 influenza pandemic in the winter of 2009–2010. All affected individuals carried the class II human leukocyte antigen (HLA) allele DQB1*06:02 and developed narcolepsy type 1 within a few weeks to months after vaccination. Similarly, many spontaneous cases of narcolepsy type 1 are preceded by infection with streptococcus or influenza, suggesting that CD4+ T cells responding to these infectious agents may cross-recognize ORX peptides presented by MHC class II molecules and secrete cytokines that could promote attack on the ORX neurons by CD8+ T cells, macrophages, and natural killer cells.[74] The loss of ORX neurons might trigger compensatory responses; for example, there are increased numbers of histaminergic neurons in the TMN in persons with narcolepsy type 1. The number of MCH neurons in these patients is normal. Treatment of EDS in narcolepsy includes stimulants that increase CNS levels of NE and dopamine, such as amphetamine, methylphenidate, modafinil, and solriamfetol. The H3 receptor inverse agonist pitolisant also reduces excessive diurnal somnolence as well as cataplectic events by promoting release of histamine and other wake-promoting signals. Gamma-hydroxybutyrate (sodium oxybate) is a $GABA_B$ receptor agonist that ameliorates sleep fragmentation, and has a moderate impact in EDS.[75,81] The medications used for cataplexy are tricyclics and selective serotonin-reuptake inhibitors that promote noradrenergic and serotonergic activity. They include clomipramine, venlafaxine, reboxetine, and fluoxetine, which are also effective for sleep paralysis and hypnagogic hallucinations.

REM SLEEP BEHAVIOR DISORDER

Rapid eye movement sleep behavior disorder (RBD) is a complex and potentially injurious parasomnia involving dream enactment behavior that often mirrors terrifying dream content of being attacked or chased. The biomarker of RBD is lack of normal loss of muscle tone as detected during polysomnography.[82–84] The cause of RBD is breakdown of the normal brainstem circuit involved in normal REM sleep.[85,86] The presence of RBD is a powerful biomarker of the presence of an underlying synucleinopathy, such a Lewy body disorder or multiple system atrophy. More than half of people with the classical form of narcolepsy also have RBD. However, RBD may also reflect a focal lesion or autoimmune disorder affecting REM sleep-controlling areas. The most common structures exhibiting neuropathology or neurodegeneration in RBD patients are the subcoeruleus, gigantocellular reticular nucleus, DR, PPT, and ventromedial medulla, and in some cases hypothalamus, substantia nigra, and limbic areas. A retrospective case series showed that the dorsal pontine tegmentum and rostral ventromedial medulla are most commonly involved in lesions associated with RBD, in some cases associated with medial temporal limbic and neocortical pathology.[87]

SLEEP MANIFESTATIONS OF OTHER AUTOIMMUNE AND NEURODEGENERATIVE DISORDERS

Autoimmune Disorders

In addition to narcolepsy, other sleep disorders have an immune pathogenesis. Sleep disorders in paraneoplastic syndromes typically coexist with limbic or brainstem encephalitis and hypothalamic disturbances. Hypersomnia has frequently been described in patients with anti-Ma2 encephalitis associated with testicular carcinoma, reflecting involvement of diencephalic, limbic, and brainstem structures in any combination. Anti-Ma2 encephalitis may manifest with a narcoleptic phenotype characterized by cataplexy and hypnagogic hallucinations. Antibodies against components of the K_v1 potassium channel complex also typically produce sleep disturbances. Morvan syndrome associated with CASPR2 antibodies in patients with malignant thymoma manifests with insomnia; limbic encephalitis related to anti-LGI1 may be associated with insomnia, hypersomnia, and RBD. There is a phenotypic overlap between these two autoimmune disorders; the common finding of hyponatremia indicates a hypothalamic target. In neuromyelitis optica spectrum disorders (NMOSDs) sleep disturbances including narcolepsy are manifestations of hypothalamic involvement by AQP4 autoantibodies. Kleine-Levin syndrome is characterized by recurrent episodes of EDS, abnormal cognition, eating abnormalities, and sexual disinhibition. The pathophysiology of this disorder remains unknown. An autoimmune basis has been considered because of its relapsing-remitting course, its triggering by infections, and its linkage to distinct DRB1–DQB1 haplotypes.

Anti-IgLON5-Associated Encephalitis

IgLON5 disease has a heterogeneous neurological presentation and is characterized by abnormal sleep architecture, RBD, serum and CSF antibodies against the neuronal protein IgLON5, a strong HLA association, and absence of coexistent autoimmune disorders.[75] The disorder is defined by tau deposits in the brainstem and hypothalamus impairing some nuclei that regulate sleep. The four main clinical phenotypes at presentation are: a sleep disorder consisting in abnormal motor sleep behaviors, RBD, insomnia, EDS, sleep attacks, and sleep breathing disturbances (including central or obstructive sleep apnea and laryngeal stridor); a bulbar syndrome that may include dysphagia, dysarthria, hypersalivation, and acute respiratory insufficiency; a progressive supranuclear palsy-like syndrome; and a Huntington disease-like syndrome with cognitive impairment and choreic movements. These manifestations may occur in variable combinations. Sleep motor manifestations in IgLON5 disease include prominent jerks, vocalizations such as talking, and purposeful behaviors such as manipulating imaginary objects. Stridor and breathing pauses are reported by the bed partners. Sleep architecture shows only a mild reduction of total sleep time but a distinctive temporal sequence of sleep abnormalities, from most abnormal at the beginning of the night to normalization at the end of the night. Initiation of sleep and re-entering of sleep after awakenings are characterized by theta activity with rapid repetitive and stereotyped leg movements distinct from periodic leg movements in sleep. Distinct sleep patterns include "undifferentiated NREM sleep" characterized by diffuse irregular theta EEG activity of 4–7 Hz and absence of vertex waves, K complexes, and sleep spindles and "poorly structured N2 sleep" characterized by scant spindles and K complexes. These patterns are commonly associated with excessive electromyographic activation linked to frequent vocalizations, simple motor activity (e.g., raising the arm, punching), and finalistic behaviors (e.g., goal-directed behaviors like sucking the thumbs while apparently eating, picking up objects, etc.). The most complex sleep behaviors in IgLON5 disease, unlike the case of RBD, occur in NREM sleep and are different from the classical NREM parasomnias (sleepwalking, sleep terrors, confusional awakenings) as they are not abrupt and do not emerge from normal N3. The sleep abnormalities in anti-IgLON5 disease are distinct from those occurring in status dissociatus. In IgLON5 disease wakefulness can be distinguished from sleep by clinical and polysomnographic features; K complexes, spindles, and delta waves are present in NREM sleep and NREM sleep can be distinguished from REM sleep. Neuropathology of this disorder showed absence of inflammatory infiltrates and presence of neuronal loss, moderate gliosis, and extensive deposits of abnormal hyperphosphorylated tau in neurons of the tegmentum of the brainstem and the hypothalamus, sparing the glia. The nuclei damaged in the brainstem are LTD, PPT, PAG, nucleus ambiguus, and gigantocellular nucleus of the medulla. The nucleus subcoeruleus is spared. The cortex, thalamus, substantia nigra, basal ganglia, and cerebellum are preserved or mildly affected.

Agrypnia Excitata

Agrypnia excitata is a sleep abnormality that occurs in the prion disorder fatal insomnia, Morvan syndrome, and delirium tremens. It is characterized by insomnia, abnormal circadian pattern, disrupted sleep architecture, motor hyperactivity, confusional-oneiric state, and prominent autonomic hyperactivity. Agrypnia excitata reflects dysfunction of the thalamus and its connections with limbic structures. The sleep abnormalities that characterize agrypnia excitata are severe insomnia and an extreme expression of status dissociatus due to breakdown of the sleep–wake boundaries. In agrypnia excitata, there is sympathetic hyperactivity and nocturnal motor overactivation characterized by simple or complex behaviors mimicking daily life activities such as eating, setting up a device, or dressing. This nocturnal finalistic activity is labeled oneiric stupor, and is nearly continuous during the entire night with quiet pauses of several minutes. Episodes of oneiric stupor can occur with open or closed eyes. Patients seem to be behaving in the context of a dream or a hallucination, but if questioned during one of these episodes they may respond that they are awake. The oneiric stupor episodes can emerge from any stage (relaxed wakefulness, NREM sleep, and REM sleep). In agrypnia excitata, the circadian rhythmicity is lost and motor activity is increased throughout the 24 h without any circadian pattern. Electrophysiological recordings show an extremely disorganized pattern with reduced sleep time, brief fragments of alpha-theta activity, reduction or absence of K complexes and spindles, loss or small amounts of N3 stage, and brief intrusions or clusters of REM sleep bursts without muscle atonia. Rapid shifts between wakefulness, NREM sleep features, and REM sleep without atonia are typical during 24 h recordings. These features differentiate agrypnia excitata from the sleep behavioral abnormalities in IgLON5 disease, where there is only mild reduction of total sleep time; K complexes, spindles, delta waves, and REM sleep are always present and do not decrease with the progression of the disease; episodes of REM sleep are not short; circadian sleep–wake pattern is normal; dysautonomia is not prominent; and neuropathology does not typically show thalamic damage.

KEY POINTS

- The control of the wake–sleep cycle depends on neurons distributed in the basal forebrain, hypothalamus, thalamus, and brainstem.

- The parabrachial nucleus contains glutamatergic neurons projecting to the forebrain that have a major role in arousal.
- The pedunculopontine tegmental nucleus contains cholinergic, glutamatergic, and GABAergic neurons that promote tonic firing in thalamocortical neurons.
- Monoaminergic arousal-promoting neurons in the locus coeruleus and rostral raphe promote arousal via several mechanisms.
- The basal forebrain contains cholinergic, glutamatergic, and GABAergic neurons that innervate the cerebral cortex and make different contributions in promoting cortical activation.
- The posterior lateral hypothalamus contains histaminergic, orexinergic, and GABAergic neurons that maintain wakefulness.
- Histaminergic neurons of the tuberomammillary nucleus promote wakefulness by direct activation of the cortex, thalamus, and several wake-promoting brainstem neurons.
- Orexin/hypocretin neurons activate several regions arousal-promoting regions, stabilize wakefulness, and regulate sleep stage transitions.
- The two primary triggers of sleep are homeostatic sleep "pressure" produced by periods of wakefulness or sleep deprivation, and circadian influences from the suprachiasmatic nucleus (SCN).
- The ventrolateral preoptic area (VLPO) and median preoptic nucleus contain GABAergic neurons that are essential for the transition from wakefulness to NREM sleep.
- Homeostatic sleep pressure following prolonged wakefulness is mediated by several somnogens, particularly adenosine.
- Adenosine is primarily secreted by neurons and to lesser extent astrocytes and promotes sleep via both A1Rs and A2Rs; the wake-promoting effect of caffeine primarily depends $A2_AR$ blockade.
- Onset of REM sleep depends on a pontine region referred to as subcoeruleus nucleus or sublaterodorsal nucleus.
- REM-on GABAergic neurons in the subcoeruleus nucleus participate in reciprocal inhibitory interactions with REM-off neurons located in the ventrolateral periaqueductal gray and lateral pontine tegmentum.
- REM-on glutamatergic neurons of the subcoeruleus nucleus project to the gigantocellular reticular nucleus of the medulla, which inhibits spinal motoneurons via direct GABA/glycinergic projections, eliciting muscle atonia.
- Cholinergic neurons increase their activity during REM sleep (REM-on) and activate the REM-on neurons of the subcoeruleus nucleus.
- Noradrenergic neurons and serotonergic neurons are REM-off neurons; they inhibit the REM-on neurons and are silent during REM sleep.
- Orexin neurons inhibit REM sleep via inputs to LC and rostral raphe neurons.
- Melanocyte-concentrating hormone neurons are intermingled with orexin neurons and promote REM sleep.
- The cellular basis of circadian timekeeping in the SCN and other tissues is a cell-autonomous clock consisting of interlocking transcriptional–translational feedback loops.
- The SCN consists of GABAergic neurons subdivided in core neurons that receive retinal inputs via the retinohypothalamic tract (RHT); and shell neurons that receive input from the core region and project to other brain areas.
- SCN neurons show a spontaneous firing cycle; they are depolarized and their firing rate peaks in the middle of day and hyperpolarized and essentially silent during the night.
- The major source of light information to the SCN is the RHT, which primarily originates in intrinsically photosensitive melanopsin-synthesizing retinal ganglion cells.
- The SCN mainly sends GABAergic projections that primarily target the subparaventricular zone, which mediates the circadian influence of the SCN on other hypothalamic targets.
- The SCN indirectly promotes arousal via inputs to the dorsomedial nucleus of the hypothalamus.
- The SCN directly inhibits the neurons of the paraventricular nucleus that activate sympathetic output to the pineal gland and melatonin secretion.
- Melatonin is released by the pineal gland during the dark period and is an internal timing signal that via MT1and MT2 receptors affects the function of the SCN and other targets.
- NREM sleep may promote memory consolidation via an active (replay) information exchange between the hippocampus and neocortex and via or local synaptic homeostasis.
- Astrocytes have a major role in brain homeostasis during sleep, in part clearance of lactate, glutamate, and amyloid β through the glymphatic system.
- Both the sleep architecture and the oscillations change during progression into older age.
- In older adults, less-robust circadian rhythms and more fragmented patterns of activity are risk factors for the development of dementia.
- A mechanism in linking sleep disturbances and dementia risk is reduced Aβ clearance via the glymphatic system.
- Narcolepsy type 1is associated with cataplexy and low or undetectable ORX levels in the CSF.

- Whereas narcolepsy type 1 is a T-cell mediated autoimmune disease, in rare cases narcolepsy results in neurodegenerative, focal, or autoimmune disorders such as neuromyelitis optica or paraneoplastic disease.
- REM sleep behavior disorder (RBD) is a biomarker of an underlying synucleinopathy but may also reflect a focal lesion or autoimmune disorder.
- Sleep disorders in paraneoplastic syndromes typically coexist with limbic or brainstem encephalitis and hypothalamic disturbances.
- IgLON5-associated disease is characterized by abnormal sleep architecture, RBD, strong HLA association, and tau deposits in the brainstem and hypothalamus.
- Agrypnia excitata occurs in fatal insomnia, Morvan syndrome, and delirium tremens, and is characterized by insomnia, abnormal circadian pattern, disrupted sleep architecture, motor hyperactivity, confusional-oneiric state, and sympathetic hyperactivity.

REFERENCES

1. Saper CB, Fuller PM. Wake-sleep circuitry: an overview. Curr Opin Neurobiol 2017;44:186–192.
2. Scammell TE, Arrigoni E, Lipton JO. Neural circuitry of wakefulness and sleep. Neuron 2017;93:747–765.
3. Adamantidis AR, Gutierrez Herrera C, Gent TC. Oscillating circuitries in the sleeping brain. Nat Rev Neurosci 2019;20:746–762.
4. Benarroch EE. Control of the cardiovascular and respiratory systems during sleep. Auton Neurosci 2019;218:54–63.
5. Luppi PH, Billwiller F, Fort P. Selective activation of a few limbic structures during paradoxical (REM) sleep by the claustrum and the supramammillary nucleus: evidence and function. Curr Opin Neurobiol 2017;44:59–64.
6. Canto CB, Onuki Y, Bruinsma B, van der Werf YD, De Zeeuw CI. The sleeping cerebellum. Trends Neurosci 2017;40:309–323.
7. Fuller PM, Sherman D, Pedersen NP, Saper CB, Lu J. Reassessment of the structural basis of the ascending arousal system. J Comp Neurol 2011;519:933–956.
8. Kaur S, Pedersen NP, Yokota S, et al. Glutamatergic signaling from the parabrachial nucleus plays a critical role in hypercapnic arousal. J Neurosci 2013;33:7627–7640.
9. Fischer DB, Boes AD, Demertzi A, et al. A human brain network derived from coma-causing brainstem lesions. Neurology 2016;87:2427–2434.
10. Chamberlin NL. Brain circuitry mediating arousal from obstructive sleep apnea. Curr Opin Neurobiol 2013;23:774–779.
11. Kaur S, Wang JL, Ferrari L, et al. A genetically defined circuit for arousal from sleep during hypercapnia. Neuron 2017;96:1153–1167 e1155.
12. Mena-Segovia J, Bolam JP. Rethinking the pedunculopontine nucleus: from cellular organization to function. Neuron 2017;94:7–18.
13. Kroeger D, Ferrari LL, Petit G, et al. Cholinergic, glutamatergic, and GABAergic neurons of the pedunculopontine tegmental nucleus have distinct effects on sleep/wake behavior in mice. J Neurosci 2017;37:1352–1366.
14. Shi G, Xing L, Wu D, et al. A rare mutation of beta1-adrenergic receptor affects sleep/wake behaviors. Neuron 2019;103:1044–1055 e1047.
15. Xu M, Chung S, Zhang S, et al. Basal forebrain circuit for sleep-wake control. Nat Neurosci 2015;18:1641–1647.
16. Scammell TE, Jackson AC, Franks NP, Wisden W, Dauvilliers Y. Histamine: neural circuits and new medications. Sleep 2019;42.
17. Krystal AD, Prather AA, Ashbrook LH. The assessment and management of insomnia: an update. World Psychiatry 2019;18:337–352.
18. Hasegawa E, Yanagisawa M, Sakurai T, Mieda M. Orexin neurons suppress narcolepsy via 2 distinct efferent pathways. J Clin Invest 2014;124:604–616.
19. Li Y, Gao XB, Sakurai T, van den Pol AN. Hypocretin/orexin excites hypocretin neurons via a local glutamate neuron: a potential mechanism for orchestrating the hypothalamic arousal system. Neuron 2002;36:1169–1181.
20. Kuwaki T, Zhang W. Orexin neurons as arousal-associated modulators of central cardiorespiratory regulation. Respir Physiol Neurobiol 2010;174:43–54.
21. Niu JG, Yokota S, Tsumori T, Qin Y, Yasui Y. Glutamatergic lateral parabrachial neurons innervate orexin-containing hypothalamic neurons in the rat. Brain Res 2010;1358:110–122.
22. Luppi PH, Peyron C, Fort P. Not a single but multiple populations of GABAergic neurons control sleep. Sleep Med Rev 2017;32:85–94.
23. Pedersen NP, Ferrari L, Venner A, et al. Supramammillary glutamate neurons are a key node of the arousal system. Nat Commun 2017;8:1405.
24. Anaclet C, Ferrari L, Arrigoni E, et al. The GABAergic parafacial zone is a medullary slow wave sleep-promoting center. Nat Neurosci 2014;17:1217–1224.
25. Garofalo S, Picard K, Limatola C, Nadjar A, Pascual O, Tremblay ME. Role of glia in the regulation of sleep in health and disease. Compr Physiol 2020;10:687–712.
26. Haydon PG. Astrocytes and the modulation of sleep. Curr Opin Neurobiol 2017;44:28–33.
27. Elmenhorst D, Elmenhorst EM, Hennecke E, et al. Recovery sleep after extended wakefulness restores elevated A1 adenosine receptor availability in the human brain. Proc Natl Acad Sci U S A 2017;114:4243–4248.
28. Lazarus M, Oishi Y, Bjorness TE, Greene RW. Gating and the need for sleep: dissociable effects of adenosine A1 and A2A receptors. Front Neurosci 2019;13:740.
29. Saper CB. The central circadian timing system. Curr Opin Neurobiol 2013;23:747–751.
30. Harding EC, Franks NP, Wisden W. The temperature dependence of sleep. Front Neurosci 2019;13:336.
31. Lazarus M, Chen JF, Urade Y, Huang ZL. Role of the basal ganglia in the control of sleep and wakefulness. Curr Opin Neurobiol 2013;23:780–785.
32. Oishi Y, Lazarus M. The control of sleep and wakefulness by mesolimbic dopamine systems. Neurosci Res 2017;118:66–73.

33. Luo YJ, Li YD, Wang L, et al. Nucleus accumbens controls wakefulness by a subpopulation of neurons expressing dopamine D1 receptors. Nat Commun 2018;9:1576.
34. Yuan XS, Wang L, Dong H, et al. Striatal adenosine A2A receptor neurons control active-period sleep via parvalbumin neurons in external globus pallidus. Elife 2017;6:e29055.
35. Castillo PR, Middlebrooks EH, Grewal SS, et al. Globus pallidus externus deep brain stimulation treats insomnia in a patient with Parkinson disease. Mayo Clin Proc 2020;95:419–422.
36. Lu J, Sherman D, Devor M, Saper CB. A putative flip-flop switch for control of REM sleep. Nature 2006;441:589–594.
37. Luppi PH, Clement O, Valencia Garcia S, Brischoux F, Fort P. New aspects in the pathophysiology of rapid eye movement sleep behavior disorder: the potential role of glutamate, gamma-aminobutyric acid, and glycine. Sleep Med 2013;14:714–718.
38. Weber F, Chung S, Beier KT, Xu M, Luo L, Dan Y. Control of REM sleep by ventral medulla GABAergic neurons. Nature 2015;526:435–438.
39. Varin C, Luppi PH, Fort P. Melanin-concentrating hormone-expressing neurons adjust slow-wave sleep dynamics to catalyze paradoxical (REM) sleep. Sleep 2018;41. doi:10.1093/sleep/zsy068 PMID 29618134
40. Young MW. Time Travels: A 40-year journey from *Drosophila*'s clock mutants to human circadian disorders (Nobel lecture). Angew Chem Int Ed Engl 2018;57:11532–11539.
41. Cox KH, Takahashi J. Circadian clock genes and the transcriptional architecture of the clock mechanism. J Mol Endocrinol 2019;63:R93–R102.
42. Albrecht U. Timing to perfection: the biology of central and peripheral circadian clocks. Neuron 2012;74:246–260.
43. Buhr ED, Takahashi JS. Molecular components of the mammalian circadian clock. Handb Exp Pharmacol 2013:3–27.
44. El Cheikh Hussein L, Mollard P, Bonnefont X. Molecular and cellular networks in the suprachiasmatic nuclei. Int J Mol Sci 2019;20:2052. doi:103390/ijms20082052
45. Lee HM, Chen R, Kim H, Etchegaray JP, Weaver DR, Lee C. The period of the circadian oscillator is primarily determined by the balance between casein kinase 1 and protein phosphatase 1. Proc Natl Acad Sci U S A 2011;108:16451–16456.
46. Shanware NP, Hutchinson JA, Kim SH, Zhan L, Bowler MJ, Tibbetts RS. Casein kinase 1-dependent phosphorylation of familial advanced sleep phase syndrome-associated residues controls PERIOD 2 stability. J Biol Chem 2011;286:12766–12774.
47. Shi G, Wu D, Ptacek LJ, Fu YH. Human genetics and sleep behavior. Curr Opin Neurobiol 2017;44:43–49.
48. Welsh DK, Takahashi JS, Kay SA. Suprachiasmatic nucleus: cell autonomy and network properties. Annu Rev Physiol 2010;72:551–577.
49. Morin LP. Neuroanatomy of the extended circadian rhythm system. Exp Neurol 2013;243:4–20.
50. Vujovic N, Gooley JJ, Jhou TC, Saper CB. Projections from the subparaventricular zone define four channels of output from the circadian timing system. J Comp Neurol 2015;523:2714–2737.
51. Borjigin J, Zhang LS, Calinescu AA. Circadian regulation of pineal gland rhythmicity. Mol Cell Endocrinol 2012;349:13–19.
52. Dubocovich ML. Melatonin receptors: role on sleep and circadian rhythm regulation. Sleep Med 2007;8 Suppl 3:34–42.
53. Jockers R, Delagrange P, Dubocovich ML, et al. Update on melatonin receptors: IUPHAR Review 20. Br J Pharmacol 2016;173:2702–2725.
54. Gobbi G, Comai S. Differential function of melatonin MT1 and MT2 receptors in REM and NREM sleep. Front Endocrinol (Lausanne) 2019;10:87.
55. Poisson A, Nicolas A, Bousquet I, Raverot V, Gronfier C, Demily C. Smith-Magenis syndrome: molecular basis of a genetic-driven melatonin circadian secretion disorder. Int J Mol Sci 2019;20:3533. doi:10.3390/ijms20143533.
56. Hida A, Kitamura S, Katayose Y, et al. Screening of clock gene polymorphisms demonstrates association of a PER3 polymorphism with morningness-eveningness preference and circadian rhythm sleep disorder. Sci Rep 2014;4:6309.
57. Born J, Rasch B, Gais S. Sleep to remember. Neuroscientist 2006;12:410–424.
58. Klinzing JG, Niethard N, Born J. Mechanisms of systems memory consolidation during sleep. Nat Neurosci 2019;22:1598–1610.
59. Tononi G, Cirelli C. Sleep and the price of plasticity: from synaptic and cellular homeostasis to memory consolidation and integration. Neuron 2014;81:12–34.
60. Hobson JA, Pace-Schott EF. The cognitive neuroscience of sleep: neuronal systems, consciousness and learning. Nat Rev Neurosci 2002;3:679–693.
61. Rasch B, Born J. About sleep's role in memory. Physiol Rev 2013;93:681–766.
62. Astori S, Wimmer RD, Luthi A. Manipulating sleep spindles—expanding views on sleep, memory, and disease. Trends Neurosci 2013;36:738–748.
63. Steriade M. Grouping of brain rhythms in corticothalamic systems. Neuroscience 2006;137:1087–1106.
64. Genzel L, Kroes MC, Dresler M, Battaglia FP. Light sleep versus slow wave sleep in memory consolidation: a question of global versus local processes? Trends Neurosci 2014;37:10–19.
65. Boyce R, Williams S, Adamantidis A. REM sleep and memory. Curr Opin Neurobiol 2017;44:167–177.
66. DiNuzzo M, Nedergaard M. Brain energetics during the sleep-wake cycle. Curr Opin Neurobiol 2017;47:65–72.
67. Iliff JJ, Wang M, Liao Y, et al. A paravascular pathway facilitates CSF flow through the brain parenchyma and the clearance of interstitial solutes, including amyloid beta. Sci Transl Med 2012;4:147ra111.
68. Tarasoff-Conway JM, Carare RO, Osorio RS, et al. Clearance systems in the brain—implications for Alzheimer disease. Nat Rev Neurol 2016;12:248.
69. Hladky SB, Barrand MA. Metabolite clearance during wakefulness and sleep. Handb Exp Pharmacol 2019;253:385–423.
70. Zhang SL, Yue Z, Arnold DM, Artiushin G, Sehgal A. A circadian clock in the blood-brain barrier regulates xenobiotic efflux. Cell 2018;173:130–139 e110.
71. Mander BA, Winer JR, Walker MP. Sleep and human aging. Neuron 2017;94:19–36.
72. Leng Y, Musiek ES, Hu K, Cappuccio FP, Yaffe K. Association between circadian rhythms and neurodegenerative diseases. Lancet Neurol 2019;18:307–318.

73. Logan RW, McClung CA. Rhythms of life: circadian disruption and brain disorders across the lifespan. Nat Rev Neurosci 2019;20:49–65.
74. Bassetti CLA, Adamantidis A, Burdakov D, et al. Narcolepsy—clinical spectrum, aetiopathophysiology, diagnosis and treatment. Nat Rev Neurol 2019;15:519–539.
75. Iranzo A. Sleep and neurological autoimmune diseases. Neuropsychopharmacology 2020;45:129–140.
76. Kallollimath P, Gujjar A, Patil M. Symptomatic narcolepsy as a presenting feature of neuromyelitis optica. Ann Indian Acad Neurol 2018;21:156–158.
77. Dauvilliers Y, Bauer J, Rigau V, et al. Hypothalamic immunopathology in anti-Ma-associated diencephalitis with narcolepsy-cataplexy. JAMA Neurol 2013;70:1305–1310.
78. Pintwala S, Peever J. Circuit mechanisms of sleepiness and cataplexy in narcolepsy. Curr Opin Neurobiol 2017;44:50–58.
79. Sakurai T. Orexin deficiency and narcolepsy. Curr Opin Neurobiol 2013;23:760–766.
80. Dauvilliers Y, Siegel JM, Lopez R, Torontali ZA, Peever JH. Cataplexy: clinical aspects, pathophysiology and management strategy. Nat Rev Neurol 2014;10:386–395.
81. Boscolo-Berto R, Viel G, Montagnese S, Raduazzo DI, Ferrara SD, Dauvilliers Y. Narcolepsy and effectiveness of gamma-hydroxybutyrate (GHB): a systematic review and meta-analysis of randomized controlled trials. Sleep Med Rev 2012;16:431–443.
82. Dauvilliers Y, Schenck CH, Postuma RB, et al. REM sleep behaviour disorder. Nat Rev Dis Primers 2018;4:19.
83. St Louis EK, Boeve BF. REM sleep behavior disorder: diagnosis, clinical implications, and future directions. Mayo Clin Proc 2017;92:1723–1736.
84. Iranzo A. Parasomnias and sleep-related movement disorders in older adults. Sleep Med Clin 2018;13:51–61.
85. Peever J, Luppi PH, Montplaisir J. Breakdown in REM sleep circuitry underlies REM sleep behavior disorder. Trends Neurosci 2014;37:279–288.
86. Iranzo A, Aparicio J. A lesson from anatomy: focal brain lesions causing REM sleep behavior disorder. Sleep Med 2009;10:9–12.
87. McCarter SJ, Tippmann-Peikert M, Sandness DJ, et al. Neuroimaging-evident lesional pathology associated with REM sleep behavior disorder. Sleep Med 2015;16:1502–1510.

28 Behavioral State Control

OVERVIEW

The spontaneous, ongoing activity in the cerebral cortex defines different cortical states, which provide a dynamic moment-to-moment regulation of cortical information processing and behavior.[1] Behavioral states such as active wakefulness, selective attention, working memory, cognitive control, and motivation are affected to various degrees by three main influences: top-down control from higher order cortex, primarily the prefrontal cortex (PFC),[2] inputs from the thalamus, and modulatory effects from ascending cholinergic and monoaminergic systems[3–5] (Figure 28.1). These modulatory systems include cholinergic neurons of the basal forebrain and mesopontine tegmentum; noradrenergic (NE) neurons of the locus coeruleus (LC), dopaminergic (DA) neurons of the ventral tegmental area (VTA) and substantia nigra pars compacta (SNc) and serotonergic (5-HT) neurons of the rostral raphe. These neurons provide widespread but functionally selective inputs to the forebrain; exhibit both tonic activity that reflects the state of arousal and burst firing in response to attentional demanding tasks or behaviorally relevant stimuli; and exert complex action via a variety of receptors expressed both in principal neurons and local interneurons in their target areas. These modulatory systems are selectively vulnerable in neurodegenerative disorders such as Alzheimer disease (AD) and Parkinson disease (PD). They also have a major role in psychiatric disorders such as anxiety, depression, and drug addiction. The aims of this chapter are to review: (1) the basic connectivity and physiology of the cholinergic and monoaminergic modulatory systems, (2) the mechanisms and their effects on attention and working memory, (3) their role in motivation and response to rewarding or aversive stimuli, and (4) examples of their involvement in neurological and psychiatric disorders.

GENERAL FEATURES OF BRAIN MODULATORY SYSTEMS

The cholinergic and monoaminergic neuromodulatory systems have several features in common.

Widespread but Functionally Selective Projections

Modulatory cholinergic and monoaminergic systems provide widespread yet selective input to several areas. Different subgroups of neurons within each nucleus target specific or functionally related areas and thus provide selective control of information processing.[5,6] The cholinergic neurons in the basal forebrain are distributed in the medial septum, diagonal band, and nucleus basalis of Meynert (NBM).[7] The density of cholinergic innervation is higher in association areas than in primary sensory cortical areas. Specific subsectors of the NBM cholinergic neurons innervate separate portions of the neocortex, which provides for functionally and spatially selective signaling.[8] For example, interconnected prefrontal and posterior cortical association areas receive their innervation from partially overlapping regions of the NBM, suggesting the presence of functional "triangles" consisting of interconnected cortical areas and common cholinergic modulatory inputs.[8] The cholinergic neurons of the mesopontine tegmentum, including pedunculopontine tegmental nucleus (PPT, PPN) and laterodorsal tegmental nucleus (LDT), participate in maintenance of active cortical state, attention, and motivation indirectly via their inputs to the thalamus, midbrain dopaminergic groups, and other brainstem nuclei.[9,10] The LC-NE system provides widespread innervation via extensive axonal arborizations that target multiple areas of the cerebral cortex and subcortical regions.[6] The most important cortical targets are association areas, including the PFC and posterior parietal cortex, as well as somatosensory and motor cortices. The main targets of dopaminergic neurons of the SNc and VTA are the striatum and the cerebral cortex.[11] The ventral tier of

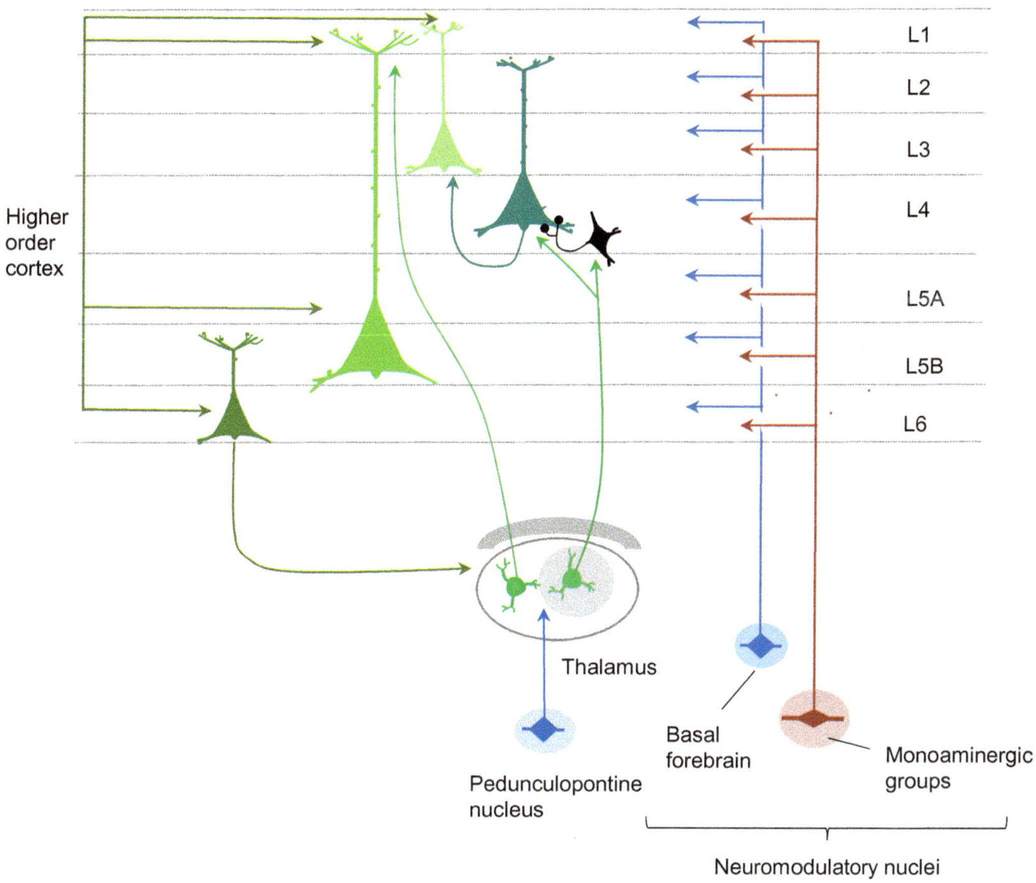

FIGURE 28.1 Influences regulating the cortical states.
Active cortical states, selective attention, and working memory are affected by three main influences: top-down control from higher order cortex, tonic inputs from the thalamus, and modulatory effects from ascending cholinergic and monoaminergic systems.

the SNc projects to the putamen; the dorsal tier projects to the caudate nucleus; and the VTA projects primarily to the nucleus accumbens (NAc).[12] Both the VTA and SNc also send projections to the cerebral cortex, where they target layer 1 throughout multiple cortical areas, and layers 5 and 6 predominantly in the PFC, motor, and posterior parietal cortex.[13] There is also a robust projection of midbrain dopaminergic neurons to the thalamus.[14] Serotonergic inputs controlling behavioral states originate in the rostral raphe nuclei, including dorsal (DR) and median (MR) raphe. Serotonergic axons densely innervate layer 1 in all cortical areas; layer 4 in primary sensory areas, particularly the primary visual cortex; and deep layers in the PFC. Many serotonergic axons target local interneurons. Neurons in the dorsolateral portion of the DR preferentially target the amygdala; those in the ventromedial portion of the DR target the orbitofrontal cortex; and those in the MR and caudal portion of the DR target the hippocampus.[15] Individual serotonergic axons typically provide collaterals to functionally interconnected areas.

All areas harboring cholinergic and monoaminergic neurons also contain intermingled populations of glutamatergic and GABAergic neurons that may project to similar targets. In addition, some VTA neurons can utilize both DA and L-glutamate as their neurotransmitter[16] and some may also release GABA.[13] The same applies to 5-HT raphe neurons.

Inputs from Areas Involved in Attention, Arousal, and Emotion

All cholinergic and monoaminergic groups receive inputs from areas of the PFC involved in attention and executive control. These inputs target both the projection neurons and local GABAergic interneurons in these nuclei. By this mechanism the PFC regulates attentional states not only via its cortico-cortical connections but also indirectly via the cholinergic and monoaminergic systems.[15,17–19]

The tonic activity of these cholinergic and monoaminergic groups during wakefulness is maintained by excitatory inputs from orexin/hypocretin neurons of the posterior lateral hypothalamus, both directly and via histaminergic neurons in the tuberomammillary nucleus. Inputs from GABAergic neurons of the ventrolateral preoptic area are responsible for the progressive reduction of the tonic activity of cholinergic neurons during NREM sleep, as discussed in the previous chapter. All cholinergic and monoaminergic groups also receive inputs from areas involved in processing of emotional and reward information, including the amygdala, hippocampus, and NAc. The parabrachial nucleus, which is involved in arousal and relays pain and other behaviorally relevant inputs, also provides inputs to these modulatory neuronal groups. Importantly, these cholinergic and monoaminergic groups are also strongly interconnected with each other.

Behavioral State-Dependent Tonic Activity

Cholinergic and monoaminergic neurons in these systems fire in two different modes: tonic and phasic. The switch between these modes regulates the different behavioral state, The tonic activity maintains an active cortical state during quiet wakefulness and progressively decreases during non-REM sleep. During REM sleep, activity of cholinergic neurons increases; for example firing of cholinergic PPT/LDT neurons is higher than during wakefulness.[10] In contrast, monoaminergic neurons become essentially silent.

The tonic activity of cholinergic and monoaminergic neurons reflects the interplay among their intrinsic electrophysiological properties; local restraint by inhibitory autoreceptors and local GABAergic interneurons; synaptic influence from wake-active or sleep-active neurons in the hypothalamus, PFC, amygdala, and other sources; and crosstalk interactions between the different neuromodulators (Figure 28.2). Inhibitory somatodendritic M2 autoreceptors in cholinergic neurons, α2 autoreceptors in LC neurons; D2 autoreceptors in midbrain dopaminergic neurons projecting to the striatum; and 5-$HT1_A$ receptors in serotonergic neurons of the DR and MR are activated in a paracrine fashion by their respective neurotransmitters released from dendrites of neighboring neurons within the nucleus. Local GABAergic neurons

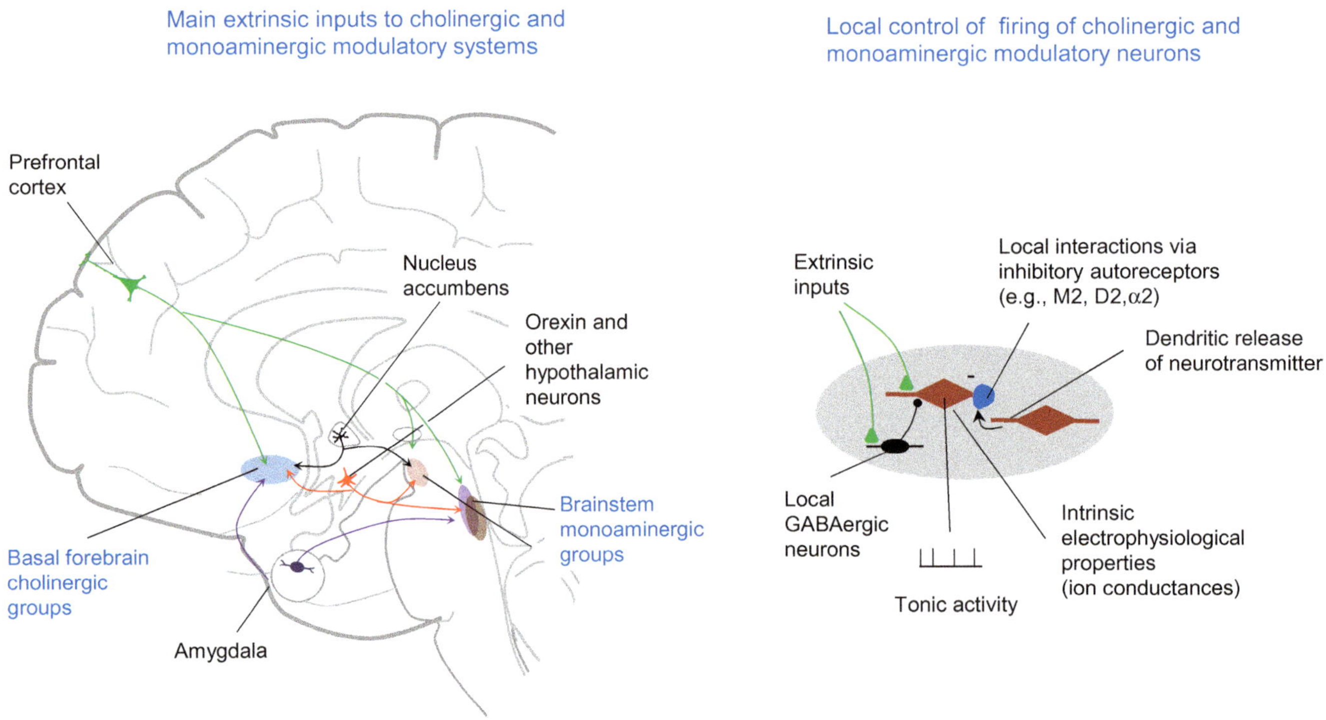

FIGURE 28.2 Influences affecting activity of modulatory cholinergic and monoaminergic neurons.
The firing of modulatory cholinergic and monoaminergic neurons is determined by the interplay among their intrinsic electrophysiological properties and synaptic influence from several sources, including local restrain by inhibitory autoreceptors and effects of local GABAergic interneurons. Their tonic activity during wakefulness is largely maintained by excitatory inputs from orexin/hypocretin neurons of the posterior lateral hypothalamus, whereas their progressively decreased activity during reduced levels of alertness and NREM sleep is triggered by inputs from sleep-promoting regions such as the preoptic area. The burst of firing of cholinergic and monoaminergic neurons in response to behaviorally salient events and attentional tasks is primarily triggered by inputs from the prefrontal cortex. These neuromodulatory systems are also important effectors of areas involved in emotional behavior and motivation, including the amygdala and the nucleus accumbens, and also participate in reciprocal interactions with each other.

in these nuclei tonically restrain the tonic firing within these nuclei. The LC-NE system is the prototype of behavioral state-dependent neuronal firing (Figure 28.3).[19,20] The tonic baseline activity of LC-NE neurons is characterized by a sustained and highly regular discharge pattern (2-5 Hz) that is related to the arousal and waking state. It is low during unaroused states that facilitate disengagement from the environment and sleep, moderate during quiet wakefulness and engagement in a focused task, and high during behavioral arousal and exploratory behavior. Transitions between these different tonic levels are facilitated by glutamatergic inputs from orbitofrontal and anterior cingulate cortices that are sensitive to task context and reward information. These transitions are also regulated by disynaptic feedforward inhibition via local GABAergic neurons that receive strong PFC input.[21]

Phasic Responses During Attention, Emotion, and Behaviorally Relevant Stimuli

The burst of firing of cholinergic and monoaminergic neurons in response to behaviorally salient events and attentional tasks is primarily triggered by inputs from the PFC. The basal forebrain cholinergic neurons are particularly active during waking states associated with locomotion or emotional stimuli. These active cortical states are associated with high-frequency, low-amplitude ("desynchronized") EEG activity.[1] Whereas the tonic activity of these neurons is related to global behavioral states, there is also a phasic release of acetylcholine (ACh) during attention-demanding tasks, reflecting their input from the PFC.[22–25] The activity of most cholinergic neurons in the PPT and LDT also correlates with patterns of thalamocortical activation. Their firing rate is highest during periods of EEG

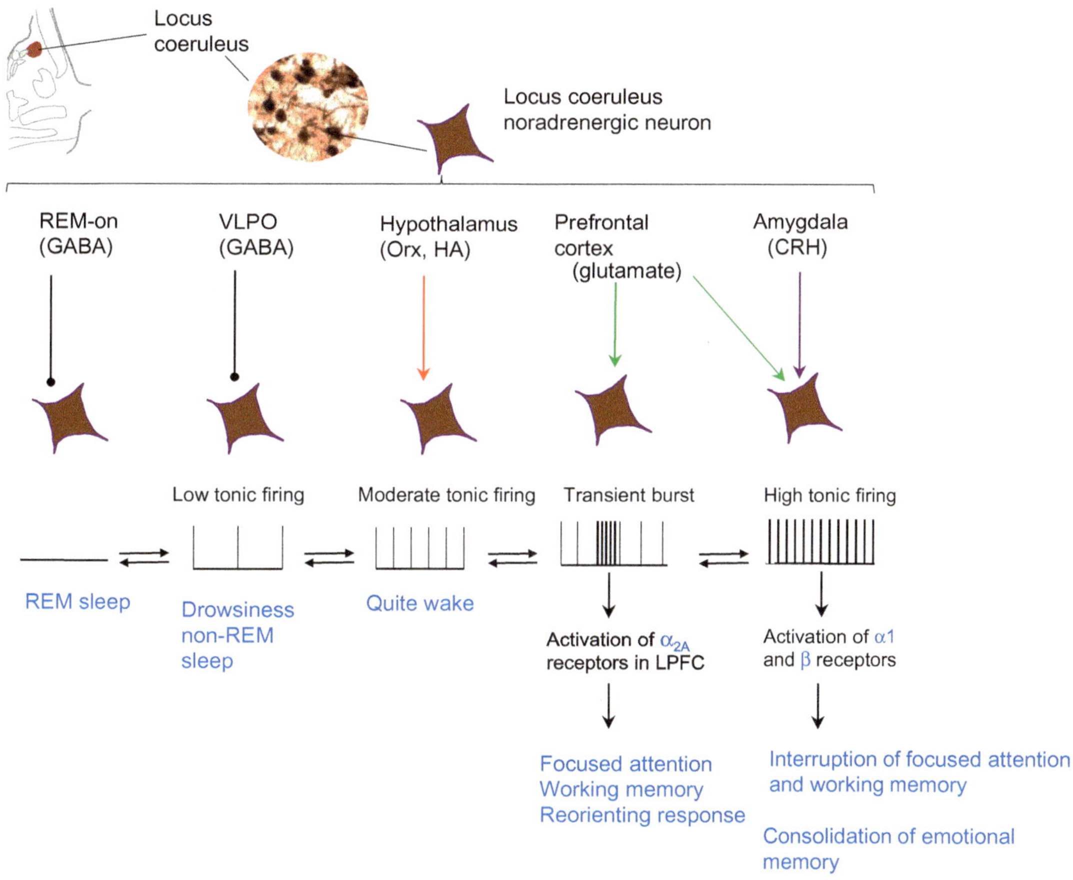

FIGURE 28.3 The locus coeruleus as a prototype of behavioral state-dependent neuronal firing.
Noradrenergic neurons of the locus coeruleus (LC) fire in two modes, tonic and phasic. Tonic baseline activity is related to the arousal and waking state. It is low during unaroused states, in part via the effects of GABAergic inputs from the ventrolateral preoptic area and silent during REM sleep. Tonic activity is moderate during quite wakefulness in part via effects of orexin (Orx) and histamine (HA) neurons of the hypothalamus. Tonic activity is high during behavioral arousal and exploratory behavior or in response to stress, in part due to corticotrophin-releasing hormone (CRH) inputs from the amygdala. During focused attention, LC neurons transiently interrupt their moderate tonic firing and respond with a phasic discharge to task-relevant stimuli. This phasic activity is triggered by inputs from the prefrontal cortex (PFC). This phasic activity promotes working memory and reorienting responses via its effects on the lateral prefrontal cortex (LPFC) and temporoparietal junction (not shown).

desynchronization, but they maintain a low level of activity during slow oscillations. This activity is temporally organized during the cortical UP states, coinciding with the presence of nested cortical gamma oscillations.[1]

During focused attention, LC neurons transiently interrupt their moderate tonic firing and respond with a phasic discharge to task-relevant stimuli. This phasic activity is triggered by PFC inputs in response to relevant targets and allows focused task performance by filtering irrelevant stimuli; they therefore help exploit current reward contingencies ("exploitation" mode). In contrast, high tonic firing of LC allows exploration of alternative behaviors ("exploration" mode). The population dynamics of the LC is characterized by sparse, dynamically regulated correlations among subsets of multiple single units over several timescales.[26] Gap junctions could contribute to brief synchrony in LC ensembles projecting to similar forebrain regions. The population of LC neurons is heterogeneous and coordinates behavioral specific responses.[27,28] For example, during Pavlovian fear conditioning, neurons connected to the basolateral amygdala are activated during fear acquisition, whereas those connected to the anterior cingulate cortex are activated during fear extinction.[29]

Dopaminergic neurons of the VTA and SNc have short latency burst responses to rewarding, aversive, or salient stimuli.[18,30] They are rapidly activated by an alerting signal for detection of potentially important sensory cues. Most midbrain DA neurons encode the motivational value of a stimulus and respond to a reward prediction error signal. They fire a burst of action potentials in response to a reward (positive reward prediction error); and pause their firing response to omission of a reward or a punishment (negative reward prediction error). These neurons therefore encode the motivational value of a stimulus. These motivational value-encoding neurons target primarily the striatum and provide an "instructive" reward signal. A second group of midbrain DA neurons increase their firing in response to both positive rewards and negative outcomes; thereby they encode the motivational salience of stimuli. These neurons primarily project to the PFC and midcingulate cortex and control attention and decision-making.

Receptor Mechanisms, Targets, and U-Curve Responses

The modulatory effects of these neurotransmitters are mediated by a variety of receptors located pre-or postsynaptically, both in principal neurons and in local GABAergic interneurons. These different receptor subtypes may drive opposite signaling events and have different affinity for their agonists. Acetylcholine elicits excitation of cortical projection cells and GABAergic interneurons, via both nicotinic receptors (nAChRs) and M1-type muscarinic receptors; and presynaptic or postsynaptic inhibition via M2-type receptors. Norepinephrine elicits synaptic excitation via α1- and β2 receptors and inhibition via α2 receptors. However, in the PFC, α2 receptors increase responsiveness of pyramidal neurons to glutamatergic inputs. The modulatory effects of DA are mediated by D1-family receptors, which exert primarily postsynaptic excitatory effects, and D2 family receptors, which produce both presynaptic and postsynaptic inhibition.[31] Serotonin also exerts complex actions on both principal neurons and local GABAergic interneurons. They include fast excitation via 5-HT2 and 5-HT3 receptors, presynaptic inhibition via $5\text{-HT1}_{B/D}$ receptors, and postsynaptic inhibition via 5-HT2_{A} receptors. The wide range of effects of neuromodulatory neurotransmitters, depending on the receptor subtype and their targets, explains why the effects of these neuromodulators follow an inverse-U-shaped dose-response curve relationship, so that too low or too high a level of neurotransmitter may be detrimental for cognition.[32]

In addition to their synaptic effects, these neurotransmitters mediate signaling via volume transmission, which provides simultaneous signals in distant brain regions on a timescale of a few seconds. This global and relatively slow neuromodulation is synchronous and controls brain states on timescales relevant to arousal and behavior. These signals affect not only distant neurons but also glial cells and blood vessels. By these mechanisms, neuromodulators coordinate synaptic and network activity with local changes in metabolism and cerebral blood flow.[33]

WAKING STATE

During quiet wakefulness there are fluctuations between activated and deactivated states, as defined by the amplitude and synchronization of network oscillations both locally and throughout the brain.[1] Arousal is a cortical state that facilitates sensory integration and neuronal computations. Active cortical states and selective attention are both characterized by reduction of low-frequency and increase in high-frequency oscillations in selected populations of neurons and facilitate local sensory processing. Acetylcholine and monoamines affect cortical states by eliciting depolarization of cortical pyramidal neurons through a reduction of K^+ currents, modulation of dendritic excitability, and control of neurotransmitter release from presynaptic terminals. Through these mechanisms, neuromodulators control excitability of cortical neurons and suppress the generation of slow oscillations. Modulatory influences may also act via GABAergic interneurons to affect cortical states and network oscillations. For example, activation of layer 2/3 GABAergic neurons expressing vasoactive intestinal polypeptide (VIP) and projecting to other inhibitory interneurons may promote active cortical states. These VIP neurons can be activated by glutamatergic inputs from higher cortical areas, cholinergic inputs via nAChRs, and serotonergic inputs via 5-HT3 receptors. There is a close correlation between transient active cortical states associated with enhanced arousal and attention and pupil diameter.[34,35]

ATTENTION

Attention is the selection of task-relevant information and strengthens neural representations of selected sensory stimuli at the expense of other, nonrelevant inputs.

General Concepts

Attentional processing may be biased by either top-down or bottom-up influences. Top-down processing reflects voluntary guidance of attention to location, objects, and features of the environment that are relevant to the current behaviors and goals. Bottom-up processing reflects the biasing of sensory processing to stimuli that are salient because of their novelty or features (such as brightness or loudness) and thus "pop-up" from their surroundings. Functional neuroimaging studies have identified two large-scale frontoparietal attention networks[36] (Figure 28.4). A dorsal network that includes the dorsolateral PFC, frontal eye fields, and superior parietal lobule is involved in goal-oriented attention and orienting responses and enables the selection of sensory stimuli based on current internal goals or expectations. A ventral frontoparietal network that includes the ventrolateral PFC, inferior parietal lobule, and temporoparietal junction is lateralized to the right hemisphere and responds to salient events in the environment. One of the main correlates of attention is the increased firing rate of neurons that represent attended locations, objects, or features, and suppression of neuronal responses to unattended stimuli. This gain change reflects the activity of both excitatory and inhibitory neurons in competing neuronal populations. The attention-driven process supports neuronal computations that enable "winner-take-all" network states. When attention biases one neuronal population over another, the winning population not only increases its firing rate but also suppresses the competitor neuronal populations, thereby increasing the signal-to-noise ratio to distinguish a relevant from an irrelevant stimulus. Increased inhibitory drive may also contribute to changes of oscillatory activity in the gamma frequency, which improves communication between selected neurons within and between brain areas. There are also changes in alpha frequency oscillations commonly associated to top-down attentional control, and beta oscillations that promote feedback influences. Neuromodulatory cholinergic and monoaminergic inputs elicit effects on sensory processing that are similar to those involved in top-down attention. This reflects the inputs from the PFC these neuromodulatory neurons. The attention network also includes the pulvinar, mediodorsal,

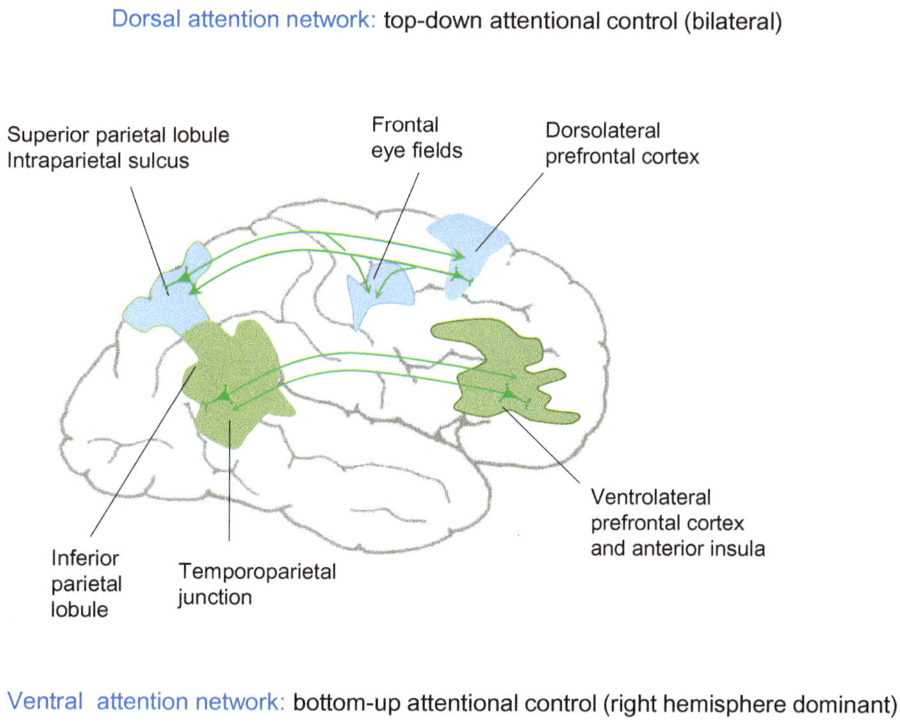

FIGURE 28.4 Attention networks.

There are two large-scale frontoparietal attention networks. A dorsal network that includes the dorsolateral PFC, frontal eye fields, and superior parietal lobule is involved in goal-oriented attention. A ventral frontoparietal network that includes the ventrolateral PFC, inferior parietal lobule, and temporoparietal junction is lateralized to the right hemisphere and responds to salient events in the environment.

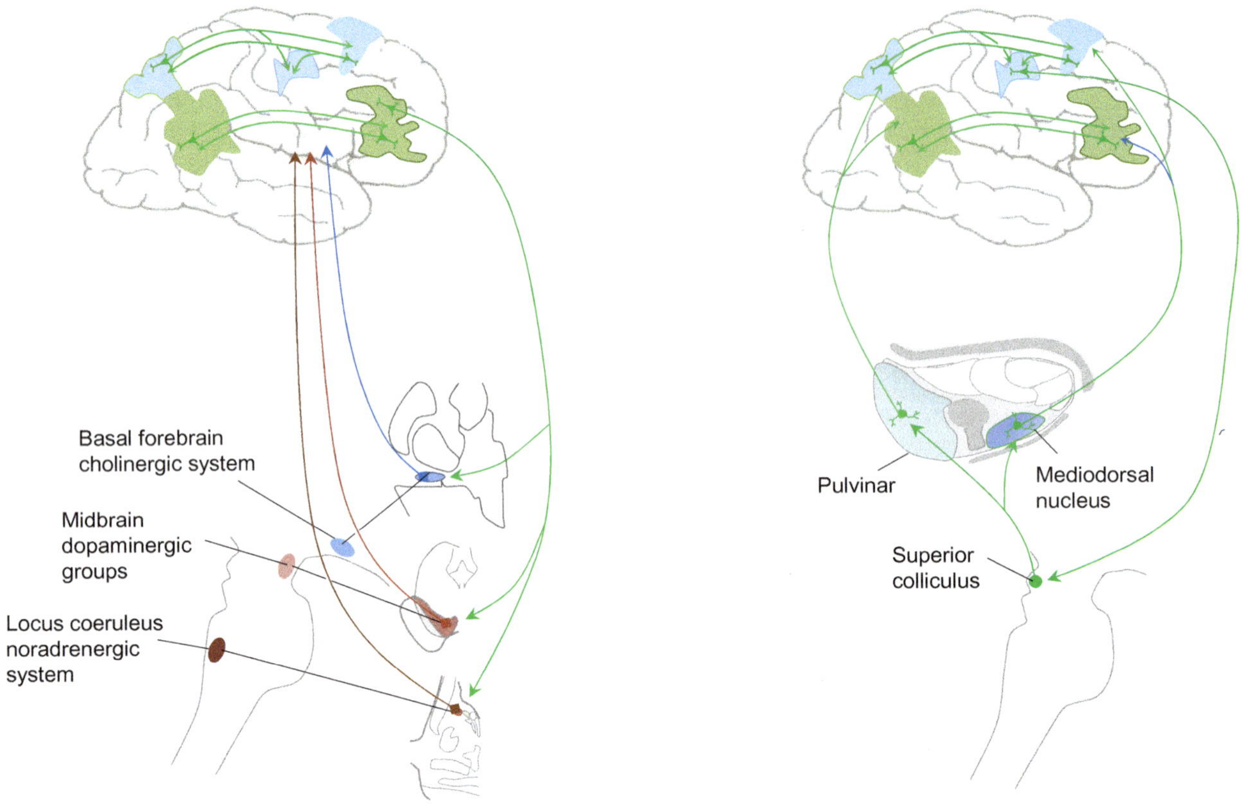

FIGURE 28.5 Subcortical connections of the attention networks.
The attention network includes the pulvinar, mediodorsal, and reticular nuclei of the thalamus, and superior colliculus. All the cortical components of the attention network are targeted by cholinergic and monoaminergic inputs.

and reticular nuclei of the thalamus, and superior colliculus (Figure 28.5).

Cholinergic Modulation of Sensory Processing

One typical example of attentional modulation of sensory processing is that of the effects of ACh action of sensory cortex (Figure 28.6). Acetylcholine has a major role in increasing signal-to-noise ratio in cortical sensory areas promoting processing of new information.[17]

Acetylcholine improves the detection of behaviorally relevant sensory stimuli by increasing evoked responses triggered by thalamic inputs while reducing background intracortical noise.[37,38] For example, in the primary visual cortex, ACh increases glutamate release from thalamocortical afferents via presynaptic nicotinic receptors while inhibiting glutamate release from recurrent cortico-cortical connections via presynaptic M2 receptors. Furthermore, activation of muscarinic M1 receptors in pyramidal neurons enhances neuronal activity to attended visual stimuli; at the same time activation of M1 receptors in GABAergic interneurons improves contrast sensitivity and orientation tuning.

Acetylcholine enhances the representation of information by desynchronization and decorrelation of neuronal activity, and promotes encoding of new memories without interference from retrieval of previous memories. This reflects the profound network effects of ACh via modulation of canonical microcircuits consisting of different subtypes of GABAergic interneurons.[39] For example, activation of nicotinic receptors depolarizes VIP-expressing neurons, leading to disinhibition of pyramidal cells and promoting their response to thalamocortical inputs. Activation of M1 receptors in fast-spiking parvalbumin neurons promotes local fast (gamma) oscillations, whereas activation of M1 receptors in somatostatin interneurons mediating lateral inhibition promotes desynchronization of background cortical activity and prevents slow oscillations.[6,19,32]

Locus Coeruleus and Reorienting Response

The LC-NE system has a major role in the reorienting response, which is the set of attentional adjustments triggered by novel and unexpected stimuli.[36] Reorienting involves the action of the right hemisphere dominant ventral frontoparietal network, which detects salient signals in the environment and then interrupts and resets the ongoing activity of the dorsal frontoparietal network, which is specialized for selecting and linking stimuli and responses.[36] Upon

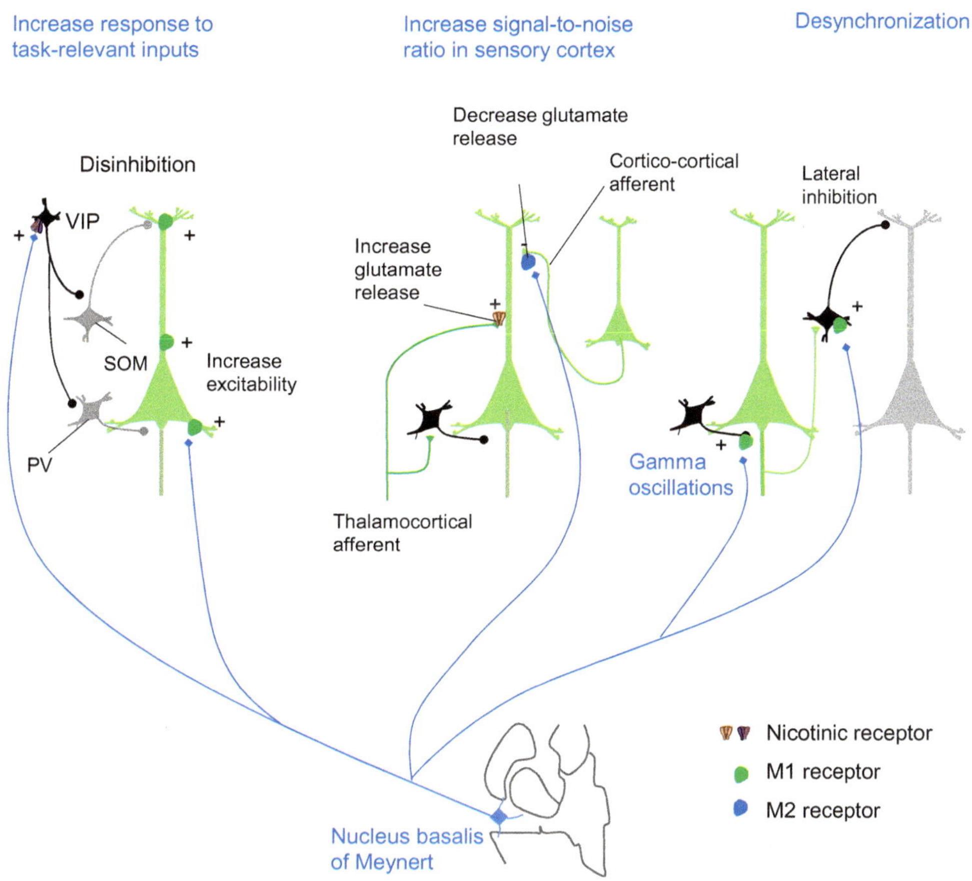

FIGURE 28.6 Effects of acetylcholine on sensory processing.
Acetylcholine (ACh) improves the detection of behaviorally relevant stimuli in sensory cortices by increasing evoked responses triggered by thalamic inputs while reducing background intracortical noise. Acetylcholine increases glutamate release from thalamocortical afferents via presynaptic nicotinic receptors (nAChRs) while inhibiting glutamate release from recurrent cortico-cortical connections via presynaptic M2 receptors (M2Rs). Activation of nAChRs depolarizes vasoactive intestinal polypeptide (VIP)-expressing neurons, leading to disinhibition of pyramidal cells and increasing their response to thalamocortical inputs. Activation of M1 receptors in fast-spiking parvalbumin (PV) neurons promotes local fast (gamma) oscillations, whereas activation of M1 receptors in somatostatin (SOM) interneurons mediating lateral inhibition promotes desynchronization of background cortical activity and prevents slow oscillations.

detection of behaviorally relevant objects or targets, attention is reoriented to the new source of information as the ventral network interrupts ongoing selection in the dorsal network, which then shifts attention toward the novel object of interest. The patterns of recruitment of the dorsal and ventral attention networks during goal-oriented behavior and reorienting responses may reflect inputs from the LC-NE system to the ventral attention network, primarily to the inferior parietal cortex and superior temporal gyrus.[19] During focused attention, LC neurons have a phasic response to target stimuli. This response shares many similarities with the P300 target-related cortical evoked potential that coincides with the response in the ventral attention network to an expected target. This activity may function as an "interrupt" or "network reset" signal that allows the flexible configuration of the cortical network once a target is detected. Whereas the high tonic activity of the LC during the exploratory mode would broaden the sensitivity of the temporoparietal junction to potentially salient environmental stimuli, the decrease in tonic LC activity during the transition from an exploratory state to a task-focused state may parallel the deactivation of temporoparietal junction when subjects engage in a demanding task and would promote engagement on the current task and filtering of distractors. Locus coeruleus neurons may function as novelty detectors, as NE released in response to novel or salient sensory stimuli may activate excitatory α1 receptors promoting bottom-up attentional processing in primary sensory cortex.[40]

Serotonin contributes both to modulation of top-down control of attention via its effects on the dorsolateral PFC and to cognitive flexibility via its effects on the orbitofrontal cortex.[41] Studies using selective pharmacological blockade indicate that both 5-HT1_A and 5HT2_A receptors modulate gamma oscillations in the PFC through fast-spiking GABAergic interneurons; activation of 5-HT1_ARs weakens cortical gamma oscillations, whereas 5-HT2_A receptors synchronize gamma waves.[41] Tonic 5-HT2 receptor activation appears to be necessary for functional coupling in cortical networks promoting goal-directed attention. Serotonin may also have a role in attentional processes during reversal learning tasks, when subjects have to inhibit a response that is no longer rewarding, shift attention to alternative stimuli, an evaluate the risk versus benefit in responding to these stimuli. This task requires evaluation of stimulus value and behavioral flexibility and is typically assessed during the Wisconsin card-sorting test. Attentional control, cognitive flexibility, and reversal learning requires adequate 5-HT levels in the dorsolateral PFC and orbitofrontal cortex. High levels of activation of 5-HT2_A receptors increases cognitive flexibility and reduces the threshold to engage in exploratory behaviors.

WORKING MEMORY

Working memory refers to the short-term maintenance of information "on-line" in the absence of sensory input. This attentional process keeps and prevents temporal decay of relevant information, maintaining its accessible state over brief periods of time for its processing, manipulation, and transformation to guide behavior.

General Mechanisms

The brain regions involved in maintaining information in working memory vary with the type of information to be maintained (Figure 28.7). The same brain regions dedicated

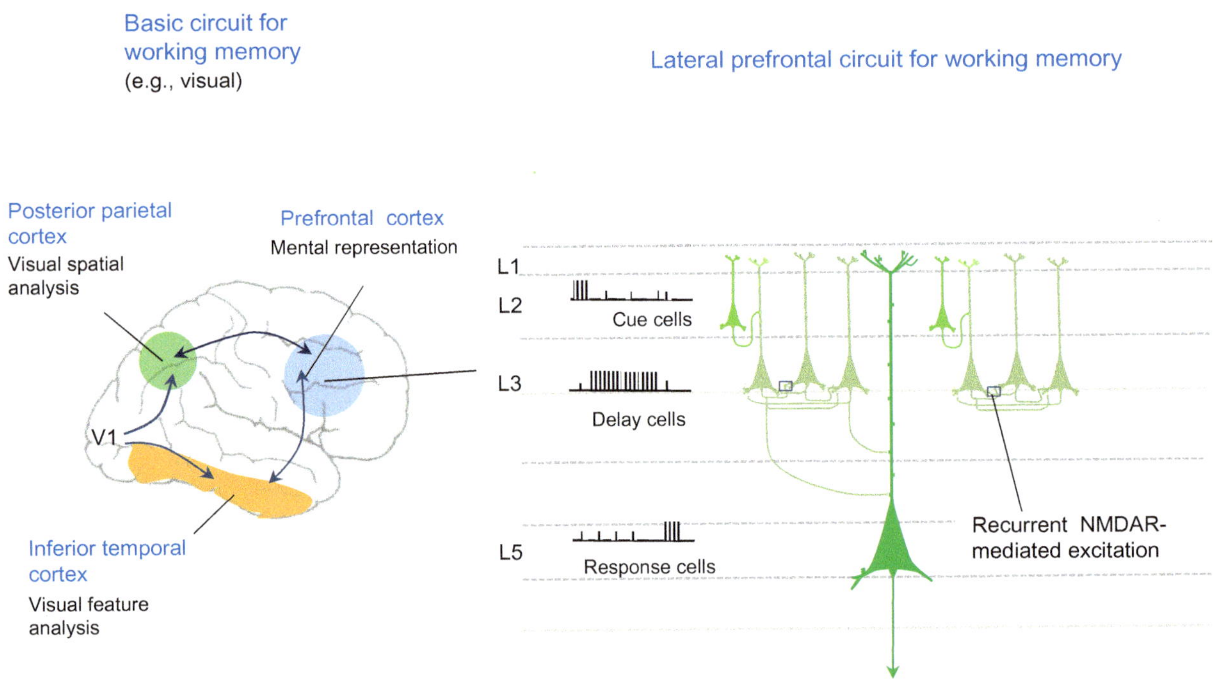

FIGURE 28.7 Mechanisms of working memory.
Working memory is the short-term maintenance of information "on-line" in the absence of sensory input. The brain regions involved in maintaining information in working memory vary with the type of information to be maintained. The regions dedicated to sensory processing are believed to store sensory information during delay periods during performance of working-memory tasks. For example, spatial visual working memory tasks activate the parietal cortex; and visual tasks involving specific stimulus categories activate category-specific regions of the ventral visual cortex. The lateral prefrontal cortex is critical for information maintenance during working-memory tasks. Electrophysiological recordings from the dorsolateral PFC in monkeys identified neurons that show persistent firing across the delay period between the presentation of a visual stimulus in a specific spatial location and the initiation of a saccade toward that stimulus during a spatial working memory task. These neurons, termed "delay" cells, exhibit persistent firing for the specific (or "preferred") spatial location during the delay period preceding the initiation of the saccade. These delay cells are pyramidal neurons located in deep layer 3 of the dorsolateral PFC that have long, thin basal dendrites and extensive horizontal projections that allow for recurrent excitation between and within columns of neurons involved in a given task. This recurrent excitation underlying persistent delay-related activity relies on N-methyl-D-aspartate receptor (NMDAR)-containing synapses.

to sensory processing are believed to store sensory information during delay periods during performance of working-memory tasks.[42] For example, spatial visual working memory tasks activate the parietal cortex; and visual tasks involving specific stimulus categories activate category-specific regions of the ventral visual cortex. Whereas during working memory tasks these posterior regions maintain sensory information (storage), the lateral PFC actively focuses attention on the relevant stimuli for the task, selects information from distractors, and processes this information according to the task.[42] Electrophysiological recordings from the dorsolateral PFC in monkeys identified neurons that show persistent firing across the delay period between the presentation of a visual stimulus in a specific spatial location and the initiation of a saccade toward that stimulus during a spatial working-memory task (Figure 28.7).[43] These neurons, termed "delay" cells, exhibit persistent firing for the specific (or "preferred") spatial location during the delay period preceding the initiation of the saccade. These delay cells are pyramidal neurons located in deep layer 3 of the dorsolateral PFC; these neurons have long, thin basal dendrites and extensive horizontal projections that allow recurrent excitation between and within columns of neurons involved in a given task.[43] This recurrent excitation underlying persistent delay-related activity relies on N-methyl-D-aspartate receptor (NMDAR)-containing synapses.[32]

The mechanisms of modulation of working memory networks in the dorsolateral PFC are fundamentally different from those involved in consolidation of long-term memory in the hippocampus or amygdala (see chapter 25). Consolidation of long-term memories depends on enduring long-term potentiation (LTP) of excitatory synapses, which requires activation of Ca^{+2} and cyclic adenosine monophosphate (cAMP) signaling. In contrast, working memory is a momentary and continuously changing pattern of recurrent activation, a process referred to as dynamic network connectivity.[32] Unlike the case of LTP, downstream signaling promoting intracellular Ca^{2+} and cAMP accumulation in the thin dendrites of layer 3 pyramidal neurons reduces the efficacy of recurrent NMDAR-mediated connections required to maintain activity of these cells during the delay period during working memory tasks. For example, opening of Ca^{2+}-activated K^+ channels or cAMP-mediated activation of hyperpolarization activated cyclic nucleotide-gated channels (HCN) leads to weakening of the recurrent synaptic interactions and thus inhibits working memory.

Cholinergic Modulation

Cholinergic and monoaminergic systems powerfully modulate attention and working-memory functions.[6,32] Cholinergic signaling in the lateral PFC is important both for top-down attention and spatial working memory. The phasic release of ACh in the PFC is triggered by glutamate, which activates presynaptic NMDARs in cholinergic terminals from the basal forebrain. Activation of α7 nAChRs present within the postsynaptic density promotes NMDAR- mediated depolarization and thus recurrent excitation of layer 3 pyramidal neurons in the PFC.[44] Acetylcholine may also promote excitability of dorsolateral PFC neurons though M1-receptor mediated closure to K_V7 (KCNQ) channels and maintain working memory via α2β4 nAChRs.[45]

Monoaminergic Modulation

Dopamine is a key modulator of lateral PFC circuits for attention and spatial working memory. Behaviorally salient stimuli elicit a burst of discharge in dopaminergic neurons, in part triggered by inputs from the superior colliculus. Activation of D1 receptors regulates the efficacy of recurrent connections in the dorsolateral PFC with a typical inverted-U-curve dose-response effect. Low-level D1 receptor activation increases excitability of PFC neurons involved in a task, while moderate D1 receptor activation improves spatial tuning by reducing the responses of neurons not involved in the current task, thus reducing noise. In contrast, excessive D1 receptor activation impairs working memory by promoting cAMP signaling in dorsolateral PFC neurons. The D2 receptors regulate the efficacy of the output of the PFC by reducing cAMP signaling. High tonic levels of extrasynaptic DA promote stability of mental representations primarily via D1 receptors, whereas phasic dopamine signals, primarily via D2 receptors, renders these circuits into a labile state so that working-memory representations can be flexibly updated to allow exploration of new behavioral strategies.[46,47]

Norepinephrine also strongly controls working memory by its effects on autoexcitatory circuits in layer 3 of the lateral PFC. Burst firing of LC neurons leads to a level of NE that activates $\alpha 2_A$ receptors and reduces Ca^{2+} and cAMP-activated currents in long-thin dendrites of layer 3 pyramidal cells of the lateral PFC, increasing the efficacy of autoexcitatory working-memory circuits. These actions may explain the beneficial effects of α2 receptor agonists such as clonidine or guanfacine in attention deficit-hyperactivity disorder (ADHD). In contrast, high levels of NE resulting from high tonic firing of LC neurons during exploration or in response to stress activate α1 and β1 receptor signaling in the lateral PFC reducing working memory performance. Activation of somatodendritic inhibitory $\alpha 2_A$ autoreceptors in LC neurons would prevent their excessive tonic activity and may thus constitute an additional mechanism for beneficial effects of clonidine or guanfacine in ADHD.

In summary, both DA and NE allow moment-by-moment changes in synaptic strength in the lateral PFC circuits and bring working-memory circuits either "on-line" or "off-line" based on the arousal state.[32,48] During reduced arousal sleep or in the setting of fatigue, low levels of DA and NE would result in low activation of D1 and $\alpha 2_A$ receptors, impairing working memory. During alert waking, moderate levels of NE would engage high-affinity $\alpha 2_A$ receptors and strengthen network connections allowing stable mental representations, while moderate levels of

DA acting via D1 receptors would sculpt these representations by weakening nonpreferred connections. In contrast, during excessive arousal or stress, high levels of NE or DA would impair recurrent excitation in the dorsolateral PFC, momentarily taking these circuits "off-line" and switching behavior to more habitual responses. In this setting, while high levels of NE or DA would weaken dorsolateral PFC top-down regulation, they would strengthen consolidation of the stressful experience through actions mediated by α1, β, and D1 receptors in the amygdala, hippocampus, and sensory cortices.[32,49]

MOTIVATION, COGNITIVE CONTROL, AND EMOTIONAL BEHAVIOR

Motivation is the process by which incentives invigorate and guide behaviors toward goals. These goal-oriented and outcome-guided responses can eventually become habits and are performed automatically. Cognitive control is required for successful pursuing of a goal, especially when it is necessary to overcome distraction or strong habitual responses. When outcomes deviate from expectations, the actions change to control future behavior. Cognitive control allocates cognitive resources such as working memory for the successful pursuing of a goal, and is a fundamental mechanism involving different neocortical networks. Cognitive control requires cognitive effort, which depends on motivation driven by incentives.

Assignation of value for decision-making, incentive-based learning, action selection, goal-oriented behavior, and cognitive control effort reflect the coordinated interaction among the orbitofrontal cortex, anterior cingulate cortex, midcingulate cortex, NAc, and ventral pallidum. Midbrain dopaminergic neurons have a major role in these processes.[12,18,30,50–56]

Dopaminergic Neurons: Motivational Value and Salience Signals

Most midbrain dopaminergic neurons exhibit a burst of action potentials in response to a positive reward prediction error and reduce or silence their firing in response to a negative reward prediction error or aversive outcome (Figure 28.8). These motivational value-coding neurons project primarily to the shell of the NAc and other portions of the striatum and are involved in novelty seeking, evaluation, and value learning. They are activated by projections from the PFC relayed via the subthalamic nucleus (STN) and PPT/ LDT. Glutamatergic and cholinergic neurons of the PPT/ LTD are activated by behaviorally relevant stimuli. Neurons of the PPT/ LD, via axon collaterals, may simultaneously trigger state transitions in midbrain dopaminergic and thalamic systems, promoting action initiation by DA effects in the striatum and facilitating high-frequency oscillations and coherence between cortical regions via the thalamus.[10] Pauses in the activity of motivation value coding midbrain dopaminergic neurons in response to a negative reward prediction error or aversive signals are triggered by neurons of the lateral habenula (LHb). These neurons are activated in response to averse outcomes or punishment and inhibit the motivational value-coding midbrain DA neurons indirectly, via a relay on GABAergic neurons in the rostromedial tegmental nucleus. The dopaminergic signal to the striatum is fundamental for reward-based action learning and selection. The burst or phasic firing of midbrain DA neurons triggers a rapid transient peak in DA levels that overwhelm reuptake by the dopamine transporter, resulting in spillover and activation of postsynaptic D1 and D2 receptors in the striatum.[57,58] In response to a reward, DA activates via D1 receptors a subpopulation striatal GABAergic projection neurons of the so-called direct pathway, promoting selection and initiation of the rewarding action. At the same time activation of D2 receptors in a second population of striatal output neurons of the so-called indirect pathway would prevent the interference with the selected action. In contrast, adverse outcomes elicit silencing of midbrain DA neurons due to the effects of the LHb resulting in fall of DA levels in the striatum. This results in interruption of the D2 receptor-mediated inhibition of the indirect pathway leading to avoidance of the action that led to that bad outcome. These pathways are further discussed in chapter 34. A second subset of midbrain dopaminergic neurons increase their firing in response to both positive or negative reward prediction errors and thus signal the motivational salience of stimuli. These neurons receive direct excitatory input from the PFC via the STN and from the LHb and project to the PFC, midcingulate cortex, and striatum. These neurons are involved in orienting, cognition, and general motivation.[30]

Dopamine, Nucleus Accumbens, and Reward-Based Action Selection

A main target of dopaminergic inputs from the VTA is the ventral striatum. The ventral striatum, particularly the NAc, provides an interface between motivation and action and is a critical component of the decision-making process for action selection, motivation, and effort. The NAc processes both appetitive and aversive incentives[59] and has a central role in incentive-based learning and development of the goal-directed behaviors.[53,54,55,59] The NAc may be primarily involved in an evaluation step during learning of motivated behavior, modulation of ongoing behavior, and willingness to expend effort in order to obtain reward.[51] The NAc receives inputs from the ventromedial PFC and projects to the ventral pallidum and substantia nigra pars reticulata, which in turn sends projections to the STN, superior colliculus, PPT, and the ventral anterior and dorsomedial nuclei of the thalamus targeting the PFC.[54,56] The NAc has two major subdivisions, core and shell, which have different connections and putative functions (Figure 28.9). Core-based circuits function in action selection and mediate

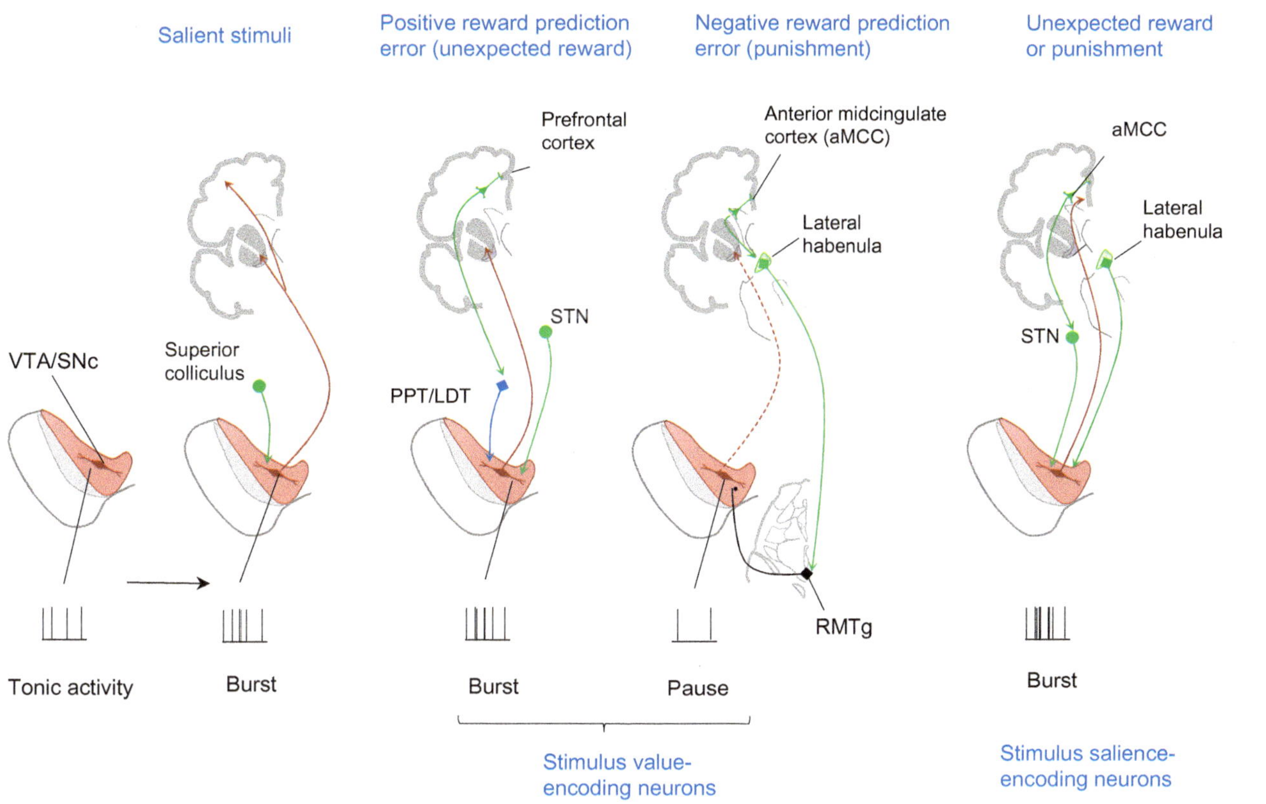

FIGURE 28.8 Firing patterns of dopaminergic neurons.
Most midbrain dopaminergic neurons produce a burst of action potentials in response to a positive reward prediction error and reduce or silence their firing in response to a negative reward prediction error or aversive outcome. They are activated by projections from the prefrontal cortex relayed via the subthalamic nucleus (STN) or pedunculopontine/laterodorsal nuclei (PPT/LDT). Pauses in the activity of motivation value-coding midbrain dopaminergic neurons in response to a negative reward prediction error or aversive signals are triggered by the lateral habenula, indirectly via a relay on GABAergic neurons in the rostromedial tegmental nucleus (RMTg). A second subset of midbrain dopaminergic neurons increase their firing in response to both positive or negative reward prediction errors and thus signal the motivational salience. These neurons receive excitatory inputs both from the PFC via the STN and directly from the lateral habenula.

conditioned emotional responses, spatial learning, and impulsive choice. The shell provides an interface between the basal ganglia, the amygdala, and other limbic areas. Shell-based circuits participate in encoding the reward value and reinforcing effects of rewards.[54,55]

Dopamine inputs from the VTA to the NAc shell are critical for Pavlovian learning based on reward-prediction error signals.[60] In addition to the "instructive" signals on striatal projection neurons, DA regulates the opposite influences of the PFC and hippocampus on reward processing in the NAc.[67] Tonically released DA, acting via D2 receptors, reduces the inhibitory effect of PFC inputs to the NAc; phasic DA transients acting via D1 receptors potentiate hippocampal activity, thus maintaining behaviors that lead to reward.[61] Dopaminergic inputs from the dorsal tier of the SNc to the head of the caudate nucleus, which interacts with the PFC, has a major role in goal-directed learning of actions guided by their outcome. Eventually, rewarding actions become habits and are performed automatically. Habit learning involves the dorsolateral striatum, particularly the posterior putamen, which receive dopaminergic inputs from the ventral tier of the SNc and interacts with the sensorimotor cortex.

There is a reciprocal GABAergic output from the striatum to the midbrain dopaminergic neurons. This reciprocal interaction varies among the different components of the striatum and provides for a "spiraling" flow of information between these components.[12] The NAc, particularly its shell region, projects to widespread territory that includes the VTA and dorsal tier of the SNc; the caudate projects to both the dorsal and ventral tiers of the SNc; and the putamen provides limited input to ventral tier of the SNc.[12] This pattern of reciprocal striato-midbrain-striatal connections provides a mechanism for information flow from limbic (NAc) to cognitive (caudate) to motor (putamen) components of the basal ganglia circuits[12] (Figure 28.10).

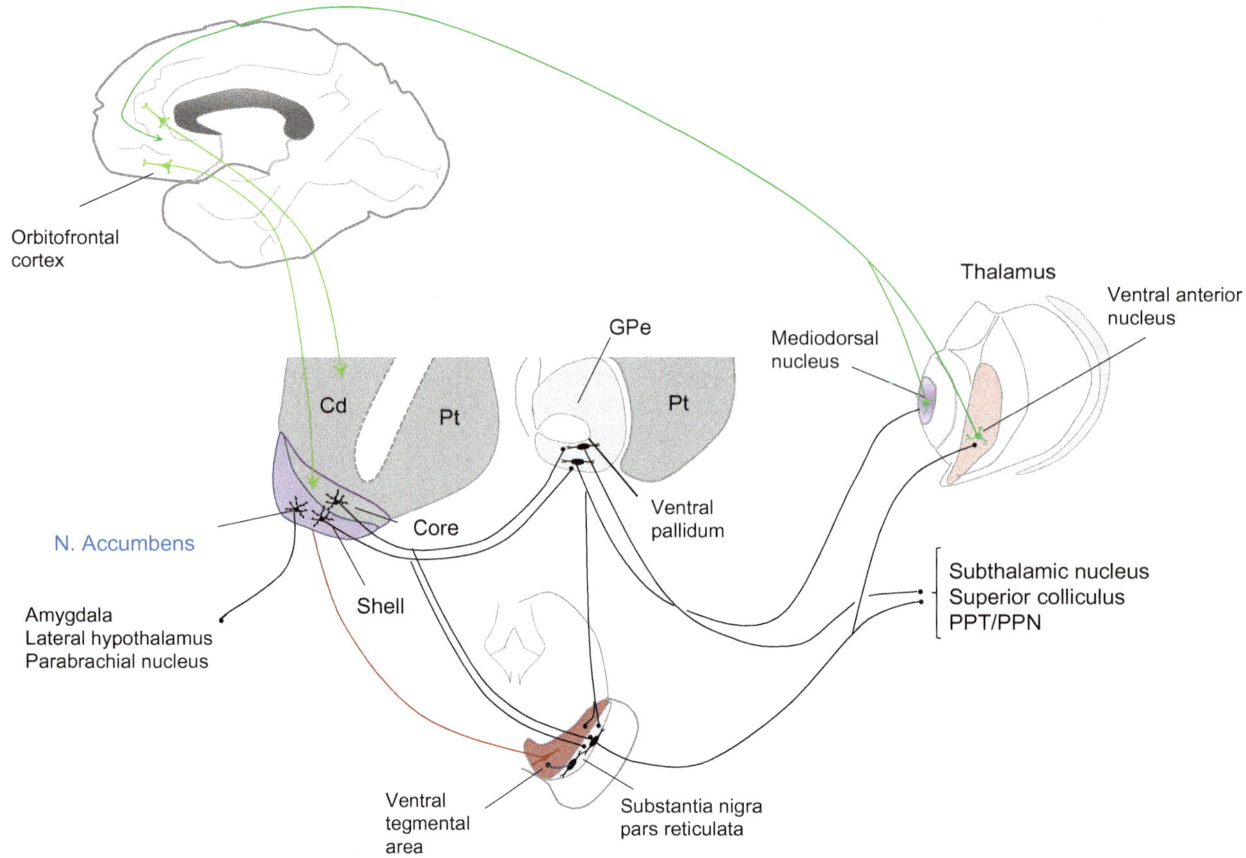

FIGURE 28.9 Nucleus accumbens.
The nucleus accumbens (NAc) has a central role in incentive-based learning and development of the appropriate goal-directed behaviors. The NAc receives excitatory inputs from the caudal ventromedial prefrontal cortex and thalamus. The NAc has two major subdivisions, core and shell, which have different connections and putative functions. The NAc core shares features with other components of the striatum. The shell provides an interface between the basal ganglia, the amygdala, and other limbic areas. The outputs of the NAc target the GABAergic neurons of the ventral pallidum and substantia nigra pars reticulata, which in turn project to the STN, superior colliculus, pedunculopontine nucleus (PPN/PPT), and the ventral anterior and dorsomedial nuclei of the thalamus. These thalamic nuclei send projections back to the orbital and medial prefrontal cortex, including the orbitofrontal and anterior and midcingulate cortex; thereby closing the so-called limbic circuit of the basal ganglia. Cd, caudate; GPe, globus pallidus pars externa; Pt, putamen.

Dopamine Signals and Allocation of Cognitive Effort

Cognitive effort is the allocation of cognitive resources, such as working memory, to the pursuit of a goal.[51] This is a motivated process driven by the behavioral relevance (affective valence) of incentives encoded by DA neurons o the VTA. Dopaminergic inputs to the NAc promote behavioral activation, exertion of effort, approach behavior, and sustained engagement in tasks.[50] In human fMRI studies, activity of the ventral striatum relates to the reward expected from the exertion of effort,[62] whereas its inactivation occurs during actions that may lead to failure.[63] The transient DA bursts and pauses of VTA neurons tracking the presence or value of a given reward can influence risky decision-making.[64] Tasks demanding cognitive control involve a conflict between the likelihood of success in obtaining a reward and the subjective effort cost required to obtain it. Phasic DA release encodes a "reward-minus effort" signal that promotes the allocation of effort by the anterior midcingulate cortex (MCC) and ventral striatum. The anterior MCC monitors action–outcome associations to determine benefits and costs and allocate cognitive effort, and then recruits the lateral PFC to implement control.[65] Electrical stimulation of the anterior MCC evoked the experience of the "will to perseverate" in response to a forthcoming challenge.[66] The anterior MCC may monitor the increased costs and incremental progress of the selected action and convey the balance between these variables to the midbrain dopaminergic neurons; the dopaminergic signal is then sent to both the lateral PFC and ventral striatum. In the lateral PFC, the increase in DA tone stabilizes the activity in recurrent working-memory networks representing the task goals. In the ventral striatum, DA release first selects sequences of

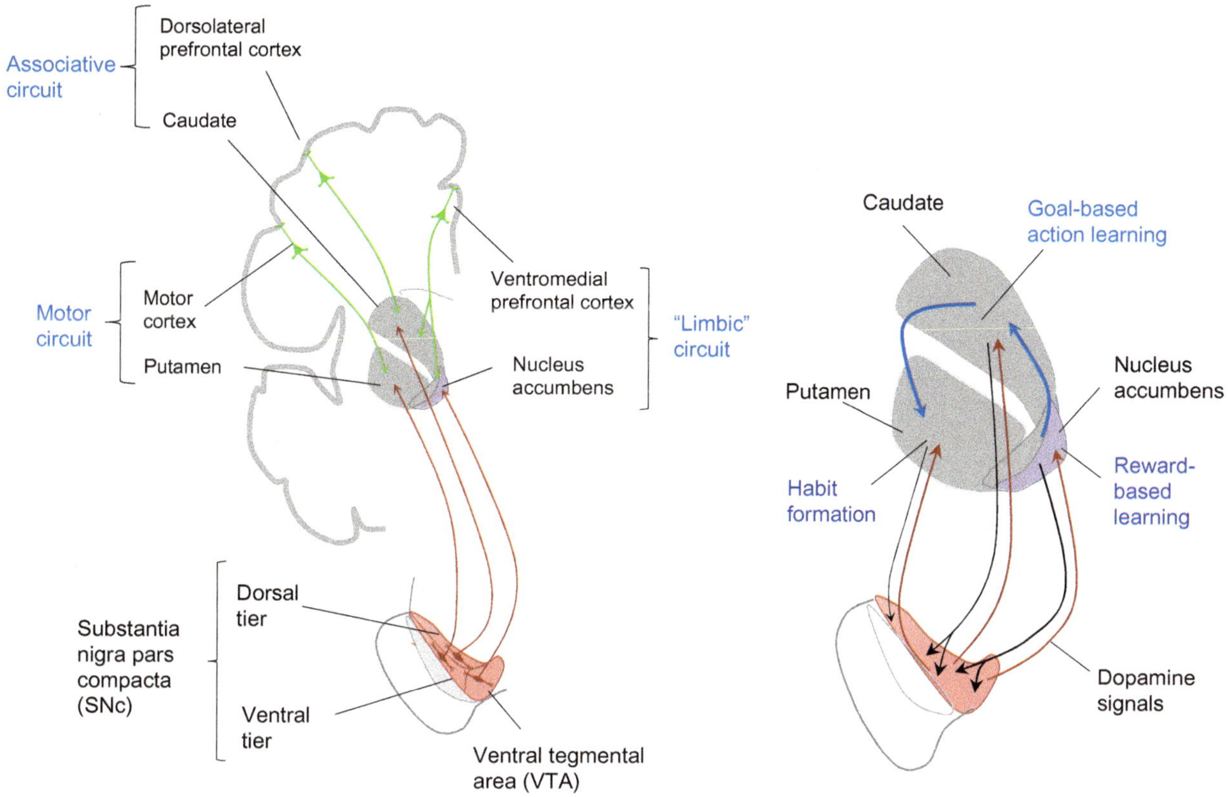

FIGURE 28.10 Dopamine signals to the striatum.
Dopamine transients in the nucleus accumbens (NAc) shell are critical for Pavlovian learning based on reward-prediction error signals. Associative learning leads to goal-oriented behavior via dopaminergic influence from the dorsal tier of the substantia nigra pars compacta on the caudate nucleus (SNc). Eventually, rewarding actions become habits primarily via the posterior putamen, which receives dopaminergic inputs from the ventral tier of the SNc. There is a reciprocal GABAergic output from the striatum to the midbrain dopaminergic neurons. This reciprocal interaction varies among the different components of the striatum and provides for a "spiraling" flow of information between these components.

goal-directed behavior and, as the goal is reached, ramping DA tone invigorates gating of action.

Anterior Midcingulate Cortex, Lateral Habenula, and Outcome Monitoring

The monitoring of the outcome of a choice is critical for behavioral adjustments. Both the anterior MCC and the LHb monitor negative outcomes[67] (Figure 28.11). The anterior MCC is activated when subjects receive negative feedback following inappropriate behaviors. In response to aversive outcome, the anterior MCC sends excitatory inputs to the LHb; the LHb elicits disynaptic inhibition of VTA/SNc dopaminergic neurons that encode motivational value and an excitatory projection of VTA neurons that encode stimulus valence. This LHb and anterior MCC can thus communicate with each other and cooperate to monitor negative outcome. Whereas the LHb quickly detects the negative outcome of an ongoing action, the anterior MCC may store information about negative past experiences to guide the appropriate behavioral adjustment during the next choice.[67]

Interactions Between Serotonin and Dopamine Signals

The activity of different subsets of serotonergic neurons of the DR regulates adaptive responses to environmental stress and rewarding or aversive stimuli. These neurons may be robustly engaged by stressful circumstances or experiences that sensitize responses to stress. Similarly to VTA neurons, serotonergic neurons of the DR may respond to the reward value or salience of stimuli. Neurons in the ventromedial DR projecting to the orbitofrontal cortex are activated by reward and inhibited by punishment and thus encode stimulus value. In contrast, neurons in the dorsolateral portion of the DR projecting to the basolateral amygdala are activated by both rewards and punishments and thus encode stimulus salience.[15]

The DR receives excitatory inputs from the PFC and LHb, both of which target serotonergic as well as local GABAergic neurons. The net effect of these inputs may thus be either excitatory or mediate feed-forward inhibition of serotonergic projection cells. Serotonergic DR and dopaminergic VTA neurons have complementary roles in response to reward and punishment. Dopaminergic VTA

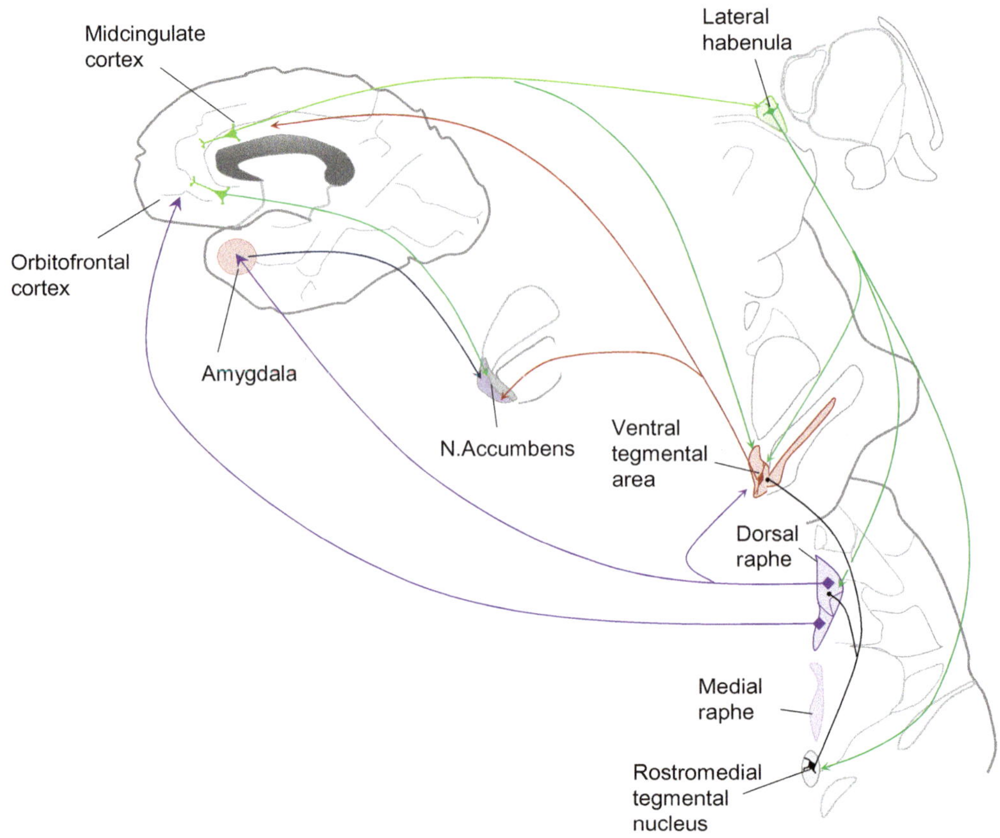

FIGURE 28.11 Pathways for cognitive effort, outcome monitoring, and dopamine-serotonin interactions.
Dopaminergic inputs to the nucleus accumbens have a major role in behavioral activation, the anterior midcingulate cortex monitors action–outcome associations to determine benefits and costs and allocate cognitive effort. Both the midcingulate cortex and lateral habenula monitor negative outcomes. The lateral habenula elicits disynaptic inhibition silencing of midbrain dopaminergic neurons that encode the motivational value of stimuli via the rostromedial tegmental nucleus, while sending excitatory projections to dopaminergic neurons that encode motivational salience. These neurons, in turn, project to the midcingulate cortex. The activity of different subsets of serotonergic neurons of the dorsal raphe regulates adaptive responses to environmental stress and rewarding or aversive stimuli. The dorsal raphe receives inputs from the prefrontal cortex and lateral habenula as well disynaptic inhibition from the lateral habenula via the rostromedial tegmental nucleus. Dopaminergic neurons projecting to the striatum receive dense excitatory projections from the dorsal raphe. Reciprocally, inhibitory GABAergic projections from the VTA and striatum regulate activity of serotonergic dorsal raphe neurons (not shown).

neurons projecting to the striatum receive dense excitatory projections from the DR; these projections are mainly glutamatergic, but also serotonergic. Activation of VTA neurons by these projections drives reward-type responses via D1 receptors in the striatum. Reciprocally, inhibitory GABAergic projections from the VTA and striatum regulate activity of serotonergic DR neurons, forming a feedback loop that intertwines DA and 5-HT systems in the reward circuitry. Serotonin may also mediate impulse control while anticipating a future reward. Serotonin may also control behavioral inhibition in an aversive context such as punishment, monetary loss, or omitted reward. Pharmacological manipulations of serotonergic neurotransmission in humans also provide evidence for an involvement of 5-HT in punishment processing.[51]

INVOLVEMENT OF NEUROMODULATORY SYSTEMS IN NEURODEGENERATIVE DISORDERS

The cognitive functions of the dorsolateral PFC decline with advancing age.[32] Studies in aging monkeys show large reductions of synapses in layer 3 with loss of synapses on long-thin dendrites of pyramidal cells that are critical for working memory. These findings may in part reflect excessive Ca^{2+} and cAMP signaling associated with decreased expression of $\alpha 2_A$ receptors. Dysregulation of neuromodulation in lateral PFC may also explain why stress and head trauma may accelerate age-related cognitive deficits.

Neuromodulatory systems are particularly vulnerable to proteinopathies such as Alzheimer disease (AD) and

Parkinson disease (PD). The vulnerability of cholinergic and monoaminergic neurons may in part be due to their intrinsic firing properties, long and highly arborized axonal projections that make them vulnerable to impaired axonal transports and thus to dying-back processes.[68] The involvement of cholinergic neurons in AD and dopaminergic neurons in PD are discussed in separate chapters of this book.

Whereas loss of basal forebrain cholinergic neurons is considered a primary mechanism for impaired attention and episodic memory in AD[69] and loss of SNc in the motor manifestations of PD, there is evidence that loss of LC noradrenergic neurons may precede that of cholinergic and dopaminergic neurons in these disorders and may contribute to behavioral manifestations such as impaired attention, anxiety, depression, and sleep disruption.[70] Postmortem studies show that both tau and α-synuclein neuropathology appears in the LC at very early disease stages, preceding involvement of the transentorhinal cortex in AD[71] and that of midbrain dopaminergic neurons in PD.[72] In AD, hyperphosphorylated tau accumulation in the LC occurs many decades before neuronal loss; similarly, α-synuclein accumulation in LC noradrenergic neurons occurs at Braak stage 2 in PD, preceding involvement of dopaminergic neurons of the SNc; but there is no LC cell loss until late disease stages. In both AD and PD, there is early loss of dendrites, proximal axons, and noradrenergic axon terminals in LC target areas, including the hippocampus and PFC, consistent with a dying-back phenomenon. At early stages of disease, accumulation of hyperphosphorylated tau or α-synuclein in LC neurons, combined with other cell stressors such as oxidative stress or neuroinflammation, may lead to abnormal hyperactivity of these neurons, which has been linked to anxiety, depression, and sleep disturbances.[70,73]

At later stages, LC neuronal cell loss leads to decline in NE levels in the PFC, hippocampal formation, and other LC targets and may contribute to deficits in arousal and attention in these disorders.[70] The wide arborizations of LC neurons may promote neuron-to-neuron seeding and propagation of abnormal tau or α-synuclein neuropathology,[74] which may be promoted by increased neuronal activity.[70]

NEUROMODULATORY SYSTEMS AND PSYCHIATRIC DYSFUNCTION

Psychosis, Schizophrenia, and Hallucinations

Psychosis refers to severe impairment in reality testing (the inability to distinguish between the external reality of the environment and internal experience), which is typically associated with hallucinations, delusions, disorganized thought processing, incoherent speech, and abnormal motor behaviors.[75] Schizophrenia is characterized by psychotic symptoms such as hallucinations, delusions, and disorganized speech; negative symptoms such as decreased motivation and emotional expressiveness; and cognitive deficits involving impaired executive functions and memory.[76] Hallucinations reflect disturbances in sensory processing and occur not only in schizophrenia but also in other psychiatric disorders, as well as in several neurologic and medical disorders.[77]

Psychosis and hallucinations may have several potential basic neurochemical substrates. These include abnormalities in D2R signaling in the striatum and PFC, reduced NMDAR-mediated activation of GABAergic interneurons in the PFC, increased 5-$HT2_A$ receptor signaling in prefrontal circuits, and impaired cholinergic transmission in the cerebral cortex and thalamus. Psychosis and hallucinations may be thus be caused by (1) increased dopaminergic transmission by drugs such as cocaine, amphetamines, or dopaminergic agonists; (2) reduced NMDAR activity in the cerebral cortex due to NMDAR encephalitis or drugs such as ketamine or phencyclidine; (3) exaggerated 5-$HT2_A$ receptor activation by drugs such as lysergic acid diethylamide (LSD), mescaline, or psilocybin; and (4) impaired cholinergic signaling in thalamocortical circuits due to degeneration of cholinergic neurons or blockade of muscarinic cholinergic receptors by drugs such as amitriptyline, nortriptyline, doxepin, oxybutynin, or diphenhydramine, particularly in the elderly.

Schizophrenia is the prototype disorder producing psychosis and hallucinations. This disorder is associated with decreased DA signaling in the PFC and increased DA signaling in the striatum. There is profound PFC dysfunction in schizophrenia, beginning in adolescence and progressing into adulthood. The most common genetic abnormality associated with a schizophrenia-like phenotype is chromosome 22q11.2 deletion syndrome (also known as DiGeorge syndrome or velocardiofacial syndrome), which is also a genetic risk factor for early-onset PD.[79] In schizophrenia, impaired working memory is associated with loss of neuropil and dendritic spines in pyramidal cells and weakened lateral GABAergic inhibition in microcircuits in layer 3 of the PFC.[80] In addition disturbed D2 receptor signaling may reduce the feedback from layer 5 to layer 3 pyramidal cells. Furthermore, increased D2 receptor signaling in the caudate may weaken the inhibition of inappropriate activity by the indirect pathway in the basal ganglia circuits. Antipsychotic medications act primarily by blocking D2 receptors. They include the first-generation drugs haloperidol and perphenazine, and the second-generation drugs clozapine, risperidone, olanzapine, quetiapine, ziprasidone, aripiprazole, paliperidone, isoperidone, arsenapine, lurasidone, cariprazine, and brexiparazole.[76] In general, these drugs are sufficient to occupy approximately 70% of D2 receptors; the exceptions are clozapine and quetiapine, which are effective at lower doses. Side effects include acute extrapyramidal side effects including akathisia, drug-induced parkinsonism, acute dystonic reactions, tardive dyskinesia, and metabolic side effects such as weight gain and metabolic syndrome. First-generation antipsychotics, as well as risperidone, paliperidone, and asenapine, can elevate prolactin level. Second-generation antipsychotic agents also have a high affinity for 5-$HT2_A$ receptors. These receptors are highly expressed in pyramidal cells of the PFC, and their excessive activation suppresses attention in healthy persons apparently due to inability to suppress distracting stimuli.[81] Hallucinogenic drugs, such as LSD, mescaline, and psilocybin, are potent 5-$HT2_A$ receptor agonists. Pimavaserin, a 5-$HT2_A$ inverse agonist, is approved for the treatment of psychosis in PD.[82] Activation of 5-$H2_A$ receptors in both the PFC and VTA increases DA release in the NAc. The high affinity of atypical antipsychotic drugs for 5-$HT2_A$ receptors might contribute to the lower incidence of DA supersensitivity that normally results from chronic D2 receptor blockade, compared with that following treatment with typical antipsychotic drugs.

Neurologic disorders that may have prominent manifestations of psychosis and hallucinations include dementia with Lewy bodies (DLB), frontotemporal dementia (FTD) associated with hexanucleotide expansions in the *C9ORF72* gene, variant Creutzfeldt-Jakob disease, right hemispheric stroke affecting frontoparietal-subcortical circuits; and status epilepticus.[78] A typical disorder associated with hallucinations is DLB.[83] The hallucinations are typically visual and may reflect impaired cholinergic modulation of thalamocortical circuits involving the visual cortex. The occipital cortex, the lateral pulvinar (which projects to the parieto-occipital association cortex) and the intralaminar nuclei (involved in perceptual arousal and awareness) are prominently affected in DLB. There is marked reduction of cholinergic innervation in both the thalamus and cerebral cortex in this disorder. Hallucinations may be related to inadequate arousal signals to the thalamus and cortex, diminishing appropriate integration of bottom-up and top-down inputs. As top-down influences modulate perception by building expectations about sensory stimuli, disruptions in ACh signaling may alter the relative certainty between bottom-up sensory information and top-down expectations. Several neuroimaging studies show increased thalamic activity during hallucinations. Hallucinations in DLB have several characteristic features. They involve mundane objects such as persons or animals and are typically nonfrightening. They do not provoke fear and anxiety as those seen in schizophrenia and related to NMDAR impairment or D2 receptor hyperfunction, and they are not distorted versions of reality as are those associated with the effects of muscarinic drugs or 5-$HT2_A$ hallucinogen agonists. Hallucinations seen in deafferentation states (such as Charles Bonnet syndrome or tinnitus) are simpler and represent features of objects rather than whole objects as in the DLB. Hallucinations in FTD are typically rare and strongly associated with a hexanucleotide C9ORF72 expansions with degeneration in the medial pulvinar.

As thalamic activity is tightly coupled to the fine balance of bottom-up and top-down information, any sensory system that relies on perceptual inference may be prone to hallucinate when the balance is shifted due to changes in excitatory or inhibitory tone. It has been proposed that impaired cholinergic α7 receptor-mediated activation of the thalamic reticular nucleus or cortical inhibitory interneurons may have a role in visual hallucinations in DLB, which could explain the beneficial effect of cholinesterase inhibitors in this disorder.[84]

Drug Addiction

Addiction is a chronic disorder of the brain reward, motivation, memory, and related circuitry and is characterized by compulsive drug seeking and use, despite harmful consequences. Addiction has been viewed as a gain-of-function disease resulting in excessive DA release in the mesolimbic system. All drugs of addiction promote burst firing of midbrain DA neurons and increase DA release in the NAc. Nicotine directly increases activity of VTA neurons and DA release from their terminals in the NAc. Nicotine also increases release of glutamate, which indirectly facilitates DA release. With long-term nicotine exposure nAChRs in GABAergic neurons become desensitized, whereas glutamatergic excitation persists. Psychostimulants such as cocaine, amphetamine, and methylphenidate inhibit presynaptic DA uptake by the DA transporter. These drugs also increase DA cell firing and trafficking and exocytosis of DA-containing vesicles. Opioids (acting via mu-type receptors), endocannabinoids (acting via CB1 receptors), benzodiazepines (acting via $GABA_A$ receptors), and γ-hydroxybutyrate (acting via $GABA_B$ receptors) indirectly promote dopaminergic VTA neuron activity by inhibiting local GABAergic interneurons. Whereas both GABAergic interneurons and dopaminergic cells in the VTA express $GABA_A$ receptors, benzodiazepines more strongly promote GABAergic inhibition of α1 subunit-containing receptors expressed in local interneurons as opposed to α2/α3 subunit-containing receptors in dopaminergic cells.

In normal conditions, DA provides learning signals in the NAc, and once the reward is fully predictable the VTA neurons are no longer activated, learning stops, and the behavior is optimized to obtain the reward. Addictive drugs can override this system, generating an inappropriate learning signal that eventually leads to compulsive drug intake at the expense of all other behaviors. Drugs of addiction, as well as natural rewarding stimuli, such as food, trigger LTP glutamatergic synapses on VTA dopaminergic neurons projecting to the shell of the NAc, promoting D1 receptor-mediated synaptic plasticity in NAc neurons.[85] The reciprocal feedback between the striatum and midbrain DA neurons results in a ventromedial-to-dorsolateral progression of the striatal region involved in behavioral learning and motivation. There is progressive engagement of the NAc core, the caudate involved in goal-oriented behavior, and eventually the putamen supporting habitual and compulsive behavior.[12,86]

A heightened ("sensitized") motivation to seek drugs may be due to impairment of cognitive processes involved in executive function. This would lead to impaired ability to update behavior according to the increasingly nonrewarding effects of drug intake, attentional bias toward drug-related cues, and compulsive behavior. A disrupted PFC function likely accounts for impaired response inhibition and salience attribution in patients with drug addiction. Reduced plasticity in the orbitofrontal cortex may lead to impairment in reversal learning and faulty functional coupling between the orbitofrontal and amygdala.

Anxiety and Depression

Multiple brain areas including the hypothalamus, amygdala, PFC, LC, and NAc are active during both stress and anxiety.[87,88] Studies in experimental animals show that neurons in the basolateral amygdala activated by predicted rewards and projecting to the shell and medial core of the NAc support reward seeking, whereas those activated by stimuli that predict an aversive outcome elicit avoidance responses. The LC is linked to both physical and emotional responses to stress as well as aversive memory consolidation.[89,90] The increase in tonic activity of the LC-NE neurons during stress is triggered by inputs from the amygdala containing corticotrophin-releasing hormone and results in β-adrenergic receptor-mediated signaling in the basolateral amygdala.[91] Norepinephrine primarily activates neurons of the basolateral amygdala that project to the anterior hippocampus, which encode negative valence and trigger anxiety-like behaviors. The ventromedial and dorsolateral DR serotonergic systems functionally oppose one another.[15] Activation of neurons in the ventromedial DR projecting to the orbitofrontal cortex decreases anxiety and promotes coping behavior in mice; in contrast, activation of neurons in the dorsolateral portion of the DR projecting to the basolateral produces anxiety-like behaviors. Thus, globally targeting the serotonergic system using SSRI treatment is likely to activate antagonistic pathways that could contribute to adverse acute effects or to resistance to SSRI treatment. Additional important targets of antidepressant treatment are 5-$HT1_A$ receptors, which function as somatodendritic autoreceptors located on 5-HT neurons and as postsynaptic heteroreceptors on target neurons. Furthermore, serotonin released in the raphe activates 5-$HT1_A$ autoreceptors to negatively regulate the firing of the serotonin system

KEY POINTS

- Behavioral states, such as active wakefulness, selective attention, working memory, cognitive control, and motivation, are affected by top-down control from higher-order cortex and modulatory effects from ascending cholinergic and monoaminergic systems.
- Neuromodulator systems include cholinergic neurons of the basal forebrain and mesopontine tegmentum; noradrenergic (NE) neurons of the locus coeruleus (LC), dopaminergic (DA) neurons of the ventral tegmental area (VTA) and substantia nigra pars compacta (SNc), and serotonergic (5-HT) neurons of the rostral raphe.
- These neuromodulatory systems provides widespread yet functionally selective inputs to the forebrain.
- The modulatory effects of these neurotransmitters are mediated by a variety of receptors located pre- or postsynaptically, both in principal neurons and in local GABAergic interneurons.
- The tonic activity of cholinergic and monoaminergic neurons maintains an active cortical state during quiet wakefulness and progressively decreases during non-REM sleep.
- Cholinergic and monoaminergic neurons exhibit burst of activity during attentional demanding tasks and in response to behaviorally relevant stimuli driven by inputs from the prefrontal cortex (PFC).
- The basal forebrain cholinergic neurons are particularly active during active cortical states associated with high-frequency, low-amplitude EEG activity.
- The tonic baseline activity of LC-NE neurons is low during unaroused states, moderate during quiet wakefulness and engagement in a focused task, and high during behavioral arousal and exploratory behavior.
- During focused attention, LC neurons transiently interrupt their moderate tonic firing and respond with a phasic discharge to task-relevant stimuli.
- Midbrain DA neurons of the VTA and SNc have short latency burst responses to rewarding, aversive, or salient stimulus.
- Most midbrain DA neurons encode the motivational value of a stimulus and respond to a reward-prediction error signal.
- Attention involves two frontoparietal networks, a dorsal network for goal-directed attention and a right-lateralized ventral network for stimulus-driven attention.
- Acetylcholine increases signal-to-noise ratio in cortical sensory areas promoting processing of new information.
- The LC-NE system has a major role in the reorienting response and may function as a novelty detector.
- Serotonin contributes both to modulation of top-down control of attention and to cognitive flexibility.
- Working memory maintains information "on-line" in the absence of stimuli, and depends on recurrent excitatory activity lateral in layer 3 of the lateral PFC networks.
- Cholinergic inputs promote excitability of the lateral PFC recurrent activity in working-memory networks.
- Both DA and NE allow moment-by-moment changes in synaptic strength in the lateral PFC circuits and

bring working-memory circuits either "on-line" or "off-line" based on the arousal state.

- In response to a rewarding stimulus, a DA peak in the striatum, acting via D1Rs, promotes activity of neurons that trigger selection of the rewarding action.
- In response to an adverse outcome, a fall of DA level in the striatum interrupts the D2R-mediated inhibition of neurons that suppressed the action that resulted in the bad outcome.
- Phasic DA release encodes a "reward-minus-effort" signal that promotes the allocation of effort by the anterior midcingulate cortex (MCC) and ventral striatum.
- Both the anterior MCC and lateral habenula (LHb) monitor negative outcomes.
- Different subsets of serotonergic neurons of the dorsal raphe regulate adaptive responses to environmental stress and rewarding or aversive stimuli.
- Neuromodulatory neuron systems are particularly vulnerable to neurodegeneration.
- Loss of LC-NE neurons precedes that of cholinergic neurons in Alzheimer disease and dopaminergic neurons Parkinson disease.
- Excessive activity of 5-HT2A in the dorsolateral PFC may impair attention due to inability to suppress distracting stimuli.
- Hallucinations are prominent features in several neurologic disorders, including dementia with Lewy bodies.
- All drugs of addiction promote burst firing of midbrain DA neurons and increase DA release in the NAc.
- Increased activity of the LC-NE neurons during stress promote consolidation of emotional memories.
- Serotonergic neurons in the rostral raphe projecting to distinct targets have opposite effects on anxiety-related behaviors.

REFERENCES

1. Poulet JFA, Crochet S. The cortical states of wakefulness. Front Syst Neurosci 2018;12:64.
2. Zagha E, Casale AE, Sachdev RN, McGinley MJ, McCormick DA. Motor cortex feedback influences sensory processing by modulating network state. Neuron 2013;79:567–578.
3. Steriade M, Timofeev I, Grenier F. Natural waking and sleep states: a view from inside neocortical neurons. J Neurophysiol 2001;85:1969–1985.
4. Saper CB, Fuller PM, Pedersen NP, Lu J, Scammell TE. Sleep state switching. Neuron 2010;68:1023–1042.
5. Marder E. Neuromodulation of neuronal circuits: back to the future. Neuron 2012;76:1–11.
6. Thiele A, Bellgrove MA. Neuromodulation of attention. Neuron 2018;97:769–785.
7. Mesulam MM. Cholinergic circuitry of the human nucleus basalis and its fate in Alzheimer's disease. J Comp Neurol 2013;521:4124–4144.
8. Zaborszky L, Gombkoto P, Varsanyi P, et al. Specific basal forebrain-cortical cholinergic circuits coordinate cognitive operations. J Neurosci 2018;38:9446–9458.
9. Gut NK, Winn P. The pedunculopontine tegmental nucleus: a functional hypothesis from the comparative literature. Mov Disord 2016;31:615–624.
10. Mena-Segovia J, Bolam JP. Rethinking the pedunculopontine nucleus: from cellular organization to function. Neuron 2017;94:7–18.
11. Fu Y, Paxinos G, Watson C, Halliday GM. The substantia nigra and ventral tegmental dopaminergic neurons from development to degeneration. J Chem Neuroanat 2016;76:98–107.
12. Haber SN. The place of dopamine in the cortico-basal ganglia circuit. Neuroscience 2014;282C:248–257.
13. Yetnikoff L, Lavezzi HN, Reichard RA, Zahm DS. An update on the connections of the ventral mesencephalic dopaminergic complex. Neuroscience 2014;282C:23–48.
14. Garcia-Cabezas MA, Rico B, Sanchez-Gonzalez MA, Cavada C. Distribution of the dopamine innervation in the macaque and human thalamus. Neuroimage 2007;34:965–984.
15. Ren J, Friedmann D, Xiong J, et al. Anatomically defined and functionally distinct dorsal raphe serotonin sub-systems. Cell 2018;175:472–487 e420.
16. Morales M, Root DH. Glutamate neurons within the midbrain dopamine regions. Neuroscience 2014;282C:60–68.
17. Picciotto MR, Higley MJ, Mineur YS. Acetylcholine as a neuromodulator: cholinergic signaling shapes nervous system function and behavior. Neuron 2012;76:116–129.
18. Schultz W. Updating dopamine reward signals. Curr Opin Neurobiol 2013;23:229–238.
19. Aston-Jones G, Waterhouse B. Locus coeruleus: from global projection system to adaptive regulation of behavior. Brain Res 2016;1645:75–78.
20. Atzori M, Cuevas-Olguin R, Esquivel-Rendon E, et al. Locus ceruleus norepinephrine release: a central regulator of CNS spatio-temporal activation? Front Synaptic Neurosci 2016;8:25.
21. Breton-Provencher V, Sur M. Active control of arousal by a locus coeruleus GABAergic circuit. Nat Neurosci 2019;22:218–228.
22. Parikh V, Kozak R, Martinez V, Sarter M. Prefrontal acetylcholine release controls cue detection on multiple timescales. Neuron 2007;56:141–154.
23. Gritton HJ, Howe WM, Mallory CS, Hetrick VL, Berke JD, Sarter M. Cortical cholinergic signaling controls the detection of cues. Proc Natl Acad Sci U S A 2016;113:E1089–1097.
24. Howe WM, Gritton HJ, Lusk NA, et al. Acetylcholine release in prefrontal cortex promotes gamma oscillations and theta-gamma coupling during cue detection. J Neurosci 2017;37:3215–3230.
25. Sarter M, Kim Y. Interpreting chemical neurotransmission in vivo: techniques, time scales, and theories. ACS Chem Neurosci 2015;6:8–10.
26. Totah NKB, Logothetis NK, Eschenko O. Noradrenergic ensemble-based modulation of cognition over multiple timescales. Brain Res 2019;1709:50–66.

27. Seo DO, Bruchas MR. Polymorphic computation in locus coeruleus networks. Nat Neurosci 2017;20:1517–1519.
28. Chandler DJ, Jensen P, McCall JG, Pickering AE, Schwarz LA, Totah NK. Redefining noradrenergic neuromodulation of behavior: impacts of a modular locus coeruleus architecture. J Neurosci 2019;39:8239–8249.
29. Uematsu A, Tan BZ, Ycu EA, et al. Modular organization of the brainstem noradrenaline system coordinates opposing learning states. Nat Neurosci 2017;20:1602–1611.
30. Bromberg-Martin ES, Matsumoto M, Hikosaka O. Dopamine in motivational control: rewarding, aversive, and alerting. Neuron 2010;68:815–834.
31. Beaulieu JM, Espinoza S, Gainetdinov RR. Dopamine receptors—IUPHAR Review 13. Br J Pharmacol 2015;172:1–23.
32. Arnsten AF, Wang MJ, Paspalas CD. Neuromodulation of thought: flexibilities and vulnerabilities in prefrontal cortical network synapses. Neuron 2012;76:223–239.
33. Lecrux C, Bourourou M, Hamel E. How reliable is cerebral blood flow to map changes in neuronal activity? Auton Neurosci 2019;217:71–79.
34. Reimer J, McGinley MJ, Liu Y, et al. Pupil fluctuations track rapid changes in adrenergic and cholinergic activity in cortex. Nat Commun 2016;7:13289.
35. Joshi S, Li Y, Kalwani RM, Gold JI. Relationships between pupil diameter and neuronal activity in the locus coeruleus, colliculi, and cingulate cortex. Neuron 2016;89:221–234.
36. Corbetta M, Patel G, Shulman GL. The reorienting system of the human brain: from environment to theory of mind. Neuron 2008;58:306–324.
37. Pinto L, Goard MJ, Estandian D, et al. Fast modulation of visual perception by basal forebrain cholinergic neurons. Nat Neurosci 2013;16:1857–1863.
38. Minces V, Pinto L, Dan Y, Chiba AA. Cholinergic shaping of neural correlations. Proc Natl Acad Sci U S A 2017;114:5725–5730.
39. Schmitz TW, Duncan J. Normalization and the cholinergic microcircuit: a unified basis for attention. Trends Cogn Sci 2018;22:422–437.
40. Sara SJ, Bouret S. Orienting and reorienting: the locus coeruleus mediates cognition through arousal. Neuron 2012;76:130–141.
41. Aznar S, Hervig Mel S. The 5-HT2A serotonin receptor in executive function: implications for neuropsychiatric and neurodegenerative diseases. Neurosci Biobehav Rev 2016;64:63–82.
42. D'Esposito M, Postle BR. The cognitive neuroscience of working memory. Annu Rev Psychol 2015;66:115–142.
43. Goldman-Rakic PS. Cellular basis of working memory. Neuron 1995;14:477–485.
44. Galvin VC, Arnsten AFT, Wang M. Evolution in neuromodulation: the differential roles of acetylcholine in higher order association vs. primary visual cortices. Front Neural Circuits 2018;12:67.
45. Sarter M, Lustig C, Blakely RD, Koshy Cherian A. Cholinergic genetics of visual attention: human and mouse choline transporter capacity variants influence distractibility. J Physiol Paris 2016;110:10–18.
46. Puig MV, Antzoulatos EG, Miller EK. Prefrontal dopamine in associative learning and memory. Neuroscience 2014;282C:217–229.
47. Durstewitz D, Seamans JK. The dual-state theory of prefrontal cortex dopamine function with relevance to catechol-o-methyltransferase genotypes and schizophrenia. Biol Psychiatry 2008;64:739–749.
48. Berridge CW, Spencer RC. Differential cognitive actions of norepinephrine a2 and a1 receptor signaling in the prefrontal cortex. Brain Res 2016;1641:189–196.
49. Xing B, Li YC, Gao WJ. Norepinephrine versus dopamine and their interaction in modulating synaptic function in the prefrontal cortex. Brain Res 2016;1641:217–233.
50. Salamone JD, Correa M. The mysterious motivational functions of mesolimbic dopamine. Neuron 2012;76:470–485.
51. Westbrook A, Braver TS. Dopamine does double duty in motivating cognitive effort. Neuron 2016;91:708.
52. Lee D. Decision making: from neuroscience to psychiatry. Neuron 2013;78:233–248.
53. Haber SN, Behrens TE. The neural network underlying incentive-based learning: implications for interpreting circuit disruptions in psychiatric disorders. Neuron 2014;83:1019–1039.
54. Salgado S, Kaplitt MG. The nucleus accumbens: a comprehensive review. Stereotact Funct Neurosurg 2015;93:75–93.
55. Humphries MD, Prescott TJ. The ventral basal ganglia, a selection mechanism at the crossroads of space, strategy, and reward. Prog Neurobiol 2010;90:385–417.
56. Root DH, Melendez RI, Zaborszky L, Napier TC. The ventral pallidum: subregion-specific functional anatomy and roles in motivated behaviors. Prog Neurobiol 2015;130:29–70.
57. Grace AA. Physiology of the normal and dopamine-depleted basal ganglia: insights into levodopa pharmacotherapy. Mov Disord 2008;23 Suppl 3:S560–569.
58. Tsai HC, Zhang F, Adamantidis A, et al. Phasic firing in dopaminergic neurons is sufficient for behavioral conditioning. Science 2009;324:1080–1084.
59. van der Meer MA, Redish AD. Ventral striatum: a critical look at models of learning and evaluation. Curr Opin Neurobiol 2011;21:387–392.
60. Stuber GD. Cortical operation of the ventral striatal switchboard. Neuron 2013;78:6–7.
61. Goto Y, Grace AA. Limbic and cortical information processing in the nucleus accumbens. Trends Neurosci 2008;31:552–558.
62. Schmidt L, Lebreton M, Clery-Melin ML, Daunizeau J, Pessiglione M. Neural mechanisms underlying motivation of mental versus physical effort. PLoS biology 2012;10:e1001266.
63. Schmidt L, Lebreton M, Clery-Melin ML, Daunizeau J, Pessiglione M. Neural mechanisms underlying motivation of mental versus physical effort. PLoS Biol 2012;10:e1001266.
64. Stopper CM, Tse MT, Montes DR, Wiedman CR, Floresco SB. Overriding phasic dopamine signals redirects action selection during risk/reward decision making. Neuron 2014;84:177–189.
65. Kennerley SW, Behrens TE, Wallis JD. Double dissociation of value computations in orbitofrontal and anterior cingulate neurons. Nat Neurosci 2011;14:1581–1589.
66. Parvizi J, Rangarajan V, Shirer WR, Desai N, Greicius MD. The will to persevere induced by electrical stimulation of the human cingulate gyrus. Neuron 2013;80:1359–1367.
67. Kawai T, Yamada H, Sato N, Takada M, Matsumoto M. Roles of the lateral habenula and anterior cingulate cortex in

negative outcome monitoring and behavioral adjustment in nonhuman primates. Neuron 2015;88:792–804.
68. Roselli F, Caroni P. From intrinsic firing properties to selective neuronal vulnerability in neurodegenerative diseases. Neuron 2015;85:901–910.
69. Hampel H, Mesulam MM, Cuello AC, et al. The cholinergic system in the pathophysiology and treatment of Alzheimer's disease. Brain 2018;141:1917–1933.
70. Weinshenker D. Long road to ruin: noradrenergic dysfunction in neurodegenerative disease. Trends Neurosci 2018;41:211–223.
71. Braak H, Alafuzoff I, Arzberger T, Kretzschmar H, Del Tredici K. Staging of Alzheimer disease-associated neurofibrillary pathology using paraffin sections and immunocytochemistry. Acta Neuropathol 2006;112:389–404.
72. Del Tredici K, Braak H. Dysfunction of the locus coeruleus-norepinephrine system and related circuitry in Parkinson's disease-related dementia. J Neurol Neurosurg Psychiatry 2013;84:774–783.
73. Borodovitsyna O, Flamini M, Chandler D. Noradrenergic modulation of cognition in health and disease. Neural Plast 2017;2017:6031478.
74. Braak H, Del Tredici K. Alzheimer's pathogenesis: is there neuron-to-neuron propagation? Acta Neuropathol 2011;121:589–595.
75. Lieberman JA, First MB. Psychotic disorders. N Engl J Med 2018;379:270–280.
76. Marder SR, Cannon TD. Schizophrenia. N Engl J Med 2019;381:1753–1761.
77. Waters F, Fernyhough C. Hallucinations: a systematic review of points of similarity and difference across diagnostic classes. Schizophr Bull 2017;43:32–43.
78. Joyce EM. Organic psychosis: the pathobiology and treatment of delusions. CNS Neurosci Ther 2018;24:598–603.
79. Butcher NJ, Marras C, Pondal M, et al. Neuroimaging and clinical features in adults with a 22q11.2 deletion at risk of Parkinson's disease. Brain 2017;140:1371–1383.
80. Selemon LD, Mrzljak J, Kleinman JE, Herman MM, Goldman-Rakic PS. Regional specificity in the neuropathologic substrates of schizophrenia: a morphometric analysis of Broca's area 44 and area 9. Arch Gen Psychiatry 2003;60:69–77.
81. Lopez-Gimenez JF, Gonzalez-Maeso J. Hallucinogens and serotonin 5-HT2A receptor-mediated signaling pathways. Curr Top Behav Neurosci 2018;36:45–73.
82. Espay AJ, Guskey MT, Norton JC, et al. Pimavanserin for Parkinson's disease psychosis: effects stratified by baseline cognition and use of cognitive-enhancing medications. Mov Disord 2018;33:1769–1776.
83. McKeith IG, Ferman TJ, Thomas AJ, et al. Research criteria for the diagnosis of prodromal dementia with Lewy bodies. Neurology 2020;94:743–755.
84. Esmaeeli S, Murphy K, Swords GM, Ibrahim BA, Brown JW, Llano DA. Visual hallucinations, thalamocortical physiology and Lewy body disease: a review. Neurosci Biobehav Rev 2019;103:337–351.
85. Luscher C. The emergence of a circuit model for addiction. Annu Rev Neurosci 2016;39:257–276.
86. Everitt BJ, Belin D, Economidou D, Pelloux Y, Dalley JW, Robbins TW. Review. Neural mechanisms underlying the vulnerability to develop compulsive drug-seeking habits and addiction. Phil Trans R Soc Lond B Biol Sci 2008;363:3125–3135.
87. Takagi Y, Sakai Y, Abe Y, et al. A common brain network among state, trait, and pathological anxiety from whole-brain functional connectivity. Neuroimage 2018;172:506–516.
88. Daviu N, Bruchas MR, Moghaddam B, Sandi C, Beyeler A. Neurobiological links between stress and anxiety. Neurobiol Stress 2019;11:100191.
89. Berridge CW, Waterhouse BD. The locus coeruleus-noradrenergic system: modulation of behavioral state and state-dependent cognitive processes. Brain Res Brain Res Rev 2003;42:33–84.
90. Sara SJ. Locus coeruleus in time with the making of memories. Curr Opin Neurobiol 2015;35:87–94.
91. McCall JG, Al-Hasani R, Siuda ER, et al. CRH engagement of the locus coeruleus noradrenergic system mediates stress-induced anxiety. Neuron 2015;87:605–620.

29 Sensory Processing

OVERVIEW

Cortical processing of sensory information is a critical initial step in cognition, including spatial orientation, object recognition, semantic knowledge, episodic memory, and emotion. Sensory modalities include exteroception (touch, vision, hearing, and olfaction), proprioception (kinesthesia, effort, and balance), and interoception (pain, temperature, visceral, and taste sensation). These different modalities are conveyed via different sensory channels that lead to activation of primary cortical sensory areas. From primary sensory cortex, information is subsequently processed via two distinct processing streams. A dorsal stream conveys spatial information (such as position and movement) to the posterior parietal cortex (PPC). A ventral stream conveys object feature information (such as shape and color, sound, tactile qualities) to the anterolateral temporal cortex. Higher-order parietal and temporal sensory areas, together with the prefrontal cortex (PFC), provide feedback attentional modulatory inputs to early cortical sensory processing areas. Cognitive sensory processing involves predictive coding, learning intermodal associations, mental imagery, multisensory integration, and multimodal integration for self-awareness and adjudication of value to sensory stimuli.

The different sensory pathways are well known to the neurologists and will only be briefly discussed here. The main aims of this chapter are to review: (1) the pathways by which sensory information reaches primary sensory areas; (2) the dorsal and ventral streams of sensory processing, with emphasis on the visual system; (3) cognitive aspects of sensory processing; and (4) cortical disorders affecting perception. The processing of pain and temperature information is discussed in other chapters of this book.

GENERAL FEATURES OF THE SENSORY SYSTEMS

The sensory systems have several features in common. They include the presence of submodality-specific channels for transduction and relay of information to the cerebral cortex; local mechanisms within each relay station that promote sensory discrimination; descending cortical modulation of sensory relay at subcortical level; modulation of sensory processing by the level of arousal, attention, behavioral relevance, and expectation; cortical information processing via a dorsal pathway for spatial information and a ventral pathway object feature representation; and multimodal sensory integration.

Receptors, Pathways and Relay Stations

In all sensory systems, the transduction of a stimulus into an electric response in the primary afferent fiber depends on specific receptors and cation channels. The peripheral region from which a stimulus can affect the central sensory neuron is known as its receptive field. At all levels, relay of sensory inputs is mediated by L-glutamate; at each relay station, sensory processing is controlled by local GABAergic circuits. With the exception of olfaction, all sensory pathways have their final relay station in first-order relay nuclei of the thalamus, which provide inputs to layer 4 of their respective primary cortical areas. Cortical areas send descending modulatory inputs to their respective relay stations to modulate transmission of information. Important sources of descending modulation include layer 6 corticothalamic neurons and layer 5 pyramidal tract neurons that target brainstem and spinal relay stations.

Attentional Modulation and Attentional Blink

As discussed in the previous chapter, both "top-down" (goal-driven) or "bottom-up" (stimulus salience-driven) attentional influences promote a "winner-takes-all" strategy that favors transmission of behaviorally relevant sensory stimuli at the expense of less relevant stimuli. One of the main correlates of attention is the increased firing rate of neurons that represent attended features or locations of objects and suppression of neuronal responses to unattended stimuli. This gain change reflects the activity of both excitatory and inhibitory neurons in competing neuronal populations. These attentional influences originate from the lateral PFC and PPC, which are components of attention networks and send feedback projections to areas involved in initial stages of sensory processing. The emotional salience of a stimulus can also bias sensory processing via projections of the amygdala. Both the PFC and amygdala modulate sensory processing via their influences on cholinergic and monoaminergic systems that target primary as well as association sensory areas.

In the presence of multiple sensory stimuli packed in time, attentional selection involves brief perceptual episodes. Two episodes of attentional selection cannot occur very close in time. When two items are presented briefly and in close succession, observers can usually report the first but often fail to report the second. This phenomenon is known as the *attentional blink*.[1–3] There are several hypotheses regarding the basis of the attentional blink. Evidence indicates that both cognitive control and emotion strongly influence the duration of the perceptual episodes and thus attentional blink.

Dorsal and Visual Streams of Sensory Processing

The processing of information downstream from early cortical sensory areas proceeds along two streams, dorsal and ventral, which have been most intensely characterized for the visual modality[4,5] but also apply to other sensory modalities. The dorsal stream proceeds toward areas of the PPC containing multimodal neurons that respond to combinations of visual, somatosensory, and other modalities. These PPC neurons provide a tridimensional representation of space that is used for programming of movements via interactions with the premotor cortex, for spatial attention and working memory via interactions with the lateral PFC, and for visual navigation via interactions with the hippocampus. The ventral stream proceeds toward areas in the anterolateral temporal cortex, which processes multimodal object feature information for object recognition, semantic knowledge, and attribution of affective relevance. Information from the dorsal and ventral streams in integrated in prefrontal cortical areas to guide attentional processes, decision-making, and executive control of behavior.

SOMATOSENSORY SYSTEM

There are two separate exteroceptive pathways, one for touch-pressure required for tactile discrimination, and the second for joint position and movement (proprioception) (Figure 29.1).

Receptor Mechanisms

Low-threshold mechanoreceptors and proprioceptors are large dorsal root ganglion (DRG) neurons (or trigeminal ganglion neurons) with fast-conducting Aβ afferents and specialized peripheral processes. These receptors provide for discriminative touch and include four types.[6,7] Two such receptors are located superficially in the skin and have small receptive fields. Merkel cells innervated by slowly adapting (SA-I) afferents provide information about locations of edges and Braille-like dot patterns, whereas Meissner corpuscles innervated by rapidly adapting (RA-I) afferents provide the sensations of texture and flutter. Two other receptors are located deeper in the skin and other tissues and have larger receptive fields. Ruffini end-organs innervated by slowly adapting (SA-II) afferents in the skin and joints respond to skin stretch across the fingertips; Pacinian corpuscles innervated by rapidly adapting (RA-II) afferents detect distal events via transmission of high-frequency vibrations through objects and surfaces, which may be important for use of tools. Tactile experience depends on various combinations of activity of these four sensory channels. Proprioception includes the sense of position and movements of the limbs and trunk (kinesthesia), the sense of effort, the sense of force, and the sense of heaviness.[8] Proprioceptors include muscle spindle receptors with IA and IB afferents sensitive to muscle length; Golgi tendon organs with Ib afferents sensitive to muscle tension; and Ruffini-like endings with SA-II afferents sensitive to skin, ligament, and joint stretch. Proprioceptive afferents have a role in conscious perception of joint movements and provide feedback inputs that guide finger movements during active touch.[6] Information about limb position and movement is not generated by individual receptors but by populations of afferents.[6] Transduction of low-threshold tactile and proprioceptive stimuli involves mechanically gated cation channels of the Piezo family.[7] Patients with *Piezo2* loss-of-function mutations have profound tactile and proprioceptive deficits.[8] Other ion channels sensitive to mechanical tactile and proprioceptive stimuli are two-pore potassium channels activated by asymmetric tension in the lipid membrane. Mechanical stimuli also directly depolarize the keratinocyte membrane.[9,10]

Parallel Somatosensory Pathways

Inputs from low threshold tactile mechanoreceptors and proprioceptors carried by primary afferents from DRG neurons predominantly ascend via the gracile and cuneate tracts in the dorsal columns to terminate in different portions of their respective dorsal column nuclei (DCN). The gracile nucleus (activated by tactile afferents from the lower limb) and the cuneate nucleus (activated by afferents from the upper limb) project via the contralateral medial lemniscus to target different portions of the ventroposterior (VP) complex of the thalamus (Figure 29.1). Low-threshold tactile mechanoreceptor afferents from individual digits terminate

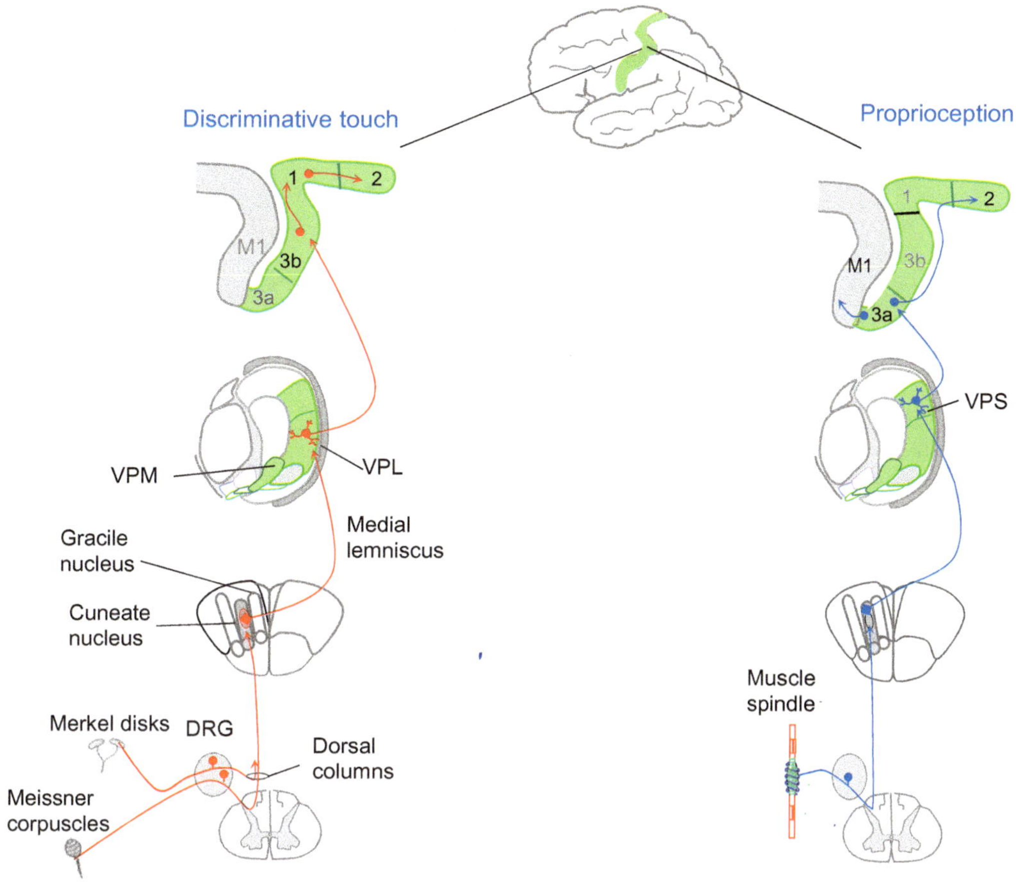

FIGURE 29.1 Somatosensory pathways for touch and proprioception.
Information from low-threshold tactile mechanoreceptors and proprioceptors largely ascends via first-order axons of dorsal root ganglion (DRG) neurons in the gracile and cuneate tracts in the ipsilateral dorsal (posterior) columns to reach the dorsal column nuclei (DCN) in the lower medulla. Inputs from low-threshold tactile mechanoreceptors from individual digits terminate in clusters located in a core region the DCN that project to the ventral posterolateral nucleus (VPL) of the thalamus; trigeminal tactile afferents terminate in the ventral posteromedial nucleus. The VPL and VPM project to area 3b and 1 in the primary somatosensory cortex (S1). Proprioceptive inputs from muscle spindle receptors, Golgi tendon organs, and Ruffini corpuscles terminate in the rostral reticular and shell regions of the DCN, which projects to the ventral posterosuperior nucleus (VPS), which conveys these inputs primarily to areas 3a and 2.

in clusters located in a core region the DCN, which project to the ventroposterolateral subnucleus (VPL), which contains a somatotopic representation of the body. Low-threshold tactile inputs from the face with relay in the principal trigeminal nucleus terminate in the ventroposteromedial nucleus (VPM).[11] Proprioceptive inputs from muscle spindle receptors, Golgi tendon organs, and Ruffini corpuscles terminate in the rostral reticular and shell regions of the DCN and project primarily to the ventroposterior superior nucleus (VPS). Large DRG neurons also provide inputs to second-order dorsal horn neurons that project both via postsynaptic dorsal column pathways to the DCN and via the spinothalamic tract (STT) to terminate primarily in the ventroposteroinferior nucleus (VPI). Proprioceptive information also reaches the ipsilateral cerebellum via the dorsal spinocerebellar tract from Clarke's column for the lower limb, and via cuneocerebellar tract from the external cuneate nucleus for the upper limb. Axons of the DCN also send collaterals to the inferior olivary nucleus and to the superior colliculus. Somatosensory inputs also reach association nuclei of the thalamus, including the inferior pulvinar and the posterior nucleus.

Primary Somatosensory Cortex

The primary somatosensory cortex (S1) is located in the postcentral gyrus and includes four subdivisions, areas 3a, 3b, 1, and 2, each containing a complete somatotopic map of the contralateral body (Figure 29.2). Areas 3b and 1 receive

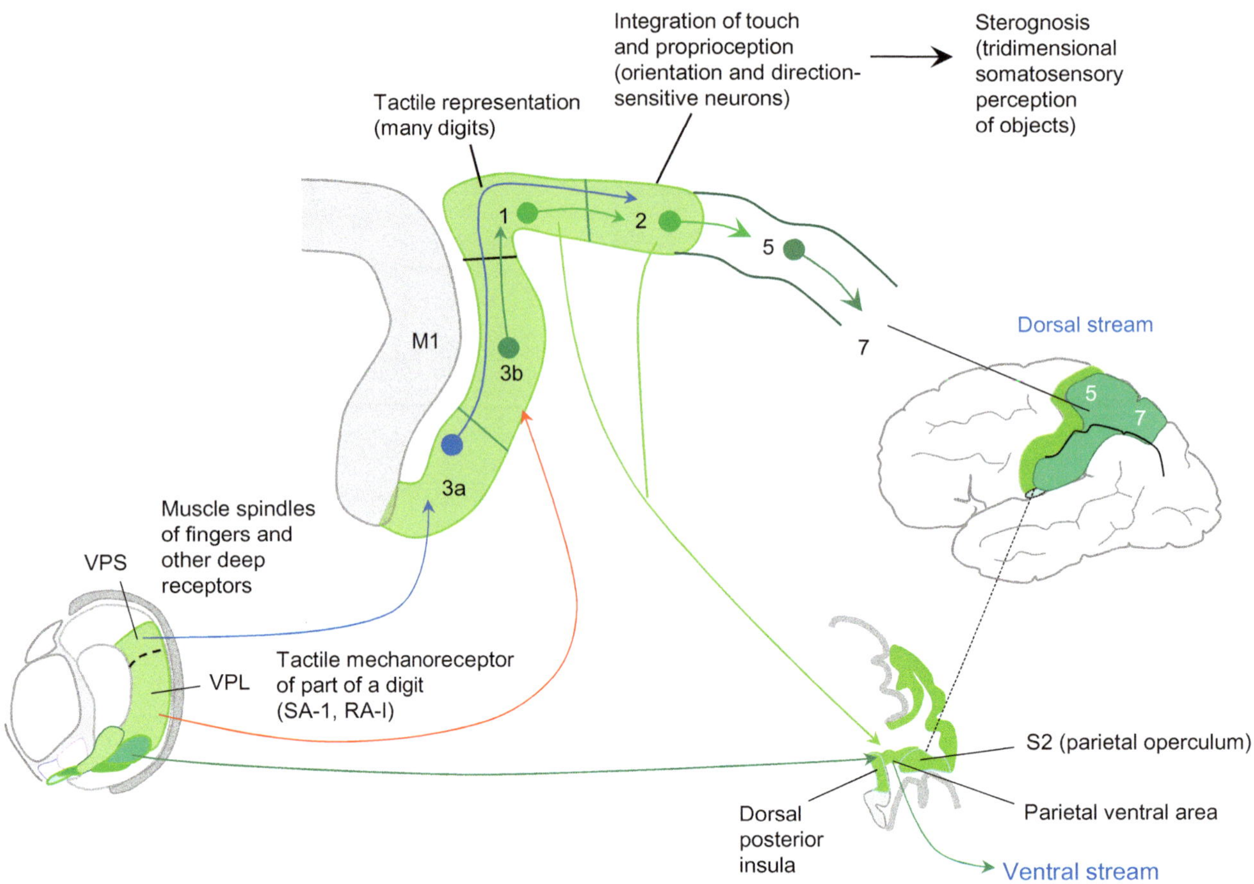

FIGURE 29.2 Somatosensory processing.

Whereas the primary somatosensory cortex receives segregated inputs from touch receptors via the ventroposterolateral (VPL) as well as ventroposteromedial nucleus (not shown) and inputs from deep receptors via the ventroposterosuperior nucleus (VPS). Cortical areas in the upper bank of the lateral (Sylvian) sulcus, including the second somatosensory area (S2) in the parietal operculum, the parietal ventral area, and dorsal posterior insula receive somatosensory information from areas 3a, 3b, 1, and 2 as well as the ventroposteroinferior (VPI) nucleus. Neurons of these areas correspond to the ventral stream for somatosensory processing and have a major role in tactile discrimination and identification via connections with the lateral temporal cortex. The posterior parietal cortex is a critical station of the dorsal pathway for sensory processing. Somatosensory inputs from S1 are processed in areas 5 (5a and 5b) and 7a in the superior parietal lobule. Areas 5a, 5b, and 7 have primarily somatosensory function; area 7a contains neurons involved in both visual and visuomotor activity.

inputs from the VPL and VPM (in the case of the face) conveying information from SA-I, RA-I, and SA-II afferents. Area 3b contains alternate columns responding to inputs from either rapidly or slowly adapting receptors with a separate and independent representation of the functionally distinct parts of the digits. These inputs converge and are integrated in area 1, which contains representation of several fingers.[12] Area 3a is located in the fundus of the central sulcus and contains neurons that respond to inputs from the muscle spindles and other deep receptors. These neurons are activated during movements, and provide outputs both to the primary motor cortex and to area 2. Area 2 contains a complex representation of both cutaneous and deep receptors from muscle spindles; many of its neurons respond to certain shapes or direction of movement, indicating a role of area 2 in combining tactile and proprioceptive information from the fingers during active touch for tactile recognition of objects (sterognosis). All the four fields of S1 are connected with those in the contralateral hemisphere via callosal connections. Information from the primary somatosensory cortex sensation is elaborated along unimodal somatosensory sensory areas. The primary sensory cortex also provides feedback to thalamic relay nuclei, pulvinar, DCN, spinal cord, and striatum.

Ventral and Dorsal Stream for Somatosensory Processing

The cortex in the upper bank of the lateral (Sylvian) sulcus, including the second somatosensory area (S2) in the parietal operculum, the parietal ventral area, and the dorsal posterior insula, receives input from areas 3a, 3b,1, and 2 as well as the VPI, and relays these inputs to lateral temporal areas involved in object recognition by touch. These areas thus correspond to the ventral stream of sensory processing.[13] Somatosensory inputs from S1 are also processed in areas 5 and area 7 in the superior parietal lobule of the PPC corresponding to the dorsal stream for somatosensory representation.[14,15] Area 5 has primarily somatosensory function and receives inputs from area 2 conveying information of cutaneous and deep receptors from many digits of both hands. Neurons of area 7b receive inputs from areas S1 and S2, anterior pulvinar, and ventral lateral nucleus of the thalamus and respond to touching of the skin, particularly the face, hand, and arm. Somatosensory inputs from areas 5 and 7b, together with inputs of area 7a receiving visual information, are conveyed to other areas of the PPC to contribute to spatial representation.

VISUAL SYSTEM

The visual system consists of the intrinsic circuits of the retina that convey inputs from photoreceptors to bipolar cells and then ganglion cells; retinal ganglion cells project via the optic nerve to the dorsal lateral geniculate nucleus of the thalamus (LGN), which relays these inputs to the primary visual cortex.

Retina

The retinal circuitry consists of parallel radial glutamatergic pathways modulated by two sets of lateral interactions (Figure 29.3). The radial pathways consist of photoreceptors, including rods and cones that synapse on bipolar cells in the outer plexiform layer. Bipolar cells then convey these visual inputs to ganglion cells in the inner plexiform layer. The

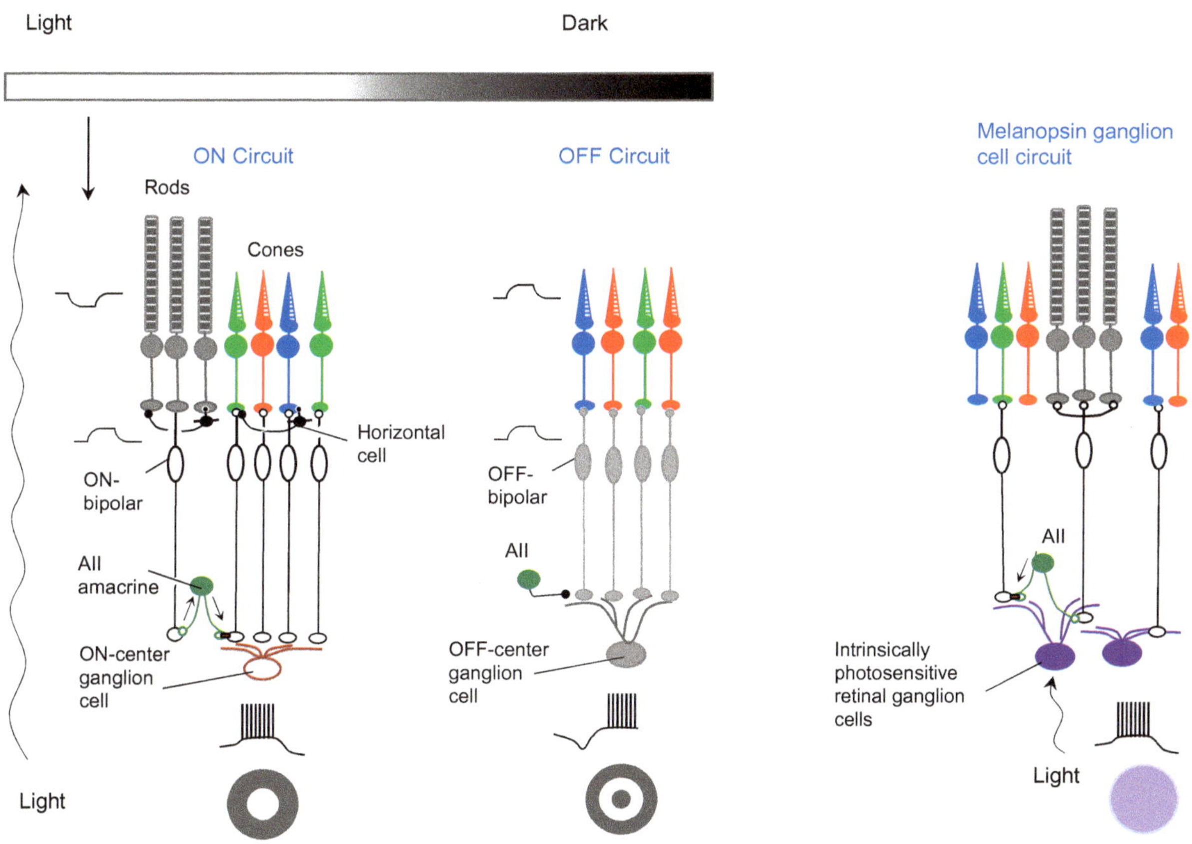

FIGURE 29.3 Circuits of the retina.
Photoreceptors synapse on bipolar cells; visual input is then passed via bipolar cells to ganglion cells in the inner plexiform layer. The ganglion cells have a circular receptive field with a center-surround organization. The lateral interactions are mediated horizontal GABAergic cells at the outer plexiform layer. Inputs from photoreceptors are conveyed to ON- and OFF bipolar cells. ON bipolar cells receive inputs from rods or cones and synapse on ON-center ganglion cells. OFF bipolar receive inputs only from cones and synapse on OFF-center ganglion cells. AII amacrine cells receive inputs from ON-rod bipolars, activate ON cone bipolar terminals via gap junctions and inhibit OFF cone bipolar terminals via glycinergic synapses. Via these mechanisms, AII amacrine cells allow activation of ON-ganglion cells under dim light. Intrinsically photosensitive retinal ganglion cells synthesize melanopsin and respond to variations in brightness. They are directly activated by light and also respond to inputs from photoreceptors.

ganglion cells have a circular receptive field with a center-surround organization: ON-center ganglion cells respond to a dot of light and are inhibited by darkness; OFF-center ganglion cells respond to a dot of darkness and are inhibited by light.

Photoreceptors have an outer segment harboring visual photopigments and tonically release glutamate at their synapses with bipolar cells. Rods are located in the peripheral retina, contain rhodopsin, and have exquisite sensitivity to single photons, so they are used for vision in dim light. Cones are concentrated in the fovea, respond to higher light intensity, and are responsible for visual acuity and color vision. Cones include different types, expressing opsins that absorb light with highest sensitivity to red (L cones), green (M-cones), or blue (S-cones) wavelengths. Opsins are G protein-coupled receptors (GPCRs) linked to the chromophore retinal. During darkness, photoreceptors carry a depolarizing current that is mediated by Na^+ and Ca^{2+} influx via a cyclic guanosine monophosphate (cGMP)-gated cation channel; this current maintains a tonic release of glutamate at their ribbon synapses with bipolar cells. Upon photon absorption, the chromophore isomerizes from 11-*cis* retinal to all-*trans*-retinal; this drives a conformational change of the opsin receptor and activation of the G protein transducin, which stimulates a cGMP phosphodiesterase. This results in cGMP hydrolysis, closure of the cGMP-gated cation channel, and photoreceptor hyperpolarization interrupting the glutamate signal at the photoreceptor-bipolar cell synapse. Recovery from light involves regeneration of 11-cis-retinal at the pigmentary epithelium of the retina, inactivation of the rhodopsin transduction pathway, and other mechanisms.

The photoreceptors convey the influences of light via ON- and OFF-bipolar cells. ON-bipolar cells receive inputs from either rods or cones and activate ON-center ganglion cells. During darkness, glutamate released from photoreceptors tonically inhibits the ON-bipolars via a metabotropic glutamate receptor (mGluR6) that elicits chloride influx; light interrupts this inhibitory signal, resulting in ON-bipolar activation. ON-cone bipolars directly activate the ON-center ganglion cells. ON-rod bipolars do so indirectly via AII amacrine cells in the inner plexiform layer. These amacrine cells activate ON-cone bipolar terminals via gap junctions and send a glycinergic inhibitory input to the OFF-cone bipolar synapse on ganglion cells (Figure 29.3). Another important group of amacrine cells are interplexiform cells that release dopamine, which inhibits coupling between AII amacrine cells. The progressive decrease of dopamine during darkness promotes AII cell coupling and thus feedforward transmission of ON-bipolar signals during starlight. OFF-bipolar receive inputs only from cones, are tonically activated by glutamate during darkness, inhibited by light, and project to OFF-center ganglion cells. Horizontal cells located at the outer plexiform later are GABAergic, collect signals from photoreceptors, are interconnected by gap junctions, and synapse on dendrites from bipolar cells located at a distance. By these mechanisms, horizontal cells have a major role in shaping the size of the receptive field in the retina. The ON- and OFF-ganglion cells primarily project to the lateral geniculate nucleus (LGN). The ON- and the OFF-photoreceptor-bipolar-ganglion cell circuits are image-forming circuits. The retina also contains a third, non-image-forming circuit mediated by a unique type of ganglion cell that synthesizes melanopsin and directly responds to light and thus are referred to as intrinsically photosensitive retinal ganglion cells. Contrary to photoreceptors, these intrinsically photosensitive melanopsin ganglion cells are directly activated by light. They also collect inputs from the rod and cone pathways and respond to variations of luminescence (brightness) and do not project to the LGN but to other targets.

Parallel Pathways from Ganglion Cells to the Lateral Geniculate Nucleus

Most retinal ganglion cells project via the optic nerve and optic tract to the dorsal LGN, which relays these inputs to the primary visual cortex (V1). The dorsal LGN consist of six layers that alternatively receive different input from either eye. The two ventral layers are magnocellular (M, large-cell) layers, the four dorsal layers are parvocellular (P, small-cell) layers, and the intercalated layers are koniocellular (K, very small-cell) layers. There are three major image-forming visual pathways from the retina that remain segregated from the retina to the LGN and then up to V1 (Figure 29.4). The P-pathway involves small ganglion cells (midget cells) that are abundant in the central retina and receive inputs from bipolar cells collecting from single cones; these small ganglion cells have small receptive fields, high spatial resolution, and color sensitivity and provide fine detail about visual object features. These small ganglion cells project to the P layers of the LGN. The M-pathway involves parasol- and garland-type ganglion cells that collect information from five to ten rods via bipolar cells; they have large receptive fields and thus poor spatial resolution but have high sensitivity to contrast; these cells are especially suited for processing of spatial information and project to the M-layers of the LGN. A third group of ganglion cells, called small bistratified cells, receive inputs from the S cones and send their small-diameter axons to the thin intercalated, or K-layers of the LGN.

Primary Visual Cortex

The different layers of the dorsal LGN provide segregated inputs to the primary visual cortex (V1, area 17, striate cortex), which has a retinotopic representation of the opposite visual hemifield. Area V1 has a prominent layer 4, commonly referred to as layer 4C, which is subdivided into three sublayers that receive inputs from different LGN layers (Figure 29.4). One of the crucial events in coding of visual stimuli is the transformation of an orientation-insensitive representation in the retina and LGN to an orientation-selective representation in V1. The so-called simple cells in V1 respond to the linear spatial summation of responses to

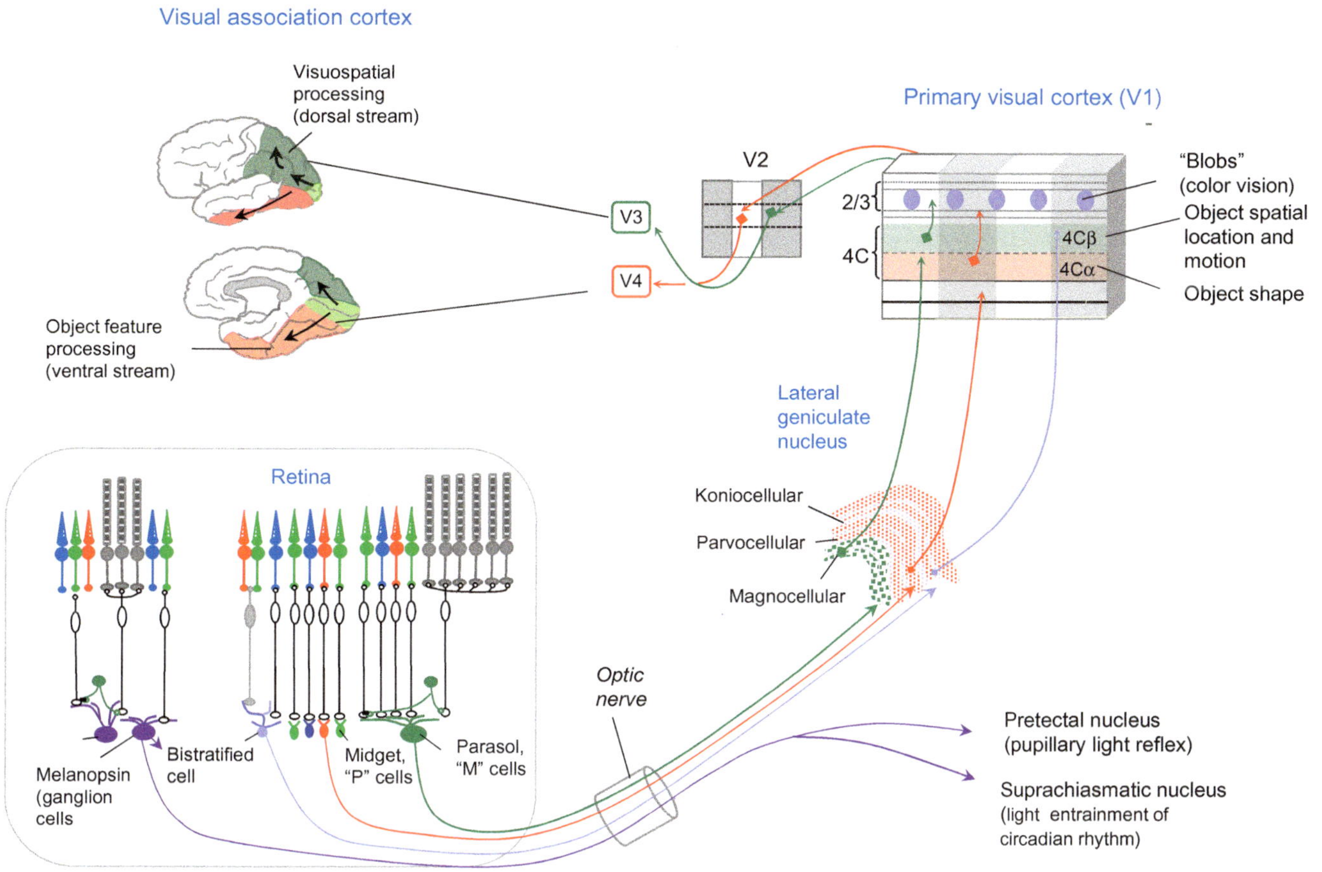

FIGURE 29.4 Parallel visual pathways.

There are three major pathways from the retina that remain partially segregated and provide different types of information to different layers of the dorsal portion of the lateral geniculate nucleus (LGN). The parvocellular (P) pathway involves small ganglion cells (midget cells) that receive inputs from single cones, provide for color vision and fine detail about visual object features, and project to the P layers of the LGN. The M (magnocellular) pathway involves parasol- and garland-type ganglion cells that have large receptive fields, are suited for processing of spatial information, and project to the M layers of the LGN. A third group of ganglion cells, called small bistratified cells, receive inputs from the S cones send their small diameter axons to the thin intercalated, or koniocellular (K), layers of the LGN. The different layers of the dorsal LGN provide segregate inputs to the primary visual cortex (V1, area 17), which is characterized by a prominent layer 4C. Sublayer 4Ca receives inputs from the M layers of the LGN and sublayer 4Cb from the P layers of the LGN. Neurons of layer 4C project to the more superficial layers 2 and 3, which in turn project to the extrastriate visual areas. Layers 3A and 2 in V1 contain functional compartments referred to as blobs, which receive direct inputs from both the P- and K layers of the LGN. Area V1 projects to the second visual area V2, which connects to the contralateral V2 via callosal connections and has a characteristic structure consisting of thick bands or stripes, thin bands, and interbands (or pale stripes), which relay to downstream extrastriate visual pathways that initiate the dorsal and ventral stream of visuospatial processing.

small light or dark dots conveyed by the LGN; complex cells in V1 respond to oriented contours over a range of positions and thus integrate information from several simple cells. Area V1 has a pattern of alternating ocular dominance bands or stripes that are best activated by one eye or the other, and is also organized into columns that are best activated by stimuli having a particular orientation. Area V1 projects to the second visual area V2, which connects to the contralateral V2 via callosal connections. Area V2 has a characteristic structure consisting of three compartments that receives distinct inputs from the M and P pathways via different sublayers of layer 3 of V1. The processing of information from early cortical visual areas occurs via the dorsal and the ventral streams.[4,5] Early visual areas activated via the M-system provide inputs via the dorsal (occipitoparietal) stream to the PPC for processing of visuospatial information (object location and movement); early visual areas activated by the P-system provide inputs via the ventral (occipitotemporal) stream to the temporal lobe for object feature identification. Where these pathways remain segregated at early stages of processing, they eventually become integrated at higher hierarchical levels.

Dorsal Stream for Visuospatial Processing

The dorsal visual stream includes several areas involved in the transformation of a retinotopic representation into a representation of space in an egocentric (body-centered) frame of reference. Portions of area V1 project to an area located in the anterior wall of the parieto-occipital sulcus that projects to the PPC via a medial pathway that targets bimodal (visual and somatosensory) areas located in the intraparietal sulcus and a lateral pathway that reaches the lateral intraparietal area (LIP, parietal eye field), medial temporal area (MT), and medial superior temporal area (MST) containing motion-sensitive neurons. All components of this circuit also receive visual information from the retina and superior colliculus via the pulvinar. This occipital-parietal circuit is the common origin of the three distinct pathways: parieto-prefrontal, parieto-premotor, and parieto-medial temporal (Figure 29.5). The parieto-prefrontal pathway involves the LIP/parietal eye field and targets the fontal eye field (area 8) and posterior middle frontal gyrus in the lateral PFC (area 46). This pathway is involved visuospatial attention, visual working memory, and top-down control of eye movements. The parieto-premotor pathway encodes space and body representations for visually guided motor actions and comprises two parallel projections. One such projection originates in the anterior parieto-occipital sulcus and medial intraparietal area (referred to as the parietal reach region) and targets the dorsal premotor cortex to control reaching movements. The second originates in the ventral intraparietal area and inferior parietal lobule and projects to the ventral premotor cortex to control grasping and movements toward the peripersonal space. Finally, the parieto-medial temporal pathway connects the posterior portions of the inferior parietal lobule, primarily the angular gyrus, to the parahippocampus and hippocampal formation via the precuneus, posterior cingulate, and retrosplenial cortex. This pathway is involved in transmission of information about spatial landmarks for navigation.

Ventral Visual Stream for Object Recognition

The ventral visual stream courses through the occipitotemporal cortex, including the fusiform gyrus and constitutes a complex recurrent and interactive network linking early visual areas with the anterior temporal cortex along multiple routes for visual information processing[5,16] (Figure 29.6). The

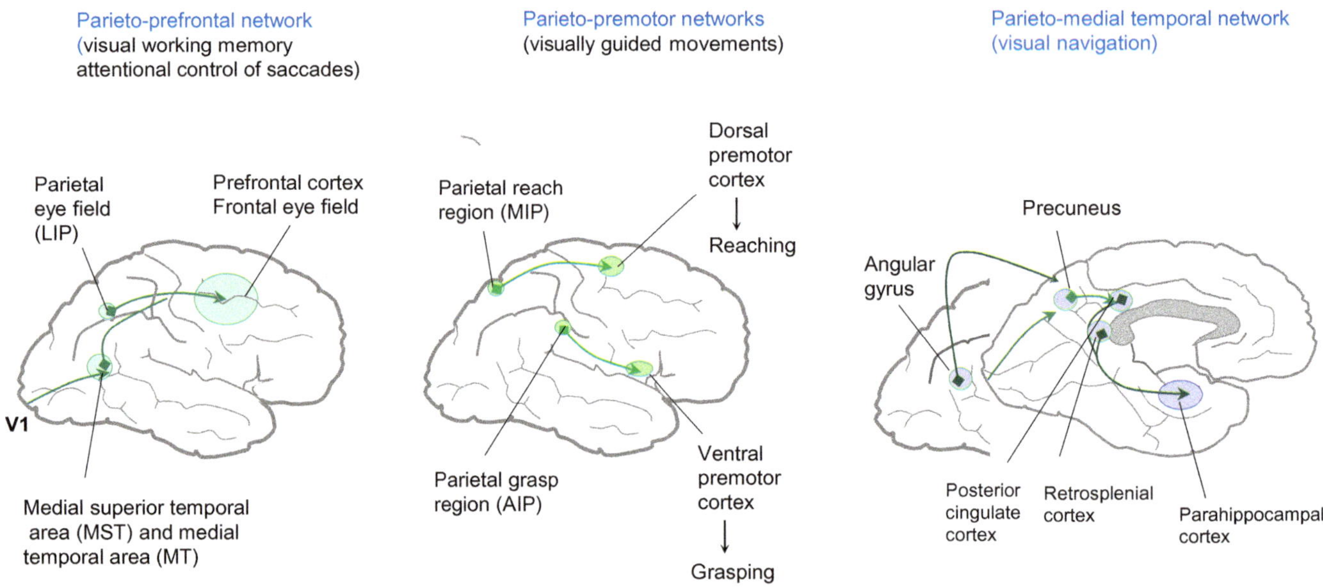

FIGURE 29.5 Dorsal visual stream.

The dorsal visual stream is initiated by a occipitoparietal circuit that transforms a retinotopic representation from early visual areas into a space representation in an egocentric reference frame. Portions of area V1 and anterior wall of the parieto-occipital sulcus project to the intraparietal sulcus and to the lateral intraparietal area (LIP), medial temporal (MT), and medial superior temporal (MST) areas, containing motion-sensitive neurons. This circuit is the common origin of three distinct pathways: parieto-prefrontal, parieto-premotor, and parieto-medial temporal. The parieto-prefrontal pathway originates in the lateral intraparietal area (LIP), which targets the posterior middle frontal gyrus in the lateral prefrontal cortex (PFC) and the fontal eye field (FEF) and is involved in visual working memory and top-down control of eye movements. The parieto-premotor pathway comprises two parallel projections; one originates in the anterior parieto-occipital sulcus and medial intraparietal area (parietal reach region) and targets the dorsal premotor cortex to control reaching movements, the second originates in the ventral intraparietal area and inferior parietal lobule and projects to the ventral premotor cortex to control grasping and. Finally, the parieto-medial temporal pathways connects the angular gyrus to the medial temporal lobe either directly or via the precuneus, posterior cingulate cortex, and retrosplenial cortex.

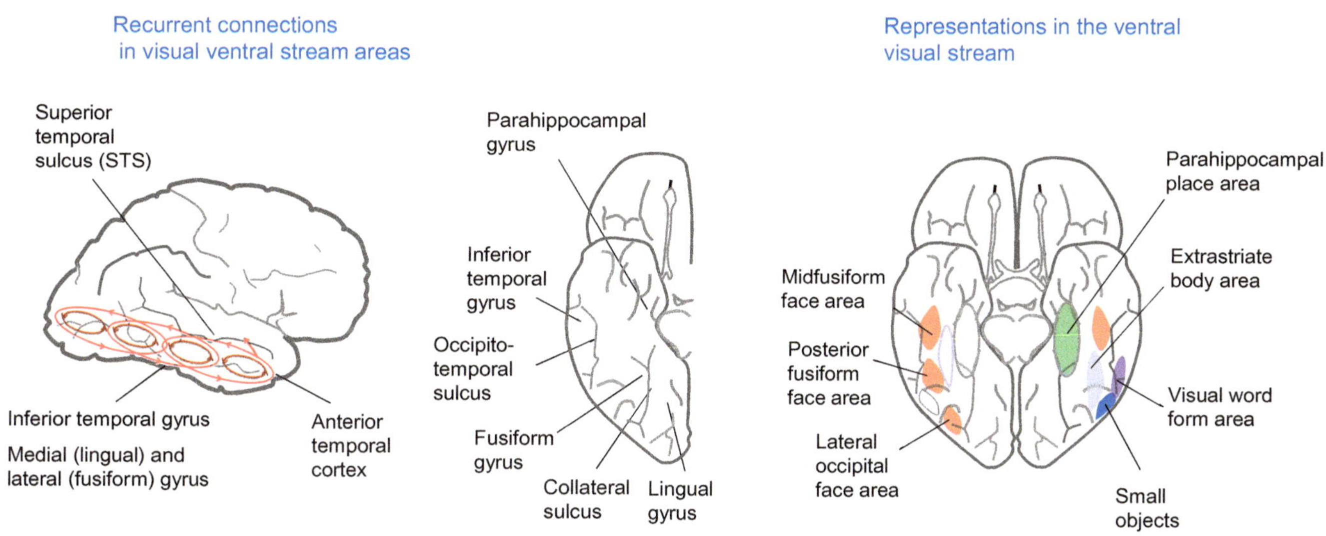

FIGURE 29.6 Object representation in the ventral visual stream.
The ventral visual stream courses through the occipitotemporal cortex to the anterior temporal cortex and constitutes a complex recurrent and interactive network linking early visual areas with the anterior temporal cortex along multiple routes for visual information processing. Areas within this network contain representations of faces, body parts, objects, and scenes. There is a functional clustering in the inferior temporal lobe with selectivity for particular objects including faces, body parts, word forms, tools, large objects, and scenes. Clusters representing faces and words receive inputs from the fovea and are represented more laterally; clusters representing scenes or landmarks receive inputs from the peripheral visual field and are located medially, in the parahippocampal place area. In the fusiform gyrus there are regions that respond selectively to faces (fusiform face area), bodies (fusiform body area), and objects (posterior fusiform gyrus). The posterior lateral occipital cortex contains areas selective for faces (occipital face area), bodies (extrastriate body area), and objects (lateral occipital area). There is a stronger representation of faces in the right than in the left hemisphere. An area that selectively responds to word forms (visual word form area) is located in the left lateral occipitotemporal sulcus.

occipitotemporal pathway represents the contralateral visual field and has a retinotopic organization; portions of the visual cortex that represent the fovea project via a central pathway to reach the anterior temporal pole; those that represent the peripheral visual field project to the parahippocampal cortex. Studies in experimental animals and fMRI studies in humans show that there is a functional clustering in the inferior temporal lobe with selectivity for particular objects including faces, body parts, word forms, tools, large objects, and scenes. Object representations can be differentiated along the ventral temporal cortex by their real-world size.[17] Clusters representing faces and words are represented more laterally, whereas clusters representing scenes or landmarks are located medially. Many of these selective regions are found in pairs. There are several regions that respond more selectively to faces, two located in the fusiform gyrus, one in the lateral inferior occipital cortex, and one in the superior temporal sulcus. The fusiform and the lateral occipital face areas are more sensitive to static features of faces that signal face identity; areas in the superior temporal sulcus are sensitive to dynamic aspects of faces, such as facial expression. There is a stronger representation of faces in the right than in the left hemisphere.[18,19] An area that selectively responds to word forms (visual word form area) is located in the left lateral occipitotemporal sulcus.[20] However, the functional specialization of these regions is graded rather than absolute. Many regions in the inferior temporal cortex may participate in the representation of multiple classes of stimuli.

The ventral visual network primarily projects to three subcortical and three cortical targets (Figure 29.7). The three major subcortical outputs target the neostriatum (caudate and putamen), ventral striatum (nucleus accumbens), and amygdala. The output to the neostriatum participates in learning of specific rules for goal-oriented behavior and then development of habits; the output to the ventral striatum is involved in reward-based learning and motivated behavior; and the output to the amygdala provides the source for visually dependent emotional regulation. The three major cortico-cortical outputs of the ventral visual stream originate in the anterior inferior temporal cortex; target the perirhinal, orbitofrontal, and inferior lateral PFC; and are bidirectional. Inputs to perirhinal cortex carry information necessary for object recognition based on familiarity; those to the orbitofrontal cortex provide information related to reward processing and stimulus-reward associations; and those to the inferior lateral frontal gyrus participate in visual working memory and integration between all forms of information.

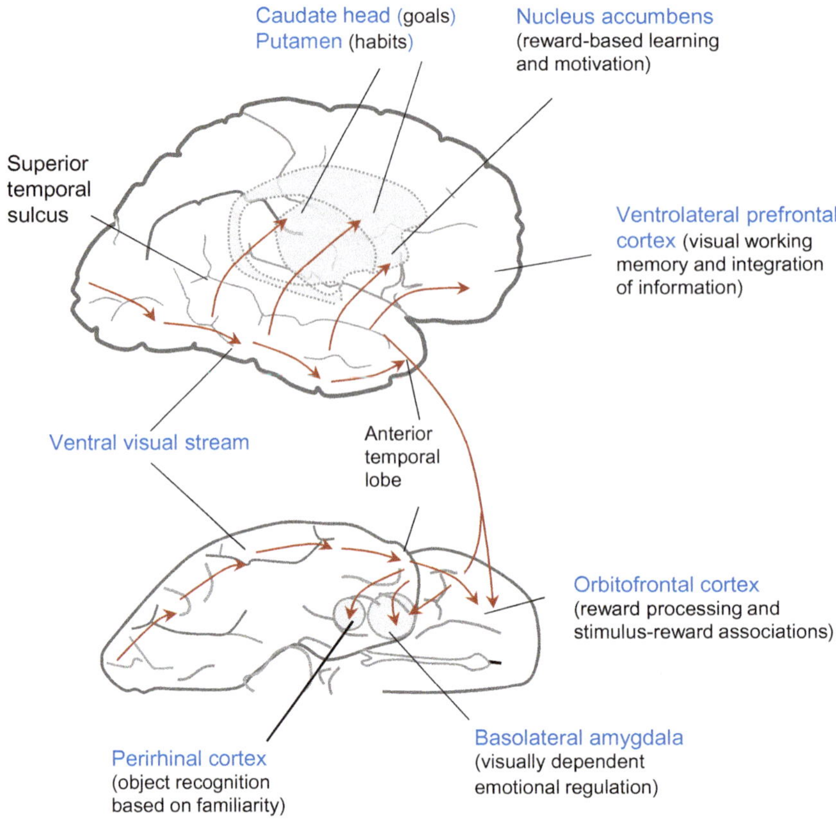

FIGURE 29.7 Targets of the ventral visual stream.
The ventral visual network primarily projects to three subcortical and three cortical targets. The three major subcortical outputs target the neostriatum, ventral striatum, and amygdala. The major cortical outputs target the perirhinal cortex, orbitofrontal cortex, and ventrolateral prefrontal cortex.

Extrageniculate Visual Pathways

The projections from retinal ganglion cells to the LGN comprise 90% of the fibers of the optic nerve and constitute the classical visual (image-forming) pathway. Other axons terminate in the superior colliculus, which has a critical role in attention and orienting responses.[21,22] The superior colliculus has a laminated structure with superficial layers that receive retinotopically organized afferents from the retina and visual cortex representing the contralateral visual field; these layers also receive inputs from brainstem auditory relay nuclei and from somatosensory pathways. The intermediate and deep layers are organized into a motor map for orientation of the eyes, head, and rest of the body toward novel stimuli located in the contralateral hemispace. The superior colliculus provides inputs to the pulvinar, which projects to visual areas in the PPC to subserve visual attention. This extrageniculate pathway is responsible for the phenomenon of "blindsight" after bilateral lesions of the primary visual cortex.

A second major extrageniculate pathway involves intrinsically photosensitive melanopsin ganglion cells that respond to changes in luminescence.[23] These cells project to the suprachiasmatic nucleus via the retinohypothalamic tract and are critical for entrainment of circadian rhythms. Melanopsin cells also provide the major light input to the pretectal nuclei and are primarily responsible for the pupillary light reflex.

AUDITORY SYSTEM

The auditory system includes the inner hair cells of the cochlea, ventral and dorsal cochlear nuclei, superior olivary nucleus, inferior colliculus, and medial geniculate nucleus (MGN), which targets the auditory cortex.

Transduction in the Cochlea

The hair cells of the cochlear organ of Corti contain apical stereocilia surrounded by endolymph, which is characterized by its high K^+ concentration. Stereocilia are interconnected by tip-links that control the opening of mechanosensitive transduction channels, including Piezo 2 channels.[24] Deflection toward the tall end of the stereocilia bundle embedded in the tectorial membrane opens K^+ channels, leading to depolarization of hair cells. Inner hair cells receive nerve afferents with cell bodies in the spiral ganglion of Corti and are the source of the auditory pathway. Outer hair cells express the motor protein prestin, receive cholinergic input from the superior olivary nucleus (olivocochlear tract) and are involved in amplification and frequency tuning of the cochlea. There is a strict tonotopic organization in the cochlea; high frequencies activate the hair cells in the basal portion of the basilar membrane and low frequencies those in apical portion; each auditory nerve fiber is most sensitive to a particular frequency, called best frequency. This tonotopic organization is maintained at all stations of the auditory pathway.

Parallel Pathways for Auditory Processing

The cochlear nerve terminates in the cochlear nuclear complex, which consists of two subdivisions, ventral and dorsal, each containing different cell types that project via separate parallel pathways that ascend via the lateral lemniscus. These pathways project bilaterally with contralateral predominance via decussating fibers from the ventral cochlear nucleus via the trapezoid body and from the dorsal cochlear nucleus via the dorsal acoustic stria. One pathway from the ventral and one from the dorsal cochlear nuclei relay tonotopic information to the contralateral inferior colliculus (central nucleus) and continue via the ventral subdivision of MGN to the primary auditory cortex (area A1). There are also several parallel pathways that are involved in binaural processing and modulation of auditory inputs to the inferior colliculus. They include direct projections from ventral cochlear nucleus to the ipsilateral or contralateral superior olivary complex and projections from the ventral and dorsal cochlear nuclei to the contralateral nucleus of the lateral lemniscus. Neurons of the medial and lateral superior olivary nucleus receive bilateral inputs from both ears and are involved in sound localization.

Auditory Cortex

The primary auditory cortex (A1, area 41), located in the transverse gyri of Heschl in the upper bank of superior temporal gyrus, receives tonotopically organized inputs from the ventral MGN and contains two tonotopic maps that are mirror images of each other.[25] The auditory cortex sends modulatory projections to lower relay stations within the auditory pathway. Tinnitus may reflect reduced inhibition in the auditory pathway due to a decrease in thalamocortical and cortico-cortical connectivity with loss of frequency selectivity both at the level of the MGN and the primary auditory cortex.[26] There are multiple higher-order auditory areas surrounding the primary auditory cortex.[27,28] They are located in the temporal plane (*planum temporale*, area 42) located just caudal to the primary auditory cortex, and in the posterior two-thirds of the superior temporal gyrus (area 22); these areas are involved in the perception of complex sounds. Whereas early stages of auditory processing recruit areas in the superior temporal gyrus bilaterally, the processing streams then diverge into a dorsoposterior stream involved in mapping sound into representation for articulation and a ventrolateral stream involved in mapping of sound into meaning.[29] The auditory cortex is subdivided into core, belt, and parabelt regions participating in sequential processing of auditory information.[30–32] Information from the primary auditory cortex proceeds sequentially either to the posterior superior temporal gyrus (dorsal stream) or to the anterior superior temporal gyrus (ventral stream).[31,32]

VESTIBULAR SENSATION

Vestibular sensation is involved in detection of self-motion, including heading direction, traveled trajectory, and traveled distance or time, which is critical for efficient spatial navigation.[33,34]

Vestibular Organs and Vestibular Nuclei

The receptive cells of the vestibular organs are hair cells that tonically release glutamate. Deflection of the stereociliary bundle toward the longer stereocilia depolarizes the hair cells and increases the release of glutamate, activating the vestibular afferents. The vestibular organs include the semicircular canals, which predominantly encode angular velocity; and the otolith organs, utricle, and saccule, which sense linear acceleration. Vestibular afferents terminate in the vestibular nuclear complex, including the superior, medial, lateral, and inferior nuclei. Signals from the otolith organs and semicircular canals converge onto single neurons in the vestibular nuclei to triggered vestibuloocular and vestibulospinal reflexes. Vestibular nuclei also convey these signals to the thalamus and then to the cerebral cortex. Vestibular acceleration signals are particularly relevant for estimating the direction of self-motion; velocity signals may be more important for estimating traveled distance or maintaining stable gaze. Vestibular signals interact with other sensory signals such as visual optic flow typically experienced during motion in the environment. The representations of self-motion, speed and direction, current heading, and location in space are mediated by various neuronal subsystems. For example, location in space is encoded by hippocampal place cells; head rotation by angular head velocity cells; heading direction by head direction cells; and distance by grid cells of the entorhinal cortex. The integration of velocity to direction is necessary to update awareness of body position in space. The velocity cells, which mainly mediate the sensation of rotation, are primarily found in the lower brainstem, whereas the head direction cell system is distributed in a network covering the anterior thalamus, hippocampal formation, and cerebral cortex.

Vestibulo-Thalamocortical Pathways

Vestibular input enters its specific thalamic nuclei via multiple projections from the vestibular nuclei and the

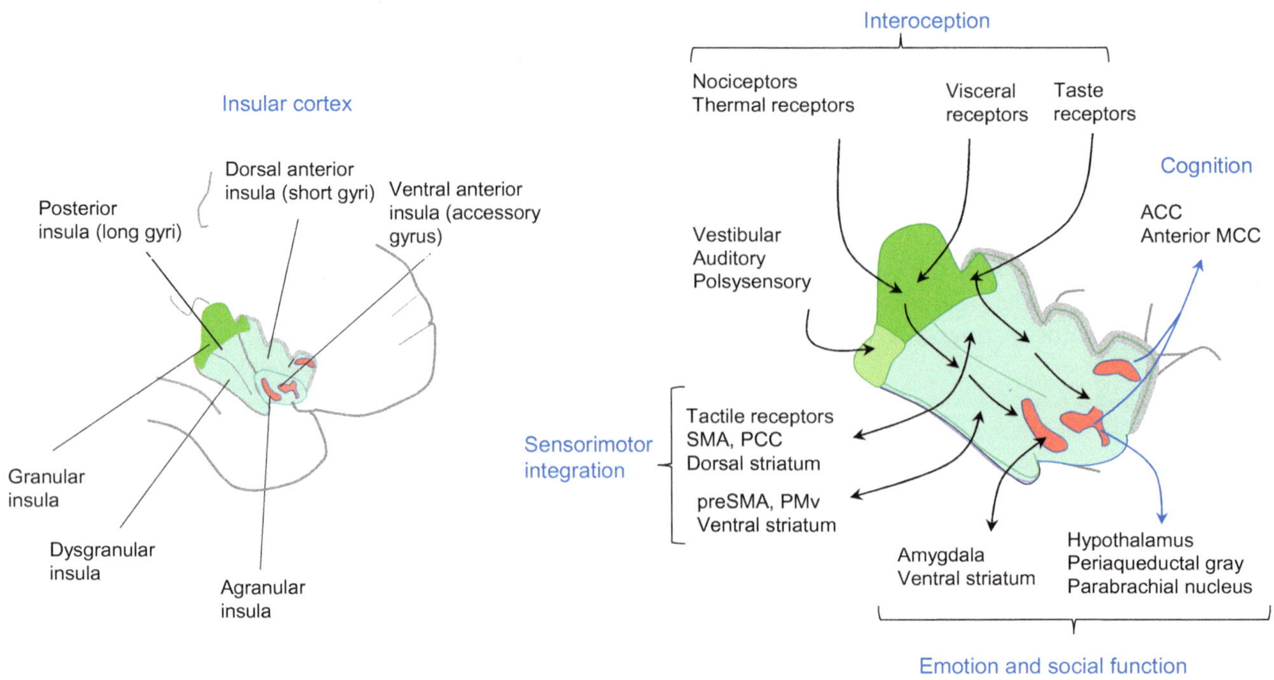

FIGURE 29.8 Connections of the insula.
Based on cytoarchitectonic analyses the insula has been subdivided into granular, dysgranular, and agranular sectors. The dorsal fundus of the granular posterior insula is the primary interoceptive area that receives pain, temperature, visceral, and taste sensation information. The dysgranular insula receives a somatotopic representation and has extensive connections with the amygdala, anterior cingulate cortex, and motor areas. The anterior agranular insula is interconnected with the anterior cingulate cortex, and amygdala, and projects to the ventral striatum, lateral hypothalamus, periaqueductal gray and brainstem autonomic nuclei.

cerebellum. There is a bilateral vestibular circuitry running from the brainstem via the thalamus to the parieto-insular vestibular cortex (PIVC), which is the core of the vestibular cortical network.[35] Five distinct and separate vestibular pathways have been identified. Three originate primarily in the superior vestibular nucleus and run ipsilaterally via the ascending tract of Deiters; two originate primarily in the medial vestibular nucleus, cross either in the pons or the midbrain, and ascend via the median longitudinal fasciculus. Two of the ipsilateral projections terminate in the posterolateral or paramedian thalamic subnuclei, whereas the third bypasses the thalamus to reach the inferior insula directly. Both contralateral pathways project to the posterolateral thalamus.

There is no single specific thalamic nucleus for vestibular sensation. Thalamic neurons conveying signals to the cerebral cortex are distributed through and near the VP and intralaminar nuclei, particularly in the centromedian/parafascicular complex. Large clusters are located at the borders of the VPL and VPM; one of these clusters, located at the intersection between the VPL, lateral pulvinar, and MGN, projects to the PIVC. Vestibular projections also terminate in scattered cell clusters in the anterior portion of the VPL, VPI, and other subnuclei of the posterolateral thalamus. The thalamus is directly involved in the differentiation between passive and active body motions.

Vestibular Cortex

The PIVC including the parietal operculum, insula, and retroinsular cortex is the primary component of the vestibular cortical network.[36] This network is present in both hemispheres and both sides are interconnected via the splenium of the corpus callosum. The central vestibular system is characterized by a hemispheric dominance that is located in the right hemisphere in right-handed and in the left hemisphere in left-handed humans. This indicates the presence of two different frames of reference, one for the egocentric manipulation of objects (handedness) and another for the allocentric localization of the self in the environment (multisensory vestibular system); these two processes of hand performance and spatial orientation could thus operate largely independently.[35] In addition to the PIVC, vestibular inputs reach somatosensory areas and areas of the posterior parietal and temporal cortex that process visual spatial and motion information and control eye movements.[37,38]

OLFACTORY SYSTEM

Olfactory Receptors and Olfactory Bulb

The neurons of the olfactory epithelium are bipolar cells with dendritic ends containing cilia that project into the overlying mucus and send their unmyelinated axons through the cribriform plate to the olfactory bulb. Of note, the sustentacular cells of the olfactory epithelium, but not or to a much lesser extent olfactory neurons, express the surface protein ACE2 (angiotensin-converting enzyme 2) and the serine protease TMPRSS2, which are involved in SARS-CoV-2 virus entry and impairment of the sense of smell in Covid-19 patients.[39,40] Odorants bind to GPCRs coupled to $G_{\alpha olf,}$ which stimulates adenylyl cyclase 3, production of cyclic adenosyl monophosphate (cAMP), opening of a cyclic nucleotide-gated Ca^{2+} channel, depolarization, and subsequent opening of Ca^{2+}-activated Cl^- channels that amplify depolarization. There are about 400 types of receptors expressed in human olfactory neurons, and an individual olfactory sensory neuron typically responds to more than one odorant type.

The olfactory bulb is an important site of information processing. Axons from olfactory receptor neurons expressing identical olfactory receptor genes coalesce and synapse on second-order projection neurons, called mitral and tufted cells, within structures called glomeruli.[41] The incoming axons from the olfactory receptor neurons also synapse on local GABAergic periglomerular interneurons that mediate feedback or feedforward inhibition within the glomerulus; some periglomerular cells also utilize dopamine, which inhibits glutamate release from olfactory receptor terminals. A second level of olfactory processing involves inhibitory GABAergic granule cells that participate in reciprocal dendrodendritic interactions with the mitral cells, resulting in lateral inhibition that enhances contrast responses to different odorants.[42] The olfactory bulb may constitute the "olfactory thalamus," as it is the final stage of processing of sensory information before reaching the cerebral cortex.[43] Whereas the olfactory bulb is affected by α-synuclein neuropathology at early stages of Lewy body disorders, the cellular mechanism underlying anosmia in Parkinson disease is still poorly defined.[44]

Olfactory Cortex

The olfactory cortex encompasses different areas. The piriform cortex, located at the junction between the caudolateral portion of the frontal lobe and the dorsomedial portion of the temporal lobe is the largest cortical olfactory area and may also function as an olfactory association area. Functional magnetic MRI studies indicate that the piriform cortex is functionally heterogeneous; its temporal lobe portion may be involved in more basic level of processing, such as odorant identification and discrimination, whereas the frontal portion is influenced by attentional state and the hedonic quality of the odorant.[45,46] The piriform cortex has widespread connections with the orbitofrontal cortex, both via a direct route and indirectly via the mediodorsal nucleus of the thalamus.[47] The posterior orbitofrontal cortex and adjacent anterior insular cortex integrate olfactory information with other sensory modalities. Other cortical primary olfactory areas include the anterior cortical nucleus of the amygdala, the periamygdaloid cortex, and the entorhinal cortex. All these areas send feedback projections back to the olfactory bulb and provide olfactory information to the amygdala and hippocampus.

TASTE SENSATION

Receptor Mechanisms

The sense of taste involves the five basic qualities of sweet, sour, salty, bitter, and umami (savory).[48] The taste receptors for sweet, umami, and bitter are GPCRs coupled to the phospholipase C-transduction pathway culminating in the activation of the Ca^{2+}-responsive transient receptor potential melastatin type (TRPM)-4 and -5 channels, which depolarize the cells and generate an action potential via voltage-gated Na^+ channels. For example, umami sense depends on activation of metabotropic glutamate receptors coupled to this pathway. This explains the coexistence of dysgeusia in patients with autoimmune cerebellar ataxia associated with mGluR1 antibodies. Transduction of sour involves the influx of protons (H^+) through an apical ion channel, which depolarizes taste cells directly and by inhibiting K^+ channels. Salt taste involves the amiloride-sensitive epithelial sodium channel (ENaC). Taste receptor cells release ATP, which activates P2X/P2X3 receptors, and 5-HT, which activate 5-HT3 receptors that depolarize the primary afferents.

Taste Pathway

Information processed in the taste buds is relayed to afferent fibers from facial (CN VII), glossopharyngeal (CN IX), and vagus (CN X) nerves that project to the nucleus of the solitary tract (NTS), where single gustatory neurons typically encode information about multiple taste qualities.[49] The NTS relays gustatory inputs to the parvocellular portion of the ventroposteromedial thalamic nucleus (VPMpc), which is the main thalamic gustatory relay to the gustatory cortex. The gustatory cortex occupies a portion of the insular cortex and part of the operculum. Neurons in the gustatory system also process nongustatory information related to the experience of food and eating, including texture, temperature, and odor and are also sensitive to visceral and homeostatic signals. These areas also integrate information from several sources to process the affective value of taste and their cognitive states. Together with the olfactory cortex, the insular gustatory cortex is a site of representation of and integration of taste, olfaction, and somatic sensation, and is part of network involved in processing of flavor (Figure 29.8).

FEATURES OF SENSORY PROCESSING

Predictive Coding

As mentioned in chapter 24, one emerging concept on sensory processing is that the brain actively constructs explanations to make inferences about the causes of its sensory inputs.[50–52] According to this view, the brain would anticipate incoming sensory inputs based on previous experience, and implement predictions that modulate activity of the appropriate sensory cortical areas in anticipation to receiving the actual sensory input from the environment. Cortical top-down predictions are compared with bottom-up representations of the actual incoming sensory information from lower levels. In this model, bottom-up feedforward connections convey prediction errors that are used to update the higher-level representations; top-down feedback projections from higher cortical areas would then suppress prediction errors in lower areas. All cortical sensory areas send descending projections to their corresponding thalamic relay nuclei, as well as to the brainstem and spinal sources of their thalamic input. Feedback inhibitory predictions can coexist with top-down attentional enhancement of sensory processing.

Learned Intermodal Associations

Learned associations between sensory stimuli provide information about statistical regularities in the environment, such as association between car and highway or fork and plate. These associations may help to predict and interpret future sensory inputs and to learn their meaning. Associative learning can occur with or without an observer's awareness. In the case of vision, this pair-coding mechanism involves interactions of neurons in the inferior temporal cortex with the hippocampus through connections via the perirhinal and lateral entorhinal cortex. These neurons respond selectively to complex objects with behavioral significance, such as faces, and participate in object recognition and long-term storage of associative visual memories. Associative learning also occurs in high-level processing areas of the dorsal visual stream. For example, neurons in the PPC may learn to associate the image of a stationary arrow pointing down with a downward movement of a pattern of dots; this associative learning depends on the memory of the motion.

The principles of associative perception and recall also apply to other sensory modalities, as well as interactions between modalities. For example, the visibility of the lips improves auditory word recognition; individuals are faster and more accurate in identifying a visual target when an auditory cue is presented at the same location. Synesthesia is a special form of intermodal interaction in which a stimulus originating from a sensory modality or submodality elicits a concurrent sensory experience in another modality. For example, grapheme-color synesthesia is characterized by the perception of specific color upon viewing a special graphic character (e.g., the number 3 may generate the perception of red). Mirror-touch synesthesia is a phenomenon in which individuals experience somatosensory sensations when seeing someone else being touched.[53] Synesthesia can be developmental or acquired. Experimental studies show that early auditory, somatosensory, or visual deprivation increases multisensory connections via an axonal reorganization process mediated by multimodal nonlemniscal thalamic nuclei and the primary sensory areas; spared senses functionally recruit deprived cortical areas by an altered development of sensory thalamocortical and cortico-cortical connections.[54] Acquired forms of synesthesia commonly arise from ingestions of drugs, including serotonergic hallucinogens, such as lysergic acid diethylamide (LSD) activating 5-HT2_A receptors,[55] thalamic lesions, and sensory deprivation (e.g., blindness).[56]

Mental Imagery

Mental imagery refers to the representation and associated experience of sensory information without a direct external stimulus.[57,58] Volitional or explicit imagery recalled from memory may serve cognitive and behavioral goals and may be either retrospective or prospective ("imagining the future"). Automatic or implicit imagery is externally driven based on learned association cues. Mental imagery shares with perception a common representation in the corresponding sensory areas. For example, fMRI studies confirm that visual imagery activates similar distributed representations in the visual cortex as the actual perception for the same content. Imagery content may be encoded several seconds before the voluntary decision of imagery; the activity in the primary visual cortex predicts future imagery vividness. Visual imagery may reflect activation of sensory areas by top-down connections from frontoparietal areas. High-level representations in anterior visual areas may be activated first, after which activity is propagated down to more low-level visual areas to fill in the visual details. However, some studies suggest that, unlike perception, the entire visual representation is activated at once at the onset of imagery. The ability to distinguish between a perception of a visual stimulus and visual imagery in part depends on the strength and ambiguity of the stimulus (bottom-up influence) and the judgment about the probability that the stimulus is the source of the perceptual experience (top-down assessment). Whereas imagery has been explored primarily in the visual modality, it can also occur in other sensory modalities.

Multisensory Integration and Perception

The brain integrates sensory inputs from several sources to eventually form a multimodal percept.[59] Several bottom-up influences affect multisensory integration, including the relative strength (salience), spatial location, and timing of different stimuli. The better spatial resolution of vision compared to audition explains the ventriloquism effect, an illusory sound localization induced by the apparent visual stimuli in space. In some cases, audition dominates vision due to the higher temporal resolution in audition than vision. One example is the sound-induced flash illusion, in which auditory inputs from beeping sounds generate illusory visual perception of a flashing light.

The cross-modal projections between unimodal sensory cortices may allow fast temporal integration of multisensory inputs. Output projections from these sensory cortices reach to higher association cortices, where multisensory integration also occurs. Important areas involved in multimodal representations include the PPC, which creates representation of space in an egocentric (individual-centered) reference frame, and the retrosplenial cortex, which processes spatial information in an allocentric (scene-based) reference frame. Several top-down factors can influence multisensory integration. These include learning of task-relevant sensory stimuli and engagement of attention during a task.

Bodily Self-Awareness

Conscious perception is not only a multisensory experience of an object but also includes the perception of the self,[60] Bodily self-consciousness is based on multisensory information. It has been studied, for example, by using visuo-tactile stimuli to induce illusory body ownership or self-attribution. A typical example is the rubber hand illusion: repeatedly touching a rubber hand placed in the participant's field of view, while simultaneously touching the participant's real hand hidden from the participant's view, creates the illusory ownership of the fake hand. These illusions rely on processing of information from the peripersonal space, which is roughly defined as the space to which one can reach. Multisensory integration of bodily signals requires integration of visual and tactile cues with proprioceptive signals that define the position of the body in space. Stimuli originally processed in sensory-dependent reference frames (eye-centered for visual, head-centered for auditory, and skin-centered for tactile stimuli) are realigned and integrated into a common proprioceptive reference frame within the peripersonal space. Neuroimaging studies show that multisensory integration for bodily self-consciousness recruits a network of multisensory cortical areas located in the inferior parietal lobule and ventral premotor cortex. These areas are involved in representation of the peripersonal space and are connected with areas related to temporo-occipital cortex (processing high-level visual and multisensory information); the posterior insula and parietal operculum (receiving vestibular projections); and the insular cortex (processing interoceptive body signals).

Insular Cortex: Multimodal Representations for Bodily Awareness

The insular cortex functions as a cortical hub involved in interoception, multimodal sensory processing, autonomic control, perceptual self-awareness, and emotional guidance of social behavior.[61,62] It includes a posterior (granular), middle (dysgranular), and anterior (agranular) regions, each with different connectivity and functions (Figure 29.8). The posterior insula receives and integrates inputs from multiple sources via the thalamus. These include pain, temperature, and visceral sensation carried via the STT and taste and visceral conveyed by the NTS, either directly or via the parabrachial nucleus in the pons. The main thalamic target of these interoceptive inputs are the ventromedial posterior and ventroposteromedial parvocellular nuclei, which project to the dorsal posterior insula. There is a topographic representation of these interoceptive inputs in the dorsal fundus of the insular cortex; the posterior portion responds to both noxious and innocuous thermal and mechanical stimuli, whereas more anterior portions respond to visceral and taste inputs. The posterior insula also receives somatosensory, visual, and vestibular information, as well as inputs from the superior colliculus, superior temporal sulcus, and auditory cortex. This multimodal sensory representation is further elaborated in the midinsular (dysgranular) cortex, which has extensive connection areas involved in high-order sensorimotor processing, emotion, and motivated behavior.[62] Information from the midinsular cortex finally reaches the anterior (agranular) insula, which further processes this information and interacts with areas involved in cognitive and emotional control, including the orbitofrontal cortex, anterior cingulate cortex amygdala, ventral striatum, lateral hypothalamus, periaqueductal gray, and brainstem autonomic nuclei. Functional neuroimaging studies indicate that there is a dorsoventral functional division in the anterior insular cortex, with a dorsal sector associated with cognitive tasks and the ventral sector involved in emotional responses. The anterior insula harbors von Economo neurons that project to the contralateral anterior insular cortex, ipsilateral anterior cingulate cortex, and brainstem nuclei involved in visceral sensation and autonomic control.[63]

The insula thus provides an interface between bodily sensation and emotion and may have a key role in perceptual awareness, social behavior, and decision-making.[62] It has been proposed that the anterior insular cortex may have a major role in awareness of oneself as a sentient (feeling) individual.[64,65] According to computational models of interoceptive predictive coding, the posterior insula would function as a comparator between expected and actual interoceptive sensation, thereby encoding an "error signal," whereas the agranular visceromotor cortices, including the anterior insula and anterior cingulate cortex, would update interoceptive predictions based on inputs received from the posterior insula.[62] Descending projections from von Economo neurons located in the anterior insula and anterior cingulate cortex may then convey "interoceptive error attenuation" commands either via top-down sensory gating or regulation of autonomic control via the periaqueductal gray.[51,66,67] A recent study showed an almost complete interruption of functional connectivity between the parabrachial nucleus and the anterior insular cortex in a comatose patient.[68] This finding supports the existence of a robust functional relation between these two regions and the link between awareness and arousal.

DISORDERS OF CORTICAL SENSORY PROCESSING

Neglect

Neglect is the acquired asymmetry in the ability to process information from one side of the space or the body; it is typically contralesional and is more common, severe, and persistent with right-sided hemispheric lesions.[69,70] Neglect can involve one side of the body, peripersonal space, or extrapersonal space. Hemispace is defined on the basis of three frames of reference, body midline, head midline, and visual field; these coordinates may influence neglect. Lesion mapping and transcranial magnetic stimulation studies show that the insula and temporoparietal junction are crucial for visual vertical perception. Neglect may occur for all objects on one side of the space or be stimulus-centered, involving one side of an object or word independently of its spatial location. Damage of the inferior parietal lobule (particularly on the right side), produces egocentric hemispatial neglect, whereas lesions in ventral cortical areas, including the medial temporal lobe, produce allocentric hemispatial neglect relative to objects. Neglect may also occur in mental imagery. Manifestations associated with neglect include extinction (tendency to report one of two stimuli presented simultaneously); somatoparaphrenia (denial of ownership of the body part, typically left upper limb); and anosognosia for hemiparesis.[71] Some patients with anosognosia will recognize their hemiparesis when their paretic hand is placed into ipsilesional hemispace suggesting that deafferentation and inattention-neglect may be important mechanisms. Some patients with anosognosia have asomatognosia and are then unaware that their paretic arm belongs to them; they do not recognize that they have a deficit. The feedforward hypothesis posits that without an attempt to move, there is no expectation of movement and in the absence of arm movement there will be no discord that leads to discovery of a mismatch.

Agnosias

Agnosia is a failure of object recognition that cannot be attributed to low-level visual or other sensory deficits. Classically, agnosia has been subdivided into aperceptive agnosia (impaired integration of form and feature information to form an internal representation of an object) and associative agnosia (normal perception stripped of its meaning). The most typical example is visual agnosia.[72] Visual agnosia may be category-specific. It may affect more the ability to name living than nonliving entities, or different semantic categories. Prosopagnosia is the inability to recognize a face as a face, extract meaning from the facial expression, or identify the person.[73–75] Prosopagnosia typically reflects involvement of right fusiform gyrus (fusiform face area) and the lateral occipital cortex (occipital face area). Functional imaging studies show fusiform activation in these patients despite the perceptual impairment. This area can be activated without exposure to the face, for example by the context of the visual scene or by listening to the person's voice, attention, or imagery processes that provide a top-down activation despite deafferentation resulting in impaired face identification. Prosopagnosia may or may not be associated with problems recognizing other types of objects. Patients with prosopagnosia patients may have difficulty distinguishing between types of birds, or flowers, or cars, what has been referred to as "within-category discrimination."

Astereognosia (astereognosis) or somatosensory agnosia, is the inability to identify objects by tactile manipulation (or by mouth) due to impaired discrimination of the size, texture, weight, and shape of the objects. Primary (apperceptive) astereognosia is the inability to discriminate shape and size by touch; associative asterognosis, or tactile agnosia is the inability to recognize objects by touch. The deficits in discrimination are most commonly seen with lesions in the primary somatosensory area and its connections; tactile agnosia is due to lesions in the parietal somatosensory association areas. Astereognosia indicates a lesion of the contralateral parietal lobe; bilateral astereognosia can occur with left postcentral lesions if there is dominance for stereognosis in the left hemisphere.

Auditory agnosia is the inability to recognize any type of sounds. Pure word deafness is a disorder where patients can identify environmental sounds but cannot understand speech despite ability to speak, write, and read. This disorder is associated with lesions affecting the primary auditory cortex bilaterally or the left superior temporal gyrus.

Pure Alexia

Pure alexia (agnosic alexia) is the specific inability to recognize words. It typically results from lesion in the left midfusiform gyrus or left occipitotemporal sulcus. The core deficit in pure alexia is loss of parallel letter recognition, resulting in letter-by-letter reading strategies. The key diagnostic feature of pure alexia is the word-length effect. The more letters in a word, the longer it takes to read it. In normal readers, the word-length effect is only about 10–20 milliseconds per letter. In alexia, it can be several seconds per letter. Pure alexia may be associated with surface dysgraphia, which is the difficulty spelling irregular words (e.g., yacht, colonel). Optic aphasia is a visual-modality-specific inability to recognize objects and words; patients are able to show the use of an object but unable to name it. It is distinguishable from anomia, as the patients are able to describe the object presented in another sensory modality, such as palpation, or can recognize an object from description.

Hallucinations

Visual hallucinations may reflect alterations in sensory processing in which the imagined content predominates regardless of its likelihood. This indicates a competitive advantage of the imaginal over the external stimulus component. Hallucinations often occur as part of a general cognitive failure, as in delirium or Lewy body disorders. In contrast, release hallucinations are rare and occur in the setting of sensory deafferentation. One typical example is Charles Bonnet syndrome, characterized by richly detailed visual imagery from pathology of the retina or optic nerve. Visual input not only relays new information but also suppresses spontaneous background activity in the visual cortex. Without that input, the background activity is released. The hallucinatory content varies with the cortical region, it does not reflect the site of the problem causing visual loss, and its content has no localizing clue. With ocular disorders, hallucinations often do not start until the second eye loses vision. Peduncular hallucinations have content that is quite similar to that of release hallucinations, but are attributed to brainstem lesions. They are usually accompanied by inversion of the sleep–wake cycle and may reflect altered function of the arousal or attention systems.

Patients with migraine may experience visual snow syndrome, which is characterized by continuous television static–like tiny flickering dots in the entire visual field and additional visual symptoms such as palinopsia (prolonged experience of the just-seen) or photophobia. These symptoms, together with hypermetabolism in the visual association area of the lingual gyrus but not in the primary cortex suggest an impairment of higher-order visual cortex function. A study using visual evoked potentials showed reduced amplitude of the N75-P100 (which reflects processing in the primary visual cortex) and a latency prolongation of the N-145 latency, which reflects impaired visual postprocessing in the higher-order visual system such as the fusiform gyrus.[76]

Disorders of Vestibular Processing

Imbalance of vestibular tone due to lesions in the ascending pathways from the otolith organs and the vertical semicircular canals result in a tilt of the subjective visual vertical, which is ipsilateral in unilateral pontomedullary lesions and contralateral with pontomesencephalic lesions. Unilateral lesions at thalamic or cortical level may also manifest with tilts of the subjective visual vertical less severe than those ocurrying after brainstem lesions; the direction of the tilts in the acute stage is constant in the single patient but varies between patients (50% ipsilateral, 50% contralateral). Thalamic astasia is a transient postural imbalance and body lateropulsion with a tendency to fall that occurs in acute lesions of the posterolateral or centromedian thalamic subnuclei. The pusher syndrome is characterized by an apparent tilt of the perceived body position in space, which the patients attempt to counteract by actively pushing or tilting the body to the contralesional side. It may be caused by lesions in the thalamus or, more commonly, in the posterior insula containing components of the multisensory vestibular network. The dominance of the right hemisphere explains the significantly higher frequency of pushing behavior in right-hemispheric strokes. Disorders of higher vestibular function involve cognition and more than one sensory modality leading to deficits of orientation and spatial memory. Disorders of higher vestibular function may occur lesions involving the multisensory vestibular cortex lesions (e.g., pusher syndrome or neglect) or with peripheral vestibular dysfunction (room tilt illusion or spatial disorientation in bilateral vestibulopathy). Even patients with chronic incomplete bilateral vestibulopathy may have anatomical and functional changes in the hippocampal formation, including hippocampal atrophy as well as subjective and objective navigational deficits.[35]

Phantom Limb

A phantom limb represents the inability to remove the amputated limb from the "off-line" representation of the body constructed in part from current sensory inputs and in part from stored memories. A similar phenomenon occurs when subjects become unaware of paralysis of a limb in hemiplegia (anosognosia). One way to eliminate these phenomena temporarily is by mirror therapy or virtual reality approaches.[77] In phantom limb the sensation of movement does not appear to originate from the periphery but is generated centrally, although it can be modified by peripheral input depending on stump muscle nerve activity. The more distal parts of a phantom limb, such as hands or feet, particularly digits, are more strongly perceived than proximal segments, which reflects the denser peripheral innervation and cortical representation. Perception of the phantom limb fades with time; more weakly perceived parts fade from awareness, leading to a telescoping of the limb. This reflects reorganization of the somatosensory cortex, where areas deprived of peripheral input are invaded by adjacent areas.[78]

Effects of Insular Lesions

Insular seizures may manifest with somatosensory, viscerosensory or visceromotor symptoms in various combinations. Somatosensory symptoms include paresthesia, thermal sensations, or pain; viscerosensory symptoms include epigastric or abdominal pain, throat tightness, and nausea. Other manifestations include olfactory, gustatory, auditory, and vestibular sensations. In humans, lesions involving the dorsal portion of the right insula have been associated with an alteration of the sense of body ownership that is necessary for self-agency.[79] Large lesions affecting the anterior insula may also be associated with alexithymia, which is impaired emotional awareness.[80] These findings led to a proposal that the anterior insular cortex is critical for awareness of oneself.[64,65] However, some patients with almost complete or complete bilateral destruction of the insula may still be able to experience everyday emotions and feelings and retain self-awareness.[81,82]

KEY POINTS

- Cortical processing of sensory information is a critical initial step in cognition, including spatial orientation, object recognition, semantic knowledge, episodic memory, and emotion.

- The sensory modalities are conveyed via parallel channels to primary cortical sensory areas.
- At each sensory nuclei, local mechanisms mediated by GABAergic interneurons promote sensory discrimination.
- Descending inputs from cortical sensory areas modulate sensory relay at their corresponding subcortical stations.
- Arousal, attention, behavioral relevance, and emotion strongly modulate sensory processing.
- Cortical processing of sensory information involves a dorsal stream to for spatial representation and a ventral stream for object feature representation.
- Transduction of low-threshold tactile and proprioceptive stimuli involves mechanically gated cation channels of the Piezo family.
- Low-threshold skin mechanoreceptors project via the dorsal columns to the core region of the dorsal column nuclei (DCN), which projects to the contralateral ventroposterolateral nucleus (VPL) of the thalamus.
- Proprioceptive inputs terminate in the rostral reticular and shell regions of the DCN, which project to the ventroposterior superior nucleus (VPS).
- The primary somatosensory cortex (S1) includes areas 3b and 1, which receive VPL inputs conveying tactile information; area 3a, which receives VPS inputs conveying information from deep receptors; and area 2, which contains representation of both cutaneous and deep receptors.
- The second somatosensory area (S2), the parietal ventral area, and the dorsal posterior insula provide somatosensory inputs to the lateral temporal cortex for tactile object recognition (ventral stream).
- Areas 5 and 7b in the superior parietal lobule integrate somatosensory information for spatial representation (dorsal stream).
- The retinal circuitry consists of photoreceptors that synapse on bipolar cells which then convey visual inputs to ganglion cells.
- Rods are located in the peripheral retina, contain rhodopsin, have exquisite sensitivity to single photons, and are used for vision in dim light.
- Cones are concentrated in the fovea; contain red, green, or blue opsins; and are responsible for visual acuity and color vision.
- During darkness, photoreceptors carry a depolarizing (dark) current via a cyclic guanosine monophosphate (cGMP)-gated cation channel that maintains a tonic release of glutamate at their synapses with bipolar cells.
- Light triggers closure of the cGMP-gated cation channel and thus photoreceptor hyperpolarization.
- ON-bipolar cells are activated by light, receive inputs from rods and cones, and activate ON-center ganglion cells; the ON-rod bipolars activate ganglion cells indirectly via AII amacrine cells.
- OFF-bipolar receive inputs from cones, respond to darkness, and send input to OFF-center ganglion cells.
- Lateral interactions mediated by horizontal cells shape the receptive fields and light responsiveness of the retinal ganglion cells.
- Ganglion cells of the ON- and OFF circuit convey image-forming inputs to the lateral geniculate nucleus (LGN), which then projects to the primary visual cortex (V1).
- Intrinsically photosensitive melanopsin ganglion cells respond to variations of luminescence (brightness) and are involved in entraining the circadian rhythm and triggering the pupillary light response.
- The parvocellular (P) pathway involves small ganglion cells that have high spatial resolution and color sensitivity and project to the P layers of the LGN.
- The M (magnocellular) pathway involves ganglion cells that are suited for processing of spatial information and project to the M-layers of the LGN.
- The dorsal stream includes a parieto-prefrontal pathway involved with visuospatial attention and control of eye movements; a parieto-premotor pathway that encodes space and body representations for visually guided motor actions, and a parieto-medial temporal pathway providing spatial landmarks for navigation.
- The ventral visual stream courses through the occipitotemporal cortex, including the fusiform gyrus, and constitutes a complex recurrent and interactive network.
- There is a functional clustering in the inferior temporal lobe with selectivity for faces, body parts, word forms, tools, large objects, and scenes.
- There is a stronger representation of faces in the right hemisphere; an area that selectively responds to word forms (visual word form area) is located in the left lateral occipitotemporal sulcus.
- The ventral visual network provides visual information for action selection, emotional responses, recognition memory, value-based decision-making, and visual working memory.
- There is a strict tonotopic organization in the cochlea; this tonotopic organization is maintained at all stations of the auditory pathway.
- There is also a sequential processing of auditory information from the primary auditory cortex to the posterior superior temporal gyrus (dorsal stream) and to the anterior superior temporal gyrus (ventral stream).

- Vestibular sensation is critical for detection of self-motion required for efficient spatial navigation.
- The olfactory bulb is an important site of information processing and constitutes the "olfactory thalamus."
- Information processed in the taste buds is conveyed to the nucleus of the solitary tract.
- The gustatory cortex occupies a portion of the insular cortex and part of the operculum.
- The brain may anticipate incoming sensory inputs based on previous experience.
- Learned associations between sensory stimuli may help to predict and interpret future sensory inputs and to learn their meaning.
- Mental imagery shares with perception a common representation in the corresponding sensory areas.
- There is a multimodal sensory representation in the cerebral cortex, which is important for self-awareness.
- The insular cortex is a richly connected structure that functions as a cortical hub involved in interoception, multimodal sensory processing, autonomic control, perceptual self-awareness, and emotional guidance of social behavior.
- Prosopagnosia typically reflects involvement of the right fusiform gyrus (fusiform face area) and the lateral occipital cortex (occipital face area).
- Pure alexia typically results from a lesion in the left midfusiform gyrus or left occipitotemporal sulcus.
- Release hallucinations are rare and occur in the setting of sensory deafferentation.
- A phantom limb represents the inability to remove the amputated limb from the "off-line" representation of the body.
- In humans, lesions involving the dorsal portion of the right insula have been associated with an alteration of the sense of body ownership.

REFERENCES

1. Dux PE, Marois R. The attentional blink: a review of data and theory. Atten Percept Psychophys 2009;71:1683–1700.
2. Snir G, Yeshurun Y. Perceptual episodes, temporal attention, and the role of cognitive control: lessons from the attentional blink. Prog Brain Res 2017;236:53–73.
3. Goodbourn PT, Martini P, Barnett-Cowan M, Harris IM, Livesey EJ, Holcombe AO. Reconsidering temporal selection in the attentional blink. Psychol Sci 2016;27:1146–1156.
4. Kravitz DJ, Saleem KS, Baker CI, Mishkin M. A new neural framework for visuospatial processing. Nat Rev Neurosci 2011;12:217–230.
5. Kravitz DJ, Saleem KS, Baker CI, Ungerleider LG, Mishkin M. The ventral visual pathway: an expanded neural framework for the processing of object quality. Trends Cogn Sci 2013;17:26–49.
6. Proske U, Gandevia SC. The proprioceptive senses: their roles in signaling body shape, body position and movement, and muscle force. Physiol Rev 2012;92:1651–1697.
7. Moehring F, Halder P, Seal RP, Stucky CL. Uncovering the cells and circuits of touch in normal and pathological settings. Neuron 2018;100:349-360.
8. Parpaite T, Coste B. Piezo channels. Curr Biol 2017;27:R250–R252.
9. Ranade SS, Woo SH, Dubin AE, et al. Piezo2 is the major transducer of mechanical forces for touch sensation in mice. Nature 2014;516:121–125.
10. Saotome K, Murthy SE, Kefauver JM, Whitwam T, Patapoutian A, Ward AB. Structure of the mechanically activated ion channel Piezo1. Nature 2018;554:481–486.
11. Patel S, Ohara S, Dougherty PM, Gracely RH, Lenz FA. Psychophysical elements of place and modality specificity in the thalamic somatic sensory nucleus (ventral caudal, vc) of awake humans. J Neurophysiol 2006;95:646–659.
12. Blankenburg F, Ruben J, Meyer R, Schwiemann J, Villringer A. Evidence for a rostral-to-caudal somatotopic organization in human primary somatosensory cortex with mirror-reversal in areas 3b and 1. Cereb Cortex 2003;13:987–993.
13. Eickhoff SB, Grefkes C, Zilles K, Fink GR. The somatotopic organization of cytoarchitectonic areas on the human parietal operculum. Cereb Cortex 2007;17:1800–1811.
14. Mountcastle VB. The parietal system and some higher brain functions. Cereb Cortex 1995;5:377–390.
15. Fogassi L, Ferrari PF, Gesierich B, Rozzi S, Chersi F, Rizzolatti G. Parietal lobe: from action organization to intention understanding. Science 2005;308:662–667.
16. Behrmann M, Plaut DC. Distributed circuits, not circumscribed centers, mediate visual recognition. Trends Cogn Sci 2013;17:210–219.
17. Konkle T, Oliva A. A real-world size organization of object responses in occipitotemporal cortex. Neuron 2012;74:1114–1124.
18. Schwarzlose RF, Swisher JD, Dang S, Kanwisher N. The distribution of category and location information across object-selective regions in human visual cortex. Proc Natl Acad Sci U S A 2008;105:4447–4452.
19. Grimaldi P, Saleem KS, Tsao D. Anatomical connections of the functionally defined "face patches" in the macaque monkey. Neuron 2016;90:1325–1342.
20. Dehaene S, Cohen L. The unique role of the visual word form area in reading. Trends Cogn Sci 2011;15:254–262.
21. May PJ. The mammalian superior colliculus: laminar structure and connections. Prog Brain Res 2006;151:321–378.
22. Basso MA, May PJ. Circuits for action and cognition: a view from the superior colliculus. Annu Rev Vis Sci 2017;3:197–226.
23. Do MTH. Melanopsin and the intrinsically photosensitive retinal ganglion cells: biophysics to behavior. Neuron 2019;104:205–226.
24. Wu Z, Grillet N, Zhao B, et al. Mechanosensory hair cells express two molecularly distinct mechanotransduction channels. Nat Neurosci 2017;20:24–33.
25. Formisano E, Kim DS, Di Salle F, van de Moortele PF, Ugurbil K, Goebel R. Mirror-symmetric tonotopic maps in human primary auditory cortex. Neuron 2003;40:859–869.
26. Berlot E, Arts R, Smit J, et al. A 7 Tesla fMRI investigation of human tinnitus percept in cortical and subcortical auditory areas. Neuroimage Clin 2020;25:102166.
27. Morosan P, Schleicher A, Amunts K, Zilles K. Multimodal architectonic mapping of human superior temporal gyrus. Anat Embryol (Berl) 2005;210:401–406.

28. Rademacher J, Burgel U, Zilles K. Stereotaxic localization, intersubject variability, and interhemispheric differences of the human auditory thalamocortical system. Neuroimage 2002;17:142–160.
29. Poeppel D. The neuroanatomic and neurophysiological infrastructure for speech and language. Curr Opin Neurobiol 2014;28:142–149.
30. Kaas JH, Hackett TA. "What" and "where" processing in auditory cortex. Nat Neurosci 1999;2:1045–1047.
31. Inui K, Okamoto H, Miki K, Gunji A, Kakigi R. Serial and parallel processing in the human auditory cortex: a magnetoencephalographic study. Cereb Cortex 2006;16:18–30.
32. Barrett DJ, Hall DA. Response preferences for "what" and "where" in human non-primary auditory cortex. Neuroimage 2006;32:968–977.
33. Cheng Z, Gu Y. Vestibular system and self-motion. Front Cell Neurosci 2018;12:456.
34. Cullen KE. Vestibular processing during natural self-motion: implications for perception and action. Nat Rev Neurosci 2019;20:346–363.
35. Brandt T, Dieterich M. Thalamocortical network: a core structure for integrative multimodal vestibular functions. Curr Opinion Neurobil 2019;32:154–164.
36. Frank SM, Greenlee MW. The parieto-insular vestibular cortex in humans: more than a single area? J Neurophysiol 2018;120:1438–1450.
37. Baier B, Conrad J, Stephan T, et al. Vestibular thalamus: two distinct graviceptive pathways. Neurology 2016;86:134–140.
38. Kirsch V, Keeser D, Hergenroeder T, et al. Structural and functional connectivity mapping of the vestibular circuitry from human brainstem to cortex. Brain Struct Funct 2016;221:1291–1308.
39. Baxter BD, Larson ED, Feinstein P, et al. Transcriptional profiling reveals TRPM5-expressing cells involved in viral infection in the olfactory epithelium. bioRxiv 2020. doi:10.1101/2020.05.14.096016
40. Bilinska K, Jakubowska P, Von Bartheld CS, Butowt R. Expression of the SARS-CoV-2 entry proteins, ACE2 and TMPRSS2, in cells of the olfactory epithelium: identification of cell types and trends with age. ACS Chem Neurosci 2020;11:1555–1562.
41. Chen WR, Shepherd GM. The olfactory glomerulus: a cortical module with specific functions. J Neurocyt 2005;34:353–360.
42. Shepherd GM, Chen WR, Willhite D, Migliore M, Greer CA. The olfactory granule cell: from classical enigma to central role in olfactory processing. Brain Res Rev 2007;55:373–382.
43. Kay LM, Sherman SM. An argument for an olfactory thalamus. Trends Neurosci 2007;30:47–53.
44. Fullard ME, Morley JF, Duda JE. Olfactory dysfunction as an early biomarker in Parkinson's disease. Neurosci Bull 2017;33:515–525.
45. Weismann M, Yousry I, Heuberger E, et al. Functional magnetic resonance imaging of human olfaction. Neuroimaging clinics of North America 2001;11:237–250, viii.
46. Gottfried JA, Winston JS, Dolan RJ. Dissociable codes of odor quality and odorant structure in human piriform cortex. Neuron 2006;49:467–479.
47. Tham WW, Stevenson RJ, Miller LA. The functional role of the medio dorsal thalamic nucleus in olfaction. Brain Res Rev 2009;62:109–126.
48. Kinnamon SC, Finger TE. Recent advances in taste transduction and signaling. F1000Res 2019;8. doi:10.12688/f1000reserch.21099.1 PMID32185015
49. Vincis R, Fontanini A. Central taste anatomy and physiology. Handb Clin Neurol 2019;164:187–204.
50. Adams RA, Shipp S, Friston KJ. Predictions not commands: active inference in the motor system. Brain Struct Funct 2013;218:611–643.
51. Barrett LF, Simmons WK. Interoceptive predictions in the brain. Nat Rev Neurosci 2015;16:419–429.
52. Bastos AM, Usrey WM, Adams RA, Mangun GR, Fries P, Friston KJ. Canonical microcircuits for predictive coding. Neuron 2012;76:695–711.
53. Linkovski O, Katzin N, Salti M. Mirror neurons and mirror-touch synesthesia. Neuroscientist 2017;23:103–108.
54. Henschke JU, Oelschlegel AM, Angenstein F, et al. Early sensory experience influences the development of multisensory thalamocortical and intracortical connections of primary sensory cortices. Brain Struct Funct 2018;223:1165–1190.
55. Kometer M, Vollenweider FX. Serotonergic hallucinogen-induced visual perceptual alterations. Curr Top Behav Neurosci 2018;36:257–282.
56. Safran AB, Sanda N. Color synesthesia: insight into perception, emotion, and consciousness. Curr Opin Neurol 2015;28:36–44.
57. Albright TD. On the perception of probable things: neural substrates of associative memory, imagery, and perception. Neuron 2012;74:227–245.
58. Pearson J, Naselaris T, Holmes EA, Kosslyn SM. Mental imagery: functional mechanisms and clinical applications. Trends Cogn Sci 2015;19:590–602.
59. Choi I, Lee JY, Lee SH. Bottom-up and top-down modulation of multisensory integration. Curr Opin Neurobiol 2018;52:115–122.
60. Blanke O, Slater M, Serino A. Behavioral, neural, and computational principles of bodily self-consciousness. Neuron 2015;88:145–166.
61. Benarroch EE. Insular cortex: functional complexity and clinical correlations. Neurology 2019;93:932–938.
62. Evrard HC. The organization of the primate insular cortex. Front Neuroanat 2019;13:43.
63. Allman JM, Tetreault NA, Hakeem AY, Park S. The von Economo neurons in apes and humans. Am J Hum Biol 2011;23:5–21.
64. Craig AD. How do you feel—now? The anterior insula and human awareness. Nat Rev Neurosci 2009;10:59–70.
65. Craig AD. Significance of the insula for the evolution of human awareness of feelings from the body. Ann N Y Acad Sci 2011;1225:72–82.
66. Seth AK, Critchley HD. Extending predictive processing to the body: emotion as interoceptive inference. Behav Brain Sci 2013;36:227–228.
67. Seth AK, Friston KJ. Active interoceptive inference and the emotional brain. Philos Trans R Soc Lond B Biol Sci 2016;371:20160007.
68. Fischer DB, Boes AD, Demertzi A, et al. A human brain network derived from coma-causing brainstem lesions. Neurology 2016;87:2427–2434.
69. Rode G, Pagliari C, Huchon L, Rossetti Y, Pisella L. Semiology of neglect: an update. Ann Phys Rehabil Med 2017;60:177–185.

70. Langer KG, Piechowski-Jozwiak B, Bogousslavsky J. Hemineglect and attentional dysfunction. Front Neurol Neurosci 2019;44:89–99.
71. Heilman KM. Possible mechanisms of anosognosia of hemiplegia. Cortex 2014;61:30–42.
72. Barton JJS. Vision: it is about the brain. J Neuroophthalmol 2018;38:271–275.
73. Bartolomeo P, Vuilleumier P, Behrmann M. The whole is greater than the sum of the parts: distributed circuits in visual cognition. Cortex 2015;72:1–4.
74. Barton JJ. Higher cortical visual deficits. Continuum (Minneap Minn) 2014;20:922–941.
75. Albonico A, Barton J. Progress in perceptual research: the case of prosopagnosia. F1000Res 2019;8.
76. Eren O, Rauschel V, Ruscheweyh R, Straube A, Schankin CJ. Evidence of dysfunction in the visual association cortex in visual snow syndrome. Ann Neurol 2018;84:946–949.
77. Richardson C, Kulkarni J. A review of the management of phantom limb pain: challenges and solutions. J Pain Res 2017;10:1861–1870.
78. Buonomano DV, Merzenich MM. Cortical plasticity: from synapses to maps. Annu Rev Neurosci 1998;21:149–186.
79. Karnath HO, Baier B. Right insula for our sense of limb ownership and self-awareness of actions. Brain Struct Funct 2010;214:411–417.
80. Jones CL, Ward J, Critchley HD. The neuropsychological impact of insular cortex lesions. J Neurol Neurosurg Psychiatry 2010;81:611–618.
81. Damasio A, Damasio H, Tranel D. Persistence of feelings and sentience after bilateral damage of the insula. Cereb Cortex 2013;23:833–846.
82. Feinstein JS. Lesion studies of human emotion and feeling. Curr Opin Neurobiol 2013;23:304–309.

30 Motor Cortex

OVERVIEW

Motor control is the control of postures and movements by central commands and segmental reflexes.[1] Voluntary movements are organized to perform a purposeful task. Motor plans are strategies aimed to perform a task and are implemented according to goals or needs. The overall strategy is then organized into motor programs before the beginning of the motor action. The control of voluntary movement involves interactions among frontal motor areas, parietal cortex, and prefrontal cortex (PFC)[2] (Figure 30.1). The frontal motor cortex includes the primary motor cortex (M1), several divisions of the lateral premotor cortex (PM), supplementary motor area (SMA), presupplementary motor area (preSMA), cingulate motor areas, and frontal eye field (FEF) and supplementary eye field. The PFC provides executive control required for decisions as to whether and when to move and how to modify movements according to changing circumstances. The posterior parietal cortex (PPC) provides a multimodal representation of space, which is conveyed to the premotor cortex to implement motor programs. The expectation of the sensory consequences of movement preserves the intended programmed action. Motor planning, motor programs, and motor execution involve cortical interactions with basal ganglia and cerebellar circuits via the thalamus. The cortical motor areas are also involved in cognitive processes, such as spatial attention, recognition of intentions of others, and suppression of inappropriate actions. The aims of this chapter are to review: (1) general features of goal-directed motor control, (2) the functional organization of the frontal motor areas, (3) the role of the PPC in representation of space and its interactions with premotor cortical areas cortex in control of visually guided movements, (4) the role of medial frontal motor areas, (5) cognitive aspects of motor control, and (6) examples of disorders of cortical motor control.

GOAL-DIRECTED MOTOR CONTROL

Motor planning, motor programs, and motor execution involve interconnected areas of the frontal and parietal cortex.

Motor Plans, Motor Programs, and Predictive Motor Control

Motor plans are strategies aimed to perform a particular task and consist of sets of feedforward commands for motor actions learned from previous successful performance.[3] Motor plans are implemented according to goals or needs. Once a motor action is planned, the overall strategy is organized into motor programs that control various parts of the performance. These programs are a set of commands structured by premotor areas before the beginning of the motor action. The brain predicts the sensory consequences of motor actions and anticipates the resulting incoming sensory inputs based on previous experience. The expectation of the sensory consequences of movement preserves the intended programmed action. According to the forward model of motor control, the motor cortex sends both a command to the motor nuclei to elicit movement and a predictive feedforward signal, known as efference copy (or corollary discharge), to the parietal cortex and cerebellum, predicting the probable sensory consequences of the commanded motor action (Figure 30.1). This sensory prediction is compared with sensory feedback resulting from the ongoing action and its effects on the external environment. This comparison generates a prediction error signal that is used to adjust the current motor command, attenuate predictable self-produced sensations, and attribute agency (self-initiation) to actions and their effects on the environment. Proprioceptive prediction errors computed by the somatosensory cortex and cerebellum are fed back to the motor cortex, which then functions as a controller to correct the motor commands. In this setting, motor behavior suppresses proprioceptive prediction errors by changing proprioceptive sensations. Planned programmed movements

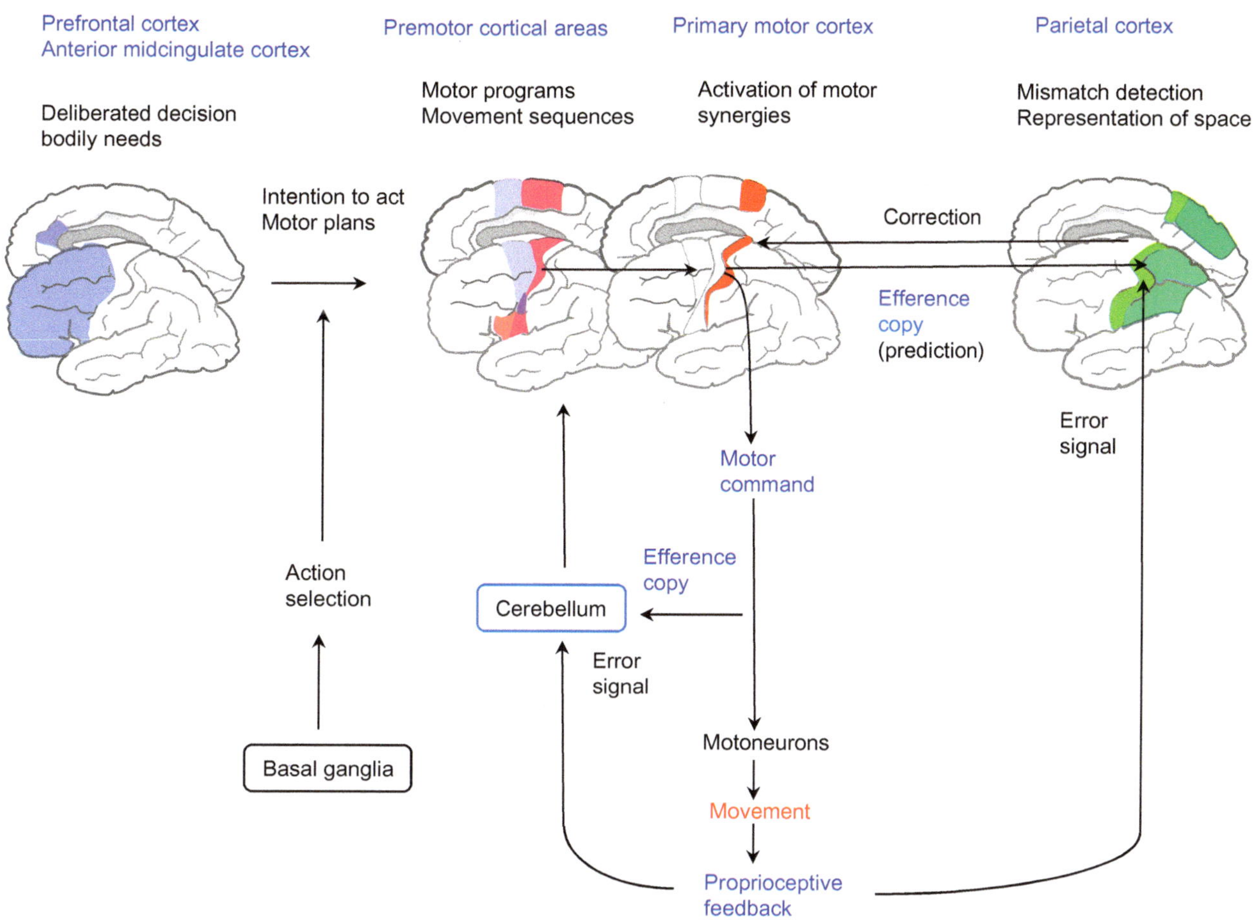

FIGURE 30.1 Cortical areas involved in motor control.
Planning, motor programs, and motor execution involve interconnected areas of the frontal and parietal cortex and their interactions with basal ganglia and cerebellar circuits via the thalamus. Motor plans are implemented by interactions between the prefrontal and midcingulate cortex. The overall strategy is organized into motor programs by premotor cortical areas. The motor cortex sends a command to motor nuclei to elicit movement, and a predictive feedforward signal to the parietal cortex and cerebellum. The motor cortex sends two simultaneous signals, a command to the motor nuclei to elicit movement, and a predictive feedforward signal, to the parietal cortex and cerebellum predicting the probable sensory consequences of the motor action.

can be made without feedback if speed is the critical element, as occurs with saccadic eye movements.

Motor Learning and Adaptation

Learning and programming of movements optimize motor skill and depend on experience. Continued use of the same programs for the performance of a task increases the accuracy of motor memory and therefore task execution. Motor adaptation is the ability to reprogram sequences of movement sequences in response to changes in the external circumstances. Motor learning and adaptation are manifestations of use-dependent plasticity of the motor system. The reciprocal connectivity among the cerebral cortex, cerebellum, and basal ganglia provides for distributed processing modules that support different forms of learning, the cerebellum is involved in supervised (error-based) learning, whereas the striatum is critical for reward-based (reinforcement) learning. Both the cerebellar and basal ganglia loops via the thalamus target the same cortical areas that send the inputs to these loops. This drives the motor cortex to perform actions learned subcortically and promotes unsupervised associative learning based on practice and associative long-term potentiation.

Decision-Making and Motor Control

Decision-making guides motor control by determining whether or not to make a movement, which movement to make next, when to initiate and how to control the selected movements, and how to update movements in response to contingencies.[3,4] Interactions between decision-making and motor control occur at the level of both planning and action programming and execution. Before target selection, the motor system prepares competing movement plans for potential targets and specifies contingency plans in order to accomplish the task goal in the setting of unexpected changes in the environment. Movements directed to a single goal, such as reaching for a target, involve a planning phase that specifies the parameters of the upcoming action and readiness for its implementation, and a control phase that provides online corrections that fine-tune the movement for its successful completion. External perturbations of the intended positions or movements of a limb result in both a short-latency spinal-generated response mediated by muscle stretch reflexes and a longer latency response produced by transcortical reflexes. These long-loop responses can control and regulate intended limb postures and trajectories by adjusting joint stiffness, and are part of the motor program. Visual feedback also has an important role in rapid movement corrections.

FUNCTIONAL ANATOMY OF THE FRONTAL MOTOR CORTEX

The frontal motor cortex is characterized by a prominent pyramidal cell layer 5 and includes several interconnected areas with partially segregated but overlapping functions (Figure 30.2).

Subdivisions and Connectivity

The primary motor cortex (M1) located in the precentral gyrus (area 4) contains large pyramidal tract cells (Betz cells) and is the main source of descending commands to α-motor neurons (motoneurons) and interneurons in the ventral (anterior) horn. The lateral premotor cortex (lateral area 6) is subdivided into dorsal (PMd), ventral (PMv), predorsal (prePMd) and the transition hub zone between PMd and PMv (PM-tr). The medial frontal motor areas include the SMA and preSMA and two cingulate motor areas, anterior (rostral cingulate zone) and posterior (caudal cingulate zone).[2,5] The frontal lobe also harbors the FEF in the precentral gyrus and sulcus and the supplementary eye field in the posteromedial portion of the superior frontal gyrus. Based on their cortico-cortical connectivity and projections, the frontal motor areas have been subdivided into the caudal "parieto-dependent" and rostral "prefronto-dependent" groups[6] (Figure 30.3). The caudal or posterior areas include M1, PMd, PMv, SMA, and caudal cingulate motor area. These regions receive prominent input from the parietal cortex, are reciprocally interconnected, and contribute to the corticospinal tract (CST). The rostral or anterior group includes the prePMd, the transitional connector hub between PMd and PMv (PM-tr), the preSMA,

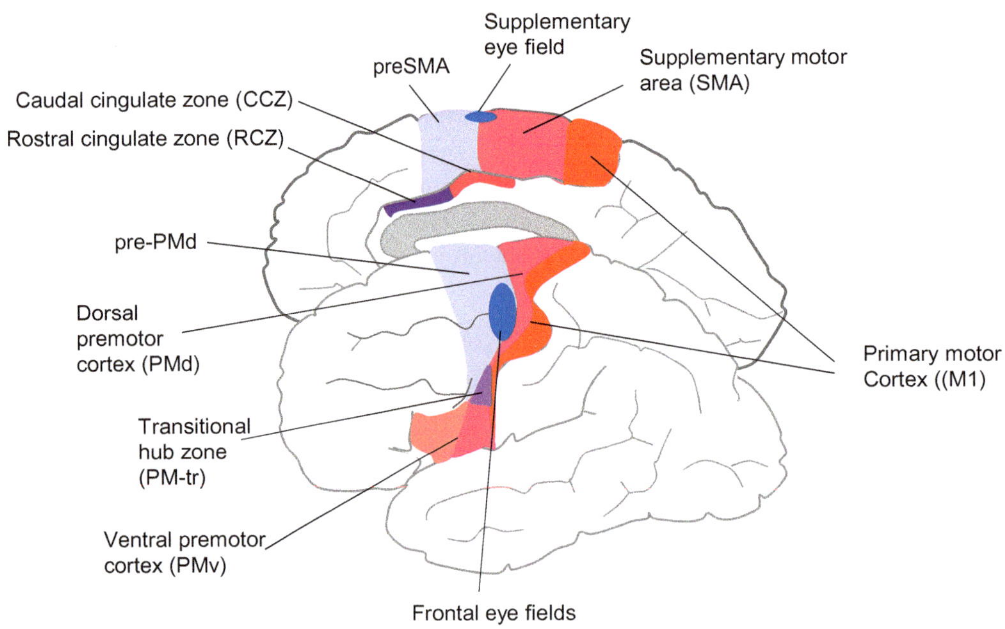

FIGURE 30.2 Frontal motor areas.
In humans, the primary motor cortex (M1) is located in the precentral gyrus (area 4). The lateral premotor cortex, or lateral area 6, is subdivided into dorsal (PMd), ventral (PMv), predorsal (prePMd), and in humans an intermediate or transition zone between PMd and PMv (PM-tr) The medial frontal motor areas include the supplementary motor area (SMA), the presupplementary motor area (preSMA); and two cingulate motor areas, anterior or rostral (RCZ) and posterior or caudal (CCZ). The frontal lobe also harbors the frontal eye field (FEF) and supplementary eye field (SEF).

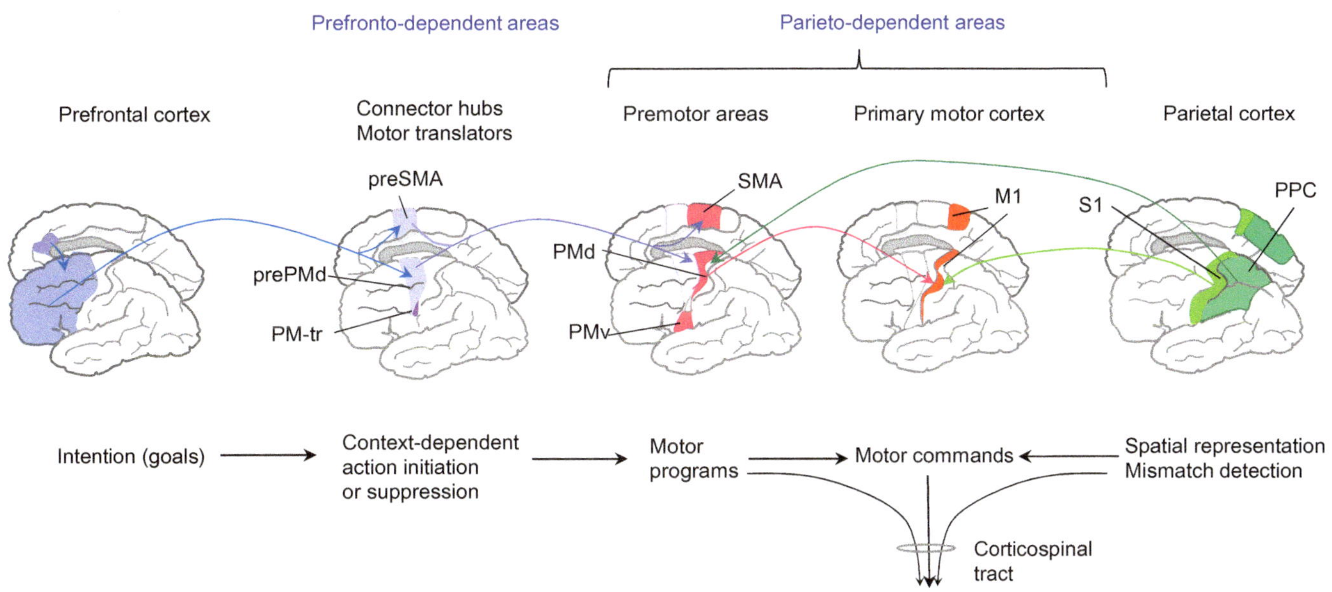

FIGURE 30.3 Connectivity of cortical motor areas.
The frontal motor areas are divided into a caudal and a rostral group based on their connectivity. The caudal or posterior premotor areas include the primary motor cortex (M1), dorsal PMd and ventral (PMv) premotor cortex, SMA, and caudal cingulate motor area (CCZ). These regions are reciprocally interconnected, receive cortical input from the parietal lobe, and contribute to the corticospinal tract. The rostral or anterior group functions as connector hubs and motor translators between the prefrontal cortex (PFC) and premotor areas. They include the prePMd, the dorsal transitional connector hub between PMd and PMv (PM-tr), preSMA, and rostral cingulate motor areas. These areas do not project via the corticospinal tract but are interconnected with each other, with premotor areas, and other cortical areas and mediate the prefrontal (cognitive) control on motor function.

and the rostral cingulate motor area. These areas receive their main input from the PFC and convey information related to motivation and long-term motor plans, including context-dependent action initiation or suppression, to the caudal premotor areas.

Representation of Muscle Synergies and Action Maps

The traditional view of the human motor cortex is that it contains an overlapping sequence of body part representations. This constitutes the classical motor homunculus defined by the pioneering studies of Penfield and Rasmussen.[7] However, high-resolution functional MRI showed some violations of the typical somatotopic representation. For example, the arm is represented in two areas, one dorsal and another ventral to a region representing the fingers.[8] Instead, both fMRI in humans and electrophysiological studies in monkeys show that different areas of M1 control different muscle synergies or "action maps." These synergies may comprise a single muscle or several combinations of agonist and antagonist muscles; and when variably combined generate the majority of natural movements.[9,10] Within M1 the representation of different muscle synergies is not topographically ordered; each synergy is represented multiple times over widespread areas, and different synergies are localized adjacent to one another in various combinations. This "fractured somatology" facilitates the combination of multiple synergies to produce complex movements. The control of muscle activation is organized into patterns of muscle coactivation, or spatial synergies, which are sequentially recruited according to muscle commands for a given action as spatiotemporal synergies. Each functional zone or action map in the motor cortex represents a complex, meaningful category of behavior, such as interactions between the hand and the mouth, actions that defend the body surface, and reach-to-grasp.[9]

Relative Role of M1 and Lateral Premotor Cortex in Action Control

Microstimulation studies in monkeys and fMRI in humans indicate that different areas of lateral frontal motor cortex have selective as well as overlapping roles in motor control (Figure 30.4). Neurons in M1 emphasize actions that focus on individual body parts, such as position and movement of the fingers during manipulation of objects, and their activity correlates with velocity and force of executed movements. Neurons in PMd participate in programming, preparation, and coordination of proximal limb movements, such as those involved in reaching. Neurons in the area just anterior to the PMd (prePMd) may be involved in the association between a visual cue and the selection and direction of movement of the hand. The PMv

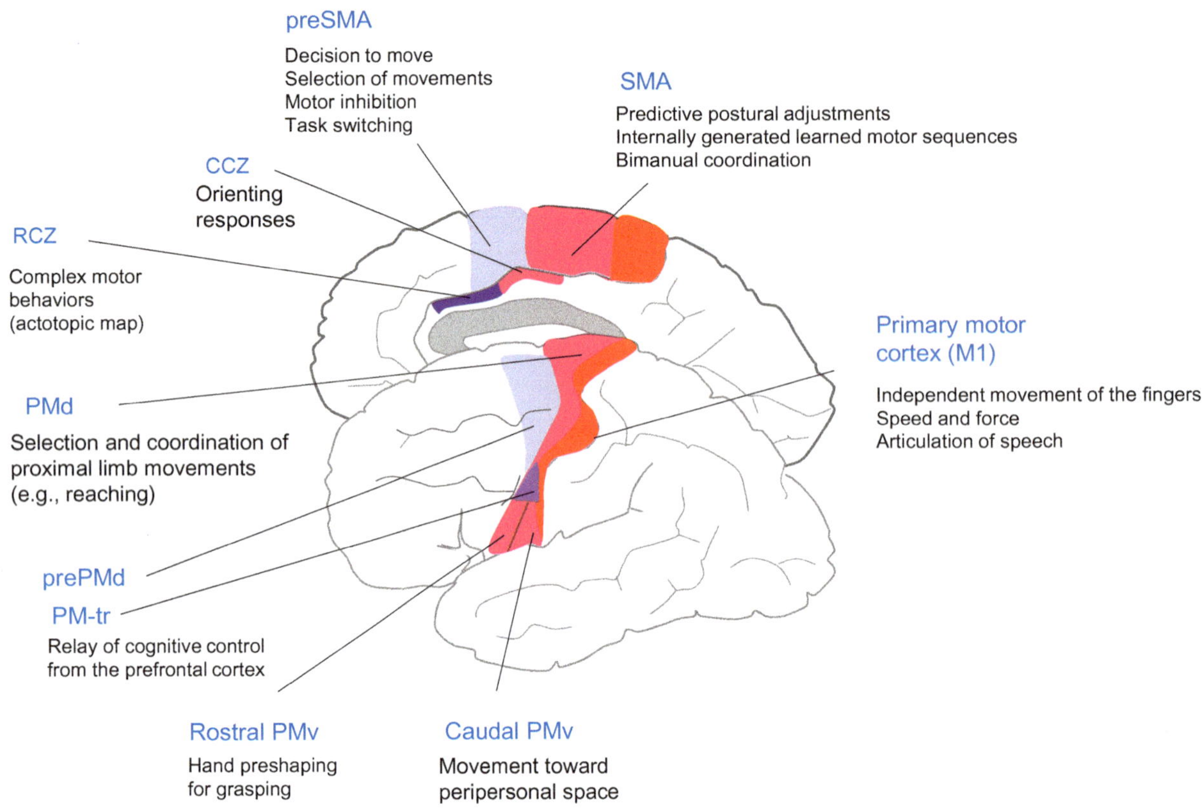

FIGURE 30.4 Main functions of frontal motor areas.
The precentral motor cortex (M1, area 4), dorsal premotor cortex (PMd), and ventral premotor cortex (PMv) participate in different aspects of motor control. Neurons in M1 have a major role in movement of the fingers during manipulation of objects. Neurons in PMd participate in programming, preparation, and coordination of proximal limb movements. The rostral PMv has a representation of hand movements such as grasping and manipulation of objects. The caudal PMv is activated during goal-directed movements toward the peripersonal space. The medial frontal motor areas include the supplementary motor area (SMA), preSMA, and cingulate motor areas. The SMA has a major role in predictive postural adjustments, internally generated learned motor sequences, and bimanual coordination. The preSMA contributes to selection and preparation of movements and decision as to when to start a movement The rostral cingulate motor area may function in conflict monitoring and the caudal cingulate motor area primarily in association with orienting.

includes a rostral subdivision that has a representation of hand movements such as grasping and manipulation of objects. This portion of the PMv also contains neurons that are activated in response to observation of actions similar to those they encode and form part of the so-called mirror motor system. In monkeys, the posterior (caudal) portion of PMv contains neurons that represent arm, neck, face, and mouth movements and are activated during goal-directed movements toward the peripersonal space. Recordings in patients during epilepsy surgery showed two neural representations of hand/mouth actions within the precentral gyrus, one representing self-feeding and a second likely associated with perioral exploration.[11]

Medial Frontal Motor Areas

The medial frontal motor areas, including the SMA, preSMA, and cingulate motor areas are involved in cognitive and executive aspects of motor planning and programming on the basis of experience, goals, or motivation[12] (Figure 30.4). The SMA contains a complete representation of body movements, typically affecting multiple proximal and distal joins. The SMA has a major role in setting motor programs for internally generated learned motor sequences, movement preparation, and modulation of interhemispheric interactions, including bimanual coordination.[13] The preSMA contributes to "cognitive" aspects of motor control, including selection and preparation of movements, decision as to when to start a movement according to contingencies or motivation, organization of motor sequences, motor inhibition, and task switching. The preSMA may also be activated in the delay period between presentation of a stimulus and movement in working memory tasks. This activity may be related to a state of preparedness for selecting a motor response based on spatial and object information held in working memory. The rostral cingulate motor area may function in either conflict monitoring (evaluative function) or attention and selection for action; the caudal cingulate motor area is activated primarily in association with execution of orienting movements.[6] A study in patients undergoing evaluation for epilepsy surgery showed that stimulation of the anterior midcingulate cortex (MCC) elicited a feeling of expectation of an imminent challenge and experience of effortful motor action that was associated with complex motor behaviors with an "actotopic" organization.[14] Stimulation of ventral portions elicited whole-body behaviors directed to the extrapersonal space, such as getting-up impulses; stimulation of the intermediate portion elicited hand actions in the peripersonal space; and stimulation of the dorsal portion elicited body-directed actions.

PHYSIOLOGY OF THE MOTOR CORTEX

The physiology of the microcircuit of the motor cortex has been investigated with both cellular approaches and high-resolution neuroimaging.[15]

Microcircuit and Outputs of the Motor Cortex

The connectivity in area M1 comprises two interconnected circuits. An upper closed-loop circuit spanning layers 2 to 5A receives thalamocortical excitatory input via layer 3; a lower closed loop circuit spanning layers 5B and 6 receives inputs from layers 2 and 3. The intratelencephalic (IT) neurons of layers 3 strongly project to the pyramidal tract (PT) neurons in layer 5B that send output to the spinal cord and the striatum. Layers 2/3 of the motor cortex receive somatosensory projections and combine sensory feedback with existing motor representations; layer 5A neurons show plastic changes in dendritic spines during motor learning and thus encode evolving motor representations driven by sensorimotor integration at the level of layers 2/3.[15] The primary motor cortex and the primary somatosensory cortex (S1) are interconnected both anatomically and functionally and both contain PT neurons that contribute to the CST. The PT neurons in in M1 fire before movement onset and their discharge correlates with the direction and force of the movement. These PT neurons function as "command" neurons that provide collaterals to subcortical motor structures and send an efference copy of motor commands to the cerebellum. Projections from area 4 signal starts and stops of movements by setting the level of activity of the spinal motoneurons and interneurons. These command PT neurons make powerful direct cortico-motoneuronal connections to motoneurons, particularly those innervating distal hand and digit muscles, loss of which produces a characteristic weakness of the thenar musculature (the "split-hand" syndrome).[16] Most corticomotoneuronal projections originate from PT neurons located in the most posterior portions of area 4, where there is a large representation of each hand muscle that overlaps extensively with that of other hand muscles and to a lesser extent with muscles acting at the elbow and shoulder; this allows for close interactions of upper limb musculature during complex reach-and-grasp tasks. These posterior M1 cortico-motoneurons respond to cutaneous inputs and may use tactile feedback for movements involved in exploratory touch. In contrast, PT neurons in the most anterior regions of M1 project to the spinal intermediate zone and to brainstem targets such as the cells of origin of the reticulospinal tracts. Some of these CST neurons receive strong central drive and are primarily involved in advanced calculations for movement; others receive inputs from moving joints and use kinesthetic feedback for execution and guidance of movements. Projections from parietal areas 2 and 5 and portions of area 4 carry descending preparatory messages for adjusting sensory input, and reach the spinal cord before movement onset. Small CST neurons provide tonic inputs to spinal motoneurons recruited early during a motor task and are used for fine gradations of force. In contrast, large CST neurons discharge phasically in association with large movements and control large spinal motoneurons that are recruited late in the buildup of muscle force.

Coding of Movement Parameters by Cortical Motor Neurons

Neural populations in the motor cortex with shared response properties may act at different times as two separate circuits, one for preparation and the second for execution of movement.[17] Movement in a particular direction is determined by the net action of a large population of cortical motor neurons.[14,18,19] This activity encodes an evolving reaching movement by applying a population code that predicts both the direction of movement and the upcoming movement trajectory.[18] The activity of neurons involved in grasping is modulated by the grasp width of the object. Different populations of M1 neurons are engaged during a power grip with all digits and during precision grip used to hold and pick up objects. The ability to record from the human motor cortex for control of a prosthetic limb has shown that the activity of single motor cortical cells could relate to both reaching and grasping.[18] Local inhibitory mechanisms may control the directional accuracy and speed of the reaching. During active behavior, the motor cortex may initiate or suppress motor programs. Command M1 neurons may not only increase but also decrease their activity before and during precision movements, indicating that they in part control the pattern of muscle activity by disfacilitating the excitatory drive to motoneurons. Movement is often associated with increases in activity of fast-spiking GABAergic neurons. Spasticity and clonus in chronic motor cortex lesions point to a net loss of inhibitory control of motor neurons. The loss of fractionated movements and the inability to independently move one body part without others indicates also that a prime role for descending influences from the motor cortex is to suppress and inhibit undesirable movements. These abnormalities may also reflect loss of cortical input to the reticulospinal system.

Cortico-Thalamo-Cortical Interactions

The motor cortex exerts direct modulatory influence on the motor thalamus (ventrolateral nucleus, VL) via layer 6 corticothalamic (CT) neurons.[20] These CT neurons are primarily driven by inputs from other cortical areas. The VL receives weak feedback input from CT neurons compared to other thalamic nuclei. In contrast, there is a strong CT output from M1 to the thalamic reticular and the posterior nuclei. The CT input from the motor cortex to the thalamic reticular nucleus, which sends inhibitory projection to the VL, could have a primary inhibitory effect on the sensitivity of VL neurons to excitatory input from the cerebellar nuclei. The excitatory output from CT neurons of M1 on the posterior nucleus, which is a high-order sensory thalamic nucleus, may enhance transfer of sensory-related activity.

Descending Gating of Sensory Information During Movement

Descending inputs from the sensorimotor cortex control information processing at the dorsal column nuclei and dorsal horn. The primary function of this corticonuclear descending control is to select certain somatosensory inputs at the expense of others; these effects are in part mediated by local interneurons. For example, projections from areas 3a and 4 target proprioceptive zones of the dorsal column nuclei and influence the tactile receptive cells. One group of corticonuclear projections is tonically active during movement and has a general inhibitory influence, preventing weak sensory inputs triggered by movement from reaching the cortex. Only those dorsal column nuclei neurons that receive strong sensory input during movement would be able to overcome this inhibition. A second group consists of collaterals of CST axons that innervate the cervical cord motoneurons controlling the upper limb. These collaterals facilitate sensory transmission through disinhibition of dorsal column nuclei, particularly during distal upper limb muscles, thus favoring the transmission of sensory feedback initiated by the movement during manipulative and exploratory behavior.

Sensory Feedback, Long-Loop Reflexes, and Beta Oscillations

The continuous sensory feedback input to the sensorimotor cortex during active movement is fundamental for smooth voluntary movements, including the fractionated movement of the digits. Inputs from proprioceptors and tactile afferents are important for manipulating objects for object recognition, a process known as "active touch." The activity of cortical motor neurons during voluntary movements also depends on long-loop transcortical reflexes. These reflexes involve descending CST predictive commands from M1 and ascending instructive sensory feedback signals via the dorsal column-lemniscal system to S1. Long-loop responses are emitted predictively in programmed postural adjustments as part of the motor program and motor set, and are important for the steady maintenance and corrections of intended postures by adjusting M1 output. They regulate skilled voluntary movements automatically and continuously, compensating for sudden unexpected load changes that may interfere with movement. Long-loop reflexes are also important for adjustment of precision grip and tactile exploration, show task-related adaptations to changing circumstances, and are susceptible to instructions given to the subject. These responses increase when the central set calls for an extra effort.

Beta-frequency oscillations (13–30 Hz) are prominent in the cortical sensorimotor areas. They reflect the tight input-output coupling and close correspondence between the motor and somatosensory receptive fields. Beta oscillations represent the periodic and synchronous activity in essentially all elements of the sensorimotor control system, including the premotor cortex, M1, S1, muscles, dorsal root ganglia, deep cerebellar nuclei, and striatum. They are prominent during postural holds when muscles are tonically active and joints remain stationary or during anticipation of somatosensory stimulation in preparation for movement. Beta oscillations disappear during movement, when activity in M1 becomes faster and desynchronized. It has been proposed that beta-oscillations reflect recurrent activity within closed loops involving M1, muscles, and somatosensory feedback, which maintain the accurate and discrete representations of motor synergies in M1.[21] For example, EEG and MEG demonstrate that the generation of beta oscillations in the motor cortex is associated with motor-related decisions, which supports the role of beta frequencies in feedback activity.

Voluntary movement suppresses beta frequencies followed by a postmovement beta rebound. The transient increase in beta oscillations seen following voluntary movement, postmovement beta rebound, has been localized to the motor cortex and involves pyramidal tract neurons in layer 5B of M1.

Assessment of Motor Cortex Excitability

Motor cortex physiology in humans has been studied using electroencephalography (EEG), magnetoencephalography (MEG), transcranial electrical stimulation and, particularly, transcranial magnetic stimulation (TMS).[22,23] TMS over the motor cortex elicits excitatory postsynaptic potentials in motoneurons that produce an EMG response called motor evoked potential (MEP), which can be recorded from a peripheral nerve, or most commonly from thenar or tibialis anterior muscles. The amplitude of the MEP reflects motor cortex excitability and can be enhanced by lower-level voluntary activation that partially depolarizes the cell body and axon hillock of PT neurons before application of the stimulus. However, there are critical differences between evoked and naturally initiated movements.[16] Studies in monkeys show that electrical or magnetic stimulation of the motor cortex induces an intense transsynaptic bombardment of pyramidal output neuron leading to high-frequency (~600 Hz) repetitive discharge. However, during natural movements, pyramidal neurons rarely exhibit these high-frequency discharges, typically firing below 100 Hz. The latency of response in hand muscles elicited by synchronous stimulation of the motor cortex is much shorter than that occurring between the onset of M1 activity and the onset of muscle activity during voluntarily generated movements.[16]

Intracortical inhibitory mechanisms are studied by paired-pulse stimulation paradigms. In normal conditions, application of a conditioned subthreshold cortical stimulus reduces the magnitude of a MEP response elicited by TMS; there is also an increase in latency of a second EMG response, called a "silent period," after a motor response induced by TMS. These changes are thought to reflect intracortical GABAergic inhibitory mechanisms. When applied in repetitive trains (repetitive TMS, rTMS) or in specific patterns, TMS can produce plastic changes in corticomotor excitability, which are reflected by changes in MEP amplitude. Another approach to studying cortical excitability is recording of event-related desynchronization of the mu rhythm (10–20 Hz) recorded over the Rolandic (sensorimotor) cortex on EEG. The desynchronization of the mu rhythm begins about 1.5 s before onset of self-paced movement and likely reflects activation of movement-related areas in preparation for movement initiation. Studies using TMS during simple reaction time and self-paced thumb-movement paradigms indicate that there is an increase in corticospinal excitability in the first 160 ms after EMG offset; this may reflect residual activity of the motor cortex followed by the effects of sensory feedback. After movement, there is also a decrease in corticospinal excitability that may last 0.5 to 1 s after EMG offset.

Human neuroimaging modalities, such as MEG and ultra-high-field (UHF) MRI and magnetic resonance spectroscopy (MRS), allow study of layer-specific activation and associated neurochemical changes in the motor cortex.[15] For example, in normal volunteers, tasks involving somatosensory input to the motor cortex elicited high fMRI signal in the superficial layers of M1, consistent with recurrent connectivity between IT neurons in layers 2/3, whereas tasks involving corticospinal output elicited high fMRI signal in the deep layers, consistent with activation of Betz cells in layer 5B. Studies using anatomically specific MEG show that alpha and beta frequencies localize to the gray–white matter boundary corresponding to infragranular layers, whereas the gamma frequency localizes to the pial surface close to supragranular layers in the motor cortex.[24] Ultra-high-field MRS at 7 T allows the detection of glutamate, glutamine, and GABA concentrations in vivo, which provides an indirect measure of neuronal excitation and inhibition that can be linked to pyramidal and interneuron cells, respectively. For example, where GABA concentration in M1 correlates with movement-related gamma synchrony.

Preparatory Activity in the Motor Cortex

In preparation to respond to a stimulus, the baseline firing of cortical motor neurons changes hundreds of milliseconds before the actual movement takes place. These preparatory changes are frequently assessed with movement-related cortical potentials recorded with scalp EEG and time-locked to movement onset. For self-initiated movements, the process of getting ready is reflected by a cortical readiness potential that is recorded as a slow negativity on the EEG long before EMG activity. This preparatory potential or *Bereitschaftspotential* starts 1 to 2 s before the actual movement; approximately 400–650 ms before movement onset, the slope of negativity turns more sharply upward (negative slope) and terminates approximately 90–100 ms before movement onset. The *Bereitschaftspotential* has classically been taken as a marker of volition, reflecting the feedforward processing of motor commands upon the intent to perform a movement and waiting for a signal to move. Recordings with subdural electrodes show that the preparatory potential originates in the SMA bilaterally and a wide area of the contralateral precentral gyrus, whereas the movement potential is generated focally in the motor representation in the contralateral precentral gyrus. In simple reaction time paradigms, the normal reaction time to a go-signal is approximately 200 ms; motor cortex excitability increases above baseline 80 ms before EMG onset and continues to increase up to the time of movement onset. Contingent negative variation is a slow negative potential recorded bilaterally from the PFC when movements are to be made in response to a known warning signal; this signal appears in the 1- to 2-s interval between a stimulus that warns the subject to prepare to move and a second stimulus that signals the subject to begin moving. Event-related potentials recorded cortical activity evolved by attention to a behaviorally relevant stimulus. The most common potential is P300, which is a measurement of attention to a novel or infrequent stimulus and is typically recorded bilaterally from the midparietal cortex.

POSTERIOR PARIETAL LOBE AND MOTOR CONTROL

The PPC is an extensive region of the human brain and its disproportionate expansion compared to other primates coincides with the development of binocular stereopsis and a prehensile hand, which are critical for tool use and tool making.[25–27] The PPC is a multimodal association area that includes several functionally distinct subdivisions containing neurons that integrate visual, somatosensory, vestibular, and auditory information to provide a tridimensional representation of space. This information is then conveyed to lateral premotor areas as coordinates that are used to program and direct visually guided motor actions. In humans, the PPC contains additional areas and hemispheric

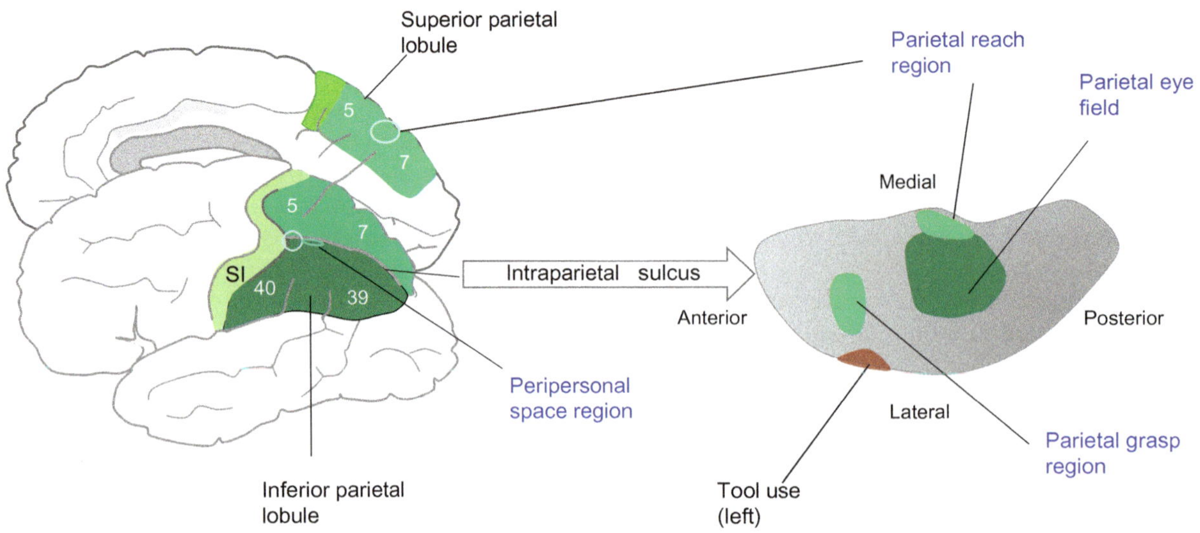

FIGURE 30.5 Functional organization of the posterior parietal cortex.
The posterior parietal cortex is subdivided into superior parietal lobule (areas 5 and 7), inferior parietal lobule (angular gyrus and supramarginal gyrus), intraparietal sulcus, and the medial parietal cortex (including the precuneus). The intraparietal sulcus contains anatomically defined areas: lateral (LIP) involved in saccadic eye movements, medial (MIP) involved in reaching, anterior (AIP) involved in grasping, and ventral (VIP) involved in movements toward the peripersonal space. In humans, the PEF (LIP homolog) occupies both the lateral and the medial banks of the intraparietal sulcus; the parietal reach region (MIP homolog), the medial superior parietal lobule and precuneus, and the parietal grasp region (AIP homolog) are located at the intersection of the anterior intraparietal sulcus and postcentral sulcus, and a homolog of area VIP is present in the ventral portion of the intraparietal sulcus and responds to stimuli directed to the peripersonal space. A human-specific region in the left inferior parietal lobe has tool-related responses.

asymmetries underlying cognitive functions such as tool use, gestures, and language.

Functional Anatomy and Connectivity

The PPC includes a superior parietal lobule, inferior parietal lobule, intraparietal sulcus, and the medial parietal cortex (Figure 30.5). The superior parietal lobule contains the somatosensory association areas 5a, 5b, and 7a and the heteromodal somatosensory and visual association area 7b. The inferior parietal lobule includes the supramarginal gyrus (area 39) and the angular gyrus (area 40). The intraparietal sulcus has sensorimotor connections anteriorly and visuospatial connections posteriorly.[25] The medial parietal cortex, including the precuneus, contains somatosensory association cortex anteriorly and heteromodal cortex posteriorly. The PPC contains multisensory neurons and is a fundamental component of the dorsal stream for visuospatial processing. The main input to the PPC is visual and originates from neurons of the dorsal stream of sensory processing that respond to object location and movement. Multimodal neurons in the PPC integrate visual with somatosensory, vestibular, and auditory inputs from other cortical areas to provide a tridimensional representation of space. Whereas the PPC primarily processes spatial information, it also contains neurons that are tuned to the shape of the objects. The PPC projects to the prefrontal and premotor cortical areas, superior colliculus, striatum, and to the cerebellum via the pontine nuclei. The primary driving thalamic input to the PPC originates from the pulvinar.

Functional Domains

Electrophysiological and tracing studies in monkeys showed that the PPC contains multiple subdivisions harboring neurons involved in multisensory integration and sensorimotor transformation for control of visually guided actions. These studies indicated that the intraparietal sulcus contains anatomically defined areas, lateral (LIP), medial (MIP), anterior (AIP), and ventral (VIP), which harbor neurons with different response patterns and connectivity with the lateral premotor cortex (Figure 30.5). Area LIP, or parietal eye field (PEF), is associated with saccadic eye movements; MIP (parietal reach area) with reaching; AIP (parietal grasp region) with grasping; and VIP with movements directed toward the peripersonal space. Functional MRI studies have identified functionally similar areas in the human PPC, with a slightly different representation.[26,27] In humans, the PEF (corresponding to LIP) occupies both the lateral and the medial banks of the intraparietal sulcus; the parietal reach region (corresponding to MIP) is typically found outside the intraparietal sulcus in the medial superior parietal lobule and precuneus, and the parietal grasp region (corresponding to AIP) is located at the intersection of the anterior intraparietal sulcus and postcentral sulcus. There is a functional gradient for representation of reaching and grasping movements, spanning posterior-medial (reaching) to anterior-lateral (grasping) in the PPC, which is consistent with the necessary interactions between reaching and grasping networks. A homolog of monkey area VIP is present in the ventral portion of the intraparietal sulcus and responds to stimuli directed to the peripersonal space. A human-specific region in the left inferior parietal lobe has tool-related responses.[26,27] Areas of the PPC also have representation of object-based information such as shape and size that activates neurons in areas involved in grasping, movement toward the peripersonal space, or saccades independently of action planning. Functional MRI studies show that viewing pictures of tools, which have strong and specific action associations, activates a left-lateralized network including the anterior intraparietal sulcus and regions in the inferior parietal lobe, along with regions in frontal and temporal cortex. This left-lateralized parietal network has been associated with viewing, hearing, executing, planning, and pantomiming tool use. This network may integrate spatial information about the two- and three-dimensional aspects of tools (dorsal visual stream) with semantic knowledge related to tool recognition and actions (ventral stream) and with a frontoparietal action-to-perception system.

Parieto-Frontal Circuits for Motor Control

The connectivity of different portions of the PPC with frontal premotor areas provides for the formation of distinct modules or networks to mediate visually guided action.

The different areas of the PPC receiving inputs from the dorsal visual stream project to frontal cortical areas via three groups of pathways.[28] A parieto-prefrontal pathway originates in the LIP and projecting to the FEF and lateral PFC is involved in attentional control of eye movements and spatial visual working memory. Separate parieto-premotor pathways to the PMd and PMv participate in sensorimotor transformations using an egocentric spatial reference frame to encode reaching, grasping, and movements toward the peripersonal space (Figure 30.6). A parieto-medial temporal pathway from the angular gyrus via the precuneus contains an allocentric representation of space required for spatial navigation.

Reaching, Grasping, and Movements Toward the Peripersonal Space

Reaching requires the use of both visual information about target location and proprioceptive information about upper limb position to specify the upcoming arm movement. Neurons in the parietal reach region respond to either or both of these inputs, code the targets in visual coordinates relative to the direction of gaze, and project to the PMd to initiate reaching movements. Grasping requires information about the tridimensional features of the object in order to reshape the hand.[29] Neurons in the anterior intraparietal area sensitive to the shape, size, and orientation of three-dimensional visual objects and forward this information to the rostral PMv.[1,29] The rostral PMv contains two types of visually responsive neurons. One group, referred to as "canonical" neurons, discharge in response to the size, shape, and orientation of an object to select the most appropriate preshaping of the hand for grasping, holding, or manipulating the object. A second group of neurons, located at the hub transitional area between PMv and PMd are "mirror

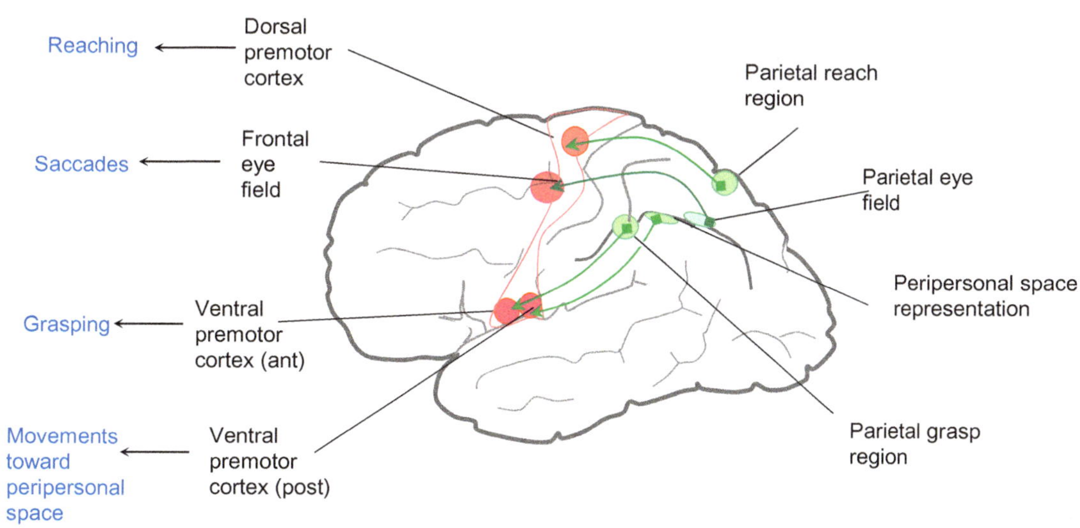

FIGURE 30.6 Parietofrontal circuits controlling visually guided movements.
Information from different areas of the PPC is conveyed to lateral premotor areas as coordinates that are used to program and direct visually guided motor actions. The tridimensional representation of space in the posterior parietal cortex based in different coordinate systems provide sensorimotor transformations for visually guided reaching, grasping, movement toward the peripersonal space, or saccades via parallel parietofrontal pathways.

neurons," that selectively discharge upon observation of an action similar to the one they encode. Finally, movements toward the peripersonal space involve a separate parieto-frontal pathway. This includes neurons in the ventral intraparietal area that respond to both visual and tactile stimuli restricted to the head and face and neurons in the posterior portion of PMv that encode movements directed toward the peripersonal space such as such those directed to the mouth or defensive responses to protect the head or body for an approaching object.

The interactions between the PPC and the FEF contribute to control of eye movements. This topic, together with motor control of speech, is discussed in chapter 32.

LEARNING AND PLASTICITY IN THE MOTOR CORTEX

Studies in experimental animals as well as fMRI and TMS studies in humans indicate that there are plastic changes in body representation in M1 both during motor learning and adaptation to injury.

Acquisition of Motor Skills

Plastic changes in the motor cortex are responsible for improvement in performance of voluntary movements with practice. The motor representations in M1 are sensitive to short- and long-term experience. Whereas simple motor tasks activate primarily the contralateral M1, performance of newly acquired complex tasks also activates the lateral PMC and SMA bilaterally. The more complex and challenging the task, the more cortical motor areas are recruited. Simple repetition of an individual movement or rapid finger movement sequences can elicit changes in M1 representation within 20 to 40 minutes. These changes include rapid enlargement of representation for newly acquired sequences and decreased representation of a previously learned sequence or a sequence practiced infrequently. As the movement is learned and executed more efficiently, there is a progressive decrease in the area of motor cortex activated. Event-related fMRI studies show that activity of the dorsolateral PFC and anterior midcingulate cingulate cortex also increases early during learning and then returns rapidly to baseline. Within hours of completing training on a motor task, the peaks of neuronal activation move away from prefrontal regions to premotor, parietal, and cerebellar regions. Motor performance and cortical activity may continue to change for weeks if there is further practice. In humans, the direct and uncrossed corticospinal pathways from M1 to ipsilateral motoneurons accounts for 10% to 15% of pyramidal fibers and primarily control trunk and proximal upper limb muscles. Studies of cortical inactivation using low frequency rTMS show that the left M1 has greater influence than the right M1 on the control of the ipsilateral hand.

Motor Cortex Plasticity Following Injury

There is a rapid and long-lasting reorganization of the motor cortex after cortical or peripheral lesions.[30] This reorganization appears within hours and persists for months. Amputations, spinal cord injury, transient differentiation, immobilization, or inhibitory rTMS modify the representation of movements in M1. For example, when the M1 arm area is impaired, the face area is activated during upper extremity movements. The most likely substrate for rapid M1 plasticity is the system of horizontal connections that functionally associate M1 neurons into neuronal assemblies to form dynamic motor maps. The existence of occult motor maps can be revealed experimentally by blockade of GABAergic receptors that mediate the feedforward inhibitory mechanisms. More persistent changes require activity-dependent synaptic modifications via mechanisms of long-term potentiation and long-term depression similar to those in the hippocampus, and eventually the development of new connections via use-dependent sprouting of dendritic spines and axon terminals.

COGNITIVE ASPECTS OF MOTOR CONTROL

The cortical areas involved in motor control are also involved in cognitive functions, including understanding the intention of others, inhibition of inappropriate responses, and the senses of free will and agency. The areas of the PFC involved in cognitive aspects of motor behavior are indirectly connected to premotor areas via connector hub regions such as the preSMA. Motor translation areas such as prePMd and rostral cingulate motor cortex mediate reciprocal output from premotor areas to the PFC.[2]

Mirror Motor System and Action Observation Network

The mirror motor system consists of neurons that are activated by the observation of a motor behavior similar to the ones that they encode.[31] An observed action produces activation in sensorimotor cortical areas of the observer as if these areas were actually programming the execution of that action. The major components of the classical mirror system are the inferior parietal lobule and anterior PMv, as well as adjacent inferior frontal gyrus, dorsal and the ventral banks of the superior temporal sulcus, and posterior medial temporal gyrus. Whereas neurons in PMv respond to action observation, a subset of these neurons that fire during execution may have a suppression of their discharge during action observation; this inhibitory effect might have a role in preventing the occurrence of movement during action observation. Functional MRI studies in humans show that observation of grasping actions activates areas the inferior parietal lobule, PMv, and caudal sector of the inferior frontal gyrus. Neurons with mirror properties may also be present in the SMA, middle cingulate gyrus, somatosensory area, and hippocampus. Goal encoding might occur not only when an action should be performed but also when the agent must refrain from performing it. The human mirror system is not only activated by observation of actions but also by representation of goals. The mirror system encodes the goal rather than the body part. For example, both the PMv and inferior parietal lobule are similarly activated upon observation of either a human or a robot arm grasping objects. Whereas the representation of the observed action in PMv is encoded somatotopically, in the inferior parietal lobule it is clustered according to its behavioral valence, regardless of the effector. Since the mirror motor system encodes goal-directed motor acts, it appears to have a fundamental role in understanding actions and intentions of others. The mirror system is also involved in imitation. Immediate imitation refers to online replication of an observed behavior. Imitation learning consists in building new motor memories based on action observation and may involve a first step of "mirror" activation of motor act representations in the inferior parietal cortex and PMv and a second step of recombination of these motor acts via interactions of the dorsolateral PFC with rostral premotor areas.

There is also a relation between personal expertise in performing some specific actions and the mirror responses to the observation of the same acts.[32] Functional MRI studies show that observation of actions performed by others also activates a second group of cortical structures that includes the superior parietal lobule and PMd. This action observation network has a strong role in representing previously acquired motor skills. Subjects with a specific motor skill show increased activation of this network during observation of the same skill. This shows that during action observation, the observer's brain tends to activate more strongly for actions that already belong to its own motor repertoire.

Response Inhibition and Response Switching

A major role of the PFC is inhibition of inappropriate or unintended motor behavior. This may be needed, for example, in the setting of a sudden change in the goal of an ongoing movement, or for stopping a movement in favor of another in response to changes in environmental cues. Two cortical regions have a major role in providing stop signals to the motor system to allow response inhibition, the inferior frontal gyrus, particularly in the right side, and the preSMA. The inferior fontal gyrus is connected to the preSMA and SMA via the frontal aslant tract.[33] This connection modulates the excitatory influence of the preSMA on the subthalamic nucleus, which has a major role in stopping ongoing movements via the so-called hyperdirect pathway. Studies using rTMS confirm the important role of the preSMA both in motor inhibition and task switching when there is change in the rules for selecting the appropriate response out of competing responses.

Free Will and Sense of Agency

Free will is the perception of choosing to make a movement. This perception includes both the sense of willing and the sense of self-agency.[34,35] The sense of willing is that of the decision to initiate a movement; self-agency is the sense that oneself is responsible for the movement that just occurred. Movement is generated subconsciously and conscious awareness of this intention occurs late in the process, even possibly after the movement itself. The "motor set" indicates both the readiness to perform a planned motor action and the completion of preparation to implement the intention. For self-initiated movements this process is reflected by the preparatory potential recorded on the scalp EEG long before EMG activity. An early study showed that whereas the cortical readiness potential begins 1–2 s before the actual movement, the perception of willing to perform the movement occurred about 200–300 ms before the movement, and the sense of movement occurred prior to the movement recorded by EMG.[36] However, recent studies show that the experience of the first wish to move is rather experienced, at least partially, from the previous impression of the movement itself.[37] This suggests that the time of intention is inferred from the time of movement.[38] The sense of willing is not time-locked to any feature of movement initiation and can be manipulated experimentally, for example with TMS.[34] Thus the perception of willing is not fully processed until after the movement; likely reflecting an interaction between frontal and parietal areas.[34] The sense of willing to perform a movement is typically followed by the sense of self-agency, which is the experience of controlling one's own actions.[35] The sense of agency includes both sense of ownership of the experience of body movement ("my body moved"), and the cognitive experience of voluntary control over that body movement ("I voluntarily made it move"). The connectivity between the frontal areas that develop motor plans for voluntary action and the parietal areas that monitor outcomes may have a key role part in computing sense of agency. The sense of agency can also be modulated experimentally using rTMS. Inhibitory rTMS applied to the preSMA reduced the ability to judge the temporal relationship between a voluntary action and a subsequent sensory stimulus, which is used to test the sense of self-agency. This would be consistent with the "comparator" model by which the sense of agency arises from the comparison between predictive motor planning signals and the actual sensory consequences of the action. Lack of prediction error would create a sense of agency. Neuroimaging studies show strong activation of the temporoparietal junction, including the angular gyrus, as the neural correlate of "nonagency." Damage to both preSMA and inferior parietal cortex can alter the experience of agency. A recent study showed that multiple brain regions are involved in the development of the sense of agency; the right supramarginal gyrus was found to be the most sensitive area involved in self-other attribution, while the bilateral precentral gyri and left inferior parietal lobule predominantly reflected sensorimotor information.[39]

DISORDERS OF CORTICAL MOTOR CONTROL

Hemispheric Stroke

Hemispheric stroke results in several changes in reaching and grasping movements. The affected limb typically exhibits paresis, spasticity, deficits in the angular trajectories of the elbow, stereotypic movement patterns or synergies, incorrect timing of components within a movement pattern, loss of interjoint functional coordination, and loss of fine, skilled movements. The stereotyped movement patterns caused by abnormal cortical control lead to muscle coactivation and high antagonist muscle activity; this result in reaching movements characterized by low and insufficient force production, low movement amplitudes, long movement times, and segmented, inaccurate trajectories. Functional neuroimaging and rTMS studies show that there is reorganization of the motor cortex following stroke.[40] These studies also show that in patients with chronic stroke there is a persistent premovement interhemispheric inhibition from the contra- to the ipsilateral motor cortex before movement execution. This led to the proposal that imbalanced inhibitory interaction between the intact and the lesioned hemisphere may contribute to impaired motor recovery. Several advanced neurotechnologies are extensively investigated to help motor recovery after stroke or other forms of injury.[41] Recent study using inhibitory rTMS of the intact hemisphere did not support the concept of interhemispheric inhibition as a mechanism of poor recovery after stroke.[42] Premovement interhemispheric inhibition does not correlate with poor motor recovery in the long term, and may rather be the consequence than the cause of impaired recovery.[43] The targeting of secondary motor areas for neuromodulation with transcranial direct current stimulation under EEG guidance might be a promising approach.[44] Neuromuscular electrical stimulation and robotics have also been investigated regarding their role in plasticity and motor recovery.[41] However, the benefits of neuromodulation on recovery may be restricted to specific subgroups of patients; this may reflect individual and specific alterations in neuronal networks during the recovery from stroke such as the microstructural integrity of the CST and its influence on cortical and subcortical targets.[45] Multivariate fMRI analyses offer the potential to serve as markers for endophenotypes of functional impairment and potential for recovery; these include ipsilesional connectivity of M1 with medial premotor areas and reorganization of the contralateral undamaged hemisphere and cerebellum.[46] Ipsilesional CST remodeling may occur with disuse; improvement of functional anisotropy in the CST 3–12 months post-stroke predicts motor recovery.[47] Other cortical motor pathways, including the cortico-cerebellar and premotor-motor pathways influence motor recovery after stroke.[48] Several biomarkers have been identified as possible predictors of motor recovery following stroke.[41] For example, the presence of upper limb MEP in response to TMS in the first three days poststroke strongly predicts good motor outcome.[49] Assessment of the effects of stroke not only in the damaged area but also in the associated network is crucial to understand the stroke-induced deficits, predict recovery, and determine options for treatment strategies; these interventions can target different areas in this network (e.g., primary motor cortex and secondary motor regions) based on individual factors of the patient.[50]

Apraxia

Praxis is the ability to perform skilled and purposeful learned voluntary movements. It may involve two components, the conceptual knowledge of the functions of tools or actions dependent on tools, and the ability to organize single actions into sequences. Functional MRI studies show that these processes are associated with activation of Broca area (area 44), anterior temporal pole, inferior parietal lobule, PMC, and SMA in the left hemisphere for the control of the right arm; and crosses via the corpus callosum to motor areas of the right hemisphere to control the left arm. Lesions affecting these regions impair the ability to either generate motor imagery or translate it into a motor program, resulting in apraxia.[51] Ideomotor apraxia is the inability to translate the observed or instructed movement into appropriate motor pattern. The two core manifestations are deficits in performing tool-use pantomimes and symbolic communicative gestures either on verbal command or imitation. Patients with lesions in the left PPC can grasp and manipulate objects, but fail to grasp tools in a manner that is consistent with their function. Lesions involving the inferior parietal lobule may also produce deficits in producing and understanding gestures. Unilateral ideomotor apraxia is an early sign of corticobasal syndrome that may occur in the setting of 4-repeat tauopathies such as corticobasal degeneration and progressive supranuclear palsy, but can also occur in other disorders such as Alzheimer disease. Ideational apraxia is the inability to retrieve the movement schema typical for certain object. Patients may use a comb for a toothbrush or a toothbrush as a fork despite their preserved ability to name and comprehend the name of the misused object or tool. Ideational apraxia is typically associated with diffuse or bilateral posterior cerebral lesions but also with damage to the posterior left hemisphere (or, in left-handed patients, with lesions in the right hemisphere). Limb kinetic apraxia is the inability to perform purposeful learned skilled movement (such as rolling a coin between the fingers). In most cases, it is associated with left hemisphere lesions; rare cases of apraxia in right-handed individuals occur with right hemisphere lesions (crossed apraxia). Some patients with callosal lesions have callosal dyspraxia, characterized by the inability to carry out commands with the left hand.

Akinesia

Bilateral lesions affecting the SMA and cingulate motor areas result in inability to initiate voluntary movement and manifest with abulia or, in extreme cases, akinetic mutism. Akinesia is a dysfunction of movement initiation, ranging from delayed response, paucity of movements (hypokinesia), and slowness of movements (bradykinesia), to freezing or even total abolition of movement and is a typical manifestation of parkinsonism including Parkinson disease (PD). Akinesia is associated with prolonged motor reaction time due to reduced buildup of cortical excitability, as reflected by reduction in the amplitude of the preparatory (readiness) potential before both self-paced movements and mental imagery. In PD movement preparation is abnormally prolonged due to a delay in muscle activation reflecting a failure of motor programming. One feature of bradykinesia is the so-called sequence effect, which refers to the decrement of amplitude and velocity with repetitive and continuing movements. Patients with PD are unable to generate an adequate initial agonist burst so that the exerted force is insufficient to reach the desired target; the movement is completed by a series of small amplitude movements indicating that bradykinesia reflects an inappropriate scaling of the dynamic muscle forces, the so-called scaling effect. Experimental models of PD indicate a role of M1 in bradykinesia. In parkinsonian models, dopamine depletion increases burst-firing in PT neurons of M1; decreases the magnitude and the temporal pattern of movement-related M1 activity; interferes with the encoding of movement parameters; and leads to plastic changes in M1, including reduction of dendritic spines in PT neurons.

Magnetoencephalographic studies show that in early PD there is greater beta power at rest and reduced beta suppression during isometric contraction in M1 compared with controls; lower M1 beta power is seen in the later disease stages. Transcranial magnetic stimulation studies indicate that patients with PD have an increased M1 excitability and reduced plasticity. Excitability abnormalities correlated with motor slowness, while plasticity alterations correlated with sequence effect. These results reproduce findings in experimental models of PD, showing reduced firing rate, increased irregular firing patterns, and abnormal beta oscillations in layer 5B in M1; this activity is driven by hyperpolarization of pyramidal cells due to synaptic inputs from GABAergic interneurons. During movement, dysfunction of PT neurons causes abnormal kinematic encoding and motor timing. These studies show layer-specific circuit dysfunction in the motor cortex is associated with either hypokinesia or levodopa-induced dyskinesia.[15] Similar layer-specific dysfunction affecting PT, IT, or local interneurons in the motor cortex can occur in Huntington disease and amyotrophic lateral sclerosis (ALS).[15]

Several fMRI studies show that akinesia in PD is associated with decreased activity in the SMA and dorsolateral PFC during voluntary action. This may reflect executive dysfunction associated with abnormal proactive inhibitory control on the SMA by a network involving the caudate nucleus, precuneus, and thalamus.[52] A review of such neuroimaging studies show that akinesia in PD is multidimensional and is associated with abnormalities not only within but also outside the motor and dopaminergic pathways.[53] Deep brain stimulation produced more robust activation of the SMA in PD patients with akinetic/rigid phenotype than in those with postural instability/gait disorder and tremor predominant phenotype.[54]

Disorders of Volitional Control and Agency

Many disorders are characterized by inability to recognize the volitional aspect of movement.[32,55] For example, patients with chorea often do not recognize that their abnormal movements are involuntary, whereas patients with tics often cannot determine whether their movements are voluntary or involuntary. Unlike normal voluntary movements, tics are often not preceded by a readiness potential in the motor cortex. In contrast, psychogenic movements are believed by the patients to be involuntary but are preceded by a normal motor cortex readiness potential. Resting-state fMRI in patients with functional movement disorders shows that impaired self-agency is associated with decreased functional connectivity between the right temporoparietal junction and the right sensorimotor cortex, cerebellar vermis, and bilateral SMA.[56] This supports a model whereby impaired motor feedforward together with altered sensory feedback to the right temporoparietal junction contributes to patients' impaired sense of self-agency.

The alien hand phenomenon is the feeling that the hand does not belong to the person and often produces unwanted movements without any sense of their being willed. The posterior variant of alien hand phenomenon typically results from damage to the nondominant (right) parietal lobe and affects the left upper limb; these patients have a strong sense of lack of ownership of the upper limb, which executes simple movements, such as arm levitation. This may reflect impaired ability of the inferior parietal lobule to process sensory feedback or be secondary to spatial neglect. The frontal variant of alien hand phenomenon, known as anarchic hand, typically results from damage to the dominant (usually left) SMA, anterior cingulate gyrus, or medial PFC. In this variant, the affected limb tends to produce complex goal-oriented movements such as reaching and grasping for objects located in their visual field; the patients are aware that the alien limb belongs to them but are unable to suppress its unwanted movements, which are experienced as involuntary. The callosal variant of alien hand phenomenon exclusively affects the nondominant (left hand) in right-handed patients; it is mostly caused by isolated corpus callosum injury and is characterized by intermanual conflicts. Mesial frontal lobe lesions may also result in diagonistic dyspraxia; the left hand performs actions contrary to actions performed by the right hand. In patients with amputations, there can often be the phantom limb phenomenon; patients can have the sense of moving their phantom limb while there is no actual movement. Anosognosia is another situation where patients may believe that they are making movement when none is performed. These situations indicate that there can be a sense of volition without feedback from an actual movement.

Disorders of Mirror Motor Function and Mirror Movements

The mirror mechanism is more represented in the left than in the right hemisphere. Therefore, patients with ideomotor apraxia may also have difficulty in recognizing and understanding the actions done by others due to impaired mirror system.[31] For example, patients with buccofacial ideomotor apraxia, who are typically impaired in carrying out face and mouth actions, may show impairment in identifying the goals of mouth-related actions, whereas patients with limb ideomotor apraxia, who are typically impaired in producing hand actions, may show impairment in identifying the goals of hand-related actions. These deficits may reflect extension of their lesions in parietal and frontal areas endowed with mirror properties.

In contrast, some lesions may lead to hyperactivity of the mirror mechanism and the release of automatic imitative behaviors. Patients with damage to the PFC may have exhibit forced motor behavior triggered by external stimuli. This condition is broadly referred to as "environmental dependency syndrome," which may manifest with "imitation behavior." Echopraxia is the forced imitation of the movements of others and results in its perseveration. Malfunctioning of the mirror mechanism is one of the factors underlying the manifestations of autism spectrum disorder, which includes impaired communication and social interactions, and restricted repetitive and stereotyped behaviors.

Lesions affecting the medial frontal motor areas may also result in mirror movements of the hand contralateral to the hand executing a specific motor act. Mirror movements refer to the unintended movement of a body part that mirrors the intentional movements of the homologous body part on the opposite site. Normal mirror movements may occur transiently in children up to 10 years of age due to insufficient development of the corpus callosum, which restricts activation to one hemisphere during execution of unilateral motor tasks. Persistence of mirror movements into adulthood occurs in hereditary disorders,[57] neurodegenerative diseases such as PD, ALS and corticobasal degeneration; and in patients with hemiparesis due stroke.[58] Congenital mirror movements may occur with mutation affecting genes controlling the normal CST decussation at the medulla or central pattern generators in the spinal cord.[57] Examples include mutations of the *DCC* (deleted in colorectal cancer) gene that encodes a receptor for the chemoattractant netrin-1, Kallmann syndrome (an X-linked disorder of neuronal migration characterized by absence of olfactory bulbs hypogonadotropic hypogonadism and persisting ipsilateral corticospinal tracts), and Jouvert syndrome (a ciliopathy characterized by abnormal development of the brainstem and cerebellar vermis).

Dystonia

Dystonia is characterized by sustained or intermittent muscle contractions causing abnormal and often repetitive movements, postures, or both. Dystonic movements are typically patterned, are often initiated or worsened by voluntary action, and are associated with overflow muscle activation. Specific movements or sensory stimuli (sensory tricks) may temporarily ameliorate the dystonic movements. Dystonia is a complex phenomenon that may reflect abnormal processing in the sensorimotor cortex, abnormalities in the intrinsic striatal circuits, or cerebellar dysfunction.[59,60] The three major pathophysiological substrates are loss of inhibition, sensory dysfunction, and derangement of synaptic plasticity. Loss of inhibition is reflected by EMG evidence of co-contraction of antagonistic muscles and overflow of activity to muscle groups not involved in the task. Abnormal intracortical inhibition occurs in both hemispheres, as shown in TMS studies. Abnormal sensorimotor integration and derangement of somatotopic representation in the sensory cortex may underlie some of the sensory phenomena associated with dystonia. Disruption of homeostatic synaptic plasticity may have an important role in dystonia. In normal conditions increased activity of the postsynaptic neuron renders stimuli inducing long-term potentiation (LTP) less effective and those inducing long-term depression (LTD) more effective; reduced postsynaptic activity has the opposite effects. In normal subjects rTMS protocols that enhance excitability downregulate practice-dependent cortical plasticity, whereas rTMS protocols that reduce excitability increase plasticity. These changes are impaired in patients with focal hand dystonia. Functional neuroimaging showed increased activity in the PFC and lateral PMC but reduced activity in M1, S1, and SMA in these patients. Task-specific focal dystonias selectively affect highly learned and complex motor behaviors associated with excessive practice and overuse. This is associated with abnormal recruitment of parietal and premotor cortices.[61]

Myoclonus

Increased motor cortex excitability may manifest with focal motor seizures or cortical myoclonus.[62] Simultaneous recording of the EEG and the EMG with the use of jerk-locked back-averaging is the most important test for the clinical study of myoclonus. Cortical myoclonus is characterized by a large, well-defined biphasic spike preceding the myoclonic jerk, usually originating from the contralateral motor cortex, and preceding the myoclonic jerk by 15 to 30 ms for the upper limb and 25 to 40 ms for the lower limb. Cortical myoclonus is further classified into spontaneous, cortical reflex myoclonus, and epilepsia partialis continua. Cortical myoclonus is typically stimulus-sensitive and may be restricted to a particular muscle group such as hand muscles, as occurs in epilepsia partialis continua, but most often is generalized. In cortical myoclonus, there is a rostrocaudal direction of muscle activation down the brainstem. This type of myoclonus usually occurs irregularly but may appear rhythmic, as occurs in patients with corticobasal degeneration. In Creutzfeldt-Jakob disease myoclonus occurs continuously or quasiperiodically at rest, with intervals ranging from 600 to 1,500 ms. Minipolymyoclonus consists of frequent independent contractions of multiple small muscles of distal limbs. Patients with cortical reflex myoclonus often have giant somatosensory evoked potentials recorded in the hemisphere contralateral to the jerking limb as well as marked enhancement of long-loop reflexes.

KEY POINTS

- Voluntary movements are organized to perform a purposeful task.
- The control of voluntary movement involves interactions among frontal motor areas, prefrontal cortex (PFC), and parietal cortex.
- Motor plans are strategies aimed to perform a particular task and are implemented according to goals or needs by PFC.
- The overall strategy is then organized into motor programs before the beginning of the motor action by premotor areas.
- The posterior parietal cortex (PPC) contains multisensory representation of space, which is conveyed to the premotor cortex to implement motor programs.
- The motor cortex sends a command to the motor nuclei to elicit movement, and a predictive feedforward signal (efference copy) predicting the probable sensory consequences of the commanded motor action.
- Sensory predictions are compared with sensory feedback signals to generate a prediction error signal that is used to adjust the current motor command.
- Learning and programming of movements optimize motor skill and depend on experience.
- Motor adaptation is the ability to reprogram sequences of movement sequences in response to changes in the external circumstance.
- The frontal motor cortex includes the primary motor cortex (M1), several divisions of the lateral premotor cortex (PM), supplementary motor area (SMA), presupplementary motor area (preSMA), cingulate motor areas, frontal eye fields (FEF), and supplementary eye fields.
- Parieto-dependent premotor areas, such as M1, PM, and SMA, receive inputs from the parietal cortex and project via the corticospinal tract (CST).
- Prefronto-dependent areas, such as the preSMA, receive inputs from the PFC, mediate cognitive control of movements, and project to the parieto-prefrontal areas.
- The motor cortex controls different muscle synergies or "action maps" that when variably combined generate the majority of natural movements.
- Neurons in M1 emphasize actions that focus on individual body parts; those in the dorsal premotor cortex (PMd) participate in programming, preparation, and coordination of proximal limb movements such as reaching; those in the anterior ventral premotor cortex (PMv) in grasping; and those in the posterior PMv in goal-directed movements toward the peripersonal space.
- The SMA has a major role in setting motor programs for internally generated learned motor sequences, movement preparation, and interhemispheric interactions.
- The preSMA contributes to selection and preparation of movements, decision as to when to start a movement, organization of motor sequences, and motor inhibition.
- The cingulate motor areas are involved in value- and outcome-based action control and orienting motor responses.
- Direct cortico-motoneuronal connections from M1 connections to motoneurons innervating distal hand and digit muscles is fundamental for dexterity.
- Movement in a particular direction is determined by the net action of a large population of cortical motor neurons.
- A prime role for descending influences from the motor cortex is to suppress and inhibit undesirable movements.
- Long-loop transcortical reflexes are important for the steady maintenance and corrections of intended postures and movement.
- The posterior parietal cortex (PPC) is a multimodal association area that includes functionally distinct subdivisions that provide a tridimensional representation of space.
- Information from different areas of the PPC is conveyed to lateral premotor areas as coordinates that are used to program and direct visually guided motor actions via parallel pathways for reaching, grasping, movement toward the personal space, and eye movements.
- There are plastic changes in body representation in M1 both during motor learning and adaptation to injury.
- There is a rapid and long-lasting reorganization of the motor cortex after cortical or peripheral lesions.
- Neurons in the mirror motor system respond to the observation of a motor behavior similar to the one that they encode and have a major role both in imitation and understanding of the intentions or goals of others.
- A major role of the PFC is inhibition of inappropriate or unintended motor behavior.
- Free will is the perception of willing (the decision to initiate a movement) and self-agency (the sense that oneself is responsible for the movement that just occurred).

- Movement is generated subconsciously, and conscious awareness of this intention occurs late in the process, even possibly after the movement itself.
- Activation of the temporoparietal junction, may be a neural correlate of "nonagency."
- Lesions affecting networks that include the left inferior parietal lobule, PMC, and SMA produce ideomotor apraxia.
- Akinesia is a dysfunction of movement initiation and primarily results from abnormal excitability and firing in M1, and reduced activation of the SMA.
- Psychogenic movements are preceded by a normal motor cortex readiness potential; impaired self-agency may be associated with decreased functional connectivity of right temporoparietal junction.
- Patients with damage to the PFC may exhibit forced motor behavior triggered by external stimuli.
- Lesions affecting the medial frontal motor areas may result in mirror movements.
- Congenital mirror movements may occur with mutations affecting genes controlling the normal CST decussation at the medulla.
- Dystonia may reflect abnormal processing in the sensorimotor cortex or in the intrinsic striatal circuits, or cerebellar dysfunction.
- Dystonia is characterized by impairment in both intracortical inhibition and synaptic homeostatic plasticity.

REFERENCES

1. Rizzolatti G, Cattaneo L, Fabbri-Destro M, Rozzi S. Cortical mechanisms underlying the organization of goal-directed actions and mirror neuron-based action understanding. Physiol Rev 2014;94:655–706.
2. Grafton ST, Volz LJ. From ideas to action: the prefrontal-premotor connections that shape motor behavior. Handb Clin Neurol 2019;163:237–255.
3. Ebbesen CL, Brecht M. Motor cortex—to act or not to act? Nat Rev Neurosci 2017;18:694–705.
4. Gallivan JP, Chapman CS, Wolpert DM, Flanagan JR. Decision-making in sensorimotor control. Nat Rev Neurosci 2018;19:519–534.
5. Vogt BA. Midcingulate cortex: structure, connections, homologies, functions and diseases. J Chem Neuroanat 2016;74:28–46.
6. Rizzolatti G, Luppino G. The cortical motor system. Neuron 2001;31:889–901.
7. Rasmussen T, Penfield W. Further studies of the sensory and motor cerebral cortex of man. Fed Proc 1947;6:452–460.
8. Meier JD, Aflalo TN, Kastner S, Graziano MS. Complex organization of human primary motor cortex: a high-resolution fMRI study. J Neurophysiol 2008;100:1800–1812.
9. Overduin SA, d'Avella A, Roh J, Carmena JM, Bizzi E. Representation of muscle synergies in the primate brain. J Neurosci 2015;35:12615–12624.
10. Graziano MSA. Ethological action maps: a paradigm shift for the motor cortex. Trends Cogn Sci 2016;20:121–132.
11. Desmurget M, Richard N, Harquel S, et al. Neural representations of ethologically relevant hand/mouth synergies in the human precentral gyrus. Proc Natl Acad Sci U S A 2014;111:5718–5722.
12. Nachev P, Kennard C, Husain M. Functional role of the supplementary and pre-supplementary motor areas. Nat Rev Neurosci 2008;9:856–869.
13. Welniarz Q, Gallea C, Lamy JC, et al. The supplementary motor area modulates interhemispheric interactions during movement preparation. Hum Brain Mapp 2019;40:2125–2142.
14. Caruana F, Gerbella M, Avanzini P, et al. Motor and emotional behaviours elicited by electrical stimulation of the human cingulate cortex. Brain 2018;141:3035–3051.
15. McColgan P, Joubert J, Tabrizi SJ, Rees G. The human motor cortex microcircuit: insights for neurodegenerative disease. Nat Rev Neurosci 2020;21:401–415.
16. Lemon R, Kraskov A. Starting and stopping movement by the primate brain. Brain Neurosci Adv 2019;3:2398212819837149.
17. Elsayed GF, Lara AH, Kaufman MT, Churchland MM, Cunningham JP. Reorganization between preparatory and movement population responses in motor cortex. Nat Commun 2016;7:13239.
18. Georgopoulos AP, Carpenter AF. Coding of movements in the motor cortex. Curr Opin Neurobiol 2015;33:34–39.
19. Johnson MT, Ebner TJ. Processing of multiple kinematic signals in the cerebellum and motor cortices. Brain Res Brain Res Rev 2000;33:155–168.
20. Yamawaki N, Shepherd GM. Synaptic circuit organization of motor corticothalamic neurons. J Neurosci 2015;35:2293–2307.
21. Aumann TD, Prut Y. Do sensorimotor beta-oscillations maintain muscle synergy representations in primary motor cortex? Trends Neurosci 2015;38:77–85.
22. Hallett M. Transcranial magnetic stimulation: a primer. Neuron 2007;55:187–199.
23. Burke MJ, Fried PJ, Pascual-Leone A. Transcranial magnetic stimulation: neurophysiological and clinical applications. Handb Clin Neurol 2019;163:73–92.
24. Bonaiuto JJ, Meyer SS, Little S, et al. Lamina-specific cortical dynamics in human visual and sensorimotor cortices. Elife 2018;7:e33977.
25. Kaas JH, Stepniewska I. Evolution of posterior parietal cortex and parietal-frontal networks for specific actions in primates. J Comp Neurol 2016;524:595–608.
26. Kastner S, Chen Q, Jeong SK, Mruczek REB. A brief comparative review of primate posterior parietal cortex: a novel hypothesis on the human toolmaker. Neuropsychologia 2017;105:123–134.
27. Konen CS, Mruczek RE, Montoya JL, Kastner S. Functional organization of human posterior parietal cortex: grasping- and reaching-related activations relative to topographically organized cortex. J Neurophysiol 2013;109:2897–2908.
28. Kravitz DJ, Saleem KS, Baker CI, Mishkin M. A new neural framework for visuospatial processing. Nat Rev Neurosci 2011;12:217–230.
29. Janssen P, Scherberger H. Visual guidance in control of grasping. Annu Rev Neurosci 2015;38:69–86.
30. Jones TA. Motor compensation and its effects on neural reorganization after stroke. Nat Rev Neurosci 2017;18:267.

31. Rizzolatti G, Sinigaglia C. The mirror mechanism: a basic principle of brain function. Nat Rev Neurosci 2016;17:757–765.
32. Errante A, Fogassi L. Parieto-frontal mechanisms underlying observation of complex hand-object manipulation. Sci Rep 2019;9:348.
33. Dick AS, Garic D, Graziano P, Tremblay P. The frontal aslant tract (FAT) and its role in speech, language and executive function. Cortex 2019;111:148–163.
34. Hallett M. Physiology of free will. Ann Neurol 2016;80:5–12.
35. Haggard P. Sense of agency in the human brain. Nat Rev Neurosci 2017;18:196–207.
36. Libet B, Gleason CA, Wright EW, Pearl DK. Time of conscious intention to act in relation to onset of cerebral activity (readiness-potential). The unconscious initiation of a freely voluntary act. Brain 1983;106 (Pt 3):623–642.
37. Dominik T, Dostal D, Zielina M, Smahaj J, Sedlackova Z, Prochazka R. Libet's experiment: a complex replication. Conscious Cogn 2018;65:1–26.
38. Sanford P, Lawson AL, King AN, Major M. Libet's intention reports are invalid: a replication of Dominik et al. (2017). Conscious Cogn 2020;77:102836.
39. Ohata R, Asai T, Kadota H, Shigemasu H, Ogawa K, Imamizu H. Sense of agency beyond sensorimotor process: decoding self-other action attribution in the human brain. Cereb Cortex 2020;30:4076–4091.
40. Sharma N, Cohen LG. Recovery of motor function after stroke. Dev Psychobiol 2012;54:254–262.
41. Micera S, Caleo M, Chisari C, Hummel FC, Pedrocchi A. Advanced neurotechnologies for the restoration of motor function. Neuron 2020;105:604–620.
42. Harvey RL, Edwards D, Dunning K, et al. Randomized sham-controlled trial of navigated repetitive transcranial magnetic stimulation for motor recovery in stroke. Stroke 2018;49:2138–2146.
43. Xu J, Branscheidt M, Schambra H, et al. Rethinking interhemispheric imbalance as a target for stroke neurorehabilitation. Ann Neurol 2019;85:502–513.
44. Elsner B, Kugler J, Mehrholz J. Transcranial direct current stimulation (tDCS) for upper limb rehabilitation after stroke: future directions. J Neuroeng Rehabil 2018;15:106.
45. Koch PJ, Hummel FC. Toward precision medicine: tailoring interventional strategies based on noninvasive brain stimulation for motor recovery after stroke. Curr Opin Neurol 2017;30:388–397.
46. Rehme AK, Volz LJ, Feis DL, et al. Identifying neuroimaging markers of motor disability in acute stroke by machine learning techniques. Cereb Cortex 2015;25:3046–3056.
47. Lin LY, Ramsey L, Metcalf NV, et al. Stronger prediction of motor recovery and outcome post-stroke by cortico-spinal tract integrity than functional connectivity. PLoS One 2018;13:e0202504.
48. Guder S, Frey BM, Backhaus W, et al. The influence of cortico-cerebellar structural connectivity on cortical excitability in chronic stroke. Cereb Cortex 2020;30:1330–1344.
49. Stinear CM, Byblow WD, Ackerley SJ, Smith MC, Borges VM, Barber PA. PREP2: a biomarker-based algorithm for predicting upper limb function after stroke. Ann Clin Transl Neurol 2017;4:811–820.
50. Hummel FC. [The importance of neuronal networks for motor rehabilitation after a stroke]. Nervenarzt 2017;88:850–857.
51. Park JE. Apraxia: review and update. J Clin Neurol 2017;13:317–324.
52. Criaud M, Poisson A, Thobois S, et al. Slowness in movement initiation is associated with proactive inhibitory network dysfunction in Parkinson's disease. J Parkinsons Dis 2016;6:433–440.
53. Spay C, Meyer G, Welter ML, Lau B, Boulinguez P, Ballanger B. Functional imaging correlates of akinesia in Parkinson's disease: still open issues. Neuroimage Clin 2019;21:101644.
54. DiMarzio M, Madhavan R, Joel S, et al. Use of functional magnetic resonance imaging to assess how motor phenotypes of Parkinson's disease respond to deep brain stimulation. Neuromodulation 2020;23:515–524.
55. Kranick SM, Hallett M. Neurology of volition. Exp Brain Res 2013;229:313–327.
56. Maurer CW, LaFaver K, Ameli R, Epstein SA, Hallett M, Horovitz SG. Impaired self-agency in functional movement disorders: a resting-state fMRI study. Neurology 2016;87:564–570.
57. Welniarz Q, Dusart I, Roze E. The corticospinal tract: evolution, development, and human disorders. Dev Neurobiol 2017;77:810–829.
58. Jiang S, Zhong D, Yan Y, et al. Mirror movements induced by hemiballism due to putamen infarction: a case report and literature review. Ann Transl Med 2020;8:19.
59. Quartarone A, Hallett M. Emerging concepts in the physiological basis of dystonia. Mov Disord 2013;28:958–967.
60. Lozeron P, Poujois A, Richard A, et al. Contribution of TMS and rTMS in the understanding of the pathophysiology and in the treatment of dystonia. Front Neural Circuits 2016;10:90.
61. Bianchi S, Fuertinger S, Huddleston H, Frucht SJ, Simonyan K. Functional and structural neural bases of task specificity in isolated focal dystonia. Mov Disord 2019;j34:555–563.
62. Caviness JN. Myoclonus. Continuum (Minneap Minn) 2019;25:1055–1080.

31 Spinal Motor Control

OVERVIEW

Motor neurons located in the ventral horn of the spinal cord and in cranial nerve nuclei, also known as lower motor neurons or motoneurons, are the final common effector of central motor commands. They provide excitatory cholinergic nicotinic output to skeletal muscle fibers forming motor units. The activity of motoneurons is controlled by segmental afferents, premotor interneurons, and descending inputs from the cerebral cortex and brainstem. With few exceptions, activity of spinal and lower brainstem motoneurons is controlled by excitatory or inhibitory interneurons that form local circuits, or functional units (modules), that control patterns of motoneuron activation eliciting motor synergies. These synergies can be flexibly modified in response to cortical and brainstem motor commands interacting with afferent feedback. Central pattern generators (CPGs), such as those involved in locomotion, respiration, and swallowing, can autonomously generate activation of motoneurons. Disturbances of segmental and descending control of motoneurons provide the basis for many neurologic disorders, including motor neuron disease and spasticity. The aims of this chapter are to briefly review: (1) the properties of spinal motoneurons and motor units; (2) the subtypes of spinal interneurons and their role in segmental reflexes; (3) the corticospinal and brainstem control of the segmental motor apparatus; (4) the mechanisms controlling muscle tone, posture, and locomotion; and (5) mechanisms and examples of disorders affecting these functions.

MOTOR NEURONS AND MOTOR UNITS

The segmental motor apparatus include motor neurons (motoneurons) and interneurons, both of which receive segmental afferent and descending inputs (Figure 31.1). In the spinal cord, motoneurons segregate into pools within lamina IX of the ventral horn. Motoneurons controlling progressively more proximal muscles are located progressively more ventrally; those innervating antagonist muscles within a given joint are segregated along the mediolateral axis.[1,2] The two major types of motoneurons are alpha (α) motoneurons that drive muscle contraction and force and gamma (γ) motoneurons that innervate the muscle spindles and maintain their sensitivity to stretch in the setting of muscle shortening.[3] The premotor interneuronal circuits are located in laminae VII and VIII of the intermediate gray matter and ventral horn.

Electrophysiological Properties of Motoneurons

Spinal motoneurons have several unique electrophysiological properties that are affected by multiple synaptic influences. They undergo sustained depolarizations referred to as plateau potentials that depend on inward currents mediated by voltage-gated sodium (Na^+) and calcium (Ca^{2+}) channels. Activation of Ca^{2+} conductances is followed by activation of Ca^{2+}-activated potassium (K^+) channels that elicit afterhyperpolarization. The biophysical properties of α-motoneurons are plastic and adapt to both increases and decreases in chronic activation, reflecting both structural changes and changes in protein synthesis and ion channel expression. Motoneurons are activated by glutamatergic inputs originating from cortical and brainstem projections, local interneurons, and primary afferents. Fast excitation involves α-amino-3-hydroxy-5-methyl-4 isoxazole propionic acid receptors (AMPARs), many of which lack or contain unedited GluA2 subunits and are therefore permeable to Ca^{2+}. Motoneurons are also activated via N-methyl-D-aspartate receptors (NMDARs) and class I metabotropic glutamate receptors (mGluRs). Fast inhibition of motoneurons is mediated by GABA, glycine, or both[4] released from local interneurons and in some cases descending projections from the brainstem. The excitability of motoneurons and interneurons is modulated by cholinergic, monoaminergic, and other signals. One important example is serotonin, which is released from projections from the medullary

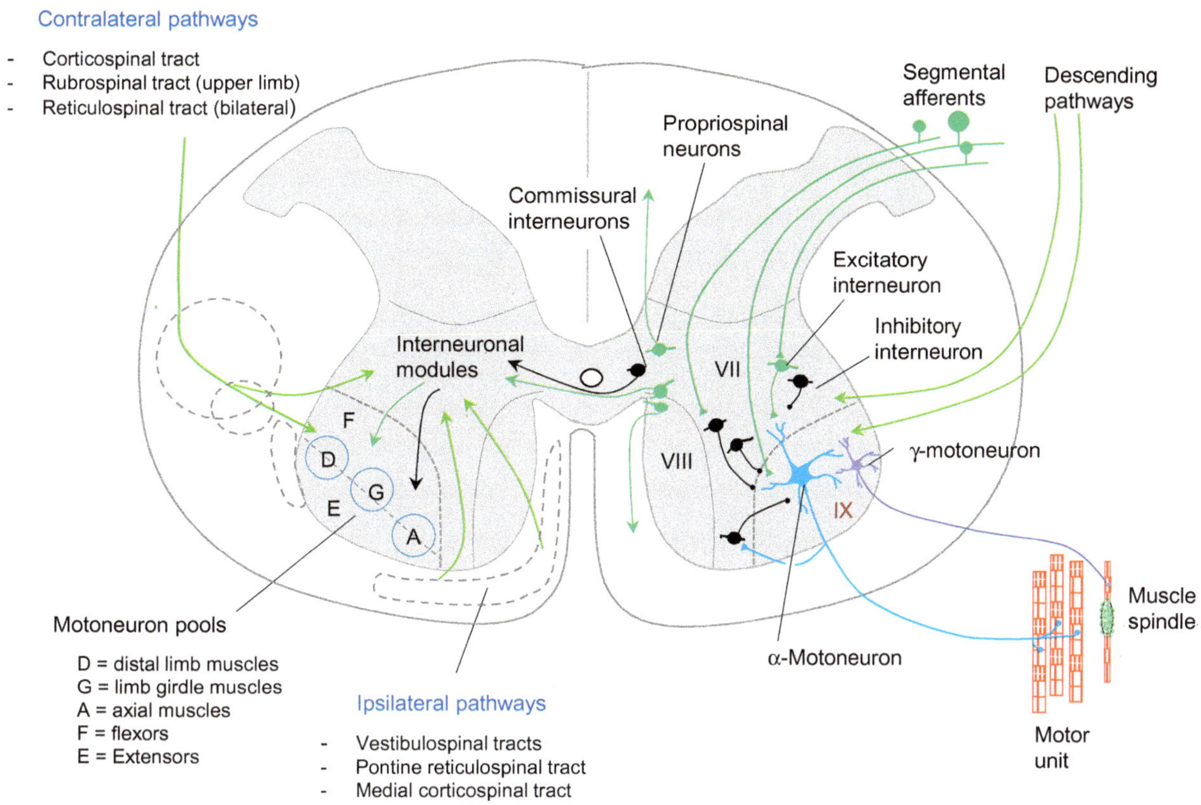

FIGURE 31.1 Segmental motor apparatus.
The segmental motor apparatus includes spinal motor neurons (motoneurons) and interneurons that receive segmental afferent and descending inputs. Spinal motoneurons segregate into pools within lamina IX and include α-motoneurons that drive muscle contraction and γ-motoneurons that innervate the muscle spindles. Motoneurons controlling progressively more proximal muscles are located progressively more ventrally. The premotor interneuronal circuits are located in laminae VII and VIII of the intermediate gray matter and ventral horn.

raphe.[5] Activation of somatodendritic 5-HT2 receptors increases α-motoneuron excitability and amplitude of responses to spinal reflexes. In contrast, prolonged release of 5-HT during excessive muscle activity decreases excitability via 5-HT1_A receptors located in their axon initial segment; this may constitute a mechanism of central fatigue.[4]

Heterogeneity of Motor Units

Individual α-motoneurons innervate a variable number of muscle fibers forming a motor unit.[6]

There are three main types of muscle fibers, each innervated by a different subtype of motoneuron and thus forming different types of motor units. Slow-twitch, fatigue-resistant (type I) fibers are oxidative and generate relatively weak contractions. These fibers are innervated by small (S) motoneurons characterized by high excitability and slow axonal conduction velocity. These S-type motor units predominate in muscles that require almost constant tone, such as those required for posture maintenance. Type S neurons have repetitive firing that amplifies and prolongs the excitatory inputs. Fast-twitch (type II) fibers include type IIb fibers that are mixed oxidative and glycolytic and fatigue resistant (FR), and IIb fibers that are glycolytic and generate strong contractions, but fatigue easily (FF). These muscle fibers are innervated by large motoneurons with lower excitability but higher conduction velocities than those in S-type motor units. Type FF motor neurons have shorter afterhyperpolarization so that their firing frequency matches the contractile speed of the target muscle. Because of their lower threshold of activation by synaptic input, S-type motoneurons are recruited earlier than those innervating FR and FF fibers. This sequential recruitment of motor units is known as the "size principle" but is violated in some specific physiological contexts. Skeletal muscles have a single point of contact between the incoming axon and each muscle fiber called the motor endplate; at this level muscle nicotinic acetylcholine receptors are clustered at the junctional folds. This clustering is one of the critical determinants of the safety margin of neuromuscular transmission, so that each action potential arriving to the motor axon and triggering a quantal release of acetylcholine produces endplate potential, leading to an all-or-none twitch in the muscle fiber.

SPINAL SEGMENTAL MOTOR APPARATUS

Segmental Afferent Inputs and Basic Reflexes

Segmental afferent inputs critically affect the spinal motor apparatus; the three main sources are the muscle spindles, innervated by Ia (dynamic) and II (static) afferents; the Golgi tendon organs innervated by type Ib afferents; and the flexor reflex afferents, which include groups III and IV muscle afferents, cutaneous afferents, and group II spindle afferents (Figure 31.2). For the most part, spinal interneurons mediate these segmental reflexes, integrate descending influences to generate motor synergies; and may initiate rhythmic activity and alternate pattern of motoneuron activation during locomotion.[7] The muscle stretch reflex is a fundamental mechanism of control of excitability of the α-motoneurons and is required to sustain maximal muscle contraction. This reflex is a length-feedback mechanism triggered by elongation of tension-activated nuclear bag muscle spindle receptors innervated by Ia afferents. Rapid elongation of the spindle triggers a rapid Ia afferent input that provides a robust monosynaptic excitation of the α-motoneurons innervating the homonymous and synergistic muscles.[8] The γ-motoneurons innervating the muscle spindles, known as fusimotor neurons, modulate the degree of spindle feedback. Activity of γ-motoneurons is necessary to maintain Ia afferent input to servo-assist the α-motoneuron during muscle shortening. In relaxed muscle, there is no fusimotor activity; in contrast, maximal muscle contraction

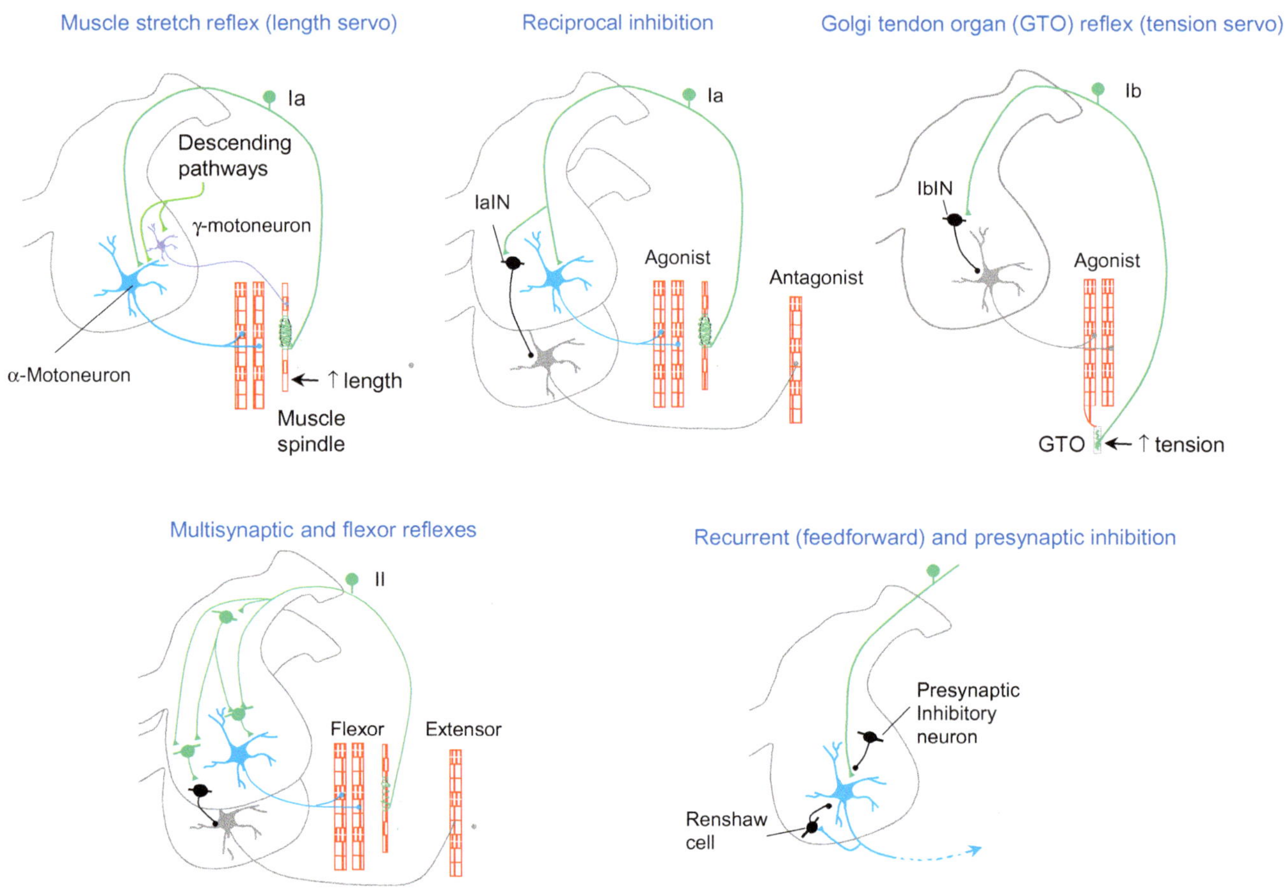

FIGURE 31.2 Basic spinal reflex motor circuits.

There are three main sources of segmental afferents to α-motoneurons. The muscle spindles, innervated by Ia (dynamic) and II (static) afferents; the Golgi tendon organs innervated by type Ib afferents; and the flexor reflex afferents, which include groups III and IV muscle afferents, cutaneous afferents, and group II spindle afferents. Rapid elongation of the spindles triggers a rapid Ia excitatory input to the α-motoneurons innervating the homonymous and synergistic muscles. The γ-motoneurons innervating the muscle spindles (fusimotor neurons) modulate the degree of spindle feedback. Ia afferent input also activates inhibitory interneurons (IaINs) that mediate reciprocal inhibition of the α-motoneurons innervating the antagonist muscles. Golgi tendon organ Ib afferents are activated by muscle tension and elicit disynaptic inhibition of the corresponding α-motoneurons via Ib inhibitory interneurons (IbINs). Flexor reflex afferents target excitatory or inhibitory interneurons and trigger polysynaptic reflexes, Renshaw cells receive a collateral excitatory input from α-motoneurons and provide a recurrent feedforward inhibitory input to the originating motor neuron. Presynaptic inhibitory neurons make axo-axonic synapses with primary Ia afferents and reduce glutamate release.

during voluntary effort requires coactivation of γ- and α-motoneurons by descending inputs. Loss of excitatory Ia proprioceptive feedback in disorders such as large fiber neuropathies or ganglionopathies deprives α-motoneurons of Ia inputs required to sustain maximal muscle contraction. A second major effect of the Ia afferent input is activation of inhibitory GABAergic interneurons (IaIN) that mediate reciprocal inhibition of the α-motoneurons innervating the antagonist muscles. Reciprocal inhibition is critical for smooth voluntary movements and appropriate control of muscle tone. The second major source afferents to the segmental motor apparatus is the Golgi tendon organ innervated by Ib afferents. These afferents are activated by muscle tension during active muscle contraction and trigger a tension-feedback reflex that results in disynaptic inhibition of the corresponding α-motoneurons via Ib inhibitory interneurons (IbINs). The third major segmental input to the spinal motor apparatus is provided by flexor reflex afferents from muscle and skin receptors. These afferents target excitatory or inhibitory interneurons and trigger two main types of polysynaptic reflexes: proprioceptive reflexes that coordinate activity of the limbs during locomotion, and nociceptive reflexes mediating limb withdrawal responses to noxious stimuli.

Interneuron Circuits and Spinal Premotor Units

All interneurons participate in networks that flexibly mediate segmental reflexes and coordinate the activity of multiple motoneuron pools dedicated to the control of individual limbs or segments across multiple joints.[1] For example, in addition to inputs from Ia afferents, IaINs receive inputs from other types of inhibitory interneurons and facilitatory inputs from high-threshold muscle afferents. Similarly, IbINs receive convergence of multimodal inputs not only from group Ib afferents but also from corticospinal, rubrospinal, and reticulospinal pathways; propriospinal neurons; and muscle spindle, cutaneous, and joint afferents. Group Ib INs project to both α- and γ-motoneurons, to other IbINs, and to cells of the ventral and dorsal spinocerebellar tracts. Renshaw cells are an important group of inhibitory glycinergic neurons located in lamina VII. They receive a collateral excitatory input from α-motoneurons and provide a recurrent feedforward inhibitory input to the originating motoneuron. The comparison between feedforward Renshaw cell-mediated inhibition and feedback Ia afferent excitation allows the α-motoneuron to compare their predictive motor commands and their consequences, thereby providing a mechanism for motor learning in spinal circuits. Recurrent inhibition appears to primarily affect motoneurons that participate in stereotypical movements, and is absent in motoneurons innervating the digits, which are used during skilled motor activity. Another major group of inhibitory interneurons are presynaptic inhibitory neurons (Figure 31.2). These GABAergic neurons have a major role in controlling the gain of the monosynaptic stretch reflex and other segmental reflexes. They make axo-axonic synapses with primary Ia afferents and reduce glutamate release by eliciting primary afferent depolarization via $GABA_A$ receptors, which in primary afferents promote efflux of chloride. Presynaptic inhibition via GABAergic interneurons is an important mechanism by which descending inputs control segmental spinal reflexes.

In addition to inhibitory interneurons, the segmental motor apparatus contains excitatory interneurons. These interneurons typically form part of multisynaptic circuits that coordinate activity of several pools of motoneurons and other interneurons. Interneurons contacted by secondary (group II) muscle spindle afferents are distributed both in the intermediate gray matter and in the dorsal horn. Those located in the intermediate zone synapse directly onto motoneurons and may be activated by group II afferents either directly or via dorsal horn interneurons. Other inputs to these interneurons include Golgi tendon organ afferents and low-threshold cutaneous and joint afferents. Group II interneurons may exert disynaptic excitatory (via other excitatory interneurons) or inhibitory (via GABAergic interneurons) actions on motoneurons, and tri- or polysynaptic actions on motoneurons via dorsal horn neurons, thus evoking widespread actions to the motoneurons. The dominating effect of group II afferents is excitation of flexor and inhibition of extensor muscles. However, they are likely to be involved in various types of reflex circuits, including the flexor reflex and transcortical-mediated stretch reflex.

Spinal Central Pattern Generator for Locomotion

Spinal interneurons form central pattern generator (CPG) networks that are responsible for the coordinated activity during locomotion. These CPGs can generate rhythmic motor activity in absence of descending and afferent inputs to the spinal cord. The basic unit of locomotion is a step cycle that includes a swing phase and a stance phase; the speed of locomotion is related to the burst frequency and cycle of rhythmic activity of extensor and flexor motor neurons on either lower limb. The cycle period is primarily regulated by the duration of the stance phase and can be altered by supraspinal control and proprioceptive feedback from stretch-sensitive muscle spindle and tension-sensitive Golgi tendon organ lower limb receptors. The presence of locomotor CPG in humans is reflected by the ability to elicit a locomotor pattern of activity in the lower limbs of patients with complete spinal cord injury (SCI), the automatic stepping in infants, and the locomotor-like pattern of activity during periodic leg movement of sleep. Humans also have a cervical CPG controlling the alternating movement of the upper arms during locomotion.[9,10]

The spinal locomotor CPG consists of rhythm-generating and pattern-generating circuits involving different types of interneurons. Rhythm-generating circuits involve excitatory glutamatergic interneurons that drive ipsilateral excitatory interneurons innervating extensor or flexor motoneurons as well as commissural interneurons with axons crossing the midline. The pattern-generating circuits drive the different pools of motor neurons via inhibitory interneurons and include a flexor-extensor pattern circuit that coordinates muscles of the ipsilateral limbs, and a left-right pattern-generating circuit that coordinates the activity between limbs. Interneurons in these pattern-generating circuits include Ia inhibitory interneurons mediating reciprocal inhibition between flexor and extensor muscles, and commissural interneurons mediating crossed inhibition between the outputs to the left and right lower limbs.

Commissural interneurons are located in laminae IV–VIII and X and include short-range (segmental) and long-range (intersegmental) neurons that project either rostrally or caudally. They receive inputs from descending motor pathways and may be either inhibitory or excitatory and project to different classes of inhibitory interneurons or directly to motoneurons. Segmental and descending afferents activate ipsilateral and contralateral projecting interneurons in parallel, coordinating the activity of motoneurons on both sides of the spinal cord. Several spinal circuits, including the muscle stretch reflex, reciprocal inhibition, and recurrent inhibition, contribute to maintenance of posture and locomotion and are differentially modulated at the different phases of locomotion. For example, during walking in humans, recurrent inhibition and reciprocal inhibition are modulated in a phase-dependent manner.

Propriospinal interneurons are located in all laminae, except lamina IX, and form ascending and descending connections between multiple spinal cord segments throughout the spinal cord. A substantial population connect the caudal cervical and the rostral lumbar segments and may synchronize the lumbar and cervical CPGs mediating interlimb coordination during locomotion. Propriospinal interneurons are more resistant to injury than outer spinal cord neurons and may have an important role in motor recovery after SCI in humans.

Spinal Interneurons and Motoneurons as Integrative Units

Spinal interneurons and their target motoneurons are components of multifunctional circuits. These circuits have a modular organization and form functional units that generate specific motor outputs by imposing specific patterns of muscle activation, or muscle synergies.[11–14] These circuits are multifunctional, as individual neurons can variably be involved in more than one motor behavior; the specific elementary motor outputs are then combined to produce coherent movements. Sensory feedback contributes up to 30% of net excitatory drive to interneurons. The gain of segmental reflexes and the activity of the spinal locomotor CPG are also regulated by a variety of neuromodulators, including l-glutamate acting via NMDAR and mGluR1 receptors. Sacral cholinergic neurons send ascending projections to the lumbar spinal cord, where they innervate both the CPG and downstream interneurons and motoneurons. Serotonin increases excitability of α-motoneurons and commissural neurons and modulates both sensory and descending inputs to spinal interneurons. Norepinephrine inhibits excitability flexor reflexes via α2-adrenoceptors while increasing excitability of α-motoneurons via α1-adrenoceptors. Astrocytes also modulate neuronal networks involved in locomotion via release of ATP, which is hydrolyzed to adenosine leading to activation of neuronal adenosine A_1 receptors; the net effect is a reduction in locomotor-like activity of motoneurons.

CORTICAL CONTROL OF VOLUNTARY LIMB MOVEMENTS

The descending motor systems have the ability to either respect or override the specific spinal motor programs according to the motor task or goal.[15] For example, reaching requires the transition from alternation to synchrony in the activation of muscles controlling a single joint. This state switch requires overriding of the reciprocal inhibitory pattern between flexors and extensors during the early stages of limb extension to permit co-contraction antagonistic muscles to help stiffen and stabilize the arm at the end of extension.

Corticospinal Tract

The descending cortical commands are conveyed to the spinal motor microcircuits via the corticospinal tract (CST), or pyramidal tract (PT) (Figure 31.3). Cortical control of brainstem motor circuits is mediated by the corticobulbar pathways and by collaterals of the CST.[16,14] The CST includes direct and indirect pathways that provide flexible, behavioral-specific control of spinal motoneurons. Two fundamental functions of the CST are to provide a general background excitation for recruitment of motoneuron pools in response to increased effort, and to control fractionated movements of the fingers. Approximately 80% of the pyramidal fibers in humans originate from the motor cortex, including the primary motor cortex (M1, area 4), premotor cortex (lateral area 6), and supplementary motor area (medial area 6); the remaining originate from the anterior cingulate motor area and somatosensory areas 3, 2, 1, and 5. The CST projections originate from large pyramidal tract (PT) neurons located in deep layer 5. They include fast-conducting PT neurons that discharge phasically before and during large and fast movements and are partially insensitive to peripheral feedback, and slow-conducting PT neurons that fire tonically during movement and are highly sensitive to peripheral feedback. Approximately 80% to 90% of corticospinal axons decussate at the lower medulla (lateral CST) and descend in the dorsolateral quadrant of the spinal cord. The rest of CST axons descend without crossing either in the ventral funiculus (anterior CST) or in the dorsolateral quadrant (uncrossed CST). Corticospinal fibers innervate multiple segments of the spinal cord; at each segment, CST terminals make diverging contacts with several pools of premotor interneurons and motoneurons. Therefore, each cortical PT neuron controls many spinal motoneurons and each spinal motoneuron is controlled by inputs from multiple cortical

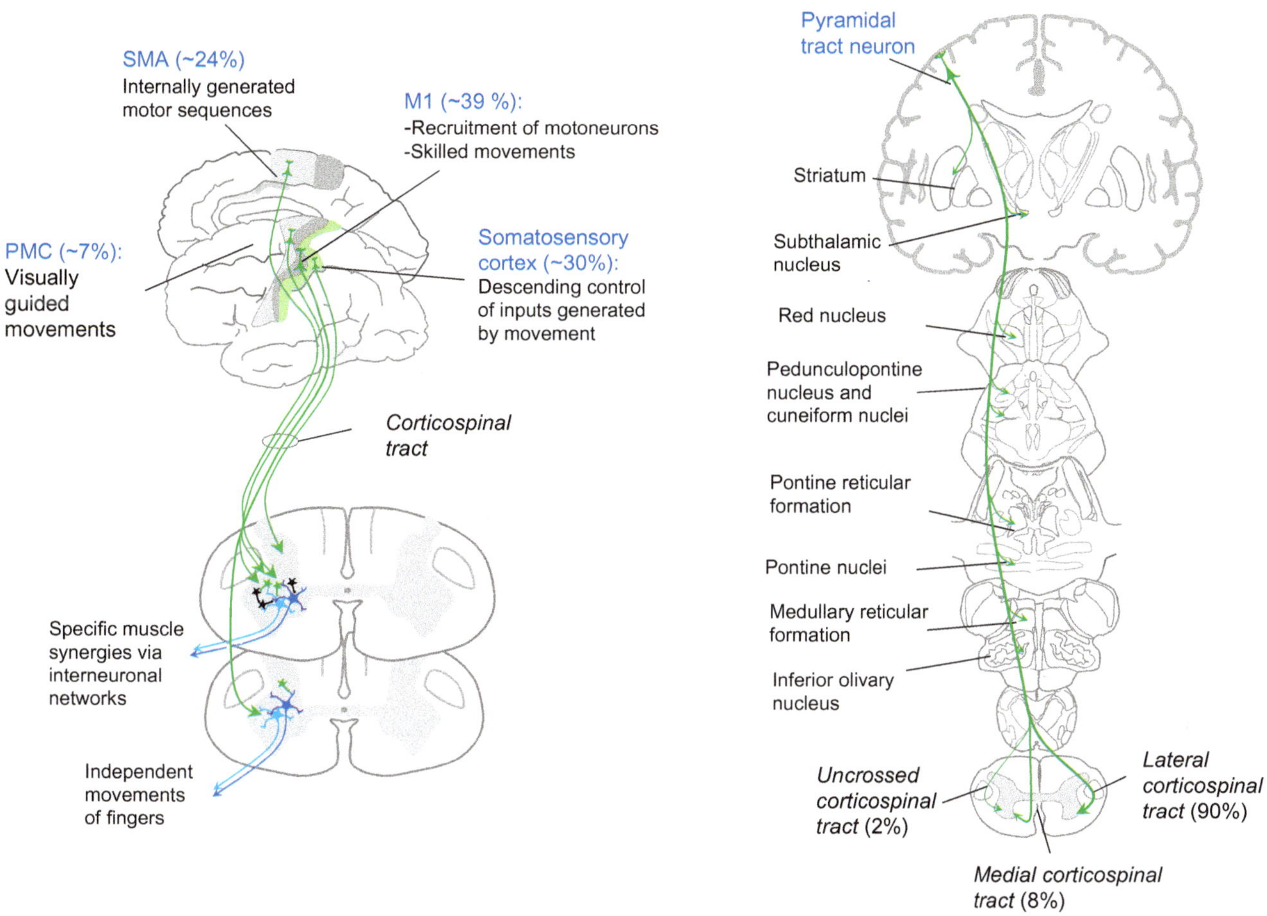

FIGURE 31.3 Cortical control of the segmental motor apparatus.
The main source of descending control of segmental motor neurons and interneurons is the corticospinal tract (CST), also known as pyramidal tract (PT). Approximately 70%–80% of the pyramidal fibers in humans originate from the motor cortex, including areas 4 (primary motor area, M1) and 6 (supplementary motor area and the lateral premotor cortex); the remainder originate from the cingulate motor area and somatosensory areas 3, 2, 1, and 5. Much of the corticospinal control is exerted via interneurons intercalated in reflex pathways that terminate on α- and γ-motoneurons. However, many M1 neurons provide direct monosynaptic projections to motoneurons innervating the distal hand muscles (cortico-motoneuronal system). Many PT neurons send collateral branches to the striatum, subthalamic nucleus, red nucleus, superior colliculus, pedunculopontine tegmental nucleus, pontine nuclei, inferior olivary nucleus, and pontomedullary reticular formation.

PT neurons. Much of the corticospinal control is exerted via interneurons intercalated in reflex pathways that terminate on α- and γ-motoneurons. Corticospinal axons also activate presynaptic inhibitory neurons; this allows the motor cortex to influence complex patterns of muscle activity by controlling segmental spinal reflexes. Many PT cells of M1 also provide direct monosynaptic projections to motoneurons innervating the distal hand muscles (cortico-motoneuronal system); fast-conducting CST axons providing these connections constitute approximately 8% of the PT in humans. These direct cortico-motoneuronal connections contribute different proportions of excitatory input to different motoneuron pools, primarily those controlling opposition of the thumb and skilled hand function. Hand motoneurons receive matched densities of monosynaptic corticospinal and Ia afferent inputs; this provides a mechanism for balancing central feedforward and peripheral feedback commands for fine motor control. The uncrossed corticospinal axons originate primarily from area 6 and terminate on propriospinal neurons and interneurons that control axial and proximal limb muscles. They may be important for ipsilateral postural adjustments when fine movements are performed with the contralateral hand. Corticospinal inputs also control locomotion over uneven ground or challenging terrains and skill walking (agility).

Efference Copy, Priming, and Breaking Effects of the Corticospinal Tract

Many PT neurons send collateral branches to the striatum, subthalamic nucleus (STN), red nucleus, superior colliculus, pedunculopontine tegmental nucleus (PPT, PPN), pontine nuclei, inferior olivary nucleus, and pontomedullary reticular formation (Figure 31.3). Via these projections, the motor cortex provides feedforward information about motor commands. Pools of spinal interneurons integrate descending cortical and brainstem motor command signals with local sensory feedback and send inputs to the cerebellum, either directly via the ventral spinocerebellar tract or via the medullary lateral reticular nucleus. The cerebellum uses this spinocerebellar system to be informed about the relative excitatory drive on specific spinal modules controlling motor synergies. Neurons in the Clarke column located in the intermediate gray matter of the thoracic spinal cord and projecting via the dorsal spinocerebellar tract and those in the external cuneate nucleus in the lower medulla projecting via the cuneocerebellar tract provide feedback information about the actual movement.

During preparation of movement excitatory and inhibitory process at the spinal level provide for mechanisms of "priming" and "braking" of motoneuron output. Excitation is aimed at priming a specific response, whereas inhibition acts to prevent this overt excitation from causing a premature movement.[17] Corticospinal inhibition may reflect both the recruitment of cortical excitatory and inhibitory interneurons and the existence of parallel pathways from the premotor cortex to the spinal cord. The main pathway for motor commands originates in the premotor cortex, which targets the primary cortex and then the spinal cord and specifies the movement parameters. There is a second pathway from the premotor cortex to the reticular formation and then to the spinal cord. This control mechanism may depend on a robust premotor-reticulospinal pathway that affects both proximal and distal muscles.[18] This premotor activity that dominates during the preparatory phase of movement cancels the excitatory command derived from M1 at that time. Soon after movement begins premotor cortical activity decreases and the spinal inhibition is lifted, revealing a circuit that is already at threshold level required for muscle activation.

CONTROL OF POSTURE AND MUSCLE TONE

The control of postural balance, muscle tone, and generation of the locomotor rhythm are integrated at the level of the brainstem. Brainstem motor pathways have been classically subdivided into three groups: medial, lateral, and "emotional" or "limbic"[19](Figure 31.4). The medial motor pathways control posture, muscle tone, and locomotion. They include the reticulospinal and vestibulospinal tracts, which descend bilaterally to all levels of the spinal cord and innervate interneurons and motor neurons controlling axial and proximal limb muscles. The medial vestibulospinal tract (VST), together with the tectospinal tract (from the superior colliculus) and the interstitiospinal tract (from the interstitial nucleus of Cajal) innervate cervical motoneurons to control head movements for head–eye coordination. The lateral VST descends more laterally throughout the spinal cord to control postural reflexes. Neurons that contribute the reticulospinal tracts are located in the pontine and medullar reticular formation and receive direct input from the motor cortex and midbrain areas and exert complex effects on regulation of muscle tone and locomotion. The lateral brainstem motor pathway is the rubrospinal tract, which controls movements of the contralateral upper limb. This pathway originates in the magnocellular portion of the red nucleus and in humans does not extend beyond the cervical cord. Whereas its function has been largely overtaken by the crossed CST, the rubrospinal tract contributes to flexor movements of the arm and wrist and has a role in recovery of some motor function following stroke.[20] The emotional motor pathways originate in several regions involved in emotion and behavioral state control, including the periaqueductal gray (PAG), nucleus retroambiguus, and monoaminergic neurons from the locus coeruleus and medullary raphe. The PAG has a major role in processes such as emotional activation of locomotion and vocalization.[21]

Vestibular System and Control of Posture

Posture is the ability to adjust both the position of the body to the direction of gravity and parts of the body in relation to each other. Postural adjustments are preprogrammed, begin in the joints closest to the support surface, and are followed by a series of interactive, internally triggered stretch reflexes. The integration of vestibular, proprioceptive, and visual information is critical for control of balance and posture. The vestibular system encodes self-motion information by detecting head movement in space and time and has a fundamental major role in orientation in space, navigation, and stabilization of gaze during head motion, in part via close interactions with the proprioceptive and visual systems. The vestibular organs include the three semicircular canals (SCCs), lateral (horizontal), anterior, and posterior, which sense angular acceleration; and the otolith organs, utricle and saccule, which sense linear acceleration (gravity and translational movements). Vestibular hair cells have similar structure, physiology and sensitivity to hair-bundle displacement in response to endolymph movement as do cochlear hair cells. Whereas the vestibular labyrinth protects the SCCs from being activated by air-conducted sound or bone conducted vibration, the otoliths have very sensitive responses to these stimuli. A defect in the wall of the bony canal, as occurs with superior canal dehiscence, impairs the protective effect on the SCCs, rendering both SCC neurons and otolith neurons sensitive to bone-conducted vibration and air-conducted sound. In this disorder, sound and vibration provide a pulsing stimulus to the endolymph that causes an activation of the SCC cupula similar to that caused by an angular acceleration. This activates SCC neurons and result in vertigo and nystagmus triggered by sound (the Tullio phenomenon) or Valsalva maneuver.

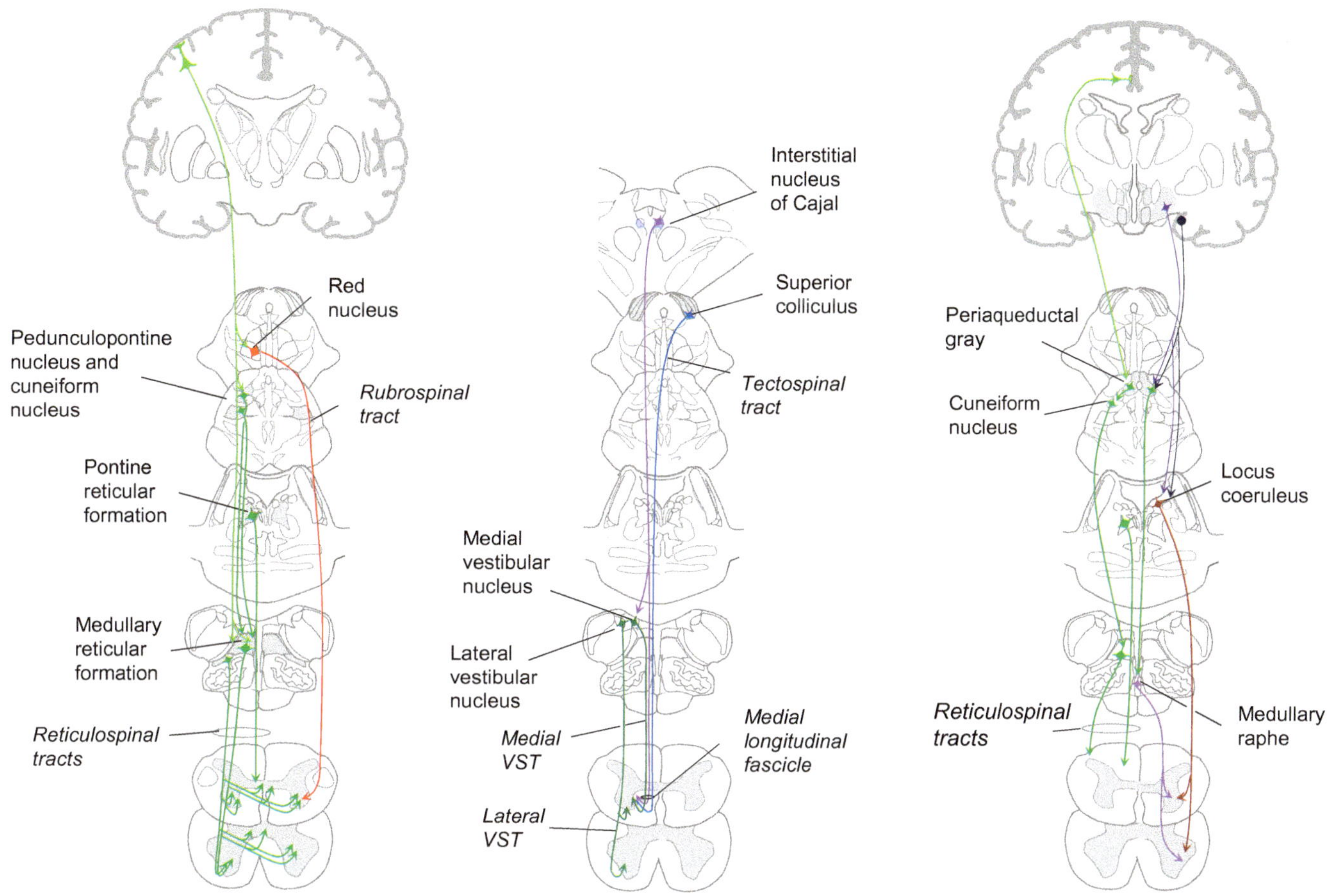

FIGURE 31.4 Descending brainstem motor pathways.
Brainstem motor pathways have been classically subdivided into three groups: medial, lateral, and "emotional." The medial motor pathways control posture, muscle tone, and locomotion. They include the reticulospinal and vestibulospinal tracts (VST), which descend bilaterally to all levels of the spinal cord and innervate interneurons and motor neurons controlling axial and proximal limb muscles. The lateral brainstem motor pathway is the rubrospinal tract, which controls movements of the contralateral upper limb. The "emotional" motor pathways originate in several regions involved in emotion and behavioral state control, including the periaqueductal gray and monoaminergic neurons from the locus coeruleus and medullary raphe nuclei.

Vestibular afferents terminate in the vestibular nuclear complex, including the superior, medial, lateral and inferior nuclei (Figure 31.5). Whereas the SCC provides inputs to all vestibular nuclei, the utricle projects primarily to the medial vestibular nucleus and the cerebellar nodulus and flocculus, whereas the saccule projects to the lateral vestibular nucleus, nodulus, and uvula. The vestibular nuclei contain two main categories of neurons. Vestibulo-ocular reflex (VOR) neurons stabilize gaze and hold the image steady to assure clear vision during brief head rotation as discussed later in the next chapter. Vestibular-only neurons project to the spinal cord and mediate the vestibulospinal reflexes. These reflexes are crucial for coordinating head and neck movements with the trunk and body to maintain the head in an upright position and maintain postural extensor tone against gravity. There are two main vestibulospinal pathways. Projections from the medial vestibular nucleus (medial VST), together with those from the superior colliculus and interstitial nucleus of Cajal descend via the medial longitudinal fasciculus to innervate motoneurons that control neck muscles and thus participate in coordination of head and eye movements. The lateral vestibular nucleus projects via the lateral VST, which increases activity of interneurons and motoneurons mediating antigravity extensor vestibulospinal reflex, which is the main mechanism by which the otolith organ controls the extensor musculature of the body. Whereas the vestibulospinal reflex may be helpful to stabilize the head and body to compensate for unexpected movements, these stabilizing command reflexes may be counterproductive during voluntary actions. The vestibular nuclei receive robust proprioceptive inputs that control vestibular responses; the interactions between the proprioceptive and vestibular systems are typically antagonistic. For example, during voluntary head movements, neck proprioceptive inputs markedly attenuate the activity of vestibulospinal neurons. The integration of vestibular and

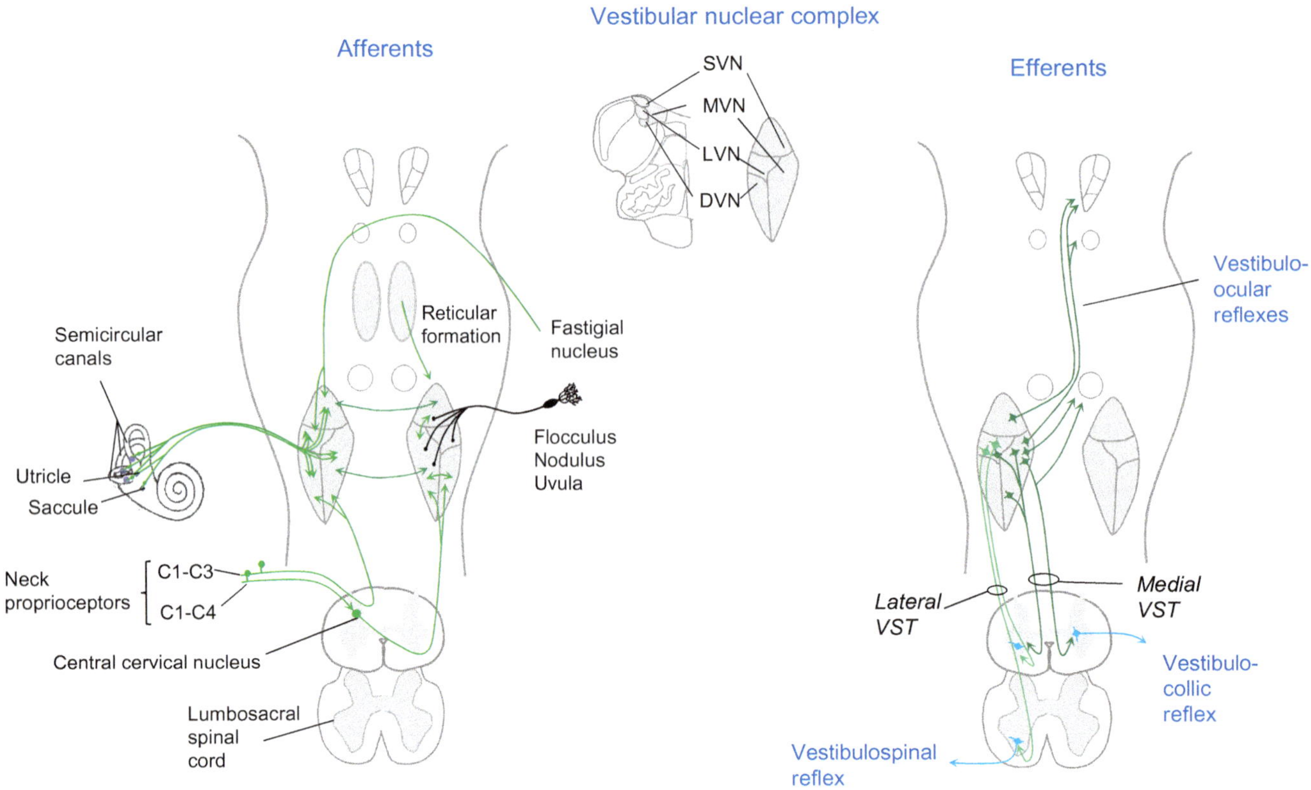

FIGURE 31.5 Main connections and functions of the vestibular nuclei.
The vestibular organs include the three semicircular canals (SCCs), which sense angular acceleration, and the otolith organs (utricle and saccule), which sense linear acceleration. Vestibular afferents terminate in the vestibular nuclear complex, including the superior (SVN), medial (MVN), lateral (LVN), and inferior (IVN) nuclei. In addition, the vestibular nuclei receive afferents from the spinal cord, reticular formation, cerebellum, and nuclei involved in control of eye movements. There also are commissural connections between the vestibular nuclei that mediate both excitatory and inhibitory interactions. Many of the individual nuclear groups in the vestibular nuclear complex on each side are interconnected either by reciprocal or unidirectional projections. The vestibular nuclei contain two main categories of neurons. The vestibulo-ocular reflex (VOR) assures clear vision during brief head rotation. Vestibulospinal reflexes coordinate head and neck movements with the trunk and body to maintain the head in an upright position and maintain postural extensor tone against gravity. The MVN together with the superior colliculus and interstitial nucleus of Cajal projects via the medial longitudinal fasciculus to innervate motoneurons that control neck muscle. The LVN projects via the lateral vestibulospinal tract, which increases activity of interneurons and motoneurons mediating the antigravity extensor vestibulospinal reflex.

proprioceptive inputs at the rostral fastigial nucleus is critical for accurate control of posture and balance. Vestibular neurons known as vestibulo-oculo-collic neurons project both rostrally to the oculomotor nuclei and caudally to the cervical spinal cord. These neurons participate in the vestibulocollic reflex, which is a compensatory response of neck muscles that stabilizes a position of the head in space and thus the direction of the gaze during head rotation. As in the case of the VOR, both angular acceleration (coded by the SCC) and linear acceleration (coded by the otolith organs) trigger this reflex. The angular vestibulocollic reflex stabilizes the head in space during head-on body movement; the linear vestibulocollic reflex compensates for vertical and lateral body translation. Otolith function is assessed clinically by vestibular-evoked myogenic potentials (VEMPs) evoked by brief repeated air-conducted sound or bound-conducted vibration. The ocular VEMP is recorded over the tensed contralateral inferior oblique muscle and originates predominantly from afferents from the utricular macula. The cervical VEMP is an inhibitory potential recorded over the tensed sternocleidomastoid muscle and originates predominantly from afferents from the ipsilateral saccular macula.

Pontomedullary Reticular Formation and Control of Muscle Tone

The reticular formation extends through the mesencephalon, pons, and medulla. The reticulospinal neurons involved in limb movement occupy the medial column of the reticular formation in the pons and medulla (Figure 31.6). It comprises the oral pontine reticular nucleus (nucleus reticularis pontis oralis, PnO); the caudal pontine reticular nucleus (nucleus reticularis pontis caudalis, PnC); and the rostral portion of the medial medullary reticular formation comprising the gigantocellular reticular nucleus (Gi), the dorsal paragigantocellular nucleus, and the lateral paragigantocellular nucleus (LPGi). The pontomedullary reticular formation receives inputs from the motor cortex, mesencephalic locomotor region, contralateral cerebellum, and ipsilateral lateral hypothalamic area. Neurons of the pontine and medullary reticular formation project to the spinal motor apparatus via reticulospinal tracts.[22,23] Reticulospinal axons branch extensively from the cervical to the lumbosacral segments and provide for synergistic control of neck, trunk, and limb muscles for control of muscle tone, posture, and locomotion.[24] Reticulospinal neurons function as command neurons that are organized to coordinate multiple movements involving excitation and inhibition across joints and across limbs. These neurons have divergent projections that may monosynaptically excite motoneuron and interneurons, facilitate or inhibit postural reflexes, and activate polysynaptic pathways via ipsilateral and contralateral descending spinal commissural interneurons. In contrast to the vestibulospinal and corticospinal

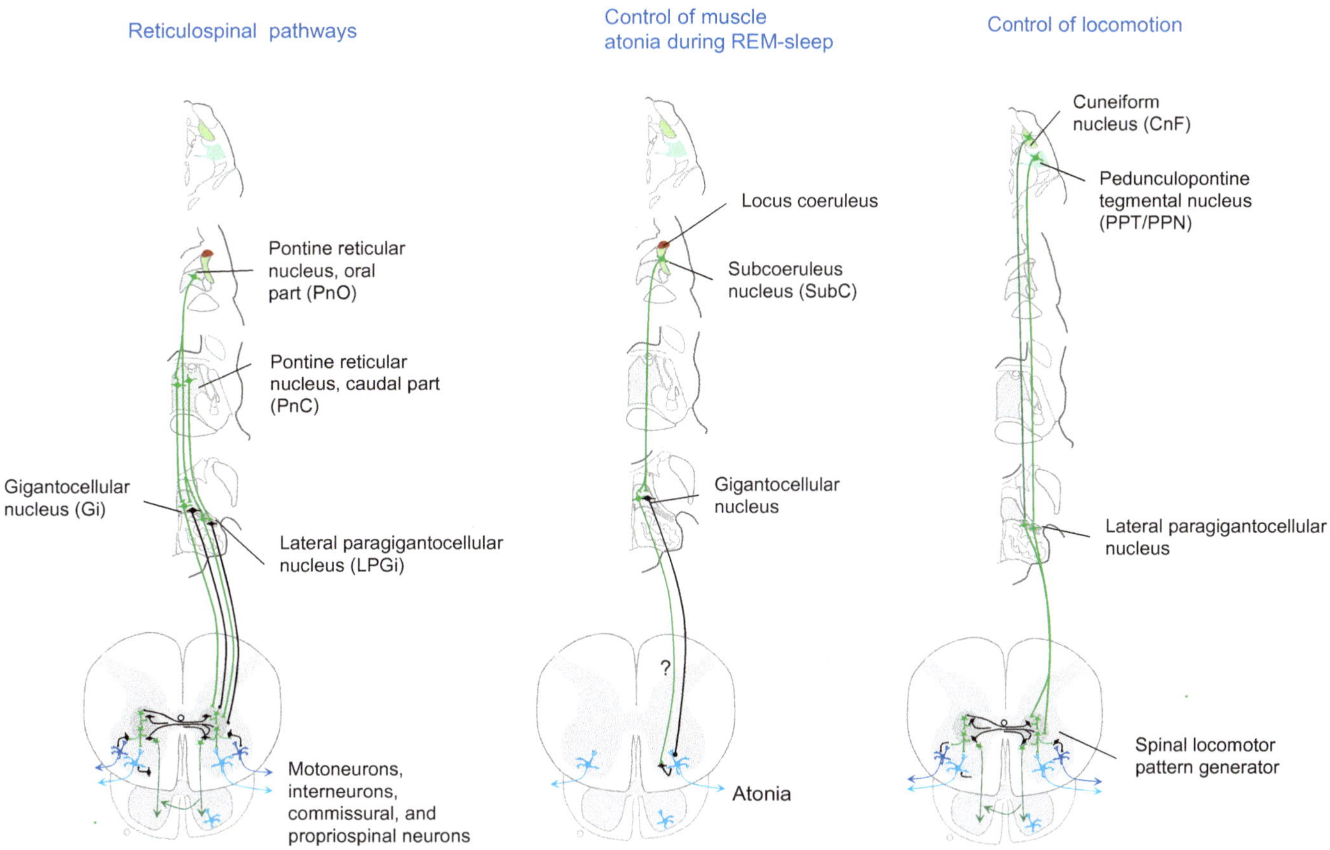

FIGURE 31.6 Reticulospinal systems and regulating muscle tone and locomotion.
The reticular formation comprises the oral pontine reticular nucleus (nucleus reticularis pontis oralis, PnO); the caudal pontine reticular nucleus (nucleus reticularis pontis caudalis, PnC), and the medullary gigantocellular reticular nucleus (Gi), lateral paragigantocellular nucleus (LPGi), and dorsal paragigantocellular nucleus Neurons of the pontine and medullary reticular formation project to the spinal motor apparatus via reticulospinal axons that branch extensively from the cervical to the lumbosacral segments and have divergent projections to motoneuron and interneurons; these projections may utilize glutamate or inhibitory transmitters such as GABA, glycine, or both. During wakefulness, reticulospinal neurons integrate postural and locomotor commands via shared pathways. The prototypical "stop" command is that associated with muscle atonia during REM sleep and originates from glutamatergic REM-on neurons located in the subcoeruleus (sublaterodorsal) nucleus projecting both to the Gi and to inhibitory interneurons in the spinal cord. GABA/glycinergic neurons in the Gi projecting to spinal motoneurons are primarily responsible for atonia in REM sleep. Medullary reticulospinal neurons also control locomotion under the control of the so-called mesencephalic locomotor region (MLR). This includes two groups of glutamatergic neurons, one located in the cuneiform nucleus and the second in the adjacent pedunculopontine tegmental nucleus (PPT/PPN). Descending signals from the MLR reach spinal circuits by recruiting glutamatergic neurons in the LPGi that target intermediate gray matter of the spinal cord.

systems, the reticulospinal system also includes descending GABAergic and glycinergic projections that target propriospinal and spinal commissural interneurons.

Reticulospinal neurons are primarily active during wakefulness and rapid eye movement (REM) sleep. During wakefulness, reticulospinal neurons integrate postural and locomotor commands and activate neural circuits in the spinal locomotor pattern generator. Simultaneous control of postural tone and locomotion involves shared pathways. While descending commands from the reticular formation can stop locomotion, the prototypical "stop" command is that associated with muscle atonia during REM sleep. This command originates from glutamatergic REM-on neurons located in the subcoeruleus (sublaterodorsal) nucleus, which contains glutamatergic neurons that project both to the Gi and to inhibitory interneurons in the spinal cord. Recent evidence indicates that GABA/glycinergic neurons in the Gi projecting to spinal motoneurons are primarily responsible for atonia in REM sleep.[25]

The reticulospinal system mediates the startle reflex, which is an involuntary whole-body jerk that commonly occurs in response to sensory stimuli such as a sudden unexpected noise or touch. In response to loud noise, there is a progressive recruitment of the different muscle groups with the orbicularis oculi starting after 30–40 milliseconds, followed by sternocleidomastoid, upper limb, and finally leg muscles. This reflex originates in the neurons in the caudal pontine reticular nucleus,[26] which receives fast input from sensory pathways and project to cranial and spinal motoneurons, and is controlled by glycinergic inhibition in the spinal cord. Synaptic depression in the sensory synapses in the PnC has been indicated as an underlying mechanism of short-term habituation of startle. Normal startle represents a form of physiological myoclonus.

CONTROL OF GAIT

Brainstem Control of Locomotion

Control of locomotion depends on separate neuronal groups located in the so-called mesencephalic locomotor region (MLR) and their effector neurons in the medullary reticular formation projecting to the spinal locomotor CPG circuits.[27,28] Recent optogenetic studies in rodents indicate that the MLR includes two groups of glutamatergic neurons, one located in the cuneiform nucleus and the second in the adjacent PPN/PPT[29] (Figure 31.6). Glutamatergic neurons in the cuneiform nucleus increase postural muscle tone and promote high-speed during ongoing locomotion. These neurons receive input from structures implicated in escaping behavior, including the PAG and may mediate defensive locomotion. Glutamatergic MLR neurons receive inhibitory GABAergic inputs from the substantia nigra pars reticulata (SNr) and globus pallidus pars interna (GPi) and excitatory inputs from hypothalamic orexin/hypocretin neurons, which promote locomotion and maintain muscle tone via orexin 2 receptors. The PPN/PPT is a hub for integration of arousal, motivation, and motor control.[30,31] In contrast to those in the cuneiform nucleus, glutamatergic PPN/PPT neurons promote phasic muscle activity but do not trigger locomotion. These neurons integrate inputs from several areas contributing to action selection and voluntary movements. The PPN/PPT also contains cholinergic neurons that have a modulatory rather than a driver role in locomotion. This effect is at least partially mediated by direct regulation of dopaminergic midbrain neurons, promoting behavioral reinforcement and action initiation via the basal ganglia circuits and may thus mediate exploratory locomotor behaviors. Both cholinergic and glutamatergic PPN neurons also project to the thalamus and basal forebrain, promoting cortical gamma oscillations consistent with a cortical active state.

The effects of the MLR on spinal locomotor CPG are mediated by reticulospinal neurons located in the caudal medulla, including subdivisions of the Gi and LPGi, which contain intermingled populations of excitatory and inhibitory neurons.[32] Descending signals from the MLR reach spinal circuits by recruiting glutamatergic neurons in the LPGi that target the intermediate gray matter of the spinal cord. The LPGi may have two separate glutamatergic populations that provide for two separate pathways, one controlling locomotor frequency through activation of rhythm-generating circuits and a second regulating gait pattern via commissural interneurons and long propriospinal neurons.[29] Glutamatergic LPGi projections also connect to glycinergic spinal neurons that are likely mediators to execute behavioral arrest during ongoing locomotion.[33]

Forebrain and Cerebellar Control of Muscle Tone and Locomotion

Locomotion has been conceptually subdivided into three categories. Exploratory locomotion is selected by volition through the basal ganglia; primary appetitive locomotion is promoted by the lateral hypothalamus, and defensive locomotion is regulated by the medial hypothalamus and the PAG. Medium spiny neurons of the striatum, via the direct pathway and indirect pathways controlling the output of the GPi/SNr, elicit opposing influence on neuronal activity in glutamatergic MLR neurons of the PPN/PPT. Movement-related dopaminergic SNc neurons display phasic bursting activity shortly before the onset of locomotion and have a role in movement initiation as their activity provides a motivational "go"-signal that encodes the vigor of an upcoming exploratory, goal-directed movement. GABAergic inputs from the nucleus accumbens to the putative MLR via the ventral pallidum may regulate reward-based locomotor behavior. In contrast, high-speed locomotion intended to escape from a threat is produced by activation of glutamatergic neurons in dorsolateral PAG, in part via projections to the cuneiform nucleus, LPGi, or both. Orexin neurons promote maintenance of muscle tone via neurons in the putative MLR. In the waking state, the emotional signals mediated by orexin may increase the level of muscle tone to facilitate locomotion.

Inputs from the cerebral cortex are important for gait initiation and visuomotor coordination of foot placement when subjects encounter an obstacle. The supplementary motor area contributes to anticipatory postural control of step initiation, in part via connections to the vermis of the cerebellum. The dorsal medial cerebellum controls locomotion via the fastigial nucleus and its connections with the reticular formation. The fastigial nucleus receives an efference copy of the spinal CPG in addition to peripheral feedback sensory information via the spinocerebellar tracts and its activity is also affected by visual and head-movement related vestibular and proprioceptive inputs. This multisensory integration may allow the fastigial nucleus to coordinate postural responses during locomotion.

MOTOR NEURON DISEASE

Amyotrophic lateral sclerosis (ALS) is the prototypical motor neuron disease. Converging mechanisms of motor neuron degeneration in this disorder include excitotoxicity and Ca^{2+} overload, mitochondrial dysfunction resulting in reduced ATP production, oxidative stress, misfolded protein accumulation triggering apoptosis; impaired ubiquitin-proteasome system and autophagy; dysregulation of RNA metabolism; reactive gliosis involving both astrocytes and microglia; and disturbance of lipid metabolism.

Mechanism of Selective Motoneuron Vulnerability

There is a selective motoneuron vulnerability in ALS.[34] The FF-type motoneurons are more vulnerable than S-type motoneurons, whereas ocular motoneurons are not affected. The reason for this selective vulnerability is unknown. Increased vulnerability of FF motoneurons may in part result from their higher firing rate, larger dendritic trees, and axon diameters compared to S-type motoneurons. The α3 subunit of the Na^+/K^+ ATPase is selectively expressed in FF-type motoneurons and binds misfolded superoxide dismutase 1. In α-motoneurons, sigma 1 receptors (Sig1Rs) are expressed in the endoplasmic reticulum located close to postsynaptic cholinergic densities expressing M2 muscarinic receptors and enriched of K^+ channels; activation of Sig-1R reduces motor neuron excitability. Studies in knockout mouse models and cases of familial ALS indicate that loss of Sig1R function constitutes a risk factor for motoneuron degeneration. The relative resistance of S-type motoneurons may reflect their expression of endoplasmic reticulum chaperones that prevent accumulation of misfolded proteins. In contrast, selective expression of matrix metalloproteinase-9 in FF-type neurons was proposed as a vulnerability factor.[35] The presence of Ca^{2+}-permeable AMPARs may increase motoneuron vulnerability proteins; the selective resistance of ocular motoneurons in ALS may in part reflect their higher intrinsic Ca^{2+}-buffering capacity due to the expression of calbindin. The pattern of protein expression may affect vulnerability to motoneuron degeneration. In ALS, as in spinal muscular atrophy, there is early involvement of the muscle spindles and a dying-back pathology pattern beginning at the neuromuscular junction and preceding axonal degeneration and motoneuron loss. This is reflected by the finding of decreased amplitudes of miniature endplate potentials, increased jitter, and a decrease in twitch force of muscle units. S-type motor neurons can temporarily compensate for the loss of FF motor neurons by axonal sprouting and reinnervation of denervated endplate. Reinnervation of the neuromuscular junction is regulated by transcription factors, For example, increased expression of the transcription factor peroxisome proliferator-activated receptor gamma coactivator 1-alpha, which drives the formation of oxidative type I (slow-twitch) muscle fibers, promotes sprouting.

Basis of the Clinical Manifestations

A typical feature of ALS and other lower motor neuron syndromes is the presence of fasciculations, which are the manifestation of spontaneous motor unit activity. Fasciculations may originate peripherally due to membrane instability in proximal or distal portions of the motor axon, or from intrinsically hyperexcitable motoneurons. In ALS, complex unstable fasciculations originate in abnormally innervated surviving motor units, likely from a generator site located in distal axonal branches. Axons in ALS patients have increased persistent Na^+ currents and reduction in K^+ currents, which contributes to membrane instability and ectopic activity. In addition, regenerating motor end plates are more sensitive to acetylcholine. Fasciculations may also be triggered by inputs from the motor cortex. Transcranial magnetic stimulation studies suggest that the cortico-motoneuronal input is probably strongest for the lower threshold, early recruited S-type motor units, which are the first producing fasciculations. However, fasciculations are more likely to occur in larger, faster conducting axons that are more excitable. Cortical influences may drive both the manifestations neuropathology in ALS.[36] Disruption of cortical control on the spinal motor apparatus is reflected by impairment of fractionated hand control and skill walking. The split hand syndrome reflects the vulnerability of the direct cortico-motoneuronal connections controlling pincer and precision grips; in this syndrome atrophy initially affects the thenar and first interosseous muscles while hypothenar muscles are unaffected. A clumsy, hesitant gait with a subtle foot drop reflects the more robust cortico-motoneuronal drive to ankle dorsiflexes than plantar flexors in ALS and other upper motor neuron syndromes. Disturbances of this corticobulbar system manifest with prominent disturbances in phonation and articulation.

FOCAL LESIONS AFFECTING THE CORTICOSPINAL SYSTEM

Hemispheric Stroke

Damage to the cortical motor areas due to stroke disrupts the orchestration of spinal modules, resulting in abnormal motor control. Abnormal patterns of muscle activity include merging and fractionation of muscle synergies that vary as a function of both the severity of impairment and time from stroke onset. Diffusor tensor imaging shows plastic changes in the red nucleus of stroke patients with severe CST injury, suggesting that the rubrospinal pathway may have a role in the recovery of hand function in some cases. The startle response, which is mediated by the pontine reticulospinal system, integrates with voluntary movements in humans and may thus provide a potential therapeutic approach for regaining volitional movement after cortical stroke.[37] In this condition, non-crossed cortico-reticular inputs could possibly allow the unaffected ipsilateral cortex to promote reticular formation plasticity and motor functional recovery. Such reticulospinal-mediated functional recovery many not only be important for axial and proximal muscles; studies in nonhuman primates indicate that this pathway is also involved in hand function and could thus be a substrate for functional recovery of hand movements.[20] The startle response can also enhance motor performance in disorders such as Parkinson disease (PD).[38]

Spinal Cord Injury

Following spinal cord injury (SCI) there are many changes in segmental motor circuits that affect both motoneurons and interneurons and reflect interruption of descending corticospinal inputs.[39] After SCI, spasticity results both from increased α-motoneuron excitability due to altered membrane channel and receptor properties and from an imbalance between excitatory and inhibitory influences on motoneurons and interneurons. One fundamental mechanism involves plateau potentials that amplify the response to segmental afferents leading to hyperreflexia. There is downregulation of the potassium chloride cotransporter 2 (KCC2), which reduces the efficacy of $GABA_A$-and glycine receptor mediated inhibition. There is also constitutive activity of excitatory 5-$HT2_C$ receptors due to interruption of descending serotonergic projections from the medullar raphe, as well as increase in the number of glutamatergic inputs to motoneurons from terminals of local interneurons. These plastic changes produce abnormalities in both the intensity and combination of muscle contractions, which are generated involuntarily. Spasticity after SCI is characterized by inability to voluntarily modulate the level of activity of a given motor pool, and to recruit the appropriate combination of motor pools. In addition, numerous anatomical abnormalities in the musculoskeletal architecture can contribute to passive stiffness. One mechanism of hyperreflexia has been attributed to the reduction in presynaptic Ia inhibition. In normal persons low-frequency stimulation of the peroneal nerve produces a short latency inhibition of the soleus H-reflex, which is attributed to presynaptic inhibition of tibial nerve afferents via $GABA_B$ receptors. This inhibitory response is markedly reduced in patients with SCI.

Spasms in SCI are a manifestation of partially recovered function in spinal locomotor CPG circuits and involve activation of commissural and propriospinal neurons that coordinate crossed and reciprocal intersegmental activity responsible for limb coordination during locomotion. These commissural neurons receive strong activation by sensory afferents via NMDARs. Group II muscle afferents may contribute to the enhanced stretch reflexes associated with spasticity. Both levodopa and α2 agonists such as clonidine and tizanidine have been used in attempts to control spasticity. These agents mimic the effects of endogenous norepinephrine in inhibiting these afferents and thus both flexor and extensor reflexes. Baclofen, a $GABA_B$ receptor agonist that reduces glutamate release from primary spinal afferents, is the most common agent used for treatment of spasticity. Gabapentin, which acts by similar mechanism, and riluzole, which inhibits glutamatergic transmission, have also been used with variable success. Botulinum toxin has been used successfully for local, short-term antispastic effects. A decrease in the gap junction protein connexin-36 has been found in SCI, suggesting a decreased electrical coupling in spinal circuits affecting the firing of motoneurons and/or interneurons that may lead to hyperreflexia. Consistent with this possibility, modafinil, which increases electrical coupling between GABA neurons, normalizes the loss of frequency-dependent depression of the H-reflex and thus attenuates hyperreflexia. Locomotor training, which provides instructive proprioceptive signals to the spinal cord, can lead to improvement of function via changes in synaptic transmission in and signaling mechanisms, including KCC2 upregulation in extensor α-motoneurons. Electrical stimulation of afferent inputs can also change the spinal circuitry and promote improvement of motor functions after SCI. In a phase I/II trial, a combined compound consisting of levodopa, carbidopa, and the 5-HT1 agonist buspirone elicited rhythmicity, flexor-extensor reciprocity, and left–right alternation in the lower limbs in some, but not all patients with complete SCI. The reticulospinal system may be involved in recovery of gross hand function after SCI.[40]

DISORDERS AFFECTING MOTOR PATTERN GENERATORS

Freezing of Gait

Patients with PD or atypical parkinsonism often experience episodes of freezing of gait (FOG). This disorder consists of a sudden unpredictable brief episode during which the patients cannot generate an effective forward stepping movement and the feet feel "glued to the ground.[41,42] There are three subtypes of FOG: shuffling with small steps, trembling in place without stepping forward or total akinesia. Most commonly FOG in PD occurs during the OFF state and may be initially L-dopa responsive; however FOG episodes eventually become L-dopa unresponsive or can even be worsened by dopaminergic medication. This could reflect maladaptive plastic changes induced by levodopa therapy, increasing the threshold for dopaminergic stimulation not only in the motor but also in the cognitive and limbic circuits of the basal ganglia that participate in control of gait.[42,43] Overactive GABAergic output from the SNr/GPi to upper brainstem locomotor pattern generators may contribute to gait disturbances in PD. Functional imaging studies support the role of this region in control of locomotion; lesions in this mesopontine region may result in inability to stand and walk or in gait incoordination ("midbrain ataxia"). There is loss of cholinergic PPT/PPN neurons in PD brains, which correlates with the degree of gait difficulties. Loss of cholinergic PPT/PPN output may affect gait by several mechanisms, including reduced ability to regulate muscle tone via descending pathways or loss of ascending projections to the thalamus affecting integration of sensory with attentional signals for postural control.[44] However, deep brain stimulation of the region that includes the PPT/PPN and lateral pontine locomotor areas has yielded heterogeneous results, without consistent improvement in terms of FOG and falls. Recent evidence points to a role of the cerebellum in FOG. Lesion mapping studies show that lesions causing FOG affect a common network involving a focal area of the dorsal medial cerebellum.[45]

Gait festination is one of the most characteristic gait disturbances in patients with PD or atypical parkinsonism. There may be two phenotypes of festination. The first reflect a primary locomotion disturbance due to the so-called sequence effect: a progressive shortening of step length, accompanied by a compensatory increase in cadence. This phenotype strongly relates to FOG with alternating trembling of the leg. The second phenotype results from a postural control problem (forward leaning of the trunk) combined with a balance control deficit (inappropriately small balance-correcting steps).[46]

REM Sleep Behavior Disorder

The biomarker of REM sleep behavior disorder (RBD) is lack of normal loss of muscle tone during REM sleep detected during polysomnography. The cause of RBD is breakdown of the normal brainstem circuit involved in normal REM sleep.[47] The most common structures exhibiting neuropathology or neurodegeneration in RBD patients are the subcoeruleus, gigantocellular reticular nucleus, DR, PPT, and ventromedial medulla. A retrospective case series provided further evidence that the dorsal pontine tegmentum and rostral ventromedial medulla are most commonly involved in lesions associated with RBD.[47] Recent studies indicate that loss of inhibitory projections from the ventromedial reticular formation to the spinal cord as the primary substrate for loss of muscle atonia during REM sleep cause of RBD.[25]

Restless Legs Syndrome (RLS) and Periodic Leg Movements of Sleep

Restless legs syndrome (RLS) manifests as an urge to move and is commonly associated with periodic limb movements of sleep (PLMS). Loss of supraspinal inhibitory modulation, or increased excitability in spinal circuits, or both are possible underlying mechanisms.[48] Studies have shown increased F wave duration, decreased tibialis anterior cutaneous silent period, and increased excitability of motor axons in RLS patients. Transcutaneous spinal direct weak current stimulation over the thoracic spinal cord via surface electrodes reduced RLS symptoms, indicating a spinal source of hyperexcitability, perhaps due to interruption of descending supraspinal inhibition. The periodic leg movements are possibly generated by the spinal CPG for gait, which generates rhythmic, repetitive, and stereotyped movements that are characteristic of PLMS. There is also similarity in movement and muscle recruitment patterns between these movements, the spinal flexor withdrawal reflex, and the Babinski response. In patients with RLS there is increased excitability of the flexor withdrawal reflex compared to controls, whereas crossed extensor reflex responses are similar, and patellar and plantar reflex responses are decreased. Impaired D2 receptor-mediated dopaminergic inhibition of spinal cord circuits could explain the beneficial effect of dopaminergic agonists in RLS. Studies show decreased dopamine reuptake, D2 receptor downregulation, and increased D1 receptor mediated excitatory effects. It has also been hypothesized that iron deficiency may produce up regulation of adenosine A2A and downregulation of adenosine A1 receptors, leading to increase in synaptic glutamate concentrations in the spinal cord. Currently, the first-line treatment for RLS are the $\alpha 2\delta$ ligands gabapentin (including gabapentin enacarbil) and pregabalin, which are particularly useful in patients with coexistent pain or insomnia. The main complication of dopaminergic agonists such as pramipexole, ropinirole and to a lesser extent rotigotine is augmentation, which is characterized by worsening of RLS with increased doses, earlier onset of RLS, and spreading of symptoms to other body parts. Augmentation may reflect downregulation of inhibitory D2/D3 and/or upregulation of excitatory D1 receptors. Iron supplementation in patients with serum ferritin levels ≤ 75 μg/L is also recommended. Opioids such as oxycodone/naloxone may be carefully considered in selected refractory cases.

Disorders of Central Nervous System Hyperexcitability

Autoimmune disorders affecting GABAergic or glycinergic transmission in the brainstem or spinal cord may manifest with excessive excitability in motor circuits leading to muscle stiffness and exaggerated startle responses. These include stiff person syndrome due to autoantibodies against glutamic acid decarboxylase, and progressive encephalomyelitis with rigidity and myoclonus due to autoantibodies against glycine receptors.[49,50] Exaggerated startle may also occur in inflammatory or anoxic injuries of the brainstem, drug intoxication, and hereditary disorders such as hereditary hyperekplexia. Disorders of inhibitory neurotransmission are discussed in another chapter of this book.

Another manifestation of excessive brainstem or spinal excitability is myoclonus.[51] Reticular reflex myoclonus manifests as generalized jerks that occur at rest, are stimulus sensitive, and are characterized by bilateral rostral-to-caudal recruitment that originates from the medullary reticular formation and primarily involves axial and proximal limb muscles. Propriospinal myoclonus primarily affects axial muscles and is characterized by simultaneous bilateral rostral and caudal recruitment originating from the spinal cord. Segmental myoclonus is generated at the particular segment or contiguous segments of the brainstem and or spinal cord. The most common type is palatal myoclonus, which is characterized by rhythmic or semi-rhythmic activation of the affected muscles in the range of 0.5–3 Hz. Essential palatal myoclonus involves the tensor veli palatini, symptomatic palatal myoclonus is due to contractions of the levator veli palatini

KEY POINTS

- The segmental motor apparatus includes motor neurons (motoneurons) and interneurons, both of which receive segmental afferent and descending inputs.
- Spinal motoneurons undergo sustained depolarizations referred to as plateau potentials.
- Motoneurons are activated by glutamatergic inputs originating from cortical and brainstem projections, local interneurons, and primary afferents, and inhibited by GABA and/or glycinergic inputs from local interneurons and descending reticulospinal pathways.
- Cholinergic, monoaminergic, and other signals modulate motoneuron excitability.
- Small (S) motoneurons innervate velocity slow-twitch, fatigue-resistant (type I) fibers.
- Large motoneurons innervate fast-twitch (type II) fibers including fatigue-resistant (FR) and fatiguable (FF) units.
- S-type motoneurons are typically recruited earlier than those innervating FR and FF fibers.
- The three main sources of segmental reflexes are the muscle spindles, innervated by Ia (dynamic) and II (static) afferents; the Golgi tendon organs, innervated by type Ib afferents; and the flexor reflex afferents.
- Spinal interneurons mediate segmental reflexes generate motor synergies, and initiate the motor pattern for locomotion.
- Propriospinal interneurons may have an important role in motor recovery after SCI in humans.
- Descending cortical commands conveyed via the corticospinal tract provide flexible control of spinal interneurons and motoneurons.
- The reticulospinal and vestibulospinal tracts control posture, muscle tone, and locomotion.
- The rubrospinal tract may contribute to recovery of some motor function of the upper limb following stroke.
- Vestibulospinal reflexes coordinate head and neck movements with the trunk and body to maintain the head in an upright position and postural tone against gravity.
- Reticulospinal neurons coordinate multiple movements involving excitation and inhibition across joints and across limbs.
- The gigantocellular reticular nucleus receives inputs from the subcoeruleus nucleus and via projections to the spinal cord elicits muscle atonia during REM sleep.
- Control of locomotion depends on separate neuronal groups located in the so-called mesencephalic locomotor region (MLR) which includes glutamatergic neurons of the cuneiform and pedunculopontine tegmental nuclei.
- Descending signals from the MLR reach spinal circuits by recruiting glutamatergic neurons in the medullary lateral paragigantocellular nucleus.
- Locomotion is regulated by inputs from the cerebral cortex, basal ganglia, and cerebellum.
- There is selective motoneuron vulnerability to degeneration in ALS.
- Spasticity following spinal cord injury (SCI) results from plastic changes that result both from increased α-motoneuron excitability and from an imbalance between excitatory and inhibitory influences on motoneurons and interneurons.
- The mechanisms of freezing of gait in Parkinson disease are probably multifactorial.
- Lack of muscle atonia during REM sleep in REM sleep behavior disorder may reflect neurodegeneration of the subcoeruleus and gigantocellular reticular nucleus.
- Autoimmune disorders affecting GABAergic or glycinergic transmission in the brainstem or spinal cord may manifest with excessive excitability in brainstem and/or spinal motor circuits, leading to muscle stiffness and exaggerated startle responses.

REFERENCES

1. Miri A, Azim E, Jessell TM. Edging toward entelechy in motor control. Neuron 2013;80:827–834.
2. Jessell TM, Surmeli G, Kelly JS. Motor neurons and the sense of place. Neuron 2011;72:419–424.

3. Kanning KC, Kaplan A, Henderson CE. Motor neuron diversity in development and disease. Annu Rev Neurosci 2010;33:409–440.
4. Rekling JC, Funk GD, Bayliss DA, Dong XW, Feldman JL. Synaptic control of motoneuronal excitability. Physiol Rev 2000;80:767–852.
5. Perrier JF, Cotel F. Serotonergic modulation of spinal motor control. Curr Opin Neurobiol 2014;33C:1–7.
6. Burke RE. Sir Charles Sherrington's the integrative action of the nervous system: a centenary appreciation. Brain 2007;130:887–894.
7. Cote MP, Murray LM, Knikou M. Spinal control of locomotion: individual neurons, their circuits and functions. Front Physiol 2018;9:784.
8. Pierrot-Deseilligny E. Assessing changes in presynaptic inhibition of Ia afferents during movement in humans. J Neurosci Methods 1997;74:189–199.
9. Klarner T, Zehr EP. Sherlock Holmes and the curious case of the human locomotor central pattern generator. J Neurophysiol 2018;120:53–77.
10. Minassian K, Hofstoetter US, Dzeladini F, Guertin PA, Ijspeert A. The human central pattern generator for locomotion. Neuroscientist 2017:1073858417699790.
11. Bizzi E, Cheung VC. The neural origin of muscle synergies. Front Comput Neurosci 2013;7:51.
12. Briggman KL, Kristan WB. Multifunctional pattern-generating circuits. Annu Rev Neurosci 2008;31:271–294.
13. Roh J, Cheung VC, Bizzi E. Modules in the brain stem and spinal cord underlying motor behaviors. J Neurophysiol 2011;106:1363–1378.
14. Nielsen JB. Human spinal motor control. Annu Rev Neurosci 2016;39:81–101.
15. Lemon RN. Descending pathways in motor control. Annu Rev Neurosci 2008;31:195–218.
16. Lemon RN. Descending pathways in motor control. Annu Rev Neurosci 2008;31:195–218.
17. Cohen O, Sherman E, Zinger N, Perlmutter S, Prut Y. Getting ready to move: transmitted information in the corticospinal pathway during preparation for movement. Curr Opin Neurobiol 2010;20:696–703.
18. Riddle CN, Edgley SA, Baker SN. Direct and indirect connections with upper limb motoneurons from the primate reticulospinal tract. J Neurosci 2009;29:4993–4999.
19. Holstege JC, Kuypers HG. Brainstem projections to spinal motoneurons: an update. Neuroscience 1987;23:809–821.
20. Kim H, Lee H, Jung KI, Ohn SH, Yoo WK. Changes in diffusion metrics of the red nucleus in chronic stroke patients with severe corticospinal tract injury: a preliminary study. Ann Rehabil Med 2018;42:396–405.
21. Holstege G, Bandler R, Saper CB. The emotional motor system. Prog Brain Res 1996;107:3–6.
22. Brownstone RM, Chopek JW. Reticulospinal systems for tuning motor commands. Front Neural Circuits 2018;12:30.
23. Takakusaki K, Chiba R, Nozu T, Okumura T. Brainstem control of locomotion and muscle tone with special reference to the role of the mesopontine tegmentum and medullary reticulospinal systems. J Neural Transm (Vienna) 2016;123:695–729.
24. Kim LH, Sharma S, Sharples SA, Mayr KA, Kwok CHT, Whelan PJ. Integration of descending command systems for the generation of context-specific locomotor behaviors. Front Neurosci 2017;11:581.
25. Valencia Garcia S, Brischoux F, Clement O, et al. Ventromedial medulla inhibitory neuron inactivation induces REM sleep without atonia and REM sleep behavior disorder. Nat Commun 2018;9:504.
26. Schmid S, Simons NS, Schnitzler HU. Cellular mechanisms of the trigeminally evoked startle response. Eur J Neurosci 2003;17:1438–1444.
27. Sherman D, Fuller PM, Marcus J, et al. Anatomical location of the mesencephalic locomotor region and its possible role in locomotion, posture, cataplexy, and parkinsonism. Front Neurol 2015;6:140.
28. Ferreira-Pinto MJ, Ruder L, Capelli P, Arber S. Connecting circuits for supraspinal control of locomotion. Neuron 2018;100:361–374.
29. Ausborn J, Shevtsova NA, Caggiano V, Danner SM, Rybak IA. Computational modeling of brainstem circuits controlling locomotor frequency and gait. Elife 2019;8.
30. Gut NK, Winn P. The pedunculopontine tegmental nucleus: a functional hypothesis from the comparative literature. Mov Disord 2016;31:615–624.
31. Mena-Segovia J, Bolam JP. Rethinking the pedunculopontine nucleus: from cellular organization to function. Neuron 2017;94:7–18.
32. Capelli P, Pivetta C, Soledad Esposito M, Arber S. Locomotor speed control circuits in the caudal brainstem. Nature 2017;551:373–377.
33. Danner SM, Wilshin SD, Shevtsova NA, Rybak IA. Central control of interlimb coordination and speed-dependent gait expression in quadrupeds. J Physiol 2016;594:6947–6967.
34. Nijssen J, Comley LH, Hedlund E. Motor neuron vulnerability and resistance in amyotrophic lateral sclerosis. Acta Neuropathol 2017;133:863–885.
35. Comley L, Allodi I, Nichterwitz S, et al. Motor neurons with differential vulnerability to degeneration show distinct protein signatures in health and ALS. Neuroscience 2015;291:216–229.
36. Eisen A, Braak H, Del Tredici K, Lemon R, Ludolph AC, Kiernan MC. Cortical influences drive amyotrophic lateral sclerosis. J Neurol Neurosurg Psychiatry 2017;88:917–924.
37. Rothwell JC. The startle reflex, voluntary movement, and the reticulospinal tract. Suppl Clin Neurophysiol 2006;58:223–231.
38. Anzak A, Tan H, Pogosyan A, et al. Subcortical evoked activity and motor enhancement in Parkinson's disease. Exp Neurol 2016;277:19–26.
39. Roy RR, Edgerton VR. Neurobiological perspective of spasticity as occurs after a spinal cord injury. Exp Neurol 2012;235:116–122.
40. Baker SN, Perez MA. Reticulospinal contributions to gross hand function after human spinal cord injury. J Neurosci 2017;37:9778–9784.
41. Giladi N, Nieuwboer A. Understanding and treating freezing of gait in parkinsonism, proposed working definition, and setting the stage. Mov Disord 2008;23 Suppl 2:S423–425.
42. Nonnekes J, Bereau M, Bloem BR. Freezing of gait and its levodopa paradox. JAMA Neurol 2019;77(3):287–288.
43. Lewis SJ, Shine JM. The next step: a common neural mechanism for freezing of gait. Neuroscientist 2016;22:72–82.

44. Snijders AH, Takakusaki K, Debu B, et al. Physiology of freezing of gait. Ann Neurol 2016;80:644–659.
45. Fasano A, Laganiere SE, Lam S, Fox MD. Lesions causing freezing of gait localize to a cerebellar functional network. Ann Neurol 2017;81:129–141.
46. Nonnekes J, Giladi N, Guha A, Fietzek UM, Bloem BR, Ruzicka E. Gait festination in parkinsonism: introduction of two phenotypes. J Neurol 2019;266:426–430.
47. Iranzo A. Parasomnias and sleep-related movement disorders in older adults. Sleep Med Clin 2018;13:51–61.
48. Dafkin C, McKinon W, Kerr S. Restless legs syndrome: clinical changes in nervous system excitability at the spinal cord level. Sleep Med Rev 2019;47:9–17.
49. Carvajal-Gonzalez A, Leite MI, Waters P, et al. Glycine receptor antibodies in PERM and related syndromes: characteristics, clinical features and outcomes. Brain 2014;137:2178–2192.
50. McKeon A, Vincent A. Autoimmune movement disorders. Handb Clin Neurol 2016;133:301–315.
51. Caviness JN. Myoclonus. Continuum (Minneap Minn) 2019;25:1055–1080.

32 Brainstem Mechanisms of Motor Control

OVERVIEW

The control of brainstem motor function has a major role in essentially all activities of daily living, and some of these are critical for survival. The brainstem gaze-control mechanisms maintain optimal visual acuity during binocular vision by ensuring that the images of objects remain steady and stimulate corresponding areas of the retina. Control of eye movements depends primarily on feedforward commands from the vestibular nuclei and cerebral cortex under the control of the cerebellum. Vocalization, speech, swallowing, and control of the upper airway during respiration are periodic or rhythmic motor acts that require coordinated motor plans integrated at the level of pons and medulla. These activities involve central pattern generator (CPG) networks driven by afferent inputs under the control of the cerebral cortex. Disorders affecting brainstem motor function are commonly encountered in clinical practice. The main aims of this chapter are to review: (1) the brainstem mechanism regulating eye movements, (2) the cortical and cerebellar influence on these circuits, and (3) the mechanism involved in swallowing and speech.

BRAINSTEM OCULOMOTOR NETWORKS

The brainstem gaze-control mechanisms are integrated at the levels of the pons and midbrain (Figure 32.1).These systems are involved in (1) fixation, which holds the image of a stationary object on the fovea by minimizing ocular drifts; (2) vestibulo-ocular reflexes (VORs) that hold the images of the world steady during brief head rotations or linear movements; (3) optokinetic responses that hold the visual images steady on the retina during sustained head rotation (4) short-latency ocular following responses to motion of the visual scene; (5) smooth pursuit that holds the image of a small moving object target on the fovea; (6) quick phase of nystagmus that reset the eyes during prolonged rotation and direct gaze toward the oncoming visual scene; (7) saccades that rapidly bring image of object of interest on to the fovea; and (8) vergence that move the eyes in opposite directions so that the images of a single object are placed and held simultaneously in the fovea of each eye. There are excellent reviews regarding the brainstem mechanisms underlying these functions,[1,2,3] and only few basic concepts will be emphasized in this chapter.

Ocular Motoneurons

The motoneurons innervating the extraocular muscles are located in the abducens (cranial nerve-CN VI), trochlear (CN IV), and oculomotor complex (CN III) nuclei. The abducens nucleus contains both the motoneurons that innervate the ipsilateral lateral rectus and internuclear neurons that send axons via the medial longitudinal fasciculus (MLF) to activate contralateral medial rectus motoneurons in the ventral cell column of the oculomotor complex. The abducens nucleus also contains a third group of neurons, the paramedian tract neurons that project to the flocculus and contribute to gaze-holding. Vertical eye movements are controlled by the trochlear nucleus innervating the contralateral superior oblique and by subnuclei of the oculomotor complex innervating the ipsilateral inferior rectus (dorsal nucleus), ipsilateral inferior oblique (intermediate nucleus), and contralateral superior rectus (medial cell column). Ocular motoneurons are active even when the eye is in primary position; they are recruited in a fixed sequence and their discharge frequency is proportional to the velocity and position of the eye in the orbit. Ocular motoneurons receive excitatory glutamatergic and inhibitory glycinergic or GABAergic inputs. During eye movements, ocular motoneurons exhibit a pulse and a step of firing. The pulse drives the globe to an eccentric position in the orbit whereas the step maintains this new position. Most extraocular muscle fibers are fast-twitch-generating fibers innervated by a single axon terminal. The remainder are innervated by multiple axon terminals and mediate small, slow contractions that may modulate eye movement for more stable vision. Twitch motoneurons receive premotor inputs involved in generation of movements, such as vestibular neurons or saccadic burst neurons; nontwitch motoneurons receive inputs from premotor nuclei involved in gaze-holding.

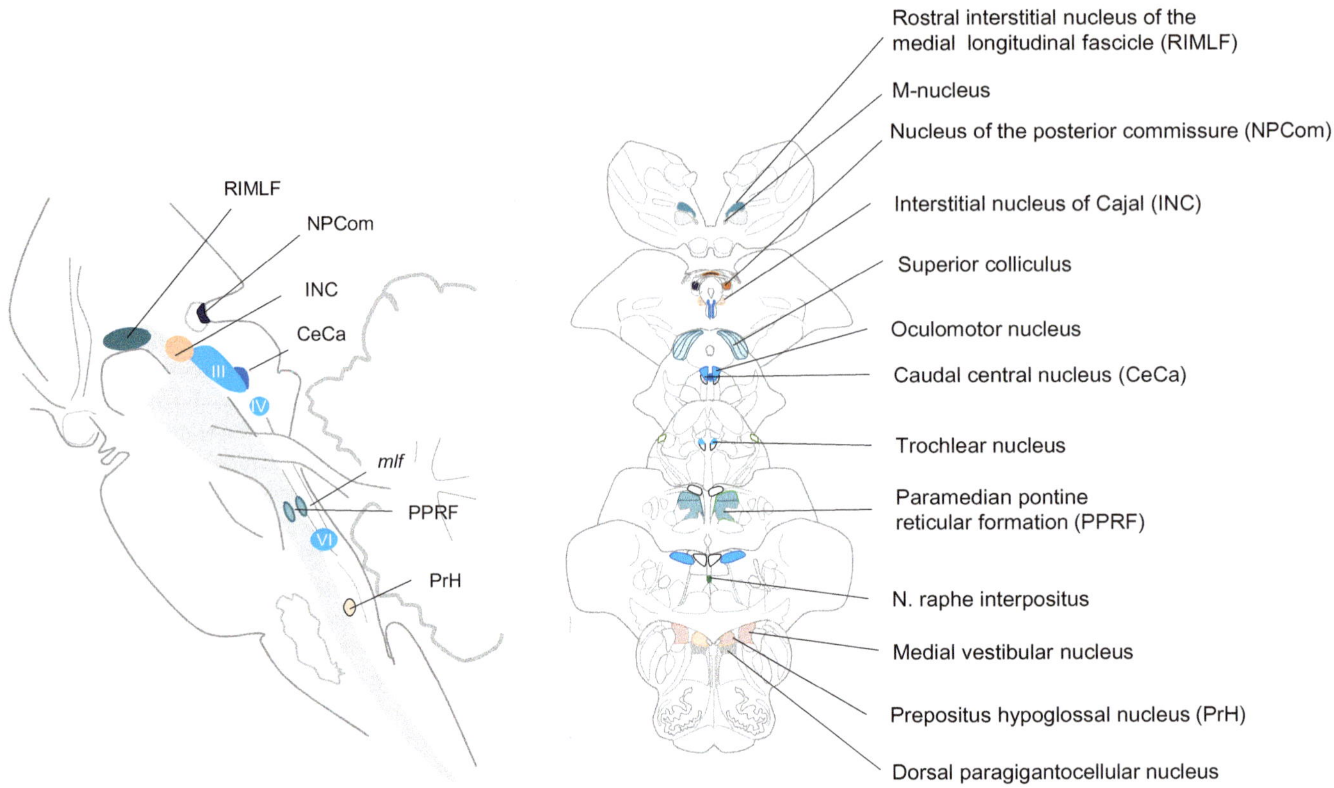

FIGURE 32.1 Brainstem control of eye movements.
The motoneurons innervating the extraocular muscles are located in the abducens (cranial nerve VI) nucleus, trochlear (cranial nerve IV) nucleus, and oculomotor complex (cranial nerve III). The abducens nucleus contains both the motoneurons that innervate the ipsilateral lateral rectus and internuclear neurons that send axons via the contralateral medial longitudinal fasciculus (mlf) to activate medial rectus motoneurons in the contralateral oculomotor complex. Horizontal saccades are triggered by excitatory burst neurons located in the paramedian pontine reticular formation (PPRF); the excitatory burst neurons for vertical and torsional saccades are located in the rostral interstitial nucleus of the median longitudinal fasciculus (RIMLF). Omnipause neurons are located in the nucleus raphe interpositus (NRi). The neural integrator network for horizontal gaze-holding primarily involves the prepositus hypoglossal nucleus (PrH). The neural integrator for vertical gaze holding is the interstitial nucleus of Cajal (INC). This nucleus, via interactions with the medial vestibular (MVN) and superior vestibular nuclei also participates in the vertical vestibulo-ocular reflex (VOR) and the ocular tilt-reaction. The premotor neurons for vergence eye movements are located in the medial mesencephalic reticular formation (not shown). The superior colliculus contains saccadic burst neurons that discharge before both reflex and voluntary saccades that mediate the visual grasp reflex in response to salient or novel stimuli. Its rostral pole harbors fixation neurons that increased their activity during visual fixation. Vertical eye movements are associated with synchronous movements of the upper eyelid. The levator palpebrae motoneurons are located in the central caudal nuclear nucleus, dorsal to the caudal pole of the oculomotor nuclear complex. The common premotor command for both eyelid elevation and upward eye movement originates from a small group of neuron, referred to as the M group, located in the rostral midbrain. The nucleus of the posterior commissure (NPCom) located in the pretectal region, participates in eyelid elevation.

Vestibulo-Ocular Reflexes

The vestibular system detects head movement in space and has a fundamental role in stabilization of gaze during head motion. The three semicircular canals (SCCs), lateral (horizontal), anterior, and posterior, sense angular acceleration and provide inputs to all vestibular nuclei. The otolith organs, utricle and saccule, sense linear acceleration including gravity and translational movements. The utricle projects primarily to the medial vestibular nucleus and the saccule projects to the lateral vestibular nucleus. The vestibular nuclei contain two main categories of neurons. Vestibulo-ocular reflex (VOR) neurons stabilize gaze and hold the image steady to assure clear vision during brief head rotation. Vestibular-only neurons project to the spinal cord and mediate the vestibulospinal reflexes as discussed in the previous chapter.

The angular and linear VORs are important for clear vision during locomotion. The angular VOR triggered by SCC input generates eye movements at short-latency to compensate for rotational head perturbations. The translational or linear VOR depends on the otolith organs and compensates for linear head movements by generating eye movements that are highly dependent on the subject's viewing distance. Whereas the angular VOR usually generates eye movements that hold the line of sight on the target, the eye movements generated by the linear VOR during viewing of a near target minimizes the relative motion between the near target and the distant background; this strategy is used to determine the relative distances of objects as the subject walks through the environment. The most direct VOR pathway involves vestibular afferents projecting to VOR neurons in the medial and superior vestibular nuclei, which send both excitatory projections to contralateral ocular motoneurons eliciting conjugate gaze deviation opposite to the direction of head movement, and inhibitory ipsilateral projections to antagonist motoneurons (Figure 32.2). The horizontal VOR is largely mediated by neurons of the medial vestibular nucleus, which send excitatory projections to the contralateral abducens nucleus. Abducens motoneurons activate the ipsilateral lateral rectus, whereas internuclear neurons in the abducens nucleus project via the contralateral MLF to activate contralateral medial rectus motoneurons in the oculomotor complex.

Vertical and torsional VORs are driven by inputs from the medial and superior vestibular nuclei projecting via the MLF to the trochlear and oculomotor nuclei. During sustained head rotation, the vestibular signal for the VOR is prolonged by a mechanism of velocity storage, which depends on the tonic discharge of the vestibular afferents. Most regions of the vestibular nuclear complex are connected bilaterally by commissural fibers. These connections support interaction between reciprocal SCC pairs and are also important for the velocity storage mechanism. While the utricular pathways to the medial vestibular nucleus are thought to be involved in the horizontal linear VOR and vestibulo-ocular motor learning functions, the saccular pathways are considered a component of the vestibulospinal system and might be more involved with the vertical linear VOR.

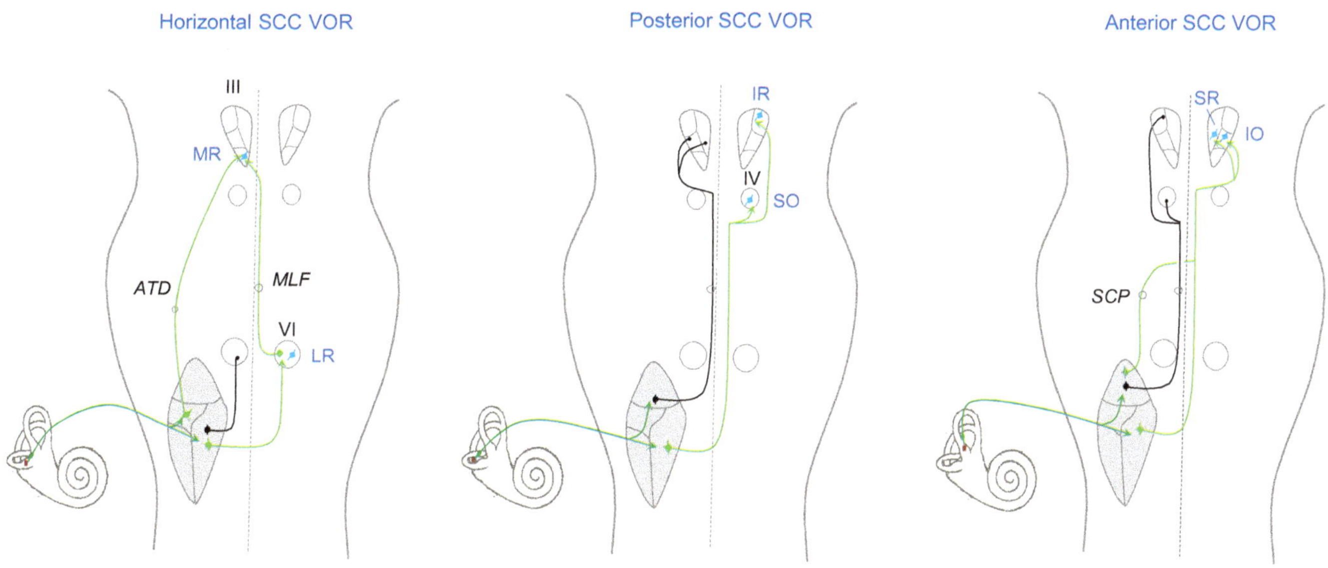

FIGURE 32.2 Pathways for the vestibulo-ocular reflexes.
The three semicircular canals (SCCs), lateral (horizontal), anterior, and posterior, sense angular acceleration and provide inputs to all vestibular nuclei. The otolith organs, utricle and saccule, sense linear acceleration including gravity and translational movements. The most direct vestibulo-ocular reflex (VOR) pathway involves vestibular afferents projecting to VOR neurons in the medial and superior vestibular nuclei, which send both excitatory projections to contralateral ocular motoneurons, eliciting conjugate gaze deviation opposite to the direction of head movement, and inhibitory ipsilateral projections to antagonist motoneurons. The horizontal VOR is largely mediated by neurons of the medial vestibular nucleus, which send excitatory projections to the contralateral abducens nucleus (VI). Abducens motoneurons activate the ipsilateral lateral rectus (LR), whereas internuclear neurons in the abducens nucleus project via the contralateral median longitudinal fasciculus (MLF) to activate contralateral medial rectus (MR) motoneurons in the oculomotor complex (III). Vertical and torsional VORs are driven by inputs from the medial and superior vestibular nuclei projecting via the MLF the trochlear (IV) and oculomotor nuclei. The posterior SCC VOR elicits conjugate downward movements by activating the contralateral superior oblique (SO) and inferior rectus (IR). The anterior SCC triggers upward gaze by activating the contralateral superior rectus (SR) and inferior oblique (IO) motoneurons.

Smooth Ocular Tracking Movements

Motion of images across the retina, known as retinal slip, is the primary stimulus to a range of smooth ocular tracking movements, including the ocular following response, optokinetic nystagmus, and smooth pursuit. The ocular following responses represent an early, low-level response of the visual system to a moving stimulus. The vestibular nuclei provide the drive to ocular motoneurons during optokinetic and smooth-pursuit movements. Optokinetic nystagmus is a response to sustained self-rotation, such as occurs during locomotion, when vestibular eye movements are progressively less able to stabilize images on the retina. Optic flow information during visual navigation generates optokinetic eye movements that complement the VOR to ensure gaze stability during self-motion. VOR neurons integrate visual and vestibular input to generate premotor commands required to drive these optokinetic responses. Optokinetic responses are conventionally tested as a large visual surround (such as moving stripes in a rotating drum) rotates about the subject for up to a minute, which induces a strong percept of self-rotation.

Smooth pursuit makes it possible to track small targets that move across the stationary background and depends on decoding visual motion, selecting a target of interest and keeping the image of the target on or near the fovea. An essential component of smooth pursuit is that attention be paid to the moving target relative to the background. Since the latency for smooth pursuit initiation is over 100 ms, perfect tracking implies that the brain must use a prediction mechanism to achieve tracking without phase shift between the eye and target. Smooth pursuit directs gaze to the object moving toward the ipsilateral hemispace. The pathway for smooth pursuit is initiated by neurons located in the medial superior temporal cortex and ventral intraparietal area, as discussed later. These neurons encode motion of visual objects and project to the dorsolateral pontine nuclei, which relay this information to the contralateral flocculus and paraflocculus and caudal vermis of the cerebellum. These cerebellar regions project to the vestibular nuclei to drive smooth pursuit. Retinal inputs conveyed via the accessory optic tract when the gaze is slipping from the fixation point (retinal slip) are also used for correction of eye movements.

Saccades

Saccades are rapid eye movements that redirect the fovea toward features of interest. Quick phases of nystagmus are the evolutionary forerunners of saccades, and reset eye position during sustained vestibular or optokinetic stimulation upon spontaneous drift of the eyes. Microsaccades are continuous small eye movements that occur upon attempt to fixate the eyes on a stationary visual target and are important for preventing visual adaptation (fading) of peripheral retinal images. Saccades, quick phases of nystagmus, and microsaccades are generated by the same brainstem machinery. Other types of saccades include random, spontaneous saccades; reflexive saccades generated by a novel stimulus that unexpectedly appears in the environment; voluntary saccades that are part of a goal-oriented behavior or a response to a command; predictive saccades generated in anticipation of or search of the appearance of a target; memory -guided saccades generated to a location where the target was previously present; and antisaccades generated in the opposite direction to the sudden appearance of a target. Horizontal saccades are triggered by excitatory burst neurons located in the paramedian pontine reticular formation (PPRF), including neurons of the caudal pontine nucleus and dorsomedial tegmental nucleus (Figure 31.7). Excitatory PPRF burst neurons provide the velocity command (pulse) to the ipsilateral abducens nucleus motoneurons and internuclear neurons; and drive inhibitory burst neurons located in the dorsal paragigantocellular that project to the motoneurons of the contralateral abducens nucleus. The excitatory burst neurons for vertical and torsional saccades and quick phases of vertical nystagmus are located in the rostral interstitial nucleus of the median longitudinal fasciculus (RIMLF) located in the rostral midbrain. Burst neurons for upward saccades project bilaterally to motoneurons supplying elevator extraocular muscles; burst neurons for downward saccades project ipsilaterally to motoneurons supplying depressor extraocular muscles. Saccades are triggered by descending inputs from the cerebral cortex, either directly or via the superior colliculus, as described later.

Visual Fixation

Omnipause neurons located in the nucleus raphe interpositus tonically inhibit the saccadic premotor neurons during fixation and slow eye movements. These omnipause neurons receive excitatory inputs from the fixation area of the superior colliculus and from the fastigial oculomotor region and send glycinergic, largely crossed inhibitory projections to the saccadic burst neurons in the PPRF and RIMLF. The initiation of a saccade requires transient inhibition and pause of firing of these omnipause neurons.

Gaze-Holding

The maintenance of eccentric eye position after a saccade requires the activity of a neural integrator network that provides a step command to ocular motoneurons. The neural integrator network for horizontal gaze-holding primary involves the prepositus hypoglossal nucleus (Figure 32.1). This nucleus is a key constituent of a vestibular-cerebellar-brainstem neural network that ensures that the eyes are held steady in all positions of gaze.[4] It projects to the extraocular motor nuclei, cerebellum, brainstem reticular formation, inferior olivary nucleus, and superior colliculus. The neural integrator for vertical gaze holding is the interstitial nucleus of Cajal (INC). This nucleus, via interactions with the medial and superior vestibular nuclei also participates in the vertical VOR and the ocular tilt-reaction. The INC also contributes to inhibition of vertical saccades The INC sends intestitiospinal projections that together with projections from the vestibular nuclei(medial vestibulospinal tract) and superior colliculus (tectospinal tract) travel in the descending portion of the MLF to reach the cervical spinal cord and participate in coordination of head and eye movements.

Vergence

The premotor neurons related to vergence eye movements are located in the medial mesencephalic reticular formation dorsal to the oculomotor complex at the level of the tectum, and provide commands to the medial rectus subdivisions of the ocular motor nuclei. During horizontal head acceleration the command for vergence is provided by the ascending tract of Deiters originating in the rostral portions of the vestibular nuclear, particularly the lateral vestibular nucleus, which project ipsilaterally to activate medial rectus motoneurons. The nucleus reticularis tegmenti pontis, which conveys saccadic signals to the cerebellum, also contains phasic-tonic cells that increase their firing during the near response, including convergence and accommodation.[5]

Superior Colliculus as an Integral Component of the Attention and Orienting Systems

The superior colliculus is a fundamental component of the attention and orientation systems. Its superficial layers receive retinotopically organized afferents from the retina and visual cortex representing the contralateral visual field; from brainstem auditory relay nuclei; and from somatosensory pathways. The intermediate and deep layers of the superior colliculus are organized into a motor map and are involved in sensorimotor transformations for orientation of the eyes, head, and the rest of the body toward novel stimuli in the contralateral hemispace. The deep layers contain saccadic burst neurons that discharge before both reflex and voluntary saccades and project to the burst neurons of the PPRF and RIMLF. These connections mediate the visual grasp reflex, which is a component of an integrated orienting response to salient or novel stimuli. In contrast, the rostral pole of the superior colliculus contains a map of the contralateral fovea and harbors fixation neurons that increased their activity during visual fixation. These neurons suppress saccades both via local inhibition of saccadic burst neurons in the intermediate and deep layers and via projections to the brainstem omnipause neurons. The superior colliculus also projects via the crossed tectospinal tract and then descending portion the MLF to upper cervical motoneurons controlling neck muscles, thus participating in head-eye coordination.

Eyelid Movement and Blinks

The oculomotor system interacts with the eyelid system. Vertical eye movements are associated with synchronous movements of the upper eyelid; blink-eliciting stimuli trigger not only transient eye closure but also eye movements. The eyelids are moved by interaction between the levator palpebrae and the orbicularis oculi muscles. The smooth superior tarsal muscle, innervated by sympathetic fibers from the superior cervical ganglion, contributes to retraction of the upper eyelid. The levator palpebrae motoneurons are located in the central caudal nucleus, located dorsal to the caudal pole of the oculomotor nuclear complex. In the awake state these neurons receive a tonic excitatory input that decreases with fatigue. The common premotor command for both eyelid elevation and upward eye movement originates from a small group of neurons, referred to as the M group, which is located in the rostral midbrain immediately medial to the caudal one-third of the RIMLF (Figure 31.7). These premotor neurons project both to the central caudal nucleus innervating the levator palpebrae muscle and to motoneurons innervating the superior rectus and inferior oblique muscles that elevate the eyes; a weaker projection targets neurons of the facial nucleus that innervate the frontalis muscle. The M group receives excitatory input from the superior colliculus, the medial and superior vestibular nuclei, and the INC, and an efference copy from collaterals of vertical saccade burst neurons of the RIMLF. The blink reflex is triggered by trigeminal afferents both via oligosynaptic pathways through the sensory trigeminal nucleus (R1) and polysynaptic pathways through the medullary reticular formation (R2). There is also a pontine lateral tegmental blink motor area ventral to the motor trigeminal nucleus; and a medullary medial tegmental blink area may contribute to the R2 response. Other stimuli such as auditory, tactile, or visual stimuli can also trigger reflex blink responses via pathways that project on premotor neurons for the orbicularis oculi muscle in the trigeminal nucleus, in the lateral pontine reticular formation, and in the medullary reticular formation and red nucleus.

Cortical Control of Eye Movements

The brainstem gaze control apparatus receives inputs from several areas of the cerebral cortex (Figure 32.3). They include the frontal eye field (FEF), parietal eye field (PEF), dorsolateral prefrontal eye field, supplementary eye field, medial temporal visual area (MT), and adjacent medial superior temporal area (MST) as well as a cingulate eye field and a medial parietal area corresponding to the precuneus.[6,7] The FEF is the primary cortical area for execution of saccades and is a fundamental component of the dorsal frontoparietal attention network for goal-driven attention. The FEF targets the deep layers of the superior colliculus and activates saccadic burst neurons both directly and via indirect pathways that involve the caudate nucleus and substantia nigra pars reticulata. The FEF also projects directly to saccadic burst neurons in the PPRF and RIMLF, to omnipause neurons of the nucleus raphe interpositus, and to the nucleus reticularis tegmentum pontis, which targets the oculomotor cerebellum. Functional MRI studies revealed a superior FEF subdivision associated with saccades and smooth pursuit and an inferior subdivision activated during combined eye and head movements.[7] The

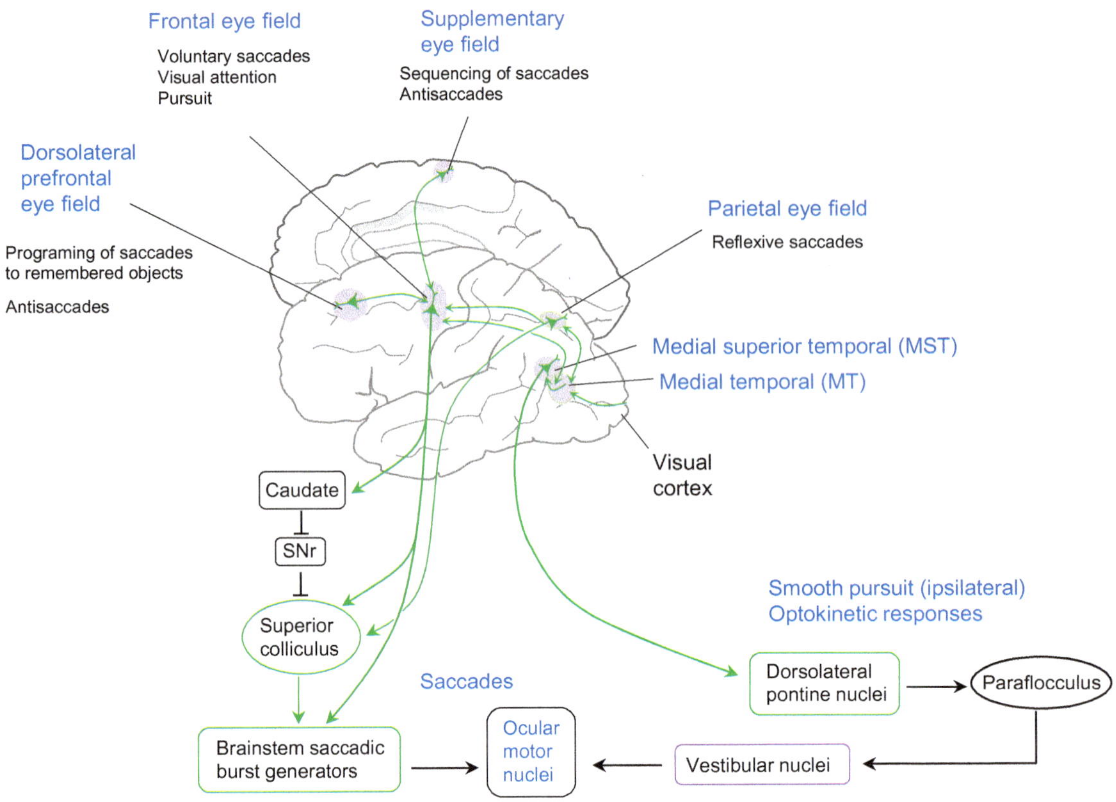

FIGURE 32.3 Cortical control of eye movements.
Neurons in the parietal eye field receive convergence of visual, auditory, and eye position signals and trigger reflexive saccades toward the contralateral visual field. This involves strong projections from the parietal eye field to the frontal eye field (FEF), superior colliculus, and other areas. The FEF is the primary cortical area for execution of saccades and contributes to smooth pursuit. The dorsolateral prefrontal eye field has a role in programming saccades to remembered locations. The supplementary eye field contains neurons that are active during learning motor sequences for successive saccades and antisaccades and may also participate in smooth pursuit. The medial temporal visual area (MT) and adjacent medial superior temporal area (MST) initiate smoot pursuit movements toward the ipsilateral visual field.

PEF is primarily involved in triggering reflexive saccades toward suddenly appearing visual stimuli in the contralateral hemifield. Neurons in the PEF receive convergent visual, auditory, and eye position signals; code the location of the visual target in eye-centered coordinates; and fire during planning of a saccadic eye movement to a target. The activity of PEF neurons is strongly modulated by the salience of the stimulus. The dorsolateral prefrontal eye field is located in areas 9 and 46 in the middle frontal gyrus and has a role in programming saccades to remembered locations. The supplementary eye field contains neurons that are active during learning motor sequences for successive saccades. Both the dorsolateral PFC and the supplementary eye fields are involved in inhibition of reflexive misdirected saccades that are inappropriate to the current goals. This function is assessed by using the antisaccade paradigm, which requires the inhibition of reflexive, visually guided saccades toward a target before performing a correct intentional saccade in the opposite direction.

Areas MT and MST contain neurons that encode the direction and velocity of moving visual stimuli and initiate smooth-pursuit movements toward the ipsilateral visual field. Area MT receives inputs from the primary visual cortex and projects to area MST. Both areas are reciprocally connected with the pursuit and saccadic regions of the FEF and PEF and send descending projections target the dorsolateral pontine nuclei, which relay oculomotor commands to the vestibulocerebellum. In turn the vestibulocerebellum projects to the medial and superior vestibular nuclei, which relay pursuit and optokinetic commands to the ocular motor neurons.

Cerebellar Control of Eye Movements

The cerebellum either directly or indirectly controls all brainstem oculomotor systems. This function involves two main components: (1) the vestibulocerebellum, including the flocculus/paraflocculus and the nodule (flocculonodular lobe), and (2) the oculomotor cerebellum encompassing the dorsal vermis (oculomotor vermis) and caudal fastigial nucleus (fastigial oculomotor region) (Figure 32.4). The vestibulocerebellum controls of the long-term adaptation of the VOR and optokinetic responses, has a major role in gaze holding mechanisms, and together with the oculomotor vermis participates in control of smooth pursuit. Purkinje cells in the flocculus/ventral paraflocculus and nodule receive both direct and second-order vestibular input, as well as projections from the prepositus hypoglossal nucleus and from the medial reticular formation (cell groups of the paramedian tracts) that relay inputs from all ocular premotor structures. These Purkinje cells control eye movements via direct inhibitory projections to the vestibular nuclei. The flocculonodular lobe modulates the VOR on the basis of visual inputs, which is crucial for a long-term adaptive mechanism to reduce visual image motion during head turns. The cerebellum contains two pursuit representations, one in the paraflocculus/flocculus region and a second in the posterior vermis. The pursuit representation in the paraflocculus is involved in the coordination of pursuit and the VOR. There is a normal functional asymmetry in the control of vertical pursuit. Purkinje cells of the flocculus are more active during downward than during upward pursuit and tonically inhibit neurons of the superior vestibular nucleus mediating upward VORs. The flocculus/paraflocculus

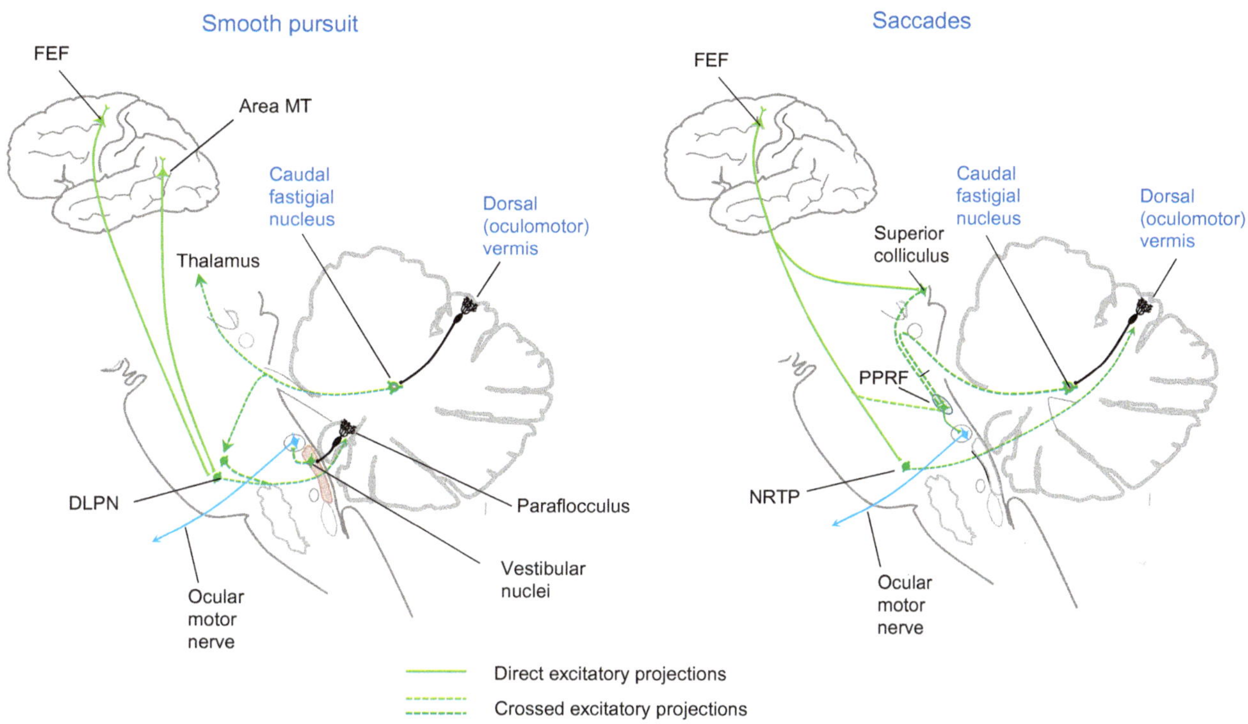

FIGURE 32.4 Cerebellar control of eye movements.

The cerebellum either directly or indirectly controls all brainstem oculomotor systems. This function involves the vestibulocerebellum, including the flocculus/paraflocculus, and the oculomotor cerebellum, encompassing the dorsal vermis (oculomotor vermis) and caudal fastigial nucleus (fastigial oculomotor region). Purkinje cells in the flocculus/ventral paraflocculus control eye movements via direct inhibitory projections to the vestibular nuclei. The ventral paraflocculus is a critical relay in the smooth pursuit pathway. The medial temporal visual area (MT) and adjacent medial superior temporal area (MST), as well as the frontal eye field (FEF) initiate smoot pursuit movements toward the ipsilateral visual field. These areas project to the dorsolateral pontine nucleus (DLPN), which relays input to the paraflocculus. Purkinje cells of the dorsal vermis control both smooth pursuit and saccades via an inhibitory input to the caudal fastigial nucleus. The caudal fastigial nucleus controls saccades via inputs to saccadic burst neurons and omnipause neurons. For example, the caudal fastigial nucleus provides a presaccadic burst that facilitates contraversive saccades via projections to the pontine paramedian reticular formation (PPRF) for horizontal saccades or to the rostral interstitial nucleus of the medial longitudinal fasciculus for vertical saccades (not shown), and "braking" discharge that terminates ipsiversive saccades via projections to inhibitory burst neurons in the dorsal paragigantocellular nucleus (not shown). The command for voluntary saccades originates in the frontal eye field (FEF), which provides excitatory input to saccadic burst neurons in the superior colliculus and conveys saccadic commands to the oculomotor cerebellum in part via the nucleus reticularis tegmentum pontis (NRTP). The pathway by which the caudal fastigial nucleus controls smooth pursuit is not yet well defined. It may include an input to the thalamus, which relays cerebellar influence to the FEF, or input to the NRTP projecting to the paraflocculus.

also participate in a brainstem neural integrator network that generates a tonic eye position command to hold gaze in eccentric positions to assure steady fixation. The nodulus and adjacent ventral uvula control the low-frequency (sustained) components of the VOR via projections to a "velocity-storage" mechanism within the vestibular nuclei; this mechanism extends the duration of the VOR during a constant-velocity rotation of the head.

The oculomotor cerebellum, including the dorsal vermis and underlying posterior (caudal) fastigial nucleus is important for the adjustment of eye movements during smooth pursuit and saccades.[8,9] The oculomotor vermis controls both visually guided saccades and smooth-pursuit eye movements by mapping retinal information onto motor vectors.[10] Purkinje cells send an inhibitory input to the fastigial oculomotor region, which in turn sends excitatory inputs to brainstem neurons that control saccades. Neurons in the fastigial oculomotor region provide both a presaccadic burst that facilitates contraversive saccades via projections to burst neurons in the PPRF (for horizontal saccades) and in the RIMLF (for vertical saccades), and "braking" discharge that terminates ipsiversive saccades via projections to inhibitory burst neurons in the dorsal paragigantocellular nucleus. Projections of the fastigial oculomotor region to omnipause neurons, either directly or via the fixation zone of the rostral pole of the superior colliculus, inhibit saccadic excitatory burst neurons. Purkinje cells in the oculomotor vermis receive information about performance during saccades and adjust their inhibition on the fastigial oculomotor region to assure the saccade arrives on target. Due to its inhibitory effect on fastigial oculomotor neurons, the dorsal vermis facilitates ipsiversive saccades and contributes to the termination of contralateral saccades. Neurons of the fastigial oculomotor region also facilitate initiation of contraversive pursuit and termination of ipsiversive pursuit. The pathways by which the caudal fastigial nucleus controls smooth pursuit have not been completely defined. They may include an input to the thalamus, which relays cerebellar influence to the FEF, or input to the pontine tegmental reticular nucleus projecting to the paraflocculus. The majority of Purkinje cells in the oculomotor vermis also modulate their activity during vergence, especially convergence.

LOWER BRAINSTEM CONTROL OF SWALLOWING AND SPEECH

Vocalization, speech, chewing, swallowing, and control of the upper airway during respiration are periodic or rhythmic motor acts that require coordinated motor plans integrated at the level of pons and medulla[11] (Figure 32.5). They involve CPGs that integrate inputs from primary afferents with descending commands and control the motoneurons of the trigeminal, facial, ambiguus, and hypoglossal nuclei. The coordination both within and between orofacial functions may involve local interactions between potentially coactive CPG circuits; central commands controlling the execution and amplitude of different actions; and peripheral feedback ensuring the appropriate timing between the different muscle groups.

Medullary Central Pattern Generators for Swallowing, Vocalization, and Speech

The control of swallowing involves complex network interactions within a medullary CPG. This CPG is located in the dorsal and ventral medulla and provides for the spatiotemporal coordination of a series of sequential contractions of the oral, pharyngeal, and laryngeal muscles that allow food transport through the pharynx and across the upper esophageal sphincter without entering the airway. The swallowing CPG can be separated into two groups: a dorsal swallowing group located in the nucleus of the solitary tract (NTS) and around the medullary reticular formation, and a ventral swallowing group located near the nucleus ambiguus.[12] The dorsal swallowing group governs the reflex control of swallowing and the generation of rhythmic activities that drive complex sequential oropharyngeal motor patterns. Neurons of the ventral swallowing group may provide the direct command to the motoneurons. The premotor neurons controlling swallowing and speech are located in the parvocellular reticular formation and ventral portion of the intermediate reticular zone near the nucleus ambiguus in the ventrolateral medulla. These regions are located in close relationship to the respiratory pattern generator for inspiration and receive cortical inputs primarily from the frontal operculum via the corticobulbar tract. Swallowing is a sequential motor event and not a rhythmic behavior such as mastication or respiration but in appropriate circumstances, such as drinking, it may acquire the properties of a rhythmic motor behavior. Most swallowing-related neurons are silent at rest but produce a burst of low-frequency spikes correlated with the timing of motor activity. Neurons in the NTS organize the sequential or rhythmic motor pattern for swallowing in response to inputs from oropharyngeal afferents particularly those carried by the superior laryngeal branch of the vagus nerve. Neurons in the reticular formation of the ventrolateral medulla distribute and coordinate the drive to the various pools of motoneurons. Swallowing, speech, and vocalization require coordination with respiration. The preBötzinger complex of the ventrolateral medulla is the inspiratory respiratory pattern generator and has extensive connections with neurons of the putative CPGs for orofacial movements, with the NTS and with motor cranial nerve nuclei involved in swallowing. The swallowing network also receives descending inputs from the sensorimotor cortex, anterior insula, frontal operculum, prefrontal, premotor, anterior cingulate, posterior parietal, and superior temporal cortices. The cortical representation of swallowing muscles is plastic; for example, in patients with right hemispheric stroke and dysphagia, recovery of

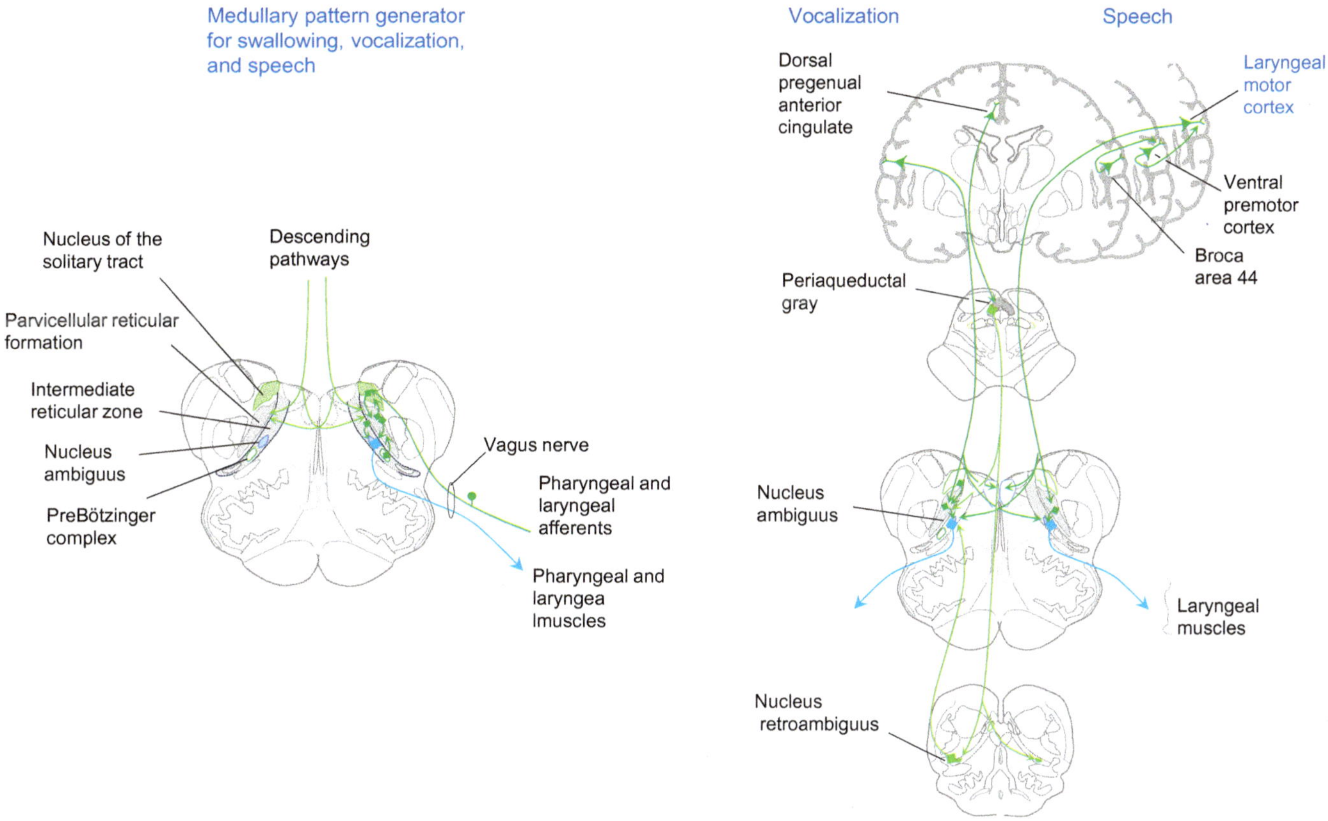

FIGURE 32.5 Medullary circuits for swallowing, vocalization, and speech.
The control of swallowing, vocalization, and speech involves complex network interaction within the central pattern generator (CPG). The swallowing CPG can be separated into: a dorsal group located in the nucleus of the solitary tract (NTS) and and a ventral group located in the ventrolateral medullary reticular formation. The premotor neurons controlling swallowing and speech are located in the parvocellular reticular formation and ventral portion of the intermediate reticular zone near the nucleus ambiguus in the ventrolateral medulla. These regions are located in close relationship to the respiratory pattern generator for inspiration and receive cortical inputs primarily from the frontal operculum via the corticobulbar tract. The preBötzinger complex is the inspiratory respiratory pattern generator and has extensive connections with neurons of the putative CPGs for orofacial movements. Control of vocalization involves the periaqueductal gray (PAG), which has strong projections to the nucleus retroambiguus. This nucleus projects to motoneurons involved in vocalization, including not only cranial but also respiratory motoneurons. Vocal control requires input from the anterior midcingulate cortex to the PAG.

swallowing function was associated with an enlarged representation of the pharynx.

Vocalization

Control of vocalization, including laughter and crying, involves the emotional motor system, primarily the periaqueductal gray (PAG), parabrachial nucleus, and ventrolateral pontine reticular formation. The PAG receives strong projections from the amygdala, anterior cingulate, insular, and orbitofrontal cortices and has strong projections to the nucleus retroambiguus in the caudal medulla. This nucleus is the only cell group that has direct access to all motoneurons involved in vocalization, including not only motoneurons innervating soft palate, pharynx, and larynx but also those innervating the diaphragm, intercostal, abdominal, and pelvic floor muscles that together determine the intraabdominal, intrathoracic, and subglottic pressure necessary for generating vocalization.[13] Diffusion tractography and fMRI studies show a functional connectivity between the PAG and the ventral laryngeal motor cortical area during vocalization.[14] This level of control is responsible for production of genetically preprogrammed innate vocalizations, including the cry or laugh of an infant. Stretch reflexes from muscle spindles may provide proprioceptive feedback assisting in voice control, but sensory afferents from the internal branch of the superior laryngeal nerve are more sensitive to activation by mucosal stretch caused by repeated mechanical perturbations of the vocal folds caused by phonation. As children develop and become capable of learning and mimicking vocal utterances, innate vocalizations become increasingly more voluntary; for example crying can be produced without an emotional stimulus or suppressed despite the presence of discomfort. This level of vocal control requires inputs from the dorsal pregenual anterior cingulate cortex to the PAG, which are responsible for the control of emotional vocalizations, voice initiation, and modulation of its intensity. This area, together with the lateral hypothalamus, may participate in the uncontrollable laughter that occurs in gelastic seizures.[15] However, lesions in other cortical areas connected with the PAG may result in similar manifestations.[16] Lesions affecting either the anterior midcingulate cortex or PAG may result in akinetic mutism.[17] A study in monkeys showed that unilateral disinhibition of the nucleus accumbens (NAc) generates vocal tics associated with bilateral activation and abnormal coupling between the nucleus accumbens and anterior cingulate cortex.[18]

Speech

The ability of humans to speak requires projections from the lateral component of the volitional or somatic motor system, which enables to modulate vocalization into words and sentences. This system originates in the motor cortex, which, via its corticobulbar fibers, has direct access to the motoneurons innervating the muscles of face, mouth, tongue, larynx, and pharynx. The corticobulbar input is largely bilateral, which allows bilateral synchronization of orofacial movements. In humans, there is also a direct connection between the motor cortex and the nucleus ambiguus controlling laryngeal muscles.

The voluntary motor articulation network includes the left inferior frontal gyrus (Broca areas 44 and 45), ventral premotor cortex (PMv), ventrolateral portion of the primary motor cortex (M1), supplementary motor area (SMA), preSMA, inferior parietal and superior temporal cortex, striatum, and cerebellum. However, the left inferior frontal gyrus is the only frontal cortical area selectively activated during articulation, whereas others are also activated during nonarticulatory movements. Direct cortical surface recordings in neurosurgical patients showed that during the cued production of words, Broca area becomes silent while motor cortex is activated.[19] Broca area is activated during production of articulatory gestures, indicating that it coordinates the transformation of information across large-scale cortical networks and formulates an appropriate articulatory code to be implemented by motor cortex. The anterior PMv integrates sensorimotor signals from the posterior parietal cortex with cognitive signals from the ventrolateral prefrontal cortex, preSMA, and anterior midcingulate cortex and projects to the ventral portion of M1 containing the representation of the larynx and orofacial muscles.

Corticobulbar Pathway

The speech motor cortex has a dorsal-to-ventral somatotopic representation controlling the movements of the lips, jaw, tongue, and pharynx/larynx along the central sulcus.[20] There is a partially overlapping representation of articulators and two separate representations of the larynx, one ventral to the tongue and a second dorsal to the lips. The corticobulbar input is largely bilateral, which allows bilateral synchronization of orofacial movements. The brainstem swallowing pattern generator receives descending inputs from the sensorimotor cortex, anterior insula, frontal operculum, prefrontal, premotor, anterior cingulate, posterior parietal, and superior temporal cortices. In addition to a bilateral projection from the motor cortex to orofacial motor nuclei, in humans there is a direct projection from the laryngeal motor cortex to the nucleus ambiguus, which enables fast and direct coordination of complex laryngeal, orofacial, and respiratory movements that facilitates learning and voluntary vocal control. The volitional articulatory motor network may exert a modulatory control on the nonverbal vocalization network; nonverbal emotional vocalizations may emerge as the voluntary articulatory control vanishes.[21] The lateral frontal cortex may gain control over articulation via disinhibition of articulatory motor activity briefly before the vocal output. For example, experimental studies indicate that vocal tics emerge as a consequence of dysrhythmic alpha coupling between critical nodes in the limbic and motor networks, including the nucleus accumbens, and anterior midcingulate cortex.[18]

DISORDERS OF EYE MOVEMENTS

There are comprehensive reviews on the disorders of eye movements resulting from lesions affecting the vestibular system, cerebellum, and brainstem gaze-control mechanisms.[22–24]

Disturbance of Cortical Gaze Control

Acute lesions of one cerebral hemisphere often result in conjugate deviation of the eyes toward the side of the lesion; this occurs more commonly after large right-sided strokes. Patients with unilateral lesions in the FEF, upon recovery from the acute effect, show only subtle deficits such as increased reaction time for memory-guided saccades and increased failure rate in antisaccadic tasks. Unilateral lesions of the PEF, particularly on the right, cause bilateral prolongation of reflex visually guided saccades. Chronic unilateral lesions affecting the FEF cause bilateral increase in reaction time and hypometria of saccades made to remembered target locations and to imagined targets, reduced ability to make anticipatory saccades to predictable movement, and impaired ability to inhibit inappropriate saccades to a novel visual stimulus. Lesions of the supplementary eye fields reduce accuracy of memory-guided saccades. Patients with lesions affecting the dorsolateral PFC have deficits in memory-guided saccades, predictive saccades, and antisaccades. Imbalance in the pursuit system manifests with low horizontal pursuit gain for targets moving toward the side of the lesion; eye movements may be too fast for targets moving toward the intact hemisphere, requiring backup saccades.

Acquired oculomotor apraxia is characterized by loss of voluntary control of saccades and pursuit, with preservation of reflex eye movements. It occurs as a consequence of acute bilateral frontal or frontoparietal lesions, particularly infarcts after cardiopulmonary bypass, or as a component of Balint syndrome due to bilateral posterior parietal lesions. Oculomotor apraxia is also a major feature of ataxia with oculomotor apraxia syndromes, typically associated with disorders of DNA repair. Some patients with oculomotor apraxia may show spasm of fixation, which is the inability to generate a voluntary eye movement to shift the gaze when a fixation target is continuously present. In patients with dementia, most of the disorders of eye movements reflect an inability to focus or to shift visual attention. Patients with Alzheimer disease, Huntington disease, or frontal lobe dementia are unable to suppress inappropriate reflexive visually triggered saccades during disrupt maintenance of steady fixation; this has been called a visual grasp reflex.

Disturbance of Cerebellar and Brainstem Control

Vestibular and cerebellar lesions manifest with a wide range of nystagmus and other oscillatory eye movements.[22,23] A comprehensive discussion of this topic is beyond the scope of this chapter, and only few examples are summarized in Table 32.1.

Several studies have defined distinct oculomotor and vestibular findings in lesions affecting specific vestibular structures in the brainstem and cerebellum. For example, lesions involving the MLF produce, in addition to classical internuclear ophthalmoplegia (INO) other abnormalities such as upbeat or jerky seesaw nystagmus, impairment of the vertical VOR and vertical smooth pursuit, contraversive ocular tilt reaction, subjective visual vertical tilt, and loss of angular VOR gain during the head impulse test for the contralesional posterior SCC. Lesions affecting the prepositus hypoglossal nucleus produce a unique syndrome characterized by ipsilesional-beating spontaneous nystagmus, horizontal gaze-evoked nystagmus more intense on looking toward the ipsilesional side, impaired pursuit more to the ipsilesional side, contralateral eye deviation, and decreased VOR gain during contralesional head-impulse test. Lesions of the flocculus/paraflocculus impair ipsilateral smooth pursuit, and VOR adaptation, and gaze-holding, resulting in gaze-evoked nystagmus and downbeat nystagmus; those affecting the nodulus produce periodic alternating nystagmus. Lesions affecting the fastigial oculomotor region produce hypometric contraversive and hypermetric ipsiversive saccades; the opposite occurs with lesions in the oculomotor vermis. Impaired function of the fastigial oculomotor regions also produce saccadic intrusions and opsoclonus due impaired activity of omnipause neurons, as typically occur in association with myoclonus in paraneoplastic brainstem encephalitis associated to neuroblastoma or anti-Ri/NOVA antibodies. Opsoclonus following cardiac bypass may result from disruption of the perineuronal net leading to impaired function of inhibitory saccadic burst neurons. The recognition of specific abnormalities in eye movements has not only localizing value but also therapeutic implications.[24] For example, downbeat nystagmus due to lesions of the flocculonodular lobe may response to 3,4-diaminopyridine; periodic alternating nystagmus due to lesions in the nodule may respond to baclofen; and acquired pendular nystagmus may respond to gabapentin or memantine.[25]

In some disorders, prominent disturbances of eye movement control are associated with markedly impaired control of posture and locomotion. One prototypical example is progressive supranuclear palsy (PSP), a neurodegenerative 4-repeat tauopathy that manifests with varied clinical presentations.[26,27] The typical phenotype is Richardson syndrome, characterized by prominent disturbances of gaze, posture, and gait. The predominant oculomotor disturbances in PSP include slow and hypometric vertical saccades (both up and down), impaired vergence, and inability to modulate the linear VOR appropriately for viewing distance.[28] These vertical and vergence eye movements normally work in concert to enable visuomotor skills that are important during locomotion and free use of the hands. The major site of early pathology in PSP is the midbrain, as manifested with the typical MRI finding of midbrain atrophy producing the characteristic "hummingbird" sign. The RIMLF and INC are affected early in the disease course, which may account for the limited range of voluntary upward or downward saccades. Whereas the angular VOR is relatively preserved until late disease stages, the linear VOR is markedly impaired; this probably reflects loss of neurons in the vestibular nuclei responding to inputs from the saccule. Patients with PSP often show head turns opposite to the direction of intended gait; this may reflect apparent functional overactivity of the vestibulo-collic reflexes and contribute to postural instability.

The prominent saccadic intrusions in PSP, including square-wave jerks upon attempted fixation lack a vertical component and may reflect involvement of the cerebellum and its output, as they also occur in disorders such as Friedreich's ataxia. Impaired inhibition of the superior colliculus by the substantia nigra pars reticulata may also be contributory.

BIOPERCULAR SYNDROME AND PSEUDOBULBAR PALSY

Bilateral lesions of the laryngeal and orofacial motor cortex results in speech loss as a manifestation of the biopercular (Foix-Marie-Chavany) syndrome, which is characterized by cortical pseudobulbar facio-labio-pharyngo-glosso-masticatory paralysis. A salient aspect of this syndrome is voluntary-automatic dissociation preserving only the nonverbal emotional vocalizations such as grunting, crying, and laughing controlled through the

TABLE 32.1 *Oculomotor Manifestations of Disorders Affecting the Brainstem or Cerebellum*

Nucleus/Area	Function	Manifestation of Impairment
Abducens nucleus	Horizontal gaze generator	Ipsilateral conjugate gaze palsy
Trochlear nucleus	Input to contralateral superior oblique	Vertical or oblique diplopia worse upon gaze toward the inferior and medial quadrant
Oculomotor nucleus	Innervation of contralateral superior rectus; ipsilateral inferior and medial rectus, and superior oblique, and levator palpebrae bilaterally	Bilateral superior rectus palsy (nuclear plus decussating fiber lesion), ipsilateral medial and superior oblique palsy, and ptosis
MLF	Contralateral connections between ocular motor and vestibular nuclei	Internuclear ophthalmoplegia
RIMLF	Vertical saccades	Impairment of vertical saccades, either downward (discrete bilateral lesions) or both upward and downward gaze (severe bilateral lesion or unilateral lesion often associated with lesion in the posterior commissure)
INC	Vertical gaze holding	Unilateral: contralateral head tilt (unilateral lesion) with torsion to the contralateral side and ipsilesional torsional nystagmus Bilateral: upbeat nystagmus and neck retroflexion
PPRF	Burst for horizontal saccades	Slowing of ipsilateral gaze
NPCom	Coordination of upward gaze and lid elevation	Vertical gaze palsy and lid retraction
Superior colliculus	Orienting saccadic responses Visual fixation	Difficulty orienting toward alerting stimuli
Prepositus hypoglossal nucleus	Key constituent of the vestibular-cerebellar-brainstem neural integrator network the holding eye steady in all positions of gaze.	Unilateral: ipsilesional-beating spontaneous nystagmus, horizontal gaze-evoked nystagmus more intense on looking toward the ipsilesional side, impaired pursuit more to the ipsilesional side, central patters of head-shaking nystagmus, contralateral eye deviation, and decreased VOR gain during contralesionally directed head impulses.
Flocculus/ paraflocculus	Adaptation of the VOR Smooth pursuit Gaze holding (neural integrator)	Impaired smooth pursuit Postsaccadic drift and gaze-evoked nystagmus toward the ipsilesional side Rebound nystagmus Downbeat nystagmus*
Nodulus	Control of velocity storage mechanism for VOR	Periodic alternating nystagmus**

TABLE 32.1 *(Continued)*

Nucleus/Area	Function	Manifestation of Impairment
Fastigial oculomotor region	Facilitation of contraversive and interruption of ipsiversive saccades Maintenance of fixation via omnipause neurons Facilitations of contraversive and inhibition of ipsiversive smooth pursuit	Hypometric contraversive and hypermetric ipsiversive saccades Saccadic intrusions*** Opsoclonus
Dorsal vermis	Facilitation of ipsiversive and interruption of contraversive saccades	Hypometric ipsiversive and hypermetric contraversive saccades

INC, interstitial nucleus of Cajal; MLF, median longitudinal fascicle; NPCom, nucleus of the posterior commissure; PPRF, pontine paramedian reticular formation; RIMLF, rostral interstitial nucleus of the medial longitudinal fascicles; * may respond with 3,4-diaminopyridine; ** may respond to baclofen; *** may respond to memantine.

midcingulate-PAG circuitry. Biopercular syndrome is a cortical form of pseudobulbar palsy. Pseudobulbar palsy is characterized by the inability to control facial movements due to bilateral upper motor neuron lesions affecting the corticobulbar tract. One salient feature is pseudobulbar affect. This refers to a disorder of emotional expression characterized by sudden, unpredictable, and involuntary episodes of crying, laughing, or other emotional displays that are exaggerated relative to or incongruent with the mood and feelings of the patients.[29] This manifestation occurs in motor neuron disease, traumatic brain injury, multiple sclerosis, stroke, multiple system atrophy-cerebellar type, Alzheimer disease, and Parkinson disease. A classical hypothesis is that pseudobulbar affect involves a loss of descending control of brainstem motor systems that control emotional expression. However, recent evidence indicates that pseudobulbar affect reflects a disruption within a widely dispersed network of emotional control including the brainstem, bilateral inferior parietal, and medial frontal regions as well as impaired modulatory control by the cerebellum. The only therapy approved so far for pseudobulbar affect is dextromethorphan/quinidine. The mechanism of action is not well understood but is postulated to be in part related to reduced reuptake of serotonin and dopamine activation of sigma-1 receptors that inhibits NMDA receptors.[30]

KEY POINTS

- The brainstem gaze-control mechanisms maintain optimal visual acuity by ensuring that the images of objects remain steady and stimulate corresponding areas of the retina.
- Ocular motoneurons are active even in primary position of gaze and are recruited in a fixed sequence; and discharge proportionally to the velocity and position of the eye.
- Horizontal eye movements are integrated in the pons via the abducens nucleus.
- Vertical and torsional eye movements are integrated in the midbrain by the trochlear nucleus and by subnuclei of the oculomotor complex.
- The vestibulo-ocular reflex (VOR) stabilizes gaze during head.
- The VOR pathway involves vestibular afferents projecting to VOR neurons in the medial and superior vestibular nuclei, which send both excitatory projections to contralateral ocular motoneurons and inhibitory ipsilateral projections to antagonist motoneurons.
- During sustained head rotation, the vestibular signal for the VOR is prolonged by a mechanism of velocity storage.
- Retinal slip triggers ocular following response, optokinetic nystagmus, and smooth pursuit.
- The vestibular nuclei provide the drive to ocular motoneurons during optokinetic and smooth-pursuit movements.
- Saccades are rapid eye movements that redirect the fovea toward features of interest.
- Horizontal saccades are triggered by excitatory burst neurons located in the paramedian pontine reticular formation (PPRF).
- The excitatory burst neurons for vertical and torsional saccades are located in the rostral interstitial nucleus of the median longitudinal fasciculus (RIMLF).
- Omnipause neurons located in the nucleus raphe interpositus tonically inhibit the saccadic premotor neurons during fixation and slow eye movements.
- Maintenance of eccentric eye position after a saccade requires the activity of a neural integrator network that provides a step command to ocular motoneurons.

- The main neural integrator for horizontal gaze-holding is the prepositus hypoglossal nucleus; the neural integrator for vertical gaze holding is the interstitial nucleus of Cajal.
- The premotor neurons related to vergence eye movements are located in the medial mesencephalic reticular formation dorsal to the oculomotor complex.
- The superior colliculus is a fundamental component of the attention and orientation system.
- The frontal eye field (FEF) is critical for execution of saccades as a component of the dorsal frontoparietal attention network for goal-driven attention.
- The FEF targets the superior colliculus and activates saccadic burst neurons both directly and via a basal ganglia circuit that involves the caudate and substantia nigra pars reticulata.
- The parietal eye field (PEF) is involved in triggering reflexive saccades toward suddenly appearing visual stimuli in the contralateral hemifield.
- The dorsolateral prefrontal eye field, together with the supplementary eye fields, inhibits reflexive misdirected saccades that are inappropriate to the current goals.
- The medial temporal (MT) and adjacent medial superior temporal (MST) areas encode the direction and velocity of moving visual stimuli and initiate smoot pursuit movements.
- The vestibulocerebellum (flocculus/paraflocculus, nodulus, and uvula) controls of the long-term adaptation of the VOR and optokinetic responses, gaze holding, and smooth pursuit via projections to the vestibular nuclei.
- The oculomotor cerebellum (dorsal oculomotor vermis and fastigial oculomotor region) controls saccades via projections to brainstem saccadic burst neurons, onmipause neurons, and superior colliculus.
- The premotor neurons controlling swallowing and speech are located in the parvocellular reticular formation and ventral portion of the intermediate reticular zone near the nucleus ambiguus.
- Neurons in the nucleus of the solitary tract organize the sequential or rhythmic motor pattern for swallowing.
- The swallowing network receives descending inputs from the sensorimotor cortex, anterior insula, and frontal operculum.
- Control of vocalization involves the pregenual cingulate cortex, periaqueductal gray, and nucleus retroambiguus.
- The corticobulbar input is largely bilateral, which allows bilateral synchronization of orofacial movements.
- Oculomotor apraxia is also a major feature of oculomotor apraxia syndromes, typically associated with disorders of DNA repair.
- Lesions of the flocculus/paraflocculus impair ipsilateral smooth pursuit, VOR adaptation, and gaze-holding, resulting in gaze-evoked nystagmus and downbeat nystagmus.
- Lesions of the nodulus produce periodic alternating nystagmus.
- Lesions affecting the fastigial oculomotor region produce hypometric contraversive and hypermetric ipsiversive saccades; the opposite occurs with lesions in the oculomotor vermis.
- Lesions of the fastigial oculomotor regions also produce saccadic intrusions and opsoclonus due impaired activity of omnipause neurons.
- Downbeat nystagmus may respond to 3,4 diaminopyridine, periodic alternating nystagmus to baclofen, and saccadic intrusions to memantine.
- Progressive supranuclear palsy (PSP) typically manifests with Richardson syndrome, characterized by prominent disturbances of gaze, posture, and gait.
- The predominant oculomotor disturbances in PSP include slow and hypometric vertical saccade), impaired vergence, and inability to modulate the linear VOR.
- Unilateral lesion of the corticobulbar pathway results in temporary dysarthria that improves with time.
- Bilateral lesions of the laryngeal and orofacial motor cortex result in the biopercular (Foix-Marie-Chavany) syndrome, which is characterized by cortical pseudobulbar facio-labio-pharyngo-glosso-masticatory paralysis.

REFERENCES

1. Ramat S, Leigh RJ, Zee DS, Optican LM. What clinical disorders tell us about the neural control of saccadic eye movements. Brain 2007;130:10–35.
2. Patel VR, Zee DS. The cerebellum in eye movement control: nystagmus, coordinate frames and disconjugacy. Eye (Lond) 2015;29:191–195.
3. Horn AK, Leigh RJ. The anatomy and physiology of the ocular motor system. Handb Clin Neurol 2011;102:21–69.
4. Kim SH, Zee DS, du Lac S, Kim HJ, Kim JS. Nucleus prepositus hypoglossi lesions produce a unique ocular motor syndrome. Neurology 2016;87:2026–2033.
5. Serra A, Chen AL, Leigh RJ. Disorders of vergence eye movements. Curr Opin Neurol 2011;24:32–37.
6. Pierrot-Deseilligny C, Milea D, Muri RM. Eye movement control by the cerebral cortex. Curr Opin Neurol 2004;17:17–25.
7. Muri RM. MRI and fMRI analysis of oculomotor function. Prog Brain Res 2006;151:503–526.
8. Ilg UJ, Thier P. The neural basis of smooth pursuit eye movements in the rhesus monkey brain. Brain Cogn 2008;68:229–240.
9. Bourrelly C, Quinet J, Goffart L. Pursuit disorder and saccade dysmetria after caudal fastigial inactivation in the monkey. J Neurophysiol 2018;120:1640–1654.

10. Thier P, Markanday A. Role of the vermal cerebellum in visually guided eye movements and visual motion perception. Annu Rev Vis Sci 2019;5:247–268.
11. Moore JD, Kleinfeld D, Wang F. How the brainstem controls orofacial behaviors comprised of rhythmic actions. Trends Neurosci 2014;37:370–380.
12. Jean A. Brain stem control of swallowing: neuronal network and cellular mechanisms. Physiol Rev 2001;81:929–969.
13. Subramanian HH, Huang ZG, Silburn PA, Balnave RJ, Holstege G. The physiological motor patterns produced by neurons in the nucleus retroambiguus in the rat and their modulation by vagal, peripheral chemosensory, and nociceptive stimulation. J Comp Neurol 2018;526:229–242.
14. Galgano J, Pantazatos S, Allen K, Yanagihara T, Hirsch J. Functional connectivity of PAG with core limbic system and laryngeal cortico-motor structures during human phonation. Brain Res 2019;1707:184–189.
15. Egea-Lucas I, Martinez-Mondejar E, Piqueres-Vidal CF, Frutos-Alegria MT. [Gelastic seizures as the presenting symptom of infarction of the cingulate gyrus]. Rev Neurol 2015;61:211–214.
16. Tran TP, Truong VT, Wilk M, et al. Different localizations underlying cortical gelastic epilepsy: case series and review of literature. Epilepsy Behav 2014;35:34–41.
17. Nagaratnam N, Nagaratnam K, Ng K, Diu P. Akinetic mutism following stroke. J Clin Neurosci 2004;11:25–30.
18. McCairn KW, Nagai Y, Hori Y, et al. A primary role for nucleus accumbens and related limbic network in vocal tics. Neuron 2016;89:300–307.
19. Flinker A, Korzeniewska A, Shestyuk AY, et al. Redefining the role of Broca's area in speech. Proc Natl Acad Sci U S A 2015;112:2871–2875.
20. Simonyan K. The laryngeal motor cortex: its organization and connectivity. Curr Opin Neurobiol 2014;28:15–21.
21. Lauterbach EC, Cummings JL, Kuppuswamy PS. Toward a more precise, clinically-informed pathophysiology of pathological laughing and crying. Neurosci Biobehav Rev 2013;37:1893–1916.
22. Eggers SDZ, Bisdorff A, von Brevern M, et al. Classification of vestibular signs and examination techniques: nystagmus and nystagmus-like movements. J Vestib Res 2019;29:57–87.
23. Kheradmand A, Colpak AI, Zee DS. Eye movements in vestibular disorders. Handb Clin Neurol 2016;137:103–117.
24. Strupp M, Thurtell MJ, Shaikh AG, Brandt T, Zee DS, Leigh RJ. Pharmacotherapy of vestibular and ocular motor disorders, including nystagmus. J Neurol 2011;258:1207–1222.
25. Zwergal A, Strupp M, Brandt T. Advances in pharmacotherapy of vestibular and ocular motor disorders. Expert Opin Pharmacother 2019;20:1267–1276.
26. Hoglinger GU, Respondek G, Stamelou M, et al. Clinical diagnosis of progressive supranuclear palsy: the movement disorder society criteria. Mov Disord 2017;32:853–864.
27. Boxer AL, Yu JT, Golbe LI, Litvan I, Lang AE, Hoglinger GU. Advances in progressive supranuclear palsy: new diagnostic criteria, biomarkers, and therapeutic approaches. Lancet Neurol 2017;16:552–563.
28. Chen AL, Riley DE, King SA, et al. The disturbance of gaze in progressive supranuclear palsy: implications for pathogenesis. Front Neurol 2010;1:147.
29. Finegan E, Chipika RH, Li Hi Shing S, Hardiman O, Bede P. Pathological crying and laughing in motor neuron disease: pathobiology, screening, intervention. Front Neurol 2019;10:260.
30. Taylor CP, Traynelis SF, Siffert J, Pope LE, Matsumoto RR. Pharmacology of dextromethorphan: relevance to dextromethorphan/quinidine (Nuedexta(R)) clinical use. Pharmacol Ther 2016;164:170–182.

33 Cerebellar Circuits

OVERVIEW

The cerebellum has a critical role in control of timing and coordination of motor, cognitive, and affective function.[1] The fundamental feature of cerebellar connectivity is the presence of multiple closed-loop circuits that interconnect the cerebral neocortex with the cerebellum via segregated input-output channels. Functional distinct areas of the cerebral cortex provide segregated input to the contralateral cerebellum via the pontine nuclei and receive reciprocal outputs from the cerebellum via the thalamus. The cerebellum also has direct interactions with the basal ganglia and with spinal and brainstem areas involved in postural and oculomotor control. The intrinsic cerebellar circuit includes the Purkinje cells that control activity of the cerebellar nuclei, which provide the cerebellar output to the rest of the central nervous system (CNS). Inputs from several sources via the mossy fiber–parallel fiber and from the inferior olivary nucleus (ION)–climbing fiber system control the inhibitory influence of Purkinje cells on the cerebellar nuclei and thus shape the cerebellar output. Cerebellar disorders manifest with oculomotor abnormalities, postural imbalance, gait ataxia, dysmetria, and tremor, as well as affective and cognitive manifestations. Impaired pacemaking activity of Purkinje cells or altered plasticity of the parallel fiber-Purkinje cell synapses are fundamental mechanisms underlying ataxia. Disturbances in the circuits linking the ION, Purkinje cells, cerebellar nuclei, and thalamus provide the pathophysiological bases for different types of tremor. The aims of this chapter are to review: (1) the extrinsic connectivity of the cerebellum, (2) the components of the intrinsic cerebellar circuits, (3) the electrophysiology of Purkinje cells and the influence of parallel and climbing fiber inputs, (4) the regulation and function of the cerebellar output via the cerebellar nuclei, and (5) emerging concepts on the pathophysiology of cerebellar ataxia and tremor.

EXTRINSIC CONNECTIVITY OF THE CEREBELLUM

The cerebellum is classically subdivided into a flocculonodular lobe and the body of the cerebellum, which includes the cerebellar vermis and hemispheres forming an anterior lobe (lobules I–V/VI) and a posterior lobe (lobules VI/VII–IX) (Figure 33.1).The different regions of the cerebellum receive their major input from the vestibular system, spinal cord, or cerebral cortex via the pontine nuclei. Except for the flocculonodular lobe, which participates in direct reciprocal interactions with the vestibular system, the cerebellum interacts with the CNS via outputs mediated by the cerebellar nuclei.[2] Based on the patterns of outputs, the anterior and posterior lobes are subdivided into a vermis, a paravermis, and a lateral cerebellar hemisphere.[3] The medial vermis projects via the fastigial nucleus to the brainstem reticular formation and to the thalamus, whereas the lateral vermis projects to the superior vestibular nucleus. The paravermis projects via the interposed nuclei, which include anterior (globose) and posterior (emboliform) subdivisions. These nuclei target the red nucleus and motor nuclei of the thalamus. The lateral cerebellar hemisphere projects via the dentate nucleus primarily to the thalamus. The dorsal dentate targets thalamic nuclei that project to the motor cortex, the ventral dentate targets thalamic nuclei that project to the association cortex. All the extrinsic connections of the cerebellum are excitatory and mediated by L-glutamate, with two important exceptions: the projection from the cerebellar nuclei to the ION which originates from GABAergic neurons, and the direct GABAergic projections from Purkinje cells of the vestibulocerebellum (flocculonodular lobe) to the vestibular nuclei.

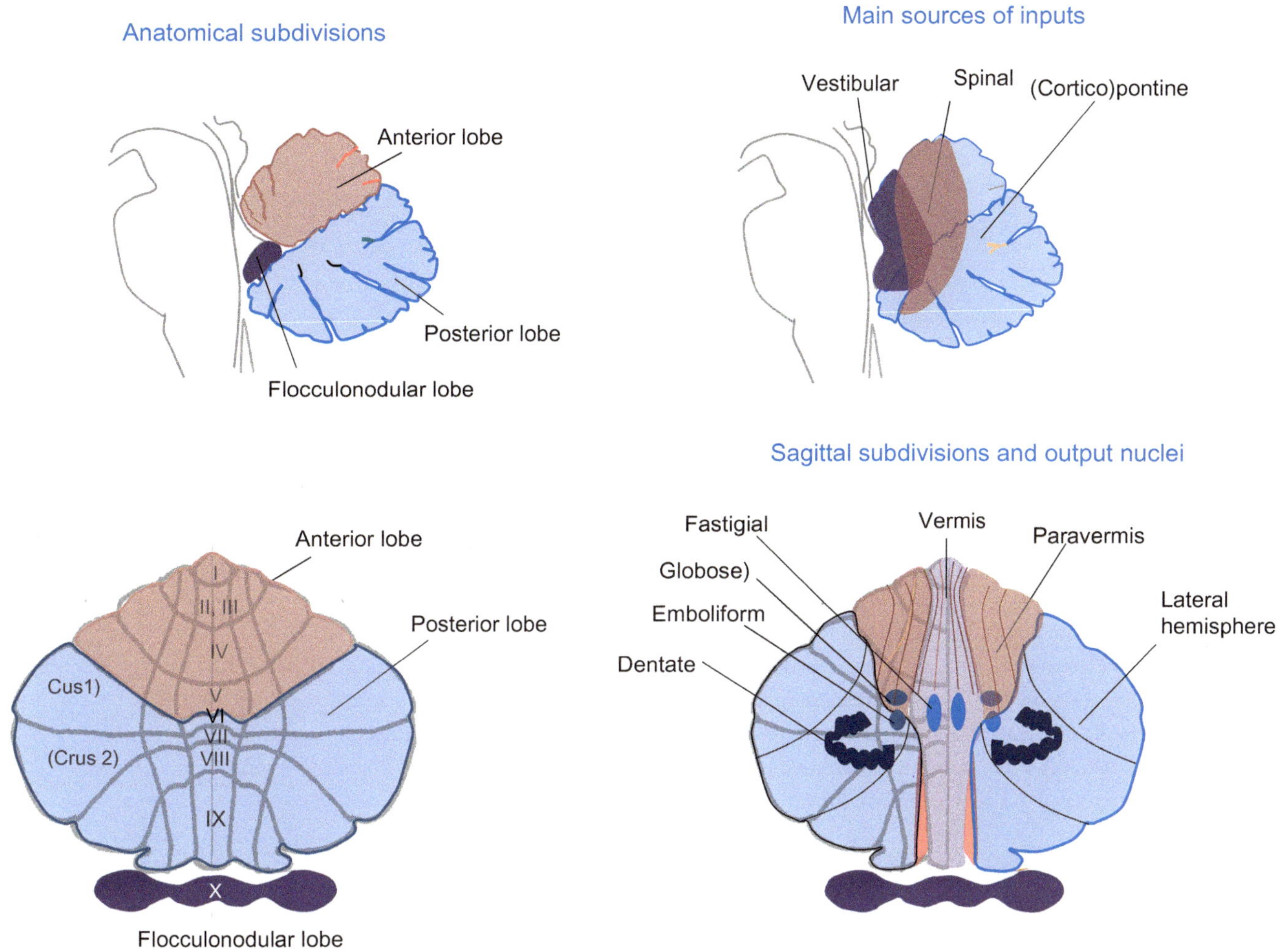

FIGURE 33.1 Anatomical subdivisions of the cerebellum.
The cerebellum is classically subdivided into a flocculonodular lobe (vestibulocerebellum) and the body of the cerebellum, which includes the cerebellar vermis and hemispheres forming an anterior lobe (lobules I–V/VI) and a posterior lobe (lobules VI/VII–IX), separated by the primary fissure. Except for the flocculonodular lobe, which participates in direct reciprocal interactions with the vestibular nuclei, the cerebellum interacts with the rest of the CNS via outputs mediated by the cerebellar nuclei. The anterior and posterior lobes are subdivided into a vermis, a paravermis, and a lateral cerebellar hemisphere. The vermis includes a medial vermis that projects to its targets via the fastigial nucleus and a lateral vermis that projects directly to the lateral vestibular nucleus. The paravermis projects to its targets via the anterior (globose) and posterior (emboliform) nucleis. The lateral cerebellar hemisphere projects to its targtes via the dentate nucleus.

Connections with the Cerebral Cortex

Based on fMRI and connectivity studies, the cerebellum can be subdivided into motor and nonmotor domains (Figure 33.2).[4–6] The motor domain includes two regions, the anterior lobe and a region in the paramedian lobule. Each contains a somatotopic representation that is a mirror image of each other. The extensive nonmotor domain includes portions of the posterior vermis and hemispheres. In humans, fMRI studies show that most of the cerebellum interacts with associative portions of the neocortex.[5–7] The fundamental feature of the interactions between the cerebellum and the cerebral cortex is the presence of multiple closed-loop circuits that interconnect the cerebral neocortex with the contralateral cerebellum via the thalamus though functionally segregated input-output channels[8] (Figure 33.3). Inputs from the cerebral cortex relayed via the pontine nuclei provide topographically organized mossy fiber projections to both the cerebellar nuclei and cerebellar cortex (cortico-ponto-cerebellar connections). For example, the visual cortex projects to the dorsolateral pontine nuclei innervating the flocculonodular lobe; the sensorimotor cortex to caudal pontine nuclei innervating the anterior lobe, and the prefrontal, cingulate, and posterior parietal cortex, to ventrally located pontine nuclei largely targeting the posterior lobe.

The cerebellum provides output to the neocortex via the deep cerebellar nuclei, which project to several territories of

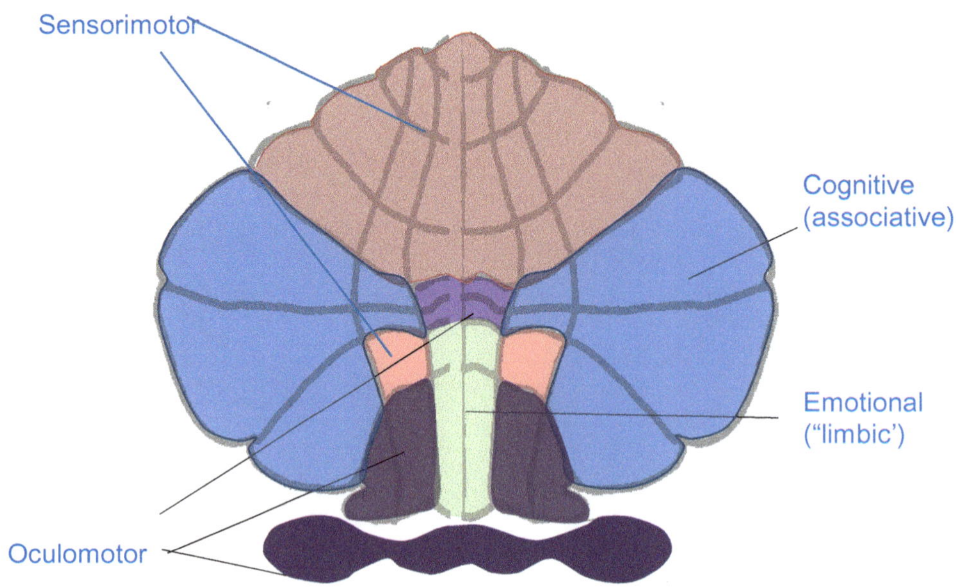

FIGURE 33.2 Motor and nonmotor domains of the cerebellum.
Based on fMRI and connectivity studies, the cerebellum can be subdivided into motor and nonmotor domains. The motor domain includes two regions, the anterior lobe and a region in the paramedian lobule; each contains a somatotopic representation that is a mirror image of the other. Most of the cerebellum interacts with associative portions of the neocortex. The extensive nonmotor domain includes portions of the posterior vermis and hemispheres. The oculomotor domains include the flocculonodular lobe (vestibulocerebellum) and the dorsal oculomotor vermis.

the contralateral thalamus. The thalamic territories of the cerebellum include the posterior portion of the ventral lateral nucleus—VL, also referred to as ventral lateral posterior—VLp or ventral intermedius—Vim), which targets motor and premotor cortical areas, and portions of the mediodorsal and intralaminar nuclei that target the prefrontal, parietal, and other association areas. The dorsal (motor) portion of the dentate nucleus relays inputs from the anterior lobe to motor territories of the thalamus that project to the cortical motor areas. The ventral (associative) portion relays inputs from the posterior lobe to thalamic territories that target the dorsolateral prefrontal cortex, posterior parietal cortex, and lateral temporal cortex (Figure 33.4).

Connections with the Basal Ganglia

There are also reciprocal connections between the cerebellum and the basal ganglia[4,9] (Figure 33.5). The basal ganglia provide input to the cerebellum via the subthalamic nucleus (STN), which projects to the pontine nuclei targeting the contralateral cerebellum. The cerebellar nuclei provide output to the basal ganglia via the intralaminar nuclei, particularly the centrolateral nucleus, which project to the striatum. Like the case of cortico-cerebellar connections, the reciprocal basal ganglia–cerebellar connections are segregated into motor and nonmotor domains. The dorsal (motor) dentate interacts with the putamen whereas the ventral (associative) dentate interacts with the caudate. The high topographic specificity of the pathways linking the different regions of the cerebral cortex, thalamus, basal ganglia, and cerebellum creates separate motor, oculomotor, associative, and limbic channels. Tactography studies in humans also show that there are also direct pathways from the dentate nucleus to the putamen and globus pallidus pars externa (GPe), and from the dentate nucleus to the globus pallidus pars interna (GPi) and substantia nigra.[10] This direct input from the dentate nucleus interact with those from the cerebral cortex to shape the basal ganglia output.

Connections with the Vestibular Nuclei, Reticular Formation, and Spinal Cord

The connectivity of the cerebellum with the motor cortex, brainstem, and spinal cord provides for control of eye movements, posture, muscle tone, and locomotion. The motor cortex sends simultaneously a command to the segmental motor apparatus to elicit a movement and predictive feedforward signal (efference copy) to the cerebellum about the expected sensory consequences of the movement. The main targets of this motor and somatosensory information are the vermis and paravermis of the anterior lobe (motor cerebellum). These regions also receive mossy fiber input from the spinal cord. One source of such spinocerebellar pathways are spinal interneurons that integrate descending

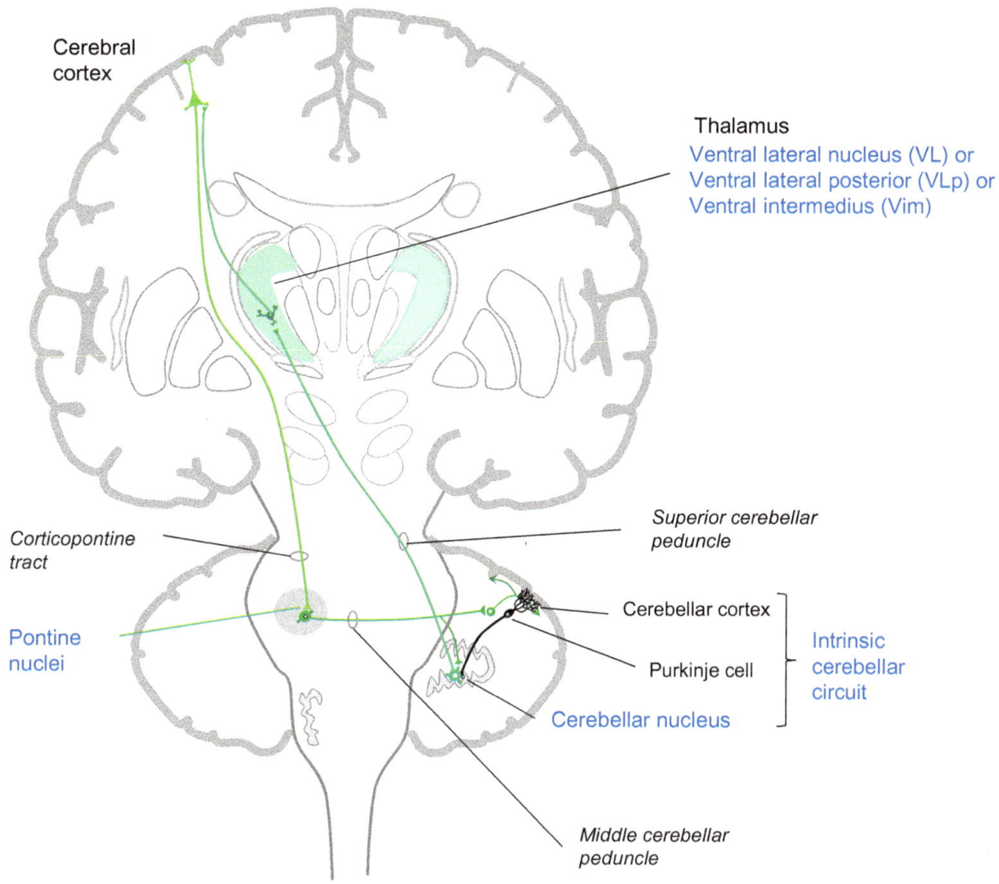

FIGURE 33.3 Basic cortico-cerebellar connections.
Inputs from the cerebral cortex are relayed to the contralateral cerebellum via the pontine nuclei, which project to contralateral cerebellum (cortico-ponto-cerebellar connections). The cerebellum provides output to the neocortex via the deep cerebellar nuclei, which project to several territories of the contralateral thalamus. The thalamic territories of the cerebellum include the posterior portion of the ventral lateral nucleus (VLp, also referred to as ventral intermedius, Vim), which targets motor and premotor cortical areas, and portions of the mediodorsal and intralaminar nuclei that target the prefrontal, parietal, and other association areas (not shown).

motor commands with local sensory feedback, as discussed in chapter 31. These interneurons send feedforward information about their relative excitatory drive both directly via the ventral spinocerebellar tract or through a relay in the lateral reticular nucleus (spino-reticulo-cerebellar tract). Feedback information about the actual movement is conveyed by neurons of the Clarke column via the dorsal spinocerebellar tract for the lower limb from the external cuneate nucleus in the medulla via the cuneocerebellar tract for the upper limb. Both feedforward and feedback signals from the spinal cord reach the ION via the spino-olivary tract and then from the ION to the cerebellum via the climbing fibers.

The cerebellum controls posture, muscle tone, and locomotion via direct projections to the lateral vestibular nucleus (source of the lateral vestibulospinal tract), medial and inferior vestibular nuclei, and pontine and medullary reticular formation (source of the reticulospinal tracts). As discussed in the previous chapter, the cerebellum has a critical role in the control of brainstem oculomotor circuits. The vestibulocerebellum, including the flocculus/paraflocculus, nodulus, and uvula (tonsil), controls the vestibulo-ocular reflex and smooth pursuit via projections to the medial and superior vestibular nuclei. The oculomotor cerebellum, including the dorsal oculomotor vermis (lobules VI–VII) and the posterior portion of the fastigial nucleus (fastigial oculomotor region) receives visual puts and inputs signaling oculomotor commands from the frontal eye fields and superior colliculus via pontine nuclei. The oculomotor cerebellum controls saccadic eye movements via fastigial projections to both saccadic burst neurons and onmipause neurons of the brainstem and superior colliculus. The oculomotor cerebellum also controls smooth pursuit.

Connections with the Inferior Olivary Nucleus

The ION is the sole origin of the climbing fibers and projects to all subdivisions of the contralateral cerebellum

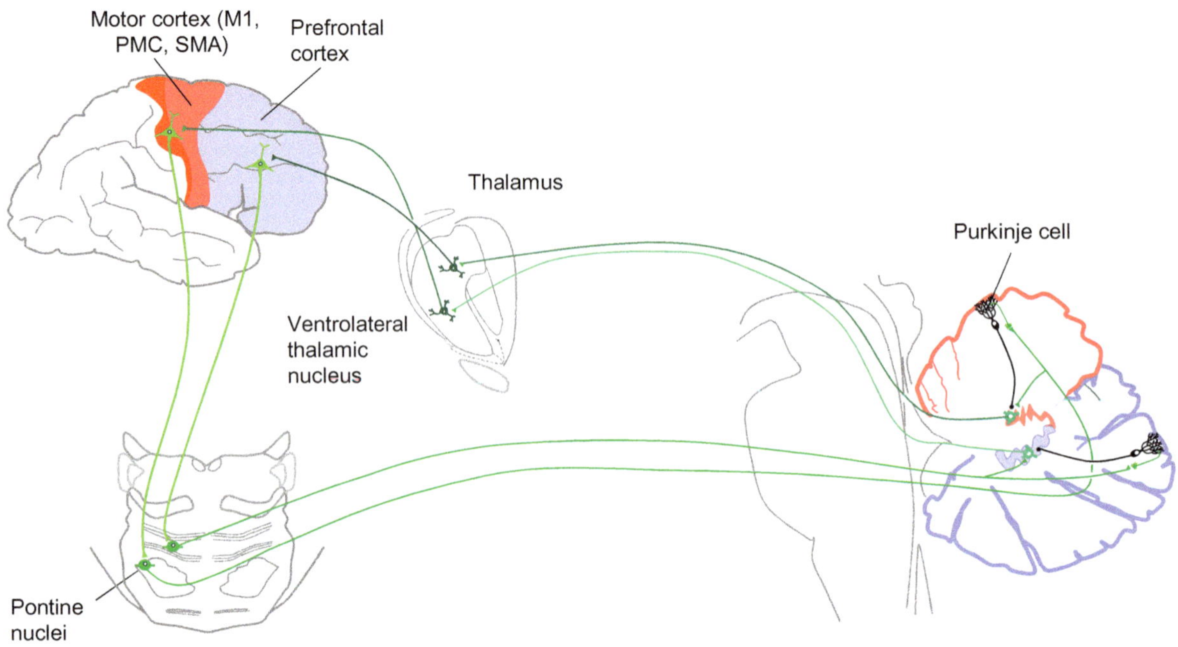

FIGURE 33.4 Functional segregation of the cerebellar outputs.
The cerebellar output to cerebral cortex via the thalamus is functionally segregated into parallel channels. For example, the dorsal (motor) portion of the dentate nucleus relays inputs from the anterior lobe to motor territories of the thalamus that project to the primary motor cortex (M1), premotor cortex (PMC), and supplementary motor area (SMA). In contrast, the ventral (associative) portion relays inputs from the posterior lobe to thalamic territories that target the dorsolateral prefrontal cortex, posterior parietal cortex, and lateral temporal cortex.

via the olivocerebellar system traveling in the inferior cerebellar peduncle. Climbing fibers target both the cerebellar nuclei and the cerebellar cortex in a regular somatotopic fashion.[11] The ION receives collateral inputs from all spinal, reticular, vestibular, and cortico-pontine pathways that target the corresponding portion of the cerebellum. The ION and the cerebellum are interconnected via several functional loops (Figure 32.6). The inhibitory olivo-nucleo-olivary loop involves a collateral projection from climbing fibers to the cerebellar nuclei (olivonuclear connection) targeting a unique population of cerebellar nuclear GABAergic neurons that send a reciprocal inhibitory nucleo-olivary output the corresponding ION neurons. This pathway provides a feedback inhibition that suppresses climbing fiber input to the related area of the cerebellar cortex. The olivo-cortico-nucleo-olivary loop involves a climbing fiber input to Purkinje cells that target the inhibitory nucleo-olivary neurons; in this the loop Purkinje cell functions as an inhibitory interneuron that disinhibits the ION. A third loop consists of an excitatory disynaptic connection, via a projection of the cerebellar nuclei to nuclei of the meso-diencephalic junction, particularly the parvocellular portion of the red nucleus, which in turn sends an excitatory projection to the ION. Both the inhibitory and excitatory loops involve ascending crossed projections from the deep cerebellar nuclei via the superior cerebellar peduncle and a descending projection via the central tegmental tract to the ION. Together with the olivocerebellar connection via the inferior cerebellar peduncle, this constitutes the so-called Guillain-Mollaret triangle.

INTRINSIC CIRCUITS OF THE CEREBELLUM

The intrinsic circuits of the cerebellum include several types of excitatory and inhibitory neurons distributed in the cerebellar cortex and cerebellar nuclei (Figure 33.7).

Cerebellar Cortex

The cerebellar cortex includes three layers, granular cell layer, Purkinje cell layer, and molecular layer. The granule cells are the most abundant neuronal type in the CNS (an estimate of 80 billion in humans).[12] Of note, granule cells are particularly susceptible to the JC virus (JCV) infection responsible for progressive multifocal leukoencephalopathy (PML); one distinct phenotype of PML is granule cell neuronopathy, characterized by exclusive or predominant cerebellar atrophy.[13] Granule cells are glutamatergic, receive excitatory inputs from mossy fibers and send ascending unmyelinated axons toward the superficial molecular layer.

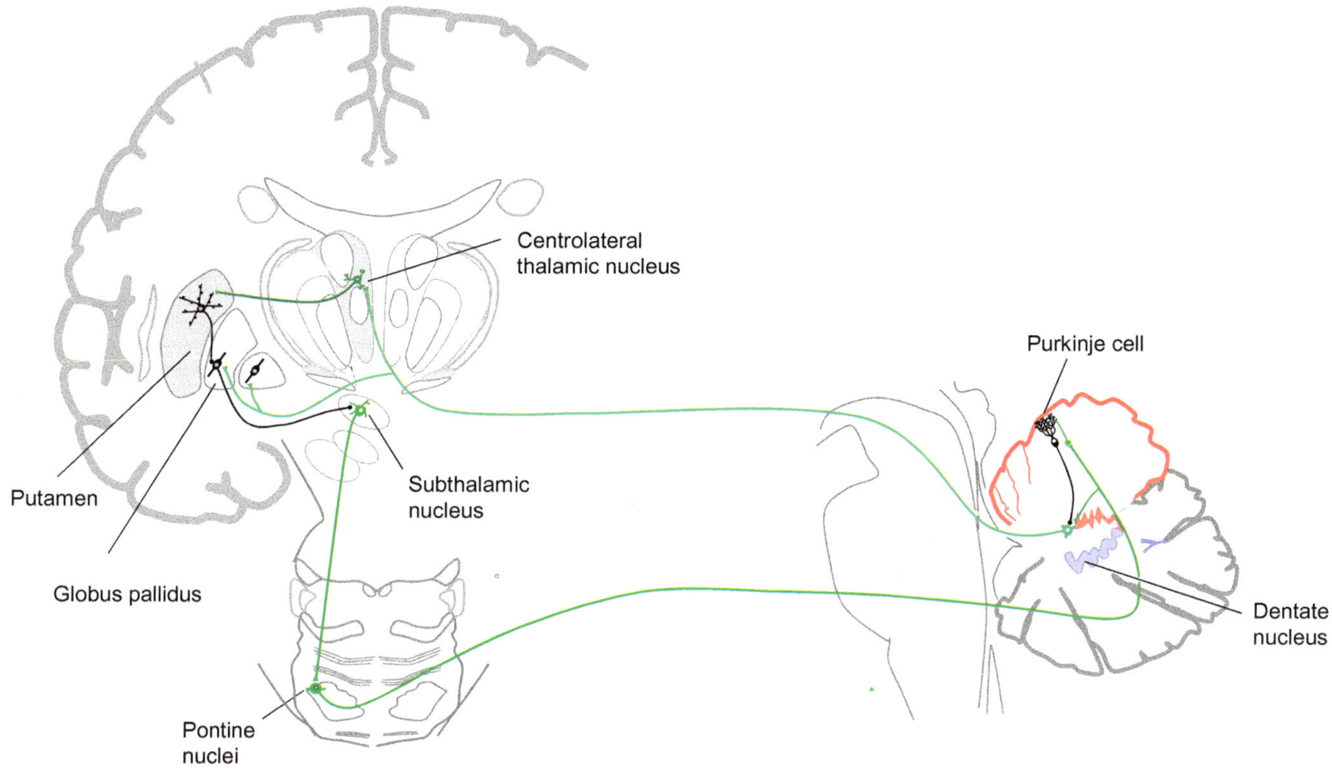

FIGURE 33.5 Reciprocal connections between the cerebellum and the basal ganglia.
The basal ganglia provide input to the cerebellum via the subthalamic nucleus (STN), which projects to the pontine nuclei that then relay basal ganglia information to the contralateral cerebellum. The cerebellar nuclei provide the main output to the basal ganglia via the intralaminar nuclei, that project to the striatum. There are also direct pathways from the cerebellar nuclei to the basal ganglia bypassing the thalamus. These include a pathway from the dentate nucleus terminating in the putamen and globus pallidus pars externa (GPe), and a pathway from the dentate nucleus to the globus pallidus pars internal (GPi) and substantia nigra (not shown).

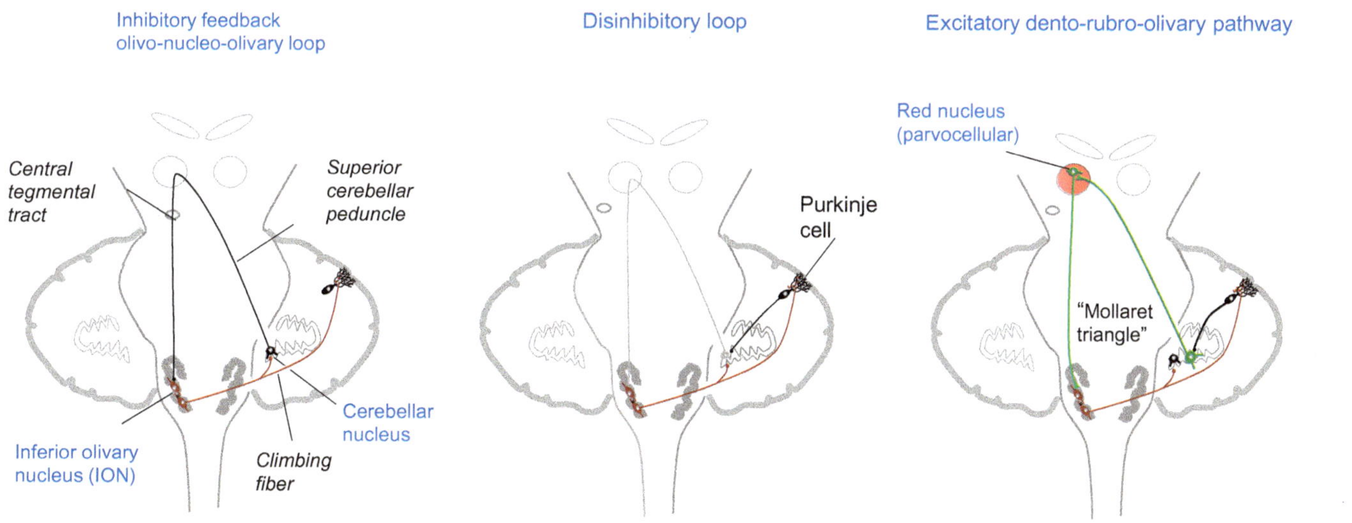

FIGURE 33.6 Inferior olivary nucleus and olivo-cerebellar interactions.
The inferior olivary nucleus (ION) provides climbing fibers to all subdivisions of the contralateral cerebellum. The ION and the cerebellum are interconnected via several functional loops, an inhibitory olivo-nucleo-olivary loop, a disinhibitory olivo-cortico-nucleo-olivary loop and an excitatory loop via nuclei in the mesodiencephalic junction and known as dento-rubro-olivary pathway (Guillain-Mollaret triangle).

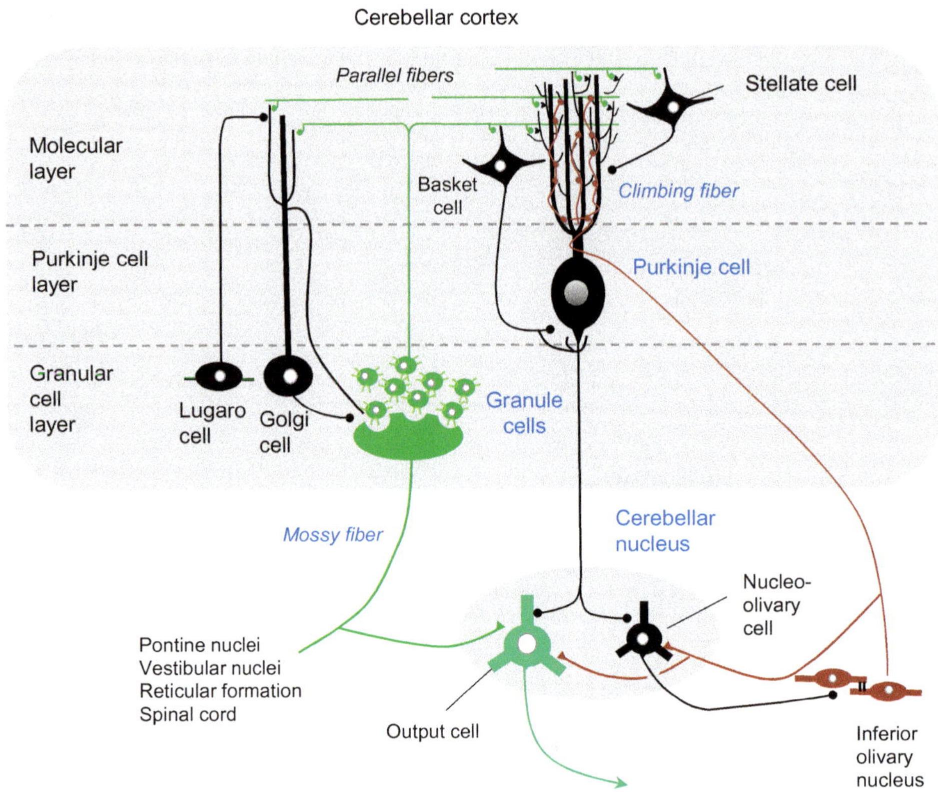

FIGURE 33.7 Intrinsic circuit of the cerebellum.
The cerebellar cortex includes three layers: the granular cell layer, Purkinje cell layer, and molecular layer. Granule cells are glutamatergic, receive excitatory inputs from mossy fibers, and send ascending unmyelinated axons toward the superficial molecular layer; these axons bifurcate into parallel fibers that target the dendrites of Purkinje cells, Golgi cells, stellate cells, basket cells, and Lugaro cells. Purkinje cells send inhibitory projections to the deep cerebellar nuclei. The climbing fibers, which originate from the ION, provide a robust input to individual Purkinje cells. The cerebellar nuclei contains glutamatergic neurons that send excitatory projections to the thalamus, red nucleus, vestibular nuclei, and reticular formation and thus are the main output system of the cerebellum, as well as and smaller GABAergic neurons that send inhibitory projections to the ION. The output neurons of the cerebellar nuclei receive excitatory input from collaterals of both mossy and climbing fibers. The cerebellar nuclei also contain several types of interneurons (not shown).

These axons bifurcate into parallel fibers that extend in each direction along the plane of the folia in the molecular cell layer, targeting the dendritic spines of Purkinje cells as well as several inhibitory interneurons. The mossy-parallel fiber system is strikingly divergent. Mossy fibers provide synaptic inputs to the short claw-like dendrites of granule cells in complex synapses called glomeruli. A single mossy fiber makes synaptic contacts with the dendrites of up to ~500 granule cells. Purkinje cells have large dendritic trees that on average may be intersected by as many as 200,000 parallel fibers, thereby collecting information from as many as a million granule cells. Parallel fibers also provide input to Golgi cells, which inhibit transmission of mossy fiber input to the granule cells. Parallel fibers also activate local GABAergic interneurons in the molecular layer, including stellate cells that contact the dendrites of nearby Purkinje cells and basket cells that innervate the cell body and axon initial segment of Purkinje cells and powerfully control Purkinje cell output. An important target of parallel fibers are Lugaro cells, which extend dendrites at a distance within the molecular layer in the plane of the parallel fibers and inhibit the Golgi cells.

The second major excitatory input to the Purkinje cells is provided by the climbing fibers from the ION. In contrast to the divergent parallel fiber system, the climbing fibers provide a robust input to individual Purkinje cells. Each ION neuron may provide up to 10 climbing fibers. Each Purkinje cell receives branches of only one climbing fiber that forms a distributed synapse along entire dendritic tree of making ~1,500 synaptic contacts primarily on proximal dendrites of Purkinje cells, thus constituting one of the most powerful synapses in the CNS.[14]

Deep Cerebellar Nuclei

Purkinje cells are GABAergic and target the deep cerebellar nuclei. The cerebellar nuclei contain two types of projection neurons.[15] Approximately one-half of them are large glutamatergic neurons that send excitatory projections to the thalamus, red nucleus, vestibular nuclei, and reticular formation. The second half consists of smaller GABAergic neurons that send inhibitory projections to the ION. In addition to strong inhibition from Purkinje cells, neurons of the cerebellar nuclei receive excitatory input from collaterals of both mossy and climbing fibers. There is convergence of Purkinje cell input to the cerebellar nuclei, with a Purkinje cell: nuclear cell ratio of ~ 20:1. A single Purkinje cell may target both large glutamatergic and small GABAergic projection neurons.[15] The cerebellar nuclei also contain several types of interneurons, including glutamatergic and GABA/glycinergic interneurons.

ORGANIZATION AND FUNCTION OF THE MOSSY AND CLIMBING FIBER SYSTEMS

Mossy Fiber Input: Multimodal Widespread Input to Purkinje Cells Populations

Granule cells receive a multimodal convergence of inputs and respond to specific combinations of sensory and motor signals.[16] These signals are conveyed by parallel fibres to provide a continuous modulation of Purkinje cell activity. The drive to Purkinje cells also comes from synapses formed by the granule cell axon as it ascends radially to the molecular layer before bifurcating into parallel fibers. Processing of mossy fiber input at the granular cell layer is closely regulated by Golgi cells. These cells are interconnected by gap junctions and make inhibitory axo-axonic and axodendritic GABAergic synapses at the glomeruli, thereby regulating the transfer of inputs from the mossy fiber to the granule cells.[17,18] As Golgi cells receive both direct excitatory input from mossy fibers and excitation from parallel fibers at their dendrites in the molecular layer, they provide both feedforward and feedback inhibition to granule cells. Feedforward inhibition from Golgi cells enhances the temporal precision of granule cell responses by narrowing their window for synaptic integration of mossy fiber input.[17,18]

Inferior Olivary-Climbing Fiber System: Timing and Error Signal

The climbing fiber input to the cerebellum is organized in strictly sagittal bands, so that nearby ION neurons target Purkinje cells localized in narrow rostrocaudal bands in the cerebellar cortex. At each sagittal zone, climbing fibers give off collaterals to the portion of the cerebellar nuclei that receives inputs from the Purkinje cells of the same zone. This sagittal organization complements the topographically arranged input from the mossy-parallel fiber system, and together these two types of inputs subdivide the cerebellar cortex into multiple functional zones, each dedicated to processing signals originating from a certain area of the body or sensory modality. The ION consists of spiny excitatory neurons that have oscillatory properties, fire spontaneously at 1–10 Hz, and are electronically coupled by dendrodendritic gap junctions so that they tend to fire in groups or clusters.[14] The efficacy of this electronic coupling is negatively modulated by GABAergic input from the cerebellar nuclei via the nucleo-olivary pathway, which thereby reduces the size of the clusters of synchronously oscillating ION neurons. Synchronization of ION may involve other circuit interactions, including common synaptic excitatory inputs.

The olivocerebellar system has a critical role in timing function for motor coordination. Climbing fibers synchronically activate different parasagittal bands of Purkinje cells at irregular intervals at a frequency of 1 to 3 Hz.[14] Simultaneous activation of several ION clusters and the degree of synchronization of ION oscillations generates timing sequences, such as observed both in the organization of coordinated movements and in physiologic tremor. The ION may also function as a comparator between predictive (feedforward) commands issued by the cerebral cortex (motor efference copy) and feedback signals from sensory receptors activated by the actual movement. This comparison generates an "error signal" that is used to adjust the motor command. For example, while learning to play the piano, predictive feedforward commands from the motor cortex to motor neurons are compared with feedback input from finger proprioceptors to generate error signals that allow the cortex to readjust the commands and thus improve performance. When a movement error occurs, neurons of the ION increase their firing rate; resetting of the oscillatory phase in the ION reorganizes the motor pattern.[19]

PHYSIOLOGY OF PURKINJE CELLS

Purkinje cells critically regulate the cerebellar output. The function of Purkinje cells is shaped by four main factors: (1) pacemaking activity reflecting their intrinsic electrophysiological properties; (2) tonic excitatory inputs from parallel fibers on their dendritic spines; (3) phasic and strong input to climbing fibers at the proximal dendrites; and (4) inhibitory influences from basket and stellate cells, as well as collaterals from other Purkinje cells.[20]

Pacemaker Activity

The hallmark of Purkinje cells is their intrinsic, regular pacing activity at ~40 Hz in the absence of synaptic inputs. Under normal conditions these cells can sustain firing at a large dynamic range; in vivo, their firing frequency is between 40–100 Hz. Purkinje cells express a unique repertoire of ion channels that regulate their pacing activity[21,22] (Figure 33.8). Fast spiking and modulation of Purkinje cells primarily depends on resurgent sodium (Na^+) currents via $Na_v1.6$ and $Na_v1.1$ channels and rapid repolarization via fast inactivating potassium (K^+) channels, particularly $K_v3.3$ channels. Depolarization activates voltage-gated calcium (Ca^{2+})

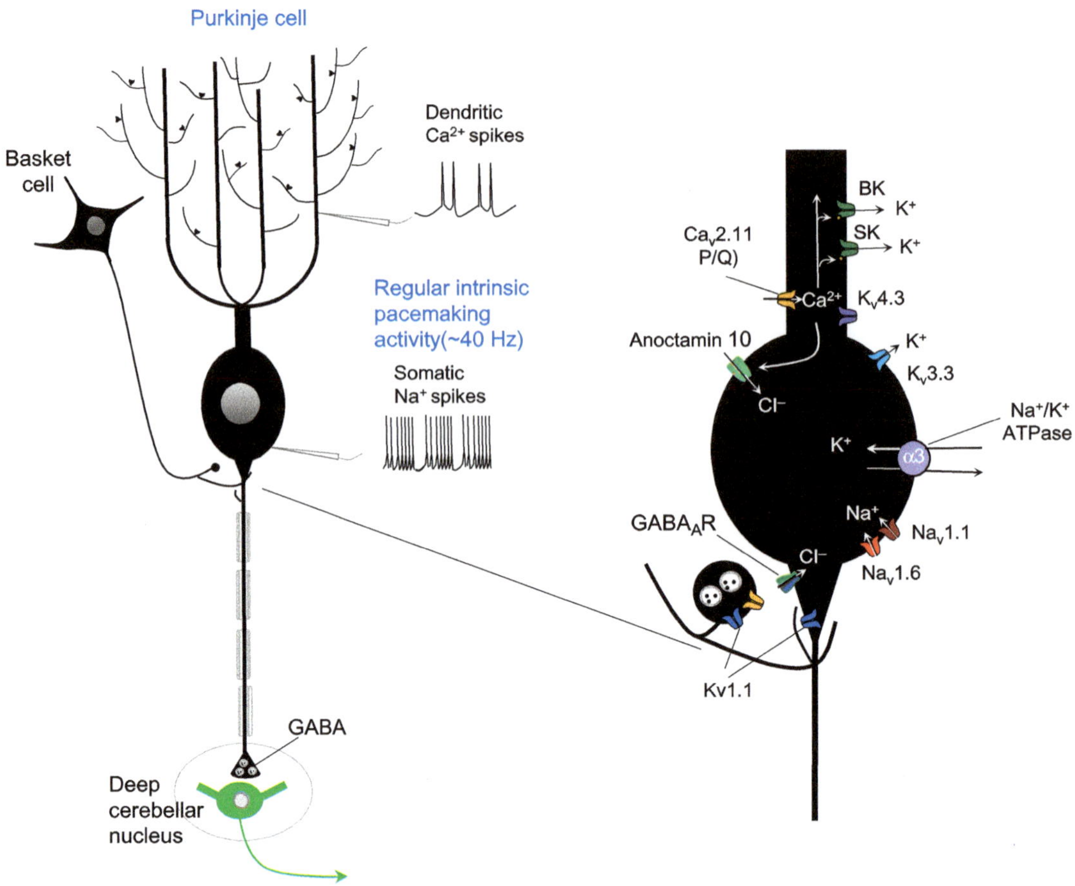

FIGURE 33.8 Electrophysiological activity and ion channels in Purkinje cells.
Fast firing of Purkinje cells depends on resurgent sodium (Na^+) currents via Na_v1.6 and Na_v1.1 channels and rapid repolarization via K_v3.3 channels. Depolarization also activates voltage-gated calcium (Ca^{2+}) channels, particularly Ca_v2.1 (P/Q) and Ca_v3 (T) channels. These voltage-gated Ca^{2+} channels are tightly coupled to calcium-activated potassium channels (K_{Ca}), primarily the large-conductance (BK, K_{Ca}1.1) and the small-conductance (SK, K_{Ca}2.2) channels. The depolarization necessary for autonomous spiking is regulated by subthreshold-(A-type) potassium channels active during that time. Ion gradients in Purkinje cells are maintained by activity of the α3 subunit containing Na^+/K^+ ATPase. Anoctamin (ANO) 2 channels are involved in calcium-dependent ionic plasticity that reduces the efficacy of GABAergic synapses by increasing the postsynaptic Cl^- concentration.

channels, particularly Ca_v2.1 (P/Q) and Ca_v3 (T) channels, which allow Ca^{2+} influx first in the fine dendritic branches, followed by the dendritic trunk. These voltage-gated Ca^{2+} channels are tightly coupled to calcium-activated potassium channels including large-conductance (BK, K_{Ca}1.1) and the small-conductance (SK, K_{Ca}2.2) channels, which generate an afterhyperpolarization that is essential for deinactivation of Na_v channels, allowing the generation of a subsequent action potential and thus promoting pacemaker activity. Ion gradients in Purkinje cells are maintained by activity of the α3 subunit containing Na^+/K^+ ATPase. Purkinje cells also express anoctamin (ANO) 2 channels in their dendritic trees; these Ca^{2+}-activated chloride (Cl^-) channels are involved in synaptic plasticity by increasing the postsynaptic Cl^- concentration and thus reducing the efficacy of GABAergic synapses.[23]

Synaptic Control of Purkinje Cells

Purkinje cells contain three synaptic domains: the distal branches covered by dendritic spines that receive synapses from parallel fibers; the proximal dendritic ramifications innervated by a single excitatory climbing fiber; and the cell body and axon hillock receiving GABAergic inputs from inhibitory basket interneurons. The glutamatergic inputs from the parallel and climbing fibers generate fast excitatory postsynaptic currents via α-amino-3-hydroxy-5-methyl-4-isoxazolepropionic acid receptors (AMPARs) and slower signals via metabotropic glutamate type 1 receptors (mGluR1s). These signals elicit depolarization and increase in intracellular Ca^{2+}, which is critical for the normal function of the Purkinje cells (Figure 33.9). Activation of AMPARs at the parallel fiber-Purkinje cell synapse triggers Na^+ influx leading to a fast excitatory potential called simple

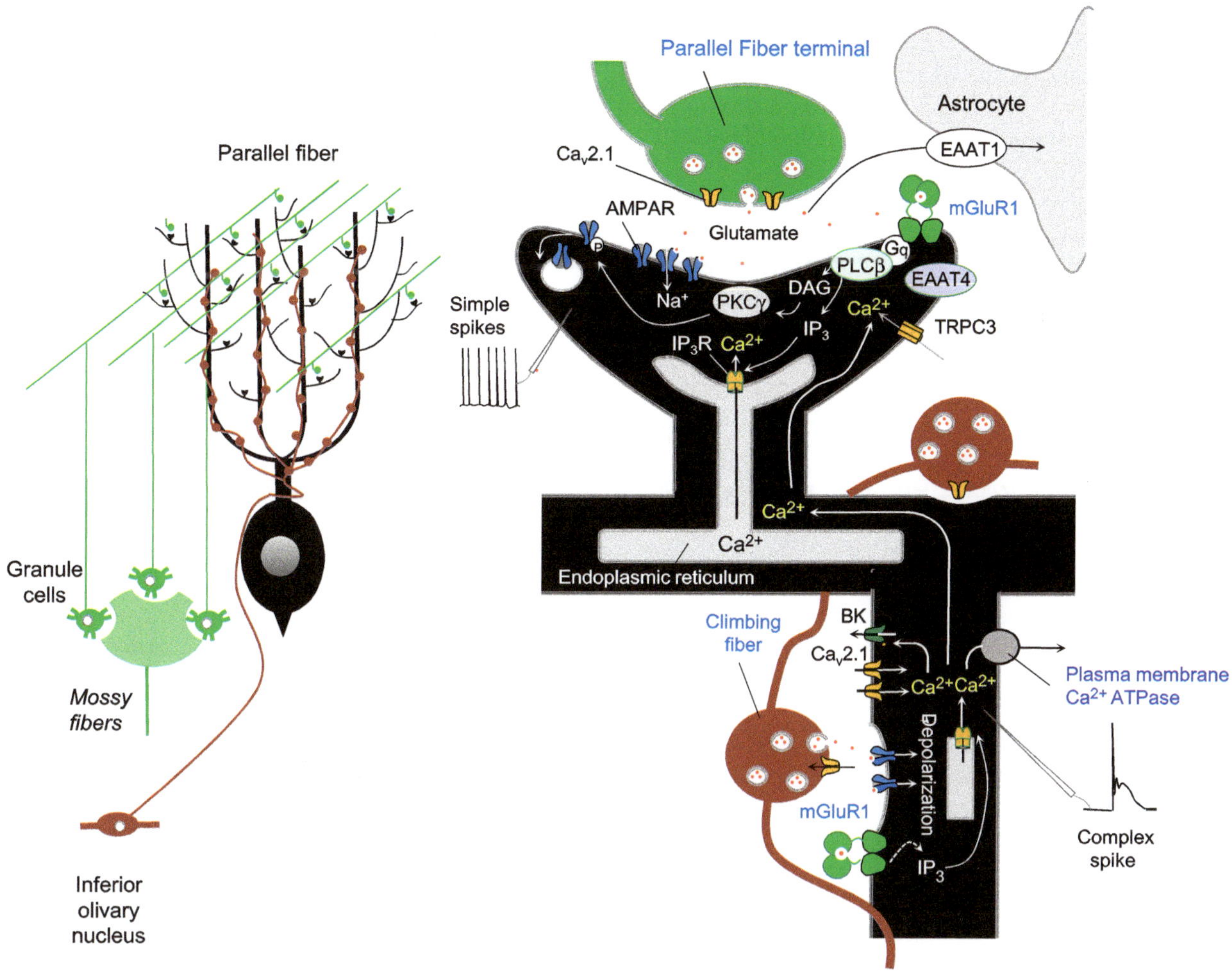

FIGURE 33.9 Synaptic control of Purkinje cells.

The glutamatergic inputs from the parallel and climbing fibers generate fast excitatory postsynaptic currents via α-amino-3-hydroxy-5-methyl-4-isoxazolepropionic acid receptors (AMPARs) and slower signals via metabotropic glutamate type 1 receptors (mGluR1s). Activation of AMPARs at the parallel fiber–Purkinje cell synapse triggers a fast excitatory potential called a simple spike. In contrast, each action potential in the climbing fiber generates a complex spike that depends on P/Q-type channels, leading to a large increase in intracellular Ca^{2+} concentration that spreads throughout the dendritic tree. The magnitude of intracellular Ca^{2+} signal is in part regulated by Ca^{2+} extrusion via the plasma membrane Ca^{2+} transporter. The glutamate signal is terminated in part via reuptake by the excitatory amino acid transporter (EAAT)-1 present in astrocytes and the EAAT4 present in Purkinje cells. The parallel fiber–Purkinje cell synapse is a site of plasticity. Activation of mGluR1 receptors coupled to the G_q, initiates a signal transduction cascade that involves phospholipase C β (PLC β) and hydrolysis of membrane phosphatidylinositol biphosphate, yielding inositol triphosphate (IP_3) and diacylglycerol (DAG). Purkinje cells express high levels of IP_3 receptors (IP_3Rs, ITPRs), which allows Ca^{2+} release from the endoplasmic reticulum (ER). This generates a localized increase in Ca^{2+} accompanied by an excitatory postsynaptic potential mediated by a member of the canonical transient receptor potential 3 (TRPC3) channels. Calcium acts synergistically with DAG to activate protein kinase Cα (PKCα), which phosphorylates GluA2 subunits of the AMPAR in the dendritic spines resulting in receptor endocytosis. The mGluR1 signal may also trigger presynaptic LTD via Ca^{2+}-triggered production of endocannabinoids and retrograde signal via inhibitory presynaptic cannabinoid 1 receptors (not shown).

spike; the high discharge rates of simple spikes (50–300 Hz) provides continuous and dynamic information about direction, amplitude, position, and speed of movement.

In contrast, because of the 1:1 relationship with Purkinje cells, multiple synaptic contacts and extensive coverage of the dendritic tree climbing fiber input provides a powerful influence. Each action potential generates a large depolarization in the dendrites of Purkinje cells called a complex spike, which primarily depends on activation of $Ca_v2.1$ (P/Q) channels.[24] These Ca^{2+} transients have a fundamental role in dendritic integration and synaptic plasticity and their magnitude is in part regulated by Ca^{2+} extrusion via the plasma membrane Ca^{2+} transporter. The glutamate signal is terminated in part via reuptake by the excitatory amino acid transporter (EAAT)1 present in astrocytes and the EAAT4 present in Purkinje cells.

Inhibitory GABAergic interneurons, including stellate cells and basket cells form small local networks synchronized by electrical coupling, and participate in mechanisms of lateral inhibition within the cerebellar cortex. The axoaxonic synapse from basket cells in the axon initial segment of the Purkinje cell strongly regulates the timing of firing of action potentials.

Plasticity at the Parallel Fiber–Purkinje Cell Synapse

Synaptic plasticity at the parallel fiber–Purkinje cell synapse has a major role in controlling Purkinje cell activity.[25–27] Activation of perisynaptic mGlu1Rs located at some distance to the site of glutamate release triggers a G_{q}- phospholipase C β cascade that results in production of inositol triphosphate (IP_3) and diacylglycerol. Purkinje cells express high levels of IP_3 receptor (IP_3R, ITPR), which allows Ca^{2+} release from the endoplasmic reticulum. This generates a localized increase in Ca^{2+} in a portion of the dendritic tree, which is accompanied by an excitatory postsynaptic potential mediated by canonical transient receptor potential 3 (TRPC3) channels. The mGluR1 signal is critical for induction of long-term depression (LTD) at the parallel fiber–Purkinje cell synapse.[25] The coincident activation of parallel and climbing fibers leads to a substantial increase in Ca^{2+} concentration at the dendrites. Calcium acts synergistically with diacylglycerol to activate protein kinase Cα (PKCα), which phosphorylates GluA2 subunits of the AMPAR in the dendritic spines resulting in receptor endocytosis. The mGluR1 signal may also trigger presynaptic LTD via Ca^{2+}-triggered production of endocannabinoids. In addition to LTD, the parallel fiber–Purkinje cell synapse may also undergo both presynaptically and postsynaptically expressed long-term potentiation.[26]

CEREBELLAR NUCLEI

The cerebellar output via the cerebellar nuclei is determined by the intrinsic electrophysiological features of their neurons, collateral excitatory inputs from mossy and climbing afferents, and strong inhibition from Purkinje cells (Figure 33.10).

Electrophysiological Activity

Neurons in the deep cerebellar nuclei have a tonic activity that is characterized by silent pauses followed by rebound excitation that is sent as a signal to the rest of the CNS. The projection of the Purkinje cell delivers a tonic inhibition of cerebellar nuclear cells; synchronous pauses in Purkinje cell firing result in a temporary lift of this tonic inhibition and generate a rebound activity in cerebellar nuclear cells. During postural adjustments, neurons of the cerebellar nuclei are initially depolarized by excitatory inputs from mossy and climbing fiber collaterals; this is followed by disynaptic feedforward inhibition via Purkinje cells activated by the same afferents, resulting in hyperpolarization and silencing ("down state") of the nuclear cells. Upon pauses of the inhibition by Purkinje cells, cerebellar nuclei cells undergo rebound depolarization generating bursts of action potentials via low-threshold Ca^{2+} channels ("up state"). The synchronous activation of a sagittal band of Purkinje cells by the climbing fibers produces synchronous inhibition of a band of cerebellar nuclear cells; this is followed by a rebound burst of activity that is transmitted as a timing signal to the cerebral cortex and subcortical premotor nuclei. This pulse-step sequence would allow prompt starting and stopping of movement.

Output of the Cerebellar Nuclei

Compared to the hundreds of thousands of separate processing units in the cerebellar cortex, the excitatory output of the deep cerebellar nuclei is coarsely organized. A single axon from a cerebellar nuclear neuron can branch and project to various brainstem and spinal targets. Thus the cerebellar output is more related to broad aspects of behavior, such as timing, planning, and execution rather than being modality- and topographically specific like the input to the cerebellum. A group of inhibitory neurons of the cerebellar nuclei project back to the cerebellar cortex targeting Golgi cells.[28] The projections from the cerebellar nuclei to the cerebral cortex via the thalamus, and those to the reticular formation and vestibular nuclei provide the substrate for the cerebellar control of coordinated and skilled limb movements, muscle tone, posture, locomotion, and eye movements. The cerebellar output is stronger to the ventral lateral nucleus (VLp/Vim) than to other thalamic nuclei.[29]

The cerebellum has a critical role both in the temporal planning of movement parameters and in error-driven online adjustments necessary to optimize motor performance. The ability to perform accurate reaching depends on the functional connectivity between the cerebellum and the primary motor cortex (M1). The cerebellum controls the excitability of M1; transcranial magnetic stimulation (TMS) of the cerebellar cortex reduces M1 excitability. This may reflect the TMS triggered activation of Purkinje cells with inhibition of the dentate nucleus and reduced excitatory

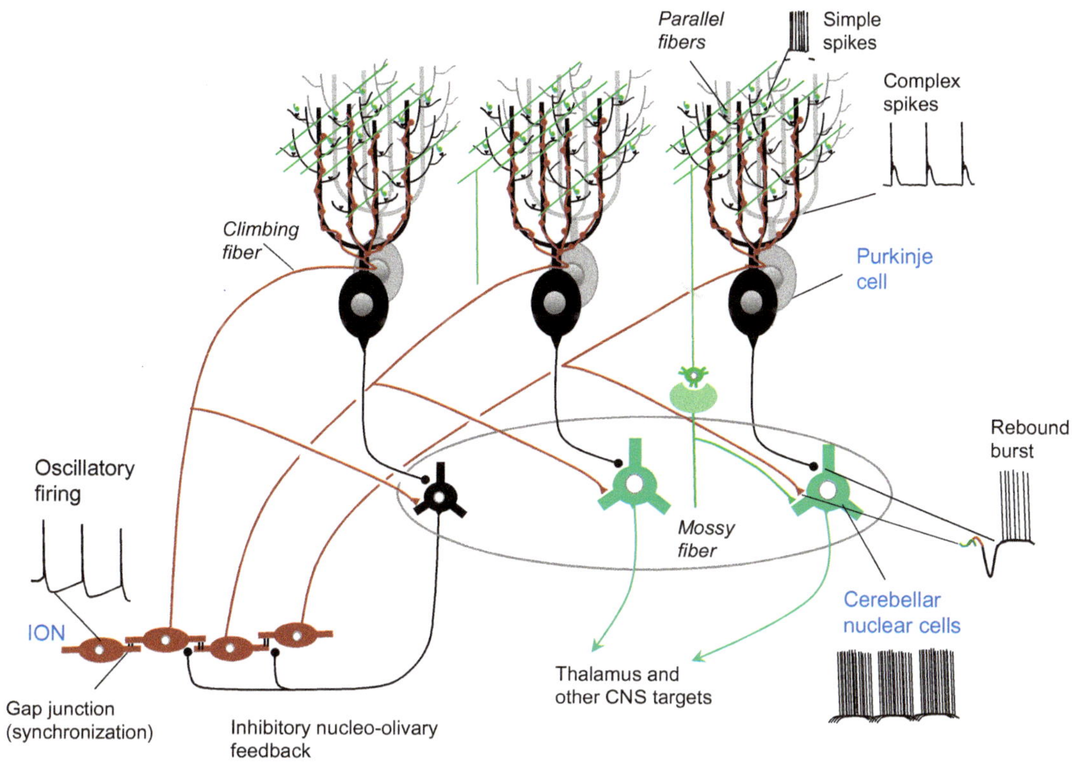

FIGURE 33.10 Physiology of the cerebellar nuclei.
The activity of neurons in the cerebellar nuclei depends on the interplay between their intrinsic membrane properties and synaptic influences, including monosynaptic excitatory inputs from collaterals of climbing fibers and mossy fibers and powerful disynaptic GABAergic inhibition from Purkinje cells. Neurons in the deep cerebellar nuclei have a tonic activity that is characterized by silent pauses followed by rebound excitation. Synchronous pauses in Purkinje cell firing results in a temporary lift of this tonic inhibition, and generates a rebound activity in cerebellar nuclear cells. The synchronous activation of a sagittal band of Purkinje cells by the climbing fibers produces synchronous inhibition of a band of cerebellar nuclear cells; this is followed by a rebound burst of activity that is transmitted as a timing signal to the rest of the brain.

effect of the dentothalamic projection on M1. Functional neuroimaging studies show that cerebellar activation, particularly in the anterior lobe, is strongly correlated with the frequency, quantity, speed, and spatial and temporal complexity of movements. During motor learning, activity of the cerebellar cortex progressively decreases while dentate nucleus activity increases in relation to movement intent, slightly before the discharge of M1. This anticipatory dentate nucleus discharge shortens the reaction time by providing a trigger signal for the motor cortex to start the intended movement in response to a relevant stimulus. This signal is further elaborated to specify the direction, timing, intensity, and patterns of muscles to use. Once the sequence is learned, dentate activation decreases and is partially superseded by activity in the striatum for automatic execution of the movement. The cerebellum is also involved in sensorimotor synchronization, in which an action, such as tapping, is temporarily locked to a predictable external event. This process involves sensory processing and time perception to allow the motor commands to anticipate the sensory input in order to synchronize the action. Accurate motor control of the limb also requires extracting both kinesthetic information from the moving limb and visual information for online correction of an action in response to continuous change in the location of a target. Functional MRI studies that the cerebellum is coupled to the inferior parietal cortex during processing of visuokinesthetic information. It has also been suggested that the primary function of the cerebellum may be to coordinate the acquisition of sensory information that can be used by the motor cortex and brainstem motor areas to initiate smooth and accurate movements.

The reciprocal interactions among the cerebellum, cerebral cortex, and basal ganglia have implications for the different forms of learning.[4,30] The cerebellum is involved in supervised (error-based) learning based on plasticity of the parallel fiber–Purkinje cell synapse under the influence of the ION. In contrast, the striatum is critical for reward-based (reinforcement, trial-and-error) learning based on dopamine signals from the midbrain, as discussed in the next chapter. Error correction signals from the climbing fibers train the Purkinje cells to control the transitions between a down-state and up-state state in cerebellar nuclei, much alike the dopaminergic signals that control the up- and down-state transitions of medium spiny neurons of the striatum for reward learning. Of note, the substantia nigra pars compacta sends dopaminergic inputs to the nucleo-olivary pathway and may control its activity according to the behavioral context. Supervised learning in the cerebellum can create a "forward model" that predicts the result of the expected actions. Both the cerebellar and basal ganglia loops via the thalamus target the same cortical areas that send the inputs to these loops. This promotes unsupervised associative learning in the motor cortex.

PURKINJE CELL DYSFUNCTION AND MECHANISMS OF ATAXIA

The functions of the cerebellum and the clinical manifestation of cerebellar disorders are well known by clinical neurologists and have been the subject of comprehensive reviews,[7,31,32] and thus only some salient features will be reemphasized in this chapter. The role of the cerebellum in oculomotor control, speech, and cognitive-affective functions are briefly reviewed in other chapters of this book. The cardinal feature of limb ataxia is the breakdown of temporal patterning of coordinated movement. This reflects the inability to precisely control timing, which is essential both to produce rapid movements and coordinate dynamic muscle interactions during multijoint movements. In patients with acute focal cerebellar lesions, upper limb ataxia correlates with damage of lobules IV–VI and lower limb ataxia with damage of lobules III–IV in the anterior lobe. In cases of cerebellar cortical atrophy, these deficits relate to involvement of the intermediate and lateral cerebellum. Patients with cerebellar lesions also have difficulties in predictive grip force control, and for movements which are time-locked to specific events that require anticipation within a millisecond range. This indicates the role of the cerebellum in alerting the cerebral cortex to incoming sensory stimuli. The main long-term consequences of cerebellar impairment are generalized slowness of movement and impaired acquisition of sensory inputs.

Purkinje cells have a major role in the pathophysiology of ataxia and are prominently involved in channelopathies and spinocerebellar ataxias (SCA). Evidence from experimental models indicate that there are at least two basic pathophysiological mechanisms underlying ataxia in these disorders: (1) impaired pacemaking activity of Purkinje cells and (2) dysregulated intracellular Ca^{2+}calcium signaling.[21,22,33–35] Genetic disorders affecting these functions are typically, but not always, autosomal dominant and manifest with episodic ataxia (EA) or SCA phenotypes. In general, channelopathies tend to present as pure cerebellar ataxia as opposed to more complex phenotypes observed in most polyglutamine repeat-associated SCAs or in autosomal recessive ataxias.

Impaired Pacemaker Activity of Purkinje Cells

Impaired pacemaker activity of Purkinje cells may result from mutations that affect ion channels or proteins regulating their expression (Table 33.1). Many of these mutations manifest with episodic ataxia. One typical example is episodic ataxia type 1 (EA1) due to *KCNA1* mutations affecting K_v1 channels; these channels regulate release of GABA from inhibitory synapses between basket and Purkinje cells. EA1 is commonly associated with neuromyotonia and occasionally seizures. Another typical example is EA2 caused by loss-of-function mutations of the *CACNA1A* gene encoding the α1 subunit the $Ca_v2.1$ (P/Q) channels. Between attacks patients with EA-2 often have downbeat nystagmus or other cerebellar oculomotor dysfunctions. Some patients may develop slowly progressive ataxia and atrophy of the vermis.[36] Findings in a mouse model suggest that the attacks of episodic ataxia in this disorder may reflect reduced Ca^{2+} influx into presynaptic terminals at excitatory parallel-Purkinje cell synapses, abnormal intrinsic pacemaker firing of Purkinje neurons, or both. In transgenic mouse models of SCA6 due to *CACNA1A* gene CAG repeat expansion, Purkinje cells show reduced spike frequency and increased spike irregularity. Acetazolamide and the nonselective potassium channel blockers 4-aminopyridine (4-AP) and 3,4-diaminopyridine (3,4-DAP) are effective in treating downbeat nystagmus in both EA2 and SCA6. Both 4-AP and 3, 4-DAP indirectly activate K_{Ca} channels and restore regularity of Purkinje cell spiking. Another form of episodic ataxia, EA5, is caused by mutations in the *CACNB4* gene encoding the auxiliary β_4 subunit of Cav2.1. EA6 is caused by heterozygous mutations in SLC1A3, which encodes a subunit of a glial excitatory amino acid transporter EAAT1, which controls availability of glutamate at excitatory synapses on Purkinje cells. Individuals with EA3, EA5, and EA6 can also respond to acetazolamide.[37]

As in the case of SCA6, other disorders affecting ion channels may manifest with progressive ataxia with a SCA phenotype. Point mutations of *KCNC3* gene encoding $K_v3.3$ are linked to SCA13. Purkinje cells of $K_v3.3$ knockout mice have reduced firing frequency due to reduced speed of repolarization, which is required for generation of the next action potential. Loss of function mutations in the *KCND3* gene encoding the Kv4.3 subunit have been linked to SCA19/22. High-frequency firing of Purkinje cells depends on resurgent sodium currents through Nav1,1 and $Na_v1.6$ channels. *SCAN1A* mutations affecting $Na_v1.1$ channels typically cause Dravet syndrome but may also be associated with ataxia. Mutations of the *FGF14* gene encoding fibroblast growth factor 14 result in SCA27. FGF14 interacts with $Na_v1.6$ channels to regulate neuronal excitability and resurgent sodium currents. These mutations suppress both sodium and calcium currents in granule cells and reduce AMPAR mediated excitation in Purkinje cells.[21]

TABLE 33.1 *Channelopathies Associated with Ataxia*

Gene	Channel Protein	Function	Syndrome
KCNA1	K_v1.1	Presynaptic control of GABA release at the basket cell--Purkinje cell synapse	Episodic ataxia 1
CACNA1A	Ca_v2.1 (P/Q) calcium (Ca^{2+}) channel pore subunit	Ca^{2+}current coupled to KCa channels to regulate spike frequency and regularity	Episodic ataxia 2 Spinocerebellar ataxia (SCA) 6
KCNC3	K_v3.3 voltage-gated potassium (K^+) channel	Potassium entry during depolarization, causes hyperpolarization	SCA13
KCND3	K_v4.3 voltage-gated K^+ channel	Potassium entry during depolarization, causes hyperpolarization	SCA19, SCA22
SCN1A	Na_v 1.1. voltage-gated sodium (Na^+) channels pore subunit	Na^+ entry and membrane depolarization during the action potential	Dravet syndrome
FGF14	Fibroblast growth factor 14	Interacts with Na_v to influence excitability	SCA27
ITPR1	Inositol 1,4,5 triphosphate (IP_3) receptor	Ca^{2+} release from the endoplasmic reticulum upon IP_3 binding	SCA15, SCA16, SCA29
TRPC3	Transient receptor potential canonical channel type 3	Essential for mGluR1-mediated synaptic transmission, long-term depression	SCA41
CACNA1G	Ca_v3.1 voltage-gated Ca^{2+} channel	Inward Ca^{2+} current (T-type) upon depolarization	SCA42
KCNMA1	K_{Ca}1.1 large conductance Ca^{2+}-activated K^+ channels (BK)	Outward K $^+$ current upon activation. Regulates spike frequency and regularity	Unnamed SCA

Dysregulation of Potassium Channels in Polyglutamine-Associated Ataxias

With the exception of SCA6, in polyglutamine-associated ataxias the disease-causing proteins are not directly associated with ion channel function. Ataxin-1 (*ATXN1* gene affected in SCA1) is associated with transcriptional regulation and RNA splicing; ataxin-2 (*ATXN2* gene affected in SCA2) is involved in RNA metabolism and control of translation; ataxin-3 (*ATXN3* gene affected in SCA3) is a deubiquitinating enzyme; ataxin-7 (*ATXN7* gene affected SCA7) is a subunit of a transcriptional coactivator acetyltransferase complex; and TATA box-binding protein (*TDP* gene affected in SCA17) is an essential component of the transcription initiation complex. Studies in transgenic mouse models show that transcriptional dysregulation of mRNA transcripts, including those encoding ion channels, particularly K^+ channels, has a major role in impaired Purkinje cell pacing and ataxia.[22] In a mouse model of SCA1 (ATXN1[82Q] mice) there is both increased dendritic excitability and reduced spiking of Purkinje cell dendrites; this is associated with reduced expression of BK and G protein-coupled inward rectifying K^+ channels. In this model, dendritic degeneration and reduced cell size resulting in increased density of K^+ channels may be a compensatory process to restore Purkinje cell spiking.[38] A combination of chlorzoxazone (an activator of subthreshold K^+ channels) and baclofen (a $GABA_B$ receptor agonist) improved Purkinje spiking and motor function in these ATXN1 mutant mice. Similarly, altered K^+ channel function have also been shown in transgenic models of SCA2.[39] In the ATX2N [127Q] model there is reduced expression of the genes encoding BK and K_v3.3 channels; reduced Purkinje cell firing frequency, dendritic degeneration, and motor impairment preceding Purkinje cell loss. SCA3 affects not only Purkinje cells but also neurons of the cerebellar nuclei and brainstem. Purkinje cells in transgenic (ATXN3 [84Q]) mice exhibit increased intrinsic excitability resulting in depolarization block and the loss of the ability to sustain spontaneous repetitive firing; in transfected cells, mutant ataxin-3 increased inactivation of Kv3.1 channels and reduced activation of Kv1.2 channels;

and administration of an activator of SK channels partially corrects abnormal Purkinje cell firing and improves motor function in SCA3 mice.[40]

Disturbances in Calcium Homeostasis and Synaptic Plasticity

Impaired intracellular Ca^{2+} signaling and progressive Ca^{2+} accumulation may contribute first to dysfunction and then to loss of Purkinje cells in some forms of SCA.[27,33] For example, abnormal interaction between mutated ataxin-2 or mutated ataxin-3 with the IP_3R results in abnormal Ca^{2+} signaling that may alter the function SK type channels, which normally provide a critical brake on Purkinje cell excitability. Normalizing intracellular Ca^{2+} signaling with drugs such as dantrolene may both improve Purkinje neuron pacemaking and reduce Ca^{2+}-induced excitotoxicity.[41] Intracellular Ca^{2+} dysregulation may also affect the mGluR1-triggered circuit plasticity in SCA. Mutations of the *ITPR1* gene encoding IP_3R1 results in SCA15/16 and congenital ataxia SCA29. These mutations may result of loss-of-function of the IP_3R but in some cases may result in increased Ca^{2+} release from intracellular stores. Mutations of the *TRPC3* gene encoding the TRPC3 Ca^{2+} channel have been associated with SCA41. Mutations of the *CACNA1G* gene encoding $Ca_v3.1$ (T) channel cause SCA42, which may be due to reduced Ca^{2+} availability to activate K_{Ca} channels. Mutations of the *KCNMA1* gene encoding the $K_{Ca}1.1$ (BK) channel have also been linked to ataxia associated with cerebellar atrophy. Impaired intracellular Ca^{2+} regulation may also occur in Friedreich ataxia, in this case affecting cerebellar granule cells, as well as cardiomyocytes.

CEREBELLAR CIRCUIT DYSFUNCTION AND TREMOR

The cerebello-thalamo-cortical circuit is a key pathophysiological component in many tremor types.[42] In addition to the cerebellum, there is also involvement of the supplementary motor area (SMA) in essential tremor; of the basal ganglia in resting tremor associated with Parkinson disease (PD) and in dystonic tremor; of both the SMA and brainstem in orthostatic tremor; and the dento rubro-olivary loop in Holmes tremor.[42]

Essential Tremor

Essential tremor is defined as bilateral upper limb action tremor (4–12 Hz) in the absence of other neurologic manifestations.[36] It is characterized by higher stability of tremor frequency than rest tremor in PD, suggesting its source in a single oscillator or tightly coupled multiple oscillators.[43] Essential tremor reflects abnormal oscillatory activity in the cerebello-thalamocortical circuit[44,45] and can be entrained by transcranial magnetic stimulation (TMS) applied on the cerebellum.[46] One potential mechanism of essential tremor is dysfunction of Purkinje cells resulting in impaired GABAergic inhibition of the deep cerebellar nuclei. This may result in motor network disruption, with both increased functional coupling between the motor cerebellum and the thalamus and decreased functional connectivity between the posterior cerebellum and the primary motor cortex (M1) during motor tasks.[47] This suggests a pathological entrainment of the cerebello-dentothalamic system with engagement of the pacemaker-like activity of the dentate nucleus.[47] Perturbed cerebellar output could generate abnormal thalamic activity and disrupt motor-related connectivity on the motor cortex, for example by amplifying inhibitory mechanisms in the motor cortex. The fundamental role of the dentothalamic system in essential tremor is supported by the beneficial effects of deep brain stimulation (DBS) in the cerebellar territory of the thalamus (VLp/Vim) in these patients. There is still controversy as to whether essential tremor is a neurodegenerative disorder. In some cases, there is Purkinje cell loss and axonal swelling (torpedoes) in their axons. Patients with essential tremor also show increased functional resting state connectivity in cognitive networks (such as the default mode network and frontoparietal networks) and decreased connectivity in the visual networks,[48] emphasizing the role of the cerebellum in nonmotor functions.

Tremor in Parkinson Disease

Resting tremor in PD is associated with abnormal oscillatory activity within the basal ganglia and the cerebello-thalamocortical circuit as well as abnormal intercircuit interactions.[49,50] Unlike essential tremor, resting tremor in PD shows alteration in tremor frequency, which points to its generation from multiple uncoupled oscillator generators with different frequencies.[43] According to the "switch-dimmer" model of tremor in PD, the basal ganglia may work as a light switch that triggers tremor initiation and the cerebellum as light-dimmer that modulates tremor amplitude.[49] In PD, the strong inhibitory output from the basal ganglia would initiate rhythmic activity in thalamocortical neurons projecting to the SMA and premotor cortex; oscillatory cortical activity would engage the cortico-ponto-cerebellar and then the dento-thalamocortical pathway. The strong rhythmic activity of the cerebello-thalamo-cortical circuit, which is related to motor timing, may enable this circuit to estimate limb position in relation to movement goals and would both sustain tremor activity and modulate tremor amplitude. The STN interacts with both the basal ganglia and the thalamocortical circuits and may participate in triggering activity in the cerebello-thalamocortical circuit producing the tremor.[49,50] This explains why DBS in the cerebellar territory of the thalamus as well as stimulation of the GPi or STN are effective in treating resting tremor in PD. Dopamine reduces tremor amplitude by increasing thalamic inhibition in the cerebellar target nucleus.[51]

Palatal Myoclonus/Tremor and Holmes Tremor

Hypertrophic olivary degeneration is a very rare type of transsynaptic degeneration caused by a lesion affecting the dento-rubro-olivary pathway (Guillain-Mollaret triangle). This results in neuronal cytoplasmic vacuolization, hypertrophy of astrocytes, gliosis and demyelination of the ION, and macroscopic hypertrophy. The classical manifestation is palatal myoclonus-tremor as occurs, for example, in disorders such as Alexander disease. Rarely olivary hypertrophy is associated with Holmes tremor, which is typically caused by lesions in brainstem, thalamus, or cerebellum. Holmes tremor is a low frequency (<4.5 Hz) resting tremor that generally involves the upper extremities, is exacerbated by posture, accentuated with intention, and lacks the very regular rhythm characteristic of other tremors. Combined injury of the dopaminergic nigrostriatal pathway and the cerebello-thalamic/cerebello-olivary pathways are necessary for development of Holmes tremor. Interruption of the Guillain-Mollaret triangle occurs in most patients with Holmes tremor after brainstem stroke. While degeneration of the disynaptic dentato-rubro-olivary tract is associated with tremor, degeneration of the monosynaptic tract is related to hypertrophic olivary degeneration. Holmes tremor can manifest approximately 4 weeks to 2 years after an insult. The reason for the delayed onset is still unclear but could reflect the new development of pathologic pathways after the initial recovery period.

MOLECULAR MECHANISMS OF AUTOSOMAL RECESSIVE CEREBELLAR ATAXIAS

Autosomal-recessive cerebellar ataxias (ARCAs) comprise a heterogeneous group of rare degenerative and metabolic genetic diseases that share the hallmark of progressive damage of the cerebellum and its associated tracts.[52] In most ARCAs, ataxia is associated with involvement of other neural systems such as peripheral nerves, retina, cerebral cortex, or basal ganglia, as well as non-neurologic tissues, such as the muscle, heart, and pancreas. This leads to severe, multisystemic phenotypes, often starting before the age of 40.[53] Next-generation sequencing has allowed identification of an increasing number of mutations associated with ARCAs. Whereas Friedreich's ataxia (FA, due to GAA intronic expansion of the *FXN* gene) is the most common ARCA (up to 25% of cases), other relatively frequent ARCAs include autosomal-recessive spastic ataxia of Charlevoix-Saguenay (ARSACS, due to *SACS*-sacsin gene mutations), spectrin repeat-containing nuclear envelope protein (*SYNE1*) ataxia, and hereditary spastic paraplegia type 7 (*SPG7*, due to mutations of the paraplegin gene). Recent evidence indicates that AAGGG expansions in the *RFC1*(replication facilitation complex 1), which are typically associated with cerebellar ataxia, vestibular arreflexia, and sensory neuropathy syndrome (CANVAS), may represent a frequent cause of late-onset ataxia in the general population.[54] The emerging common pathways underlying ARCAs include three main clusters: mitochondrial dysfunction, impaired DNA repair, and complex lipid homeostasis[52] (Table 32.2). There is major interaction between these three mechanisms. For example, disorders of mitochondrial metabolism lead to oxidative stress and oxidative DNA damage and mutations affecting DNA repair may also affect repair of mitochondrial DNA.

From the clinical standpoint, common causes of ARCAs have been subdivided into three categories:[52] The first is that of cerebellar ataxias associated with prominent sensory neuronopathy, such as Friedreich ataxia, sensory ataxia, dysarthria, and ophthalmoparesis (SANDO), associated with polymerase gamma (POLG) mutations, and CANVAS. Important differential diagnoses include treatable ataxias such as ataxia with isolated vitamin E deficiency due to *TTPA* (α-tocopherol transfer protein) mutations; abetalipoproteinemia due to *MTP* (*MTTP*, microsomal triglyceride transfer protein) mutations, and Refsum disease due to *PHYH* (phytanic acid hydrolase) mutations. The second major group are cerebellar ataxias with sensorimotor peripheral neuropathy. This phenotype is typical of disorders of DNA repair, such as ataxia telangiectasia due to *ATM* (ataxia telangiectasia mutated) mutations, ataxia with oculomotor apraxia (AOA) type 1 due to *APTX*-(aprataxin) mutation, and AOA2 due to *SETX* (senataxin) mutations. Other features in these disorders are oculomotor apraxia, chorea or dystonia, and in many cases elevation of alpha fetoprotein and other non-neurologic features. Cerebrotendinous xanthomatosis (CTX) due to CYP27A1 (cytochrome P27A1) mutations is also characterized by sensorimotor neuropathy as well typical non-neurologic manifestations, MRI and laboratory findings, and potential response to treatment. The third group of ARCAs include disorders with no prominent neuropathy and are heterogeneous, including ARCA type 1 due to *SYNE-1-* mutations, ARCA type 2 due to *COQ8* (coenzyme Q8) mutations, and Niemann-Pick type C disease due to *NPC1* or *NPC2* mutations. Several autosomal-dominant ataxia genes can also cause autosomal-recessive ataxia in case of biallelic inheritance, often giving rise to very severe, and early-onset recessive ataxia syndromes.

AUTOIMMUNE CEREBELLAR ATAXIAS

Cerebellar ataxia is a common manifestation of autoimmune disorders, particularly paraneoplastic disorders. As in the case of ARCAs, cerebellar ataxia is typically associated with other neurologic manifestations that may help establish the causal diagnosis[55,56] (Table 32.3). In some cases, for example in the case of mGLuR1signaling pathway, antibodies target molecules affected in genetic ataxic syndromes.

TABLE 33.2 *Representative Example of Autosomal Recessive Cerebellar Ataxias (ARCAs)*

Disorder	Gene (protein)	Function	Salient Clinical Features
Mitochondrial causes of ARCA (examples)			
Friedreich ataxia (FA)	*FXN* (frataxin)	Fe-S biogenesis	No cerebellar atrophy Cervical spinal cord atrophy Sensory neuronopathy Pyramidal signs Square wave jerks Cardiomyopathy, diabetes
ARSACS	*SACS* (sacsin)	Facilitate mitochondrial fission and intracellular localization	Spasticity Peripheral neuropathy Linear T2 signal in the pons
SPG7	*SPG7* (paraplegin)	Quality control mitochondrial protease	Spasticity Neuropathy Ragged red fibers
AFG3L2/SPAX5	*AFG3L2*	Mitochondrial protease	Dystonia myoclonus Epilepsy
COQ8A/ADCK3	*COQ8A* (coenzyme Q8)	CoQ10 biogenesis	Exercise intolerance Intellectual disability Seizures
SANDO/SCAE	*POLG* (polymerase G)	Replication of mtDNA	Sensory axonal neuropathy External ophthalmoparesis Deafness Epilepsy
Mitochondrial DNA depletion syndrome	*TWNK* (Twinkle)	Mitochondrial helicase associated	Sensory ataxia External ophthalmoparesis Hypogonadism
Defects of DNA repair			
Ataxia telangiectasia (AT)	*ATM* (ataxia telangiectasia mutated)	Double-strand DNA repair	Oculomotor apraxia Choreoathetosis Dystonia Sensorimotor Neuropathy, Telangiectasias Immunodeficiency Cancer susceptibility Increased α-fetoprotein
AT-like disorder 1 (ATLD)	*MRE11A*	Double-strand DNA repair	Childhood-onset Oculomotor apraxia Myoclonus Normal α-fetoprotein
Ataxia with oculomotor apraxia type (AOA) type 1	*APTX* (aprataxin)	Single-strand DNA break repair	Childhood onset Oculomotor apraxia Sensorimotor PN Mild increase in AFP and cholesterol and decreased albumin
AOA2 type 2	*STX* (senataxin)	Resolution of RNA: DNA hybrids	Oculomotor apraxia Chorea, dystonia Sensorimotor PN

TABLE 33.2 *(Continued)*

Disorder	Gene (protein)	Function	Salient Clinical Features
AOA4	*PNKP*	Single-strand DNA break repair	Microcephaly SZ, DDD
Spinocerebellar ataxia with axonal neuropathy (SCAN1)	*TDP1*	Single-strand DNA break repair	Axonal sensorimotor PN Seizures,
XRCC1-associated apraxia with oculomotor apraxia	*XRCC1*	Single-strand DNA break repair	Adult onset Oculomotor apraxia Sensorimotor PN
CANVAS	*RFC1* (replication factor complex subunit 1 intronic AAGG expansion)	DNA polymerase accessory protein; for replication and DNA repair	Cerebellar ataxia Vestibular arreflexia Sensory neuropathy Chronic cough Autonomic dysfunction
ARCA associated with disorders of complex lipid metabolism			
Niemann-Pick type C	*NPC1, NPC2*	Processing of endocyted cholesterol	Vertical faze palsy Cataplexy Dystonia Cognitive/behavioral Hepatosplenomegaly Increased oxysterols
Cerebrotendinous xanthomatosis (CTX)	*CYP27A1*	Sterol-27 hydroxylase	Spasticity Sensorimotor PN Chronic diarrhea Cataracts Tendon xanthomas Increase T2 signal in MCP Increase cholestenol
Refsum disease	*PHYH* (PEJ)	Phytanic acid hydroxylase	Sensorimotor PN Pigmentary retinopathy Anosmia Hearing loss Ichthyosis Increase phytanic acid
PLA2G6	*PLA2G6* (phospholipase A2 group 6)	Deacylation of phosphatidycholine	Dystonia, parkinsonism Optica atrophy Cognitive/psychiatric
PNPLA6	*PNPLA6*	Esterification of phosphatidylcholine	Spasticity Choriretinal dystrophy
Metachromatic leukodystrophy	ARSA (arylsulfatase A)	Hydrolysis of ceramide sulfate	Variable phenotype Ataxia in juvenile form

TABLE 33.3 *Autoantibodies Associated with Cerebellar Ataxia*

Antibody	Associated Cancer	Typical Associated Features
Hu (ANNA-1)	SCLC (small cell lung carcinoma)	Limbic encephalitis Sensory and autonomic ganglionopathy Intestinal pseudo-obstruction
Ri/ NOVA (ANNA-2)	SCLC, breast CA	Opsoclonus/myoclonus Brainstem encephalitis Jaw dystonia Laryngeal stridor
PCA-1	Breast, Müllerian ACA	Vertigo Nystagmus
MAP1b (PCA-2)	SCLC	Brainstem encephalitis
CRMP-5	SCLC, thymoma	Optic neuritis Retinitis Myelopathy (tractopathy) Neuropathy
Ma-1	Testicular carcinoma	Narcolepsy Vertical gaze palsy
Kelch-1	Seminoma	Vertigo Hearing loss Polyradiculopathy
mGluR1PCA-Tr	Lymphoma	Dysgeusia
PCA-Tr (DNER)3	Hodgkin	None
GAD-65	Rare in isolation	Seizures, Stiff-person syndrome
P/Q channel	SCLC	Lambert-Eaton myasthenic syndrome Seizures
Neuronal intermediate filament (NIF)	Neuroendocrine SCLC, Merkel, pancreas	Encephalopathy, myelopathy
AP3B2	Rare	Spinocerebellar ataxia Myeloneuropoathy
Septin-5	None recorded	Prominent oscillopsia

KEY POINTS

- The cerebellum has a critical role in control of timing and coordination of movement, acquisition of skills, and cognitive and affective functions.
- The cerebellar circuits consist of multiple closed-loop circuits that interconnect the neocortex with the cerebellum via functionally segregated input-output channels.
- There are reciprocal connections between the cerebellum and the basal ganglia.
- The intrinsic cerebellar circuit includes the Purkinje cells of the cerebellar cortex, which control the cerebellar output to the rest of the CNS via the cerebellar nuclei.
- The connectivity of the cerebellum with the brainstem and spinal cord provides for control of eye movements, posture, muscle tone, and locomotion.
- The cerebellum receives both feedforward information about cortical motor commands and feedback information about the sensory consequence of the actual movement.
- The ION and the cerebellum are interconnected via an inhibitory olivo-nucleo-olivary loop, a disinhibitory olivo-cortico-nucleo-olivary loop and an excitatory dento-rubro-olivary pathway.
- Granule cells receive multimodal convergence of inputs and respond to specific combinations of sensory and motor signals.

- Processing of mossy fiber input at the granule cell layer is closely regulated by Golgi cells.
- A single climbing fiber from the ION provides a powerful synaptic input the Purkinje cell.
- The ION contains neurons that tend to fire in groups or clusters and have a critical role in timing function for motor coordination.
- The ION may also function as a comparator between predictive and feedback signals and generates an error signal that is used to adjust the motor command.
- Purkinje cells are characterized by an intrinsic pacemaker activity that depends on the interactions among several ion channels, particularly P/Q and several K^+ channels.
- Glutamatergic inputs from parallel fibers and climbing fibers activate AMPA and metabotropic type 1 (mGluR1) receptors in Purkinje cells.
- Activation of mGluR1 receptors activates downstream signals that trigger long-term depression at the parallel fiber–Purkinje cell synapse.
- Neurons in the deep cerebellar nuclei send a timing signal to the rest of the CNS.
- Purkinje cell dysfunction, including impaired pacemaking activity and dysregulated intracellular Ca^{2+}calcium signaling is a major mechanism of ataxia.
- Many mutations affecting ion channel function manifest with episodic ataxia (EA), such as EA1 due to *KCNA1* mutations and EA2 caused by *CACNA1A* mutations.
- With the exception of spinocerebellar ataxia 6 (SCA6), most polyglutamine-associated ataxias are result from transcriptional dysregulation affecting K^+ channels.
- Impaired intracellular Ca^{2+} signaling and progressive Ca^{2+} accumulation may contribute first to dysfunction and then to loss of Purkinje cells in some forms of SCA.
- The cerebello-thalamo-cortical circuit is a key pathophysiological component in many tremor types.
- Common mechanisms of autosomal recessive cerebellar ataxia (ARCA) include mitochondrial dysfunction, defects of DNA repair, and disorders of complex lipid metabolism, some of these disorders provide targets for treatment.
- Cerebellar ataxia is a common manifestation of autoimmune disorders, particularly paraneoplastic disorders, and is typically associated with other neurologic manifestations that may help establish the causal diagnosis.

REFERENCES

1. D'Angelo E. Physiology of the cerebellum. Handb Clin Neurol 2018;154:85–108.
2. Apps R, Hawkes R. Cerebellar cortical organization: a one-map hypothesis. Nat Rev Neurosci 2009;10:670–681.
3. Voogd J, Koehler PJ. Historic notes on anatomic, physiologic, and clinical research on the cerebellum. Handb Clin Neurol 2018;154:3–26.
4. Bostan AC, Dum RP, Strick PL. Cerebellar networks with the cerebral cortex and basal ganglia. Trends Cogn Sci 2013;17:241–254.
5. Stoodley CJ, Schmahmann JD. Functional topography in the human cerebellum: a meta-analysis of neuroimaging studies. Neuroimage 2009;44:489–501.
6. Buckner RL, Krienen FM, Castellanos A, Diaz JC, Yeo BT. The organization of the human cerebellum estimated by intrinsic functional connectivity. J Neurophysiol 2011;106:2322–2345.
7. Buckner RL. The cerebellum and cognitive function: 25 years of insight from anatomy and neuroimaging. Neuron 2013;80:807–815.
8. Adamaszek M, D'Agata F, Ferrucci R, et al. Consensus paper: cerebellum and emotion. Cerebellum 2017;16:552–576.
9. Chen CH, Fremont R, Arteaga-Bracho EE, Khodakhah K. Short latency cerebellar modulation of the basal ganglia. Nat Neurosci 2014;17:1767–1775.
10. Quartarone A, Cacciola A, Milardi D, et al. New insights into cortico-basal-cerebellar connectome: clinical and physiological considerations. Brain 2020;143:396–406.
11. Ausim Azizi S. . . . And the olive said to the cerebellum: organization and functional significance of the olivo-cerebellar system. Neuroscientist 2007;13:616–625.
12. Herculano-Houzel S. Coordinated scaling of cortical and cerebellar numbers of neurons. Front Neuroanat 2010;4:12.
13. Henry C, Jouan F, De Broucker T. JC virus granule cell neuronopathy: a cause of infectious cerebellar degeneration. J Neurol Sci 2015;354:86–90.
14. Llinas RR. Cerebellar motor learning versus cerebellar motor timing: the climbing fibre story. J Physiol 2011;589:3423–3432.
15. Uusisaari M, De Schutter E. The mysterious microcircuitry of the cerebellar nuclei. J Physiol 2011;589:3441–3457.
16. Sawtell NB. Multimodal integration in granule cells as a basis for associative plasticity and sensory prediction in a cerebellum-like circuit. Neuron 2010;66:573–584.
17. Duguid I, Branco T, Chadderton P, Arlt C, Powell K, Hausser M. Control of cerebellar granule cell output by sensory-evoked Golgi cell inhibition. Proc Natl Acad Sci U S A 2015;112:13099–13104.
18. Eyre MD, Nusser Z. Only a minority of the inhibitory inputs to cerebellar golgi cells originates from local GABAergic cells. eNeuro 2016;3.
19. Chaumont J, Guyon N, Valera AM, et al. Clusters of cerebellar Purkinje cells control their afferent climbing fiber discharge. Proc Natl Acad Sci U S A 2013;110:16223–16228.
20. Witter L, Rudolph S, Pressler RT, Lahlaf SI, Regehr WG. Purkinje cell collaterals enable output signals from the cerebellar cortex to feed back to Purkinje cells and interneurons. Neuron 2016;91:312–319.
21. Shakkottai VG, Paulson HL. Physiologic alterations in ataxia: channeling changes into novel therapies. Arch Neurol 2009;66:1196–1201.
22. Bushart DD, Shakkottai VG. Ion channel dysfunction in cerebellar ataxia. Neurosci Lett 2019;688:41–48.
23. Zhang W, Schmelzeisen S, Parthier D, Frings S, Mohrlen F. Anoctamin calcium-activated chloride channels may

modulate inhibitory transmission in the cerebellar cortex. PLoS One 2015;10:e0142160.
24. Ait Ouares K, Filipis L, Tzilivaki A, Poirazi P, Canepari M. Two distinct sets of Ca(2+) and K(+) channels are activated at different membrane potentials by the climbing fiber synaptic potential in Purkinje neuron dendrites. J Neurosci 2019;39:1969–1981.
25. Ito M, Yamaguchi K, Nagao S, Yamazaki T. Long-term depression as a model of cerebellar plasticity. Prog Brain Res 2014;210:1–30.
26. Hoxha E, Tempia F, Lippiello P, Miniaci MC. Modulation, plasticity and pathophysiology of the parallel fiber-Purkinje cell synapse. Front Synaptic Neurosci 2016;8:35.
27. Brown SA, Loew LM. Integration of modeling with experimental and clinical findings synthesizes and refines the central role of inositol 1,4,5-trisphosphate receptor 1 in spinocerebellar ataxia. Front Neurosci 2014;8:453.
28. Ankri L, Husson Z, Pietrajtis K, et al. A novel inhibitory nucleo-cortical circuit controls cerebellar Golgi cell activity. Elife 2015;4:e06262. doi:10.7554/eLife.06262
29. Gornati SV, Schafer CB, Eelkman Rooda OHJ, Nigg AL, De Zeeuw CI, Hoebeek FE. Differentiating cerebellar impact on thalamic nuclei. Cell Rep 2018;23:2690–2704.
30. Caligiore D, Pezzulo G, Baldassarre G, et al. Consensus paper: towards a systems-level view of cerebellar function: the interplay between cerebellum, basal ganglia, and cortex. Cerebellum 2017;16:203–229.
31. Manto M, Bower JM, Conforto AB, et al. Consensus paper: roles of the cerebellum in motor control--the diversity of ideas on cerebellar involvement in movement. Cerebellum 2012;11:457–487.
32. Zee DS. A neurologist and ataxia: using eye movements to learn about the cerebellum. Cerebellum Ataxias 2018;5:2.
33. Hekman KE, Gomez CM. The autosomal dominant spinocerebellar ataxias: emerging mechanistic themes suggest pervasive Purkinje cell vulnerability. J Neurol Neurosurg Psychiatry 2015;86:554–561.
34. Meera P, Pulst SM, Otis TS. Cellular and circuit mechanisms underlying spinocerebellar ataxias. J Physiol 2016;594:4653–4660.
35. Paulson HL, Shakkottai VG, Clark HB, Orr HT. Polyglutamine spinocerebellar ataxias—from genes to potential treatments. Nat Rev Neurosci 2017;18:613–626.
36. Bhatia KP, Bain P, Bajaj N, et al. Consensus statement on the classification of tremors. from the task force on tremor of the International Parkinson and Movement Disorder Society. Mov Disord 2018;33:75–87.
37. Jen JC, Wan J. Episodic ataxias. Handb Clin Neurol 2018;155:205–215.
38. Chopra R, Bushart DD, Shakkottai VG. Dendritic potassium channel dysfunction may contribute to dendrite degeneration in spinocerebellar ataxia type 1. PLoS One 2018;13:e0198040.
39. Dell'Orco JM, Pulst SM, Shakkottai VG. Potassium channel dysfunction underlies Purkinje neuron spiking abnormalities in spinocerebellar ataxia type 2. Hum Mol Genet 2017;26:3935–3945.
40. Shakkottai VG, do Carmo Costa M, Dell'Orco JM, Sankaranarayanan A, Wulff H, Paulson HL. Early changes in cerebellar physiology accompany motor dysfunction in the polyglutamine disease spinocerebellar ataxia type 3. J Neurosci 2011;31:13002–13014.
41. Liu J, Tang TS, Tu H, et al. Deranged calcium signaling and neurodegeneration in spinocerebellar ataxia type 2. J Neurosci 2009;29:9148–9162.
42. Nieuwhof F, Panyakaew P, van de Warrenburg BP, Gallea C, Helmich RC. The patchy tremor landscape: recent advances in pathophysiology. Curr Opin Neurol 2018;31:455–461.
43. di Biase L, Brittain JS, Shah SA, et al. Tremor stability index: a new tool for differential diagnosis in tremor syndromes. Brain 2017;140:1977–1986.
44. Raethjen J, Deuschl G. The oscillating central network of essential tremor. Clin Neurophysiol 2012;123:61–64.
45. Hopfner F, Helmich RC. The etiology of essential tremor: genes versus environment. Parkinsonism Relat Disord 2018;46 Suppl 1:S92–S96.
46. Brittain JS, Cagnan H, Mehta AR, Saifee TA, Edwards MJ, Brown P. Distinguishing the central drive to tremor in Parkinson's disease and essential tremor. J Neurosci 2015;35:795–806.
47. Buijink AW, van der Stouwe AM, Broersma M, et al. Motor network disruption in essential tremor: a functional and effective connectivity study. Brain 2015;138:2934–2947.
48. Benito-Leon J, Louis ED, Romero JP, et al. Altered functional connectivity in essential tremor: a resting-state fMRI study. Medicine (Baltimore) 2015;94:e1936.
49. Helmich RC, Hallett M, Deuschl G, Toni I, Bloem BR. Cerebral causes and consequences of parkinsonian resting tremor: a tale of two circuits? Brain 2012;135:3206–3226.
50. Helmich RC. The cerebral basis of Parkinsonian tremor: A network perspective. Mov Disord 2018;33:219–231.
51. Dirkx MF, den Ouden HE, Aarts E, et al. Dopamine controls Parkinson's tremor by inhibiting the cerebellar thalamus. Brain 2017;140:721–734.
52. Synofzik M, Puccio H, Mochel F, Schols L. Autosomal recessive cerebellar ataxias: paving the way toward targeted molecular therapies. Neuron 2019;101:560–583.
53. Renaud M, Tranchant C, Martin JVT, et al. A recessive ataxia diagnosis algorithm for the next generation sequencing era. Ann Neurol 2017;82:892–899.
54. Cortese A, Tozza S, Yau WY, et al. Cerebellar ataxia, neuropathy, vestibular areflexia syndrome due to RFC1 repeat expansion. Brain 2020;143:480–490.
55. Honorat JA, McKeon A. Autoimmune movement disorders: a clinical and laboratory approach. Curr Neurol Neurosci Rep 2017;17:4.
56. Damato V, Balint B, Kienzler AK, Irani SR. The clinical features, underlying immunology, and treatment of autoantibody-mediated movement disorders. Mov Disord 2018;33:1376–1389.

34 Basal Ganglia Circuits

OVERVIEW

The basal ganglia are core components of circuits involved in reward (reinforcement)-based action learning; action selection and initiation of goal-directed behaviors; and automatic execution of both learned motor plans (habit formation) and innate motor programs such as locomotion. The components of the basal ganglia circuits include the striatum, globus pallidus, substantia nigra, subthalamic nucleus (STN), and pedunculopontine tegmental nucleus (PPT/PPN)[1,2] (Figure 34.1). The striatum is a hub for the interaction among multiple afferents and local networks regulating basal ganglia function.[2] It integrates influence from excitatory inputs from the cerebral cortex and thalamus; local circuits involving GABAergic and cholinergic interneurons, and modulatory input from midbrain dopaminergic neurons. The output of the striatum is mediated by GABAergic neurons that target the globus pallidus pars externa (GPe), globus pallidus pars interna (GPi), and substantia nigra pars reticulata (SNr). The GPi/SNr provide a tonic GABAergic input to the thalamus and brainstem. The STN facilitates this output via tonic activation of the GPi/SNr. The STN receives excitatory input from the cerebral cortex and inhibitory inputs from the GPe, which is in turn activated by the STN and inhibited by the striatum. The interactions among these components of the intrinsic basal ganglia circuits provide for direct, indirect, and a hyperdirect pathways that control the inhibitory basal ganglia output mediated by the GPi/SNr.[3] Reciprocal interactions between output neurons of the striatum, local circuits within the striatum, reciprocal projections from the GPe to the striatum, and direct projections from the cerebral cortex and cerebellum to the GPe and GPi/SNr, add a new level of complexity to the basal ganglia circuits. Dopaminergic inputs to the striatum promote learning, selection, and execution of actions; dopaminergic inputs to the STN-GPe circuit prevent abnormal oscillatory activity in the basal ganglia and their targets. Loss of dopaminergic inputs lead to plastic changes and abnormal activity in basal ganglia circuits, which underlie some major motor manifestations of Parkinson disease (PD), including akinesia and levodopa-induced dyskinesias. Imbalance between dopaminergic and cholinergic influence in the striatum, as well as influences from the cerebellum have been associated with dystonia. The main aims of this chapter are to review: (1) the basic intrinsic and extrinsic connectivity of the basal ganglia, (2) current models of the basal ganglia circuits, (3) the regulation of function of the striatum, (4) the functions of the globus pallidus and STN, and (5) current views on the pathophysiology of PD and hyperkinetic disorders.

INTRINSIC BASAL GANGLIA CONNECTIVITY AND MODELS OF BASAL GANGLIA FUNCTION

The striatum, including the nucleus accumbens (NAc), caudate, and putamen receives glutamatergic inputs from the cerebral cortex. These cortical projections are topographically organized, creating separate functional networks.[4] The orbitomedial prefrontal cortex, midcingulate cortex, hippocampus, and amygdala target primarily the NAc and the ventromedial caudate; the dorsolateral PFC targets the head of the caudate; and the sensorimotor cortex targets the posterior (motor) putamen.[1,5] However, there is partial overlap between the different cortical projections to the striatum. The second major glutamatergic input to the striatum originates from the thalamus, primarily from the intralaminar nuclei.[6] The output neurons of the striatum are GABAergic medium spiny projection neurons (SPNs, also commonly known a medium spiny neurons, MSNs), which target the GABAergic neurons of the GPe, GPi, and SNr. The GPi/SNr provides the inhibitory output of the

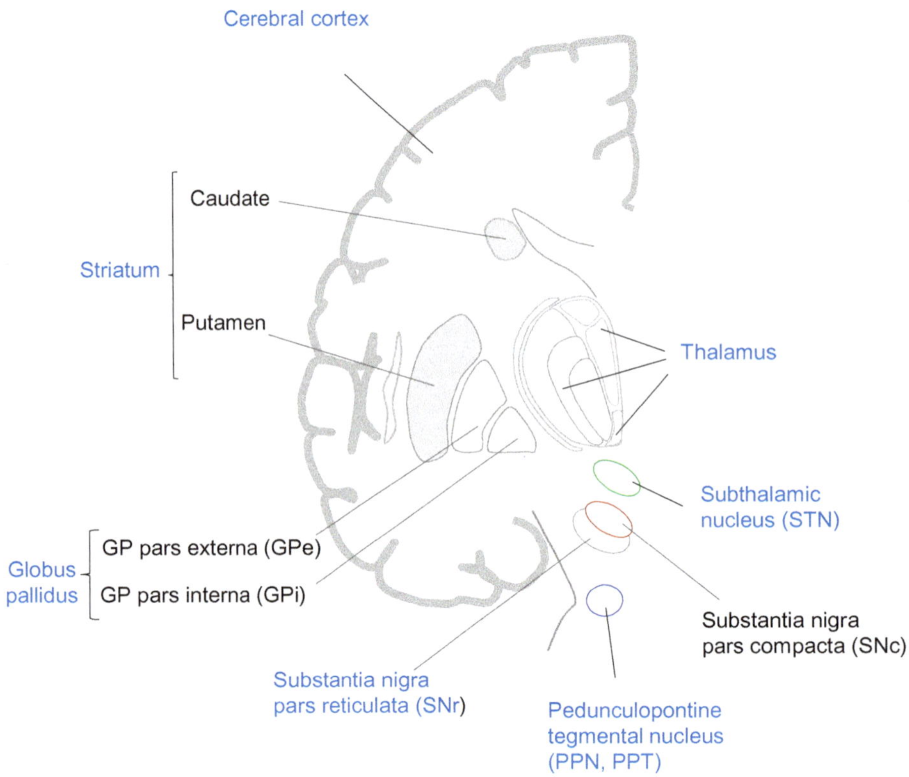

FIGURE 34.1 Basic component of the basal ganglia circuits.
The basal ganglia circuits include the striatum, globus pallidus pars interna (GPi) and pars externa (GPe), substantia nigra (SN) and subthalamic nucleus (STN), and their targets in the thalamus and brainstem. Neurons in the striatum, GPi, GPe, and SNr are GABAergic; those in the STN and thalamus are glutamatergic. The activity within the basal ganglia circuits is controlled by dopaminergic inputs from the substantia nigra pars compacta (SNc) and ventral tegmental area (VTA). The pedunculopontine tegmental nucleus (PPN/PPT) is an integral component of the basal ganglia circuits and contains cholinergic, glutamatergic, and GABAergic neurons.

basal ganglia. The STN provides tonic excitatory input to the GPe, GPi, and SNr and receives both excitatory input from the cerebral cortex and inhibitory input from the GPe.

Basic Connectivity: Direct, Indirect, and Hyperdirect Pathways

The basic intrinsic connectivity of the basal ganglia provides for the three classic pathways, direct, indirect, and hyperdirect, that regulate the output of the basal ganglia (Figure 34.2). The direct pathway involves a population of SPNs that project to the GPi and SNr. Since the GPi/SNr tonically inhibit thalamocortical and brainstem neurons initiating actions, the direct pathway transiently interrupts this tonic output and triggers initiation of a selected action ("go" signal). The indirect pathway involves a second population of SPNs that inhibit the GPe. As the GPe tonically inhibits the STN, the indirect pathway disinhibits the STN. Since the STN promotes the inhibitory output of the GPi/SNr, the indirect pathway leads to action suppression ("no-go" signal). The hyperdirect pathway consists of direct inputs from the cortex to the STN, which via its excitatory effects on the GPi/SNr both inhibits action initiation and interrupts ongoing actions ("stop" signal). These basic interactions led to development of several models of basal ganglia function. The two main examples are the parallel model and the center-surround model.[7–10]

Parallel Model of Basal Ganglia Function

According to the classical parallel model of basal ganglia function, dopamine (DA) has opposite effects on the direct and indirect pathways. This is based on evidence that direct pathway SPNs express primarily excitatory D1 to receptors (D1Rs) whereas indirect pathway SPNs primarily express inhibitory D2 receptors (D2Rs). In this model, a peak of DA in the striatum would increase activity of the D1R-expressing direct pathway SPNs while simultaneously inhibiting the activity of D2R-expressing indirect pathway SPNs (Figure 34.3). In this model, the net effect of a DA peak in the striatum due to burst activity of midbrain dopaminergic neurons in response to a reward is to promote initiation of a selected action via a direct-pathway SPN-mediated suppression of the GPi/SNr. Simultaneously DA would inhibit the SPN neurons of the indirect pathway SPNs that would interfere with the selected action.[7–10] However, both

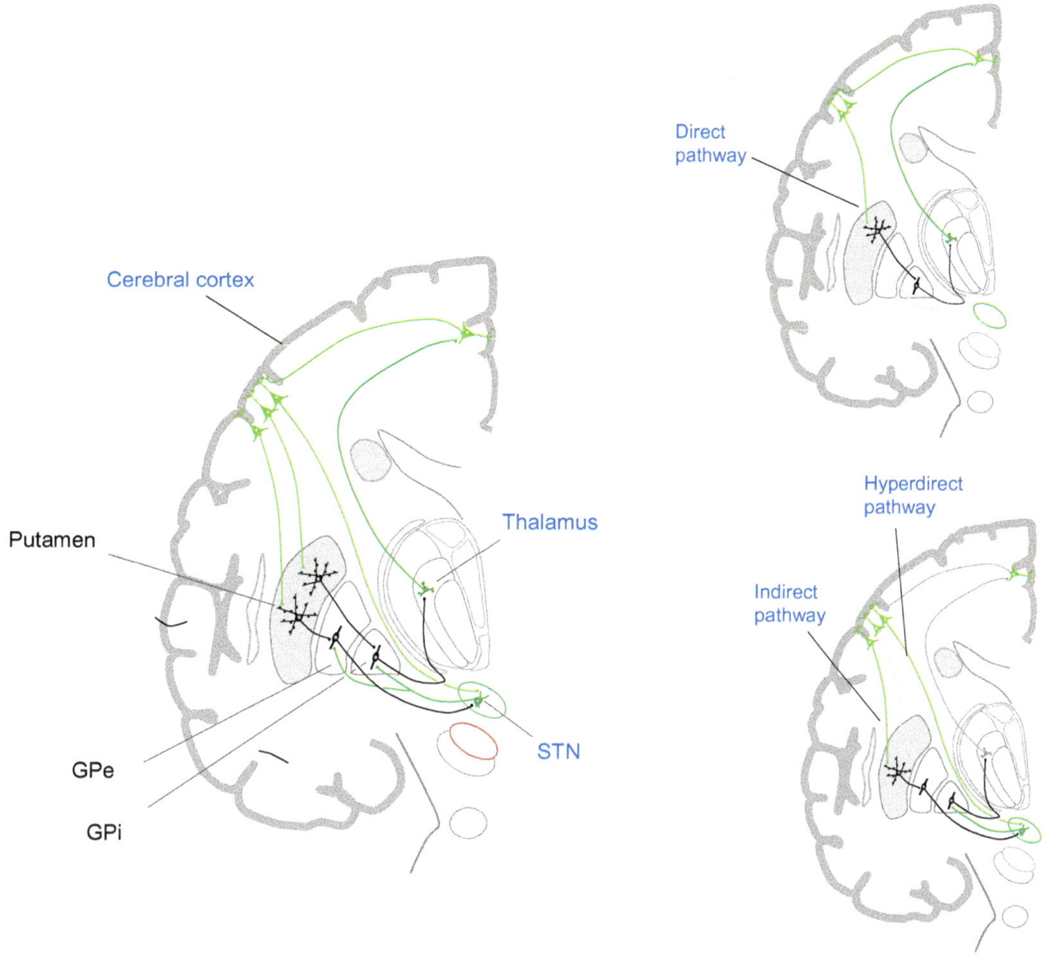

FIGURE 34.2 Direct, indirect, and hyperdirect pathways.
The output neurons of the globus pallidus pars interna (GPi) and substantia nigra pars reticulata (SNr) tonically inhibit the action pattern generators in the thalamus and brainstem. The GPi/SNr receive excitatory projections form the subthalamic nucleus (STN), which is activated by inputs from the cerebral cortex and inhibited by inputs from the globus pallidus pars externa (GPe). There are three parallel pathways by which the cerebral cortex controls the basal ganglia output via the GPi/SNr: a direct pathway from the striatum to the GPi/SNr, an indirect pathway from the striatum to the GPe and involving the STN and GPi/SNr, and a hyperdirect pathway from the cortex to the STN.

the direct and indirect pathway SPNs are coactive during movement initiation and both are engaged during execution and termination of motor sequences.[10,11] Direct pathway SPNs promote initiation of the selected action, whereas indirect pathway SPNs act simultaneously to inhibit all other competitive undesirable actions. While direct SPNs remain active with a correct action, indirect pathway SPNs signal when an action is incorrect and it is time to switch strategies. These indirect pathway SPNs become activated when the DA levels fall in the striatum due to a pause in dopaminergic neurons firing in the absence of reward, thereby leading to a suppression of the unrewarding action.[11]

Center-Surround Model of Basal Ganglia Function

The "center-surround" model is based on the pattern of connectivity within the basal ganglia circuits. The somatosensory and motor cortices project to the striatum in a somatotopic manner; information from different body parts terminates in distinct areas of the striatum without overlapping. The projections from the striatum to the GPi/SNr and GPe also maintain very precise topographical organization without convergence. In contrast, single neurons of the STN receive inputs from widespread cortical areas and convergent inputs from different portions of the GPe, and send diffuse projections to both the GPi and GPe. According to the center-surround organization model, to execute an action, other similar or competing actions must be simultaneously suppressed (Figure 34.4). This model is based on the evidence that the STN sends widespread uniform projections to the GPi/SNr and GPe, whereas the striatal projections target selected sets of GPi/SNr or GPe neurons.[12] Via these connections, the input from the cerebral cortex would

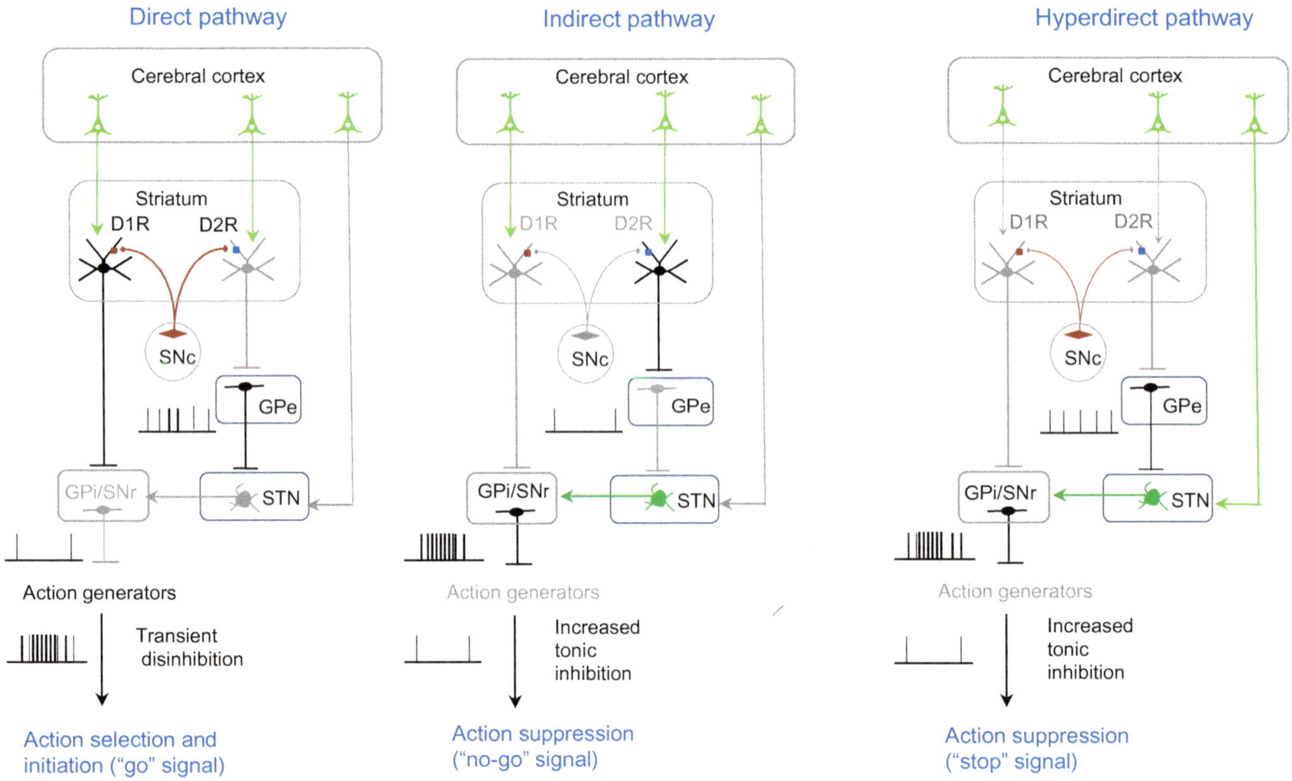

FIGURE 34.3 Parallel model of basal ganglia function.
According to the classical parallel model of basal ganglia circuits, a release of dopamine (DA) from terminals of ventral tegmental area (VTA) or substantia nigra pars compacta (SNc) neurons in response to a reward activates direct pathway striatal projection neurons (dSPNs) via D1Rs, thereby promoting action initiation via inhibition of the globus pallidus pars interna (GPi) and substantia nigra pars reticulata (SNr), while inhibiting, via D2Rs indirect pathway SPNs that may interfere with the selected action. In contrast, a fall in DA in the striatum due to a pause in midbrain dopaminergic neurons leads to disinhibition of indirect pathway SPNs (iSPNs), which in turn inhibit the globus pallidus pars externa (GPe), and disinhibit the subthalamic nucleus (STN) and action suppression via the GPi/SNr. The hyperdirect pathway from the cortex to the STN, activates the inhibitory output from the GPi/SNr.

provide for both a "global excitatory" and "local inhibitory" influence on the GPi. Activation of the hyperdirect and indirect pathway via the STN would produce broad increases in GPi firing, which in turn inhibit the thalamus to suppress all competing actions. Simultaneously, activation of the direct pathway SPNs would focally inhibit a subset of GPI neurons, thereby permitting action selection by disinhibiting the appropriate thalamic target.[10]

PARALLEL BASAL GANGLIA-THALAMOCORTICAL CIRCUITS

Different portions of the striatum and STN receive segregated inputs from the cerebral cortex and participate in parallel motor, oculomotor, cognitive, and emotional circuits. Via basal ganglia-thalamocortical connections, these circuits form parallel overlapping loops (Figure 34.5). However, these loops interact at the level of the cerebral cortex.

Motor Circuit

The motor circuit is primarily involved in habit formation and motor execution, including action sequencing. It originates in the sensorimotor cortex and is centered on the putamen (particularly its dorsocaudal region). The output is mediated by the ventrolateral portion of the GPi, which targets a thalamic territory variably referred to as the lateral portion of the ventral anterior nucleus (VAl), anterior portion of the ventral lateral nucleus (VLa), or posterior ventral oralis nucleus (VOp). This territory projects to the supplementary motor area (SMA) and lateral premotor cortex. The motor circuit includes the dorsolateral portion of the STN and the PPT/PPN, which influences muscle tone during locomotion.

Oculomotor Circuit

The oculomotor circuit is involved in triggering of saccadic eye movement in responses to internal needs (goal-driven or top-down attention) or behavioral-relevant stimuli (stimulus-driven or bottom-up attention).[13] This

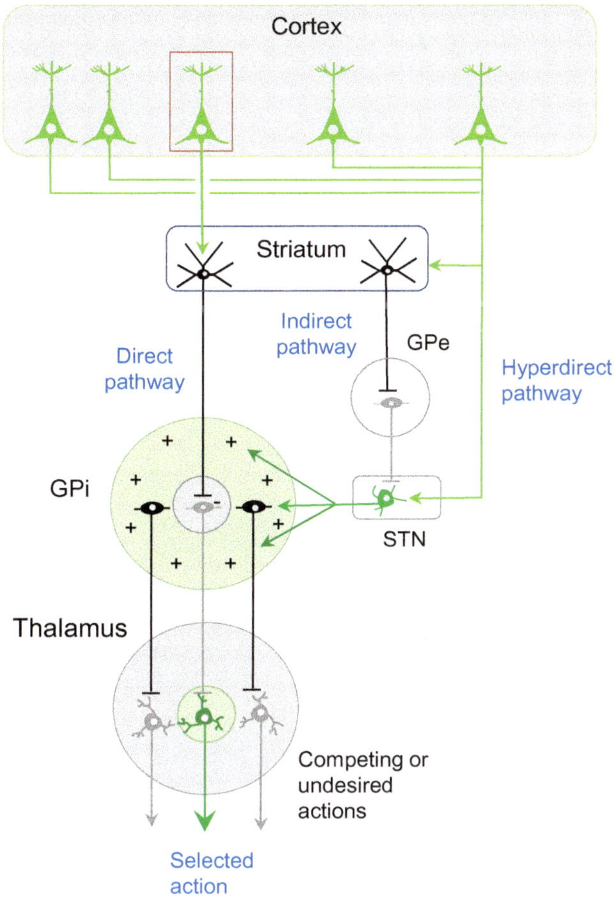

FIGURE 34.4 Center-surround model of basal ganglia function. The "center-surround" organization model is based on anatomical findings that the subthalamic nucleus (STN) sends widespread uniform projections to the globus pallidus pars interna (GPi) and pars externa (GPe), whereas the striatal projections target selected sets of the same GPi or GPe neurons. According to this model, activation of the hyperdirect and indirect pathway would produce broad increases in GPi firing, which in turn inhibit the thalamus to suppress competing actions. Simultaneously, the direct pathway would focally inhibit the GPi and permit action selection by disinhibiting the appropriate thalamic target.

circuit originates in the frontal eye field and the supplementary eye fields, which project to the head and the tail of the caudate nucleus. These portions of the caudate send GABAergic inputs to neurons in the SNr that tonically inhibit saccadic burst neurons of the superior colliculus. Activation of this circuit transiently disinhibits the superior colliculus, triggeringa saccadic eye movement toward the attended object.[13] This circuit is closed by projections to the paralaminar region of the mediodorsal nucleus (MD) which projects to the frontal eye fields and interacts with the attentional system.

Associative (Cognitive) Circuits

The associative, or cognitive, circuits control goal-initiated behavior. These circuits originate primarily in the dorsolateral and ventrolateral prefrontal cortex (PFC) and involve primarily the dorsolateral portion of the head of the caudate nucleus. The head of the caudate nucleus projects to portions of the GPi and SNr that target nuclei of the thalamus that project back to the lateral PFC; the SNr targets the medial VA and the GPi targets the lateral MD. The associative territory of the STN receives inputs from the dorsolateral PFC and frontal eye fields and projects to the SNr, and is thus involved both in oculomotor control and cognitive aspects of motor behavior.

Limbic Circuit

The limbic circuit is involved in reward-based learning and motivated behavior. It originates in the orbitofrontal, medial prefrontal, and midcingulate cortex and targets the ventral striatum, primarily the NAc, as well as rostral and ventral portions of the caudate and putamen.[14,15] The NAc consists of a shell and core regions that target the SNr and the ventral pallidum, which target different territories of the VA and MD that project back to orbitomedial, medial prefrontal, and cingulate cortex. Both the SNr and ventral pallidum also project to the STN, superior colliculus, and PPN/PPT. This connectivity provides for four parallel circuits, two from the NAc shell and two from the NAc core.[16]

Dopaminergic Input to the Basal Ganglia-Thalamocortical Circuits

The different territories of the basal ganglia receive partially segregated input midbrain dopaminergic neurons. Inputs to the putamen (motor circuit) and STN are provided by neurons located in the ventral tier of the substantia nigra pars compacta (SNc) and promote automatic execution of learned behavior (habits) via interactions with the sensorimotor cortex. Inputs to the caudate nucleus (association circuit) originate in the dorsal tier of the SNc and control goal-oriented behavior via interactions with the lateral prefrontal cortex. Inputs to the ventral striatum, including the NAc, originate in the ventral tegmental area (VTA) and support reward-based learning and motivated behavior, via interactions with the PFC and midcingulate cortex.

STRIATUM: INTRINSIC CIRCUITRY AND PHYSIOLOGY

Recent advances in cell labelling and electrophysiological recordings have provided new insights into the complex organization of the striatum.[2,17–19]

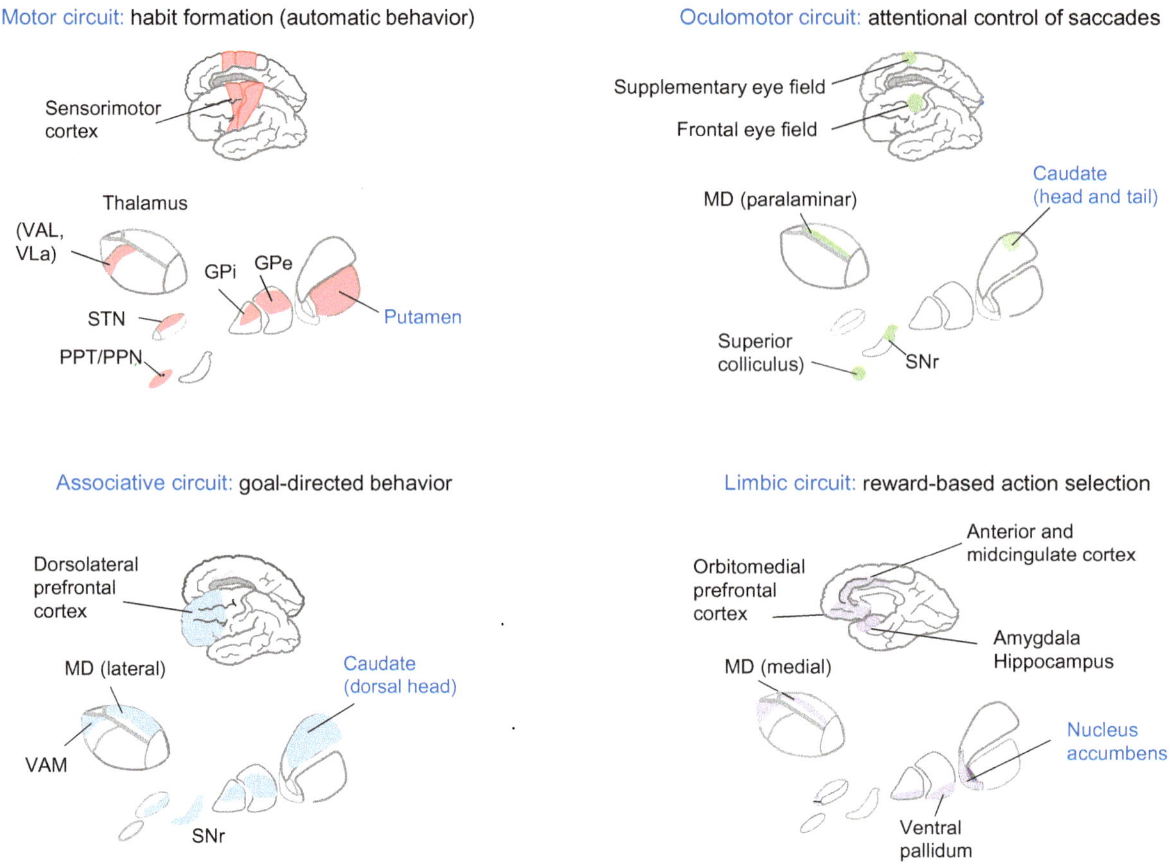

FIGURE 34.5 Parallel basal ganglia–thalamocortical circuits.
The basic organization of the basal ganglia provides for parallel cortico-basal ganglia-thalamocortical circuits. The motor circuit originates in the sensorimotor cortex and is centered on the putamen; its output is mediated by the ventrolateral portion of the globus pallidus interna (GPi), which targets the lateral portion of the ventral anterior (VA) nucleus (also known as ventral lateral anterior [VLa] or ventral oralis posterior [VOp]), which projects to the supplementary motor area (SMA) and lateral premotor cortex. This circuit includes the dorsolateral portion of the subthalamic nucleus (STN) and the pedunculopontine tegmental nucleus (PPN/PPT). The oculomotor circuit originates in the frontal eye field and the supplementary eye fields, which target portions of the head and the tail of the caudate nucleus, which project to neurons of the substantia nigra pars reticulata (SNr) that tonically inhibit saccadic burst neurons of the superior colliculus. The oculomotor circuit is closed projections to the paralaminar region of the mediodorsal nucleus (MDpl) which projects to the frontal eye fields. The associative circuits originate in the lateral prefrontal cortex (PFC) and involve primarily the head of the caudate nucleus, which projects to portions of the GPi and SNr that target portions of the thalamus that project back to the lateral PFC, including the parvicellular portions of the VA (VApc) and MD (MD pc). The associative territory of the STN receives inputs from the dorsolateral PFC and frontal eye fields and projects to the SNr. The limbic circuit originates in the orbitofrontal, medial prefrontal, and midcingulate cortex and targets the ventral striatum, primarily the nucleus accumbens (NAc). The main targets of the NAc are the SNr and the ventral pallidum, which target the magnocellular portion of the ventral anterior nucleus (VAm) and MD (MDmc), hypothalamus, and midbrain. The limbic territory of the STN receives inputs from the medial prefrontal and midcingulate cortices and projects to the ventral and medial pallidum.

Compartmentalization and Heterogeneity of Medium Spiny Output Neurons

The SPNs constitute the majority (~95%) of neurons of the striatum and the sole source of its output. These neurons are distributed into two compartments referred to as striosomes (patch) and matrix[17] (Figure 34.6).The matrix contains most of the SPNs projecting via the direct and indirect pathways and receives its major cortical input from the sensorimotor cortex. In contrast, striosomes contain SPNs that project to the SNc and VTA and receive their input from limbic cortical areas.[18] Direct pathway SPNs targeting the GPi/SNr express substance P and dynorphin and are enriched with excitatory D1Rs and inhibitory cholinergic M4 receptors (M4Rs). Indirect pathway SPNs projecting to the GPe express enkephalin and are enriched with inhibitory D2Rs, as well as excitatory adenosine $A2_A$

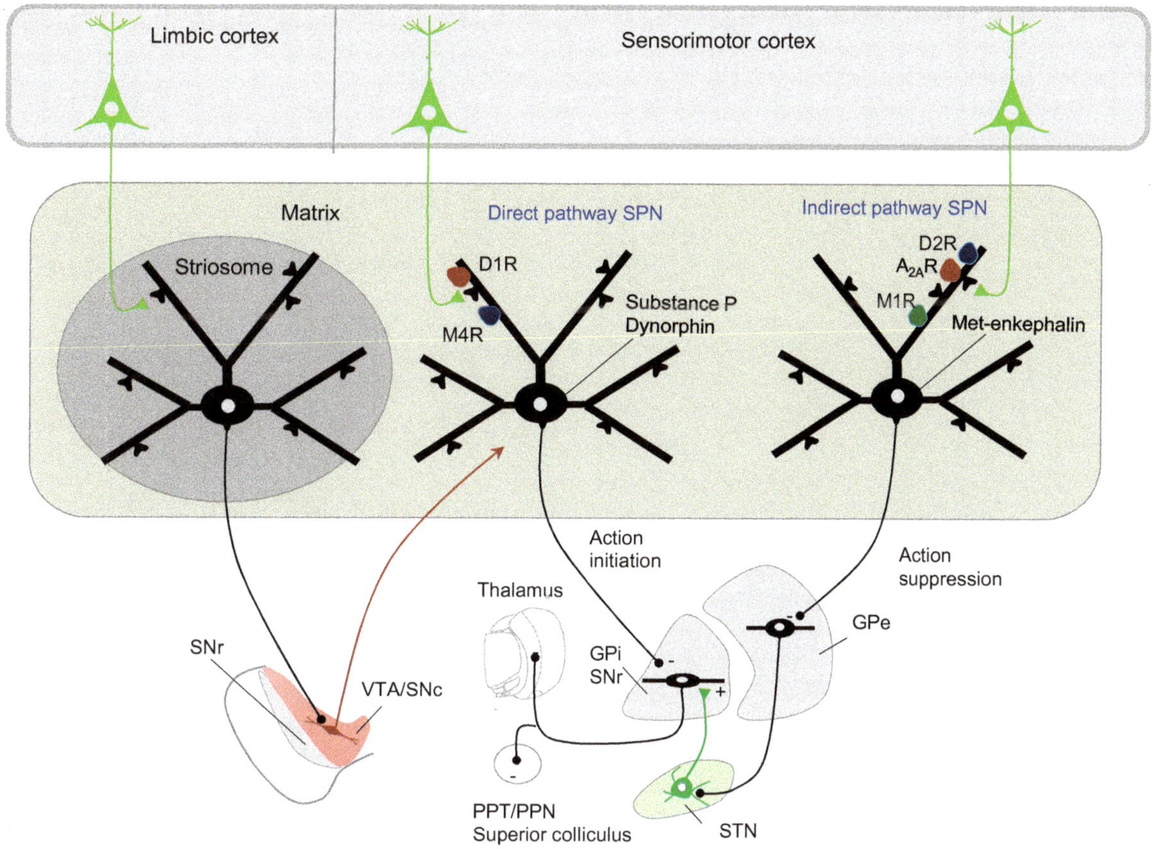

FIGURE 34.6 Compartmentalization and heterogeneity of medium spiny neurons in the striatum.
The medium spiny projection neurons (SPNs) of the striatum include several populations. Direct pathway SPNs express the D1 receptor (D1R), substance P (sP), dynorphin (Dyn), and cholinergic M4 receptors. Indirect pathway SPNs express D2 receptors (D2R), enkephalin (Enk), adenosine $A2_A$ receptors ($A2_A$), D2/$A2_A$ receptor heterodimers, M1 receptors (M1R), and metabotropic type 5 glutamate receptors. The SPNs in the striatum are distributed into two compartments referred to as striosome (patch) and matrix. The matrix contains most of the direct and indirect pathway SPNs and receives its major cortical input from the sensorimotor cortex. Striosomes contain SPNs that project to the SNc and VTA and receive their input from limbic cortical areas.

receptors ($A2_A$Rs), D2/$A2_A$receptor heterodimers, excitatory M1 cholinergic receptors (M1Rs), and metabotropic type 5 glutamate receptors (mGluR5Rs). A subset of SPNs expresses both D1Rs and D2Rs and projects to targets of both the GPi/SNr and the GPe.

Firing Patterns of Medium Spiny Neurons

The SPNs have unique electrophysiological behavior[18] (Figure 34.7). At rest, their activity is dominated by potassium (K^+) conductances that maintain a "down state," in which they are relatively silent. In response to highly convergent excitatory glutamatergic inputs from corticostriatal afferents, SPNs undergo a transition to an "up state," which promotes firing of bursts of action potentials. This up state primarily depends on calcium (Ca^{2+}) influx via Ca_v.1 (L)-type channels and N-methyl-D-aspartate receptors (NMDARs). The transitions between the "down" and the "up" states are strongly regulated by dopaminergic and cholinergic inputs. At baseline, tonic release of DA acting via presynaptic D2Rs and tonic release of acetylcholine (ACh) from local interneurons acting via presynaptic M4Rs maintain the "down state" by inhibiting glutamate release from corticostriatal afferents. In contrast, peaks of DA promote the up-state transition via D1Rs in direct pathway SPNs, whereas peaks of ACh promote the up-state transition via M1Rs in indirect pathway SPNs.

Effects of Cortical and Thalamic Inputs

The cortical input to the striatum originates from both intratelencephalic (IT) and pyramidal tract (PT) neurons in layer 5 of the cerebral cortex and target both SPNs and interneurons[19] (Figure 34.8). The IT neurons project both to the ipsilateral and contralateral striatum and typically fire in relationship to movement planning. The PT neurons project both to the ipsilateral striatum and to other subcortical areas including the STN, brainstem, and spinal cord and fire during movement execution. There is also a subpopulation of GABAergic neurons

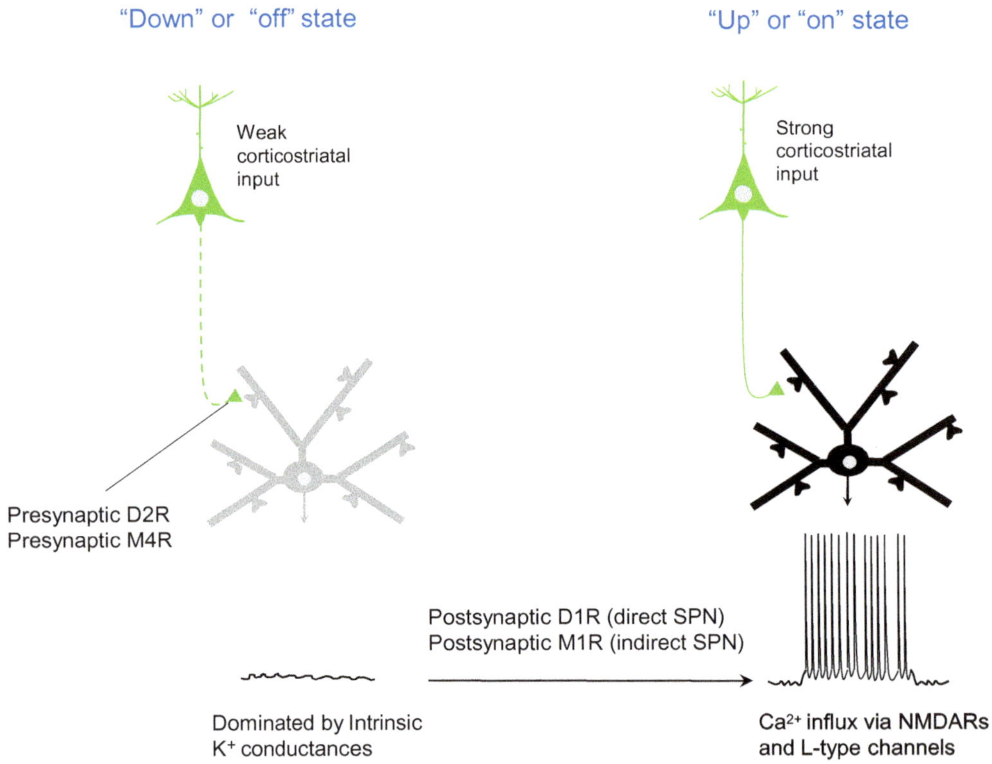

FIGURE 34.7 Firing patterns of medium spiny neurons and effects of dopamine and acetylcholine.
The striatal projection neurons (SPNs) have unique electrophysiological behavior. At rest, their activity is dominated by potassium (K^+) conductances that maintain a "down state," in which they are relatively silent. In response to highly convergent excitatory glutamatergic inputs from corticostriatal afferents, SPNs undergo a transition to an "up state," which promotes firing of bursts of action potentials via activation of N-methyl-D-aspartate receptors (NMDARs) and L-type calcium (Ca^{2+}) channels. The transitions between the "down" and the "up" states are strongly regulated by dopaminergic and cholinergic inputs. At baseline, tonically released dopamine acting via presynaptic D2 receptors (D2R)s and tonically released acetylcholine from local interneurons acting via presynaptic M4 receptors (M4Rs) maintain the "down state" by inhibiting glutamate release from corticostriatal afferents. In contrast, peaks of dopamine promote the up state in direct pathway SPNs (dSPNs) via postsynaptic D1 receptors (D1Rs), whereas peaks of acetylcholine activate the transition to the "up state" in indirect pathway SPNs (iSPNs) via M1 receptors (M1Rs).

in deep layer 5 and layer 6 that project to the striatum and also fire during movement execution. The thalamus provides the second major excitatory glutamatergic input to the striatum.[6] The main source of these thalamostriatal projections are the intralaminar nuclei, particularly the centromedian (CMn)/parafascicular (Pf) complex, which innervates SPNs as well as cholinergic and GABAergic interneurons. The CMn conveys inputs from the motor cortex to the putamen; the Pf conveys inputs from the association cortex (prefrontal and posterior parietal), to the caudate and the NAc. The CMn/Pf neurons also receive strong GABAergic projections from the GPi and SNr, as well as afferents from the cerebellar nuclei, superior colliculus, PPN, locus coeruleus, and dorsal raphe. The striatum also receives inputs from other thalamic nuclei, particularly the central lateral nucleus (CL), which conveys inputs from the cerebellum.[20]

Striatal Interneurons

Although interneurons constitute approximately 5% of the neuronal population of the striatum, they have a critical role in local processing of information and shaping SPN output. They include large aspiny cholinergic neurons and different subpopulations of GABAergic interneurons[2] (Figure 34.8). The giant aspiny cholinergic interneurons have widespread dendritic and axonal fields and integrate information from different compartments over large regions of the striatum.[4] They have a tonic activity primarily modulated by somatodendritic M2 inhibitory autoreceptors, receive strong inputs from the CMn/Pf, and have important reciprocal interactions with dopaminergic terminals. Parvalbumin-expressing fast-spiking GABAergic interneurons provide the most prominent GABAergic input to SPNs, targeting their perisomatic region. These GABAergic interneurons receive inputs from the cerebral

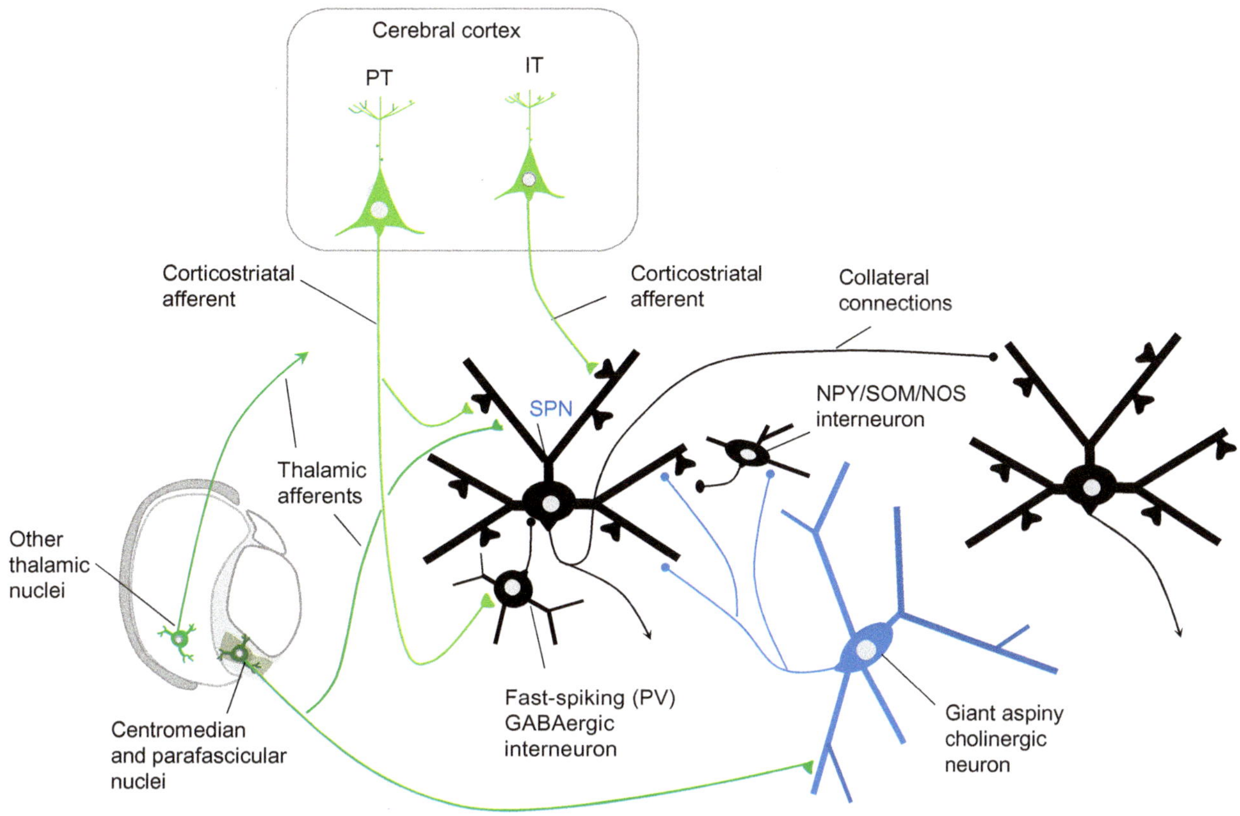

FIGURE 34.8 Intrinsic circuits in the striatum.

There are two classes of cortical neurons that provide input to the striatum, intratelencephalic (IT) neurons and pyramidal tract (PT) neurons. The main source of thalamostriatal projections are neurons in the intralaminar nuclei, particularly the centromedian/parafascicular (CMn/Pf) complex. The striatum also contains large aspiny cholinergic and different subpopulations of GABAergic interneurons. The giant aspiny cholinergic interneurons receive strong inputs from the CMn/Pf. Parvalbumin (PV)-expressing fast-spiking GABAergic interneurons receive inputs from the cerebral cortex and provide unidirectional feedforward inhibition of SPNs. Other GABAergic interneurons express somatostatin (SOM), neuropeptide Y (NPY), and nitric oxide (NO) and target the distal dendrites of SPNs. Local circuits in the striatum include collateral GABAergic connections between SPNs. These connections target the distal dendrites and mediate lateral inhibition between distant SPN populations.

cortex and provide a strictly unidirectional feedforward inhibition of SPNs; fast-spiking GABAergic interneurons are interconnected by gap junctions and each contacts most of its SPNs neighbors producing a "blanket" of inhibition. Other subpopulation of striatal GABAergic interneurons express somatostatin, neuropeptide Y and nitric oxide and target the distal dendrites of SPNs. These GABAergic interneurons are activated by cholinergic inputs and mediate feedback inhibition of SPNs. Other interneuron populations include serotonin 5-HT3 receptor-expressing neurons and tyrosine-hydroxylase-expressing neurons that release GABA but not DA.

Collateral GABAergic Connections Between SPNs

One important component of the local circuits in the striatum are collateral GABAergic connections between SPNs.[2] These connections target the distal dendrites and mediate lateral inhibition between distant SPN populations. There is a functional asymmetry in these lateral connections. Indirect pathway SPNs project strongly to both direct and indirect pathway SPNs and strongly inhibit the direct pathway SPNs. As these inhibitory terminals express D2Rs, dopamine may promote activity of direct pathway SPNs by inhibiting GABA release from these inhibitory collaterals. In contrast, collaterals from direct pathway SPNs send weaker projection to other direct pathway SPNs. Collateral interactions between SPNs provide for the organization of these neurons into sparsely distributed functional ensembles involving synchronized firing of related SPNs units located at a distance from each other.[2]

Mechanisms of Action of Dopamine in the Striatum

Tonic firing of dopaminergic neurons maintains a steady baseline level of DA that acts primarily via high-affinity extrasynaptic and presynaptic D2Rs to restrain glutamate release from corticostriatal afferents; this promotes the down state of SPNs in the absence of behavioral meaningful stimuli. Dopamine peaks during burst firing activate direct pathway SPNs via D1Rs coupled to G_{olf}, leading to activation of the adenylyl cyclase 5 (ADC5)-cyclic adenosine monophosphate (cAMP)–protein kinase A (PKA) signaling pathway. This leads to inhibition of Ca^{2+}-activated K^+ currents and thus increased excitability and transition to the up state of direct pathway SPNs. The inhibitory effect of DA on indirect pathway SPNs via D2Rs involve $G_{i/o}$ proteins, which inhibit adenylyl cyclase, activate K^+ channels, and inhibit Ca^{2+} influx both via Ca_v1 (L) and NMDAR channels, promoting the down state of these SPNs. D2R activation also inhibits GABA release from their axon collaterals innervating the direct pathway SPNs. Most midbrain dopaminergic neurons targeting the striatum encode the reward value of stimuli. They increase their discharge in response to a reward, promoting via D1R in the direct pathway the selection of the rewarding action; they pause in response to an adverse outcome, which leads to reduced D2R mediated inhibition of indirect pathway SPNs and thus suppression of the action that led to the adverse outcome.[13,18] In addition to these immediate effects, repeated exposure to DA elicits bidirectional plasticity at corticostriatal synapses[11,15] (Figure 34.9). Upon repeated exposure to a rewarding stimulus over time, the coincident activation of D1Rs and NMDARs leads to long-term potentiation (LTP) of corticostriatal synapses on direct pathway SPNs, which promotes selection of the rewarding action in the future. In contrast, activation of

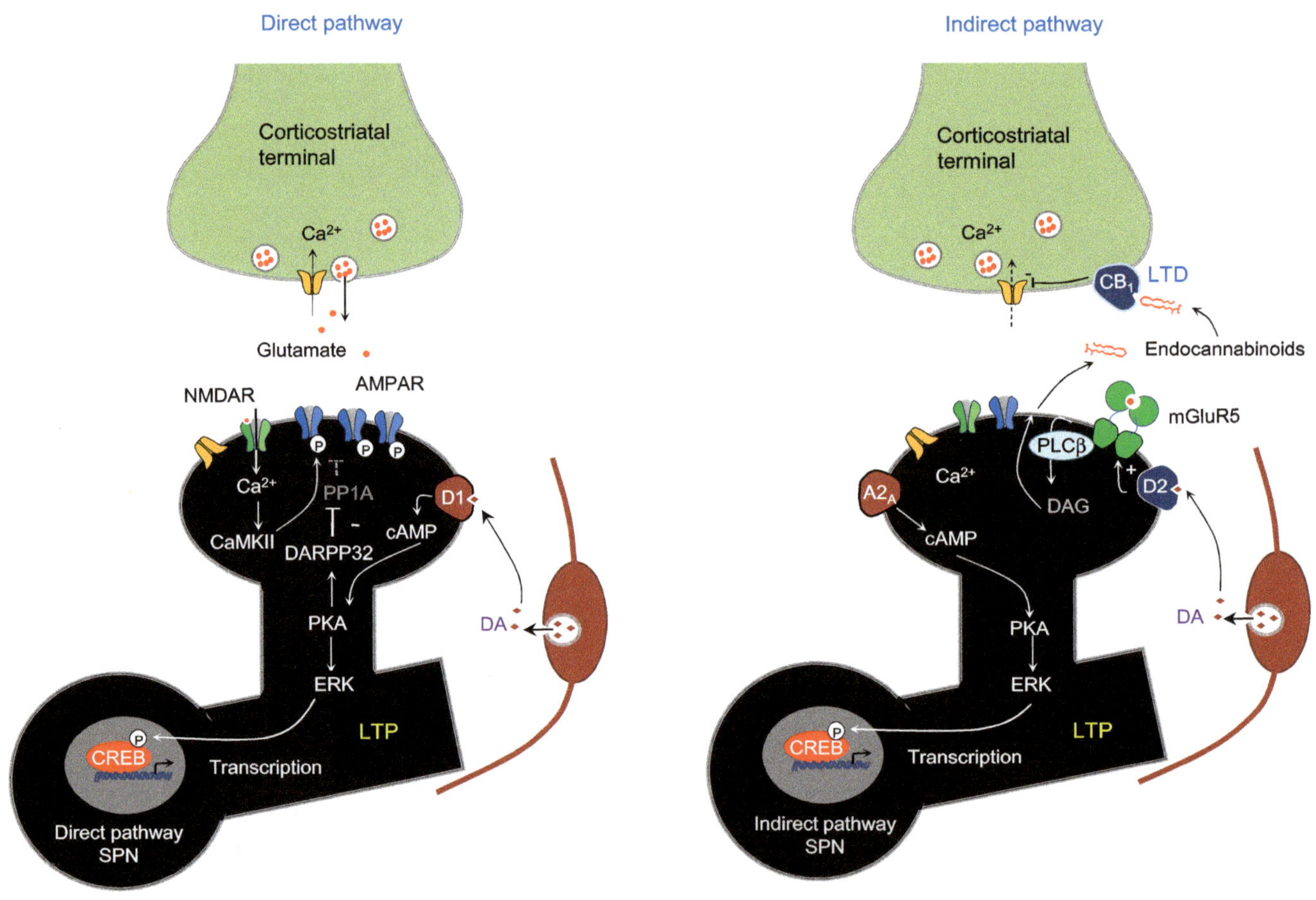

FIGURE 34.9 Effect of dopamine in synaptic plasticity in the striatum.
Upon repeated exposure to a rewarding stimulus over time, the coincident activation of dopamine D1 receptors (D1Rs) and N-methyl-D-aspartate receptors (NMDARs) leads to long-term potentiation (LTP) of corticostriatal synapses on direct pathway striatal projection neurons (dSPNs).This involves the D1R-coupled G_{olf}–cyclic adenosine monophosphate (cAMP)–protein kinase A (PKA cascade). PKA phosphorylates the dopamine- and cyclic AMP-regulated phosphoprotein of 32kD (DARPP-32), which amplifies the PKA signal by inhibiting protein phosphatase 1. D1R-induced LTP also involves activation of extracellular signal-regulated kinase (ERK) and phosphorylation of the transcription factor Ca^{2+} and cyclic AMP response element-binding protein (CREB). In contrast, activation of postsynaptic D2Rs elicits long-term depression (LTD) of corticostriatal synapses on indirect pathway SPNs (iSPNs) by promoting metabotropic glutamate receptor 5 (mGluR5) signaling and production of endocannabinoids, which acts via presynaptic CB1 receptors to inhibit glutamate release at these synapses. Adenosine released locally in response to synaptic activity acts via $A2_A$Rs coupled to cAMP signaling and antagonizes the effects D2R in iSPNs.

postsynaptic D2Rs elicits long-term depression (LTD) of corticostriatal synapses on indirect pathway SPNs. This involves mGluR5 signaling and production of endocannabinoids, which act via presynaptic CB1 receptors to inhibit glutamate release at these synapses. Adenosine released locally in response to synaptic activity acts via $A2_A$Rs coupled to the Gs-adenylyl cyclase-cAMP-PKA cascade and thus antagonizes the effects D2Rs.

Effects of Acetylcholine and Its Interactions with Dopamine

The giant aspiny cholinergic interneurons have a major role in regulation of the basal ganglia circuits (Figure 34.10). Tonic release of ACh increases the signal-to-noise ratio in striatal circuits. Alerting inputs are conveyed by the thalamic intralaminar nuclei to the striatal cholinergic interneurons, which regulate attentional set and behavioral switching. In response to an unexpected event, excitatory inputs from the thalamus trigger a transient burst of cholinergic interneuron activity, which produces an ACh peak that inhibits glutamate release from all corticostriatal synapses, interrupting ongoing behavior. This short burst is followed by a pause in cholinergic interneuron firing, which in part results from D2R-mediated inhibition by DA released in response to the peak of ACh acting via presynaptic nicotinic receptors on dopaminergic terminals. The pause of cholinergic interneurons is followed by a rebound excitation and a secondary burst, during which ACh activates postsynaptic excitatory M1Rs on indirect pathway SPNs, leading to suppression of the previous action. Acetylcholine also affects plasticity at corticostriatal synapses. Activation of M4Rs antagonizes the effects of D1Rs in direct pathway SPNs, leading to LTD of the corticostriatal synapse. The interactions among dopaminergic, cholinergic, and glutamatergic

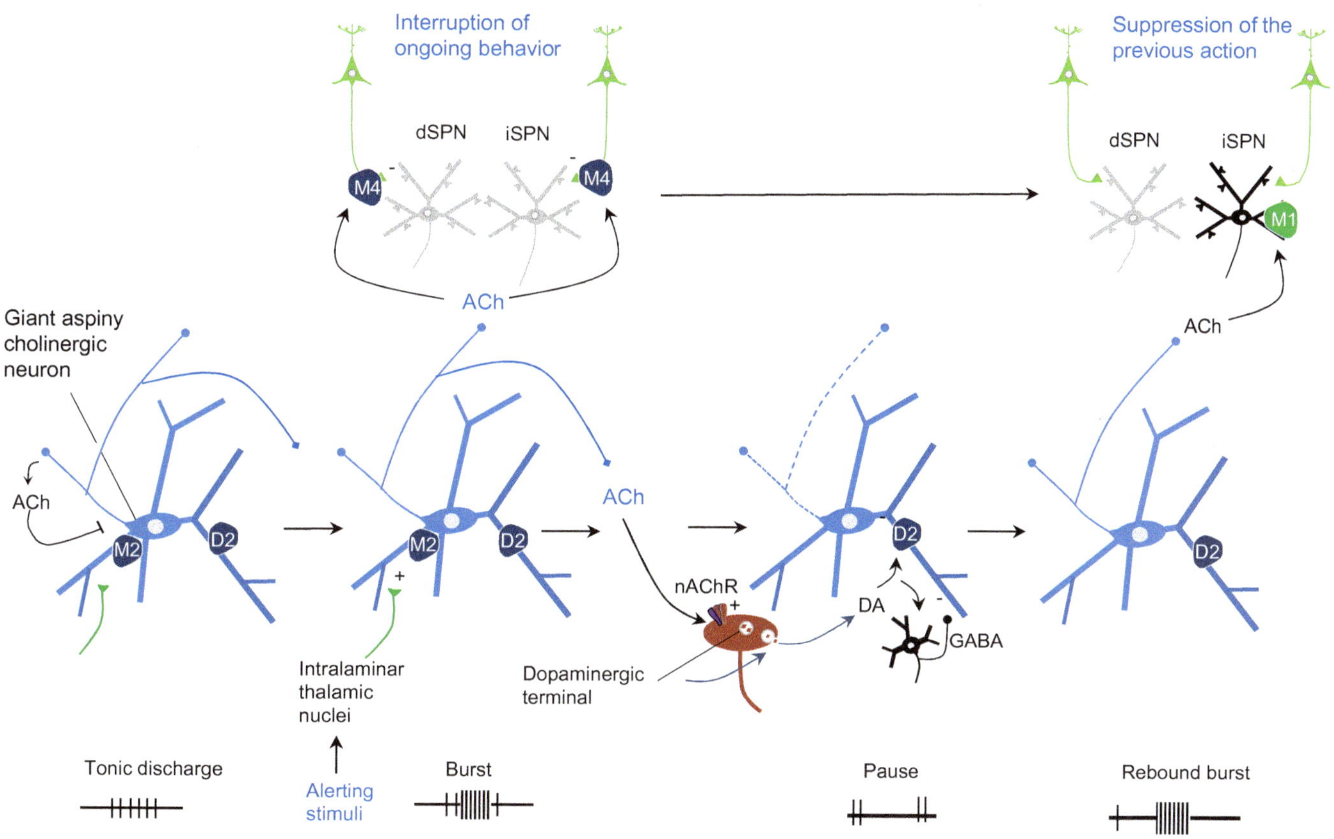

FIGURE 34.10 Alerting cholinergic signaling in the striatum.
Tonic release of acetylcholine (ACh) from giant aspiny neurons increases the signal-to-noise ratio in striatal circuits by inhibiting, via presynaptic M4 and M2 receptors, glutamate release from corticostriatal afferents innervating both direct pathway striatal projection neurons (dSPN) and indirect pathway SPNs (iSPNs). In response to an unexpected event, there is a transient burst of cholinergic interneuron activity triggered by excitatory input from the intralaminar thalamic nuclei. The short burst is followed by a pause cholinergic interneurons firing; this results from the release of dopamine triggered by cholinergic activation of presynaptic nicotinic receptors in dopaminergic terminals. Dopamine inhibits the activity of cholinergic neurons and ACh release via D2 receptors (D2Rs) and activates via D5Rs local GABAergic interneurons indirectly inhibiting the activity of cholinergic interneurons. The pause of cholinergic interneurons is followed by a rebound excitation and a secondary burst, during which ACh activates postsynaptic M1Rs preferentially expressed in iSPNs leading to suppression of the previous action.

inputs, the presence of receptor heterodimers, the cross-talk among downstream signaling, and the effects of locally released signals such as endocannabinoids makes the modulation of intrinsic striatal circuits extremely complex.[8]

GLOBUS PALLIDUS: CONNECTIVITY AND FUNCTIONS

The globus pallidus is a fundamental component of both the intrinsic and extrinsic basal ganglia circuitry. Whereas the GPi has gained most interest as a target for deep brain stimulation (DBS) for treatment of both Parkinson disease (PD) and dystonia, recent evidence indicates that the GPe is not only a fundamental component of the indirect pathway involved in the pathophysiology of akinesia but also has extrinsic connections that makes this structure a potential therapeutic target.

Extrinsic Connectivity

In the classical model, the activity of both the GPi/SNr and GPe is primarily driven by excitatory input from the STN and transiently interrupted by GABAergic inputs from the striatum. However, diffusion magnetic resonance imaging and tractography studies show that globus pallidus also receive projections from both the cerebral cortex and cerebellum[21,22] (Figure 34.11). The corticopallidal pathway targets both the GPe and the GPi. There are extensive inputs from the prefrontal, motor, and posterior parietal cortex to the GPe. Based on this connectivity, the GPe is segregated into a dorsal sensorimotor cluster, ventral associative cluster, and posterior parietal cluster. There is a smaller projection from the superior the frontal gyrus and sensorimotor cortex to the ventral posterior portion of the GPi (sensorimotor territory) and a direct cortico-nigral connection originating from the superior frontal gyrus, PFC, and motor areas. There are important reciprocal direct

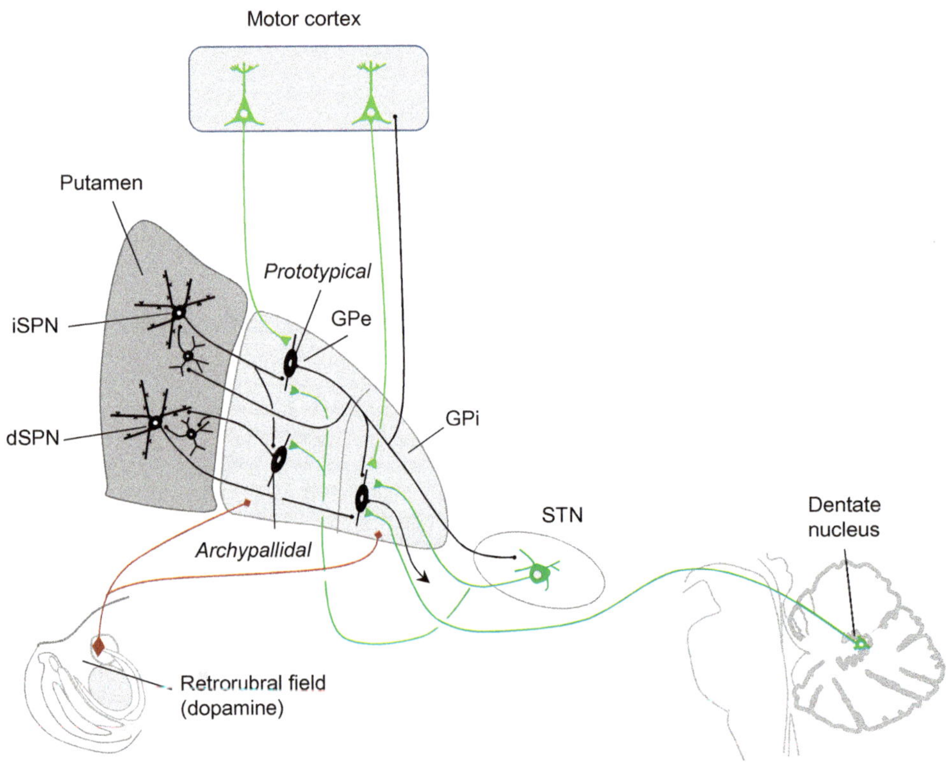

FIGURE 34.11 Connectivity of the globus pallidus.
The activity of both the GPi/SNr and GPe is primarily driven by excitatory input from the STN and transiently interrupted by GABAergic inputs from the striatum. In addition, diffusion magnetic resonance imaging and tractography studies showed direct connections from the cerebral cortex and cerebellum to the globus pallidus. The corticopallidal pathway targets both the GPe and the GPi. There are extensive inputs from the prefrontal, motor, and posterior parietal cortex to the GPe and a smaller connection from superior the frontal gyrus and sensorimotor cortex to the GPi. There is a direct connection between the dentate nucleus and the globus pallidus.

connections between the dentate nucleus and the globus pallidus. Dentato-pallidal connections cluster in the GPi, together with associative and sensorimotor corticopallidal clusters.[21,22]

Effects on Thalamic Activity

The motor thalamus integrates the tonic inhibitory inputs from the GPi/SNr with the excitatory inputs from the cortex. The pallidal territory of the thalamus (VAl/VLa) receives inputs from the GPi and targets the SMA, lateral premotor cortex, and primary motor cortex and primarily guides movements of the limb. In contrast, the SNr output primarily controls movement of proximal muscles, head, neck, and eyes. Most neurons in the thalamic motor nuclei exhibit a peak of activity preceding movement onset. The tonically active GPi/ SNr inputs elicit strong thalamic inhibition that blocks the excitatory drive form the motor cortex to the thalamus. The transient focal interruption of this tonic inhibition by the direct pathway would open the thalamic "gate" and allow transmission of excitatory corticothalamic signals in the subset of thalamocortical neurons encoding the chosen action, whereas the surrounding neurons remain inhibited. When cortical input is weak or when the GPi/SNr is pathologically exaggerated, hyperpolarization of thalamic neurons promotes a "rebound burst" mode of activity that leads to a slow rhythmic activity of thalamocortical neurons. This may trigger abnormal activity in motor circuits, as hypothesized as a mechanism for rest tremor in PD.[23,24]

Pallido-Striatal Connection

Classically, the GPe has been implicated primarily in the indirect pathway and in reciprocal interactions with the STN. However, the GPe also sends back projections to the striatum. The GPe contains two major subpopulations of GABAergic neurons.[25,26] The first population comprises the "prototypical" neurons, which are fast-spiking neurons and participate in the indirect pathway by targeting the STN and GPi/SNr. These prototypical GPe neurons also project back to the striatum, targeting primarily the fast-spiking GABAergic interneurons, thus controlling their feedforward inhibition of SPNs. The second population of GPe neurons, referred to as "arkypallidal" neurons, project massively only to the striatum, targeting both SPNs and interneurons. Arkypallidal neurons may provide a "stop" signal to the striatum to cancel evolving actions.[27] These two subpopulations of GPe neurons fire at inversed phases during both sleep and active states, and this difference is exacerbated in the setting of DA loss, as shown in experimental models. There is also a distinct population of prototypical GPe neurons target the cerebral cortex and the thalamic reticular nucleus.[28] These GPe neurons receive cortical inputs from PT neurons and may thus participate in reciprocal cortico-pallido-cortical loops.

SUBTHALAMIC NUCLEUS AND INTRINSIC CONTROL OF BASAL GANGLIA CIRCUITS

The STN is a nodal point of both the indirect and hyperdirect pathways that lead to action suppression via the GPi/SNr. The STN also participates in reciprocal interactions with the GPe, predisposing to oscillatory activity within the basal ganglia-thalamocortical circuits.

Functional Connectivity

The STN receives excitatory input from the cerebral cortex, inhibitory input from the GPe, and modulatory input from midbrain dopaminergic neurons. The cortical inputs to the STN are topographically segregated. The dorsolateral STN receives inputs from the inferior lateral PFC (predominantly from the right hemisphere) and subserves motor suppression, whereas the ventromedial STN receives inputs from the orbitomedial PFC and may thus be involved in cognitive and behavioral functions. Whereas both the indirect and the hyperdirect pathways promote activity of the STN, they may have different but complementary effects. The indirect pathway via the striatum and GPe leading to disinhibition of the STN may function to "prospectively" inhibit initiation of undesired action (no-go signal). In contrast, the hyperdirect cortico-STN pathway may rapidly and "retrospectively" interrupt ongoing action ("stop signal). The STN is also an effector in cognitive and emotional (limbic) circuits of the basal ganglia and relays excitatory inputs from the PFC to midbrain dopaminergic neurons triggering burst activity of these cells (Figure 34.12).

Regulation of STN Activity

Neurons of the STN have a spontaneous activity that is shaped by four main factors: intrinsic electrophysiological properties; driving glutamatergic inputs from the cerebral cortex; feedback GABAergic inhibition from the GPe, and modulatory effects of DA.[29] STN neurons fire spontaneously at ~5–15 Hz due to recurrent opening of subthreshold Na_v channels; the timing is controlled by hyperpolarization via SK type Ca^{2+}-activated K^+ channels. Excitatory inputs from the cerebral cortex drive STN neuron activity in the beta band (13–30 Hz) (Figure 34.12). Feedback GABAergic input from the GPe elicits a $GABA_A$ receptor-mediated hyperpolarization of STN neurons that deactivates their Na_v channels and increases their responsiveness to subsequent cortical inputs. Upon recovery from hyperpolarization, STN neurons fire a rebound burst of action potentials. This STN activity can be relayed to the GPe via feedforward excitation, and then be conveyed via the GPi/SNr to thalamocortical neurons.

In normal resting conditions, the STN, GPe, and GPi discharge at high frequency without rhythm or correlation. During movement, their discharge shows somatotopically

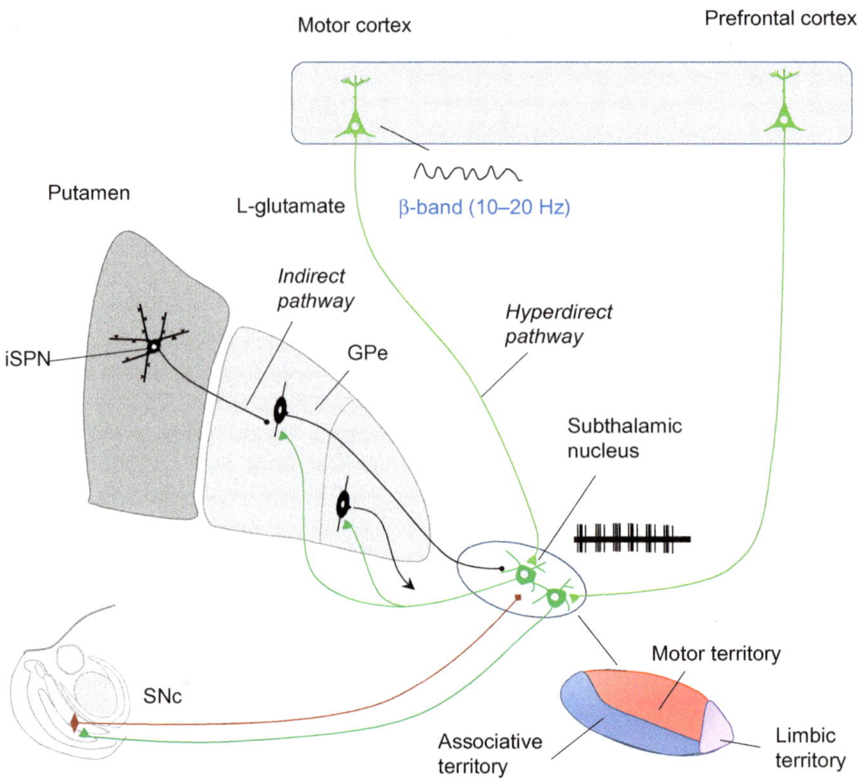

FIGURE 34.12 Connectivity and physiology of the subthalamic nucleus.
The subthalamic nucleus (STN) is a nodal point of both the indirect and hyperdirect pathways. The activity of STN neurons is shaped by their intrinsic electrophysiological properties, driving glutamatergic inputs from the cerebral cortex, feedback GABAergic inhibition from the globus pallidus pars externa (GPe), and modulatory effects of dopamine (DA). Excitatory inputs from the cerebral cortex drive STN neuron activity in the β-band; this rhythmic β-frequency activity directly imparted to the STN can be relayed to the GPe via feedforward excitation, and then be conveyed via the globus pallidus pars interna (GPi) and substantia nigra pars reticulata (SNr) GPi/SNr to thalamocortical neurons. Feedback GABAergic input from the GPe elicits a $GABA_A$ receptor-mediated hyperpolarization of STN neurons that deactivates their voltage-gated sodium channels (Na_v) and triggers a rebound burst activity of STN neurons via voltage-gated calcium channels. Dopamine regulates the activity of the STN-GPe circuit via D2 receptors.

organized activity with complex spatiotemporal patterns. These interactions promote rhythmic, coherent activity in both the STN and GPe via the powerful reciprocal connections between these two structures. Cortical inputs produce LTP at the GPe-STN synapse, thus maintaining the balance between the influence of the hyperdirect (cortical) and indirect (GPe) pathways on the STN.

Dopamine and Inhibition of Synchronized Oscillatory Activity in Basal Ganglia Circuits

In normal conditions, beta oscillations in the motor system reflect motor readiness and promote tonic, preparatory activity at the expense of voluntary movements. Beta activity in both the cortex and STN is suppressed in anticipation of a cue to initiate movement, and the latency of suppression of these beta oscillations correlates with the motor reaction time in normal subjects. In response to salient events, peak DA levels in the basal ganglia circuits would suppress beta oscillations to initiate the selected action. Dopamine sets the pattern of activity of STN neurons and prevents abnormally synchronized oscillatory in the STN-GPe circuit by several mechanisms, mediated primarily via D2Rs. They include reduced excitability of the indirect pathway SPNs and GPe neurons; presynaptic inhibition of GABA release at both the SPN-GPe and GPe-STN synapses; and presynaptic inhibition of glutamate release at the cortico-STN synapse. In addition, activation of D1Rs elicits depolarization and thus inactivation of Na_v and Ca_v channels in STN neurons, thereby reducing their intrinsic activity and preventing burst firing.[29]

OTHER RELEVANT CONNECTIONS OF THE BASAL GANGLIA CIRCUITS

Connectivity Between the Basal Ganglia and the Cerebellum

There are reciprocal connections between the basal ganglia and the cerebellar circuits via several pathways. The STN provides an excitatory projection input to the pontine nuclei, which are the primary source of mossy fiber input to the cerebellum.[30] Reciprocally, the cerebellar output via the dentate nucleus affects the basal ganglia circuits via two parallel mechanisms. One is a projection to the intralaminar thalamic nuclei, primarily the CL, which targets the striatum. The second is via direct projections from the dentate nucleus terminating in the putamen, GPe, GPi, and SNr.[21,31] The reciprocal connections between the basal ganglia and cerebellum, both between each other and with the cerebral cortex via the thalamus, provide for segregated circuits controlling both motor and nonmotor functions.[30] The prominent inputs from prefrontal association cortex to the GPe may have a role in flexible control of goal-oriented motor behavior.[31] The direct cortico-GP and substantia nigra pathways, in cooperation with those from the dentate nucleus, would give the cortex an ability to fine-tune decision-making and motor action selection, as well as more rapid flexibility to any unexpected changes in the environment.[31]

Serotonergic Modulation

All components of the basal ganglia circuits receive serotonergic inputs from the dorsal raphe nucleus.[32] The substantia nigra is the most densely innervated component of these circuits. Serotonin (5-HT) exerts multiple effects, both directly and via interaction with the dopaminergic system. They include presynaptic inhibition of glutamate or GABA release via $5\text{-HT}1_{B/D}$ receptors, postsynaptic inhibition via $5\text{-HT}1_A$ receptors, and postsynaptic excitation via $5\text{-HT}2_A$, $5\text{-HT}2_C$, and 5-HT4 receptors. Some effects are mediated by interneurons. For example, in the striatum activation of $5\text{-HT}2_C$ receptors in local cholinergic neurons indirectly elicits a decrease in activity of the SPNs. In the GP, the net effect of 5-HT in vitro is to increase neuronal activity by both presynaptic and postsynaptic mechanisms In the STN, 5-HT increases membrane excitability and firing frequency via $5\text{-HT}2_C$ and 5-HT4 receptors and reduces neuronal excitability via $5\text{-HT}1_A$ receptors. The basal ganglia, particularly components of the limbic circuit, send projections back to the dorsal and median raphe nuclei.

MECHANISMS UNDERLYING THE MOTOR MANIFESTATIONS OF PARKINSON DISEASE

Parkinson disease is characterized by neuronal loss and accumulation of α-synuclein (α-SYN) inclusions as Lewy bodies and Lewy neurites in the peripheral and central nervous systems. Levodopa-responsive motor symptoms reflect loss of dopaminergic neurons of the SNc with reduced number of dopaminergic terminals in the striatum, as reflected by reduced levels of the dopamine transporter (DAT) and vesicular monoamine transporter 2 (VMAT2).[33] Chronic loss of dopaminergic signaling triggers change in synaptic plasticity and circuit dynamics.[10]

Selective Vulnerability of Nigra Dopaminergic Neurons

Dopaminergic denervation of the striatum in PD typically progresses from the posterior putamen to more anterior regions, due to early selective vulnerability of densely packed dopaminergic neurons located in "nigrosomes" of the ventral tier of the SNc.[34] This may explain the early impairment in automatic (habitual) motor behavior, despite spared ability to learn and accurately perform complex motor sequences. Several features make SNc more vulnerable than VTA neurons to neurodegeneration in PD. Nigrostriatal dopaminergic cells are metabolically vulnerable due to their highly divergent axonal arborizations and intrinsic physiological properties that predispose to mitochondrial oxidant stress and proteostatic dysfunction. Nigrostriatal SNc neurons express L-type ($Ca_v1.3$) channels that trigger Ca^{2+} transients in the mitochondria and generate oxidative stress in dendrites;[35] they also have low expression of the buffering Ca^{2+}-binding protein calbindin; and reduced activity of aldehyde dehydrogenase 1, which normally prevents accumulation of pro-oxidant products of DA metabolism.[36] Impaired VAMT2 activity increases cytosolic availability of DA, which can then be metabolized to toxic 3,4-dihydroxyphenylacetaldehyde (DOPAL).[37] There is also an interaction among α-SYN, dysfunction of the autophagosome-lysosomal pathway, and the endoplasmic reticulum stress response that contribute to dopaminergic cell death in PD.[38]

Cortical Involvement in the Pathogenesis of PD

It has been proposed that selective vulnerability of ventrolateral tier SNc neurons innervating the putamen would reflect their input from the motor cortex.[39] One typical feature of PD is focal onset of parkinsonian signs such as reduced arm swinging or hand tremor and later in the disease course somatotopically related levodopa-induced dyskinesia (LID). Repetitive transcranial magnetic stimulation (rTMS) studies show reduced intracortical inhibition and loss of plasticity in the motor cortex contralateral to the motor symptoms. In healthy subjects, activation of the motor cortex using rTMS elicits release of striatal DA, as measured with [(^{11})C]raclopride PET. This effect may be mediated via a disynaptic cortico-STN-nigral excitation. A substantial amount of physiological α-SYN is localized at corticostriatal glutamatergic terminals in the striatum and may be secreted from these terminals in response synaptic activity. Extracellular α-SYN activates presynaptic $Ca_v2.2$ channels in nigrostriatal terminals triggering DA release.

Thus, increased corticostriatal activity may promote accumulation and increase neurotoxicity of α-SYN on dopaminergic terminals in the posterior putamen, ultimately leading to retrograde neurodegeneration of nigrostriatal neurons in the ventrolateral SNc region.[29]

Plastic Changes in Neuronal Excitability and Synaptic Activity in the Striatum

Animal models show that loss of dopaminergic inputs triggers cell-specific compensatory plastic changes in intrinsic excitability and SPNs leading to an imbalance between the activity of the indirect and direct pathways.[9] Hyperactivity of the indirect pathway reflects loss of D2R-mediated SPN inhibition; hypoactivity of the direct pathway reflects loss of D1R-mediated SPN activation. This imbalance may be exaggerated by reduced presynaptic D2R-mediated inhibition of GABA release from collaterals of indirect pathway SPNs innervating the direct pathway SPNs.[40] However, in response to loss of DA signaling, SPNs undergo homeostatic changes in their intrinsic excitability and synaptic plasticity that tend to restore the balance between these two pathways.[9] This plasticity could explain why motor manifestations of PD only occur after loss of more than one-half of dopaminergic innervation of the striatum. In the hyperactive indirect pathway, loss of D2R-mediated inhibition leads to reduced intrinsic activity of SPNs, which undergo pruning of dendritic spines secondary to increased activity-dependent Ca^{2+} influx. In contrast, loss of D1R-mediated excitation leads to a compensatory increase in excitability of direct pathway SPNs. In addition to these adaptations in intrinsic excitability, there are also homeostatic changes in synaptic plasticity [9].

Imbalance Between Dopaminergic and Cholinergic Influence in the Striatum

The classical concept of a functional antagonism between DA and ACh in the striatum led to the hypothesis that an imbalance between these two influences underlies the motor manifestations of PD. Accordingly, muscarinic receptor antagonists such as trihexyphenydil were the first accepted treatment for this disorder. However, the interactions between these two neurochemical signals in the striatum are complex. Loss of DA results in increased activity of cholinergic interneurons due to reduced efficacy of signaling from inhibitory M4 autoreceptors in cholinergic interneurons. Dopamine depletion is also associated with increased cholinergic innervation of the indirect pathway SPNs and decreased cholinergic innervation of direct pathway SPNs. Striatal dysfunction in PD may also reflect selective impairment of control of SPNs by corticostriatal and thalamostriatal afferents. Studies in monkeys with 1-methyl-4-phenyl-1,2,3,6 tetrahydropyridine (MPTP)-induced parkinsonism indicate that akinesia and hypometria in PD may reflect selective hypofunction of PT neurons innervating the striatum and subcortical structures. Postmortem studies show that there is a 30%–40% loss of CMn/Pf neurons in PD, and this is seen even in cases with mild motor deficits with no further progression with severity of motor dysfunction [34].

Circuit Dysfunction and Akinesia in Parkinson Disease

There is evidence that akinesia (hypokinesia and bradykinesia) reflects several types of circuit dysfunction in PD. These include exaggerated activity of the indirect pathway (firing rate mechanism), bursting of individual neurons, excessive synchronization, and loss of functional segregation in the basal ganglia circuits.[10,41] Consistent with the parallel model of basal ganglia function, extracellular single-unit recordings in parkinsonian primates and humans revealed increased average firing of neurons of the GPi and STN, and reduced firing in the GPe, reflecting impaired activity of the direct and hyperactivity of the indirect pathways. In addition to changes in firing rate across the basal ganglia-thalamocortical loop, parkinsonism is also characterized by substantial alterations in the pattern of single-cell firing and synchronization between nodes in the basal ganglia circuit. Bursting of individual neurons may reflect changes in intrinsic properties or synaptic input of neurons and occurs in the GPi, GPe, STN, thalamus, and motor cortex in both PD patients and in parkinsonian nonhuman primates. Levodopa reduces bursting in the GPi in parallel with improvement in motor function. Abnormal synchronized rhythmic activity occurs in both beta frequency (13–30 Hz) and tremor frequency (4–10 Hz) in the STN, GPe, GPi, thalamus, and sensorimotor cortex in PD. Abnormal, synchronous beta frequency oscillations in PD are driven by the cortical-STN-GPe loop reflecting loss of dopaminergic modulation; pallidostriatal projections may promote such oscillations by creating a positive feedback loop in the DA depleted state.[42] The power of beta oscillations correlates with bradykinesia and rigidity and is reduced by dopamine replacement therapy or DBS. The mechanisms by which high-frequency (> 60 Hz) DBS interrupts abnormal beta frequency synchrony, restores physiological beta activity in the corticospinal system and improves akinesia are not fully understood.[43]

Another circuit-level abnormality in PD is loss of functional segregation in basal ganglia circuits with loss of somatotopic organization; this may in part reflect impaired DA modulation of lateral inhibitory connection between indirect SPNs and direct SPN pairs.

Resting Tremor and Role of Basal Ganglia and Cerebellar Interactions

Patients with PD may have different types of tremor. The most common is resting tremor, which is inhibited during movement but may reoccur at a similar frequency when adopting a posture (reemergent tremor). Postural/kinetic tremor occurs at a higher frequency and is nonharmonically related to the resting tremor. Unlike bradykinesia and rigidity, resting tremor in PD does not correlate with the degree of nigrostriatal DA cell loss, which explains the wide variability in the response of resting tremor to dopaminergic therapy among patients with PD. Patients with tremor-predominant PD have more dopaminergic cell loss in the retrorubral area, which provides inputs to the STN and GP, compared to those without tremor.[44] Patients with tremor-predominant PD have been found to have lower availability of serotonin transporter but less severe deficit in striatal dopamine transporter compared to PD patients with no tremor.[45] Resting tremor in PD is associated with abnormal oscillatory activity within the basal ganglia and the cerebello-thalamocortical circuit and abnormal intercircuit interactions.[24,46] Unlike essential tremor, resting tremor in PD shows alteration in tremor frequency that points toward its generator from multiple uncoupled oscillators generators with different frequencies.[47] According to the "dimmer-switch" model, both the basal ganglia and the cerebellothalamic circuits contribute to the generation and maintenance of resting tremor in PD.[24,46] The basal ganglia may work as a light switch that triggers tremor initiation and the cerebellum as a light-dimmer that modulates tremor amplitude. The hyperactive GPi, via its strong inhibitory GABAergic input to the VA (VLa), would initiate rhythmic activity in thalamocortical neurons projecting to the SMA and premotor cortex; this oscillatory activity would engage the cerebellothalamocortical system via the cerebellar territory of the thalamus; and the cerebellar output would sustain tremor activity and modulate tremor amplitude.[24,46] This explains the beneficial effect of DBS applied either to cerebellar thalamic territory (VLp/Vim) or the basal ganglia components (GPi or STN) in treating resting tremor in PD. Dopamine also reduces tremor amplitude by increasing thalamic inhibition in the VLp/Vim.[48]

Levodopa-Induced Dyskinesia

Levodopa-induced dyskinesia (LID) in the setting of PD reflects multiple pathophysiological mechanisms.[49] LID is the consequence of severe dopaminergic denervation; relates to disease duration; and can develop independently of previous administration or duration of treatment with levodopa. Peak-dose dyskinesia manifests primarily with chorea and may be generalized or affect the more affected side or upper body during the ON state. Diphasic dyskinesia has variable distribution and may affect exclusively the legs, producing ballistic to stereotypic alternating movements. The hypothesized events leading to LID include pulsatile stimulation of DA receptors, excessive presynaptic DA fluctuations of leading to increase receptor occupancy, downstream postsynaptic signaling changes, and effects of other neurotransmitter systems.

In the setting of severe loss of dopaminergic terminals, pulsatile administration of levodopa leads to peak synaptic levels of DA that cannot be regulated either by uptake by the DAT or via D2 inhibitory autoreceptors. This sustained activation prevents normal plasticity in both direct and indirect pathway SPNs, so that synaptic strengths in these pathways become randomized. This eventually leads to changes in firing pattern and oscillatory activity in the basal ganglia-thalamocortical circuits, disinhibition of thalamocortical neurons, overactivation of the motor cortex, and random, purposeless movements that characterize LID.[49] Most of the mechanisms underlying LID have been studied in rodent models. A major element in LID is maladaptive plasticity of corticostriatal synapses due to increased D1R-mediated activation of direct pathway SPNs, as reflected by activation of downstream extracellular signal regulated kinase and mitogen and stress-activated kinase 1 pathways leading to phosphorylation of histone H3 and increased expression of ΔFosB and prodynorphin messenger RNA. There is also loss of synaptic homeostatic plasticity, with loss of synaptic depotentiation (reversal of LTP) and thus increased excitability of direct pathway SPNs.[50] Development of LID has also been associated with increased glutamatergic signaling via NMDARs, which provides the rationale for the use of the NMDAR antagonist amantadine in patients with motor fluctuations and LID. In the setting of severe loss of dopaminergic terminals, exogenously administered levodopa can undergo uptake by serotonergic terminals in the striatum, and converted to DA by the nonselective L-amino acid decarboxylase. Serotonergic terminals may then release DA as false neurotransmitter contributing to nonphysiological peak levels of DA. Both 5-HT1_A receptor agonists that reduce firing of dorsal raphe neurons and 5-HT1_B receptor agonists that reduce DA release from serotonergic terminals synergistically reduce dyskinesia in experimental LID models. There is also a potential role of cholinergic, histaminergic, noradrenergic, opioid, and endocannabinoid systems in LID.[49]

DYSTONIA

Dystonia is a network disorder that may reflect abnormalities in the basal ganglia circuits, abnormal processing in the sensorimotor cortex, or cerebellar dysfunction.[22,51,52] Evidence indicates that three major pathophysiological substrates of dystonia are loss of inhibition within the motor cortex, sensory dysfunction, and derangement of synaptic plasticity. Several potential mechanisms of dystonia affect the basal ganglia circuits.[22,51]

Striatal Dopaminergic and Cholinergic Mechanisms of Dystonia

Studies in genetic forms and experimental models indicate that potential mechanisms of dystonia include reduced dopaminergic signaling and increased cholinergic signaling in the striatum. Impaired dopaminergic signaling is responsible for several forms of dystonia.[53] The typical example is dopa-responsive dystonia, which is linked to mutations that affect genes encoding proteins involved in DA biosynthesis or downstream signaling, including *GCH1* (GTP cyclohydrolase1), *TH* (tyrosine hydroxylase), *SPR* (sepiapterin reductase), and *GNAL* (G protein α-activating polypeptide, olfactory type, G_{olf}). Striatal cholinergic dysfunction is also an important mechanism of dystonia.[54,55] Excessive activity of cholinergic interneurons may underlie DYT1 linked to mutations of the *TOR1* gene encoding torsin A. Experimental models of DYT1 showed a reversal in the inhibitory action of D2Rs on activity of cholinergic neurons, leading to paradoxical D2R activation due to increase in Ca^{2+} currents and depolarization of cholinergic neurons. In mutant *DYT1* mice activation thalamostriatal afferents cause exaggerated activity of cholinergic neurons, leading to impaired integration between corticostriatal and thalamostriatal inputs. Imbalance between the striosome- and matrix-related motor outputs may also contribute to development of dystonia.

Role of the Globus Pallidus

There is indirect evidence of abnormal plasticity of basal ganglia-thalamocortical circuits in dystonia. Excessive oscillatory corticopallidal activity between 3 and 10 Hz correlates with dystonic movements.[56] Studies using simultaneous magnetoencephalography and local field recordings in patients with idiopathic dystonia show connectivity between the GPi and the cerebral cortex via three distinct oscillatory networks: a sensorimotor corticopallidal network oscillating at beta frequency; a pallidotemporal network oscillating in the theta frequency range; and a cerebello-pallidal network oscillating at alpha frequency.[56] Excessive synchrony between the basal ganglia and the cortex could interfere with normal processing of sensory inputs and motor output. DBS of the GPi is highly effective in dystonia by desynchronizing pallidal activity thus restoring the normal plasticity in the sensorimotor loop. The slow improvement of dystonia over time suggests a process progressive plasticity and neuronal reorganization. The degree of pallido-cerebellar coupling at alpha frequency may represent a compensatory mechanism, as it was inversely correlated with the severity of dystonic symptoms.[56]

Role of the Cerebellum

There is increasing evidence of an important role of the cerebellum in dystonia [57]. Torsin A is involved in synaptogenesis and dendritic arborization, not only in the striatum but also in cerebellum; cerebellar synaptogenesis is abnormal in mouse models of DYT1. Studies in a mouse model of rapid-onset dystonia-parkinsonism (DYT12) associated with mutations of the *ATP1A3* gene showed abnormal burst firing of cerebellar nuclei, which is transmitted to the striatum via the CL thalamic nucleus.[20] The cerebellum plays a substantial role not only in dystonia but also in PD.[30,57] For example, during self-initiated movement, there is weakening of effective connectivity of the striatum with both the cerebral cortex and cerebellum and strengthening of connectivity between the motor cortex and cerebellum in PD patients. This may reflect a compensatory role of cerebellar hyperactivity to counterbalance hypoactivity in some other regions, such as the SMA and the striatum. Whereas cerebellar compensation may occur early in the disease, it may be maladaptive upon disease progression, for example by contributing to development of LID. Aberrant neuronal synchrony in PD related to LID may propagate from the STN to the cerebellum and "lock" the cerebellar cortex in a hyperactive state. DBS of the STN and GPi alleviate levodopa-induced hyperactivity in the cerebellum associated with LID; repetitive transcranial magnetic stimulation over the cerebellum reduces LID.

OTHER HYPERKINETIC MOVEMENT DISORDERS

It has been proposed that one mechanism of hyperkinetic movement disorders is loss of synaptic downscaling and excessive LTP.[50] This could be a common mechanism underlying hyperkinetic movement disorders including LID, dystonia, and Huntington disease (HD).

Huntington Disease

There is progressive disconnection between the cerebral cortex and striatum in HD.[58] Striatal degeneration is associated with altered activity at corticostriatal synapses and early loss of indirect pathway SPNs, which may contribute to chorea and other dyskinesias at early stages of the disease. Studies in mouse models show that there are early changes in the membrane properties of SPNs and loss of presynaptic and postsynaptic marker proteins.[59]

Mutant huntingtin has distinct but interacting roles in cortical and striatal neurons in HD pathogenesis, in part via huntingtin adaptor proteins. Presynaptic mechanisms in HD may reflect impaired transport of synaptic vesicles, vesicular release, and endocytosis. Mutant huntingtin also leads to mistrafficking and extrasynaptic mislocalization of NMDAR subunits, deficits in transsynaptic trophic signaling via brain-derived neurotrophic factor, and reduction in presynaptic CB1R signaling by endocannabinoids.[59] All these changes reflect the complex biology of normal huntingtin.[60] Studies in mouse models of HD show that there is inability to downscale LTP after stimulation of corticostriatal synapses, which destabilizes synaptic circuits. There is also early loss of thalamostriatal terminals followed by loss of corticostriatal terminals, even before detectable loss of SPNs. Cholinergic interneurons are largely spared in HD; however in both postmortem striatal tissue and in transgenic mice there are decreased levels of markers of cholinergic transmission.

Hyperkinetic Disorders Associated with Abnormalities in D1 Receptor Signaling

Mutations affecting proteins involving in D1R signaling in the striatum have been liked to hyperkinetic movement disorders.[61,62] Heterozygous mutations in the *GNAL* (guanine nucleotide-binding protein subunit alpha L) gene encoding the stimulatory α subunit of G_{olf} may lead to its uncoupling from D1RS in SPNs and cause cervical or cranial dystonia with a mean onset in the third decade; these mutations have also been linked to childhood-onset generalized dystonia and mild intellectual disability. Gain-of-function mutations of the *ADCY5* encoding adenylyl cyclase 5, which mediates the D1R signal in the striatum, or loss-of-function mutations of the *PDE10A* gene encoding PDE10, which turns off this signal, increase cAMP levels in the striatum and cause chorea and other hyperkinetic movement disorders. *ADCY5* mutations produce a variable phenotype, including childhood-onset paroxysmal or persistent chorea and/or dystonia, familial dyskinesia and facial myokymia; autosomal-dominant chorea and dystonia; benign hereditary chorea; and early-onset dystonia with myoclonus. Patients with *ADCY5* mutations typically present with delay of motor milestones, infantile-onset action-induced generalized choreoathetosis, dystonia, or myoclonus with characteristic episodic exacerbations during drowsiness; some may show mild improvement after treatment with clonazepam, clobazam, and bilateral pallidal DBS. Homozygous *PDE10A* mutations manifest as an early-onset hyperkinetic movement disorder. Both *PDE10A* and *ADCY5* mutations are associated with loss of DAT expression in the striatum, loss of neuromelanin-containing neurons in substantia nigra, and white and gray matter pathology within the nigrostriatal and striatocortical pathways.[61] Paraneoplastic autoantibodies targeting PDE10A may produce hyperkinetic movement disorders; some of the cases may occur in the setting of treatment with immune checkpoint inhibitors.[63]

Tourette Syndrome

Tourette syndrome is characterized by tics that are transiently worsened by stress and acute administration of dopaminergic drugs. Neuropathological studies indicate that development of tics may reflect loss of cholinergic and fast-spiking GABAergic interneurons in the caudate and the putamen. Several other neurotransmitter systems, including histaminergic inputs and local endocannabinoid system have been associated with this disorder.[64] Both targeted ablation of cholinergic interneurons[65] and knockout of the *HDAC* gene leading to depletion of histamine[66] reproduce stereotypic behaviors resembling those seen in Tourette syndrome. Studies in rodents indicate that either loss of cholinergic interneurons or blockade of $GABA_A$ receptors in the striatum can induce tic-like stereotypies. In the striatum, acute stress or administration of amphetamine or cocaine leading to increased DA level triggers a D2R-mediated inhibition of ACh release and stereotypy. Whereas postmortem studies show reduced cholinergic innervation of the striatum in this disorder, PET studies show normal levels of vesicular an acetylcholine transporter in these patients.[67]

KEY POINTS

- The basal ganglia are involved in reward-based action learning, action selection, initiation of goal-directed behaviors, and automatic execution of habits.
- The striatum integrates influence from excitatory inputs from the cerebral cortex and thalamus: local circuits involving GABAergic and cholinergic interneurons, and modulatory dopaminergic inputs.
- The medium spiny projection neurons (SPNs) of the striatum target the globus pallidus pars externa (GPe), globus pallidus pars interna (GPi), and substantia nigra pars reticulata (SNr).
- The GPi/SNr provide the tonic output of the basal ganglia to the thalamus and brainstem.
- The direct pathway from SPNs to the GPi/SNr interrupts their tonic inhibitory output and triggers action initiation ("go" signal).
- The indirect pathway from SPNs to the GPe disinhibits the STN, thereby promoting the GPi/SNr output leading to action ("no-go" signal).
- A peak of dopamine (DA) increases activity of the D1R-expressing direct pathway SPNs, promoting initiation of a selected action, while simultaneously inhibiting the activity of D2R-expressing indirect pathway SPNs.
- Both the direct and indirect pathway SPNs are coactive during movement initiation, execution, and termination.
- Direct pathway SPNs promote initiation of the selected action, whereas indirect pathway SPNs act simultaneously to inhibit all other competitive undesirable actions and signal when an action is incorrect and it is time to switch strategies.
- The hyperdirect pathway from the cortex to the STN can interrupt ongoing action by promoting the excitatory input from the STN to the GPi/SNr ("stop" signal).
- According to center-surround model, cortical activation of the hyperdirect and indirect pathways would suppress competing actions while simultaneous activation of the direct pathway would focally inhibit a subset of GPi neurons permitting action selection.
- Distinct cortical projections to different components of the striatum provide for parallel motor control, oculomotor, cognitive (associative), and emotional (limbic) circuits.
- Dopamine acting via D1Rs promotes LTP at the corticostriatal synapses on the direct pathway, and via D2Rs elicits LTD at the corticostriatal synapse on the indirect pathway via retrograde endocannabinoid signaling.

- In response to an alerting inputs from the thalamus, striatal cholinergic neurons interrupt the ongoing action and promote behavioral switching.
- In addition to inputs from the striatum, the GP also receives direct projections from both the cerebral cortex and cerebellum.
- When the GPi/SNr is pathologically exaggerated, hyperpolarization of thalamic neurons promotes a "rebound burst" mode of activity that may lead to abnormal slow rhythmic activity.
- The GPe contains two subpopulations of GABAergic neurons that project back to the striatum.
- The spontaneous activity of STN neurons depends on their interplay among intrinsic electrophysiological properties, driving glutamatergic inputs from the cerebral cortex, feedback GABAergic inhibition from the GPe, and modulatory effects of DA.
- Dopamine sets the pattern of activity of STN neurons and prevents abnormally synchronized oscillatory activity in the basal ganglia circuits.
- Dopaminergic SNc neurons are selectively vulnerable given their divergent axonal arborizations and intrinsic physiological properties.
- Loss of dopaminergic inputs triggers compensatory plastic changes in excitability of SPNs that lead to an imbalance between the indirect and direct pathways.
- Akinesia in PD may reflect exaggerated activity of the indirect pathway as well as bursting of individual neurons, excessive synchronization and loss of functional segregation in the basal ganglia circuits.
- Resting tremor in PD is associated with abnormal oscillatory activity within the basal ganglia and the cerebello-thalamocortical circuit and abnormal intercircuit interactions.
- Levodopa-induced dyskinesia (LID) is due to multiple pathophysiological mechanisms and reflects the severity of dopamine cell loss.
- Dystonia is a network disorder that may reflect abnormalities in the basal ganglia circuits, abnormal processing in the sensorimotor cortex, or cerebellar dysfunction.
- Potential mechanisms of dystonia include reduced dopaminergic signaling, increased cholinergic signaling, and activation of cerebellar inputs to the striatum.
- Mutations affecting proteins involved in D1R signaling in SPNs have been liked to hyperkinetic movement disorders.
- Paraneoplastic autoantibodies targeting PDE10A may produce hyperkinetic movement disorders.
- Development of tics in Tourette syndrome may in part reflect loss of cholinergic and fast-spiking GABAergic interneurons in the striatum.

REFERENCES

1. Alexander GE, DeLong MR, Strick PL. Parallel organization of functionally segregated circuits linking basal ganglia and cortex. Annu Rev Neurosci 1986;9:357–381.
2. Burke DA, Rotstein HG, Alvarez VA. Striatal local circuitry: a new framework for lateral inhibition. Neuron 2017;96:267–284.
3. DeLong MR, Wichmann T. Basal ganglia circuits as targets for neuromodulation in parkinson disease. JAMA Neurol 2015;72:1354–1360.
4. Choi EY, Yeo BT, Buckner RL. The organization of the human striatum estimated by intrinsic functional connectivity. J Neurophysiol 2012;108:2242–2263.
5. Haber SN, Behrens TE. The neural network underlying incentive-based learning: implications for interpreting circuit disruptions in psychiatric disorders. Neuron 2014;83:1019–1039.
6. Smith Y, Raju DV, Pare JF, Sidibe M. The thalamostriatal system: a highly specific network of the basal ganglia circuitry. Trends Neurosci 2004;27:520–527.
7. DeLong M, Wichmann T. Update on models of basal ganglia function and dysfunction. Parkinsonism Relat Disord 2009;15 Suppl 3:S237–240.
8. Calabresi P, Picconi B, Tozzi A, Ghiglieri V, Di Filippo M. Direct and indirect pathways of basal ganglia: a critical reappraisal. Nat Neurosci 2014;17:1022–1030.
9. Surmeier DJ, Graves SM, Shen W. Dopaminergic modulation of striatal networks in health and Parkinson's disease. Curr Opin Neurobiol 2014;29:109–117.
10. McGregor MM, Nelson AB. Circuit mechanisms of Parkinson's disease. Neuron 2019;101:1042–1056.
11. Grillner S. The enigmatic "indirect pathway" of the basal ganglia: a new role. Neuron 2018;99:1105–1107.
12. Beck S, Hallett M. Surround inhibition in the motor system. Exp Brain Res 2011;210:165–172.
13. Hikosaka O, Kim HF, Yasuda M, Yamamoto S. Basal ganglia circuits for reward value-guided behavior. Annu Rev Neurosci 2014;37:289–306.
14. Humphries MD, Prescott TJ. The ventral basal ganglia, a selection mechanism at the crossroads of space, strategy, and reward. Prog Neurobiol 2010;90:385–417.
15. Salgado S, Kaplitt MG. The nucleus accumbens: a comprehensive review. Stereotact Funct Neurosurg 2015;93:75–93.
16. Root DH, Melendez RI, Zaborszky L, Napier TC. The ventral pallidum: subregion-specific functional anatomy and roles in motivated behaviors. Prog Neurobiol 2015;130:29–70.
17. Crittenden JR, Graybiel AM. Basal ganglia disorders associated with imbalances in the striatal striosome and matrix compartments. Front Neuroanat 2011;5:59.
18. Gerfen CR, Surmeier DJ. Modulation of striatal projection systems by dopamine. Annu Rev Neurosci 2011;34:441–466.
19. Shepherd GM. Corticostriatal connectivity and its role in disease. Nat Rev Neurosci 2013;14:278–291.
20. Chen CH, Fremont R, Arteaga-Bracho EE, Khodakhah K. Short latency cerebellar modulation of the basal ganglia. Nat Neurosci 2014;17:1767–1775.
21. Cacciola A, Calamuneri A, Milardi D, et al. A connectomic analysis of the human basal ganglia network. Front Neuroanat 2017;11:85.

22. Quartarone A, Hallett M. Emerging concepts in the physiological basis of dystonia. Mov Disord 2013;28:958–967.
23. Llinas RR, Ribary U, Jeanmonod D, Kronberg E, Mitra PP. Thalamocortical dysrhythmia: a neurological and neuropsychiatric syndrome characterized by magnetoencephalography. Proc Natl Acad Sci U S A 1999;96:15222–15227.
24. Helmich RC. The cerebral basis of parkinsonian tremor: a network perspective. Mov Disord 2018;33:219–231.
25. Mallet N, Micklem BR, Henny P, et al. Dichotomous organization of the external globus pallidus. Neuron 2012;74:1075–1086.
26. Hegeman DJ, Hong ES, Hernandez VM, Chan CS. The external globus pallidus: progress and perspectives. Eur J Neurosci 2016;43:1239–1265.
27. Mallet N, Schmidt R, Leventhal D, et al. Arkypallidal cells send a stop signal to striatum. Neuron 2016;89:308–316.
28. Abecassis ZA, Berceau BL, Win PH, et al. Npas1(+)-Nkx2.1(+) neurons are an integral part of the cortico-pallido-cortical loop. J Neurosci 2020;40:743–768.
29. Wilson CJ, Bevan MD. Intrinsic dynamics and synaptic inputs control the activity patterns of subthalamic nucleus neurons in health and in Parkinson's disease. Neuroscience 2011;198:54–68.
30. Caligiore D, Pezzulo G, Baldassarre G, et al. Consensus paper: towards a systems-level view of cerebellar function: the interplay between cerebellum, basal ganglia, and cortex. Cerebellum 2017;16:203–229.
31. Quartarone A, Cacciola A, Milardi D, et al. New insights into cortico-basal-cerebellar connectome: clinical and physiological considerations. Brain 2020;143:396–406.
32. Kawashima T. The role of the serotonergic system in motor control. Neurosci Res 2018;129:32–39.
33. Kaasinen V, Vahlberg T. Striatal dopamine in Parkinson disease: a meta-analysis of imaging studies. Ann Neurol 2017;82:873–882.
34. Halliday G. Clinicopathological aspects of motor parkinsonism. Parkinsonism Relat Disord 2007;13 Suppl 3:S208–210.
35. Surmeier DJ, Guzman JN, Sanchez-Padilla J, Schumacker PT. The role of calcium and mitochondrial oxidant stress in the loss of substantia nigra pars compacta dopaminergic neurons in Parkinson's disease. Neuroscience 2011;198:221–231.
36. Cai H, Liu G, Sun L, Ding J. Aldehyde dehydrogenase 1 making molecular inroads into the differential vulnerability of nigrostriatal dopaminergic neuron subtypes in Parkinson's disease. Transl Neurodegener 2014;3:27.
37. Goldstein DS, Kopin IJ, Sharabi Y. Catecholamine autotoxicity: implications for pharmacology and therapeutics of Parkinson disease and related disorders. Pharmacol Ther 2014;144:268–282.
38. Michel PP, Hirsch EC, Hunot S. Understanding dopaminergic cell death pathways in Parkinson disease. Neuron 2016;90:675–691.
39. Foffani G, Obeso JA. A cortical pathogenic theory of Parkinson's disease. Neuron 2018;99:1116–1128.
40. Lemos JC, Friend DM, Kaplan AR, et al. Enhanced GABA transmission drives bradykinesia following loss of dopamine D2 receptor signaling. Neuron 2016;90:824–838.
41. Eisinger RS, Cernera S, Gittis A, Gunduz A, Okun MS. A review of basal ganglia circuits and physiology: application to deep brain stimulation. Parkinsonism Relat Disord 2019;59:9–20.
42. Corbit VL, Whalen TC, Zitelli KT, Crilly SY, Rubin JE, Gittis AH. Pallidostriatal projections promote beta oscillations in a dopamine-depleted biophysical network model. J Neurosci 2016;36:5556–5571.
43. Herrington TM, Cheng JJ, Eskandar EN. Mechanisms of deep brain stimulation. J Neurophysiol 2016;115:19–38.
44. Jellinger KA. Post mortem studies in Parkinson's disease: is it possible to detect brain areas for specific symptoms? J Neural Transm Suppl 1999;56:1–29.
45. Pasquini J, Ceravolo R, Qamhawi Z, et al. Progression of tremor in early stages of Parkinson's disease: a clinical and neuroimaging study. Brain 2018;141:811–821.
46. Helmich RC, Hallett M, Deuschl G, Toni I, Bloem BR. Cerebral causes and consequences of parkinsonian resting tremor: a tale of two circuits? Brain 2012;135:3206–3226.
47. di Biase L, Brittain JS, Shah SA, et al. Tremor stability index: a new tool for differential diagnosis in tremor syndromes. Brain 2017;140:1977–1986.
48. Dirkx MF, den Ouden HE, Aarts E, et al. Dopamine controls Parkinson's tremor by inhibiting the cerebellar thalamus. Brain 2017;140:721–734.
49. Espay AJ, Morgante F, Merola A, et al. Levodopa-induced dyskinesia in Parkinson disease: current and evolving concepts. Ann Neurol 2018;84:797–811.
50. Calabresi P, Pisani A, Rothwell J, Ghiglieri V, Obeso JA, Picconi B. Hyperkinetic disorders and loss of synaptic downscaling. Nat Neurosci 2016;19:868–875.
51. Lozeron P, Poujois A, Richard A, et al. Contribution of TMS and rTMS in the understanding of the pathophysiology and in the treatment of dystonia. Front Neural Circuits 2016;10:90.
52. Berman BD, Jinnah HA. Dystonia: five new things. Neurol Clin Pract 2015;5:232–240.
53. Goodchild RE, Grundmann K, Pisani A. New genetic insights highlight "old" ideas on motor dysfunction in dystonia. Trends Neurosci 2013;36:717–725.
54. Eskow Jaunarajs KL, Bonsi P, Chesselet MF, Standaert DG, Pisani A. Striatal cholinergic dysfunction as a unifying theme in the pathophysiology of dystonia. Prog Neurobiol 2015;127–128:91–107.
55. Deffains M, Bergman H. Striatal cholinergic interneurons and cortico-striatal synaptic plasticity in health and disease. Mov Disord 2015;30:1014–1025.
56. Neumann WJ, Jha A, Bock A, et al. Cortico-pallidal oscillatory connectivity in patients with dystonia. Brain 2015;138:1894–1906.
57. Wu T, Hallett M. The cerebellum in Parkinson's disease. Brain 2013;136:696–709.
58. Ross CA, Aylward EH, Wild EJ, et al. Huntington disease: natural history, biomarkers and prospects for therapeutics. Nat Rev Neurol 2014;10:204–216.
59. Veldman MB, Yang XW. Molecular insights into cortico-striatal miscommunications in Huntington's disease. Curr Opin Neurobiol 2018;48:79–89.
60. Saudou F, Humbert S. The biology of huntingtin. Neuron 2016;89:910–926.
61. Lohmann K, Klein C. Update on the genetics of dystonia. Curr Neurol Neurosci Rep 2017;17:26.

62. Niccolini F, Mencacci NE, Yousaf T, et al. PDE10A and ADCY5 mutations linked to molecular and microstructural basal ganglia pathology. Mov Disord 2018;33:1961–1965.
63. Zekeridou A, Kryzer T, Guo Y, et al. Phosphodiesterase 10A IgG: A novel biomarker of paraneoplastic neurologic autoimmunity. Neurology 2019;93:e815–e822.
64. Udvardi PT, Nespoli E, Rizzo F, Hengerer B, Ludolph AG. Nondopaminergic neurotransmission in the pathophysiology of Tourette syndrome. Int Rev Neurobiol 2013;112:95–130.
65. Xu M, Kobets A, Du JC, et al. Targeted ablation of cholinergic interneurons in the dorsolateral striatum produces behavioral manifestations of Tourette syndrome. Proc Natl Acad Sci U S A 2015;112:893–898.
66. Abdurakhmanova S, Chary K, Kettunen M, Sierra A, Panula P. Behavioral and stereological characterization of Hdc KO mice: relation to Tourette syndrome. J Comp Neurol 2017;525:3476–3487.
67. Albin RL, Minderovic C, Koeppe RA. Normal striatal vesicular acetylcholine transporter expression in Tourette syndrome. eNeuro 2017;4.

Section V

Survival Systems

35 Peripheral and Spinal Mechanisms of Nociception

OVERVIEW

Nociception is a mechanism that protects the organism from injury. Nociceptors can be active in the absence of pain perception. They can be activated with stimuli that are below threshold for pain perception, and many respond to nonnociceptive stimuli. As a result, nociceptor activity routinely drives behaviors in the absence of consciously perceived pain. Nociception involves unmyelinated Aδ- and unmyelinated C afferents from neurons in in the dorsal root ganglion (DRG) or trigeminal ganglion. These neurons constitute a heterogeneous population in terms of their responsiveness to stimuli, neurochemical composition, and targets in the dorsal horn. Specific molecular markers, such as transient receptor potential (TRP) channels and Mas-related G protein-coupled receptor (Mrgpr) subtypes, have allowed the identification of the different classes of primary nociceptor afferents transmitting the sensation of pain and itch. Nociceptors express a unique repertoire of ion channels and receptors that are responsible for their basic properties, including lack of spontaneous activity, high threshold of activation, and responsiveness to subthreshold stimuli and repetitive firing in pathological conditions. Different subtypes of nociceptive afferents project to separate laminae of the dorsal horn, where they activate spinothalamic tract (STT) projection neurons and different types of excitatory and inhibitory interneurons. The dorsal horn is thus a site of complex processing and gating of nociceptive information. Products of inflammation or axonal injury trigger changes in the expression and function of ion channels in nociceptors, resulting in increased excitability; this process is known as peripheral nociceptor sensitization. Genetic nociceptor channelopathies may be associated with either paroxysmal pain disorders or insensitivity to pain. Increased activity of nociceptors leads to plastic changes in the dorsal horn that result in increasing excitability of projection neurons and reduced influence of local inhibitory circuits. These findings provide new insights into the pathophysiology of the manifestations of neuropathic pain, including spontaneous pain, hyperalgesia, mechanical allodynia, and neuropathic itch. However, development of chronic pain reflects an interaction among afferent sensory inputs and brain circuits involved in attention, affect, and memory, as discussed in the next chapter. The main aims of this chapter are to review: (1) the functional heterogeneity of nociceptors, (2) the local circuits in the dorsal horn, (3) the mechanisms of peripheral sensitization, and (4) the mechanisms of central sensitization in the dorsal horn, including the role of glial cells and neuroinflammation.

NOCICEPTORS

Nociceptors are specialized high-threshold sensory afferents from DRG or trigeminal ganglion cells innervating the skin, muscle, joints, viscera, dental pulp, and dura. Nociceptors are free endings sometimes surrounded by terminal Schwann cells and respond to noxious or potentially damaging stimuli.[1] The two main types of nociceptors are small myelinated (Aδ) mechanical sensitive and unmyelinated (C) polymodal nociceptors (Table 35.1). All nociceptors use glutamate as their primary neurotransmitter and project to spinal dorsal horn or trigeminal nuclei caudalis.

Functional Diversity

Nociceptors constitute a heterogeneous population in terms of their axons, electrophysiological properties, and chemical signature (Figure 35.1). Medium diameter Aδ nociceptor afferents mediate acute, well-localized "first" or fast pain; they include type I high-threshold mechanical nociceptors (HTMs) that respond to both mechanical and chemical stimuli but are relatively insensitive to heat and type II HTM that are sensitive to heat but less so to mechanical stimuli. Unmyelinated C fibers convey poorly localized, "second" or slow pain; most are polymodal and are both heat and mechanically sensitive C-afferents; others include C-heat nociceptors and C-mechano-cold nociceptors. There is a population of C-fiber nociceptors that are insensitive to mechanical stimuli in the absence of tissue inflammation;

TABLE 35.1 *Types of Primary Cutaneous Afferents to the Dorsal Horn*

Fiber type	Diameter	Conduction Velocity	Receptor Type	Sensory Modality
Aβ-type (large myelinated)	10 μm	60 $m.s^{-1}$	Low-threshold mechanoreceptor	Discriminative touch
Aδ-type (small myelinated)	2.5 μm	12 ms^{-1}	Peptidergic nociceptor	Heat-triggered pain
			Nonpeptidergic nociceptor	Mechanical-triggered pain
			Cold receptor	Innocuous cold
C-type (unmyelinated)	1 μm	<2 ms^{-1}	Peptidergic nociceptor	Heat-triggered pain
			Nonpeptidergic nociceptor	Mechanical-triggered pain
			Warm receptor	Innocuous warmth
			Pruriceptors	Itch
			Low-threshold mechanoreceptor	Emotional touch

these "silent" or mechanically insensitive afferents constitute approximately 15%–20% cutaneous C-fiber afferents in the human skin. Nociceptors exhibit pronounced activity-dependent hyperpolarization and reduced conduction velocity in response to repetitive stimulation.[2] Pain produced by chemical stimulation of either group III or IV nociceptive some muscle nerves is experienced as deep, aching, or cramping.

Neurochemical Heterogeneity

Nociceptors can also be broadly classified into two separate populations on the basis of the absence of neuropeptides, growth factor dependence, and ion channels and receptor repertoire (Table 35.2). Peptidergic C nociceptors express substance P and calcitonin-gene related peptide (CGRP), the tyrosine kinase A receptor for nerve growth factor (NGF), and the transient receptor potential (TRP) vanilloid type 1 (TRPV1), ankyrin type 1 (TRPA1), and melastatin 8 (TRPM8) channels. The majority of heat-sensitive TRPV1 peptidergic C fibers express presynaptic μ-type receptors.[3] Nonpeptidergic C nociceptors express the c-Ret receptor for glial-derived neurotrophic factor (GDNF), purinergic $P2X_3$ receptors, and the Mas-related G protein-coupled receptor member D (MrgprD). A class of C-fibers present in in viscera and deep somatic tissues expressing the nicotinic acetylcholine receptor subunit alpha-3 are normally mechanically insensitive ("silent") but respond to mechanical stimuli after injury.

Ion Channels Regulating Nociceptor Excitability

Nociceptors express a unique repertoire of ion channels and receptors (Table 35.3, Figure 35.2).[4–8] Several voltage-gated sodium channels (Na_v) are key determinants of nociceptor excitability. They include Na_v1.7 (*SCN9A* gene), Na_v1.8 (*SCN10A* gene) and Na_v1.9 (*SCN11A* gene). The Na_v1.7 channel is expressed in both large and small diameter DRG neurons, as well as in sympathetic ganglion neurons and olfactory sensory neurons. In nociceptors, Na_v1.7 is present in the soma and axons of peptidergic and nonpeptidergic nociceptive DRG neurons and in their peripheral and central terminals. Na_v1.7 channels produce a low threshold, rapidly activating and inactivating depolarizing current that boosts subthreshold stimuli and increases nociceptor excitability. In a subset of DRG neurons, Na_v1.7 channels may also produce resurgent currents that support burst firing repolarization following a strong depolarization. Na_v1.8 channels carry most (80%–90%) of the current underlying the depolarization phase of the action potential; they are slowly inactivated by depolarization and thus support repetitive firing of DRG neurons in response to sustained depolarization. Na_v1.9 channels are almost selectively expressed in small DRG neurons and produce a persistent a Na^+ current that amplifies the response of nociceptors to subthreshold depolarizing inputs.

Nociceptors also express different subtypes potassium (K^+) channels that dampen nociceptor excitability and firing frequency. They include two-pore K^+ channels (K_{2P}), voltage-gated K^+ channels (K_v), Ca^{2+}-activated K^+ channels (K_{Ca}), Na^+-activated K^+ channels (K_{Na}), and inward-rectifying K^+ channels (K_{ir}). Many K_{2P} channels are constitutively open and generate a background "leak" current that stabilizes the resting membrane potential below firing threshold of nociceptors. DRG neurons express many members of the K_{2P} channel family, including TRESK, TREK1 and TRAAK, which are regulated by mechanical stimuli, heat, acid, and changes in the environments Nociceptors also express several voltage gated Ca^{2+} channels (Ca_v) including L-type (Ca_v1.2), N-type (Ca_v2.2), and

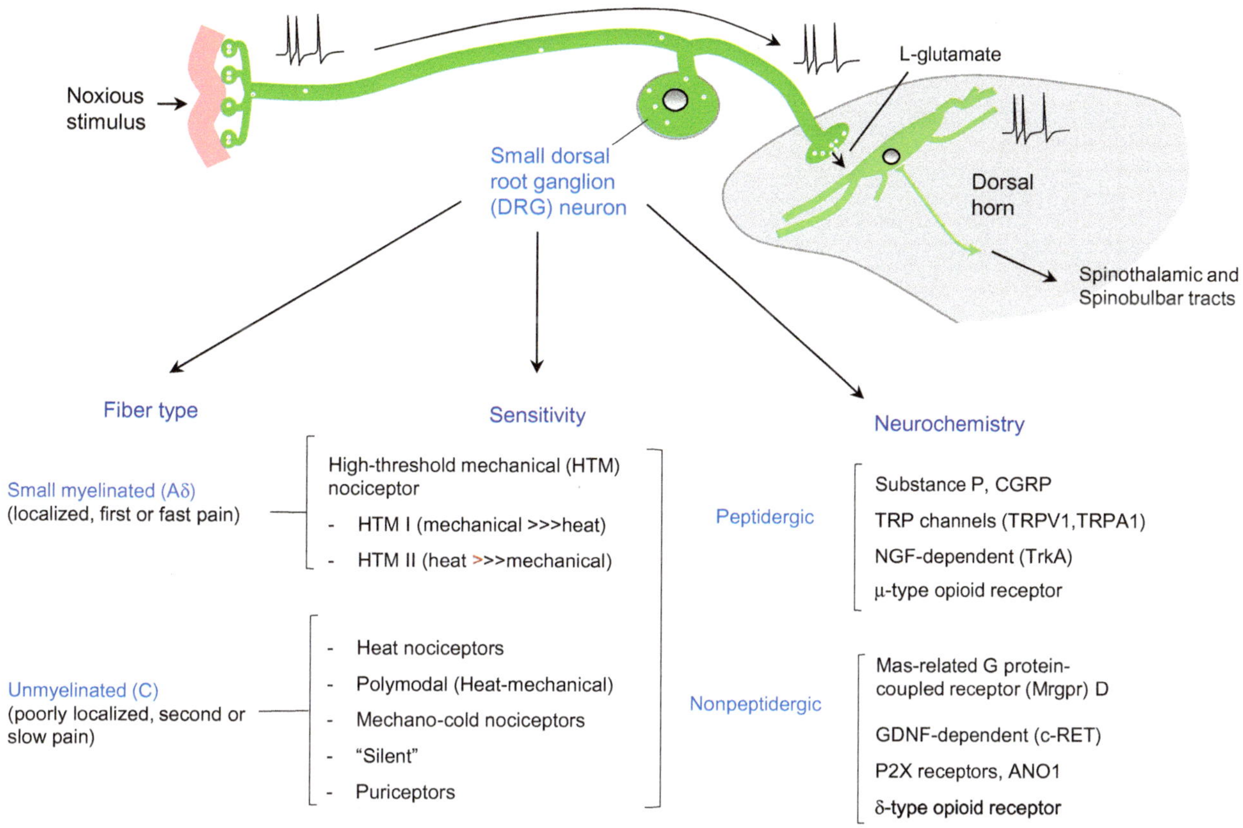

FIGURE 35.1 Heterogeneity of nociceptors

Nociceptors constitute a heterogeneous population in terms of their axons, electrophysiological properties and chemical signature. Medium-diameter Aδ nociceptor afferents mediate acute, well-localized "first" or fast pain; they include type I high-threshold mechanical nociceptors (HTMs), which respond to both mechanical and chemical stimuli but are relatively insensitive to heat, and type II HTMs, which are more sensitive to heat but less so to mechanical stimuli. Unmyelinated C fibers convey poorly localized, "second" or slow pain; most are polymodal and are both heat- and mechanically sensitive C-afferents. A population of "silent" C-fiber nociceptors are insensitive to mechanical stimuli in the absence of tissue inflammation. Nociceptors can also be broadly classified into two separate populations on the basis of the absence of neuropeptides, growth factor dependence, and ion channels and receptor repertoire. Peptidergic C nociceptors express substance P and calcitonin-gene-related peptide (CGRP), the tyrosine kinase A receptor for nerve growth factor (NGF), and the transient receptor potential (TRP) channels TRPV1 and TRPA1. The majority of heat-sensitive TRPV1 peptidergic C fibers express presynaptic μ-type receptors. Nonpeptidergic C nociceptors express the c-Ret receptor for glial-derived neurotrophic factor (GDNF), purinergic $P2X_3$ receptors, and the Mas-related G protein-coupled receptor member D (MrgprD).

T-type ($Ca_v3.2$ and $Ca_v3.3$) channels. The N-type ($Ca_v2.2$) channels are located in presynaptic terminals and trigger release of glutamate, substance P, and CGRP both at central and peripheral terminals of nociceptors. The α2δ subunit of high-voltage-gated Ca^{2+} channels, including the N-type channels, increases the membrane expression of the functional α1 subunit and is thus an important determinant of channel function. The α2δ subunit is upregulated in experimental models of inflammatory and neuropathic pain, and is the target of gabapentin and pregabalin.

Transient Receptor Potential (TRP) Channels

TRP channels are nonselective cation channel with high permeability to Ca^{2+} and are multimodal receptors. TRPV1, TRPA1, and TRPM8 define different nociceptor populations.[9,10] TRPV1 channels are activated by noxious heat (>43°C), low pH (5.2), capsaicin, and bioactive lipids such as anandamide; TRPV1-expressing nociceptors thus mediate heat-induced and inflammatory pain. TRPA1 is a molecular integrator of many exogenous and endogenous noxious stimuli, including reactive oxygen species (ROS) and other inflammatory agents released at the site of injury and is expressed in a subpopulation of TRPV1-positive neurons. TRPM8 is expressed in approximately 15%–30% of C-fibers and a minor proportion of Aδ fibers and is activated by cold stimuli ranging from innocuous cool to noxious cold temperatures (<30°C), as well as cooling agents such as menthol. TRP channels are intrinsically sensitive to phosphatidylinositol bisphosphate and are therefore modulated by G protein-coupled receptors linked to the

TABLE 35.2 *Neurochemical Markers of Nociceptors and Pruriceptors*

Receptor Type	Nonpeptidergic	Peptidergic	Pruriceptors
Neurotransmitter	Glutamate	Glutamate Substance P CGRP	Glutamate Substance P CGRP Natriuretic polypeptide B
Receptor expression (example)	c-Ret (for GDNF) P2X3 MrgprD Delta opioid receptor	TrkA (for NGF) μ-opioid receptor	Histamine H1 and H4 PAR2 MrgprA3, MrgprD TRPV1, TRPA1
Channel expression (example)	Purinergic $P2X_3$	TRPV1, TRPA1	TRPV1, TRPA1

GDNF, glial-derived neurotrophic factor; Mrgp, Mas-related G protein-coupled receptors; NGF, nerve growth factor; PAR2, proteinase-associated receptor 2; TRP, transient receptor potential; TRPA1, transient receptor potential l ankyrin type 1; TRPV1, transient receptor potential vanilloid type 1; TrkA, tyrosine kinase A.

TABLE 35.3 *Ion Channels in Nociceptors*

Channel	Function
$Na_v1.7$	Amplifies subthreshold stimuli
$Na_v1.8$	Underlies the action potential Supports repetitive firing
$Na_v1.9$	Amplifies and prolongs small subthreshold depolarizations
$Na_v1.3$	Upregulated following nerve injury, mediates action potential
$K_v1.1$	Delays onset of the action potential
$K_v2.2$	Influences repolarization and hyperpolarization during repetitive firing
$K_v3.4$	Accelerates repolarization
$K_v4.3$	Limits action potential threshold, duration, and firing frequency
K_v7 (7.2,7.3, and 7.5)	Regulates action potential threshold and accommodation
BK_{Ca}	Feedback inhibition that slows repetitive firing
K_{Na}	Contributes to a long-lasting hyperpolarization following repetitive firing
K_{2P}	Background current that stabilizes the resting membrane potential
$Ca_v1.2$ (L)	May contribute to nociceptor excitability
$Ca_v2.2$ (N)	Presynaptic release of neurotransmitters from nociceptive afferents
$Ca_v3.2$ (T)	Promotes burst firing and glutamate release
TRPV1	Activated by noxious heat, low pH, capsaicin, and as anandamide. Involved in heat-induced pain and acid-evoked sensitization
TRPA1	Integrator of many exogenous and endogenous noxious stimuli
TRMP8	Activated by both innocuous and noxious cold
ASIC	Activated by acidic pH; permeable to Na^+ and elicit cell depolarization
HCN	Constitutively open near resting membrane potential, limits excitability, modulated by cAMP.
TMEM16A(ANO1)	Ca^{2+}-activated Cl^- channel; elicits Cl^- efflux resulting in depolarization
P2X3	Activated by ATP involved in visceral sensation and inflammatory pain
5-HT3R	Activated by serotonin in the setting of inflammation

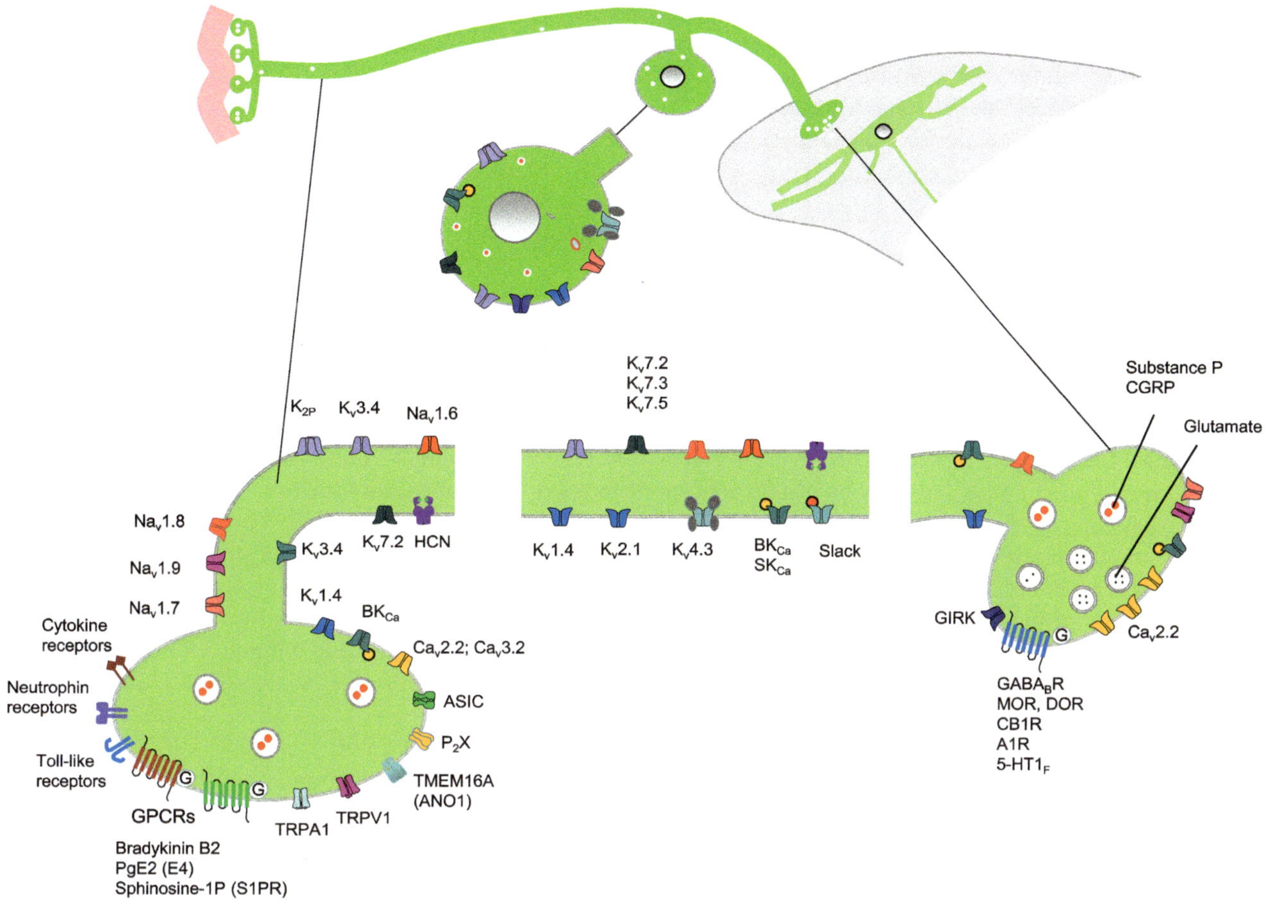

FIGURE 35.2 Ion channels in nociceptors.
Several voltage-gated sodium channels (Na_v) are key determinants of nociceptor excitability. They include $Na_v1.7$, $Na_v1.8$, and $Na_v1.9$ channels that set the threshold of activation and initiate and sustain firing of action potentials nociceptors. Different subtypes of potassium (K^+) channels, including two-pore K^+ channels (K_{2P}), voltage-gated K^+ channels (K_v), Ca^{2+}-activated K^+ channels (K_{Ca}), Na^+-activated K^+ channels (K_{Na}), and inward-rectifying K^+ channels (K_{ir}), determine excitability and firing properties of nociceptors. Several voltage-gated Ca^{2+} channels (Ca_v) including L-type ($Ca_v1.2$), N-type ($Ca_v2.2$), and T-type ($Ca_v3.2$ and $Ca_v3.3$) channels promote nociceptor excitability and neurotransmitter release. Transient receptor potential (TRP) channels are multimodal receptors and include TRP vanilloid type 1 (TRPV1), TRP ankyrin type 1 (TRPA1, and TRP melastatin 8 (TRPM8) receptors. Other channels contribute to nociceptor excitability, particularly in the setting of inflammation. They include acid-sensing ion channels (ASICs); hyperpolarization-activated cyclic nucleotide-gated (HCN) channels; anoctamin (ANO) channels (also known as transmembrane protein 16- [TMEM16] channels); ATP-sensitive ionotropic P2X and metabotropic P2Y receptors; and serotonin $5\text{-}HT_3$ receptors ($5\text{-}HT_3Rs$). Several GPCRs respond to products of inflammation such as bradykinin (B2 receptors) and prostaglandins. Nociceptive afferents also express receptors for growth factors and cytokines at both their peripheral and central terminals. The central terminals of nociceptive afferents express several presynaptic inhibitory receptors include μ- or δ-type opiate receptors, $GABA_B$ receptors, adenosine A1 receptors (A1Rs), and cannabinoid CB1 receptors (CB1Rs).

G_q-phospholipase C (PLC) pathway, which has different effects according to the TRP channel type.

Other Channels in Nociceptors

Several other channels contribute to nociceptor excitability, particularly in the setting of inflammation. Acid-sensing ion channels (ASICs) are activated by acidic pH; are primarily permeable to Na, and elicit cell depolarization leading to secondary intracellular accumulation of Ca^{2+}. For example. ASIC3 is an essential pH sensor for pain and is primarily located in nociceptive fibers innervating the skeletal and cardiac muscle, joints, and bone; in these tissues, anaerobic metabolism leads to buildup of lactic acid and protons that activate this channel.[11] Hyperpolarization-activated cyclic nucleotide-gated (HCN) channels are activated by membrane hyperpolarization; they are permeable to Na^+ and K^+ and are constitutively open at voltages near the resting membrane potential. In many cases, activation is facilitated by direct interaction with cyclic adenosine monophosphate (cAMP). Opening of HCN channels elicits membrane depolarization toward threshold for action potential generation. Nociceptive neurons express both HCN1 and HCN2 channels, HCN2 channels may have a prominent role in both inflammatory and neuropathic pain, whereas HCN1 channels may also contribute to cold hyperalgesia and allodynia in the setting of oxaliplatin-induced neuropathy.[12] Anoctamins, also known as transmembrane protein 16 (TMEM16) proteins, are involved in a variety of functions that include ion transport, phospholipid scrambling, and regulation of other membrane proteins.[13] Anoctamin 1 (ANO1, TMEM16A) is a Ca^{2+}-activated Cl^- channel that elicits Cl^- efflux resulting in membrane depolarization and triggering of action potentials in DRG neurons. It is expressed in nociceptors and is activated by products of inflammation that elicit small DRG depolarization following TRPV1 activation.[14] However, nociceptive DRG neurons also express the ANO3/TMEM16C channel, which colocalizes with Slack, the protein forming the K_{Na} channel; this interaction enhances its Na^+ sensitivity of the channel eliciting membrane hyperpolarization and reducing nociceptor firing.[15]

Receptors in Nociceptive Afferents

Nociceptive fibers express a wide range of ligand-gated (ionotropic) and G protein-coupled (metabotropic) receptors (GPCRs) (Table 34.5). Some of these receptors contribute to nociceptor sensitization in the setting of inflammation. Purinergic signaling mediated by ATP acting via ionotropic P2X and metabotropic P2Y receptors has an important role in transmission of nociceptive information.[16] P2X receptors permeable to Na^+ and Ca^2, in particular P2X2 and P2X, are abundantly expressed in nonpeptidergic nociceptive DRG neurons and are involved in mechanosensory transduction and both somatic and visceral pain.[17] The P2Y receptors including P2Y1 and P2Y2 are GPCRs that are expressed in nociceptors and may interact with TRPV1. The serotonin 5-HT3 receptor (5-HT3R) is a ligand-gated cation channel that is expressed in a minority of nociceptors; whereas they are not required for acute nociception in response to physiological stimuli they contribute to persistent nociceptive processing in the setting of injury. Several GPCRs respond to products of inflammation such as bradykinin and lipid mediators such as prostaglandins. These mediators elicit, increased nociceptor excitability via different mechanisms, including inhibition of K^+ channels downstream of G_q-PLC signaling and facilitation of TRPV1-mediated responses. The central terminals of nociceptive afferents at the dorsal horn express a variety of presynaptic inhibitory receptors that reduce release excitatory transmitters from afferent terminals. They include the μ- or δ-type opiate receptors, $GABA_B$ receptors, adenosine A1 receptors (A1Rs), and cannabinoid CB1 receptors.

Both the peripheral and central terminals of nociceptive DRG neurons also express receptors for growth factors such as NGF; cytokines such as interleukin-1β (IL-1β), tumor necrosis factor-α (TNF-α) and chemokine CCL2; and spingosine 1 phosphate (S1PRs). Upon injury or infection nociceptive neurons respond to damage/pathogen-associated molecular patterns through pattern recognition receptors such as Toll-like receptors (TLRs) which, in addition to slow-acting canonical signaling, also couple to ion channels enabling rapid modulation of nociceptive neuronal activity.

Pruriceptors

Approximately 5% of C-fibers are "itch" fibers; they respond to histamine and other pruritogens but are insensitive to mechanical stimuli.[18,19] These afferents are referred to as pruritoceptors or pruriceptors. They detect a wide variety of pruritogenic stimuli via multiple types of G protein-coupled receptors. These include the H1 and H4 receptors for histamine, the Mas-related G protein-coupled receptors MrgprA3 and MrgprD, and the proteinase-associated receptor 2, among others. Itch-sensing GPCRs trigger downstream signaling cascades that ultimately promote opening of TRP channels such as TRPV1 and TRPA1 in C-afferents. For example, histamine elicits itch in humans via mechano-insensitive C-afferents. Many these afferents are also nociceptive and express both H1 and TRPV1 receptors; the presence of TRPV1 receptors is required for histamine to elicit itch. However, activation of afferents expressing both TRPV1 and MrgprA3 receptors by the antimalarial agent chloroquine elicits itch but not pain.

Tactile Receptors and Their Potential Contribution to Pain

The sense of touch provides a moment-to-moment information about the nature of the physical environment.[20] The predominant afferents are low-mechanical-threshold tactile mechanoreceptors with large myelinated Aβ afferents; these afferents are involved in discriminative touch and express δ-type opioid receptors. There is also a subpopulation of C-fibers (C-tactile afferents) that respond to gentle touch such as low brushing or stroking with a finger. These tactile C-afferents are thought to be involved in detection of affective touch and are hypothesized to be important in social interactions and for skin-to-skin contact.

The mechanically gated cation channels of the Piezo family are critically involved in transduction of low-threshold tactile as well as proprioceptive stimuli. Loss-of-function *Piezo2* mutations result in profound mechanosensory and proprioceptive deficits but spare acute mechanical pain sensation. However, mouse and human studies indicate that Piezo2 expression in primary afferents is required for dynamic mechanical allodynia. All primary afferent subtypes terminate within or in close proximity to keratinocytes, which shape the responses of both nociceptive and nonnociceptive afferents. Mechanical stimulation of keratinocytes directly depolarizes the keratinocyte membrane (probably via Piezo 1 channels) and elicits inward currents in adjacent sensory neurons. Keratinocytes signal to sensory nerve terminals by releasing ATP, which activates sensory P2X4 receptors in primary afferents.

DORSAL HORN CIRCUITRY

The dorsal horn is subdivided into five cytoarchitectonic laminae (I–V) according to Rexed (Figure 35.3). Lamina I primarily contains different subtypes of projection neurons that contribute to both the STT and several spinobulbar pathways. Lamina II or substantia gelatinosa is subdivided into an outer (IIo) and an inner (IIi) region containing different subtypes of local excitatory or inhibitory interneurons. Laminae III to V constitute the deep dorsal horn and contain different subtypes of projection neurons as well as interneurons.[21–25]

Primary Afferent Input to the Dorsal Horn

The most superficial laminae (I and II) of the dorsal horn receive predominantly nociceptive and thermal afferent input, while more ventral laminae (III–VI) receive input from low-threshold mechanoreceptors and proprioceptors. Peptidergic nociceptors signaling heat-induced pain terminate both in layer I, targeting projection neurons expressing neurokinin 1 substance P receptors (NK1R), -and in outer lamina II targeting different subsets of inhibitory and

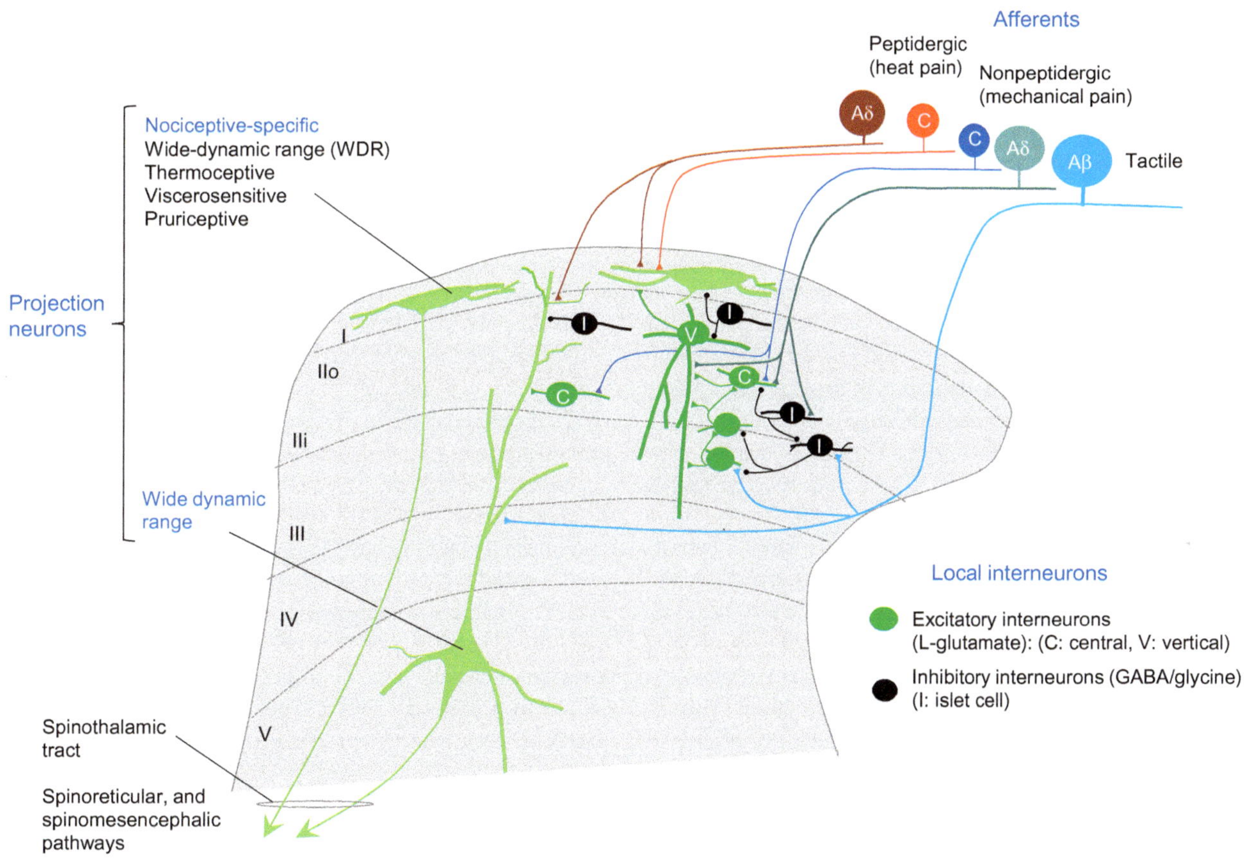

FIGURE 35.3 Dorsal horn circuitry.
Lamina I and lamina V contain different subtypes of projection neurons that contribute to both the spinothalamic tract (STT) and several spinobulbar pathways. Lamina II or substantia gelatinosa includes an outer (IIo) and an inner (Iii) region containing different subtypes of excitatory or inhibitory interneurons. Laminae I and II receive predominantly nociceptive and thermal afferent input, while laminae III–VI receive input from low-threshold mechanoreceptors and proprioceptors. Peptidergic nociceptors signal- heat-induced pain and target both STT projection neurons in lamina I and different subsets of inhibitory and excitatory interneurons in outer lamina II (IIo). Nonpeptidergic afferents signal mechanically induced pain and target excitatory interneurons of inner lamina II (Iii), which then convey noxious mechanical inputs to lamina I via polysynaptic excitatory pathways. Mechanosensitive nociceptive afferents activate STT neurons indirectly via a polysynaptic feedforward circuit mediated by excitatory interneurons, including central (C), and vertical (V) interneurons. Relay of innocuous mechanical (touch) input to the superficial dorsal horn also involves a sequential pathway of dorsally projecting excitatory interneurons in lamina II activated by excitatory interneurons in lamina III receiving inputs from low-threshold Aβ mechanoreceptors. Local GABA/glycinergic interneurons neurons, including islet cells, control excitability within dorsal horn circuits via both presynaptic and postsynaptic mechanisms.

excitatory interneurons. In contrast, nonpeptidergic afferents signaling mechanically induced pain target excitatory interneurons of inner lamina II (IIi), which then convey noxious mechanical inputs to lamina I via polysynaptic excitatory pathways. Low-threshold tactile afferents (including Aβ, Aδ, and C-type) project to inner lamina II and laminae III–IV. They transmit crude and affective aspects of touch; after injury, these afferents are recruited into nociceptive circuits and convey light touch as painful (i.e., mechanical allodynia). Low-threshold Aβ mechanosensitive afferents arborize in an area that extends from inner lamina II to laminae V and project in a columnar fashion targeting different neuronal subpopulations in specific laminae.

Projection Neurons and Their Targets

The second-order projection neurons of the dorsal horn are located in lamina I and in laminae III–V and project via the STT and several parallel pathways (Figure 35.3). Lamina I contains the majority of STT neurons. They include nociceptive-specific neurons responsive to heat- or mechanically induced pain; neurons responsive to innocuous cooling; and neurons responsive to noxious heat, noxious mechanical (pinch), or cold stimuli. Some lamina I neurons may also be activated by pruritic agents such as histamine. The majority of nociceptive lamina I neurons express the NK1R for substance P and convey discriminative aspects of pain, such as its location and quality. There are several thalamic and brainstem targets of lamina I STT neurons, as discussed in the next chapter. Lamina I also contains neurons that lack NK1R and may receive tactile inputs from low-threshold C-mechanoreceptors relaying affective touch or from TRMP8-expressing C-afferents responding to innocuous cooling. The STT neurons located in the deep dorsal horn (laminae III–V) are wide dynamic range (WDR) neurons. They have large receptive fields and respond in a graded manner to both innocuous and noxious stimuli, thus coding stimulus intensity. Innocuous inputs to these neurons are provided by large-diameter Aβ afferents. Lamina V WDRs have long dorsally directed dendrites that penetrate the superficial dorsal horn, where they may be directly activated by peptidergic afferents. Lamina V also and receive inputs from excitatory interneurons activated by nonpeptidergic nociceptive afferents in deep layer II. Lamina V neurons both contribute to the STT and target subcortical structures involved in affective processing of pain sensation, such as the amygdala and hypothalamus.

Excitatory and Inhibitory Interneurons

Dorsal horn interneurons are particularly concentrated in lamina II or substantia gelatinosa. They include several morphologically distinct excitatory and inhibitory subtypes and have a critical role in both transmission and gating of nociceptive inputs.[26,27] Excitatory interneurons include radial, vertical, and central cells and use L-glutamate. They can be subdivided into different subpopulations according to the expression of different markers.[28] Selective subpopulations of excitatory interneurons may be the target of distinct primary afferents. For example, vertical interneurons expressing somatostatin receive inputs from both low-threshold Aβ and high-threshold nociceptive A/C mechanoreceptors; those expressing protein kinase C primarily receive inputs from low-threshold Aβ mechanoreceptors; and those expressing gastrin-releasing peptide receive inputs from pruriceptors. Inhibitory interneurons constitute approximately one-third of the neuronal population in the dorsal horn. The majority are islet cells and use GABA, glycine, or both as their neurotransmitter. There are several nonoverlapping subpopulations of inhibitory neurons, which differ in their neurochemical signature, electrophysiological properties, and afferent input. For example, parvalbumin-expressing GABAergic interneurons are tonic-spiking, receive input from nonnociceptive low-threshold Aβ afferents and establish axo-axonic synapses with myelinated afferents innervating excitatory interneurons. In contrast, inhibitory neurons expressing dynorphin, galanin, neuropeptide Y, or neuronal nitric oxide synthase receive inputs from nociceptive afferents and synapse on both excitatory and other inhibitory interneurons.

Parallel Lines for Transmission of Afferent Information in the Dorsal Horn

There are several feedforward excitatory circuits for transmission of nociceptive inputs to STT neurons (Figure 35.3). Heat-sensitive peptidergic afferents monosynaptically activate lamina I STT neurons. In contrast, mechanosensitive nonpeptidergic nociceptive afferents activate STT neurons indirectly via a feedforward circuit mediated by excitatory interneurons. This circuit consists of a polysynaptic ventral-to-dorsal pathway that involves the sequential activation of excitatory interneurons from inner to outer lamina II. In this pathway, mechanosensitive C nociceptor afferents activate central interneurons in inner lamina II, which in turn excite vertical cells in outer lamina II, which then convey excitatory projections to STT neurons in lamina I. Since vertical excitatory interneurons in outer lamina II also receive direct input from Aδ nociceptors, this circuit also provides a backup excitatory drive for nociceptive transmission in lamina I. Relay of input from low-threshold Aβ mechanoreceptors (touch) to lamina I also involves a pathway sequentially mediated by three types of dorsally projecting excitatory interneurons from inner to outer lamina II. The convergence of direct Aδ/C mechanical nociceptor input and indirect, excitatory interneuron-mediated low-threshold Aβ mechanoreceptor input on vertical excitatory interneurons in outer lamina II provides a substrate for innocuous mechanical stimuli to elicit pain (mechanical allodynia). C-tactile afferents also project to inner lamina II and have access, via excitatory interneurons, to wide dynamic range projection neurons in lamina I and lamina V. There is also a labeled line for itch sensation via a serial excitatory pathway that includes C-type pruriceptive afferents releasing natriuretic peptide B and excitatory interneurons expressing gastrin-releasing peptide, which activates a third group of excitatory interneurons that target lamina I STT neurons.[18,19,22,29]

Inhibitory Circuits in the Dorsal Horn

Local GABA/glycinergic interneurons have a critical role in controlling excitability within dorsal horn circuits. In normal conditions, these interneurons prevent the access of inputs from low-threshold mechanoreceptors to nociceptive neurons by feedforward inhibition. For example, parvalbumin-expressing GABA/glycinergic islet cells receive input from low-threshold primary afferents and provide the substrate for an inhibitory gate control of nociceptive transmission in the dorsal horn via both presynaptic and postsynaptic mechanisms. These inhibitory neurons provide axo-axonic inhibitory synapse on primary myelinated afferents, thereby gating the access of low-threshold afferent input to excitatory interneurons projecting to lamina I. These inhibitory islet cells may also mediate some of the descending monoaminergic modulatory control on pain transmission. However, some inhibitory islet or central cells receive direct input from nociceptive peptidergic C-fibers and are activated by noxious stimuli; these cells could promote pain transmission by inhibiting other inhibitory islet cells.

Neurochemical Transmission in the Dorsal Horn

The primary neurotransmitter of excitatory afferents to STT and other projection neurons in the dorsal horn is L-glutamate, which acts via α-amino-3-hydroxy-5-methylisoxazole propionic acid receptors (AMPARs) to elicit a short-lasting response of the STT neurons (Figure 35.4). Burst of activity of nociceptors triggers an N-methyl-D-aspartate receptor (NMDAR)-mediated long-term potentiation (LTP) of excitatory glutamatergic synapses onto their targeted dorsal horn projection neurons. In response to burst activity, peptidergic nociceptive afferents release substance P, which acting via NK1 coupled to G_q signaling elicits membrane depolarization by reducing postsynaptic K^+ conductances in STT neurons, thereby promoting activation of NMDAR activation by glutamate. Several neurochemical signals inhibit transmission of nociceptive signal in the dorsal horn (Figure 35.5). Presynaptic receptors, including $GABA_A$ and $GABA_B$, μ-type and δ-type opioid, CB1 cannabinoid, and adenosine A1 receptors, inhibit presynaptic voltage-gated $Ca_v2.2$ (N-type) channels. $GABA_A$ receptors and glycine receptors (GlyRs) mediate fast postsynaptic inhibition, which depends on the Cl^- gradient maintained by the potassium-chloride cotransporter 2 (KCC2). Opioid and other GPCRs reduce postsynaptic excitability via G protein-activated inward-rectifying K^+ channels (GIRKs). As discussed in the next chapter, descending influences from a brainstem pain modulatory circuit strongly modulate transmission of nociceptive inputs in the dorsal horn. These influences originate in brainstem neurons expressing GABA, enkephalin, or monoamines such as serotonin and norepinephrine and modulate nociceptive processing via several mechanisms. They include presynaptic inhibition of neurotransmitter release from primary afferents, direct effect on STT neurons, or effect on interneurons. For example, norepinephrine acting via presynaptic α2 receptors and serotonin, acting via presynaptic $5\text{-HT}1_B$ receptors reduce neurotransmitter release from primary afferents. Norepinephrine may also reduce nociceptive transmission via excitatory α1 receptors located in local GABAergic and glycinergic inhibitory neurons.

ABNORMAL NOCICEPTOR ACTIVITY AND PAIN

Abnormal activity of nociceptors results from three main mechanisms: genetic channelopathies, peripheral sensitization by product of inflammation, and plastic changes resulting from axonal injury.

Nociceptor Channelopathies

Mutations affecting the sodium channels Nav1.7 (*SCN9A* gene), Nav1.8 (*SCN10A* gene), and Nav1.9 (*SCN11A* gene) in nociceptors may result in paroxysmal pain disorders, insensitivity to pain, or both, as a result of either gain-of-function or loss-of-function of these channels[30–34] (Table 35.4). Missense *SCNA9A* mutations resulting in $Na_v1.7$ channel gain-of-function produce inherited erythromelalgia. This autosomal dominant disorder is characterized by severe burning pain and erythema in the feet, hands, and occasionally the nose and ears. The pain is initially episodic and precipitated by warmth, exercise, prolonged standing, and sometimes alcohol; and is typically relieved by cooling. These gain-of-function *SCN9A* mutations make nociceptors hyperexcitable by increasing the probability of channel activation and slowing channel deactivation. Carbamazepine and mexiletine are nonselective, activity-dependent sodium channel blockers that may be efficacious in relieving symptoms in some but not all cases.[31,32] Gain-of-function *SCNA9* mutations are also associated with paroxysmal extreme pain disorder. This autosomal recessive condition with onset in infancy is characterized by paroxysmal episodes of rectal, perineal, ocular, and mandibular pain, which may be triggered by defecation, eating, or strong emotions.[33,34] In this disorder, pain is associated with autonomic manifestations including flushing, lacrimation, rhinorrhea, bradycardia, and apnea; flushing can present in a harlequin pattern that alternates between the left and right side during different episodes. These mutations impair $Na_v1.7$ fast inactivation, leading to a persistent current and generation of resurgent Na^+ currents. *SCN9A*-gene variants producing gain-of-function of $Na_v1.7$ were found in approximately 30% of a cohort of patients with idiopathic painful small fiber neuropathies. Autonomic symptoms vary in spectrum and severity according to the mutation and depending on its impact on sympathetic ganglion neurons, which also express $Na_v1.7$ channels. Increased depolarization in response to some mutations may reduce sympathetic ganglion neuron

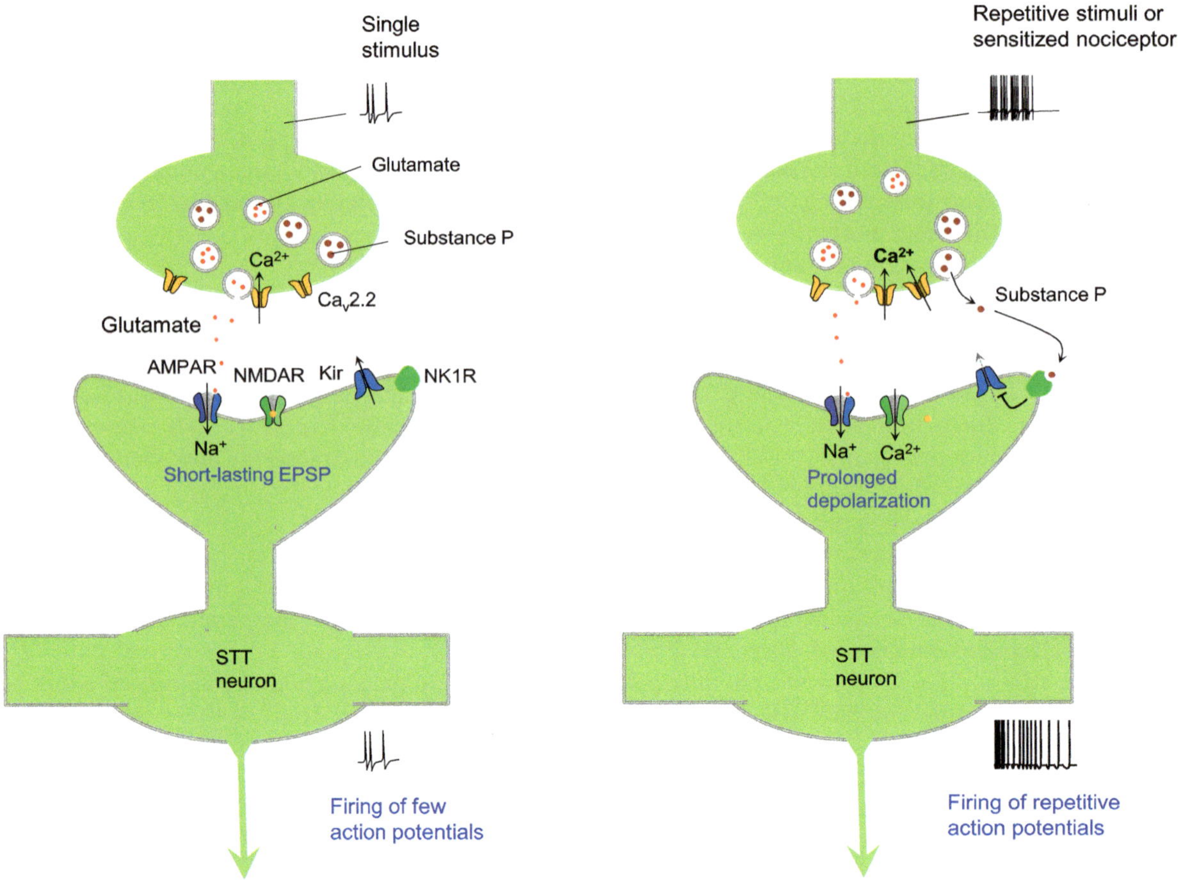

FIGURE 35.4 Neurochemical transmission in the dorsal horn.
The primary neurotransmitter of excitatory afferent input to spinothalamic tract (STT) and other projection neurons in the dorsal horn is L-glutamate, which acts via α-amino-3-hydroxy-5-methyl-isoxazole propionic acid receptors (AMPARs) to elicit a short-lasting response of the STT neurons. Burst of activity of nociceptors triggers an N-methyl-D-aspartate receptor (NMDAR)-mediated long-term potentiation (LTP) of excitatory glutamatergic synapses onto their targeted dorsal horn projection neurons. In response to burst activity, peptidergic nociceptive afferents release substance P, which acting via neurokinin-1 (NK1) receptors coupled to G_q signaling elicits membrane depolarization by reducing postsynaptic K^+ conductances in STT neurons, thereby promoting activation of NMDAR activation by glutamate, triggering repetitive discharge of STT neurons.

excitability by a mechanism of depolarization block. Gain-of-function *SCNA10* mutations, associated with increased Nav1.8 channel responses and DRG neuron hyperexcitability, have also been identified in patients with painful small fiber neuropathy that may respond to carbamazepine, but response duration varies among patients. Missense mutations of the *SCN11A* gene causing $Na_v1.9$ channel gain-of-function and DRG hyperexcitability have also been linked to autosomal dominant episodic pain syndrome. Clinical characteristics include intense pain localized principally to the distal lower extremities and occasionally in the upper body, especially in the joints of fingers and arms; episodic pain may appear late in the day and relapse once every 2–5 days, may be exacerbated with fatigue associated with excessive sweating, and relieved by application of heat or by oral anti-inflammatory analgesics.

Some nociceptor sodium channelopathies are associated with insensitivity to pain. For example, inactivating *SCNA9* mutations leading to loss of $Na_v1.7$ function produce congenital insensitivity to pain associated with congenital anosmia (due to the normal role of $Na_v1.7$ in olfactory transduction). Compound heterozygous nonsense *SCNA9* mutations have also been linked to a hereditary sensory and autonomic neuropathy type II D, which is characterized by loss of pain and temperature sensation, anhidrosis, hyposmia, hearing loss, and bone dysplasia. Congenital insensitivity to pain has also been linked to gain-of-function *SCN11A* mutations. These patients have hyperhidrosis in the absence of precipitating factors and severe gastrointestinal dysfunction, including episodes of diarrhea and constipation. Gain-of-function *SCNA11* mutations increase $Na_v1.9$ function by interfering with voltage-dependent inactivation; this results

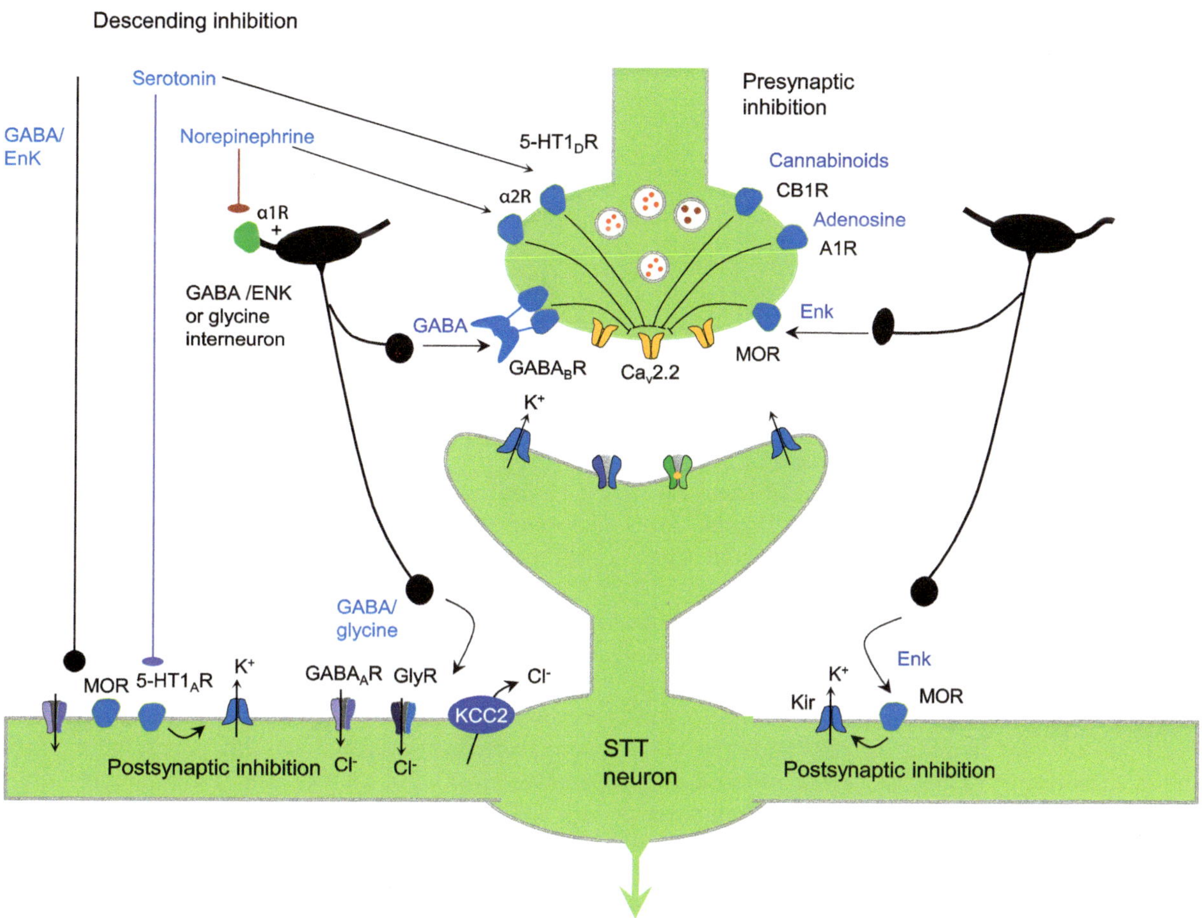

FIGURE 35.5 Inhibitory transmission in the dorsal horn.

In normal conditions, neurotransmitter release from primary afferents is inhibited by several chemical signals acting via presynaptic receptors, including $GABA_B$, μ-type and δ-type opioid, CB1 cannabinoid, and adenosine A1 receptors, which inhibit voltage-gated $Ca_v2.2$ (N-type) channels. $GABA_A$ and glycine receptors (GlyRs) mediate fast postsynaptic inhibition, which depends on the Cl^- gradient maintained by the potassium-chloride cotransporter 2 (KCC2). Opioids reduce postsynaptic excitability via G protein-coupled inward-rectifying K^+ channels (GIRKs). Descending influences mediated by GABA/enkephalin or monoamines such as serotonin and norepinephrine modulate nociceptive processing via presynaptic inhibition of neurotransmitter release from primary afferents, direct effect on STT neurons, or effect on interneurons. For example, norepinephrine, acting via presynaptic α2 receptors, and serotonin, acting via presynaptic 5-HT_{1B} receptors, reduce release of glutamate and neuropeptides from primary afferents. Norepinephrine may also elicit antinociception via excitatory α1 receptors located in local GABAergic and glycinergic inhibitory neurons.

in sustained depolarization that leads to inactivation of $Na_v1.7$ and $Na_v1.8$ channels resulting in conduction block of nociceptors, hence the insensitivity to pain.[30]

Other channelopathies have also been associated with familiar pain syndromes. Gain-of-function TRPA1 mutations causes an autosomal-dominant familial episodic pain syndrome characterized by episodes of debilitating upper body pain, triggered by fasting and physical stress.[35] TRPA1 variants have been linked to carbamazepine-responsive cramp-fasciculation syndrome.[36]

Peripheral Inflammation and Nociceptor Sensitization

Peripheral inflammation or axonal injury leads to nociceptor sensitization. This manifests with spontaneous nociceptor activity (pain), increase sensitivity to noxious stimuli (primary hyperalgesia), expansion of the receptive fields (secondary hyperalgesia), and activation by innocuous mechanical or thermal stimuli (allodynia). Inflammation and peripheral nerve injury promote nociceptor sensitization via interacting mechanisms (Figure 35.6). Peptidergic nociceptors, in addition to conveying afferent input to the dorsal

TABLE 35.4 *Nociceptor Sodium Channelopathies*

Gene	Channel Dysfunction	Consequence	Phenotype
SCNA9	Na_v 1.7 gain-of-function		Familial erythromelalgia Paroxysmal extreme pain disorder Idiopathic painful peripheral neuropathy
	Na_v 1.7 loss-of-function		Channelopathy-associated congenital insensitivity to pain Hereditary sensory and autonomic neuropathy type II D (with anosmia)
SCNA10	Na_v 1.8 gain-of-function		Idiopathic painful peripheral neuropathy
SCNA11	Na_v 1.9 gain-of-function		Autosomal dominant episodic pain syndrome

horn, have an efferent function as sensorimotor nerves. In the setting of tissue injury or in response to chemical or mechanical stimuli in visceral organs peptidergic DRG terminals antidromically release substance P and CGRP in a Ca^{2+}-dependent fashion.[1,37] These neuropeptides elicit vasodilatation, increase vascular permeability, and trigger release of local mediators (autacoids) from mastocytes and other cells. This response is referred to as neurogenic inflammation. During inflammation, peripheral nociceptors sense cytokines released by immune cells and release signals such as substance P, CGRP, CCL2 and microRNAs to activate resident immune cells such as macrophages, mast cells and dendritic cells. For example, substance P released from nociceptive terminals increase release of IL-1β, IL-6 and TNF-α from macrophages. Chemical signals released from macrophages and other local cells at the site of injury include bradykinin, histamine, prostaglandin E2 (PGE2), thromboxanes, leukotrienes, ATP, NGF, brain-derived neurotrophic factor (BDNF), endocannabinoids, proinflammatory cytokines, chemokines, proteases, and nitric oxide (NO).[1,17,37] These mediators elicit upregulation of cation channels in nociceptors, both by altering their expression or membrane trafficking and via interactions of G protein-coupled or tyrosine kinase receptors. There is redundancy of transduction pathways and targets for peripheral nociceptor sensitization. TRPV1 is a core downstream target for many inflammatory signals. For example, bradykinin, acting via B2 receptors, increases TRPV1 activity both by reducing its inhibition by phosphatidylinositol bisphosphate and by direct activation of the channel via production of eicosanoids Bradykinin also elicits pain by promoting release of intracellular Ca^{2+}, closure of M-type K^+ channels and opening TMEM16A/ANO1 channels.[38] NGF directly activates TRPV1 via several downstream kinases and promotes expression of pronociceptive proteins, such as substance P, TRPV1, and Nav1.8.[39] Activation of the protein kinase A by inflammatory mediators leads to internalization of the Na^+-activated K^+ channels and thereby sensitize primary afferent nociceptors to mechanical, thermal, and osmotic stimuli.[40]

Axonal Plasticity Following Injury

In normal conditions, the spontaneous discharge of nociceptive afferents is of low frequency and random, requiring both spatial and temporal summation at the level of the dorsal horn to elicit the experience of pain.[41] Nerve injury results in several electrophysiological abnormalities in nociceptors, including spontaneous impulse generation; sensitization to mechanical, heat, and cold stimuli; and polyspike responses.[42,43] These abnormalities reflect plastic changes in ion channel expression, including upregulation of pronociceptive $Na_v1.7$, $Na_v1.8$, Ca_v, and TRP channels and downregulation of antinociceptive K^+ channels.[44–46] For example, $Na_V1.7$ channels accumulate at nerve endings together with the axon injury signal extracellular receptor activated kinase (ERK), which phosphorylates the channel and reduces its activation threshold. In contrast, in the setting of axonal injury, there is reduced expression of several types of K^+ channels, which in part reflects epigenetic mechanisms. Axonal injury or inflammation trigger upregulation of the RE1-silencing transcription factor (REST), which elicits histone methylation and thus epigenetic silencing of expression of K^+ channels, as well as downregulation of μ-type opioid receptors.[47] Retigabine is an anticonvulsant agent that enhances $K_v7.2/K_v7.3$ activation and M currents in axotomized nociceptive fibers and reduced neuropathic pain in experimental models.[48] Sphingosine 1 phosphate released in the setting of injury promotes peripheral sensitization via S1PR1 and SP1R3 receptors resulting in activation or TRPV1 and TRPA1 and inhibition of outward Cl- and K^+ currents.

Schwann cells detect nerve injury and have a critical role in the development and maintenance of neuropathic pain.[49] After nerve injury, the former myelinating Schwann cells degrade their myelin and become nonmyelinating repair Schwann cells. There is upregulation of multiple receptors and channels in Schwann cells following nerve injury, including P2X receptors, and activation of TLRs that respond to damage-associated molecular patterns) released from necrotic sensory neurons. This leads to activation of intracellular signaling pathways and release of growth factors,

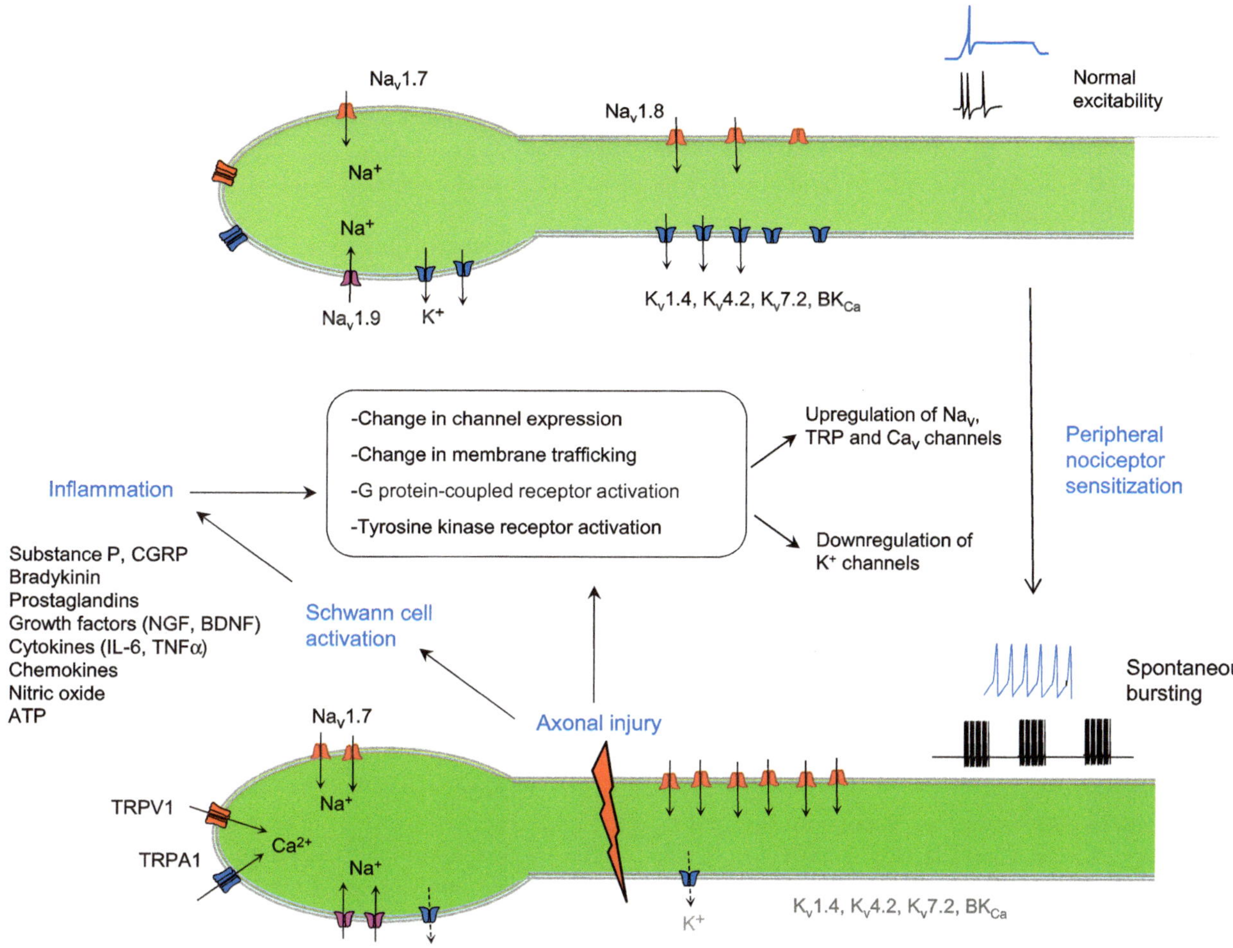

FIGURE 35.6 Nociceptor sensitization by inflammation or nerve injury.
Peripheral inflammation or axonal injury leads to nociceptor sensitization. Chemical mediators released from nerve terminals or local cells at the site of injury include substance P, calcitonin gene-related peptide (CGRP), adenosine triphosphate (ATP), bradykinin, eicosanoid and related lipids (prostaglandins, thromboxanes, leukotrienes and endocannabinoids), nerve growth factor (NGF), brain-derived neurotrophic factor (BDNF), cytokines, chemokines, proteases, and nitric oxide (NO). These mediators elicit upregulation of cation channels in nociceptors, both by altering their expression or membrane trafficking and via interactions with G protein-coupled or tyrosine kinase receptors that trigger signal transduction cascades. In normal conditions, the spontaneous discharge of nociceptive afferents is of low frequency and random. Nerve injury results in spontaneous impulse generation, and burst discharge. These abnormalities reflect plastic changes in ion channel expression, including upregulation of pronociceptive $Na_v1.7$ and $Na_v1.8$, Ca_v, and TRP channels and downregulation of antinociceptive K^+ channels. Schwann cells detect nerve injury and upregulate multiple receptors and channels, leading to activation of intracellular signaling pathways that trigger release growth factors, proinflammatory cytokines such tumor necrosis factor-α (TNF-α), chemokines, and ATP.

proinflammatory cytokines such as TNF-α, chemokines, and ATP. Activation of TRPA1 expressed in Schwann cells promotes mechanical allodynia and neuroinflammation via paracrine mechanisms.

Other Peripheral Mechanisms of Pain

Experimental models show that painful neuropathy induced by some chemotherapeutic agents involves upregulation and excessive activation of TRP channels in nociceptors. For example, TRPV1and TRPA1 are involved in thermal hyperalgesia induced by cisplatin, whereas TRPA1 and TMP8 mediate pain and cold allodynia induced by oxaliplatin.[50] Studies in mice show that activation of TLR4 in DRG neurons by paclitaxel causes increased expression of CCL2 resulting in macrophage infiltration to the DRG.

Experimental models of diabetic neuropathy show that altered Ca^{2+} homeostasis and oxidative stress associated with activation of the polyol pathway and advanced glycation endproducts promote activation of several TRP channels that are mostly responsible from diabetic neuropathic pain.[51] The concept of "autoimmune pain" originates from evidence that autoantibodies against component of voltage-gated K+ channels, such as LGI1 (leucine-rich glioma activated-1) and particularly CASPR2 (contactin-associated protein 2), are associated with pain that typically has subacute onset and is commonly associated with other manifestations of axonal hyperexcitability.[52,53]

DORSAL HORN MECHANISMS OF CENTRAL SENSITIZATION

Disturbances on the dorsal horn circuit leading to an imbalance between excitation and inhibition maintain the pain state following nerve injury. This process, called central sensitization, has a major role in the manifestations of neuropathic pain, including mechanical allodynia.[36,45,54,55] Several processes contribute to central sensitization at the level of the dorsal horn. They include LTP of excitatory synapses on STT neurons, axonal plasticity, impaired GABAergic inhibition, local microglial inflammation, and descending facilitation (Figure 35.7).

Long-Term Potentiation of Excitatory Synapses on Spinothalamic Neurons

Repeated nociceptor firing, as occurs in the setting of nerve injury, elicits a long-lasting facilitation of the responses of dorsal horn STT projection neurons, not only to nociceptive but also to innocuous stimuli. Burst of nociceptor afferent activity leading to substance P release elicits NMDAR-mediated homosynaptic LTP on the overactive synapse. There is also heterosynaptic LTP of synapses receiving innocuous inputs conveyed by C-type or low-threshold Aβ-type afferents. This allows the spread of the change in synaptic strength to neighboring nonactivated synapses, and expands the stimulus-sensitive territory outside that of the damaged nerve or area of tissue injury. This mechanism provides a substrate for both mechanical allodynia and secondary hyperalgesia. Long-term potentiation may occur at the presynaptic or postsynaptic levels and largely reflects Ca^{2+}-mediated mechanisms. Postsynaptic LTP is triggered by Ca^{2+} influx via voltage-gated $Ca_v1.2$ (L-type) channels and NMDARs, as well as Ca^{2+} release from intracellular stores. The resulting increase in intracellular Ca^{2+} triggers several downstream cascades, including those mediated by a variety of protein kinases, such as calmodulin kinase II (CAMKII) and ERK. These pathways are also activated by BDNF, which is released in an activity-dependent manner and promotes upregulation of expression of AMPARs in the postsynaptic membrane, activation of transcription and local translation of synaptic proteins, and structural changes in dendritic spines. Whereas substance P facilitates induction of NMDAR-dependent LTP, it is not necessarily for LTP maintenance. However, substance P also controls the expression of cytokines and chemokines as well as transcription factors that increase the synthesis of pro-inflammatory mediators that contribute to the development of hyperalgesia.[56] Presynaptic mechanisms may also lead to increased release of glutamate from C-afferents in the dorsal horn; this may be promoted by retrograde signals such as NO and PGE2 triggered by increase in intracellular Ca^{2+} downstream of NMDAR activation.

Plastic Changes in Primary Afferents and Excitatory Interneurons

Peripheral axotomy leads to sprouting of Aβ afferents into laminae I and outer lamina II. After nerve injury, Aβ afferent undergo a phenotypic change including upregulation of expression of substance P and other neuropeptides. Repetitive noxious stimulation also leads to downregulation of $K_v4.2$ channels in excitatory neurons, leading to increased excitability of these cells and thereby promoting neuropathic pain.[57]

Loss of Inhibition in the Dorsal Horn, Mechanical Allodynia, and Neuropathic Itch

The manifestations of neuropathic pain, such as mechanical allodynia and itch, primarily reflect impaired inhibition within dorsal horn circuits. Several mechanisms may contribute to loss of GABAergic and glycinergic inhibition in the dorsal horn in the setting of axonal injury or tissue inflammation. They include excitotoxicity damage of GABAergic neurons; long-term depression of inhibitory GABAergic transmission; and reduced efficacy of inhibitory transmission via $GABA_A$ or glycine receptor channels.[54] For example, activation of TRPV1 channels expressed in a population of GABAergic dorsal horn interneurons may produce long-term depression of excitatory input from myelinated fibers to these inhibitory neurons.[58] Peripheral axonal injury also triggers presynaptic Ca^{2+}-dependent signaling that results in global downregulation of the excitatory drive to GABAergic neurons from nociceptive Aδ- and C-fibers.[59] BDNF released from microglia activated in the setting of axonal injury downregulates the expression of the potassium-chloride cotransporter 2 (KCC2) in lamina I neurons; this leads to a depolarization shift in the equilibrium potential of chloride, thereby reducing the efficacy of $GABA_A$ and glycine receptor-mediated inhibition.[60] However, these effects are not persistent,[61] and GABAergic and glycinergic neurons may retain their inhibitory effect in the setting of neuropathy. Administration of drugs that activate $GABA_A$ receptors,[62] transplantation of GABA precursor neurons in the dorsal horn,[63] or selective activation of glycinergic neurons[27] reduces pain in experimental models. Low-threshold Aβ primary afferent fibers mediate dynamic mechanical allodynia evoked by slow brushing across the skin whereas unmyelinated C fibers may primarily mediate static allodynia evoked by indentation of the skin. The precise mechanisms through which inflammation or injuries alter the mechanical sensitivity of ion channels in skin receptors leading to allodynia are incompletely understood.

In normal conditions the pathway responsible for mechanical allodynia is inactive due to surrounding feedforward

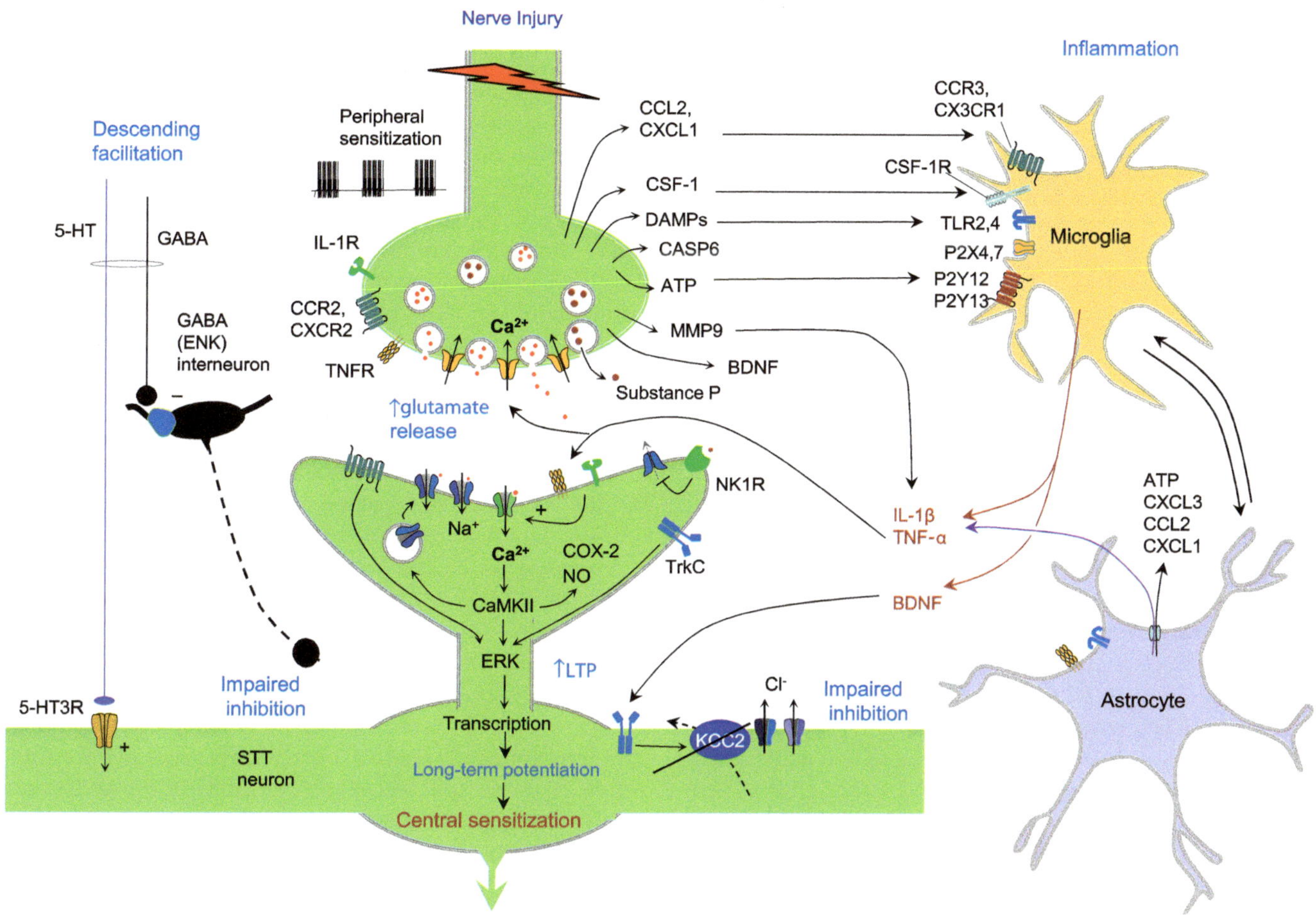

FIGURE 35.7 Mechanisms of nociceptive sensitization in the dorsal horn.

Several processes contribute to central sensitization at the level of the dorsal horn. They include long-term potentiation (LTP) of excitatory synapses on spinothalamic tract (STT) neurons, impaired GABAergic inhibition, microglial inflammation, and descending facilitation. Burst of nociceptor afferent activity leading to substance P release elicits N-methyl-D-aspartate receptor (NMDAR)-mediated LTP on the overactive synapse via Ca^{2+}-mediated mechanisms potentiated by Ca^{2+} influx via voltage-gated $Ca_v1.2$ channels and Ca^{2+} release from intracellular stores (not shown). Calcium triggers downstream cascades including activation of calmodulin kinase II (CAMKII) and extracellular signal-regulated kinase (ERK). These pathways are also activated by the depolarizing effects of substance P and action of brain-derived neurotrophic factor (BDNF) via tropomyosin kinase C (TrkC) receptors. LTP involves increased expression of α-amino-3-hydroxy-5-methyl-isoxazole propionic acid receptors (AMPARs), activation of transcription and local translation of synaptic proteins, and structural changes in dendritic spines. Several mechanisms may contribute to loss of GABAergic and glycinergic inhibition in the dorsal horn. They include reduced efficacy of inhibitory transmission due to downregulation of potassium-chloride cotransporter 2 (KCC2) in lamina I. Multiple signaling molecules released from damaged primary afferents participate in induction and maintenance of microglial activation. They include colony-stimulating factor-1 (CSF-1); chemokines such as CCL2 acting via microglial CCR2 receptors; matrix metalloproteinase 9 (MMP9), which induces cleavage and activation of interleukin 1 (IL-1)β; and caspase-6 (CASP6), which induces release of tumor necrosis factor α (TNF-α) from microglia, and damage-associated molecular patterns (DAMPs) that activate toll-like receptors (TLRs)-2 and 4. Several subtypes of purinergic receptors in microglia, including P2X4, P2X7, P2Y12, and P2Y13, promote microglial activation in response to ATP released from damaged afferents. Peripheral nerve injury also results in upregulation of the CX3CR1 chemokine receptor and upregulation of complement components C1q, C3, and C4 in spinal microglia (not shown) Signals released from microglia promote central sensitization both by increasing excitatory transmission and reducing efficacy of local inhibition in the dorsal horn. For example, IL-1 promotes glutamate release from primary afferents and activation of AMPARs while reducing glutamate uptake from astrocytes. Serotonergic inputs from the rostral ventromedial medulla via 5-HT3 and descending inhibition local GABA/Enk neurons by GABA/enkephalin neurons in the rostral ventromedial medulla may be contributory.

inhibition via GABA/glycinergic interneurons.[55,64] Both long-term depression of excitatory synapses on GABAergic neurons[58] or toxin-mediated ablation or silencing of glycinergic neurons[27] result in mechanical allodynia. Removal of glycine inhibition may also enable tactile stimuli to activate astrocytes, leading to release of D-serine and activation of NMDARs.[65] Removal of GABAergic or glycinergic inhibition may also result in neuropathic itch. The multisynaptic dorsal horn itch pathway is under tonic inhibition by specific inhibitory GABA interneurons that express galanin and the κ opioid receptor agonist dynorphin.[66,67] Depletion of glycinergic interneurons also resulted in behavioral manifestations of itch; local activation of these neurons alleviated chloroquine- and histamine-induced itch in experimental models.

Glial Activation

Peripheral nerve injury triggers a strong activation of microglia and astrocytes in the dorsal horn.[68,69] While C-fiber activation is sufficient to elicit this response, activation of large A-fibers is also important to maintain microglial activation. Multiple signaling molecules released from damaged primary afferents participate in induction and maintenance of spinal microgliosis. They include colony-stimulating factor-1 (CSF-1), chemokines such as CCL2; matrix metalloproteinase 9 that activates IL-1β; caspase-6; and damage-associated molecular patterns that activate microglial TLRs. For example, after nerve injury CSF-1 is induced in injured DRG neurons and transported to axonal terminals in the spinal cord to induce microgliosis.

Several subtypes of purinergic receptors including ionotropic P2X (P2X47 and P2X7) and metabotropic P2Y (P2Y12, P2Y13) receptors are upregulated in microglia following nerve injury and promote microglial activation in response to ATP released from damaged afferents. Peripheral nerve injury also results in upregulation of the CX3CR1 chemokine receptor and upregulation of complement components C1q, C3, and C4 in spinal microglia. Other mechanisms may trigger microglial activation in the dorsal horn, including activation of TLR4 receptors triggered by drugs such as paclitaxel[70] and even by psychosocial stress, as shown in a mouse model.[71]

Signals released from microglia promote central sensitization both by increasing excitatory transmission and reducing efficacy of local inhibition in the dorsal horn. For example, IL1-β promotes glutamate release from primary afferents and activation of AMPARs while reducing glutamate uptake from astrocytes. BDNF released by microglia potentiates substance P release from primary afferents. Studies in rodent models show that microglia activation in the dorsal horn persists for long periods following nerve injury, beyond involvement of proinflammatory cytokine and chemokine signaling. In this chronic phase, selective depletion of spinal microglia by blocking BDNF signaling almost completely reverses pain hypersensitivity.[72]

In basal conditions, astrocytes in the dorsal horn decrease nociceptive transmission by releasing ATP, which is hydrolyzed to adenosine that acts via inhibitory A1 receptors in nociceptive neurons, and also by releasing type 1 interferons, which are anti-inflammatory cytokines.[69] In the setting of nerve or spinal cord injury, spinal astrocytes respond to pro-inflammatory mediators released by activated microglia or injured DRG neurons and contribute to central sensitization and neuropathic pain by releasing TNF-α, IL-1β, chemokines CCL2 and CXCL10, matrix metalloproteinase 9, and other mediators and decreased production of the anti-inflammatory IL-10.[69] Astrocytic activation also has a major role in mechanisms of neuropathic itch.[69] Sphingolipid signaling mediated by S1P1R1 also has a role in some neuropathic pain conditions, such as that induced by paclitaxel or bortezomib or in the setting of inflammatory demyelination. Plastic changes in reactive astrocytes may also promote central sensitization; for example there is upregulation of expression of connexin-43 hemichannels and the water channel aquaporin 4; reduction of the high-affinity glutamate transporter EAAT2 (excitatory amino acid transporter 2); and increased release of D-serine, a co-agonist of NMDARs, resulting in increased glutamatergic transmission

In experimental models, microglial activation precedes and typically subsides before astrocyte activation. Whereas astrocytes contribute to nearly all persistent pain conditions, microglia appear to regulate only certain types of pain conditions. For example, nerve injury results in the activation of both microglia and astrocytes, whereas chemotherapy- or HIV-1 induced peripheral neuropathy is associated with marked astrogliosis, but little or no microgliosis.[69]

Descending Pain Facilitation

Plasticity in the descending pain modulatory system, including the rostral ventromedial medulla, may promote descending pain facilitation and perpetuate chronic pain states in the setting of nerve injury or inflammation. In experimental models, there is astrocytic activation in several regions involved in descending pain modulation, including the periaqueductal gray and rostral ventromedial medulla.[69] Experimental evidence indicates a role of serotonergic inputs from the rostral ventromedial medulla mediated by 5-HT3 receptors, which are cation channels that trigger depolarization of STT neurons. Activation of these receptors may also promote dorsal horn sensitization via neuron-glial interactions. Intrathecal administration of a 5-HT3R agonist trigger neuron-to-microglia signaling via the chemokine fractalkine, microglia-to-astrocyte signaling via IL-18; and astrocyte-to-neuron signaling via IL-1β. All these interactions lead to increased activation of NMDARs and hyperexcitability of spinal projection neurons.

KEY POINTS

- Nociceptors protect the organism from injury and can be active in the absence of pain perception.

- Nociception involves heterogeneous populations of primary unmyelinated Aδ- and unmyelinated C afferents from neurons in the dorsal root ganglion (DRG) or trigeminal ganglia that use glutamate as their primary neurotransmitter.
- Heat-sensitive DRG neurons also utilize neuropeptides such as substance P and express transient receptor potential (TRP) channels.
- Na_v1.7 channels boost subthreshold stimuli and increase nociceptor excitability; Na_v1.8 channels are responsible of the action potential and support repetitive firing; Nav1.9 channels amplify the response to subthreshold inputs.
- Nociceptors also express different subtypes of potassium (K^+) channels that dampen nociceptor excitability.
- TRPV1 channels mediate sensitivity to noxious heat; TRPA1 s respond to chemical signals including products of oxidative stress, and TRPM8 channels mediate sensitivity to cold.
- Nociceptive fibers express a wide range of receptors that contribute to sensitization in the setting of inflammation.
- The dorsal horn is a site of complex processing and gating of nociceptive information.
- There are two major types of nociceptive STT neurons; nociceptive-specific neurons concentrated in superficial lamina I, and wide dynamic range neurons concentrated in deep layer V.
- Lamina II, or substantia gelatinosa, contains different subtypes of excitatory (glutamatergic) and inhibitory (GABA/glycinergic) interneurons that have a critical role in both transmission and gating of nociceptive inputs.
- High-frequency activity of primary afferents promotes release of substance P, which via NK1 receptors elicits depolarization and allows NMDAR activation.
- Several presynaptic receptors, including $GABA_A$ and $GABA_B$, μ-type and δ-type opioid, CB1 cannabinoid, and adenosine A1 receptors, inhibit neurotransmitter release from nociceptor afferents.
- Mutations affecting Nav1.7 (*SCN9A* gene), Nav1.8 (*SCN10*A gene), or Nav1.9 (*SCN11*A gene) in nociceptors may result in paroxysmal pain disorders, insensitivity to pain, or both.
- Peripheral inflammation or axonal injury leads to nociceptor sensitization.
- Nociceptive terminals antidromically release substance P and CGRP, resulting in neurogenic inflammation.
- Inflammatory mediators elicit upregulation of sodium channels and TRPV1 channels in nociceptors.
- Nerve injury results in upregulation of pronociceptive Na_v1.7, Na_v1.8, Ca_v, and TRP channels and downregulation of antinociceptive K^+ channels, in part via epigenetic mechanisms.
- Schwann cells detect nerve injury and have a critical role in the development and maintenance of neuropathic pain.
- Antibodies against CASPR2 are associated with pain that typically has subacute onset and is commonly associated with other manifestations of axonal hyperexcitability.
- Disturbances of the dorsal horn circuit leading to an imbalance between excitation inhibition result in central sensitization that maintains the pain state following nerve injury.
- Several processes contribute to central sensitization at the level of the dorsal horn. They include LTP of excitatory synapses on STT neurons, axonal plasticity, impaired GABAergic inhibition, local microglial inflammation, and descending facilitation.
- Peripheral nerve injury triggers a strong activation of microglia and astrocytes in the dorsal horn.
- Signals released from glial cells promote central sensitization by both increasing excitatory transmission and reducing efficacy of local inhibition in the dorsal horn.
- Plasticity in the descending pain modulatory system elicits descending pain facilitation, in part via release of serotonin, which acting via 5-HT3 receptors promotes dorsal horn sensitization via neuron-glial interactions.

REFERENCES

1. Basbaum AI, Bautista DM, Scherrer G, Julius D. Cellular and molecular mechanisms of pain. Cell 2009;139:267–284.
2. Schmelz M, Schmidt R. Microneurographic single-unit recordings to assess receptive properties of afferent human C-fibers. Neurosci Lett 2010;470:158–161.
3. Bardoni R. Role of presynaptic glutamate receptors in pain transmission at the spinal cord level. Curr Neuropharmacol 2013;11:477–483.
4. Moldovan M, Alvarez S, Romer Rosberg M, Krarup C. Axonal voltage-gated ion channels as pharmacological targets for pain. Eur J Pharmacol 2013;708:105–112.
5. Dib-Hajj SD, Geha P, Waxman SG. Sodium channels in pain disorders: pathophysiology and prospects for treatment. Pain 2017;158 Suppl 1:S97–S107.
6. Du X, Gamper N. Potassium channels in peripheral pain pathways: expression, function and therapeutic potential. Curr Neuropharmacol 2013;11:621–640.
7. Tsantoulas C. Emerging potassium channel targets for the treatment of pain. Curr Opin Support Palliat Care 2015;9:147–154.
8. Lee S. Pharmacological inhibition of voltage-gated Ca(2+) channels for chronic pain relief. Curr Neuropharmacol 2013;11:606–620.
9. Julius D. TRP channels and pain. Annu Rev Cell Dev Biol 2013;29:355–384.

10. Luo J, Walters ET, Carlton SM, Hu H. Targeting pain-evoking transient receptor potential channels for the treatment of pain. Curr Neuropharmacol 2013;11:652–663.
11. Lee CH, Chen CC. Roles of ASICs in nociception and proprioception. Adv Exp Med Biol 2018;1099:37–47.
12. He JT, Li XY, Zhao X, Liu X. Hyperpolarization-activated and cyclic nucleotide-gated channel proteins as emerging new targets in neuropathic pain. Rev Neurosci 2019;30:639–649.
13. Oh U, Jung J. Cellular functions of TMEM16/anoctamin. Pflugers Arch 2016;468:443–453.
14. Takayama Y, Tominaga M. Involvement of TRPV1-ANO1 interactions in pain-enhancing mechanisms. Adv Exp Med Biol 2018;1099:29–36.
15. Evely KM, Pryce KD, Bausch AE, et al. Slack KNa channels influence dorsal horn synapses and nociceptive behavior. Mol Pain 2017;13:1744806917714342.
16. Burnstock G. Purinergic mechanisms and pain—an update. Eur J Pharmacol 2013;716:24–40.
17. Davidson S, Copits BA, Zhang J, Page G, Ghetti A, Gereau RWt. Human sensory neurons: membrane properties and sensitization by inflammatory mediators. Pain 2014;155:1861–1870.
18. LaMotte RH, Dong X, Ringkamp M. Sensory neurons and circuits mediating itch. Nat Rev Neurosci 2014;15:19–31.
19. Han L, Dong X. Itch mechanisms and circuits. Annu Rev Biophys 2014;43:331–355.
20. Moehring F, Halder P, Seal RP, Stucky CL. Uncovering the cells and circuits of touch in normal and pathological settings. Neuron 2018;100:349–360.
21. Todd AJ. Neuronal circuitry for pain processing in the dorsal horn. Nat Rev Neurosci 2010;11:823–836.
22. Braz J, Solorzano C, Wang X, Basbaum AI. Transmitting pain and itch messages: a contemporary view of the spinal cord circuits that generate gate control. Neuron 2014;82:522–536.
23. Mendell LM. Constructing and deconstructing the gate theory of pain. Pain 2014;155:210–216.
24. Steinhoff M, Scmelz M, Lorinc Szabo I, Oaklander AL. Clinical presentation, management, and pathophysiology of neuropathic itch. Lancer Neurol 2018;17:709–720.
25. Cheng L, Duan B, Huang T, et al. Identification of spinal circuits involved in touch-evoked dynamic mechanical pain. Nat Neurosci 2017;20:804–814.
26. Zeilhofer HU, Wildner H, Yevenes GE. Fast synaptic inhibition in spinal sensory processing and pain control. Physiol Rev 2012;92:193–235.
27. Foster E, Wildner H, Tudeau L, et al. Targeted ablation, silencing, and activation establish glycinergic dorsal horn neurons as key components of a spinal gate for pain and itch. Neuron 2015;85:1289–1304.
28. Azad N, Iyer AK, Wang L, Liu Y, Lu Y, Rojanasakul Y. Reactive oxygen species-mediated p38 MAPK regulates carbon nanotube-induced fibrogenic and angiogenic responses. Nanotoxicology 2013;7:157–168.
29. Mishra SK, Hoon MA. The cells and circuitry for itch responses in mice. Science 2013;340:968–971.
30. Dib-Hajj SD, Waxman SG. Sodium channels in human pain disorders: genetics and pharmacogenomics. Annu Rev Neurosci 2019;42:87–106.
31. Fischer TZ, Gilmore ES, Estacion M, et al. A novel Nav1.7 mutation producing carbamazepine-responsive erythromelalgia. Ann Neurol 2009;65:733–741.
32. Choi JS, Zhang L, Dib-Hajj SD, et al. Mexiletine-responsive erythromelalgia due to a new Na(v)1.7 mutation showing use-dependent current fall-off. Exp Neurol 2009;216:383–389.
33. Fertleman CR, Ferrie CD, Aicardi J, et al. Paroxysmal extreme pain disorder (previously familial rectal pain syndrome). Neurology 2007;69:586–595.
34. Choi JS, Boralevi F, Brissaud O, et al. Paroxysmal extreme pain disorder: a molecular lesion of peripheral neurons. Nat Rev Neurol 2011;7:51–55.
35. Kremeyer B, Lopera F, Cox JJ, et al. A gain-of-function mutation in TRPA1 causes familial episodic pain syndrome. Neuron 2010;66:671–680.
36. von Hehn CA, Baron R, Woolf CJ. Deconstructing the neuropathic pain phenotype to reveal neural mechanisms. Neuron 2012;73:638–652.
37. Gold MS, Gebhart GF. Nociceptor sensitization in pain pathogenesis. Nat Med 2010;16:1248–1257.
38. Lee B, Cho H, Jung J, Yang YD, Yang DJ, Oh U. Anoctamin 1 contributes to inflammatory and nerve-injury induced hypersensitivity. Mol Pain 2014;10:5.
39. Schaible HG. Emerging concepts of pain therapy based on neuronal mechanisms. Handb Exp Pharmacol 2015;227:1–14.
40. Nuwer MO, Picchione KE, Bhattacharjee A. PKA-induced internalization of slack KNa channels produces dorsal root ganglion neuron hyperexcitability. J Neurosci 2010;30:14165–14172.
41. Serra J, Bostock H, Sola R, et al. Microneurographic identification of spontaneous activity in C-nociceptors in neuropathic pain states in humans and rats. Pain 2012;153:42–55.
42. Kleggetveit IP, Namer B, Schmidt R, et al. High spontaneous activity of C-nociceptors in painful polyneuropathy. Pain 2012;153:2040–2047.
43. Ratte S, Prescott SA. Afferent hyperexcitability in neuropathic pain and the inconvenient truth about its degeneracy. Curr Opin Neurobiol 2016;36:31–37.
44. Campbell JN, Meyer RA. Mechanisms of neuropathic pain. Neuron 2006;52:77–92.
45. Alles SRA, Smith PA. Etiology and pharmacology of neuropathic pain. Pharmacol Rev 2018;70:315–347.
46. Fransen E. Ionic mechanisms in peripheral pain. Prog Mol Biol Transl Sci 2014;123:23–51.
47. Willis DE, Wang M, Brown E, Fones L, Cave JW. Selective repression of gene expression in neuropathic pain by the neuron-restrictive silencing factor/repressor element-1 silencing transcription (NRSF/REST). Neurosci Lett 2016;625:20–25.
48. Djouhri L, Malki MI, Zeidan A, Nagi K, Smith T. Activation of Kv7 channels with the anticonvulsant retigabine alleviates neuropathic pain behaviour in the streptozotocin rat model of diabetic neuropathy. J Drug Target 2019;27:1118–1126.
49. Wei Z, Fei Y, Su W, Chen G. Emerging role of Schwann cells in neuropathic pain: receptors, glial mediators and myelination. Front Cell Neurosci 2019;13:116.
50. Nakagawa T, Kaneko S. Roles of transient receptor potential ankyrin 1 in oxaliplatin-induced peripheral neuropathy. Biol Pharm Bull 2017;40:947–953.
51. Naziroglu M, Dikici DM, Dursun S. Role of oxidative stress and Ca(2)(+) signaling on molecular pathways of neuropathic pain in diabetes: focus on TRP channels. Neurochem Res 2012;37:2065–2075.

52. Klein CJ, Lennon VA, Aston PA, McKeon A, Pittock SJ. Chronic pain as a manifestation of potassium channel-complex autoimmunity. Neurology 2012;79:1136–1144.
53. Vincent A, Pettingill P, Pettingill R, et al. Association of leucine-rich glioma inactivated protein 1, contactin-associated protein 2, and contactin 2 antibodies with clinical features and patient-reported pain in acquired neuromyotonia. JAMA Neurol 2018;75:1519–1527.
54. Zeilhofer HU, Benke D, Yevenes GE. Chronic pain states: pharmacological strategies to restore diminished inhibitory spinal pain control. Annu Rev Pharmacol Toxicol 2012;52:111–133.
55. Peirs C, Williams SP, Zhao X, et al. Dorsal horn circuits for persistent mechanical pain. Neuron 2015;87:797–812.
56. Zieglgansberger W. Substance P and pain chronicity. Cell Tissue Res 2019;375:227–241.
57. Huang HY, Cheng JK, Shih YH, Chen PH, Wang CL, Tsaur ML. Expression of A-type K channel alpha subunits Kv 4.2 and Kv 4.3 in rat spinal lamina II excitatory interneurons and colocalization with pain-modulating molecules. Eur J Neurosci 2005;22:1149–1157.
58. Kim YH, Back SK, Davies AJ, et al. TRPV1 in GABAergic interneurons mediates neuropathic mechanical allodynia and disinhibition of the nociceptive circuitry in the spinal cord. Neuron 2012;74:640–647.
59. Leitner J, Westerholz S, Heinke B, et al. Impaired excitatory drive to spinal GABAergic neurons of neuropathic mice. PLoS One 2013;8:e73370.
60. Ferrini F, De Koninck Y. Microglia control neuronal network excitability via BDNF signalling. Neural Plast 2013;2013:429815.
61. Castro A, Li Y, Raver C, et al. Neuropathic pain after chronic nerve constriction may not correlate with chloride dysregulation in mouse trigeminal nucleus caudalis neurons. Pain 2017;158:1366–1372.
62. Knabl J, Witschi R, Hosl K, et al. Reversal of pathological pain through specific spinal GABAA receptor subtypes. Nature 2008;451:330–334.
63. Braz JM, Wang X, Guan Z, Rubenstein JL, Basbaum AI. Transplant-mediated enhancement of spinal cord GABAergic inhibition reverses paclitaxel-induced mechanical and heat hypersensitivity. Pain 2015;156:1084–1091.
64. Duan B, Cheng L, Bourane S, et al. Identification of spinal circuits transmitting and gating mechanical pain. Cell 2014;159:1417–1432.
65. Miraucourt LS, Peirs C, Dallel R, Voisin DL. Glycine inhibitory dysfunction turns touch into pain through astrocyte-derived D-serine. Pain 2011;152:1340–1348.
66. Ross SE, Mardinly AR, McCord AE, et al. Loss of inhibitory interneurons in the dorsal spinal cord and elevated itch in Bhlhb5 mutant mice. Neuron 2010;65:886–898.
67. Kardon AP, Polgar E, Hachisuka J, et al. Dynorphin acts as a neuromodulator to inhibit itch in the dorsal horn of the spinal cord. Neuron 2014;82:573–586.
68. Chen G, Zhang YQ, Qadri YJ, Serhan CN, Ji RR. Microglia in pain: detrimental and protective roles in pathogenesis and resolution of pain. Neuron 2018;100:1292–1311.
69. Ji RR, Donnelly CR, Nedergaard M. Astrocytes in chronic pain and itch. Nat Rev Neurosci 2019;20:667–685.
70. Yan X, Li F, Maixner DW, et al. Interleukin-1beta released by microglia initiates the enhanced glutamatergic activity in the spinal dorsal horn during paclitaxel-associated acute pain syndrome. Glia 2019;67:482–497.
71. Sawicki CM, Kim JK, Weber MD, et al. Microglia promote increased pain behavior through enhanced inflammation in the spinal cord during repeated social defeat stress. J Neurosci 2019;39:1139–1149.
72. Echeverry S, Shi XQ, Yang M, et al. Spinal microglia are required for long-term maintenance of neuropathic pain. Pain 2017;158:1792–1801.

36 Central Processing and Modulation of Pain

OVERVIEW

Pain is a complex sensation. The experience of pain triggers somatic and autonomic reflexes, memories, and changes in emotional state and motivation.[1] The threshold and magnitude of acute pain can be modulated by attention, expectations, and mood. A noxious stimulus does not necessarily cause pain, and different individuals respond to the same magnitude of noxious stimulation with different experiences of pain. These observations reflect the effect of pain modulation by endogenous mechanisms triggered by attention and emotion. Optogenetic studies in rodents and functional magnetic resonance imaging (fMRI) in humans have provided important insights into the central mechanisms involved in the central processing of pain sensation. These studies identified key areas activated in response to painful stimuli.[2] The brain plays an active role in both acute and chronic pain perception. Other interactive networks, including those involved in attention and motivation have major roles in modulating responses to acute pain sensation and predisposition to chronic pain.[3] These areas also provide input to a brainstem pain modulatory system that may either suppress or potentiate nociceptive transmission in the dorsal horn. One model proposes that chronic pain develops in stages, where predisposing factors in combination with an injury precipitate the transition to a stable chronic state.[4] Studies in both animal models and humans indicate that synaptic plasticity, abnormal functional connectivity within networks involved in cognitive control, emotion and motivation, and descending facilitation all contribute to the development of chronic pain.[5] The main aims of this chapter are to review: (1) the ascending pathways and relays for pain perception and responses to pain; (2) the cortical areas activated in response to acute pain; (3) the cortical areas involved in emotional, attentional, and motivational aspects of the pain sensation; (4) the influences of attention and reward in pain modulation; (5) the functional organization of the descending pain modulatory systems; and (6) mechanisms of chronic pain.

ASCENDING PATHWAYS AND RELAYS FOR PAIN PERCEPTION

Nociceptive information ascends to the contralateral thalamus via the spinothalamic tract (STT) and the trigeminothalamic tract. Ascending nociceptive pathways also target the medullary reticular formation, parabrachial nucleus, periaqueductal gray (PAG), and superior colliculus.[6] All these pathways utilize L-glutamate as their major excitatory neurotransmitter.

Spinothalamic Tract Components and Targets

The STT is functionally heterogeneous; it includes several components that target different portions of the contralateral thalamus and participate in different aspects of pain sensation[6] (Figure 36.1). The majority of STT axons originate from nociceptive-specific neurons in lamina I and wide dynamic range neurons located both in lamina I and in laminae IV–VI (primarily lamina V) of the dorsal horn. The axons of these STT neurons cross the midline and ascend in the ventrolateral quadrant of the spinal cord to reach the contralateral ventroposterolateral nucleus (VPL). A similar pathway originating in the trigeminal nucleus caudalis conveys nociceptive inputs from cranial structures via the trigeminothalamic tract to the ventroposteromedial thalamic nucleus (VPM). The VPL/VPM projects to the primary somatosensory cortex (S1). Many of the cells in this pathway are nociceptive specific, have small and somatotopically organized contralateral receptive fields, and encode stimulus intensity participating in sensory-discriminative aspects of pain sensation. A second pathway originating in deep dorsal horn neurons with larger receptive fields target the ventral posteroinferior nucleus (VPI), which projects to the secondary somatosensory cortex (S2).[6] Many STT neurons in the deep dorsal horn (layer V) also send projections or

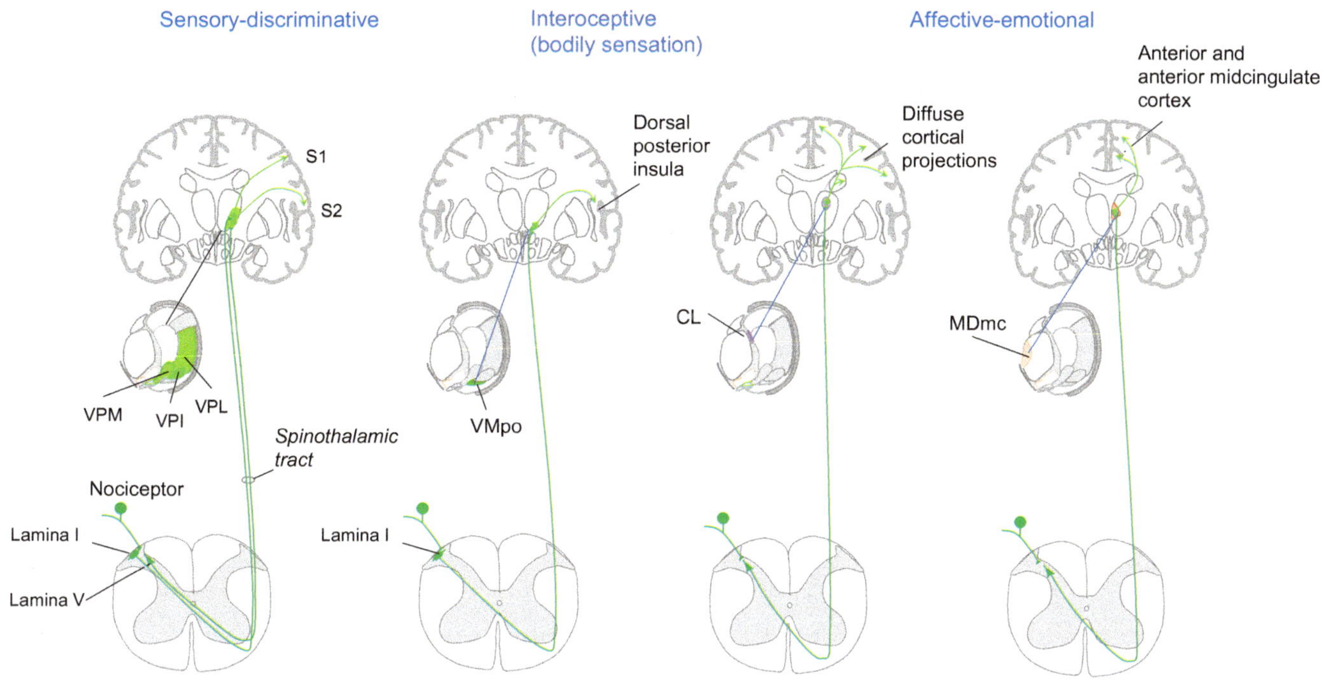

FIGURE 36.1 Components of the spinothalamic tract (STT).
The majority of STT axons originate from nociceptive-specific neurons in lamina I and wide dynamic range neurons located in lamina V; these axons cross the midline and ascend to reach the contralateral ventroposterolateral (VPL) nucleus of the thalamus. A similar pathway originating in the trigeminal nucleus terminates in the ventroposteromedial thalamic nucleus (VPM, not shown). The VPL/VPM projects to the primary somatosensory cortex (S1). STT axons also target the ventral posteroinferior nucleus (VPI), which projects to the secondary somatosensory cortex (S2). Axons collateral of STT neurons in the deep dorsal horn (layer V) terminate in the intralaminar thalamic nuclei, particularly the central lateral nucleus (CL), which projects broadly to the cerebral cortex. Other STT axons terminate in the medial (magnocellular) portion of the mediodorsal nucleus (MDmc), which together with the intralaminar nuclei provides inputs to the anterior cingulate cortex (ACC). There may be a selective STT projection from lamina I to the medial part of the posterior complex termed posterior ventromedial nucleus (VMpo), which targets insular cortex. However, the role of the VMpo in pain is controversial.

collaterals to the intralaminar complex of the thalamus; particularly the central lateral nucleus (CL).[7] Neurons in the CL have large, bilateral receptive fields and project broadly to the cerebral cortex. Some STT axons terminate in the posterior thalamic complex, which also receives inputs from other sensory modalities, whereas others terminate in the medial portion of the mediodorsal (MD) nucleus, which provides inputs to the anterior and midcingulate cortex. One important target of the STT is the anterior pulvinar.

The prototype central pain syndrome is thalamic pain due to stroke (Dejerine-Roussy syndrome).[8] It is typically impossible to predict what individual will develop such pain disorder following a thalamic stroke. Structural MRI and functional studies on STT excitability (quantitative sensory analysis and laser-evoked potentials) indicate that damage of the STT-thalamocortical system is critical for development of thalamic pain and most responsible lesions affect multiple nuclei, with maximal convergence in the anterior pulvinar; lesions affecting the VPL and lemniscal system were similarly distributed in patients with and those without pain [8].

There is some evidence for a selective STT projection from lamina I to the medial part of the posterior complex termed posterior ventromedial nucleus (VMpo) nucleus, which targets the insular cortex.[9–11] However, the specific role of the VMpo in pain is controversial.[12] Other STT neurons are located in the intermediate gray matter in laminae VII–X, especially at thoracic and sacral segments that receive inputs from visceral organs.[6] These neurons in the vicinity of the central canal project via the dorsal column to the dorsal column nuclei, which project to the VPL. Interruption of midline and posterior columns can relive visceral pain, such as pelvic and epigastric cancer pain.[13] Whereas the specific thalamic connections involved in nociceptive processing in humans are still debated, neuroimaging studies coupled to surgical investigations have confirmed the relevance of thalamic nuclei identified from animal studies.[14,15]

Spinoreticular Tract

Projections from nociceptive neurons of the spinal cord (or trigeminal nucleus caudalis) to the brainstem reticular formation are particularly important for integrating nociceptive activity with arousal, autonomic, and homeostatic responses (Figure 36.2). These pathways also trigger descending pain modulation and indirectly convey nociceptive information to forebrain regions involved in emotion and motivation.[16] The spinoreticular tract originates from lamina I, V, X, and particularly laminae VII–VIII. The axons of many of these neurons decussate, ascend in the ventrolateral quadrant, and terminate in several nuclei of the brainstem reticular formation, including serotonergic and catecholaminergic groups; lateral reticular, paragigantocellular oral, and caudal reticular pontine nuclei; and, importantly, the parabrachial nucleus (PB).[6] The PB receives an important input from lamina I of the dorsal horn (spino-parabrachial pathway) and is an important relay of nociceptive, visceral, and thermal information, which together constitute the so-called interoceptive information. The PB provides integrated interoceptive input to the hypothalamus, amygdala, and thalamus. Of relevance is a projection from calcitonin gene-related peptide (CGRP)-containing PB neurons that target the amygdala, periventricular hypothalamus, and thalamic nuclei, which project to the posterior insular cortex and other regions involved in pain processing. These thalamic nuclei include the subparafascicular nucleus of the intralaminar complex and nuclei

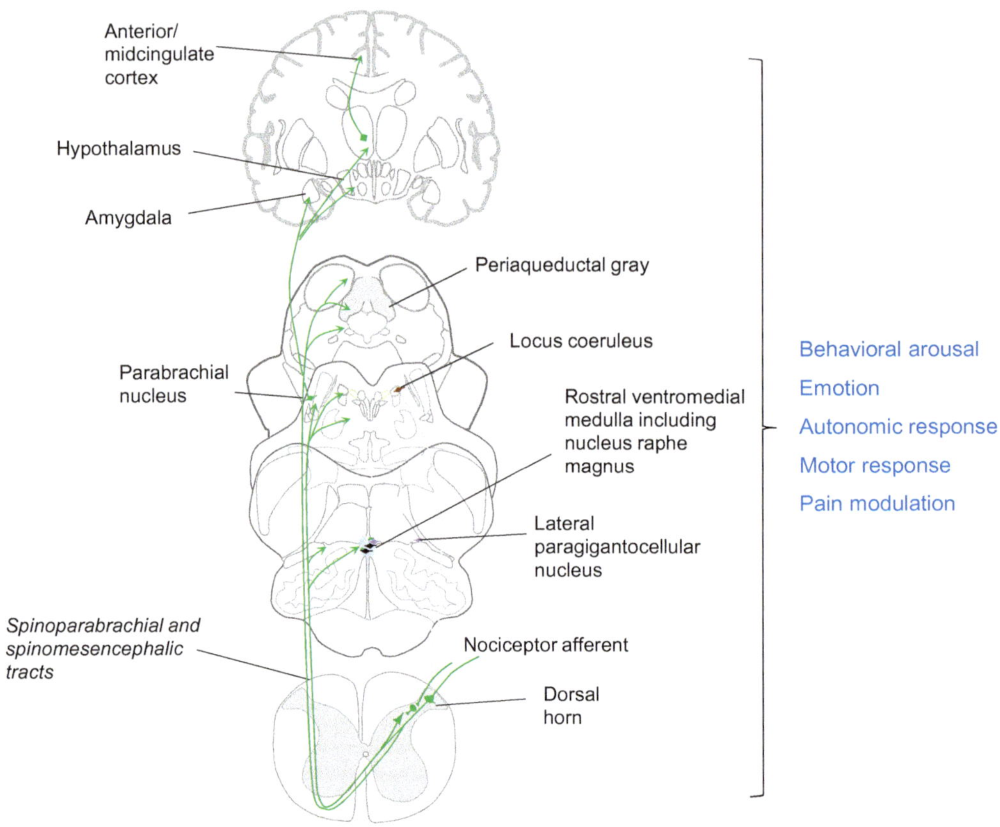

FIGURE 36.2 Spinoreticular and spinomesencephalic tracts.
Projections from nociceptive neurons of the spinal cord (or trigeminal nucleus caudalis) to the brainstem reticular formation integrate nociceptive activity with arousal, autonomic, and homeostatic responses. These pathways also trigger descending pain modulation and indirectly convey nociceptive information to forebrain regions involved in emotion and motivation. The spinoreticular tract originates particularly from laminae VII–VIII. The axons of many of these neurons decussate, ascend in the ventrolateral quadrant, and terminate in several nuclei of the brainstem reticular formation, including serotonergic and catecholaminergic groups; lateral reticular, paragigantocellular oral, and caudal reticular pontine nuclei; and, importantly, the parabrachial nucleus (PB). The PB receives an important input from lamina I of the dorsal horn (spinoparabrachial pathway) and is an important relay of nociceptive, visceral, and thermal information (interoceptive information). The PB provides interoceptive input to the hypothalamus, amygdala, and thalamus. The spinomesencephalic tract originates from laminae I and V and projects to the periaqueductal gray (PAG), cuneiform nucleus, superior colliculus, pretectal nuclei, red nucleus, and premotor oculomotor nuclei. Of particular relevance is the projection to the PAG, which is a nodal component of the central pain modulatory system.

in the ventromedial posterior portions of the thalamus.[17] The PB also sends an independent input to component of the pain modulatory circuit.

Spinomesencephalic Tract

The spinomesencephalic tract originates from laminae I and V and projects to the PAG, cuneiform nucleus, superior colliculus, pretectal nuclei, red nucleus, and premotor oculomotor nuclei. Of particular relevance is the projection to the PAG, which is a nodal component of the central pain modulatory system. The PAG consists of separate functional columns, dorsomedial, dorsolateral, lateral, and ventrolateral, which receive distinct projections from both the forebrain and ascending nociceptive pathways and initiate inputs and behavioral state-specific patterns of motor, autonomic, and pain-modulatory responses via descending projections to the brainstem.[18] The lateral and dorsolateral PAG column receives somatotopically organized inputs from superficial nociceptors (primarily Aδ type), relayed by lamina I of the spinal cord and caudal trigeminal nucleus. The ventrolateral PAG column receives convergent input from both the superficial and deep dorsal horn relaying nociceptive afferent information from visceral, muscle, and C-fiber skin nociceptors.

CORTICAL ACTIVATION DURING THE ACUTE PAIN EXPERIENCE

There is a large distributed brain network involved in nociceptive process that sustains the complex, multifactorial subjective experience of pain.

Pain Matrix

Several studies, including positron emission tomography (PET), fMRI, electroencephalography (EEG), and magnetoencephalography (MEG), have identified a common group of cortical regions activated during an acute pain experience in humans.[1,2,19] These areas comprise approximately 15% of the cortical surface and include the primary (S1) and secondary (S2) somatosensory cortex, insular cortex, and portions of the anterior cingulate cortex (ACC), midcingulate cortex (MCC), and prefrontal cortex (PFC). There areas have been defined as the "pain matrix." A large study using fMRI-based machine-learning analyses identified a pattern of fMRI activity across brain regions, or " neurologic signature," that were consistently associated with heat-induced pain. These included the secondary somatosensory cortex, posterior and anterior insula, ACC, thalamus, and PAG. This neural "pain signature" had high sensitivity and specificity in discriminating painful heat from nonpainful warmth and was also activated during pain anticipation, pain recall, and discriminating between physical pain and social pain.[2,15] These responses were substantially reduced with the administration of the μ-opioid agonist remifentanil.[2,15]

Individual Variability of Cortical Activation During the Acute Experience of Pain

The pain system has been classically thought of as having lateral (sensory-discriminatory) and medial (affective-cognitive-evaluative) neuroanatomical components.[20] However this concept is an oversimplification. Different brain regions have a more or less active role depending on the precise interplay of the factors involved in influencing pain perception, including attention and emotional state. Thus the pain matrix is an interactive and actively modulated group of brain regions that contribute to the pain experience.[2] However, almost none of the areas activated during acute pain are specific to nociception or to pain perception.[21] Both healthy individuals and patients with chronic pain report natural fluctuations in spontaneous pain that depend on attention to nociceptive stimuli and are reflected in changes of activation in several cortical areas including the medial prefrontal and anterior cingulate cortex.[4] Some of these areas are consistently activated during provoked, chronic, or imagined pain.

Insular Cortex, Interoception, and Body Feelings

The insular cortex is involved in a wide range of sensory, cognitive, affective, and motor functions and receives inputs from multiple sources. The posterior insula is involved in processing of primary sensations such as pain, temperatures, and visceral sensation as part of an interoceptive bodily representation.[11] (Figure 36.3) The dorsal posterior insula receives nociceptive inputs from contralateral lamina I of the dorsal horn or from the PB via the ventromedial posterior nucleus of the thalamus. One study suggested a specific role for the dorsal posterior insula in pain.[22] However, the specificity of the dorsal posterior insula for nociception has been questioned.[23] The posterior insula projects to the midinsula, which conveys multimodal inputs to the anterior insula. The anterior insula has reciprocal connections with the ACC, orbitofrontal cortex, and amygdala. Early fMRI studies showed that physical intensity of the pain stimulus correlates with activation of the posterior insula whereas perceived pain correlated with bilateral activation of the anterior insula.[24] According to one model, the posterior insula generates an internal cortical representation of homeostatic condition of the body by integrating pain with other interoceptive inputs and then provides this information to the anterior insula to generate the conscious "body feeling" and associated emotions.[24] The anterior insula is strongly activated when humans experience subjective feelings of the body and emotional awareness, including empathy for pain.[24–26]

Cingulate Cortex and Multiple Aspects of Pain Processing

The cingulate cortex includes three major divisions that form three different "limbic" subsystems.[27,28] The ACC is involved in emotional processing; the MCC in action-outcome learning and feedback-guided decision-making;

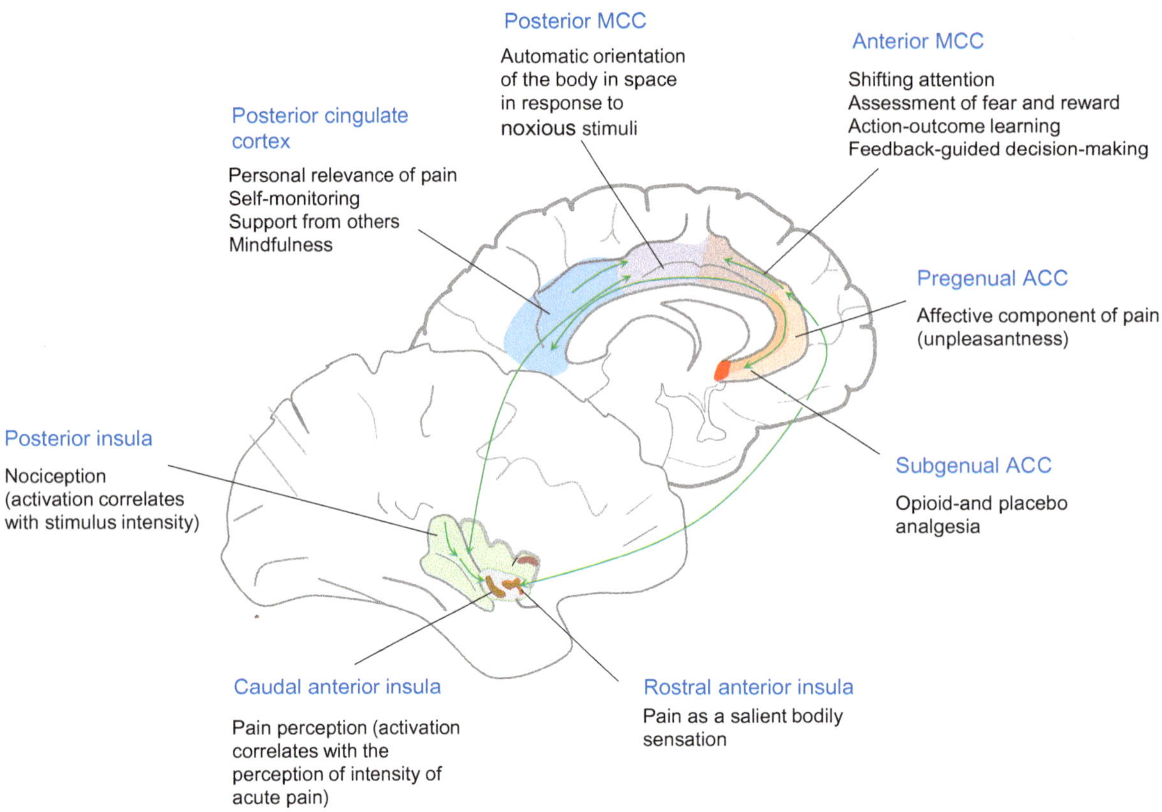

FIGURE 36.3 Cortical areas activated by acute pain.
The most common cortical regions activated during an acute pain experience in humans include the primary (S1) and secondary (S2) somatosensory cortex, insular cortex, anterior and midcingulate cortex, and prefrontal cortex (PFC) as well as the thalamus. The physical intensity of the pain stimulus correlates with activation of the posterior insula, whereas perceived pain correlates with bilateral activation of the anterior insula. The anterior insula is strongly activated when humans experience subjective feelings of the body and emotional awareness. The pregenual anterior cingulate cortex (ACC) has been linked to the emotional/affective component of pain and anxiety associated with pain anticipation. The anterior midcingulate cortex (MCC) may thus function as a hub where information about negative affective stimuli such as pain, can activate motor areas responsible for expression of affect, such as the face, and trigger execution of goal-directed behavior.

and the posterior cingulate cortex (PCC) in assessment of self-relevance of objects and events.[27,28] Each of these functional divisions has a distinct involvement in pain processing.[29] The main sources of nociceptive information to these cingulate areas are the mediodorsal, intralaminar, and midline thalamic nuclei, which convey inputs from the STT and PB.[29] The ACC is a component of the "anterior" limbic subsystem that includes the amygdala, orbitofrontal cortex, anterior insula, hypothalamus, nucleus accumbens (NAc), and PAG. The ACC includes subgenual (subcallosal) and pregenual subdivisions that are involved in emotional processing. The subgenual ACC is primarily activated by negatively valenced stimuli or episodic memories associated with sadness[30] and has direct projections to the hypothalamus and brainstem autonomic areas. The pregenual ACC has been linked to the emotional and affective components of pain, anxiety associated with pain anticipation, and learned changes in behavior in response noxious stimuli.[29,31] It is activated during acute noxious stimulation in proportion to the attention to unpleasantness of pain. Pregenual ACC activation is associated with that of other components of large-scale networks involved in experience of the bodily state; suppression of unwanted reflex-like actions; and ability to evaluate, respond to, and report bodily sensations and to share thoughts and feelings of others.[32,33] In experimental models, selective activation of pyramidal neurons in the ACC rapidly reduced the threshold for mechanical pain and hyperalgesia, whereas activation of parvalbumin GABAergic interneurons in this area had an opposite effect.[34] Neurons in the deep layers of the ACC send direct projections to subcortical areas involved in descending pain modulation.

The anterior MCC is the site most consistently activated in the response to acute noxious cutaneous stimulation and its activation primarily reflects pain-induced drive of attention.[35] It provides an interface between pain and affective and cognitive processing for action selection.[31,36] Together with the anterior insula, the anterior MCC forms the hub of an emotional/salience network that integrates interoceptive information with emotional salience to guide behavior and is also activated during empathy for pain, when individuals observed nociceptive stimulation of others.[37] The anterior MCC receives strong dopaminergic inputs from the ventral tegmental area, expresses high density of D1 receptors, and is involved in reward monitoring, action-reinforcement associations, and response selection and is thus a site of overlap between the pain (aversive) and reward systems.[31] The prediction of either pain or reward outcomes helps in selecting the appropriate action of behavior and may be in part determined by fear evoked by nociceptive inputs conveyed by the thalamus and the amygdala. Imaging studies demonstrate that physical pain, social pain, and negative affect activate an overlapping region of the anterior MCC.[36] A study using electrical stimulation during presurgical evaluation of patients with medically refractory epilepsy showed that whereas stimulation of the pregenual ACC elicited interoceptive, emotional, and autonomic responses, that of the anterior MCC elicited complex motor behaviors, but no pain.[38] The primary role of posterior MCC is the reflexive orientation of the body in space in response to noxious stimuli independent on reward or emotional value.[31] Whereas the main source of nociceptive input to the posterior MCC are the intralaminar and midline thalamic nuclei, parietal nociceptive neurons provide context for visual and spatial orientation that provide orienting, anticipatory information reaches the posterior MCC.[31]

The PCC is a core component of the default mode network involved in conscious processing of pain experience and reappraisal of pain perception by self-relevant contextual events and memories. The PCC has robust reciprocal connections with the subgenual ACC. Intracranial recordings in humans evaluated for epilepsy surgery show that both the PCC and the ACC had a delayed activation in response to nociceptive heat inputs and that this delayed response persists well after the occurrence of conscious pain perception; this response may thus underlie processes such as self-awareness and pain modulation (Fig. 36.3).[39]

ROLES OF ATTENTION, COGNITION, AND CONTEXT IN PAIN MODULATION

Attentional and emotional factors differentially influence pain sensation via descending pathways from the prefrontal cortex, ACC cingulate cortex, and amygdala to the PAG.[5]

Fluctuations of Pain and Dynamic Brain Connectome

Pain is often dynamic in nature; the experienced intensity and quality of pain sensation can vary from moment to moment. Whereas primary afferent nociceptors do not usually show spontaneous activity, nociceptive neurons in the CNS can show ongoing activity even in the absence of any overt noxious stimulus; however this spontaneous activity is not sufficient to create pain.[40] Spontaneous brain-network dynamics are thus relevant for understanding the neural substrate of acute and chronic pain, as well as individual differences in pain vulnerability and coping ability.[3,40] Background low-frequency fluctuations in functional connectivity across large-scale networks defined by fMRI strongly affect pain perception. These networks include the salience and attention networks activated during behaviorally relevant tasks, and the default mode network, which is active when a person is engaged in internal thoughts ("mind wandering") and disengaged from the environment. Resting-state fMRI studies in healthy subjects showed that intrinsic brain activity correlates with individual variability in the natural tendency to attend to pain.[3] The relevance of ongoing activity of large-scale networks in influencing subsequent pain perception led to the introduction of the term "dynamic pain connectome."[3,40] In one study, whereas most brain regions were activated by noxious stimuli, the degree of activation varied from trial to trial depending on the fluctuating degree of attention to pain.[3] Spontaneous mind-wandering away from pain was associated with activity on the default mode network and interconnected areas such as medial PFC and the PAG;[3] this predicted a reduced subsequent pain sensation in response to application of a nociceptive stimulus.[41] The structural and dynamic functional connectivity between the medial PFC and the PAG varied according to each subject's propensity to attend to or mind wander away from pain.[3] The trait-like characteristic of prioritizing attentional demands over pain versus allowing pain to interfere with attention also modifies the individual susceptibility to pain.[3] Cognitive self-regulatory mechanisms, including self-generated context and imagery can also modulate affective processes, including negative emotions associated with chronic pain. Functional resonance imaging studies show that both intensity of painful stimuli (bottom-up input) and self-regulatory strategies (top-down modulation) strongly influence the reported pain sensation in normal persons.[5] One such study showed the nociceptive/affective pain responses are dissociated from cognitive/evaluative aspects of pain.[42] Whereas the intensity of a painful stimulus (noxious heat) was encoded by the activity within the brain pain signature network, self-regulation involved functional connections between the ventromedial PFC cortex and the NAc.[42]

Nucleus Accumbens, Motivational State, and Pain Modulation

The NAc has a critical role in processing of rewards and cognitive control of decision-making, and motivation. These functions primarily depend on the influence of dopaminergic inputs from the ventral tegmental area (VTA) and interactions with the PFC and MCC. The NAc is a key structure mediating motivational processes and via its connections provides a common circuit for drug addiction and in top-down modulation of pain,[43,44] including opioid analgesia.[45] The dopamine signals in response to painful stimuli vary in the different portions of the NAc. In anesthetized rats, acute painful tail pinch triggers a time-locked release of dopamine in the NAc core signaling the salience of the aversive event; termination of the painful stimulus is associated with dopamine release in the NAc shell, indicating the rewarding effect of pain alleviation.[46] Optogenetic activation of the medial PFC produced a strong antinociceptive effect and relieved the aversive quality of pain in a rat model of chronic neuropathic pain; this antinociceptive effect was mediated by glutamatergic inputs to the NAc.[47] Functional MRI studies show that activity of the NAc correlates with that of the VTA, which signals reward and motivation, and with that of the PAG, which is involved in descending pain modulation. In one study, pain onset was associated with negative signal and pain relief with a positive signal change in the NAc; opposite changes occurred in the ACC.[48] In another study, there was increased activity in the putative shell region of the NAc upon anticipation of an impending painful stimulus presumably reflecting the prediction of the salience signal; there was increased activity in the putative NAc core at the prediction of pain offset reflecting the anticipated reinforcement value of pain relief.[49]

BRAINSTEM PAIN MODULATORY SYSTEM

The descending pain modulatory system is a network that regulates nociceptive processing within the dorsal horn to produce either facilitation or inhibition. It includes the PAG, bulbospinal neurons of the rostral ventromedial medulla (RVMM), including the serotonergic neurons of the nucleus raphe magus and adjacent lateral paragigantocellular nucleus (LPGi); caudal ventrolateral medulla; dorsal reticular nucleus; noradrenergic neurons of the locus coeruleus and adjacent A5 group; and the A11 group of the hypothalamus projecting to the spinal cord.[50] (Figure 36.4) Many of the areas of the descending pain modulatory network receive inputs both from neurons relaying nociceptive information, such as those in the dorsal horn and PB, and from forebrain regions involved in processing affective and emotional responses to pain, including medial PFC, ACC, amygdala, and hypothalamus. This system has an important roles in pain inhibition and mediates the so-called diffuse noxious inhibitory control, which involves descending inhibition of the dorsal horn neurons receiving nociceptive input when a painful input is applied to a remote body part outside of the receptive field of the recorded neurons.[51] Neurons of this network also express opioid receptors and mediate opioid-, placebo-, and acupuncture-triggered analgesia. However, the system can also promote pain facilitation, particularly in chronic pain states. The balance between inhibition and facilitation of nociception via this system is dynamic and can be altered in different behavioral, emotional, and pathologic states.[50,52]

Periaqueductal Gray

The PAG is a critical component of the so-called emotional motor system,[53,54] which is a distributed network that receives input from the medial PFC, ACC, amygdala, and hypothalamus and projects to brainstem areas that control behavior-specific patterns of motor and autonomic responses. The PAG consists of separate columns that receive different types of nociceptive inputs and trigger distinct responses to pain and other stressors. The lateral column of the PAG receives inputs from skin nociceptors; in experimental animals, stimulation of the lateral PAG triggers active copying or fight-or-flight responses, characterized by motor activation, sympathetic excitation, and opioid-independent analgesia. In contrast, the ventrolateral PAG receives inputs from visceral and muscle receptors and is also activated by repetitive stimulation of skin nociceptors. In experimental animals, activation of the ventrolateral PAG elicits a passive copying or "paying death" response characterized by immobility, sympathetic inhibition, parasympathetic activation, and opioid-dependent analgesia. These responses are mediated by distinct projections from each column of the PAG to different neuronal groups in the medulla. The connections of the PAG in humans have been studied using diffusion tractography.[55] A human study using high-resolution fMRI confirmed the functional subdivisions of the PAG identified in animals.[56] This study showed differential activation different portions of the PAG while participants were exposed to emotionally aversive images. Feeling of anger were associated with diminished activity in ventrolateral "passive-coping" columns, whereas self-reported sadness correlated with activity in the rostral lateral region suggesting and approach-oriented activity in a column involved in active-coping.[56]

The PAG has a complex neurochemical organization that includes glutamatergic, GABAergic, and dopaminergic neurons. Of relevance in the setting of pain modulation are glutamatergic neurons projecting to the RVMM and other lower brainstem modulatory regions, and local GABAergic neurons that tonically inhibit these PAG projection neurons. GABAergic neurons in the PAG express μ-opioid receptors (MORs) and are a critical target for opioid-induced analgesia.[57] Stimulation of the ventrolateral PAG elicits analgesia in humans.[58] Neurons in this region also express cannabinoid 1 receptors (CB1R) that produce analgesia.[59] Electroacupuncture has substantial antinociceptive effects both in inflammatory and neuropathic pain models, inhibits GABAergic neurons, and activates glutamatergic neurons in this CB1R expressing region of the PAG.[59]

Rostral Ventromedial Medulla

The RVMM receives a dense input from the ventrolateral PAG and sends diffuse bilateral projections that terminate at multiple levels of the dorsal horn. The RVMM exerts a bidirectional effect on nociception. It contains "OFF-cells" that show a pause in their activity upon exposure to

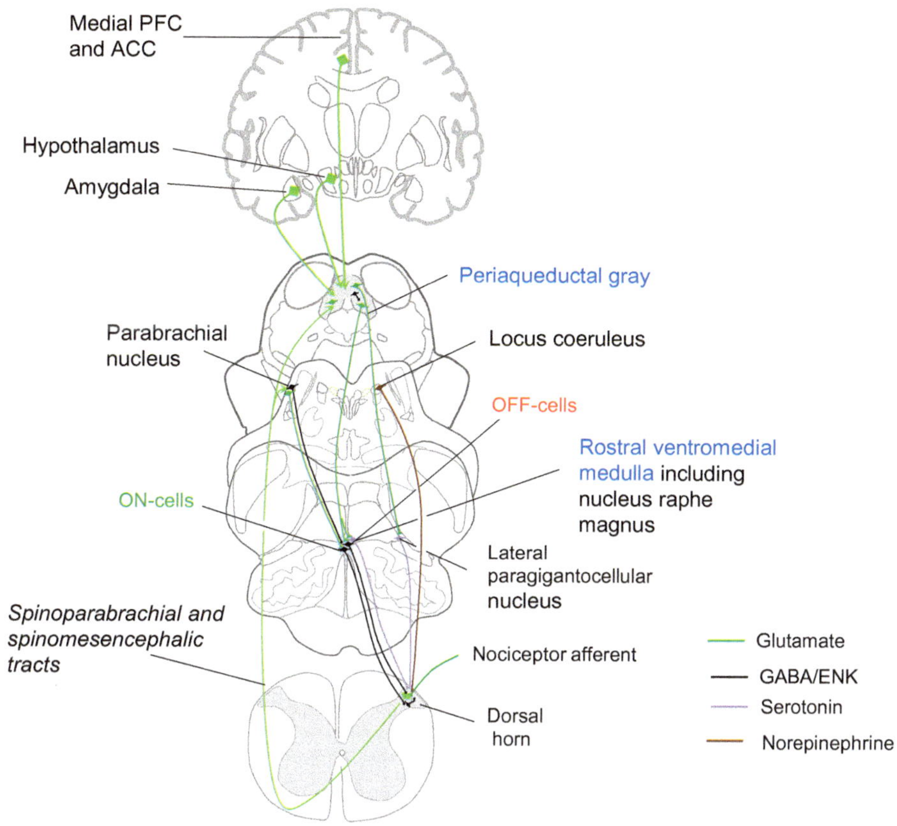

FIGURE 36.4 Descending pain modulatory system.

The descending pain modulatory system includes the periaqueductal gray (PAG) and its projection to bulbospinal neurons of the rostral ventromedial medulla (RVMM), including the serotonergic neurons of the nucleus raphe magus (RMg) and adjacent lateral paragigantocellular nucleus (LPGi); noradrenergic neurons of the locus coeruleus and adjacent A5 group; and the A11 group of the hypothalamus projecting to the spinal cord (not shown). Many of the areas of the descending pain modulatory network receive inputs both from neurons relaying nociceptive information such as those in the dorsal horn and parabrachial nucleus and from forebrain regions involved in processing affective and emotional responses to pain, including medial prefrontal cortex (PFC), anterior cingulate cortex (ACC), amygdala, and hypothalamus. The RVMM exerts a bidirectional effect on nociception. It contains "OFF-cells" that elicit analgesia and "ON-cells" that elicit hyperalgesia. The pathway by which nociceptive inputs gain access to the RVMM ON- and OFF-cells involves the parabrachial nucleus. This nucleus sends direct glutamatergic and GABAergic inputs to RVMM neurons, producing a net inhibitory input to OFF-cells and net excitatory input to ON-cells engaged by acute noxious stimulation. The majority of the RVMM output to the dorsal horn consists of dual GABA/enkephalinergic projections that exert presynaptic inhibition of nociceptive afferents. "ON-cells" of the RVMM are GABAergic and facilitate mechanical pain nociception by inhibiting dorsal horn interneurons involved in presynaptic inhibition of somatosensory neurons.[62,63,67,69] Serotonergic neurons in the nucleus raphe magnus (RMg) and lateral paragigantocellular nucleus (LPGi) are activated by noxious thermal stimuli and may participate in different mechanisms of pain modulation.

a noxious stimulus, and "ON-cells" that show a burst of activity in this condition. Stimulation of OFF-cells elicits analgesia, whereas that of ON-cells elicits hyperalgesia.[50,60] The pathway by which nociceptive inputs gain access to the RVMM ON- and OFF-cells involves the PB.[61] This nucleus sends direct glutamatergic and GABAergic inputs to the RVMM, producing a net inhibitory input on OFF-cells and activation of ON-cells. The majority of projections from the RVMM to the dorsal horn are dual GABA/enkephalinergic, but some are purely GABAergic, serotonergic, or glutamatergic. These inputs project through the dorsolateral funiculus and primarily innervate layers I, II, and V.[62] Activation of GABA/enkephalinergic cells corresponding to the "OFF" cells of the RVMM decreases sensitivity to noxious heat and mechanical stimuli.[62] Both GABA and enkephalin can exert presynaptic inhibition of the sensory afferents. However, about half of the ON-cells of the RVMM are GABAergic; they may facilitate mechanical pain nociception by inhibiting dorsal horn GABA/enkephalinergic interneurons involved in presynaptic inhibition of somatosensory neurons.[63] The dorsal reticular nucleus receives bilateral projections from lamina I, IV–VII, and X and sends excitatory projections to the dorsal horn, thus potentially participating in an excitatory spino-medullo-spinal pronociceptive circuit.

Monoaminergic Groups

Descending monoaminergic inputs also provide a complex control of nociceptive processing in the dorsal horn. Serotonergic neurons in the nucleus raphe magnus and LPGi in the adjacent ventrolateral medulla are activated by noxious thermal stimuli and may participate in different mechanisms of pain modulation.[64] The specific activation of neurons in the LPGi nucleus by intense noxious stimuli suggests its involvement in antinociceptive feedback control in response to unbearable pain that triggers a defense reaction. The LPGi receives major afferent projection from the dorsolateral PAG, which is involved in sympathetic and motor activation and analgesia associated with this defense reaction. In contrast, the serotonergic neurons of the nucleus raphe magnus receive their main input from the ventrolateral PAG and might respond to inescapable pain that induces passive coping behavior with immobility, decreased cardiac activity, and strong analgesia.[64]

The effects of monoamines on transmission in the dorsal horn are complex. They involve different receptor subtypes located at the primary nociceptive afferents, dorsal horn projection neurons, local excitatory or inhibitory interneurons, and glial cells. There is a crosstalk between descending monoaminergic and local neurochemical signals, such as adenosine, endogenous opioids, and nitric oxide. Presynaptic reuptake via selective transporters and control of release via presynaptic inhibitory autoreceptors regulates the local concentration of monoamines and thus their effects on the targets in the dorsal horn. These antinociceptive effects typically involve presynaptic inhibitory receptors that reduce release of glutamate and neuropeptides from primary afferents. These include presynaptic 5-$HT1_B$, α2 adrenergic, and D2 dopaminergic receptors. Norepinephrine may also elicit antinociception via excitatory α1 receptors located in local GABAergic and glycinergic inhibitory neurons.

Triggers of Descending Pain Modulation

Many brain areas involved in attention, motivation, emotion, fear, and mood strongly influence pain sensation via the descending brainstem modulatory network. They include the medial PFC, ACC, insula, amygdala, and hypothalamus. All these areas project to the PAG, RVMM, and other brainstem cell groups. Of particular relevance in chronic pain mechanisms are inputs from the ACC to the PAG and dorsal horn.[65] In addition, inputs from nociceptive dorsal horn neurons to the PAG, RVMM, and catecholaminergic cell groups as well as inputs from the PB to the RVMM may trigger excitatory or inhibitory spino-bulbo-spinal feedback loops that are affected by forebrain influences and may amplify the pain state.[52] The overall balance between inhibitory and excitatory supraspinal signals provides the basis for top-down modulation of pain sensation according to motivation, emotion, and other behavioral variables (Figure 36.5).[5]

OPIOID-MEDIATED ANALGESIA, TOLERANCE, AND PLACEBO EFFECTS

Opioid Signaling

Opioids have a critical role in endogenous responses to pain, reward, and motivation. There are four main types of opioid : μ (mu, MOR), δ (delta, DOR), κ (kappa, KOR), and orphan receptors. In general, MORs are activated by β-endorphin and enkephalins, DORs by enkephalins, and KORs by dynorphins. Pain therapy primarily targets the MORs, which are expressed at all levels of the pain modulatory pathway, including the ACC, PAG, RVMM, and dorsal horn. Opioid receptors are G protein-coupled receptors that are coupled to $G_{i/o}$ signaling, which triggers inhibitory transduction pathways at both postsynaptic and presynaptic sites. They include activation of G protein inward-rectifying potassium channels (GIRK) that hyperpolarize target cells, and inhibition of presynaptic calcium channels (Ca_v2) and thus neurotransmitter release. Activation of opioid receptors also inhibits adenylyl cyclase and thus cyclic adenylyl monophosphate (cAMP) production, and may activate other signaling proteins, such as protein kinase C and extracellular signal-regulated kinase via β-arrestin pathways, which are independent of G protein signaling.[57]

Mechanisms of Analgesic Effects

The MOR-expressing GABAergic neurons within the ventrolateral PAG are critical targets for the analgesic effects of opioids. Under normal conditions, these neurons have tonic activity and inhibit the ventrolateral PAG neurons projecting to the RVMM. Activation of MOR reduces tonic activity of these GABAergic neurons, which results in an increase in the output from the ventrolateral PAG to the RVMM.[66] The ventrolateral PAG targets both OFF- and ON-cells of the RVMM. Some studies suggest that whereas glutamatergic projections from the PAG excite OFF-cells the PAG also provides GABAergic projection that inhibits ON-cells. However, a major effect of opioids is disinhibition of the ventrolateral PAG promoting activity of OFF cells in the RVMM, which via GABA/enkephalinergic projections inhibit pain transmission in the dorsal horn. This has been classically referred to as supraspinal analgesia. Another important target for opioid-mediated analgesia is the ACC. Studies in rodents show that the effect of opioids within the pregenual ACC is to selectively modulate the affective qualities of neuropathic pain.[67] Opioids, acting via MORs inhibit pyramidal projection neurons of the ACC projecting to the PAG. The ACC-to-PAG projection is thought to be involved

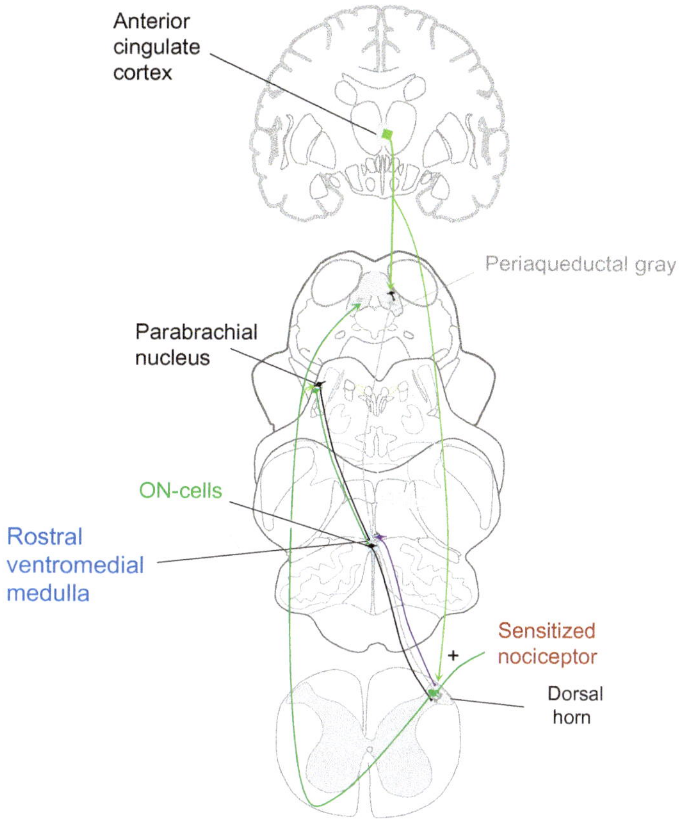

FIGURE 36.5 Descending pain facilitation.
The anterior cingulate cortex (ACC) is a key cortical control for descending facilitation systems. Increased activity of pyramidal neurons in the ACC may elicit potentiation of pain both via the periaqueductal gray (PAG)–rostral ventromedial medulla (RVMM) pathway and through direct corticospinal projection to superficial layers of the dorsal horn. Descending pain facilitation involves serotonergic inputs from the RVMM to the dorsal horn and is triggered by intense activation of the RVMM. Inputs from the parabrachial nucleus to ON-cells of the RVMM may indirectly promote pain via inhibition of dorsal horn inhibitory interneurons. The facilitatory effects of descending serotonergic inputs in nociceptive transmission in the dorsal horn are largely mediated by 5-HT3 receptors.

in hyperalgesia in the setting of chronic pain, perhaps by activating the local GABAergic neurons in the PAG.[65] Opioids also elicit spinal analgesia at the level of the dorsal horn. The inhibitory effects of local GABA/enkephalin interneurons on glutamate and substance P release from C-nociceptive afferents is mediated by presynaptic MORs.

Mechanisms of Opioid Tolerance

Long-term opioid treatment leads to adaptations in many signaling proteins that mediate the effects of MORs within the PAG-RVMM-dorsal horn pathway; this has have been proposed as a mechanism of opioid tolerance. In contrast to the acute inhibitory effect of opioids on cAMP production, chronic morphine treatment upregulates cAMP via compensatory changes in intracellular signaling. The mechanisms underlying tolerance may be dependent on the specific MOR agonist. For example, morphine does not readily recruit β-arrestin or internalize the receptor, whereas high-efficacy agonists such as fentanyl readily do both. This difference in signaling suggests differences in tolerance mechanisms.[57] Cholecystokinin, which is expressed in the PAG–RVMM–dorsal horn pathway blocks opioid activation of OFF-cells and may also regulate opioid tolerance. Many other signaling targets in the PAG and dorsal horn have been implicated in opioid tolerance.

Opioids are potent activators of microglia within the CNS, and microglial inflammation is a strong contributor to the development of opioid tolerance.[68] Activated microglia release cytokines and brain-derived neurotrophic factor, which promote excitation of STT neurons and reduce efficacy of local inhibition. These mechanisms lead to increased sensibility to pain the setting of chronic opioid use. Opioids activate the immune receptor, toll-like receptor 4 (TLR4), triggering a prominent proinflammatory signaling. The TLR4 signaling pathway involves activation of sphingomyelinase with production of ceramide, triggering downstream cascades for cell survival, apoptosis, and release of proinflammatory cytokines. Activation of TLR4 signaling can induce "naïve tolerance" to opioids whereas inhibition of TLR4, its co-activators, or ceramide biosynthesis, leads to attenuation of morphine tolerance and decreased microglial activation.

Placebo and Opioid Analgesia

Placebo and nocebo effects refer to the effects of the patient's positive and negative expectations and constitute models to understand how the psychosocial context modulates the experience of pain.[69] Placebo effects are associated with the release of endogenous opioids, endocannabinoids, dopamine, oxytocin, and vasopressin in a target-specific manner. For example, dopamine release has a role in placebo effects in Parkinson disease but not in treatment of pain. Placebo induces activation of opioid neurotransmission in the ACC, NAc, and PAG and dopaminergic activation in the NAc.[70] A negative context, for example, through verbal suggestion, elicits a nocebo effect and exacerbates pain through the activation of cholecystokinin and the deactivation of the opioid and dopamine systems.[71] Genetic influences may affect the placebo and nocebo effects mediated by these neurotransmitters. Placebo effects related to pain have only small effects on the fMRI correlates of pain.[2] However, combined psychophysical analysis and imaging studies showed changes in connectivity of the PFC and insula with components of the pain modulatory network during both placebo and nocebo responses.[72] The PAG and RVMM have consistently been shown to be activated during placebo analgesia, acupuncture analgesia, and anxiety-induced hyperalgesia.[73] The pregenual ACC has a major role in recruitment of brain modulatory areas mediating placebo- and endogenous opioid-dependent analgesia.[74] The opioid antagonist naloxone acutely reduced both placebo analgesia and associated responses in pain-modulatory cortical structures, such as the pregenual ACC, PAG, and RVMM, and their functional coupling with each other.[75] In contrast, nocebo effects can cause increased signaling from the spinal cord to the brain. Stress and memory may have a role in the expectation of the effects of treatment. The molecular events and changes in network activity are mediated by the anticipation of future outcomes. Expectations can be affected by changes in perception and cognition and may be acquired from previous experiences, verbal instruction, or social observation. Learning and classical conditioning play a role in both placebo and nocebo effects.

MECHANISMS OF CHRONIC PAIN

Emerging evidence suggests that chronic pain is associated with altered functional connectivity in areas involved in affective-emotional processing and in components of the descending pain modulatory system. In humans, the diffuse noxious inhibitory control system is studied using the "conditioned pain stimulation" paradigm, in which a painful stimulus delivered to one part of the body suppresses pain resulting from a standardized noxious stimulus applied to a remote body part. Patients with chronic pain have inability to initiate this conditioned pain modulation.[72,76]

Disrupted Functional Connectivity Within the Pain Control System

Studies have shown abnormalities in functional connectivity within the pain control system, including the PAG, in patients with chronic pain.[77–79] Brain activity in relation to subjective pain gradually shifts dynamically away from sensory to limbic cortical regions.[49] The degree of disruption of intrinsic connectivity within the pain modulatory system correlates with individual differences in pain intensity and duration. For example, in patients with chronic pain disorders, increased functional connectivity between the medial PFC and other components of the default mode network with the PAG relates to individual differences in rumination with repetitive focus on discomforting emotion or stimuli.[80] The strength of functional connectivity between the medial PFC and the NAc predicted the risk of patients with back pain to transition to chronicity.[49] This increased connectivity may in part reflect a compensatory mechanism, as activation of the PFC-NAc pathway has a beneficial effect on experimental models of pain. Abnormalities in functional connectivity in chronic pain may be partially reversible on successful treatment.[81] Functional neuroimaging studies showed that lack of conditioned pain modulation analgesia was associated with greater signal intensity in the mid-cingulate and dorsolateral prefrontal cortices and increased functional connectivity with the dorsal reticular nucleus, compared with individuals who showed normal conditioned pain modulation.

Cingulate Cortex and Descending Pain Facilitation

After injury, neurons in the periphery and brain show aberrant spontaneous activity. Nerve injury induces ectopic activity in primary afferents and abnormal bursting in the central nociceptive system, including the deafferented thalamus. Chronic pain causes long-term neuroplasticity, including dysregulation of thalamocortical oscillations in the sensory thalamus due to ectopic firing of thalamocortical neurons reflecting abnormal expression of ion channels.[82] Chronic pain states in part reflect dysfunction in descending pain modulatory systems.[83] Whereas both chronic inflammatory and neuropathic pain involve central plasticity, their mechanism and underlying pathways and central circuits are different.[84] Under pathological conditions, long-term activation of descending facilitation may contribute to chronic pain via a positive feedback mechanism. The ACC is a key cortical control for this descending facilitation. Studies in vitro show potentiation of glutamatergic synapses with increased excitability of ACC neurons in animal models of chronic pain.[85] Synaptic plasticity in the ACC includes both postsynaptic and presynaptic long-term potentiation (LTP). Postsynaptic LTP involves N-methyl-D-aspartate receptors (NMDARs) and Ca^{2+} signaling. Local activation of astrocytes may contribute to enhanced activity in the ACC.[65] Increased activity of pyramidal neurons in the ACC may elicit potentiation of pain both via the PAG-RVMM pathway and through direct corticospinal projection to superficial layers of the dorsal horn.[86] In several models of chronic pain, lesions of the ACC attenuate the affective component of the pain state. Optogenetic studies in mice showed that thalamic projections from the mediodorsal nucleus may be involved in conveying aversive information to the ACC in the setting of chronic pain.[87] In contrast, chronic pain induced strengthening of excitatory synapses from the basolateral amygdala to the ACC, which opposed the aversive aspects of chronic pain.[87] Whereas the ACC has a critical role in promoting chronic pain, recent studies in mice show that the MCC also gates sensory hypersensitivity and modulates nociceptive sensory plasticity via a direct pathway to the posterior insular cortex.[88] This pathway may amplify perception in the setting of nociception via insular projections to serotonergic neurons of the RVMM mediating descending pain facilitation.[88]

Plasticity of the Bulbospinal Pain Modulatory System

Studies in rodents indicate that the RVMM also undergoes plastic neurochemical changes that limit hyperalgesia in chronic inflammatory pain.[80] Inputs from the lateral PB to the RVMM activated by sensitized superficial dorsal horn neurons may have an important role in the transition from acute to chronic pain.[89] Descending pain facilitation involves serotonergic inputs from the RVMM to the dorsal horn and is triggered by intense activation of the RVMM.[90–92] The facilitatory effect of serotonin on spinal neural responses is more robust for visceral than for cutaneous thermal noxious stimuli and is mediated by 5-HT3 receptors. Several inputs to the RVMM may trigger serotonergic descending facilitation of nociceptive dorsal horn circuits. One possible source are inputs from superficial dorsal horn neurons, either directly or via the PB, triggering a spino-bulbo-spinal reflex that potentiates nociceptive transmission in the setting of peripheral or spinal injury. Serotonergic input may also promote dorsal horn sensitization via neuron–glial interactions. Intrathecal administration of a 5-HT3R agonist triggered neuron-to-microglia signaling via the chemokine fractalkine, microglia-to-astrocyte signaling via interleukin (IL)-18, and astrocyte-to-neuron signaling via IL-1β. All these interactions lead to increased activation of NMDARs and hyperexcitability of spinal projection neurons. Ondansetron, a 5-HT3 antagonist acutely alleviates mechanical allodynia in patients with neuropathic pain.[84–86] The reciprocal excitatory interactions between the dorsal horn and the medullary dorsal reticular nucleus may also contribute to maintenance of the chronic pain state.

Role of the Mesolimbic System and Motivation

Behavioral manifestations of chronic pain states, including avoidance behavior also involve plasticity in the NAc. Studies in transgenic mice with experimental chronic neuropathic pain showed that development of tactile allodynia is associated with increased excitability of indirect pathway medium spiny neurons in the medial shell of the NAc, reflecting reduced D2 receptor signaling in these neurons and leading to action avoidance.[93,94] Maladaptive plasticity in the NAc core may result in reduced motivation in the setting of chronic pain. In experimental mouse models, induction of chronic neuropathic or inflammatory pain was associated with reduced performance in a test measuring behavioral motivation; this as associated with altered subunit expression and kinetics of NMDARs in indirect pathway medium spiny neurons of the NAc core.[95] The recognition of the importance of the reward/motivation circuit centered in the NAc in emotional and cognitive components of chronic pain provides rationale for therapeutic approaches. For example, dopaminergic therapy aimed to modulate plasticity of the indirect pathway in the NAc may be helpful to prevent manifestations such as allodynia, reduced motivation, and depression associated with chronic pain. Consistent with this possibility, a pilot study showed that transdermal rotigotine may be beneficial for treatment of chronic pain associated with Parkinson disease.[96] Bupropion and other drugs that inhibit dopamine transporters may have analgesic effect by increasing dopamine levels in the NAc.

Therapeutic Implications

Different portions of the cingulate cortex may be distinctly involved in different aspects of opioid and placebo-induced analgesia.[29] The pregenual ACC has the highest level of opioid receptor binding and is the major site of the opioid-mediated placebo effect. The subgenual/pregenual ACC recruits descending pain inhibitory control pathways via the PAG during analgesia triggered by endogenous opioid release, placebo, distraction from pain, and habituation to pain.[35] In contrast, analgesia induced by hypnosis, which may reflect reduction of fear, primarily targets the anterior MCC, and acupuncture-induced analgesia activates the posterior MCC.[29] The ACC and PCC are activated during self-reported reduction in pain perception induced by hypnosis or by empathetic verbal feedback from others.[97] Deep brain stimulation (DBS) has long been considered for treatment of patients with intractable pain syndromes. The most common targets are the PAG/periventricular gray matter region, VPL/VPM or both, and ventral posterior lateral/posterior medial thalamus. Other targets include the ACC, anterior limb of the internal capsule, and centromedian/parafascicular nucleus of the thalamus. The most common indications have been post-stroke pain, phantom limb pain, and brachial plexus injury. Outcomes have varied between studies and across chronic pain diagnoses.[98] Deep brain stimulation or transcranial magnetic stimulation of the ACC, which provides a major input to the NAc and is key component of the reward/motivation circuit, may also provide pain relief.[99] The entry of self-relevant information into the PCC may leads the revaluation of pain intensity perception via interchange with the ACC and the sequential engagement of the descending pain control system via the PAG.[35] Stimulation of the motor cortex below the threshold of motor excitability could induce elicits changes in regional cerebral blood flow in both the ACC and anterior MCC, and these changes are correlated with the magnitude of analgesic effect and associated with activation of the endogenous opioid system.[35]

KEY POINTS

- Pain is a complex sensation that has sensory-discriminative, cognitive-, and affective-emotional dimensions.
- The experience of pain triggers somatic and autonomic reflexes, memories, and changes in emotional state and motivation.
- The spinothalamic tract (STT) is functionally heterogeneous and targets different portions of the thalamus projecting to different projections to the cortex.
- Projections from nociceptive neurons to the brainstem reticular formation trigger arousal, autonomic and homeostatic responses, and descending pain modulation.
- There is a large distributed brain network involved in nociceptive processes that sustains the complex, multifactorial subjective experience of pain.
- This network, referred to as "pain matrix or "neural pain signature," includes the primary (S1) and secondary (S2) somatosensory cortex, insular cortex, portions of the anterior cingulate cortex (ACC) and midcingulate cortex (MCC), and prefrontal cortex (PFC).
- The anterior insula is strongly activated when humans experience subjective feelings of the body and emotional awareness.
- The pregenual ACC has been linked to the emotional/affective component of pain.
- The anterior midcingulate cortex (MCC) is a hub where information about negative stimuli, including pain, can lead to activation of goal-directed behavior.
- Fluctuations in activity of the attention, salience, and default mode networks correlate with individual variability in the natural tendency to attend to and perceive acute pain.
- The reward and motivation circuit, including the dopaminergic neurons of the ventral tegmental area and the nucleus accumbens (NAc), is activated during pain cessation.
- Interactive networks involved in attention and motivation provide input to a brainstem pain modulatory system that may either suppress or potentiate nociceptive transmission.
- The descending pain modulatory network includes the periaqueductal gray (PAG), the rostral ventromedial medulla (RVMM) including serotonergic neurons of the nucleus raphe magus and adjacent LPGi, and the locus coeruleus and adjacent noradrenergic groups.
- The RVMM exerts a bidirectional effect on pain processing via OFF-cells and ON-cells projecting to the dorsal horn.
- The effects of monoamines on transmission in the dorsal horn are complex and involve different receptor subtypes located at the primary nociceptive afferents, dorsal horn projection neurons, local excitatory or inhibitory interneurons, and glial cells.
- Opioids elicit supraspinal analgesia by inhibiting local GABAergic neurons in the PAG and RVMM, thus promoting descending pain inhibition.
- Opioids elicit spinal analgesia by presynaptically and postsynaptically inhibiting transmission of nociceptive input in the dorsal horn.
- Placebo induces activation of opioid neurotransmission in the ACC, NAc, and PAG and dopaminergic activation in the NAc.
- Chronic pain alters functional connectivity in areas involved in affective-emotional processing and in components of the descending pain modulatory system.
- Synaptic plasticity in the ACC is a key component of pain facilitation.
- Descending pain facilitation involves serotonergic inputs triggered by intense activation of the RVMM.
- Behavioral manifestations of chronic pain states, including avoidance behavior and reduced motivation involve plasticity in the NAc.
- Deep brain stimulation (DBS) may provide benefit to patients with intractable pain syndromes.

REFERENCES

1. Apkarian AV, Reckziegel D. Peripheral and central viewpoints of chronic pain, and translational implications. Neurosci Lett 2019;702:3–5.
2. Wager TD, Atlas LY, Lindquist MA, Roy M, Woo CW, Kross E. An fMRI-based neurologic signature of physical pain. N Engl J Med 2013;368:1388–1397.
3. Kucyi A, Davis KD. The dynamic pain connectome. Trends Neurosci 2015;38:86–95.
4. Baliki MN, Chialvo DR, Geha PY, et al. Chronic pain and the emotional brain: specific brain activity associated with spontaneous fluctuations of intensity of chronic back pain. J Neurosci 2006;26:12165–12173.

5. Bushnell MC, Ceko M, Low LA. Cognitive and emotional control of pain and its disruption in chronic pain. Nat Rev Neurosci 2013;14:502–511.
6. Willis WD, Jr. The somatosensory system, with emphasis on structures important for pain. Brain Res Rev 2007;55:297–313.
7. Ren Y, Zhang L, Lu Y, Yang H, Westlund KN. Central lateral thalamic neurons receive noxious visceral mechanical and chemical input in rats. J Neurophysiol 2009;102:244–258.
8. Vartiainen N, Perchet C, Magnin M, et al. Thalamic pain: anatomical and physiological indices of prediction. Brain 2016;139:708–722.
9. Blomqvist A, Zhang ET, Craig AD. Cytoarchitectonic and immunohistochemical characterization of a specific pain and temperature relay, the posterior portion of the ventral medial nucleus, in the human thalamus. Brain 2000;123 Pt 3:601–619.
10. Craig AD. Retrograde analyses of spinothalamic projections in the macaque monkey: input to ventral posterior nuclei. J Comp Neurol 2006;499:965–978.
11. Craig AD. Topographically organized projection to posterior insular cortex from the posterior portion of the ventral medial nucleus in the long-tailed macaque monkey. J Comp Neurol 2014;522:36–63.
12. Willis WD, Jr., Zhang X, Honda CN, Giesler GJ, Jr. A critical review of the role of the proposed VMpo nucleus in pain. J Pain 2002;3:79–94.
13. Raslan AM, Cetas JS, McCartney S, Burchiel KJ. Destructive procedures for control of cancer pain: the case for cordotomy. J Neurosurg 2011;114:155–170.
14. Montes C, Magnin M, Maarrawi J, et al. Thalamic thermo-algesic transmission: ventral posterior (VP) complex versus VMpo in the light of a thalamic infarct with central pain. Pain 2005;113:223–232.
15. Seghier ML, Lazeyras F, Vuilleumier P, Schnider A, Carota A. Functional magnetic resonance imaging and diffusion tensor imaging in a case of central poststroke pain. J Pain 2005;6:208–212.
16. Tracey I, Mantyh PW. The cerebral signature for pain perception and its modulation. Neuron 2007;55:377–391.
17. de Lacalle S, Saper CB. Calcitonin gene-related peptide-like immunoreactivity marks putative visceral sensory pathways in human brain. Neuroscience 2000;100:115–130.
18. Keay KA, Bandler R. Distinct central representations of inescapable and escapable pain: observations and speculation. Exp Physiol 2002;87:275–279.
19. Apkarian AV, Bushnell MC, Treede RD, Zubieta JK. Human brain mechanisms of pain perception and regulation in health and disease. Eur J Pain 2005;9:463–484.
20. Albe-Fessard D, Berkley KJ, Kruger L, Ralston HJ, 3rd, Willis WD, Jr. Diencephalic mechanisms of pain sensation. Brain Res 1985;356:217–296.
21. Mouraux A, Diukova A, Lee MC, Wise RG, Iannetti GD. A multisensory investigation of the functional significance of the "pain matrix." Neuroimage 2011;54:2237–2249.
22. Segerdahl AR, Mezue M, Okell TW, Farrar JT, Tracey I. The dorsal posterior insula subserves a fundamental role in human pain. Nat Neurosci 2015;18:499–500.
23. Davis KD, Bushnell MC, Iannetti GD, St Lawrence K, Coghill R. Evidence against pain specificity in the dorsal posterior insula. F1000Res 2015;4:362.
24. Craig AD. How do you feel—now? The anterior insula and human awareness. Nat Rev Neurosci 2009;10:59–70.
25. Craig AD. Significance of the insula for the evolution of human awareness of feelings from the body. Ann N Y Acad Sci 2011;1225:72–82.
26. Critchley HD, Harrison NA. Visceral influences on brain and behavior. Neuron 2013;77:624–638.
27. Vogt BA. Cingulate cortex in the three limbic subsystems. Handb Clin Neurol 2019;166:39–51.
28. Rolls ET. The cingulate cortex and limbic systems for action, emotion, and memory. Handb Clin Neurol 2019;166:23–37.
29. Vogt BA. Pain and emotion interactions in subregions of the cingulate gyrus. Nat Rev Neurosci 2005;6:533–544.
30. Palomero-Gallagher N, Eickhoff SB, Hoffstaedter F, et al. Functional organization of human subgenual cortical areas: Relationship between architectonical segregation and connectional heterogeneity. Neuroimage 2015;115:177–190.
31. Vogt BA. Midcingulate cortex: structure, connections, homologies, functions and diseases. J Chem Neuroanat 2016;74:28–46.
32. Palomero-Gallagher N, Hoffstaedter F, Mohlberg H, Eickhoff SB, Amunts K, Zilles K. Human pregenual anterior cingulate cortex: structural, functional, and connectional heterogeneity. Cereb Cortex 2019;29:2552–2574.
33. Raichle ME. The brain's default mode network. Annu Rev Neurosci 2015;38:433–447.
34. Kang SJ, Kwak C, Lee J, et al. Bidirectional modulation of hyperalgesia via the specific control of excitatory and inhibitory neuronal activity in the ACC. Mol Brain 2015;8:81.
35. Peyron R, Quesada C, Fauchon C. Cingulate-mediated approaches to treating chronic pain. Handb Clin Neurol 2019;166:317–326.
36. Shackman AJ, Salomons TV, Slagter HA, Fox AS, Winter JJ, Davidson RJ. The integration of negative affect, pain and cognitive control in the cingulate cortex. Nat Rev Neurosci 2011;12:154–167.
37. Timmers I, Park AL, Fischer MD, et al. Is empathy for pain unique in its neural correlates? a meta-analysis of neuroimaging studies of empathy. Front Behav Neurosci 2018;12:289.
38. Caruana F, Gerbella M, Avanzini P, et al. Motor and emotional behaviours elicited by electrical stimulation of the human cingulate cortex. Brain 2018;141:3035–3051.
39. Bastuji H, Frot M, Perchet C, Magnin M, Garcia-Larrea L. Pain networks from the inside: spatiotemporal analysis of brain responses leading from nociception to conscious perception. Hum Brain Mapp 2016;37:4301–4315.
40. Kucyi A, Davis KD. The neural code for pain: from single-cell electrophysiology to the dynamic pain connectome. Neuroscientist 2017;23:397–414.
41. Tu Y, Zhang Z, Tan A, et al. Alpha and gamma oscillation amplitudes synergistically predict the perception of forthcoming nociceptive stimuli. Hum Brain Mapp 2016;37:501–514.
42. Woo CW, Roy M, Buhle JT, Wager TD. Distinct brain systems mediate the effects of nociceptive input and self-regulation on pain. PLoS Biol 2015;13:e1002036.
43. Elman I, Borsook D. Common brain mechanisms of chronic pain and addiction. Neuron 2016;89:11–36.
44. Navratilova E, Porreca F. Reward and motivation in pain and pain relief. Nature Neurosci 2014;17:1304–1312.
45. Borsook D, Upadhyay J, Chudler EH, Becerra L. A key role of the basal ganglia in pain and analgesia—insights gained through human functional imaging. Mol Pain 2010;6:27.
46. Budygin EA, Park J, Bass CE, Grinevich VP, Bonin KD, Wightman RM. Aversive stimulus differentially triggers

subsecond dopamine release in reward regions. Neuroscience 2012;201:331–337.
47. Lee M, Manders TR, Eberle SE, et al. Activation of corticostriatal circuitry relieves chronic neuropathic pain. J Neurosci 2015;35:5247–5259.
48. Becerra L, Borsook D. Signal valence in the nucleus accumbens to pain onset and offset. Eur J Pain 2008;12:866–869.
49. Apkarian AV, Baliki MN, Farmer MA. Predicting transition to chronic pain. Curr Opin Neurol 2013;26:360–367.
50. Heinricher MM, Tavares I, Leith JL, Lumb BM. Descending control of nociception: specificity, recruitment and plasticity. Brain Res Rev 2009;60:214–225.
51. Le Bars D. The whole body receptive field of dorsal horn multireceptive neurones. Brain Res Brain Res Rev 2002;40:29–44.
52. Chen Q, Heinricher MM. Descending control mechanisms and chronic pain. Curr Rheumatol Rep 2019;21:13.
53. Holstege G, Georgiadis JR. The emotional brain: neural correlates of cat sexual behavior and human male ejaculation. Prog Brain Res 2004;143:39–45.
54. Venkatraman A, Edlow BL, Immordino-Yang MH. The brainstem in emotion: a review. Front Neuroanat 2017;11:15.
55. Hadjipavlou G, Dunckley P, Behrens TE, Tracey I. Determining anatomical connectivities between cortical and brainstem pain processing regions in humans: a diffusion tensor imaging study in healthy controls. Pain 2006;123:169–178.
56. Satpute AB, Wager TD, Cohen-Adad J, et al. Identification of discrete functional subregions of the human periaqueductal gray. Proc Natl Acad Sci U S A 2013;110:17101–17106.
57. Lueptow LM, Fakira AK, Bobeck EN. The contribution of the descending pain modulatory pathway in opioid tolerance. Front Neurosci 2018;12:886.
58. Barbaro NM. Studies of PAG/PVG stimulation for pain relief in humans. Prog Brain Res 1988;77:165–173.
59. Zhu H, Xiang HC, Li HP, et al. Inhibition of GABAergic neurons and excitation of glutamatergic neurons in the ventrolateral periaqueductal gray participate in electroacupuncture analgesia mediated by cannabinoid receptor. Front Neurosci 2019;13:484.
60. Fields HL, Barbaro NM, Heinricher MM. Brain stem neuronal circuitry underlying the antinociceptive action of opiates. Prog Brain Res 1988;77:245–257.
61. Chen Q, Roeder Z, Li MH, Zhang Y, Ingram SL, Heinricher MM. Optogenetic evidence for a direct circuit linking nociceptive transmission through the parabrachial complex with pain-modulating neurons of the rostral ventromedial medulla (RVM). eNeuro 2017;4.
62. Zhang Y, Zhao S, Rodriguez E, et al. Identifying local and descending inputs for primary sensory neurons. J Clin Invest 2015;125:3782–3794.
63. Francois A, Low SA, Sypek EI, et al. A brainstem-spinal cord inhibitory circuit for mechanical pain modulation by GABA and enkephalins. Neuron 2017;93:822–839 e826.
64. Gau R, Sevoz-Couche C, Hamon M, Bernard JF. Noxious stimulation excites serotonergic neurons: a comparison between the lateral paragigantocellular reticular and the raphe magnus nuclei. Pain 2013;154:647–659.
65. Tsuda M, Koga K, Chen T, Zhuo M. Neuronal and microglial mechanisms for neuropathic pain in the spinal dorsal horn and anterior cingulate cortex. J Neurochem 2017;141:486–498.
66. Samineni VK, Grajales-Reyes JG, Copits BA, et al. Divergent modulation of nociception by glutamatergic and gabaergic neuronal subpopulations in the periaqueductal gray. eNeuro 2017;4.
67. Gomtsian L, Bannister K, Eyde N, et al. Morphine effects within the rodent anterior cingulate cortex and rostral ventromedial medulla reveal separable modulation of affective and sensory qualities of acute or chronic pain. Pain 2018;159:2512–2521.
68. Cahill CM, Taylor AM. Neuroinflammation-a co-occurring phenomenon linking chronic pain and opioid dependence. Curr Opin Behav Sci 2017;13:171–177.
69. Colloca L, Barsky AJ. Placebo and nocebo effects. N Engl J Med 2020;382:554–561.
70. Scott DJ, Stohler CS, Egnatuk CM, Wang H, Koeppe RA, Zubieta JK. Placebo and nocebo effects are defined by opposite opioid and dopaminergic responses. Arch Gen Psychiatry 2008;65:220–231.
71. Carlino E, Benedetti F. Different contexts, different pains, different experiences. Neuroscience 2016;338:19–26.
72. Damien J, Colloca L, Bellei-Rodriguez CE, Marchand S. Pain modulation: from conditioned pain modulation to placebo and nocebo effects in experimental and clinical pain. Int Rev Neurobiol 2018;139:255–296.
73. Knudsen L, Petersen GL, Norskov KN, et al. Review of neuroimaging studies related to pain modulation. Scand J Pain 2018;2:108–120.
74. Bingel U, Lorenz J, Schoell E, Weiller C, Buchel C. Mechanisms of placebo analgesia: rACC recruitment of a subcortical antinociceptive network. Pain 2006;120:8–15.
75. Eippert F, Bingel U, Schoell ED, et al. Activation of the opioidergic descending pain control system underlies placebo analgesia. Neuron 2009;63:533–543.
76. Lewis GN, Rice DA, McNair PJ. Conditioned pain modulation in populations with chronic pain: a systematic review and meta-analysis. J Pain 2012;13:936–944.
77. Harper DE, Ichesco E, Schrepf A, et al. Resting functional connectivity of the periaqueductal gray is associated with normal inhibition and pathological facilitation in conditioned pain modulation. J Pain 2018;19:635 e631–635 e615.
78. Yu R, Gollub RL, Spaeth R, Napadow V, Wasan A, Kong J. Disrupted functional connectivity of the periaqueductal gray in chronic low back pain. Neuroimage Clin 2014;6:100–108.
79. Hemington KS, Wu Q, Kucyi A, Inman RD, Davis KD. Abnormal cross-network functional connectivity in chronic pain and its association with clinical symptoms. Brain Struct Funct 2016;221:4203–4219.
80. Kucyi A, Moayedi M, Weissman-Fogel I, et al. Enhanced medial prefrontal-default mode network functional connectivity in chronic pain and its association with pain rumination. J Neurosci 2014;34:3969–3975.
81. Ceko M, Shir Y, Ouellet JA, Ware MA, Stone LS, Seminowicz DA. Partial recovery of abnormal insula and dorsolateral prefrontal connectivity to cognitive networks in chronic low back pain after treatment. Hum Brain Mapp 2015;36:2075–2092.
82. Saab CY. Pain-related changes in the brain: diagnostic and therapeutic potentials. Trends Neurosci 2012;35:629–637.
83. Yarnitsky D. Role of endogenous pain modulation in chronic pain mechanisms and treatment. Pain 2015;156 Suppl 1:S24–31.
84. Kuner R, Flor H. Structural plasticity and reorganisation in chronic pain. Nat Rev Neurosci 2016;18:20–30.

85. Bliss TV, Collingridge GL, Kaang BK, Zhuo M. Synaptic plasticity in the anterior cingulate cortex in acute and chronic pain. Nat Rev Neurosci 2016;17:485–496.
86. Chen T, Taniguchi W, Chen QY, et al. Top-down descending facilitation of spinal sensory excitatory transmission from the anterior cingulate cortex. Nat Commun 2018;9:1886.
87. Meda KS, Patel T, Braz JM, et al. Microcircuit mechanisms through which mediodorsal thalamic input to anterior cingulate cortex exacerbates pain-related aversion. Neuron 2019;102:944–959 e943.
88. Tan LL, Pelzer P, Heinl C, et al. A pathway from midcingulate cortex to posterior insula gates nociceptive hypersensitivity. Nat Neurosci 2017;20:1591–1601.
89. Chen Q, Heinricher MM. Plasticity in the link between pain-transmitting and pain-modulating systems in acute and persistent inflammation. J Neurosci 2019;39:2065–2079.
90. Cai YQ, Wang W, Hou YY, Pan ZZ. Optogenetic activation of brainstem serotonergic neurons induces persistent pain sensitization. Mol Pain 2014;10:70.
91. Zhuo M. Descending facilitation. Mol Pain 2017;13:1744806917699212.
92. Guo W, Miyoshi K, Dubner R, et al. Spinal 5-HT3 receptors mediate descending facilitation and contribute to behavioral hypersensitivity via a reciprocal neuron-glial signaling cascade. Mol Pain 2014;10:35.
93. Ren W, Centeno MV, Berger S, et al. The indirect pathway of the nucleus accumbens shell amplifies neuropathic pain. Nat Neurosci 2016;19:220–222.
94. Danjo T, Yoshimi K, Funabiki K, Yawata S, Nakanishi S. Aversive behavior induced by optogenetic inactivation of ventral tegmental area dopamine neurons is mediated by dopamine D2 receptors in the nucleus accumbens. Proc Natl Acad Sci U S A 2014;111:6455–6460.
95. Schwartz N, Temkin P, Jurado S, et al. Chronic pain: decreased motivation during chronic pain requires long-term depression in the nucleus accumbens. Science 2014;345:535–542.
96. Rascol O, Zesiewicz T, Chaudhuri KR, et al. A randomized controlled exploratory pilot study to evaluate the effect of rotigotine transdermal patch on Parkinson's disease-associated chronic pain. J Clin Pharmacol 2016;56:852–861.
97. Fauchon C, Faillenot I, Quesada C, et al. Brain activity sustaining the modulation of pain by empathetic comments. Sci Rep 2019;9:8398.
98. Frizon LA, Yamamoto EA, Nagel SJ, Simonson MT, Hogue O, Machado AG. Deep brain stimulation for pain in the modern era: a systematic review. Neurosurgery 2020;86:191–202.
99. Mohseni HR, Smith PP, Parsons CE, et al. MEG can map short and long-term changes in brain activity following deep brain stimulation for chronic pain. PLoS One 2012;7:e37993.

37 Autonomic Control and Survival

OVERVIEW

The autonomic nervous system controls the functions of visceral effectors via preganglionic sympathetic and parasympathetic neurons that activate peripheral autonomic ganglia (Figure 37.1). The autonomic output is controlled by several interconnected areas distributed throughout the neuraxis. These areas also control arousal and respiration. Preganglionic neurons receive two major influences: inputs from visceral receptors that trigger autonomic reflexes, and descending influences from the brainstem and forebrain regulating autonomic output during homeostatic, adaptive, or emotional responses. Central commands to preganglionic neurons may be sent as predictive signals to visceral organs, which in turn provide feedback visceral sensation resulting from the actual response of the target organ. The mismatch between feedforward commands and feedback signals generates an error prediction signal that is utilized in the CNS to modify the autonomic commands. The sympathetic nervous system generates patterns of response to specific physiological challenges and is critical for maintenance of arterial blood pressure, regulation of regional blood flow, thermoregulation, and response to exercise and internal or external challenges to homeostasis or survival. In contrast, the parasympathetic system mediates organ-specific reflexes such as including those control of gastrointestinal motility and micturition. The enteric nervous system (ENS) controls local peristaltic reflexes and secretion. The brainstem contains several areas that provide commands to preganglionic neurons and are critical sites of interactions between cardiovascular, respiratory, and other vital functions with behavioral arousal and the sleep–wake cycle. The brainstem and spinal autonomic areas receive descending inputs from the hypothalamus, amygdala, and cerebral cortex, which integrate reflex responses into integrated patterns for homeostasis, adaptation to stress (allostasis), emotion, and behavior. Autonomic failure is a major manifestation of many neurologic disorders and may severely impact quality of life. Brainstem disorders affecting the interactions among cardiovascular control, reparation, and arousal may be life-threatening. The aims of this chapter are to review: (1) the general organization and functions of the sympathetic and parasympathetic systems; (2) the general organization of central autonomic control; and (3) the brainstem reflexes control of cardiovascular, respiratory, bladder, and gastrointestinal functions. The organization of the hypothalamus and other forebrain areas controlling autonomic functions are discussed in the next chapter.

ORGANIZATION OF THE AUTONOMIC OUTPUT

The peripheral control of visceral organs is exerted by the sympathetic and parasympathetic systems, ENS, and visceral afferents. The sympathetic and parasympathetic outputs consist of preganglionic neurons located in the brainstem or spinal cord and autonomic ganglion neurons that innervate the target organs. Preganglionic neurons have small myelinated axons and utilize acetylcholine (ACh) as their neurotransmitter. Acetylcholine elicits fast excitation of all autonomic ganglion and enteric neurons via ganglion type (α_3/β_4) nicotinic receptors (gnAChRs). In some ganglia ACh may also have modulatory effects via muscarinic receptors. The autonomic ganglia contain several groups of neurons that innervate the visceral targets. Sympathetic neurons are located in prevertebral and paravertebral ganglia, and their effects are largely mediated by norepinephrine (NE) acting via α1, β1 (cardiac), and β2 receptors. The only exception is sympathetic neurons innervating the sweat glands, which utilize ACh. The parasympathetic ganglion neurons are located close to or at the target organs, and neurons of the ENS are located within the walls of the gut. Both types of neurons include two main groups; one that primarily utilizes ACh, which elicits excitatory effects largely via M3 receptors; and neurons that utilize nitric oxide and vasoactive intestinal peptide. Inhibitory effects of cholinergic neurons are mediated by M2 receptors. ATP

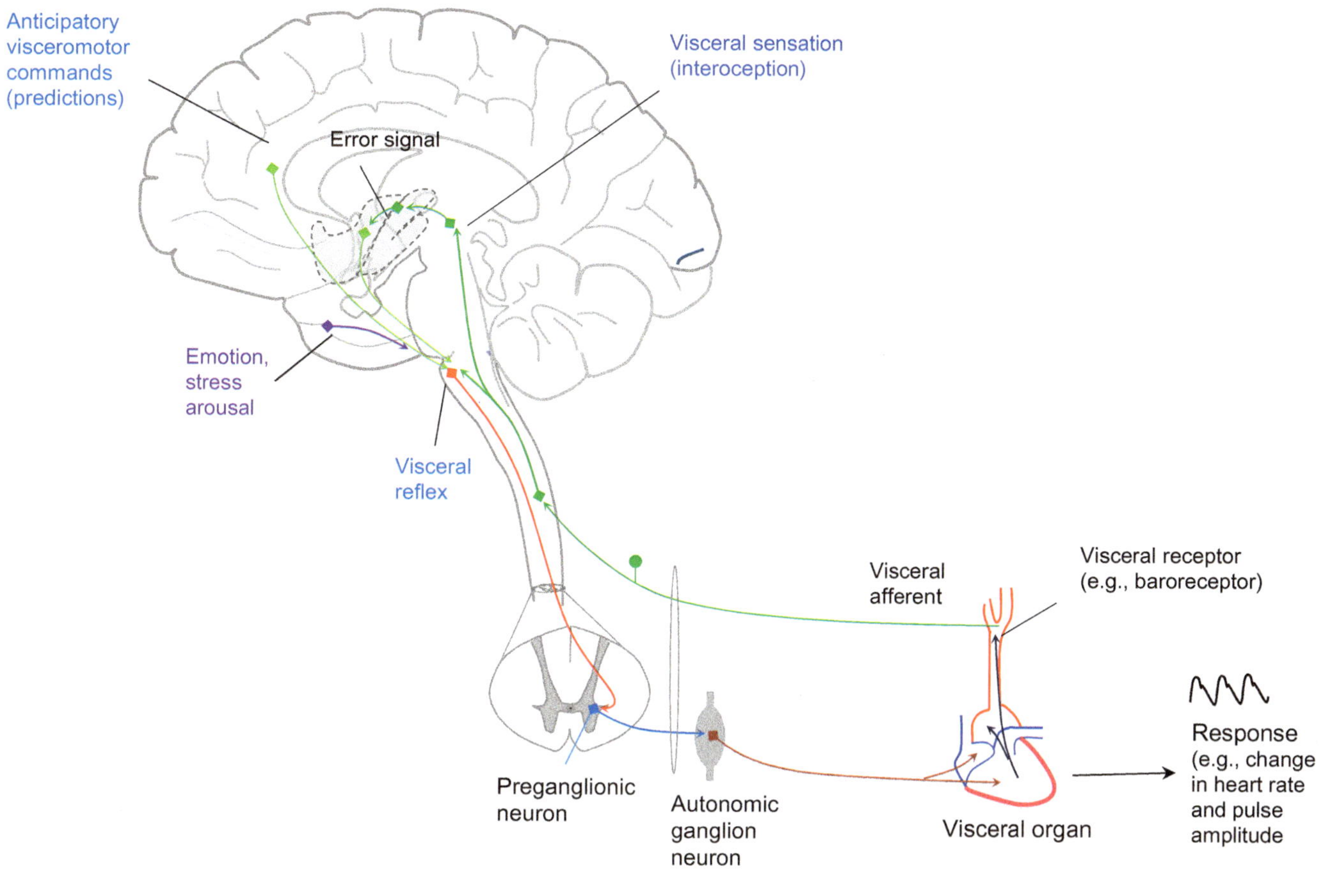

FIGURE 37.1 Organization of the autonomic output.

The autonomic output via preganglionic sympathetic and parasympathetic neurons affects visceral organs via peripheral autonomic ganglia. Preganglionic neurons receive inputs from visceral receptors that trigger autonomic reflexes, and descending influences from the brainstem and forebrain regulating autonomic output during homeostatic, adaptive, or emotional responses. The central autonomic commands to preganglionic neurons may be sent as predictive signals about the expected sensory consequences resulting from activation of the target organs. The mismatch between feedforward commands and feedback signals resulting from visceral activity generates an error prediction signal that is utilized in the CNS to modify the autonomic commands and/or the sensory predictions.

is an important cotransmitter in sympathetic, parasympathetic, and enteric neurons. The main effects of the sympathetic and parasympathetic systems are summarized in Table 37.1.

Preganglionic Sympathetic Neurons

The sympathetic nervous system has a critical role in maintenance of arterial blood pressure, regulation of regional blood flow, thermoregulation, and integrated response to exercise, disturbances in homeostasis, and external stressors. The sympathetic preganglionic neurons are located in four distinct groups in the thoracolumbar spinal cord. The majority are located in the intermediolateral cell column (intermediolateral nucleus, IML) between the T1 and L2 segments of the spinal cord.[1] The preganglionic sympathetic neurons form distinct functional subunits that provide excitatory inputs to sympathetic ganglia or adrenal gland. These neurons cluster in groups according to their function, forming different functional units, including muscle vasoconstrictor, cutaneous vasoconstrictor, cutaneous vasodilator, sudomotor, pilomotor and others[2] (Figure 37.2). Preganglionic sympathetic neurons are electrically coupled by gap junctions, which may promote synchronized activity of neurons that share similar effector function. These neurons respond to peripheral afferent inputs and receive inputs from the brainstem and hypothalamus.[3–5] Segmental inputs affect the preganglionic sympathetic neurons largely via excitatory or inhibitory interneurons.[6] These preganglionic neurons also respond to inputs from Aδ and C afferents transmitting pain, itch, temperature, and visceral sensation; these afferents terminate in layers I–V of the dorsal horn, innervate propriospinal neurons and interneurons located in the intermediate gray matter, and provide a polysynaptic influence on preganglionic sympathetic neurons.[1] In most

TABLE 37.1 *Effects of the Sympathetic and Parasympathetic Output*

Target	Sympathetic (neurotransmitter and receptor)	Parasympathetic (neurotransmitter and receptor)
Pupil	Dilation (NE, α1)	Constriction (ACh, M3)
Ciliary muscle	N/A	Accommodation (ACh, M3)
Salivary and lacrimal glands	Inhibition (NE, α2?)	Stimulation (ACh, M3, VIP)
Pineal gland	Melatonin secretion (β2)	—
Facial blood vessels	Constriction (NE, α1) Dilation (NE, E, β2?)	—
Cerebral blood vessels	Constriction (NE, α1)	Dilation (NO, VIP)
Skeletal muscle vessels	Constriction (NE, α1) Dilation (NEe, E, β2)	—
Skin vessels	Constriction (NE, α1) Dilation (NO?, ACh?)	—
Sweat glands	Stimulation (ACh, M3)	Stimulation in abnormal conditions (NE, α1)
Heart	Stimulation (NE, β1)	Inhibition (ACh, M2)
Bronchi	Dilation (NE, E, β2)	Constriction (ACh, M3)
Gastrointestinal motility	Inhibition (β2)	Contraction (ACh, M3) Relaxation (NO, VIP)
Gastrointestinal secretion	Inhibition (α2)	Gastric acid secretion (M1) Intestinal secretion (M3, VIP)
Visceral blood vessels	Constriction (NE, α1)	Dilation (NO, VIP)
Bladder detrusor	Inhibition (β2, β3)	Stimulation (M3)
Bladder neck	Stimulation (α1)	Inhibition (NO)
Rectal smooth muscle	Inhibition (β2)	Stimulation (M3)
Erectile tissue	Constriction (α1)	Dilation (NO)
Vas deferens	Contraction (α1)	—
Endocrine function and metabolism	Epinephrine (E) secretion Thyroid hormone secretion Glycogenolyis (E, β2, β3) Lipolysis (NE, E, β2, β3)	Secretion of insulin and gastrointestinal hormones (ACh, M3)

ACh, acetylcholine; NE, norepinephrine; NO, nitric oxide; VIP, vasoactive intestinal polypeptide

cases, segmental afferents cause excitation of these neurons, but in some cases they may elicit inhibition via interneurons, such as those in lamina X. Descending inputs from the brainstem and hypothalamus target different subpopulations of preganglionic sympathetic neurons or local interneurons and engage them in specific response patterns appropriate to the circumstances. Spinal interneurons receive convergent information from descending pathways and segmental afferents and may have an important role in the interplay between the sympathetic and the motor systems. For example, during exercise there is a close coordination of muscle control with sympathetically mediated redistribution of blood flow. Several brain regions send descending projections that provide collaterals to both motor neurons and preganglionic sympathetic neurons, both directly and via interneurons and propriospinal neurons. These supraspinal projections may act as a "central command" for coordination of motor and sympathetic responses.

Interruption of these supraspinal inputs, as occurs with cervical or upper thoracic spinal cord injury (SCI) unmasks the reflex drive of sympathetic preganglionic neurons by segmental visceral and somatic afferents via local excitatory interneurons. This may trigger a massive, unpatterned sympathoexcitation in response to peripheral stimuli such as bladder distension, which is the basic mechanism of autonomic dysreflexia.

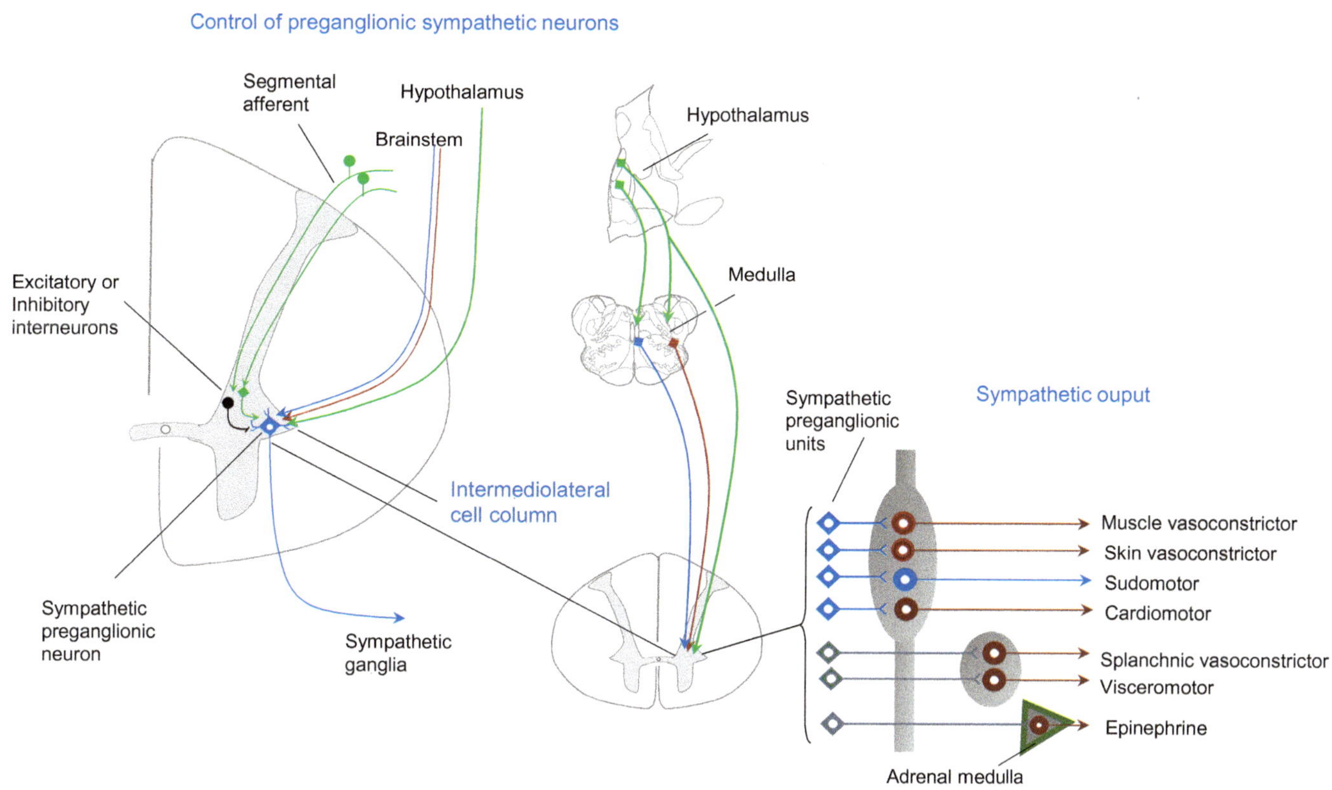

FIGURE 37.2 Preganglionic sympathetic units.
The sympathetic preganglionic neurons (SPNs) are located in four topographically distinct groups in the thoracolumbar spinal cord. The majority are located in the intermediolateral cell column between the T1 and L2 segments of the spinal cord. According to their function, SPNs form different units, including muscle vasoconstrictor, cutaneous vasoconstrictor, cutaneous vasodilator, sudomotor, pilomotor, and others. The functional heterogeneity of SPNs largely reflects their distinct descending inputs from the brainstem and hypothalamus as well as inputs from primary somatic and visceral afferents, which influence SPNs both directly and via local excitatory or inhibitory interneurons.

Sympathetic Ganglia and Their Effectors

The preganglionic sympathetic axons terminate on paravertebral, prevertebral, and terminal ganglia, as well as the adrenal medulla. Paravertebral ganglia include the superior cervical ganglion that innervates the cranial effectors including the pupil, blood vessels and sweat glands of the face, cerebral blood vessels, and pineal gland. Thoracolumbar paravertebral ganglia innervate blood vessels and sweat glands of the trunk and limbs, as well as thoracic viscera. The prevertebral ganglia, including the celiac, superior mesenteric, and hypogastric ganglia, innervate effectors in the abdomen and pelvis. The adrenal medulla receives preganglionic inputs via the splanchnic nerves and release epinephrine to the general circulation.

The effects of NE mediated by α1 receptors promote smooth muscle contraction, including vasoconstriction; β1 receptors stimulate effectors in the heart; and β2 and β3 receptors elicit visceral smooth muscle relaxation and activation of glycolysis and lipolysis. The α2 receptors function primarily as inhibitory presynaptic receptors, both in noradrenergic terminals (autoreceptors) and in parasympathetic and afferent terminals. Unlike other sympathetic ganglion neurons, those innervating the sweat glands are cholinergic.

Parasympathetic Output

The parasympathetic output can be subdivided from the functional standpoint into outputs to cranial effectors via cranial nerves III, VII, and IX; outputs to the thoracic and abdominal viscera mediated by the vagus nerve (cranial nerve X); and outputs to pelvic organs (bladder, rectum, and sexual organs) originating from sacral preganglionic neurons located at the S2–S4 segments. Cranial parasympathetic inputs originate from neurons in the Edinger-Westphal nucleus that project via the oculomotor nerve to the ciliary ganglion. Neurons of the salivatory (or salivary) nuclear complex project via the facial nerve to the sphenopalatine (pterygopalatine), submandibular and submaxillary ganglia and via the glossopharyngeal nerve to the otic ganglion. Cranial parasympathetic reflexes elicit pupil constriction and accommodation, lacrimal and salivary gland secretion, and cranial vasodilation. Vagal preganglionic neurons are located in the dorsal motor nucleus of the vagus (DMV) and ventrolateral intermediate (semicompact) portion of the nucleus ambiguus (NAmb) in the medulla. The DMV mediates all vago-vagal reflexes controlling motility and secretion in the gastrointestinal and respiratory tracts.[7] The NAmb provides vagal output to cardiac ganglion neurons controlling the sinus node.[8] Vagal reflexes are critical for beat-to-beat control of the heart rate and activation of upper gastrointestinal motility. Sacral preganglionic nucleus control micturition, defecation, and sexual function. The primary neurotransmitter of most parasympathetic ganglia and ENS is ACh, which mediates excitatory responses such as smooth muscle contraction and glandular secretion via M3 muscarinic receptors. In contrast, vagal inputs to the heart reduce automatism and conduction via inhibitory M2 receptors. Other parasympathetic effects on visceral effectors, primary smooth muscle relaxation and vasodilation, are mediated by noncholinergic neurons that utilize NO and vasoactive intestinal polypeptide.

VISCERAL AFFERENT SYSTEM

The visceral afferent system is a major source of information regulating autonomic outputs and has a fundamental role in interoception, or bodily sensations.

Visceral Afferents

Small-myelinated (Aδ) and unmyelinated (C) primary afferents innervating the viscera convey nonpainful mechanical sensation such as visceral distension, as well as nociceptive and temperature sensations. These afferents may antidromically release chemical signals that affect he functions of the blood vessels, visceral smooth muscles, and exocrine glands.

Spinal visceral afferents traveling with the sympathetic nerves (splanchnic afferents) have their cell bodies in the thoracolumbar dorsal root ganglion (DRG), and afferents traveling via the pelvic nerves have their cell bodies in the sacral DRG. Vagal afferents have their cell bodies in the nodose and adjacent jugular ganglia; glossopharyngeal afferents have their cell body in the petrosal ganglion. Most organs are innervated by two different extrinsic visceral afferents; for example, the bladder receives visceral afferents from the pelvic and splanchnic nerves. Visceral afferents convey the sensation of visceral pain and trigger the sensations of nausea, organ filling, distension, and dyspnea. Like somatic nociceptive afferents, they utilize L-glutamate as their primary neurotransmitter. At least 50% of these small DRG neurons also synthesize neuropeptides, such as substance P and calcitonin-gene related peptide (CGRP), and may also release NO and ATP.

Central Projections

Some visceral afferents remain in the peripheral organ and mediate local axon reflexes; some provide collateral input to autonomic ganglion cells and mediate ganglion reflexes. Visceral sensation reaches the central nervous system via both spinal and brainstem afferents. Viscerosensory neurons of the DRG provide primary afferent inputs that terminate in the dorsal horn (primarily lamina I) and intermediate gray matter of the spinal cord. The density of innervation of the viscera is low compared with that of the skin and deep somatic tissue, and inputs from different visceral organs converge at individual levels of the dorsal horn. Many dorsal horn neurons receiving inputs from visceral afferents also receive inputs from somatic pain afferents. This provides the basis for referred pain. Dorsal horn neurons convey visceral information both via spinothalamic tract and spinobulbar pathways. Some information is transferred by axons in the midline portion of the dorsal columns. This includes pain from midline structures of the pelvis and sensations related to micturition, defecation, and gastric distension. Most visceral sensation is unconscious and serves to trigger visceral reflexes and integrated autonomic, endocrine, and other adaptive responses. Visceral inputs are largely carried by brainstem afferents that terminate in the nucleus of the solitary tract (NTS)[9]. The NTS is subdivided into rostral, intermediate, and caudal regions. The rostral NTS receives input from taste receptors (primarily via the facial nerve), the intermediate portion from gastrointestinal afferents (via the vagus nerve), and the caudal portion from carotid baroreceptors and chemoreceptors (via the glossopharyngeal nerve) as well as cardiac, pulmonary, and upper airway receptors (via the vagus nerve). Each portion of the NTS contains subnuclei that receive organ-specific afferents participate in specific reflexes. However, some areas of the NTS receive convergent inputs from gastrointestinal, cardiovascular, and respiratory afferents and may be primarily involved in relaying this information to rostral areas of the CNS. The NTS also receives projections from lamina I of the spinal cord and from the area postrema, which lacks a blood-brain barrier (BBB) and provides signals from the blood and CSF.

The NTS sends projections to the thalamus, hypothalamus, and amygdala, both directly and via a relay in the parabrachial nuclear complex of the pons (PB). The subnuclear organization of the PB complex includes a lateral PB (with multiple subdivisions), medial PB, external medial PB, and Kölliker-Fuse subnuclei (KF). The PB complex has reciprocal connections with medullary and forebrain areas involved in autonomic, respiratory, and behavioral state control. The lateral PB and KF also receive inputs from lamina I and the trigeminal nucleus caudalis. There is convergence of inputs from the NTS and lamina I into several PB subnuclei; this provides for integration of pain and temperature sensations with gustatory, gastrointestinal, and cardiorespiratory information. The PB complex also receives inputs from the area postrema.

CENTRAL AUTONOMIC CONTROL

Central autonomic control is distributed throughout the neuraxis and is hierarchically organized (Figure 37.3).[10,11]

Components

Areas in the medulla and lower pons mediate cardiovascular, respiratory, gastrointestinal, and micturition reflexes and relay visceral information to the upper brainstem and forebrain. The upper pons and midbrain contain areas that integrate autonomic control with pain modulation, responses to stress, behavioral arousal, and motor responses. The hypothalamus functions as a pattern generator for integrated autonomic, endocrine, and behavioral responses to ensure bodily homeostasis and adaptation to environmental challenges. The core telencephalic areas controlling autonomic function are the amygdala, insular cortex, and anterior cingulate cortex. The primary excitatory transmitter in the autonomic pathways is L-glutamate; the primary inhibitory transmitters is γ-aminobutyric acid (GABA). The activity of these areas is modulated in a state-dependent function by cholinergic, monoaminergic, and peptidergic influences from the brainstem, basal forebrain, and hypothalamus. Local circuit interactions mediated by nitric oxide, purines, endocannabinoids, and other signals, both from neighboring neurons and astrocytes also regulate the activity of these central autonomic areas.

Multiple Sources of Input

The central autonomic control areas receive inputs from several sources. One fundamental source are pathways conveying inputs from visceral receptors, nociceptors, thermoreceptors, and muscle receptors relayed by spinal afferents via ascending projections to lamina I of the dorsal horn

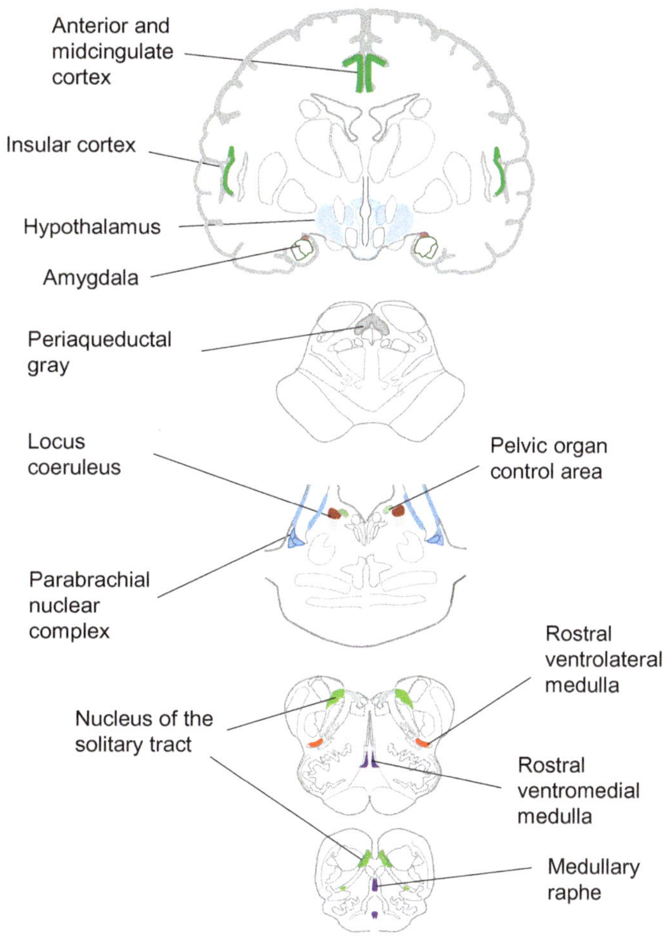

FIGURE 37.3 Central autonomic control areas.
Central autonomic control is distributed throughout the neuraxis and is hierarchically organized. Areas in the medulla and lower pons mediate autonomic reflexes and relay visceral information to the upper brainstem and forebrain. The upper pons and midbrain contain areas that integrate autonomic control with pain modulation, responses to stress, behavioral arousal, and motor responses. The hypothalamus functions as a pattern generator for integrated autonomic, endocrine, and behavioral responses to ensure bodily homeostasis and adaptation to environmental challenges. The amygdala, insular cortex, and anterior and midcingulate cortex integrate bodily sensation, emotion, and autonomic control.

or via cranial nerve afferents that relay in NTS.[9] Humoral signals from the blood (e.g., levels of glucose or cytokines) or CSF (such as pH) can reach the central autonomic areas either directly or indirectly via sensory circumventricular organs (CVOs), which lack a BBB.[12] The central autonomic control areas also receive inputs from areas involved in behavioral arousal and the sleep–wake cycle, including cholinergic neurons of the basal forebrain and mesopontine tegmentum, monoaminergic groups, and orexin (ORX) neurons in the lateral hypothalamus. Circadian signals are provided by the suprachiasmatic nucleus, indirectly via other hypothalamic nuclei. The amygdala and anterior cingulate cortex provide signals triggered by emotion or other behaviorally relevant states.

Output: Premotor Autonomic Neurons

The hypothalamus, amygdala, and cerebral cortex largely control the preganglionic sympathetic or parasympathetic output via premotor autonomic neurons located in the medulla and pons[10,11,13] (Figure 37.4). These premotor neurons project to the preganglionic neurons and mediate a variety of visceral reflexes. The NTS is the first relay station of visceral afferents that initiate cardiovascular, respiratory, and gastrointestinal reflexes.[9] The rostral ventrolateral medulla (RVLM) contains premotor sympathoexcitatory neurons that project to the IML and have a critical role in control of blood pressure. The RVLM neurons are glutamatergic and include the C1 group of neurons that also synthesizes epinephrine.[3] The C1 neurons have a major role as sensors and mediators of responses to internal stressors such as hypoxia and hypoglycemia.[14] The rostral ventromedial medulla (RVMM) and medullary raphe, including serotonergic neurons of nucleus raphe pallidus (RPa), provide sympathoexcitatory outputs that initiate responses to cold and external stressors. The PB/KF nuclear complex receives inputs from the NTS and dorsal horn, projects to the forebrain and to medullary cardiovascular and respiratory areas, and has a major role in arousal, respiratory control, and other homeostatic functions. The ventrolateral medullary reticular formation harbors the respiratory pattern-generator network and chemosensitive areas.[15] These respiratory groups are intimately linked anatomically and functionally with the NTS, PB/KF, and C1 groups and participate in coordination of respiration with autonomic control.[13] The pelvic organ-stimulating center, also known as pontine micturition center (PMC) or Barrington nucleus, is located in the dorsal pontine tegmentum and sends direct excitatory projections to the parasympathetic motoneurons in the sacral cord innervating the pelvic organs, and has a critical role in control of micturition, as well as defecation, and function of sexual organs.[16,17]

CARDIOVASCULAR CONTROL

The control of arterial blood pressure and heart rate involves two interactive mechanisms: feedback control via medullary reflexes, primarily the baroreceptor reflex (baroreflex); and feedforward, state-dependent modulation of these reflexes via descending inputs from the hypothalamus, periaqueductal gray (PAG), amygdala, insula, and cingulate cortex.[4] A fundamental mediator of both reflex and descending influences are the premotor sympathoexcitatory neurons in the RVLM (including the C1 group). The RVLM controls peripheral vascular resistance via IML neurons that trigger vasoconstriction of splanchnic and skeletal muscle blood vessels.[3] The sympathetic output to resistance vessels controlling arterial pressure can be assessed by microneurography, recording muscle sympathetic nerve activity that shows bursts time-locked with the arterial pulse. Neurons of the RVLM also promote sympathetically mediated cardiac stimulation and thus increased cardiac output. The second major effector are neurons in the preganglionic parasympathetic neurons of the NAmb that provide vagal inputs to cardiac ganglion neurons that innervate the sinoatrial and atrioventricular nodes, thus providing a beat-to-beat control of the heart rate.[8]

Baroreceptor Reflex and Control of Blood Pressure

The baroreceptor reflex is the principal buffering mechanism for short-term regulation of arterial blood pressure[4] (Figure 37.5). This reflex is triggered by activation of mechanosensitive carotid baroreceptor afferents of the glossopharyngeal nerve and aortic arch afferents of the vagus nerve. These afferents express Piezo2 channels that respond to mechanical stretch and are activated on a beat-to-beat basis by vessel wall deformation elicited by the pulse pressure.[18] Baroreceptor afferents provide a monosynaptic excitatory input to neurons located in the caudal portion of the NTS. In response to an increase in blood pressure, these barosensitive NTS neurons trigger two parallel pathways, sympathoinhibitory and cardioinhibitory, that tend to lower blood pressure back to baseline. The sympathoinhibitory pathway is mediated by GABAergic neurons in the caudal ventrolateral medulla, which inhibit the premotor sympathoexcitatory neurons of the RVLM. The baroreflex control of total peripheral resistance is the primary mechanism for maintaining arterial blood pressure[4] and preventing orthostatic hypotension (OH). Upon standing (i.e., orthostatic stress) there is venous pooling in the abdomen and lower limbs resulting in reduced venous return, cardiac output, and thus pulse pressure. This change elicits a reduced firing of carotid baroreceptors and thus their input to barosensitive NTS neurons. The reduced baroreflex inhibition of RVLM neurons allows activation of sympathetic output that triggers splanchnic and skeletal muscle vasoconstriction via $\alpha 1$ receptors. This reduces venous pooling and increases peripheral resistance thereby preventing OH. Whereas C1 neurons of the RVLM do not appear to be critical for maintenance of arterial pressure during wakefulness, they are involved in maintenance of arterial pressure during anesthesia, and mediate both the sympathoexcitatory responses to hypoxia and the increase in arterial pressure following

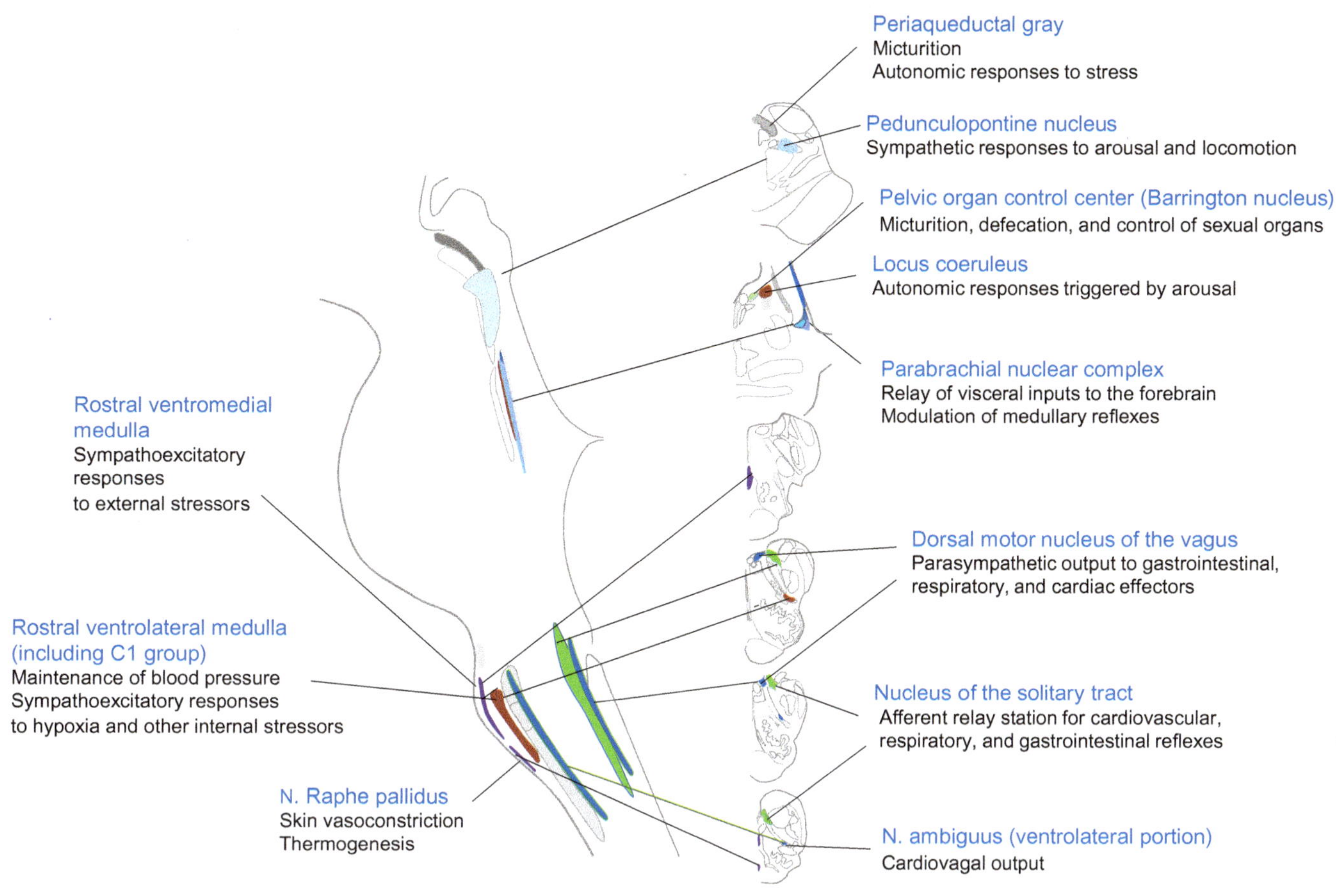

FIGURE 37.4 Brainstem control of autonomic function.
Several areas of the medulla and lower pons mediate cardiovascular, respiratory, and other reflexes critical for survival and control of visceral function. The nucleus of the solitary tract is the first relay for cardiovascular, respiratory, and gastrointestinal reflexes and relays visceral and taste information to rostral brain areas. The rostral ventrolateral medulla contains sympathetic excitatory neurons that project to the intermediolateral cell column, and trigger vasoconstriction of skeletal muscle, splanchnic, and renal vessels. The C1 neurons have a major role as sensors and mediators of responses to internal stressors such as hypoxia and hypoglycemia. The rostral ventromedial medulla and nucleus raphe pallidus (RPa) provide sympathoexcitatory outputs that trigger responses to cold and tachycardia in response to external stressors. The parabrachial nuclear complex provides an interface between medullary reflexes and forebrain mechanisms regulating cardiovascular, respiratory, and other homeostatic functions. The pelvic organ stimulating center (pontine micturition center) innervates sacral preganglionic neurons controlling the bladder, distal colon, rectum, and internal genital organs. The periaqueductal gray, locus coeruleus, and pedunculopontine tegmental nucleus coordinate autonomic with arousal and stress responses.

baroreceptor denervation.[19] The baroreflex cardioinhibitory pathway involves a direct input from the NTS to vagal preganglionic neurons to the NAmb, which project to cholinergic neurons in the cardiac ganglion that inhibit the automatism of the sinus node, resulting in bradycardia.

The efficacy of the baroreflex, or baroreflex gain, is typically tested by assessing the cardiovagal component, recording the changes in heart rate in response to changes in blood pressure elicited by either vasoconstrictor or vasodilator drugs. In the research setting, it may also be assessed by changes in muscle sympathetic nerve activity. In the clinical autonomic laboratory, the baroreflex is indirectly assessed by the beat-to-beat responses of the blood pressure and heart rate during the Valsalva maneuver or head-up tilt.[20] There is resetting of the baroreflex during exercise, mental stress, and sleep.[21] During exercise, the baroreflex resets at new operating levels of blood pressure to maintain flow to both vital organs and muscle.[22] This resetting reflects the effects of both a "central command" and muscle afferents activated during exercise.[21 22] There is

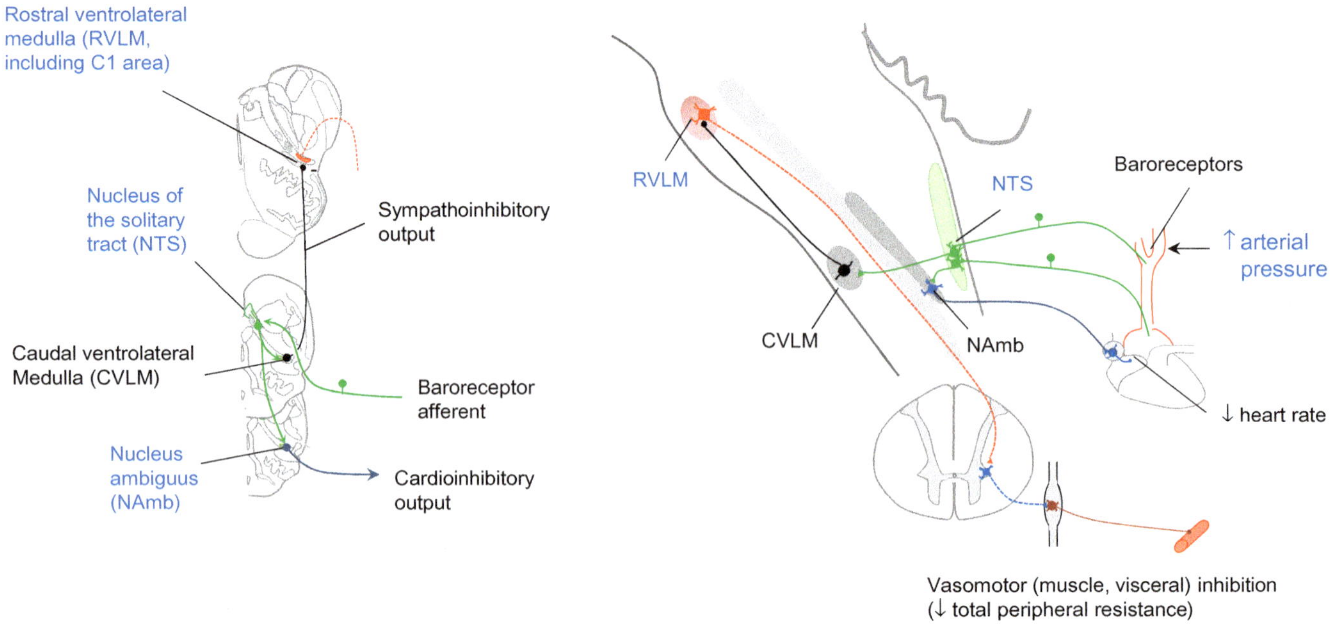

FIGURE 37.5 Baroreceptor reflex.

The baroreceptor reflex is triggered by activation of carotid baroreceptor and aortic arch afferents that provide monosynaptic excitatory input to the caudal portion of the nucleus of the solitary tract (NTS). Barosensitive NTS neurons trigger a sympathoinhibitory and a cardioninhibitory pathway. The sympathoinhibitory pathway is mediated by GABAergic neurons in the caudal ventrolateral medulla that inhibit the premotor sympathoexcitatory neurons of the rostral ventrolateral medulla (RVLM), leading to a decrease in total peripheral resistance. The cardioinhibitory pathway is mediated by a direct projection from the NTS to the cardiovagal neurons of the nucleus ambiguus (NAmb), which reduces the heart rate.

also a continuous modulation or resetting of the baroreflex during each phase of the sleep–wake cycle.[23] Baroreflex sensitivity increases during both NREM and REM sleep due to increased responsiveness of NTS neurons to baroreceptor afferents; this allows maintenance of lower arterial blood pressure compared to the waking state. In addition, the arterial baroreflex strongly modulates the state of behavioral arousal.[23] Descending inputs from the hypothalamus and PAG regulate both the baroreflex gain and sympathetic outputs in relationship to the state of arousal.[24]

Control of Cardiac Function

The control of cardiac function involves intrinsic and extrinsic components. The intrinsic cardiac nervous system consists of cardiac ganglia that contain afferent, efferent, and local circuit neurons that use ACh as their primary transmitter. These neurons are highly interconnected and have intrinsic activity that is modulated by sympathetic or vagal inputs. The sympathetic output to the heart originates in preganglionic neurons that receive influence from both the RVLM and the RVMM.[24] There is left-to-right asymmetry of cardiac sympathetic innervation, with some interindividual variability. The primary neurotransmitter of cardiac sympathetic neurons is NE, acting primarily via β1 but also via α1 receptors. The sympathetic output increases the automatism of the sinoatrial node (and thus heart rate), conduction through the atrioventricular, excitability of the His-Purkinje system, force of contraction during systole, and speed of relaxation of the cardiac muscle cells during diastole. Cardiac parasympathetic output originates primarily from the NAmb, and to a lesser extent the DMV, which via cholinergic cardiac ganglion neurons elicit M2 receptor-mediated inhibition of the pacemaker activity of the sinoatrial node, reduced atrioventricular conduction, and decreased excitability of the His-Purkinje system.

A fundamental aspect of the cardiovagal output controlling the heart rate is its modulation during the respiratory cycle. The rhythmic discharge of the cardiovagal neurons of the NAmb, driven by the baroreflex, is strongly modulated by respiration due to influences from the neighboring respiratory oscillator and from pulmonary stretch afferents via the NTS.[25] Cardiovagal neurons of the NAmb are inhibited during inspiration and excited during inspiration. This results in respiratory sinus arrhythmia (tachycardia in inspiration and bradycardia in expiration), which is an important index of the integrity of cardiovagal function and is the primary driver of heart rate variability. Heart rate variability refers to the beat-to-beat variation of the RR interval (the reciprocal of the heart rate) that results from interactions between the vagal and sympathetic influences on the sinoatrial node. Power spectrum analyses show that the high frequency component of heart rate variability reflects respiratory modulation of cardiovagal output.

Afferents from the heart, coronary, and pulmonary arteries trigger a variety of cardiovascular reflexes. Atrial distension due to volume load activates myelinated vagal afferents that synapse on the NTS and trigger reflex activation of sympathetic input to the sinoatrial node (tachycardia) and inhibition of renal sympathetic activity and release of arginine vasopressin (AVP), promoting sodium and water excretion. Unmyelinated spinal and vagal afferents from the ventricles are activated by strong mechanical or chemical stimuli, including products of ischemia or inflammation. The spinal afferents elicit cardiac pain via input to lamina I dorsal horn and excitatory cardiac reflexes via local interneurons projecting to the IML (the so-called cardio-cardiac reflex). In contrast, unmyelinated vagal afferents in the ventricles may trigger a fall in blood pressure and rate via inputs to the NTS.

BRAINSTEM CONTROL OF RESPIRATION

Breathing originates from a central pattern generator located in the lower brainstem and depends on inputs from central chemosensitive areas and afferents from chemoreceptors and mechanoreceptors via the NTS[15,26] (Figure 37.6). The control of respiration is intimately related to that of cardiovascular function.[13]

Respiratory Pattern Generators

Breathing includes an inspiratory phase followed by a passive expiratory phase. A third phase at the end of inspiration, called postinspiratory phase prolongs the contraction of the diaphragm and laryngeal adductor muscles; retards lung deflation and promotes alveolar gas exchange. Increased metabolism and oxygen consumption trigger active expiration, which increases the tidal volume. Expiration becomes intermittently active during REM sleep.[27] Inspiration, postinspiration, and active expiration are controlled by three distinct pattern generators.[28–30] The preBötzinger complex, located in the ventrolateral medulla, is the critical pattern generator of inspiration.[15] It contains glutamatergic neurons that project to pontine and medullary premotor respiratory regions that drive the motoneurons controlling the inspiratory pump and airway resistance.[28–30]

Central Chemoreceptive Zones

Central chemoreceptors sense brain interstitial fluid proton (H(+) concentration, and thereby detect and integrate information on alveolar ventilation (arterial PCO_2), cerebral blood flow and metabolism, and acid-base balance.[31–33] Studies in rodents indicate that the primary central respiratory chemosensitive zone is located close to the ventral medullary surface; this area is referred to as retrotrapezoid nucleus or ventral parafacial nucleus.[32] Glutamatergic neurons of this nucleus are activated by increased PCO_2 via intrinsic proton receptors and by paracrine mechanisms mediated by signals from astrocytes, such as ATP. These neurons also receive synaptic input from peripheral chemoreceptors activated by hypoxia via a relay in the NTS.[33] The retrotrapezoid nucleus sends excitatory inputs to the preBötzinger complex and other brainstem respiratory groups.[33] Respiratory chemosensitivity also involves serotonergic neurons of the medullary raphe.[34,35] Neurons of the nucleus raphe pallidus and raphe obscurus detect changes in pH/CO_2 and hypoxia and provide widespread innervation to all respiratory groups, exerting a global excitatory effect on the respiratory network and increasing excitability of phrenic motoneurons in the spinal cord.[34,36]

Control of Respiratory Pump and Airway

The premotor respiratory neurons innervating the spinal motor neurons controlling the respiratory muscles are located in a continuous column that extends from the rostral to the caudal portions of the ventrolateral medulla and is known as the of ventral respiratory group. This column includes, from rostral to caudal, the Bötzinger complex containing expiratory neurons, the rostral ventral respiratory group containing inspiratory neurons, and the caudal ventral respiratory group, including the nucleus retroambiguus, containing expiratory neurons. The ventral respiratory column receives inputs from the retrotrapezoid nucleus, preBötzinger complex, and NTS. Neurons of the ventral respiratory group, as well as some neurons in the NTS, send direct projections to respiratory motoneurons of the spinal cord. The cranial motor nuclei controlling airway resistance include the NAmb, which innervates innervating the larynx and pharynx via the vagus nerve, and the hypoglossal, trigeminal, and facial nuclei. The respiratory network controls the phasic activity of muscles that stiffen and open the upper airway, such as the genioglossus muscles.

Parabrachial Nuclear Complex and Control of Respiration

Components of the PB nuclear complex, including the external lateral PB, lateral crescent, and KF, constitute the so-called pontine respiratory group (the classical "apneustic" center), which has a major role in respiratory phase-switching especially in terminating inspiration. This pontine respiratory group receives inputs from the NTS, preBötzinger complex, retrotrapezoid nucleus, medullary serotonergic groups, C1 area, and lamina I. Neurons in different portions of the lateral PB/KF complex generate distinct respiratory patterns and changes in the upper airway via descending projections to the NTS and to different

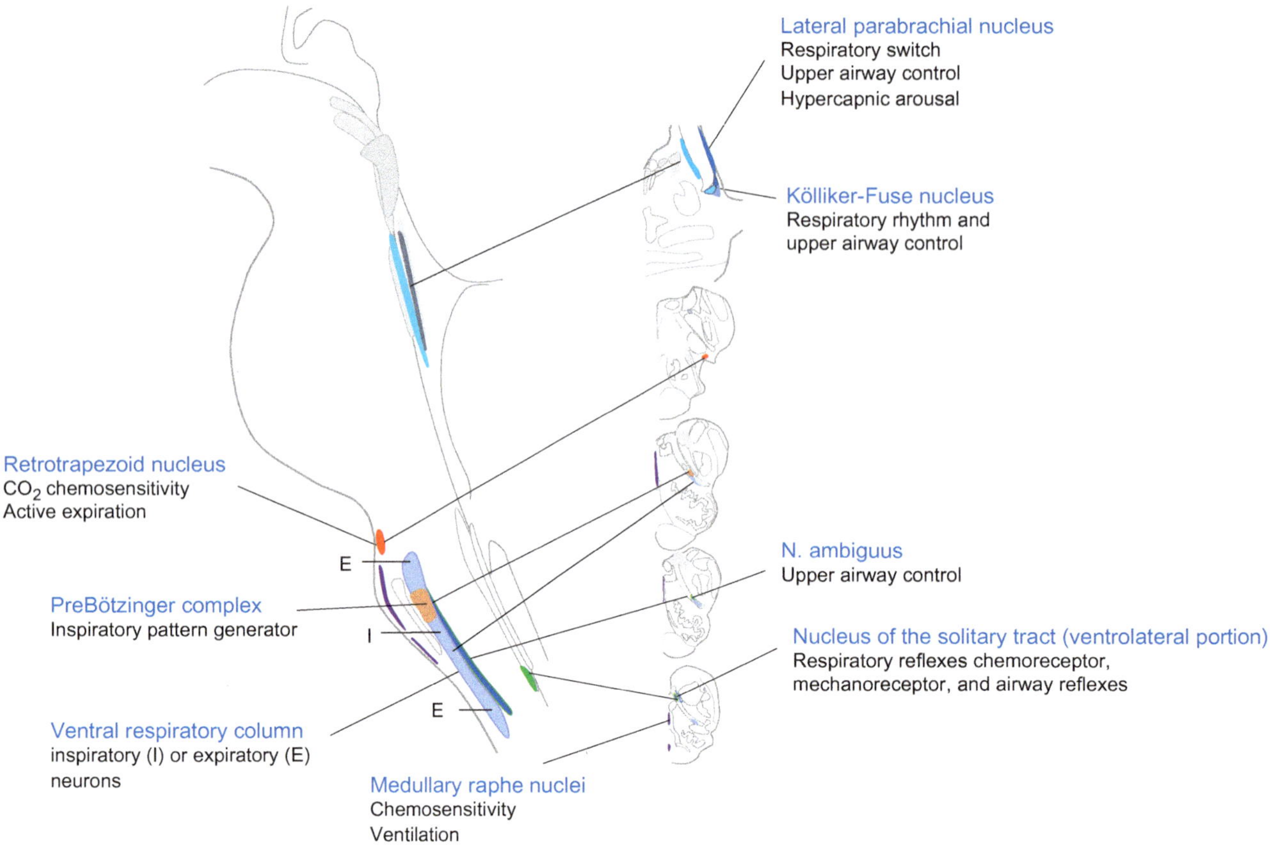

FIGURE 37.6 Brainstem areas controlling respiration.
The preBötzinger complex, located in the ventrolateral medulla, is the critical pattern generator of inspiration. The primary central respiratory chemosensitive zone is the retrotrapezoid nucleus, located close to the ventral medullary surface. Respiratory chemosensitivity also involves serotonergic neurons of the medullary raphe. The ventral respiratory group forms a continuous column of premotor respiratory neurons that extend from the rostral to the caudal portions of the ventrolateral medulla. These columns include, from rostral to caudal, the Bötzinger complex containing expiratory neurons (E), the rostral ventral respiratory group containing inspiratory (I) neurons, and the caudal ventral respiratory group, including the nucleus retroambiguus containing expiratory neurons. These neurons as well as some neurons in the NTS, send direct projections to respiratory motoneurons of the spinal cord. The cranial motor nuclei controlling airway resistance include the NAmb, which innervates innervating the larynx and pharynx via the vagus nerve, and the hypoglossal, trigeminal, and facial nuclei (not shown).

groups of premotor neurons of the ventral respiratory column.[37–39]

Coordination Between Respiratory and Cardiovascular Control

The caudal portion of the NTS has a major role in coordinating respiratory and sympathetic activities.[40–42] Neurons in the caudal NTS receive inputs from baroreceptors, cardiac receptors, and carotid chemoreceptors sensitive to hypoxia, pulmonary mechanoreceptors, and irritant receptors from the airways. The NTS is the first relay and integrative station for the arterial chemoreceptor reflex, which is the principal mechanism for maintenance of arterial PO_2 during hypoxia. Chemoreceptors are located in the carotid and aortic bodies and are stimulated by reduced PaO_2, triggering a reflex that consists of increase of respiratory rate and depth of respiration, sympathetic vasoconstriction, and reduced heart rate. These effects are mediated by projections of NTS neurons to brainstem respiratory groups, to C1 premotor sympathoexcitatory neurons of the RVLM, and to cardiovagal neurons of tie NAmb.[33] The NTS also provides inputs from cardiovascular receptors to the lateral PB, which participates in control of arterial blood pressure via projections to the NTS and RVLM.[43]

Interactions Among Arousal, Respiration, and Cardiovascular Control

The lower brainstem is a site of crucial interactions among arousal, respiration, and cardiovascular control[13] (Figure 37.7). The lateral PB contains glutamatergic and CGRP neurons that project to the basal forebrain and trigger arousal in response to hypercapnia.[44,45] The C1 neurons in

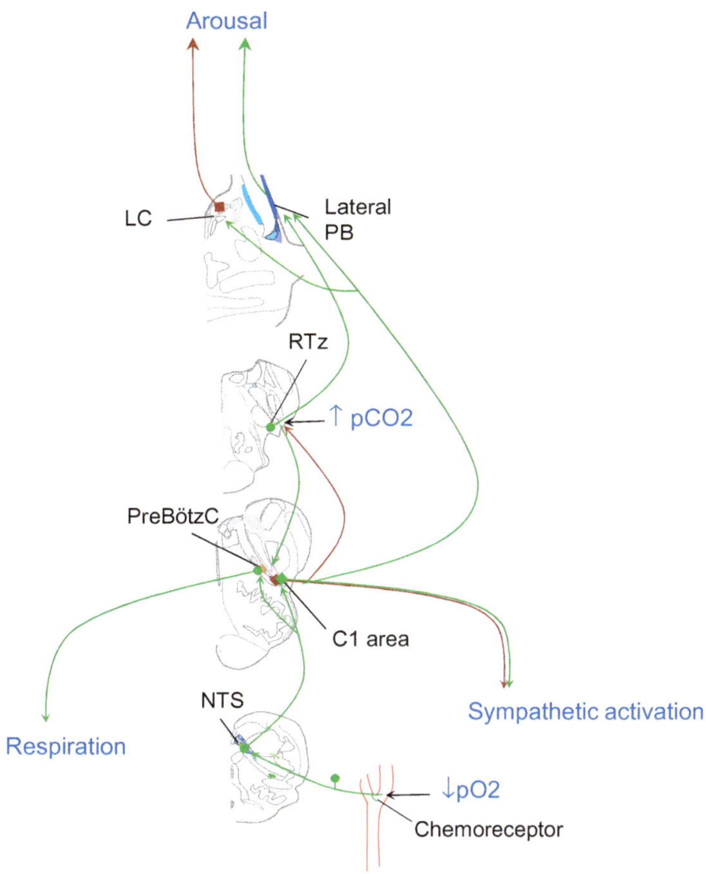

FIGURE 37.7 Brainstem integration of arousal, cardiovascular, and respiratory control.
The caudal portion of the nucleus of the solitary tract (NTS) has a major role in coordinating respiratory and sympathetic activities. The lateral parabrachial nucleus (PB) has a critical role in triggering arousal in response to hypercapnia. The C1 neurons in the rostral ventrolateral medulla respond to hypoxia and have a major role in integration of sympathoexcitatory, respiratory, and arousal responses via their widespread glutamatergic and adrenergic projections. These neurons are activated by hypoxia and promote ventilation via inputs to both the preBötzinger complex (PreBötzC) and retrotrapezoid nucleus (RTz). Several upper brainstem areas have strong interactions with lower brainstem autonomic areas and orchestrate autonomic responses associated with arousal, stress, and other behavioral states. They include the locus coeruleus (LC), which sends diffuse projections that have a major role in arousal, attention, and stress response and descending projections to autonomic areas.

the RVLM respond to hypoxia and have a major role in integration of sympathoexcitatory, respiratory, and arousal responses via their widespread glutamatergic and adrenergic projections.[14] These neurons elicit sympathetic excitation via inputs to the IML, promote ventilation via inputs to both the preBötzinger complex (inspiratory pattern generator) and retrotrapezoid/parafacial nucleus (involved in active expiration), and promote arousal via projections to the upper brainstem and hypothalamus. Several upper brainstem areas interact with lower brainstem autonomic areas and orchestrate autonomic responses associated with arousal, stress, and other behavioral states.[46] They include the locus coeruleus (LC), pedunculopontine tegmental nucleus (PPN/PPT), and PAG. The noradrenergic neurons of the LC send diffuse projections throughout the central nervous system and have a major role in arousal, attention, and stress response.[47] The LC also sends descending projections to autonomic areas such as the DMV, sacral preganglionic neurons, and central gray and dorsal horn of the spinal cord. Together with other catecholaminergic cell groups, including area A7 and the nucleus subcoeruleus region, the LC provides polysynaptic collateral projections to both the IML and the ventral horn. These catecholaminergic presympathetic-premotor protections to neurons innervating the skeletal muscle and the adrenal gland have an important role in somatomotor–sympathetic integration.[48] The PPT/PPN contains intermingled populations of cholinergic, glutamatergic, and GABAergic neurons that differentially promote thalamocortical activation and REM sleep, participate in control of locomotion, and increase dopamine release from midbrain neurons in response to reward.[49] The PPT/PPN contains functionally distinct areas affecting respiration, cardiovascular function, and activity of upper airway muscles.[50] Putative command neurons in the PPT/PPN are connected to both motor and autonomic areas and may integrate the somatomotor and sympathetic functions during different behaviors, including arousal and locomotion.[51] The PAG provides an anatomical and functional interface between the forebrain areas involved in cognitive and emotional processing and lower brainstem circuits mediating autonomic reflexes, pain modulation, and motor responses. Different columns of the PAG initiate distinct patterns of response to stress according to the types of stressor and the ability to cope to stress, as discussed in the next chapter.[52]

CONTROL OF THE BLADDER

Peripheral Innervation

The function of the lower urinary tract is regulated by the interaction among parasympathetic, sympathetic, and somatic efferents[17,53] (Figure 37.8). The preganglionic parasympathetic output originates in the sacral parasympathetic nucleus at S2-S4 segments; the sympathetic output is via SPNs located at the T11-L1 segments; and the somatomotor output to the external sphincter and pelvic floor from motoneurons of the Onuf nucleus at S1–S3 segments. The sacral parasympathetic cholinergic output is critical for normal voiding and is mediated by sacral preganglionic neurons projecting via the pelvic nerve to both cholinergic and noncholinergic neurons located in local ganglia close to or within to the bladder wall. Cholinergic output promotes detrusor contraction via muscarinic M3 receptors, whereas output from nitroxidergic neurons elicit relaxation of the bladder neck. In contrast, both the sympathetic output to the bladder and the Onuf nucleus output to the external sphincter promote urine storage. Several areas control the function of the bladder, urethra, and external urethral sphincter via these outputs. The most important is the pelvic organ control center (pontine micturition center, PMC, Barrington nucleus) located in the dorsomedial pons close to the LC. Other areas include the PAG, medullary raphe, LC, A5 noradrenergic group, and areas in the hypothalamus, anterior cingulate, and motor cortex.

Micturition Reflex

The basic micturition reflex system is a spino-ponto-spinal reflex that is triggered by high-frequency firing of A-δ fiber afferents when bladder filling and intraluminal pressure reach a threshold. These afferents activate a distinct cell group called Gert's nucleus in the sacral cord, which relays this information to the central part of the PAG.[54] In response to these inputs, neurons in the PAG send an excitatory projection to the PMC, which via descending pathways to the sacral cord allows coordinated bladder contraction and external sphincter relaxation for normal bladder emptying. These descending inputs activate the sacral preganglionic neurons innervating the bladder detrusor and inhibit, via local interneurons, the Onuf nucleus motoneurons innervating the external urethral sphincter.

Urine Storage Reflexes

The urine storage reflexes are integrated at the level of the lumbosacral spinal cord. The sympathetic storage reflex is a sacrolumbar intersegmental pathway that provides a negative feedback that allows the bladder to accommodate larger volumes during bladder filling. This reflex is elicited by low-frequency discharge vesical afferents and results in relaxation of the detrusor via β2 and β3 receptors and contraction of the bladder neck via α1 receptors. This sympathetic pathway is turned off, probably by the PMC, when bladder pressure increases to the threshold for micturition. Motoneurons of the Onuf nucleus have a tonic discharge that increases during bladder filling; this activity is mediated in part by a spinal reflex pathway (the guarding reflex) activated by low-level afferent input from the bladder. Studies in the cat showed that the pons may also contain an area located ventral and lateral to the pelvic organ control center called the pelvic urine storage center, which provides direct excitatory input to these Onuf motoneurons.[16] Contraction of the external urethral sphincter also induces firing in pudendal nerve axons that activate inhibitory interneurons in the spinal cord. These interneurons suppress reflex bladder activity by inhibiting both the pelvic parasympathetic nucleus and the interneurons on the micturition reflex pathway. This bladder-to-external urethral sphincter-to-bladder reflex pathway represents a second spinal negative feedback mechanism that promotes urinary continence. Stimulation of the pontine urine storage center located ventrolateral to the PMC not only excites the external sphincter motoneurons of Onuf nucleus but also inhibits reflex bladder activity, via a projection to the nucleus raphe magnus, which sends serotonergic projections that inhibit the sacral parasympathetic nucleus.

Several functional neuroimaging studies have explored the role of the cerebral cortex in mechanisms of voiding and continence.[53] The medial prefrontal cortex is activated during voiding but deactivated in response to bladder filling. The anterior cingulate cortex and the insula may be activated by the unpleasant sensation of bladder filling and inhibit the medial prefrontal cortex; this may reduce the effect of the medial prefrontal cortex on the PAG and thus leads to stabilization of the micturition reflex to maintain continence. The anterior midcingulate cortex may help to suppress voiding via sympathetic activity, and is usually coactivated with the adjacent supplementary motor cortex, which leads to contraction of the pelvic floor and striated sphincter muscles. This voluntary control ensures that the bladder is regularly emptied at the appropriate time and place.

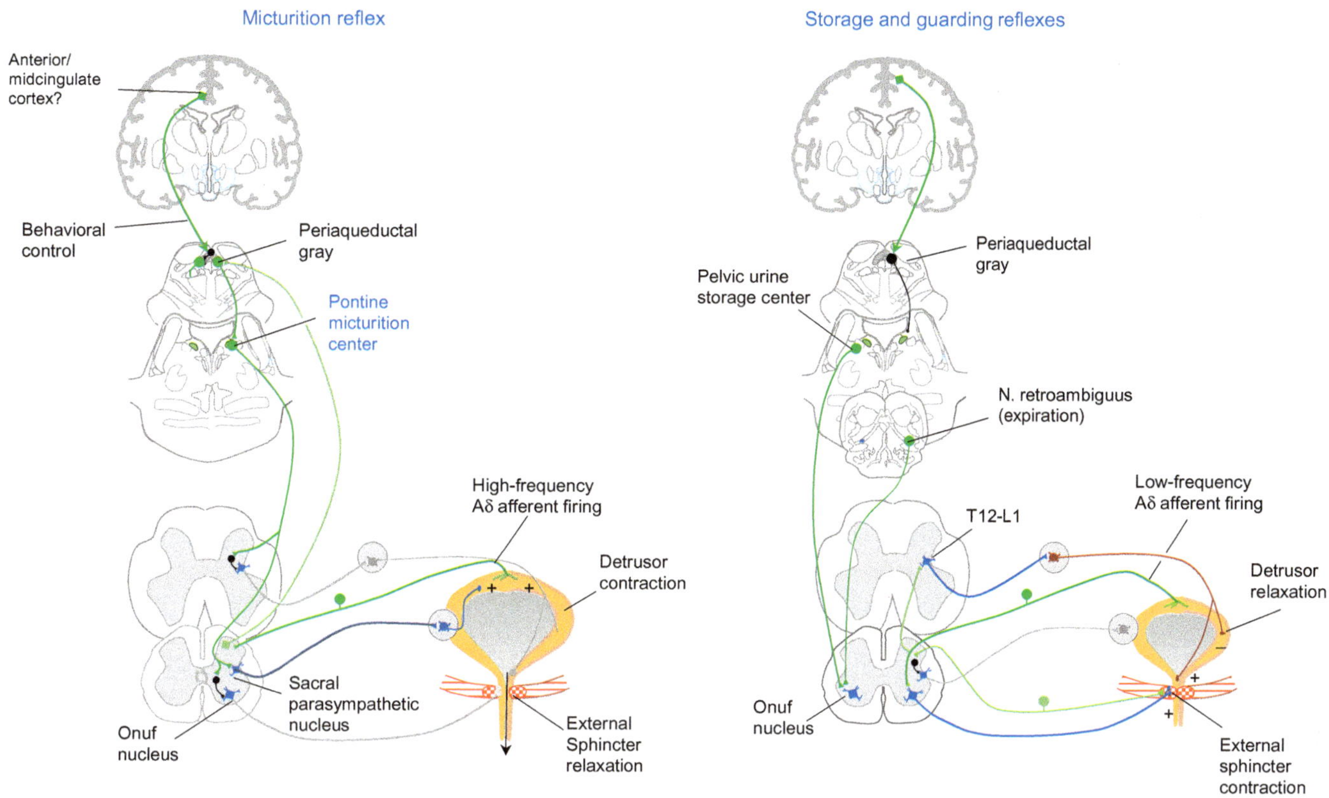

FIGURE 37.8 Control of bladder function.

The lower urinary tract receives parasympathetic, sympathetic, and somatic innervation. The sacral parasympathetic cholinergic output is critical for normal voiding. The basic micturition reflex system is a spino-ponto-spinal reflex that is triggered by high-frequency firing of bladder filling afferents that activate relay neurons in the sacral cord, which project to the periaqueductal gray (PAG). Neurons in the central PAG send an excitatory projection to the pontine micturition center (PMC), which sends projections that activate the sacral preganglionic neurons innervating the bladder detrusor and inhibit, via local interneurons, the Onuf nucleus motoneurons innervating the external urethral sphincter. Higher brain regions in prefrontal cortex and limbic system, by means of its projections to the PAG are able to interrupt this basic reflex system. In contrast, urine storage reflexes are integrated at the level of the lumbosacral spinal cord. The sympathetic storage reflex is a sacrolumbar intersegmental pathway that provides a negative feedback that allows the bladder to accommodate larger volumes during bladder filling. Motoneurons of the Onuf nucleus exhibit a tonic discharge that increases during bladder filling; this activity is mediated in part by a spinal reflex pathway (the guarding reflex). The pons may also contain an area located ventral and lateral to the pelvic organ control center called the pelvic urine storage center, which provides direct excitatory input to these Onuf motoneurons.

GASTROINTESTINAL MOTILITY

Motility and secretion in the gastrointestinal tract are controlled by several neural influences, including extrinsic innervation via the parasympathetic and sympathetic ganglion neurons; intrinsic reflexes mediated by the ENS; visceral afferents that initiate ganglion, spinal, and medullary reflexes; and somatic efferents controlling the striate muscles of the pharynx, upper esophagus, and pelvic floor.

Enteric Nervous System

Motility and secretion in the gastrointestinal tract are primarily controlled by the ENS, with additional modulatory influence from extrinsic parasympathetic and sympathetic inputs, and visceral afferents.[55] The ENS consists of two ganglionated plexuses, myenteric (of Auerbach) and submucosal (of Meissner), located within the walls of the gut. Neurons of the myenteric plexus control the activity of the smooth muscle of the gut, whereas those in the submucosal plexus regulate mucosal secretion and blood flow. They include motor neurons innervating the longitudinal and circular smooth muscle; secretomotor neurons; vasomotor neurons; interneurons coordinating the peristaltic reflexes; and intrinsic primary afferent neurons. The ENS controls gut motility and secretion via local reflexes that are triggered by local distension of the intestinal wall, distortion of the mucosa, and chemical contents in the lumen. The peristaltic reflex allows the normal orderly propulsion of the contents of the gut and involves an ascending excitatory and a descending inhibitory motor component. Sensory neurons, interneurons, and excitatory motor neurons in the ENS are cholinergic and elicit smooth muscle contraction; inhibitory motor neurons utilize VIP or NO and elicit smooth muscle relaxation; and secretomotor neurons utilize ACh and VIP.[56]

Vago-Vagal Reflexes

The DMV provides excitatory inputs to all neurons of the ENS. Vagal influence on esophagus and stomach is critical for vago-vagal reflexes integrated at the level of the NTS. These reflexes regulate the esophageal phase of swallowing and gastric emptying. The DMV provides parallel excitatory and inhibitory pathways controlling gastrointestinal motility. The excitatory pathway involves myenteric neurons that utilize ACh, which stimulates smooth muscle contraction; the inhibitory pathway is mediated by myenteric neurons that utilize VIP, NO, or ATP in various combinations. Vagal influence on gut motility is most prominent in the esophagus and stomach. The importance of vagal control decreases substantially in the small bowel and colon, where motility and secretion are primarily controlled by local ENS reflexes. The sacral parasympathetic output activates cholinergic ENS neurons that promote propulsive activity of the rectum during defecation and inhibitory neurons that initiate colonic relaxation. Anal relaxation induced by rectal distension (recto-anal inhibitory reflex) is mediated by NO.

Sympathetic Inhibition of Gastrointestinal Motility

The prevertebral sympathetic ganglia innervating the gut are the site of convergence of preganglionic inputs via the splanchnic nerves, afferents from cholinergic neurons of the ENS, and collaterals of primary dorsal root ganglion afferents. The sympathetic prevertebral reflex is a feedback mechanism that inhibits gut motility.

AUTONOMIC FAILURE

Autonomic failure may affect the sympathetic, parasympathetic, or enteric nervous system either in isolation or in various combinations.[57]

Clinical Manifestations

Sympathetic failure manifests primarily with neurogenic orthostatic hypotension (nOH) and anhidrosis; cranial parasympathetic failure with intolerance to light, dry eyes (xerophthalmia), and dry mouth (xerostomia); sacral parasympathetic failure with urinary retention and erectile dysfunction; and ENS failure with gastroparesis and constipation. Neurogenic OH is the manifestation of impaired sympathetically mediated vasoconstriction of skeletal muscle and mesenteric vessels in response to baroreceptor unloading due to orthostatic stress. It may occur as a consequence of disorders affecting the barosensitive sympathoexcitatory neurons of the RVLM, spinal preganglionic sympathetic neurons, autonomic ganglia, unmyelinated axon, NE availability, or vascular α1 adrenergic receptors (typically as a side effect of drugs). Anhidrosis in autonomic failure may reflect impairment of central thermoregulatory pathways, spinal preganglionic sudomotor units, or cholinergic sympathetic ganglion neurons or their peripheral axons. Neurogenic bladder can manifest with detrusor overactivity or underactivity. Reduced detrusor activity leads to incomplete bladder emptying, increased postvoid residual, low peak urinary flow rate, and eventually urinary retention and overflow incontinence. Impaired micturition may result from lesions affecting the bladder afferents. sacral parasympathetic neurons or their axons. or cholinergic muscarinic neurotransmission. Neurogenic bladder is commonly associated with erectile and ejaculatory dysfunction in men and poor vaginal lubrication in women. Symptoms of delayed esophageal transit include dysphagia and regurgitation; delayed gastric emptying produces early satiety, anorexia, and nausea, bloating, belching, postprandial vomiting, and pain. Lower gastrointestinal dysmotility manifests with constipation, and occasionally with diarrhea.

Main Causes

Disorders causing autonomic failure can be classified according to the presence or absence of associated neurologic manifestations, such as peripheral neuropathy or parkinsonism, and their temporal profile. Subacute isolated autonomic failure affecting sympathetic, parasympathetic, and ENS function, in various combinations, occurs in autoimmune autonomic ganglionopathy. About 50% of these cases are caused by autoantibodies against the gnAChRs. Autoimmine autonomic ganglionopathy may also be a paraneoplastic manifestation, for example due to anti-Hu antibodies associated with small cell lung carcinoma, or may be associated with sensory ganglionopathies, as in the case of Sjögren syndrome. Autonomic failure may be a major feature of small fiber neuropathies due to diabetes or, amyloidosis, Distal vasomotor and sudomotor dysfunction associated with pain may also occur in other distal painful neuropathies, such as hereditary sensory and autonomic neuropathies; Fabry disease; and sodium channelopathies.

Progressive autonomic failure occurs in neurodegenerative synucleinopathies. "Pure" autonomic failure without other neurologic manifestations may occur in isolation or may precede the development of a Lewy body disorders or multiple system atrophy (MSA). Multiple system atrophy is characterized by prominent nOH, neurogenic bladder with eventual urinary retention and incontinence and erectile dysfunction, associated with parkinsonism, cerebellar ataxia, or both. The neuropathological hallmark of MSA is the accumulation of α-synuclein containing glial cytoplasmic inclusions in oligodendrocytes and neuronal loss in nigrostriatal, cerebellar and central autonomic circuits, including the C1 area, medullary raphe, IML, and PMC and Onuf nucleus.[58] Autonomic manifestations, such as constipation, may be also be a prominent early non-motor symptom in Parkinson disease.[55] The early gastrointestinal manifestations and involvement of the ENS and DMV by Lewy body pathology has led to the hypothesis of propagation of α-synuclein pathology from the periphery to the central nervous system via the vagus nerve. However, this issue remains controversial. In Lewy body disorders, including PD, there is a selective cardiac sympathetic denervation that may allow the differential diagnosis between PD and MSA and between dementia with Lewy bodies and Alzheimer disease in the majority of cases.

Brainstem Involvement and Combined Cardiovascular and Respiratory Dysregulation

The complex interactions among brainstem areas involved in cardiovascular control, automatic respiration, and arousal provide the bases for sleep-related respiratory and cardiovascular dysfunction in many disorders.[13] For example, in patients with MSA, loss of C1 neurons may manifest not only with nOH but also with reduced respiratory chemosensitivity and arousal responses. In this disorder, loss of neurons in the preBötzinger complex, lateral PB, and medullary raphe may contribute to sleep apnea, respiratory dysrhythmia, impaired arousal responses to hypoxemia and hypercapnia, laryngeal stridor, and death during sleep. Congenital central hypoventilation syndrome is associated with mutation of the *PHOX-2B* gene encoding a transcription factor that is necessary for differentiation of carotid body afferents and neurons of several brainstem nuclei including the retrotrapezoid nucleus, NTS/dorsal vagal complex, medullary catecholaminergic (including C1) neurons, some pontine regions, and cholinergic effector neurons. These patients have loss of hypoxic or hypercapnic ventilatory reflexes abnormal fluctuations of arterial PCO2 and, in severe cases, fatal respiratory failure during sleep.[59] A defect in hypercapnia/hypoxia-induced arousal due to impaired activity of medullar serotonergic neurons may contribute to some cases of sudden infant death syndrome[60] and sudden unexplained death in epilepsy,[61] as well as sudden death in MSA.[62]

KEY POINTS

- The autonomic nervous system controls the functions of visceral effectors via several interconnected areas distributed throughout the neuraxis.
- These areas are components of a central autonomic network, but they also control many other functions including arousal, and respiration.
- The peripheral control of visceral organs is exerted by the sympathetic and parasympathetic systems, enteric nervous system (ENS), and visceral afferents.
- The preganglionic sympathetic and parasympathetic neurons are cholinergic and provide fast excitation to autonomic ganglia and ENS via ganglion-type ($\alpha_{3/}\beta_4$) nicotinic receptors.
- Preganglionic neurons receive two major influences: inputs from visceral receptors that trigger autonomic reflexes, and descending influences from the brainstem and forebrain regulating autonomic output during homeostatic, adaptive, or emotional responses.
- The sympathetic nervous system generated patterns of response critical for maintenance of arterial blood pressure, regulation of regional blood flow, thermoregulation, and integrated response to stress.
- The sympathetic preganglionic neurons form distinct functional subunits, including skin vasoconstrictor, muscle vasoconstrictor, sudomotor, and others.
- Most descending inputs to the preganglionic sympathetic neurons originate from the medulla and hypothalamus, which engage different subpopulations in specific response patterns.
- Spinal interneurons may have an important role in the interplay between the sympathetic and the motor systems.
- Most sympathetic effects are mediated by norepinephrine (NA) via α1 receptors (smooth muscle contraction), β1 receptors (cardiac stimulation) and β2 receptors. (smooth muscle relaxation).
- Sympathetic ganglion neurons innervating the sweat glands are cholinergic.
- The parasympathetic system mediates organ-specific reflexes such as pupil constriction, lacrimation, salivation, gastrointestinal motility and secretion, micturition, defecation, and erection.
- The parasympathetic output is mediated both via cholinergic neurons that trigger smooth muscle contraction and glandular secretion via M3 receptors, and by noncholinergic neurons that use VIP and NO and elicit smooth muscle relaxation.
- The dorsal motor nucleus of the vagus (DMV) mediates all vago-vagal reflexes controlling motility and secretion in the gastrointestinal and respiratory tracts.
- The nucleus ambiguus is the main source of vagal input to the heart.
- Sacral preganglionic nucleus control micturition, defecation, and sexual function.
- The central autonomic control is distributed throughout the neuraxis and is hierarchically organized.

- Areas in the medulla and lower pons mediate cardiovascular, respiratory, gastrointestinal, and micturition reflexes and relay visceral information to the upper brainstem and forebrain.
- The nucleus of the solitary tract (NTS) is the first relay station of visceral afferents.
- The rostral ventrolateral medulla (RVLM) contains sympathoexcitatory neurons (including the C1 group) that have a critical role in maintenance of blood pressure and responses to internal stressors.
- The rostral ventromedial medulla (RVMM) and medullary raphe provide sympathoexcitatory outputs in responses to cold and tachycardia in response to external stressors.
- The parabrachial nuclear complex (PB) has a major role in control of arousal, respiration, cardiovascular function, thermoregulation, and food intake.
- The baroreceptor reflex is the principal buffering mechanism for short-term regulation of arterial blood pressure and to prevent orthostatic hypotension.
- The cardiovagal neurons of the NAmb are critical for the beat to beat modulation of the heart rate during respiration.
- The preBötzinger complex is the critical pattern generator of inspiration.
- The retrotrapezoid nucleus located close to the ventral medullary surface is the primary central respiratory chemosensitive zone for ventilatory responses to hypercapnia.
- Neurons of the nucleus raphe pallidus and raphe obscurus exert a global excitatory effect on the respiratory network.
- Several brainstem areas, including the PB and the C1 area, participate in the interactions among arousal, respiration, and cardiovascular control.
- The micturition reflex involves the periaqueductal gray and pontine micturition center (PMC).
- The PMC coordinates bladder detrusor contraction and relaxation of the external urethral sphincter.
- Sympathetic output triggers relaxation of the detrusor muscle and, together with the Onuf nucleus output to the external sphincter, is involved in urine storage.
- Motility and secretion in the gastrointestinal tract are primarily controlled by the ENS.
- Vagal inputs primarily control motility of the esophagus and stomach.
- Autonomic failure may affect the sympathetic, parasympathetic, or ENS either in isolation or in various combinations.
- Sympathetic failure manifests primarily with neurogenic orthostatic hypotension and anhidrosis.
- Cranial parasympathetic failure manifests with intolerance to light, dry eyes, and dry mouth.
- Sacral parasympathetic failure manifests with urinary retention and erectile dysfunction; and ENS failure manifests with gastroparesis and constipation.
- Subacute isolated autonomic failure occurs in autoimmune autonomic ganglionopathy.
- Autonomic failure may be a major feature of diabetic or amyloid peripheral neuropathies.
- Progressive autonomic failure occurs in neurodegenerative synucleinopathies such as multiple system atrophy (MSA) or Lewy body disorders.
- Early neurogenic orthostatic hypotension and urinary retention strongly suggest the diagnosis of MSA.
- The interactions among brainstem areas involved in cardiovascular control, automatic respiration, and arousal provide the bases for sleep-related respiratory and cardiovascular dysfunction and pose a risk of death during sleep in many disorders, such as MSA.

REFERENCES

1. Deuchars SA, Lall VK. Sympathetic preganglionic neurons: properties and inputs. Compr Physiol 2015;5:829–869.
2. Janig W, Habler HJ. Neurophysiological analysis of target-related sympathetic pathways--from animal to human: similarities and differences. Acta Physiol Scand 2003;177:255–274.
3. Guyenet PG. The sympathetic control of blood pressure. Nat Rev Neurosci 2006;7:335–346.
4. Dampney RA. Central neural control of the cardiovascular system: current perspectives. Adv Physiol Educ 2016;40:283–296.
5. Barman SM, Yates BJ. Deciphering the neural control of sympathetic nerve activity: status report and directions for future research. Front Neurosci 2017;11:730.
6. Wehrwein EA, Orer HS, Barman SM. Overview of the anatomy, physiology, and pharmacology of the autonomic nervous system. Compr Physiol 2016;6:1239–1278.
7. Travagli RA, Anselmi L. Vagal neurocircuitry and its influence on gastric motility. Nat Rev Gastroenterol Hepatol 2016;13:389–401.
8. Gourine AV, Machhada A, Trapp S, Spyer KM. Cardiac vagal preganglionic neurones: an update. Aut Neurosci e: basic & clinical 2016;199:24–28.
9. Cutsforth-Gregory JK, Benarroch EE. Nucleus of the solitary tract, medullary reflexes, and clinical implications. Neurology 2017;88:1187–1196.
10. Saper CB. The central autonomic nervous system: conscious visceral perception and autonomic pattern generation. Annu Rev Neurosci 2002;25:433–469.
11. Benarroch EE. The central autonomic network: functional organization, dysfunction, and perspective. Mayo Clin Proc 1993;10:988–1001.
12. Siso S, Jeffrey M, Gonzalez L. Sensory circumventricular organs in health and disease. Acta Neuropathol 2010;120:689–705.

13. Benarroch EE. Brainstem integration of arousal, sleep, cardiovascular, and respiratory control. Neurology 2018;91:958–966.
14. Stornetta RL, Guyenet PG. C1 neurons: a nodal point for stress? Exp Physiol 2018;103:332–336.
15. Del Negro CA, Funk GD, Feldman JL. Breathing matters. Nat Rev Neurosci 2018;19:351–367.
16. Holstege G. How the emotional motor system controls the pelvic organs. Sex Med Rev 2016;4:303–328.
17. Fowler CJ, Griffiths D, de Groat WC. The neural control of micturition. Nat Rev Neurosci 2008;9:453–466.
18. Zeng WZ, Marshall KL, Min S, et al. PIEZOs mediate neuronal sensing of blood pressure and the baroreceptor reflex. Science 2018;362:464–467.
19. Wenker IC, Abe C, Viar KE, Stornetta DS, Stornetta RL, Guyenet PG. Blood pressure regulation by the rostral ventrolateral medulla in conscious rats: effects of hypoxia, hypercapnia, baroreceptor denervation, and anesthesia. J Neurosci 2017;37:4565–4583.
20. Kaufmann H, Norcliffe-Kaufmann L, Palma JA. Baroreflex dysfunction. N Engl J Med 2020;382:163–178.
21. Dampney RAL. Resetting of the baroreflex control of sympathetic vasomotor activity during natural behaviors: description and conceptual model of central mechanisms. Front Neurosci 2017;11:461.
22. Michelini LC, O'Leary DS, Raven PB, Nobrega AC. Neural control of circulation and exercise: a translational approach disclosing interactions between central command, arterial baroreflex, and muscle metaboreflex. Am J Physiol Heart Circ Physiol 2015;309:H381–392.
23. Silvani A, Dampney RA. Central control of cardiovascular function during sleep. Am J Physiol Heart Circ Physiol 2013;305:H1683–1692.
24. Coote JH, Chauhan RA. The sympathetic innervation of the heart: Important new insights. Autonomic Neuroscience: Basic & Clinical 2016;199:17–23.
25. Farmer DG, Dutschmann M, Paton JF, Pickering AE, McAllen RM. Brainstem sources of cardiac vagal tone and respiratory sinus arrhythmia. J Physiol 2016;594:7249–7265.
26. Smith JC, Abdala AP, Borgmann A, Rybak IA, Paton JF. Brainstem respiratory networks: building blocks and microcircuits. Trends Neurosci 2013;36:152–162.
27. Burke PG, Kanbar R, Basting TM, et al. State-dependent control of breathing by the retrotrapezoid nucleus. J Physiol 2015;593:2909–2926.
28. Anderson TM, Garcia AJ, 3rd, Baertsch NA, et al. A novel excitatory network for the control of breathing. Nature 2016;536:76–80.
29. Yackle K, Schwarz LA, Kam K, et al. Breathing control center neurons that promote arousal in mice. Science 2017;355:1411–1415.
30. Yang CF, Feldman JL. Efferent projections of excitatory and inhibitory preBotzinger complex neurons. J Comp Neurol 2018;526:1389–1402.
31. Nattie E, Li A. Central chemoreceptors: locations and functions. Compr Physiol 2012;2:221–254.
32. Guyenet PG, Bayliss DA. Neural control of breathing and CO2 homeostasis. Neuron 2015;87:946–961.
33. Guyenet PG, Bayliss DA, Stornetta RL, et al. Interdependent feedback regulation of breathing by the carotid bodies and the retrotrapezoid nucleus. J Physiol 2018;596:3029–3042.
34. Hodges MR, Richerson GB. The role of medullary serotonin (5-HT) neurons in respiratory control: contributions to eupneic ventilation, CO2 chemoreception, and thermoregulation. J Appl Physiol (1985) 2010;108:1425–1432.
35. Corcoran AE, Richerson GB, Harris MB. Functional link between the hypocretin and serotonin systems in the neural control of breathing and central chemosensitivity. J Neurophysiol 2015;114:381–389.
36. Morinaga R, Nakamuta N, Yamamoto Y. Serotonergic projections to the ventral respiratory column from raphe nuclei in rats. Neurosci Res 2018;143:20–30.
37. Herbert H, Moga MM, Saper CB. Connections of the parabrachial nucleus with the nucleus of the solitary tract and the medullary reticular formation in the rat. J Comp Neurol 1990;293:540–580.
38. Yokota S, Kaur S, VanderHorst VG, Saper CB, Chamberlin NL. Respiratory-related outputs of glutamatergic, hypercapnia-responsive parabrachial neurons in mice. J Comp Neurol 2015;523:907–920.
39. Chamberlin NL, Saper CB. Topographic organization of respiratory responses to glutamate microstimulation of the parabrachial nucleus in the rat. J Neurosci 1994;14:6500–6510.
40. Zoccal DB, Furuya WI, Bassi M, Colombari DS, Colombari E. The nucleus of the solitary tract and the coordination of respiratory and sympathetic activities. Front Physiol 2014;5:238.
41. Molkov YI, Zoccal DB, Baekey DM, et al. Physiological and pathophysiological interactions between the respiratory central pattern generator and the sympathetic nervous system. Prog Brain Res 2014;212:1–23.
42. Guyenet PG. Regulation of breathing and autonomic outflows by chemoreceptors. Compr Physiol 2014;4:1511–1562.
43. Davern PJ. A role for the lateral parabrachial nucleus in cardiovascular function and fluid homeostasis. Front Physiol 2014;5:436.
44. Kaur S, Pedersen NP, Yokota S, et al. Glutamatergic signaling from the parabrachial nucleus plays a critical role in hypercapnic arousal. J Neurosci 2013;33:7627–7640.
45. Chamberlin NL. Brain circuitry mediating arousal from obstructive sleep apnea. Curr Opin Neurobiol 2013;23:774–779.
46. Venkatraman A, Edlow BL, Immordino-Yang MH. The brainstem in emotion: a review. Front Neuroanat 2017;11:15.
47. Benarroch EE. Locus coeruleus. Cell Tissue Res 2018;373:221–232.
48. Nam H, Kerman IA. Distribution of catecholaminergic presympathetic-premotor neurons in the rat lower brainstem. Neuroscience 2016;324:430–445.
49. Mena-Segovia J, Bolam JP. Rethinking the pedunculopontine nucleus: from cellular organization to function. Neuron 2017;94:7–18.
50. Padley JR, Kumar NN, Li Q, Nguyen TB, Pilowsky PM, Goodchild AK. Central command regulation of circulatory function mediated by descending pontine cholinergic inputs to sympathoexcitatory rostral ventrolateral medulla neurons. Circ Res 2007;100:284–291.
51. Krout KE, Mettenleiter TC, Loewy AD. Single CNS neurons link both central motor and cardiosympathetic systems: a double-virus tracing study. Neuroscience 2003;118:853–866.

52. Bandler R, Keay KA, Floyd N, Price J. Central circuits mediating patterned autonomic activity during active vs. passive emotional coping. Brain Res Bull 2000;53:95–104.
53. de Groat WC, Griffiths D, Yoshimura N. Neural control of the lower urinary tract. Compr Physiol 2015;5:327–396.
54. Holstege G. The emotional motor system and micturition control. Neurourol Urodyn 2010;29:42–48.
55. Cersosimo MG, Raina GB, Pecci C, et al. Gastrointestinal manifestations in Parkinson's disease: prevalence and occurrence before motor symptoms. J Neurol 2013;260:1332–1338.
56. Anlauf M, Schafer MK, Eiden L, Weihe E. Chemical coding of the human gastrointestinal nervous system: cholinergic, VIPergic, and catecholaminergic phenotypes. J Comp Neurol 2003;459:90–111.
57. Benarroch EE. The clinical approach to autonomic failure in neurological disorders. Nat Rev Neurol 2014;10:396–407.
58. Coon EA, Cutsforth-Gregory JK, Benarroch EE. Neuropathology of autonomic dysfunction in synucleinopathies. Mov Disord 2018;33:349–358.
59. Moreira TS, Takakura AC, Czeisler C, Otero JJ. Respiratory and autonomic dysfunction in congenital central hypoventilation syndrome. J Neurophysiol 2016;116:742–752.
60. Duncan JR, Paterson DS, Hoffman JM, et al. Brainstem serotonergic deficiency in sudden infant death syndrome. JAMA 2010;303:430–437.
61. Massey CA, Sowers LP, Dlouhy BJ, Richerson GB. Mechanisms of sudden unexpected death in epilepsy: the pathway to prevention. Nat Rev Neurol 2014;10:271–282.
62. Tada M, Kakita A, Toyoshima Y, et al. Depletion of medullary serotonergic neurons in patients with multiple system atrophy who succumbed to sudden death. Brain 2009;132:1810–1819.

38 Homeostasis and Adaptation

OVERVIEW

Central control of homeostasis and adaptation to internal or external challenges requires the integrated activity of the hypothalamus, amygdala, insula, and anterior cingulate cortex (ACC). These areas are reciprocally interconnected and either directly or indirectly have access to brainstem areas controlling autonomic outputs and respiration. The hypothalamus receives and integrates interoceptive, humoral, and emotional signals and functions as a pattern generator for coordinated autonomic and endocrine responses to restore the internal milieu and adapt to challenges to survival.[1] The amygdala provides automatic tagging of the valence (positive or negative) and intensity of innate or conditioned environmental stimuli and thereby their behavioral relevance[2] and triggers automatic survival responses via the hypothalamus and brainstem.[3] The insula is the primary interoceptive cortex and integrates multiple sensations to generate the awareness of the state of the body.[4] The ACC provides subjective relevance to these feelings to guide behavior.[5–7] Interoception strongly influences emotion, cognition, and motivation. Central autonomic commands from the anterior insula and ACC may be sent as predictive signals about the expected sensory consequences that would result from activation of the target organs. The mismatch between feedforward commands and feedback signals conveyed to the posterior insula generates an error prediction signal that influences cognitive and emotional processing. Disorders affecting these forebrain regions, for example in the setting of stroke, seizures, or limbic encephalitis, may manifest with life-threatening disturbances such as cardiac arrhythmias and risk of sudden death. The aims of this chapter are to review: (1) the general organization of the hypothalamus; (2) the role of the hypothalamus and its connections in stress responses, control of inflammation, thermoregulation, and other homeostatic and adaptive responses; (3) the main connectivity and functions of the amygdala, insula, and ACC in autonomic control; and (4) some examples of disorders affecting these functions.

HYPOTHALAMUS

The hypothalamus has an integrative role and functions as a pattern generator of autonomic, endocrine, and behavioral responses. These functions depend on several nuclei that participate in circuits that control stress responses, fluid and electrolyte balance, body temperature, food intake and energy metabolism, and reproduction.[1] These nuclei receive and integrate information from multiple sources, project to areas controlling autonomic, endocrine, and motor output, and participate in circuits that regulate the behavioral state, circadian rhythms and wake–sleep cycle. Via these circuits and their effectors the hypothalamus functions to maintain body functions at key set points (homeostasis), or to overcome an internal or external stressor (allostasis). The functions of the hypothalamus in regulation of sleep and circadian rhythms are discussed in chapter 27.

Nuclear Organization

The hypothalamus includes a preoptic, tuberal, and posterior or mammillary region. Each of these regions can be subdivided into a periventricular, medial, and lateral zone (Figure 38.1). Nuclei in the periventricular zone surround the third ventricle and include those that control anterior pituitary secretion. The medial zone contains most of the nuclei involved in homeostasis and adaptive responses. The lateral hypothalamus contains nuclei that participate in control of arousal and reward responses. The preoptic area includes several neuronal groups that participate in thermoregulation, electrolyte-balance, wake–sleep regulation, and reproduction. The tuberal hypothalamus contains nuclei that participate in integrative circuits controlling

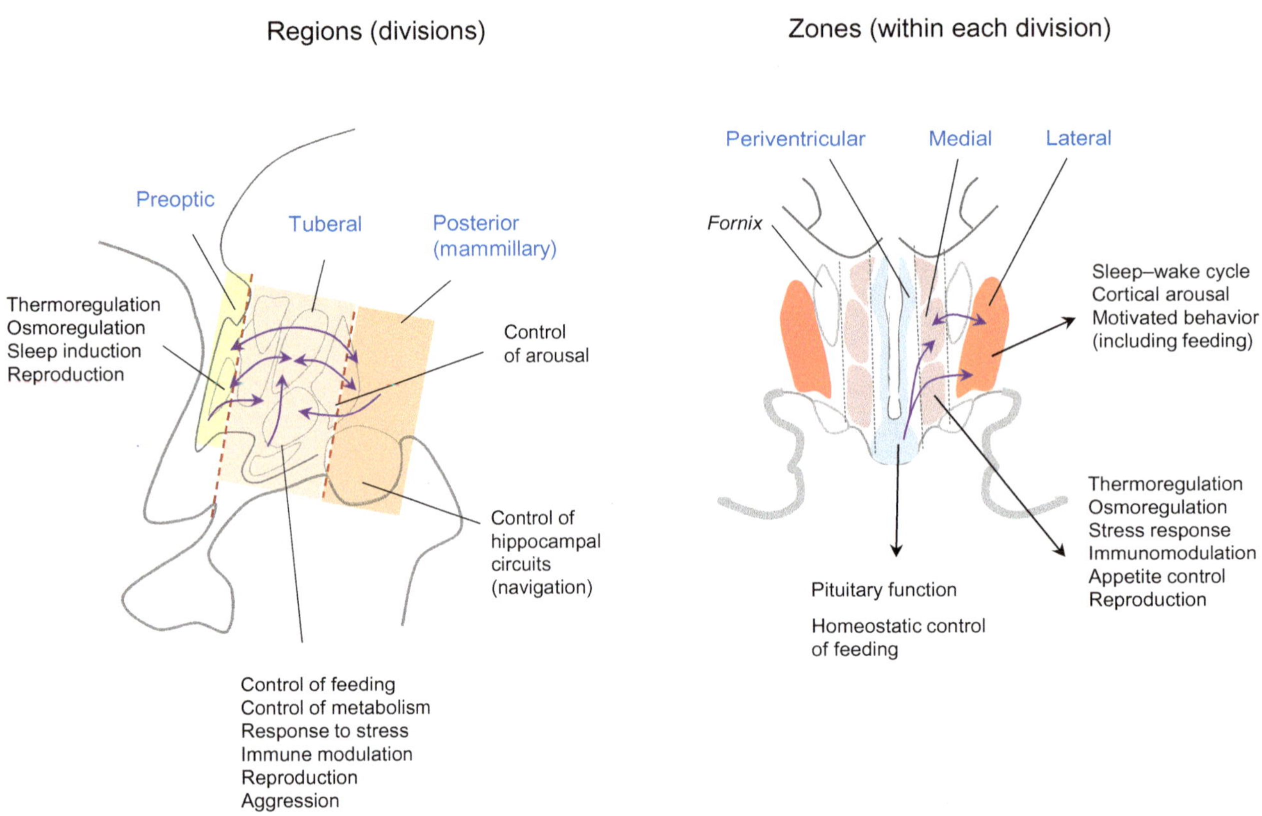

FIGURE 38.1 Anatomical and functional organization of the hypothalamus.

The hypothalamus is divided from rostral to caudal into the preoptic area, tuberal region, and posterior or mammillary region. Each of these regions can be subdivided into a periventricular, medial, and lateral zone). Nuclei in the periventricular zone control anterior pituitary secretion. The medial zone contains most of the hypothalamic nuclei involved in homeostasis and adaptive responses. The lateral hypothalamus contains nuclei that participate in control of arousal and reward responses.

of feeding, responses to stress, aggression, and sexual behavior. The posterior hypothalamus, particularly the posterior lateral hypothalamus, has a critical role in control of arousal, stress responses, and motivated behaviors. Most connections of the hypothalamus are mediated by L-glutamate or GABA.

Inputs to the Hypothalamus

The hypothalamus receives and integrates information from multiple sources (Figure 38.2). Some signals from the blood or CSF, such as temperature, osmolality, or circulating glucose or steroid hormones, may directly affect neurons of the hypothalamus sensitive to these stimuli. Circulating peptides and cytokines affect hypothalamic nuclei through paracrine mechanisms via endothelial cells or via circumventricular organs (CVOs). They include the subfornical organ (SFO) and vascular organ of the lamina terminalis (organum vasculosum of the lamina terminalis, OVLT) located along the anterior wall of the third ventricle, and the area postrema located in the fourth ventricle. These areas contain fenestrated capillaries and thus lack a blood-brain barrier (BBB).[8] Neurons and astrocytes in these areas express several receptors and channels that allow them to sense multiple blood-borne signals. Examples include the aquaporin 4 (AQP4) water channel, the transient receptor potential (TRP) channel TRPV1, sodium-gated sodium channels (Nax), and angiotensin II receptors. The ependymal lining of the circumventricular organs contains specialized cells, called tanycytes, harboring multiple microvilli or cilia that contact the CSF and express a unique repertoire of receptors for detection of levels of nutrients and hormones.[9]

The second major source of inputs to the hypothalamus involves pathways conveying temperature, visceral, and pain sensation. These pathways originate from afferents that relay on lamina I of the dorsal horn, spinal trigeminal nucleus, or nucleus of the solitary tract (NTS). Inputs from lamina I ascend directly via spinohypothalamic pathways or more commonly via a relay in the parabrachial nucleus (PB) of the pons (spinoparabrachial pathway). Similarly, the NTS may project the hypothalamus either directly or via the PB. These inputs may also reach the hypothalamus via ascending monoaminergic systems.

Inputs related to automatic survival responses originate primarily from the centromedial nucleus of the amygdala (CeM) or its functional continuum, the bed nucleus of the

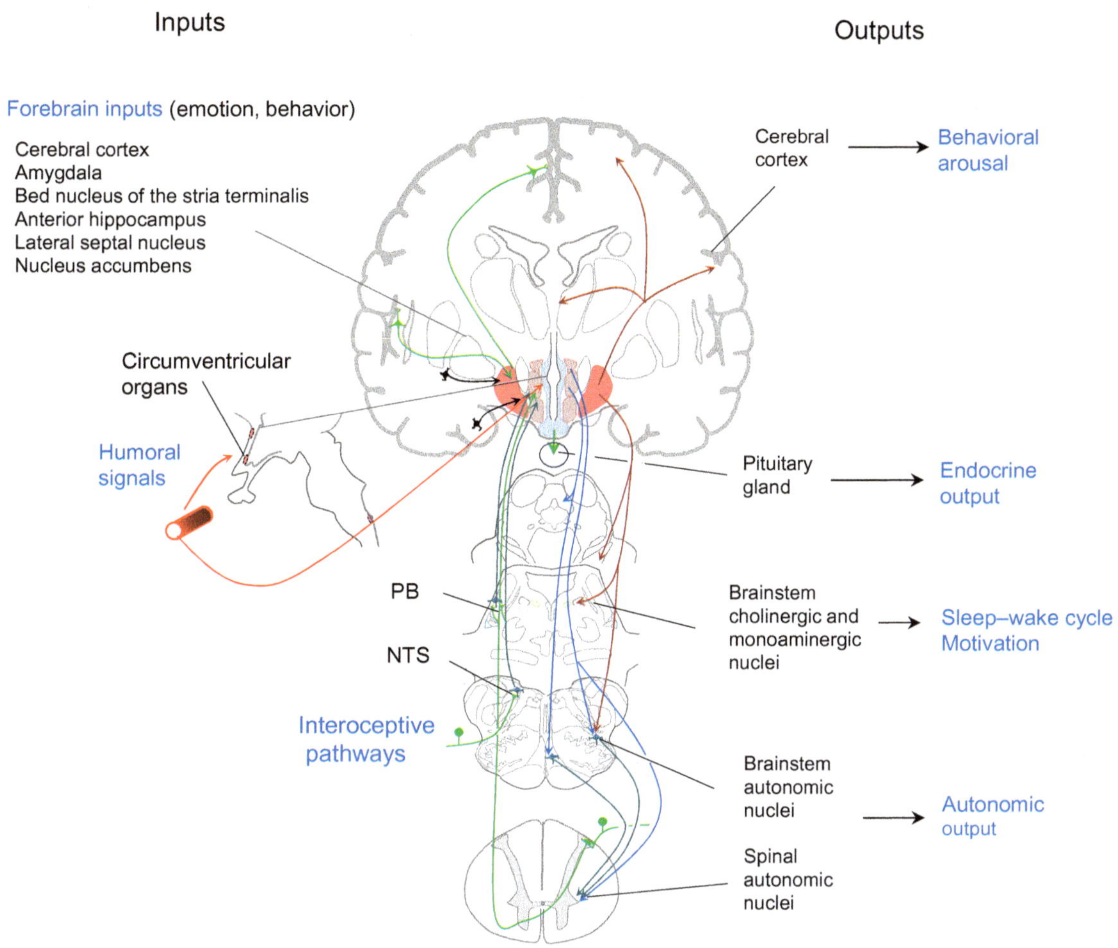

FIGURE 38.2 Main connections of the hypothalamus.

The hypothalamus receives humoral, interoceptive, circadian, and emotional influences. Some signals, such as blood osmolarity and temperature, directly affect hypothalamic neurons. Circulating peptides affect hypothalamic neurons indirectly, either through paracrine mechanisms via endothelial cells or via circumventricular organs. Interoceptive pathways conveying temperature, visceral, and pain sensation from lamina I (LI) reach the hypothalamus either directly or via a relay in the parabrachial nucleus (PB); visceral afferent information from the nucleus of the solitary tract (NTS) reaches the hypothalamus both directly and via the PB. The hypothalamus also receives important inputs from areas involved in emotional and reward processing. The output to autonomic nuclei controls the preganglionic sympathetic or parasympathetic neurons either directly or, more commonly, via brainstem preautonomic neurons. The endocrine output occurs via the pituitary gland. Hypothalamic projections to brainstem cholinergic and monoaminergic neurons potently modulate the behavioral state. Direct projections from the posterior and lateral hypothalamus to the cerebral cortex also participate in cortical arousal.

stria terminalis (BNST). Other inputs related to emotional behavior originate from the insular cortex, ACC, and shell of the nucleus accumbens (NAc).

Finally, the hypothalamus receives inputs from areas involved in behavioral arousal and motivation, including dopaminergic neurons of the ventral tegmental area (VTA), noradrenergic neurons of the locus coeruleus (LC), serotonergic neurons of the rostral raphe, epinephrine neurons of the C1 area of the rostral ventrolateral medulla (RVLM), and norepinephrine neurons of the caudal ventrolateral medulla (A1 group) or dorsomedial medulla (A2 group).

Outputs of the Hypothalamus

The hypothalamic projections control autonomic responses, endocrine function, state of arousal, and motivation (Figure 38.2).The output to autonomic nuclei originate primarily in the paraventricular nucleus (PVH), dorsomedial nucleus (DMH), and perifornical region including orexin (ORX, hypocretin) neurons.[10] These hypothalamic projections control the output of preganglionic sympathetic and parasympathetic neurons either directly or, more commonly, via a relay on brainstem preautonomic neurons located in the RVLM, rostral ventromedial medulla (RVMM), and nucleus raphe pallidus (RPa). Hypothalamic projections also target viscerosensory relay nuclei such as the NTS and PB. One important relay of hypothalamic outputs controlling autonomic, as well as pain modulatory and motor output is the periaqueductal gray (PAG).

The endocrine output of the hypothalamus includes two main neurosecretory systems. The magnocellular system consists of large neurons of the PVH and supraoptic nucleus (SON) that produce either arginine vasopressin (AVP) or oxytocin and send their axons via the pituitary stalk to the posterior pituitary, for release of these hormones into the general circulation. The parvocellular system comprises several groups of small neurons located in the periventricular zone that send axons to the median eminence, and secrete releasing or release-inhibiting hormones that reach the anterior pituitary via portal vessels and control function of endocrine cells. Important examples include neurons of the PVH secreting corticotrophin releasing hormone (CRH) in response to stress, and dopamine neurons in the arcuate nucleus (ARC, infundibular nucleus) that tonically inhibit prolactin secretion. The hypothalamus also regulates endocrine function indirectly, through inputs to autonomic nuclei innervating the adrenal gland, pancreas, and thyroid gland.

Finally, the hypothalamus provides outputs to areas involved in behavioral state control. They include brainstem cholinergic and monoaminergic groups involved in arousal and attention. The ORX neurons in the posterior lateral hypothalamus, and histaminergic neurons of the tuberomammillary nucleus send excitatory projections that maintain the wake state, whereas the ventrolateral preoptic area (VLPO) sends inhibitory projections that promote transition to NREM sleep (see chapter 27). The lateral hypothalamic area contains ORX, GABAergic, and glutamatergic neurons that send projections to the VTA and NAc, the two key components of the reward and motivation circuit.

RESPONSE TO STRESS

Stress refers to experiences that are challenging physiologically, emotionally, or both. Stress can originate from the internal environment, such as hypoglycemia, pain, or inflammatory cytokines or from external or social stressors. Internal stressors such as pain reach the stress circuits via interoceptive and brainstem catecholaminergic pathways, whereas others such inflammatory cytokines activate these circuits via the sensory CVOs or paracrine interactions through capillary endothelial cells. Psychological stressors include novelty, unpredictability, decreased sense of control, and threat. The two hypothalamic effector systems activated by stress are the sympathetic-adrenomedullary and the hypothalamic-pituitary-adrenal (HPA) axis.[11,12] Whereas the acute release of epinephrine and cortisol promotes adaptation to an acute stressor, chronic elevation of these same mediators can cause deleterious pathophysiological changes leading, for example, to cardiovascular disease. These paradoxical effects led to the introduction of the term "allostasis" to refer to the active process by which the body responds to daily events and maintains homeostasis. Allostasis means "achieving stability through change."[11]

The autonomic output both via the sympathetic ganglia and epinephrine secretion by the adrenal medulla mediates the most immediate reaction to stress. Excessive stress may also trigger vagal outputs to the gastrointestinal system, resulting in excessive gastric acid secretion or gastrointestinal dysmotility. Several hypothalamic areas trigger autonomic responses to stress, including the PVH, DMH, and lateral hypothalamus, which respond to different types of stressor and initiate different responses (Figure 38.3).[10] Autonomic PVH neurons send projections to the intermediolateral cell column (IML), RVLM, and NTS and control sympathetic outflow to the heart, kidneys, and other organs. These PVH neurons have a major role in vasomotor responses to long-term challenges, such as sustained water deprivation or chronic intermittent hypoxia, and may contribute to development of hypertension The DMH has a major role in sympathoexcitatory responses to psychological stressors via inputs to the RVMM and medullary raphe (particularly the RPa) projecting to the IML and eliciting tachycardia.[10] The ORX neurons of the lateral hypothalamus and perifornical region activate cardiovascular and respiratory responses associated with behavioral arousal, reward and motivated behavior, and stress. These neurons send excitatory projections to the PVH and to brainstem autonomic and respiratory nuclei; they trigger sympathetic cardiovascular activation and attenuation of the baroreflex, and promote respiratory responses to hypercapnia.[13,14] A group of neurons of the perifornical region also send excitatory glutamatergic inputs to RVLM neurons targeting sympathetic preganglionic neurons innervating the adrenal gland in response to hypoglycemia.

Periaqueductal Gray and Response to Stress

The responses to stress vary according not only according to the type of stressor but also according to the individual's perception and ability to cope.[15] These different responses are in part orchestrated by different columns of the PAG, which mediate inputs from different forebrain areas. The dorsolateral PAG generates increases in sympathetic activity and respiratory rate that resemble the responses naturally evoked by psychological stressors. The lateral PAG mediates responses to acute, transient challenges that trigger the so-called defense reaction. This response resembles the response to physical exercise and includes sympathetic activation, redistribution of blood flow to the limbs, and "fight" or "flight" motor responses which reflect an active coping strategy. In contrast, the ventrolateral PAG is activated in the setting of unescapable stress and deep visceral or muscle pain, and initiates a passive coping response referred to as "playing death," which includes immobility, sympathetic inhibition, and parasympathetic activation. The stress

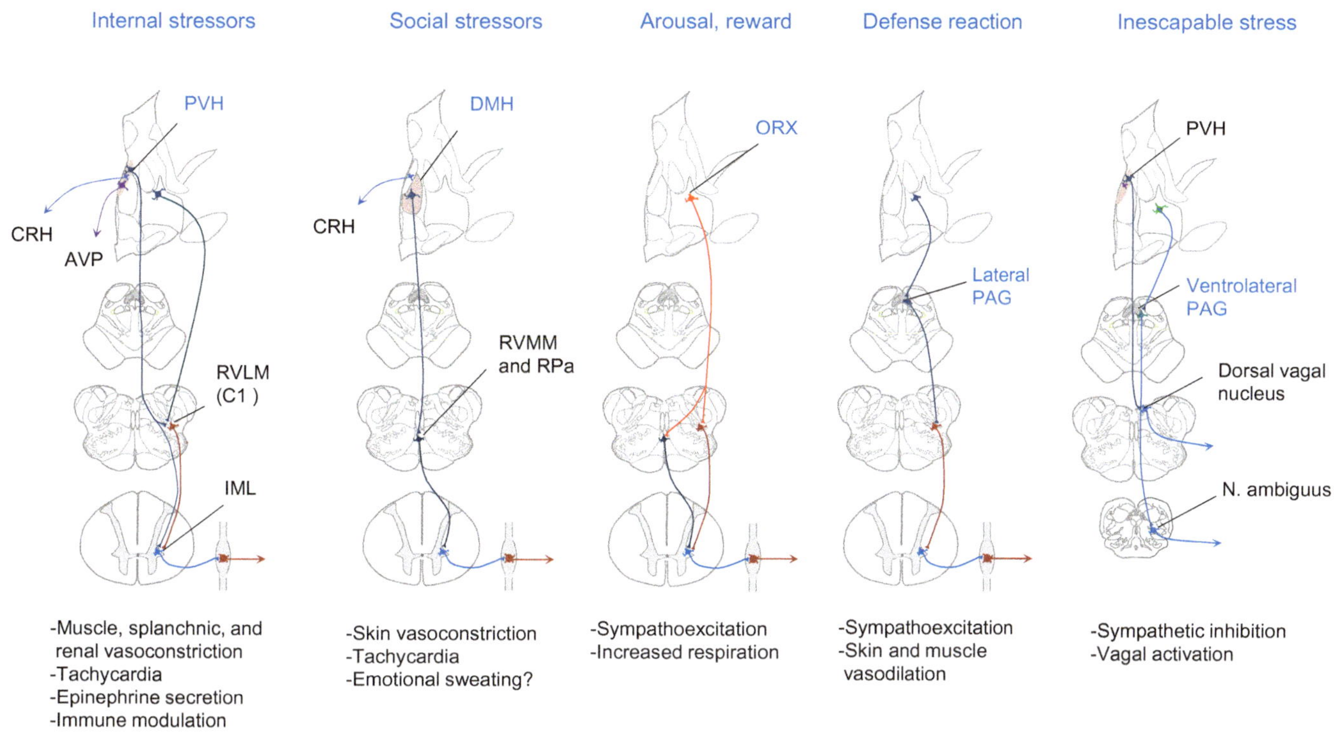

FIGURE 38.3 Responses to stress.

The responses to stress vary according to the type of stimuli and engage different hypothalamic areas. The paraventricular nucleus (PVH) is critical for integrated responses to internal stressors. Autonomic PVH neurons send projections to the intermediolateral cell column (IML) and rostral ventrolateral medulla (RVLM), including the C1 group. The PVH also releases arginine vasopressin (AVP) and corticotrophin-releasing hormone (CRH). The response to psychological and other external stressors involves primarily the dorsomedial nucleus (DMH), which triggers tachycardia via projections to sympathoexcitatory neurons in the rostral ventromedial medulla (RVMM) and medullary raphe. The orexin (ORX) neurons trigger sympathetic cardiovascular activation, attenuate baroreflex-triggered bradycardia, and promote respiratory responses to hypercapnia. The defense reaction involves the lateral periaqueductal gray (PAG) via its projections to the RVLM, and is part of an active coping strategy. Inescapable stress initiates a passive coping mechanism via the ventrolateral PAG; this includes sympathoinhibition and parasympathetic activation.

responses initiated by the PAG also trigger descending pain modulation.

Hormonal Response

The HPA response is triggered by CRH neurons of the PVH, which stimulate ACTH secretion and then release of cortisol from the adrenal cortex. In addition to its peripheral effects, CRH also promotes NE release from brainstem terminals in the PVH. Glucocorticoids bind to mineralocorticoid receptors (MR or type I) and glucocorticoid receptors (GR or type II). Type I receptors are mainly distributed in the limbic system, including the hippocampus and amygdala; type II receptors are present in subcortical and cortical structures and mediate the negative feedback that regulates the HPA axis. The amygdala activates the HPA axis, whereas the prefrontal cortex and the hippocampus have an inhibitory effect via GABAergic neurons surrounding the PVH.

Extrahypothalamic Stress System

In addition to the sympatho-adrenomedullary and HPA systems, there is a third stress system involving noradrenergic and CRH-mediating signaling in the CeM and BNST, which together form a functional unit known as extended central amygdala. This system may have particular importance in maintaining fearful states. CRH neurons in the CeM activate fast tonic activity of LC neurons, which release NE in the amygdala and promote fear conditioning. Thus, acute stress increases the level of vigilance and favors emotionally charged responses to salient information and promotes emotional memory consolidation, The LC also participates in autonomic responses to stress through its reciprocal interactions with C1 neurons of the RVLM. These neurons constitute a brain "alarm system" that responds to internal stressors such as hypoxia and inflammation and that triggers sympathoexcitatory cardiovascular responses, arousal, and respiration.

REGULATION OF IMMUNE RESPONSES

Immune Signals to the Central Nervous System

There are close reciprocal interactions between the autonomic and the immune systems.[16,17] The sympathetic, parasympathetic, and enteric nervous systems as well as primary sensory afferents receive signals from immune cells and release neurochemical transmitters that regulate immune functions. These neuro-immune interactions occur at multiple levels, including the gut, the CNS, and lymphoid organs. For example, enteric neurons and glial cells interact with enteroendocrine cells and local macrophages and can sense signals from the gut lumen, including those from the microbiota; these signals elicit local immune responses and reach the CNS. There are two pathways, humoral and neural, by which the immune system communicates with the brain. Interleukins (ILs) and other signals from immune cells can access the hypothalamus via the neurovascular unit or CVOs such as the OVLT. Cytokines also activate receptors in vagal afferents that project to the NTS, which relays these inputs, either directly or via the PB to the hypothalamus.

Neural Modulation of Immune Responses

The PVH orchestrates the immunomodulatory responses to inflammatory signals both via neural end endocrine outputs. The PVH, in part via its projections to the C1 area of the RVLM, promotes sympathetic output to lymphoid organs, including the spleen, which elicits potent anti-inflammatory responses via β2 adrenergic receptors expressed in multiple cells of the innate and adaptive immune systems.[16] The parvocellular CRH neurons of the PVH activate the HPA and cortisol exerts potent inhibitory effects on lymphoid cells, either directly or by facilitating the sympathetic effects in lymphoid organs. Psychological stress, via central catecholaminergic mechanisms, increases release of proinflammatory cytokines, such as IL-1, IL-6, and tumor necrosis factor α, from microglia within the hypothalamus, hippocampus, and prefrontal cortex. Glucocorticoids inhibit production of brain cytokines by suppression of LC activity and inhibition of proinflammatory downstream signal transduction cascades in glial cells.[17]

THERMOREGULATION

The regulation of the internal body, or core, temperature involves feedback and feedforward mechanisms integrated at the preoptic area.[18,19] These thermoregulatory responses are mediated by the sympathetic output to the skin. An increase in core temperature evokes a negative feedback that results in skin vasodilation and sweating. The primary thermoregulatory feedforward sensory signal comes from cold and warm thermoreceptors in the skin. An increase in skin temperature promotes heat dissipation. In contrast, a decrease in skin temperature triggers skin vasoconstriction and brown fat lipolysis to promote thermogenesis. These reflex thermoregulatory responses represent an early line of defense against potential threats to core temperature.

Hypothalamic Groups Involved in Thermoregulation

There are three groups of thermoregulatory neurons in the preoptic area that participate in local circuits activated by increase in blood temperature, inputs from peripheral thermal receptors, or both (Figure 38.4). Neurons in the medial preoptic (MPO) are warm-sensitive, respond to increase in core temperature, tonically inhibit cold-sensitive neurons, and initiate feedback responses for heat dissipation. Neurons in the median preoptic area (MnPO) receive inputs from warm and cold receptors and interact with other hypothalamic thermoregulatory groups. The DMH contains neurons that initiate thermoregulatory responses to cold via projections to the rostral portion of the nucleus raphe pallidus (RPa).

Inputs from Skin Thermoreceptors

The afferent input into the thermoregulatory system comes from thermosensitive dorsal root ganglion neurons that innervate the skin and viscera and project to lamina I of the spinal cord. Thermal sensation in the face is conveyed by similar neurons in the trigeminal system. Cold-sensitive neurons activated by innocuous cold (~14–30°C) express transient receptor potential melastatin type 8 (TRPM8) channels; warm-sensitive neurons responsive to innocuous warmth (~34–42°C) may express TRPM2 and perhaps TRPV1 channels. Cold- and warm-sensitive neurons in lamina I send segregated ascending glutamatergic projections to different subdivisions the lateral PB, which in turn project to the MnPO.

Responses to Heat

The preoptic area harbors warm-sensitive neurons distributed in the MnPO, MPO, and ventral portion of the lateral preoptic area. The firing of these neurons reflects core temperature and contributes to a negative feedback signaling that prevents heat production and promotes heat loss. These neurons are also activated by cutaneous warm sensation. Most of the warm-sensitive neurons are GABAergic and send projections that tonically inhibit cold-responsive neurons in DMH and RPa. In addition, glutamatergic warm-sensitive neurons in the MPO and ventral lateral preoptic region directly promote cooling by promoting skin vasodilation. In humans, heat loss involves both skin vasodilation and sweating. Sweating is mediated by sympathetic cholinergic neurons acting via muscarinic M3 receptors in sweat glands. Functional magnetic resonance imaging (fMRI) studies show that the premotor neurons for sweating appear to be located in the RVMM. The central pathways that drive cutaneous active vasodilation in human skin remain unknown.

Response to Cold

Cold-sensitive neurons of the MnPO receive input from cold receptors in the skin and inhibit the warm-sensitive neurons in the MPO, thereby disinhibiting the cold-responsive neurons of the DMH and rostral RPa. Both the

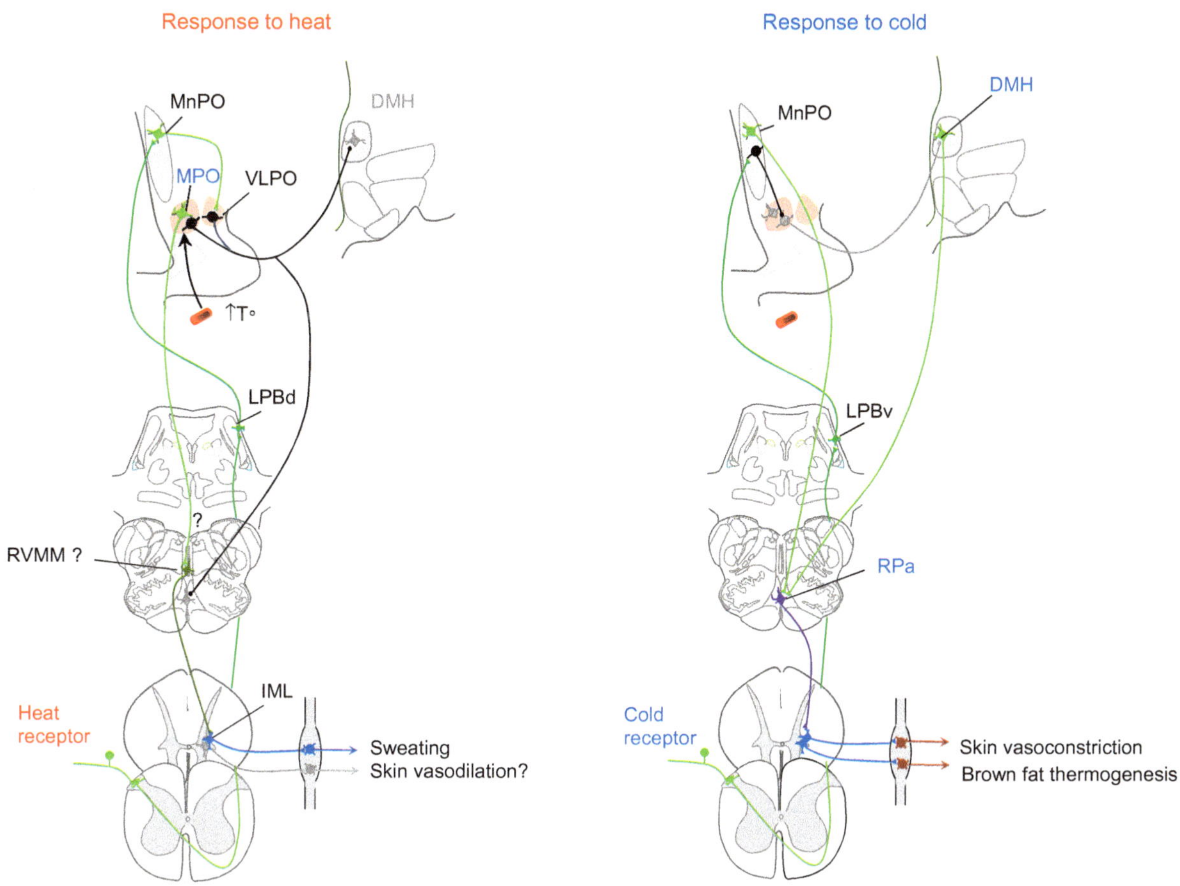

FIGURE 38.4 Mechanisms of thermoregulation.
The regulation of the internal body, or core, temperature involves feedback and feedforward mechanisms integrated at the preoptic area. An increase in core temperature activates warm-sensitive neurons distributed in the median preoptic area (MnPO), medial preoptic area (MPO), and ventral portion of the lateral preoptic area (vLPO). These neurons elicit negative feedback that results in inhibition of both thermogenesis and cutaneous vasoconstriction via inhibition of cold-sensitive neurons in the dorsomedial nucleus of the hypothalamus (DMH) and nucleus raphe pallidus (RPa). These warm-sensitive neurons also activate skin vasodilation and sweating; premotor neurons for sweating appear to be located in the rostral ventromedial medulla (RVMM). Cold-sensitive neurons activated by innocuous cold and warmth-sensitive neurons responsive to innocuous warmth project to thermosensitive dorsal horn neurons that send segregated ascending glutamatergic projections to the lateral parabrachial nucleus (PB); cold- and warmth-activated PB neurons project to the MnPO LPBd=dorsal lateral parabrachial; LPBv, ventral lateral parabrachial.

MnPO and the DMH also send direct excitatory projections to the RPa. The rostral RPa sends glutamatergic and serotonergic inputs to preganglionic sympathetic neurons in the spinal cord, triggering cutaneous vasoconstriction mediated by α1 adrenergic receptors and thermogenesis in the brown adipose tissue via β receptors.[20] Descending serotonergic inputs from the RPa to the ventral horn may also be involved in shivering. Inputs from the DMH to the rostral RPa, both directly and via the PAG also elicit tachycardia in the setting of fever or stress.

Febrile Response

The febrile response also involves neurons in the preoptic area. Cytokines such as IL-6 or activation of toll-like receptors on macrophage-like cells residing in the CVOs leads to activation of cyclooxigenase-2 within glial and endothelial cells, resulting in production of prostaglandin E2 (PGE2). Locally produced and blood-borne PGE2 acts via inhibitory EP3 receptors on warm-sensitive neurons of the MnPO and MPO, reducing their activity. This results in disinhibition of the neurons of the DMH and RPa, triggering cutaneous vasoconstriction, brown adipose tissue thermogenesis, and shivering (chills), which mimic the cold-defense responses.

Interactions Between Thermoregulation and Sleep

Sleep onset is fundamentally connected with thermoregulatory mechanisms promoting body cooling. Direct skin warming can shorten sleep-latency and promote non–rapid eye movement (NREM) sleep. The interactions between changes in body temperature and sleep onset involve a microcircuit in the preoptic area. Warm-sensitive neurons in the MnPO facilitate induction of NREM sleep via direct GABAergic projections to wake-active brainstem neurons. In addition, the MnPO contains warm-sensitive glutamatergic/nitroxidergic neurons that activate both GABA/galanin neurons of the VLPO that are critical for NREM sleep induction and neurons of the MPO that elicit body cooling. Under natural conditions, increased circulating melatonin also coincides with declining core temperature prior to sleep onset.

OSMOREGULATION AND FLUID HOMEOSTASIS

Challenges to fluid homeostasis, such as water deprivation, cause increases in plasma osmolality and plasma sodium concentration and disturbances in plasma volume and blood pressure. These stimuli trigger an integrated response that includes thirst, anorexia, and secretion of AVP (antidiuretic hormone, ADH) by magnocellular neurons of the SON and PVH, and increased sympathetic activity to maintain blood pressure (Figure 38.5).

Hypothalamic Areas Controlling Water and Sodium Metabolism

The critical areas involved in osmoregulation and fluid homeostasis are located in the lamina terminalis in the anterior wall of the third ventricle and include the SFO, OVLT, and MnPO.[21] Both the SFO and the OVLT contain osmosensitive neurons expressing TRPV1 and both neurons and astrocytes expressing sodium-gated sodium channels (Nax) that can detect extracellular sodium concentrations. The MnPO functions as an integration center.

Thirst

The lamina terminalis circuit drives drinking through negative reinforcement. The negative valence of the sensation of thirst provides a signal to cells in the SFO.[21] The

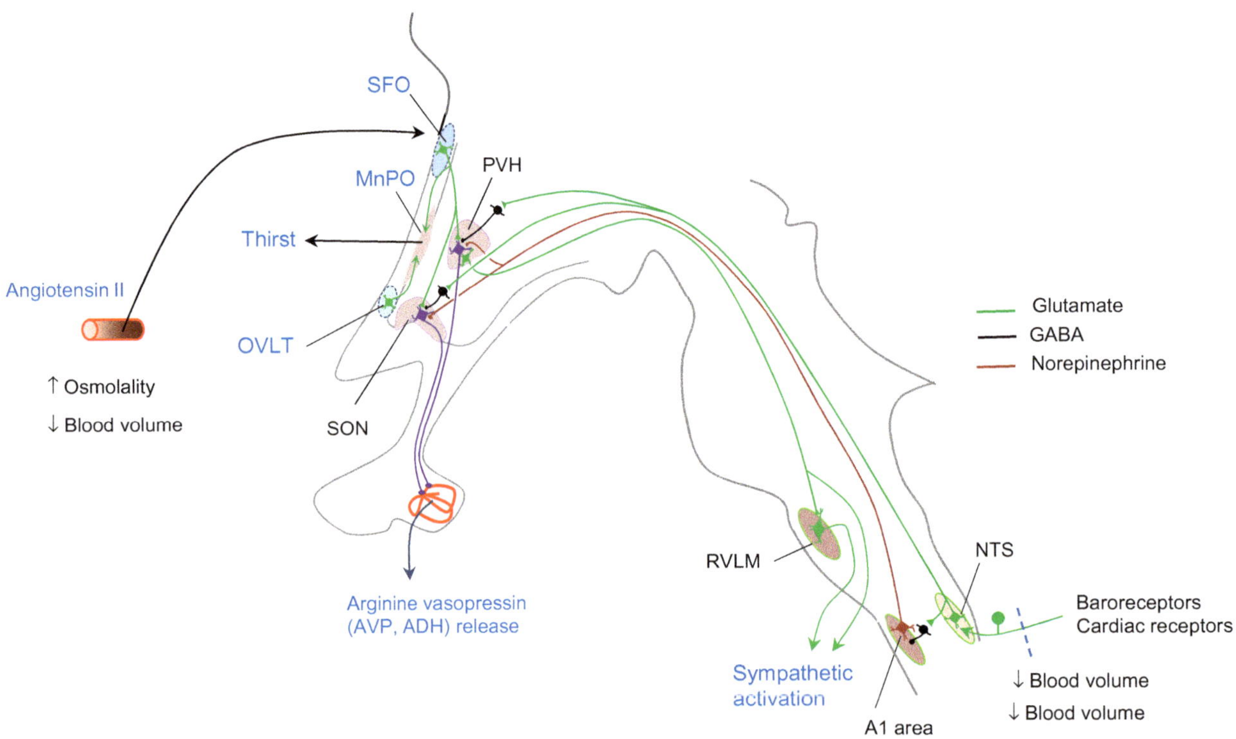

FIGURE 38.5 Control of water and sodium homeostasis.
The critical areas involved in osmoregulation and fluid homeostasis include the subfornical organ (SFO), vascular organ of the lamina terminalis (OVLT), and median preoptic nucleus (MnPO). These areas trigger thirst, anorexia, secretion of AVP (antidiuretic hormone, ADH) by magnocellular neurons of the supraoptic nucleus (SON) and paraventricular nucleus (PVH), and increased sympathetic activity to maintain blood pressure. Hypovolemia simulates renin secretion and consequently production of angiotensin II, which activates the osmosensitive neurons of the SFO and OVLT via angiotensin type 1 receptors; these receptors are also present in PVH and SON neurons and trigger AVP release. In response to a fall of blood pressure or hypovolemia, this tonic baroreceptor inhibition is lifted, leading to an increase in circulating AVP via a pathway that is in part mediated by noradrenergic inputs from A1 neurons in the caudal ventrolateral medulla. RVLM = rostral ventrolateral medulla.

SFO contains intermingled populations of glutamatergic and GABAergic neurons with opposing effects on drinking behavior. Glutamatergic neurons stimulate thirst via projections to the OVLT and MnPO whereas GABAergic neurons suppress thirst via inputs to the OVLT. In addition to stimulating drinking, SFO neurons also promote release of AVP. Soon after water drinking starts, there is a decreased firing of glutamatergic SFO neurons and inhibition of AVP release, which occur before the composition of the blood is corrected. This rapid prediction of the impending restoration of homeostasis is a feedback triggered by the detection of water in the oral cavity. The stimulation of drinking by eating, known as prandial thirst, involves glutamatergic neurons in the SFO that are rapidly activated during eating before any change in plasma osmolality. Conversely, dehydration potently suppresses food intake, which is known as dehydration anorexia. There is also a circadian regulation of thirst and drinking via projections of AVP neurons in the SCN to the OVLT, which promotes drinking in the hours immediately preceding sleep.

Control of Vasopressin Release by Angiotensin II and Cardiovascular Reflexes

Hypovolemia simulates renin secretion by the kidney and consequently production of angiotensin II (ANG II). Circulating ANG II activates neurons of the SFO and OVLT via angiotensin type 1 receptors (AT1Rs). The SFO contains glutamatergic neurons that also synthesize ANG II and send an excitatory input to magnocellular neurons of the SON and PVH secreting AVP/ADH. ANG II triggers AVP release via AT1Rs in these neurons. At the basal state, AVP/ADH release from the SON and PVH is tonically inhibited by the baroreflex and cardiac reflexes mediated by the NTS via GABAergic neurons. The NTS also inhibits noradrenergic neurons in the A1 area that provide excitatory inputs to the SON and PVN. In response to a fall of blood pressure, hypovolemia, or prolonged orthostatic stress, this tonic baroreceptor inhibition is lifted, leading to an increase in circulating AVP, in part via A1 noradrenergic inputs resulting in $\alpha 1$ receptor-mediated stimulation of magnocellular neurons.

Control of Sodium Intake

Projections from ANG II-activated SFO neurons to autonomic PVH neurons targeting the RVLM and IML increase sympathetic nerve activity and thus control blood pressure, renal blood flow, and sodium excretion. Circulating ANG II also promotes the release of aldosterone by the adrenal cortex. In addition to promoting sodium reabsorption by the kidney, aldosterone acts via mineralocorticoid receptors in a unique population of aldosterone-sensitive glutamatergic cells in the NTS to regulate sodium homeostasis. These neurons respond to sodium deprivation and activate neurons in the lateral PB and BNST to promote sodium intake. Circulating ANG II and aldosterone act synergistically to control salt appetite. Aldosterone potentiates the effects of ANG II in stimulating sodium appetite via AT1Rs in the SFO.

REGULATION OF FOOD INTAKE AND ENERGY METABOLISM

Feeding is regulated by several mechanisms. They include long-term feedback from the adipose tissue to ensure adequate energy stores; environmental cues that promote eating when food is available; balance between the drive to eat and competing survival drives; and short-term feedback from the gut that regulate meal size.[22]

Homeostatic Regulation of Food Intake

The first basic component of control of appetite is the homeostatic regulation of food intake. This depends on circulating signals, primarily leptin, which is released from the adipose tissue and provides a long-term feedback signal that reflects fat stores and inhibits food intake.[23] Leptin acts on two functionally antagonistic neuronal populations in the ARC (infundibular) nucleus of the hypothalamus. A population of neurons that express Agouti-related protein (AgRP), neuropeptide Y (NPY), and GABA promote food intake and are inhibited by leptin. Falling leptin levels signal an energy deficit, which produces a state of negative valence (hunger) that leads to food-seeking behaviors through disinhibition of these neurons. A second population of ARC neurons expresses cocaine- and amphetamine-related transcript (CART) and proopiomelanocortin (POMC). These CART/POMC neurons inhibit food intake via action of α-melanocyte-stimulating hormone (αMSH) and are activated by leptin. The antagonistic effects between orexinergic AgRP/NPY/GABA neurons and anorexinergic CART/POMC neurons reflect their opposite influences on neurons in the PVH that express the melanocortin 4 receptors (M4Rs) and are activated by αMSH. Neurons of the PVH elicit homeostatic satiety and reduce total food consumption via projections to the PB complex.

Upon a fall in leptin levels perceived as hunger, AgRP/NPY/GABA neurons initiate feeding by inhibiting the feeding suppressing signal from POMC neurons to the PVH neurons. This inhibitory effect involves several mechanisms including rapid GABAergic inhibition of POMC neurons, NPY-mediated inhibition of MC4R-expressing PVH neurons, and AgRP mediated antagonism of MC4Rs in PVH neurons. In normal conditions, activity of AgRP neurons is rapidly suppressed just as the food consumption commences, indicating that these neurons appear to be primarily involved in food seeking to avoid the unpleasant sensation of hunger.

There are interactions between signals controlling feeding and sleep. Leptin activates warm-sensitive neurons in the preoptic area when there is an increase in ambient temperature; this promotes sleep and results in inhibition of both thermogenesis and food consumption. The circuitry linking thermal sensation to appetite control and sleep may involve leptin-activated POMC neurons that inhibit local GABAergic neurons in sleep-promoting preoptic area regions. In contrast, behavioral needs of food overcome those of sleep and thermal comfort. The AgRP neurons function as "hunger sensors" and promote food-seeking behavior, even at the expense of sleep, via inhibition of POMC neurons.

Hedonic or Reward-Based Eating

The second aspect of regulation of food intake involves the lateral hypothalamus, which integrates eating behavior and reward.[24] The LHA has a strong connectivity with the reward circuit, including the VTA and NAc. Activity of some LHA neurons encodes reward, aversive, or associated conditioned stimuli. The LHA contains GABAergic neurons that promote feeding. These neurons target local GABAergic neurons of the VTA, thus promoting reward-based feeding by indirectly increasing activity of dopaminergic VTA neurons. Inputs from neurons in the NAc shell target GABAergic neurons of the LHA and thus inhibit feeding. A second population of LHA neurons are glutamatergic, and inhibit feeding via projections to the lateral habenula, which inhibits the activity of dopaminergic VTA neurons. Inputs from GABAergic neurons of the BNST promote feeding by inhibiting the glutamatergic LHA neurons. Both the GABAergic and the glutamatergic neurons of the LHA also innervate the PB, which can also serve to regulate homeostatic feeding.

Satiety Circuit

The third circuit regulating food intake is the satiety circuit, which promotes the termination of a meal. Satiety is triggered by several gut-derived hormonal signals. Information related to ingested food is transmitted from the stomach and small intestine via vagal afferents to the NTS. These afferents are activated by either luminal stretch of visceral organs or by paracrine signals secreted in response to nutrients by enteroendocrine cells located in the gut epithelium. Potential satiation signals include cholecystokinin (CCK), glucagon-like peptide 1, peptide YY, and serotonin (5-HT). In response to nutrients, CCK released by cells in the upper small intestine, or 5-HT secreted by enterochromaffin cells stimulate vagal afferents that relay gut signals to the NTS. Amylin, which is co-released with insulin by pancreatic β cells, also causes satiation via neurons in the area postrema that connect to the NTS. An important satiety circuit involves CCK neurons of the NTS that project to neurons of the lateral PB that synthesize calcitonin gene-related peptide (CGRP). These PB neurons promote meal termination via projections to the CeM. The same pathway mediates malaise-induced anorexia and conditioned taste aversion. In contrast, ghrelin is an orexinergic signal produced by enteroendocrine cells in the stomach; its release is not regulated by luminal contents or stomach stretch but rather by autonomic inputs. Ghrelin stimulates appetite; its levels are highest before a meal, fall with eating, and increase with subsequent fasting. The ghrelin receptor is expressed by neurons in many brain regions where it elicits stimulation of appetite. The main function of ghrelin is to prevent hypoglycemia.

Glucose Sensing, Endocannabinoids, and Regulation of Food Intake

The central regulation of glucose homeostasis not only involves the antagonistic effects of leptin and ghrelin but also reflects the effects of both circulating insulin and glucose in the hypothalamus.[23] Insulin activates ATP-dependent K^+ channels as well as downstream signaling pathways shared with those mediating the inhibitory effects of leptin on orexigenic AgrP/NPY/GABA neurons. By this mechanism, insulin interacts with leptin to prevent excessive feeding.

Circulating glucose is transported across the BBB via the glucose transporter 1 (GLUT1) in endothelial cells and astrocytes in an insulin-independent manner, and accesses neurons via GLUT3 and other transporters differentially distributed in the CNS. There are specialized glucosensitive neurons in the hypothalamus and brainstem, which regulate sympathetic and parasympathetic outputs to peripheral organs, including the endocrine pancreas and the liver. Both glucose-excited and glucose-inhibited neurons are present in the ARC, PVH, ventromedial nucleus, and LHA. For example, glucose-excited neurons in the ventromedial nucleus take up glucose via GLUT2 and metabolize glucose to yield ATP, which closes ATP-sensitive K^+ channels leading to neuronal activation and reducing food intake. A typical example of glucose-inhibited neurons is ORX neurons, which are activated in the setting of low levels of glucose.[23]

Endocannabinoids acting via cannabinoid 1 receptors (CB1Rs) have a major role in promoting accumulation of energy stores for future needs, a process referred to as "exostasis."[25] Activation of CB1Rs in the CNS increases sensitivity to the appetitive properties of food and stimulates food intake beyond satiety. For example, CB1R activation increases dopamine release from VTA terminals in the NAc, signaling reward and motivation, while inhibiting homeostatic hypothalamic mechanisms that control food intake according to immediate needs. These receptors inhibit the anorexigenic CART/POMC neurons and drive these neurons to synthesize β-endorphin (which is orexigenic) rather than the anorexigenic α-MSH; CBR1Rs also facilitate the activity of ORX neurons.[25]

FOREBRAIN CIRCUITS FOR FEELINGS, EMOTIONS, AND AUTONOMIC INTERACTIONS

The amygdala, insula, ACC, and anterior midcingulate cortex (MCC) participate in integrated circuits that utilize interoceptive information for emotional responses and control of behavior.[3] They form a highly interconnected network that is activated during several tasks affecting autonomic output[3,26–34] (Figure 38.6).

Amygdala, Automatic Tagging of Affective Valence, and Survival Responses

The amygdala provides automatic tagging of the valence (positive or negative) and intensity of innate or conditioned environmental stimuli and thereby their behavioral relevance.[2] The outputs of the amygdala to the hypothalamus, PAG, and brainstem autonomic nuclei trigger automatic survival responses to either unconditioned stimuli, such as pain, or conditioned stimuli, such as fear. These outputs originate in the CeM and its functional extension, the BNST. A major source of aversive information to the amygdala is the PB, which conveys pain and visceral sensation either directly to the CeM, triggering innate survival responses, or via thalamus to the lateral nucleus, triggering conditioned responses via the intrinsic amygdala circuit described in chapter 25. The CeM sends dense GABAergic and peptidergic projections to different portions of the hypothalamus, PAG, PB, NTS, RVLM, and vagal nuclei. Via these projections, the CeM initiates several survival responses.[35] They include, according to the stimulus, sympathetic, or parasympathetic activation, secretion of stress hormones, and innate motor responses, such as respiratory changes, vocalization, startle, and freezing.[36]

Interoception and Emotion

Conscious emotional experience is closely bound to changes in bodily sensations.[37] Emotions are adaptive, patterned neural responses akin to physiological drives such as thirst and hunger and are distinguished from feelings, which are the internal sensations resulting from these patterned responses.[38] The subjective experience of emotion

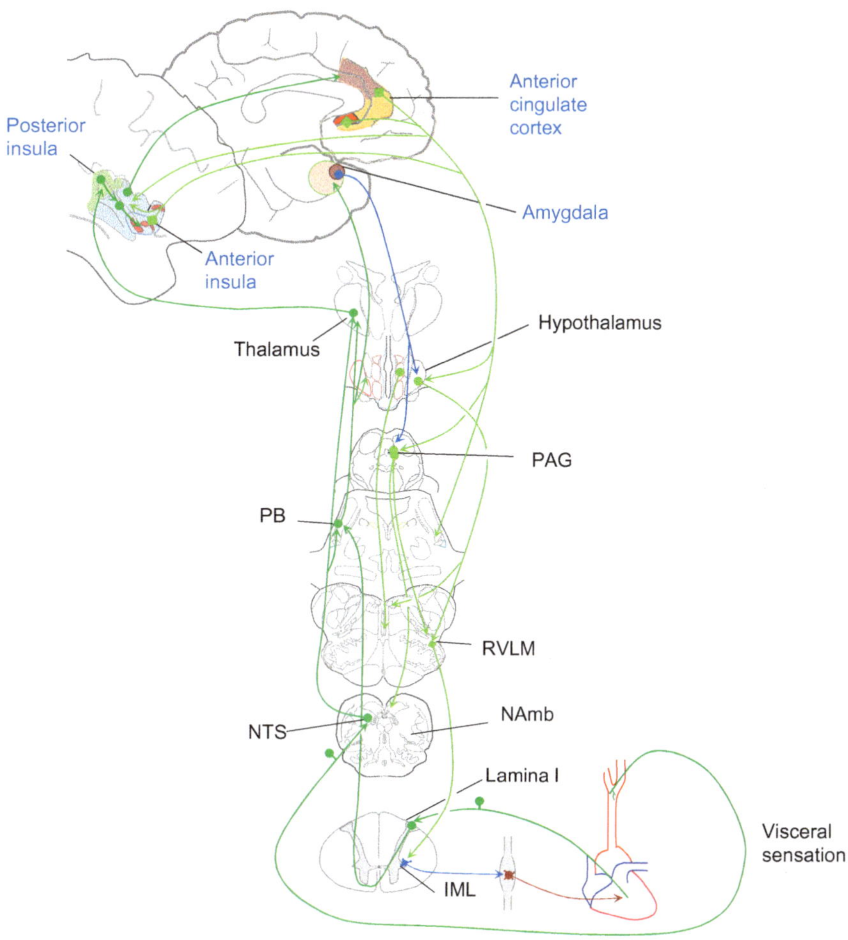

FIGURE 38.6 Predictive coding and control of autonomic function.
The amygdala, insula, anterior cingulate cortex (ACC), and anterior midcingulate cortex (MCC) are consistently activated in humans during tasks associated with sympathetic or parasympathetic responses. These areas receive visceral sensory feedback via lamina I of the dorsal horn, nucleus of the solitary tract (NTS), and parabrachial nucleus (PB) via the posterior ventromedial complex of the thalamus, which projects to the dorsal insula. The anterior insula, anterior cingulate cortex, and amygdala are interconnected and control autonomic outputs via projections to the hypothalamus, periaqueductal gray (PAG), rostral ventrolateral medulla (RVLM), nucleus ambiguus (NAmb), and spinal preganglionic neurons of the intermediolateral cell column (IML).

strongly depends on the CNS representations of afferent input from peripheral organs, which constitutes interoception.[39,40] Interoception includes information from visceral organs as well as signals from hormones, nutrients, and inflammatory mediators. Interoceptive sensations are typically more general and diffuse than somatomotor and somatosensory sensation, including pain. Ascending interoceptive signals share neural substrates and interact with descending signals that drive autonomic and humoral responses. Interoception influences not only emotions but also motivation.[41]

Many studies on interoception have focused on cardiovascular arousal.[42] Heartbeat detection tasks test the ability of individuals to perceive their own heartbeats at rest. The timing and strength of each heartbeat is signaled by the firing of arterial baroreceptors with each ventricular contraction. Cardiovascular arousal occurs through "top-down" baroreflex suppression, allowing heart rate and blood pressure to rise together. The impact of this cardiac interoception on perceptual aspects of emotion can be tested by comparing responses to brief stimuli presented around systole, when the baroreceptors are active, to stimuli presented at diastole, when the baroreceptors are quiescent.[43] Generally, baroreceptor signals inhibit sensory processing such as pain or startle responses. However, these cardiac arousal signals selectively amplify the processing of threat, including the detection and perception of fear signals. One study used an automated neck suction device to stimulate the carotid sinus mechanoreceptors synchronously with fMRI when individuals were engaged in viewing faces with different emotional expressions.[43] This study showed that both right and left carotid stimulation influenced brain activity within opercular regions, with a stronger activation within left insula during right stimulation compared to left stimulation. This study also showed that right, but not left carotid stimulation attenuated the perceived intensity of fear upon viewing a fearful face; this was associated with attenuation of amygdala activation.[43] Individual differences in basal heart rate variability predicted the extent to which right carotid stimulation attenuated amygdala responses during fear processing.[43] Interoception, emotional regulation, and social cognition may converge in the right anterior insula, orbitofrontal and inferior frontal gyri, and amygdala.[44]

Cortical Influences on Autonomic Function

The dorsal posterior insula is the primary interoceptive cortex as it receives and integrates inputs from visceral, pain, and thermal receptors.[4] The posterior insula projects via the midinsula to the anterior insula, which integrates interoceptive signals with emotional and cognitive processing and is involved in conscious experience of bodily sensation.[4] Whereas the insula is the primary viscerosensory cortical area, it is also a visceromotor area controlling both the sympathetic and parasympathetic outputs, primarily via a relay in the lateral hypothalamus.[45] The insular cortex projects to the RVLM, and its activity correlates with increase in sympathetic nerve activity.[46] There may be a lateralization of insular control of cardiovascular function, with a right-sided dominance for sympathetic activation in response to mental stress or during the Valsalva maneuver.[45] This putative lateralization of autonomic control has been linked to susceptibility to cardiac arrhythmias and other cardiovascular changes after stroke.[47] The insular cortex also appears to be involved in the top-down or perceptual components of cardiovascular control during exercise and may have a role in regulating cardiovascular responses via its contribution to central command control in this condition.[48]

The anterior insula, ACC, and anterior MCC are components of two large-scale cortical networks. The ventral anterior insula (frontoinsular cortex) and the pregenual ACC (areas 24a and b) are hub components of the salience network.[49] These areas contain large layer 5 projection neurons, called von Economo neurons, and respond to homeostatically relevant stimuli.[50] These neurons are more abundant in the right than in the left hemisphere, which may underlie some lateralization of autonomic control.[50] Stimulation of the pregenual ACC during presurgical mapping in patients with epilepsy elicited emotional face expression, interoceptive sensations and sympathoexcitatory responses that included hot flushes, cold sweats, and tachycardia; many patients explicitly interpreted these symptoms in terms of fear and anxiety.[51] Supporting the proposal of a lateralized control of autonomic function, a study on patients with behavioral variant frontotemporal dementia showed that left lateralized atrophy of the frontoinsular and ACC was associated with reduced baseline cardiovagal activity.[52] The subgenual portion of the ACC projects to autonomic areas involved in parasympathetic control of the heart and its stimulation results in a decrease in blood pressure.[53] Activation of the subgenual ACC strongly correlates with indices of cardiovagal activity, such as heart rate variability.[54] The dorsal anterior insula and anterior MCC are the hub of a cingulo-opercular task-control network that is thought to have a major role in task set initiation and maintenance in part by providing for sustained vigilance.[55] Functional neuroimaging studies have shown activation of this network during several tasks affecting autonomic output.[26–34,56]

Interoceptive Predictions and Autonomic Control

Recent models of interoception and emotion incorporate the Bayesian concepts of predictive coding.[57,58] In this model, the brain makes sense of dynamic changes of viscerosensory information by predicting the likely causes of those changes. Prior interoceptive experiences are generated as predictions that are sent to effector organs as probable interoceptive consequences. The difference between an expected internal state and the actual afferent interoceptive information generates a prediction error signal. The function of this "top-down" efferent neural drive to the peripheral autonomic system would be to change the internal bodily state and thus minimize prediction errors by changing the visceral feedback afferent input. Centrally generated predictions of physiological states are expressed in autonomic reflexes in the absence of feedback error signal. Unpredicted interoceptive inputs generate prediction errors, which trigger both emotional feelings and homeostatic responses.[57,58] The embodied predictive interoception coding model emphasizes the role of the insula in emotion generation. According to this model, pyramidal projection neurons in deep layers V and VI of the agranular cortex, including the pregenual ACC and anterior insula, generate predictions about physiological states that are sent, via cortico-cortical projections, to the midinsular and posterior insular cortex. In the posterior insula, visceromotor predictions are compared to afferent interoceptive inputs, and this comparison generates prediction errors that are sent back to agranular cortices to refine the interoceptive predictions.[57] Von Economo neurons in the inferior portion of the anterior insula and the ACC project to the contralateral anterior insular cortex, ipsilateral ACC, and particularly target brainstem nuclei involved in visceral sensation and autonomic control, including the PAG and, particularity, the PB.[59] These descending projections from von Economo neurons may thus convey "interoceptive error attenuation."[59]

The representations of interoceptive information do not need to reach conscious awareness in order to influence feelings and emotions. Interoception influences cognitive and emotional processing area by a mechanism of homeostatic feedback, particularly when psychological arousal is unexpected and there is a discrepancy between predictive and interoceptive signals, resulting in anxiety.[37]

HYPOTHALAMIC DISORDERS

Hypothalamic Involvement in Neurologic Disease

The hypothalamus may be affected in several disorders (Box 38.1). Many of these disorders are characterized by a combination of impaired thermoregulation, osmoregulation, and sleep–wake cycle regulation. For example, neuromyelitis optica spectrum disorders associated with antibodies against AQP4, which is expressed in astrocytic processes in the hypothalamus, may manifest with narcolepsy and syndrome of inappropriate secretion of antidiuretic hormone (SIADH) or galactorrhea.[60,61] AntiMa2 diencephalitis may manifest with narcolepsy/cataplexy with ORX deficiency and central hypothyroidism, which may reflect CD8+ T cell infiltration in of the hypothalamus.[62] Episodic hypothermia with hyperhidrosis is typically associated with agenesis of the corpus callosum (Shapiro syndrome) but may also occur with other lesions or functional disorders affecting the preoptic hypothalamic region, leading to a reduced set-point for heat dissipation.[63] Drugs such as oxybutynin or glycopyrrolate that reduce sweating or centrally active drugs such as clonidine, cyprohepadine, or gabapentin may be helpful in isolated cases. In contrast, hypothermia in disorders such as Wernicke encephalopathy and multiple sclerosis may reflect impairment of the pathways involved in cold-defense responses at the level of the DMH, PAG, RPa, or spinal cord.

The hypothalamus may have an important role in mechanism of migraine or cluster headache.[64] Functional neuroimaging studies show alterations in hypothalamic functional connectivity shortly before the beginning of migraine headaches. While the more posterior part of the hypothalamus seems to be important for the acute pain stage, the more anterior part seems to play an important role in attack generation and development of chronic migraine.[65] Dysfunction of the hypothalamus is also an important cause of endocrine disorders, which will not be further discussed here. Hypothalamic inflammation has been associated with metabolic syndrome, including obesity, diabetes mellitus, hyperlipidemia, and hypertension.[66] A high fat diet elicits inflammation in the hypothalamus and promotes obesity. This may reflect the effects of long-chain saturated fatty acids and activation of microglia and astrocytes by reactive oxygen species.[67]

BOX 38.1 DISORDERS AFFECTING THE HYPOTHALAMUS

Immune disorders

Neuromyelitis optica spectrum disorders (NMOSDs) due to aquaporin 4 (AQP4) antibodies
Leucine-rich glioma-inhibited (LGI1) encephalitis
Contactin-associated related protein-2 (CASPR2) encephalitis
Ma2 encephalitis associated with testicular carcinoma
Multiple sclerosis
Hypophysitis associated with immune checkpoint inhibitors

Granulomatous and infectious disorders

Sarcoidosis
Langerhans cell histiocytosis
Granulomatosis with polyangiitis (Wegener disease)
Whipple disease
Behcet disease
Chronic meningitis (e.g., tuberculosis)
Infundibulohypohysits associated with IgG4

Neoplasms

Glioma
Germinoma
Lymphoma

Others

Wernicke encephalopathy
Episodic hypothermia with hyperhidrosis
IgLON5 disease (tauopathy)

Allostatic Load as a Disease Mechanism

Because chronically increased allostasis can lead to pathophysiology, McEwen introduced the term "allostatic load or overload" to refer to the wear and tear that results from either too much stress or from inefficient management of allostasis, such as not turning off the response when it is no longer needed.[11 68] The experience of being "stressed out" is associated with elevation of cortisol, sympathetic activity, and proinflammatory cytokines, and a decline in parasympathetic activity. A typical example involves the consequences of poor or inadequate sleep. Sleep restriction to 4 hours of sleep per night increases blood pressure; decreases parasympathetic tone; promotes increased appetite (possibly through elevation of ghrelin and decreased levels of leptin); increases evening cortisol and insulin levels; and increases circulating proinflammatory markers. Studies in animal models show that allostatic overload resulting from chronic stress causes atrophy of neurons in the hippocampus and PFC. Allostatic brain plasticity mechanisms and allostatic hormonal influences provide both the developing and adult brain with ability to adapt via structural and functional plasticity in response to stressful experiences, including neuronal replacement, dendritic remodeling, and synapse turnover. Allostatic responses also produce continuous changes in gene expression via epigenetic mechanisms. In the setting of chronic stress, there is shrinkage on the dendritic trees in the hippocampus and prefrontal cortex and expansion of dendritic trees in neurons of the basolateral amygdala.[69]

AUTONOMIC HYPERACTIVITY

Autonomic hyperactivity is typically characterized by excessive activation of the sympathetic system and manifests with hypertension, tachyarrhythmia, hyperhidrosis, peripheral vasoconstriction, and hyperthermia or hypothermia. The most common causes of sympathetic hyperactivity are head trauma, hypoxic brain injury, subarachnoid hemorrhage, autonomic dysreflexia in the setting of spinal cord injury, Guillain-Barré syndrome, and iatrogenic disorders such as neuroleptic malignant syndrome and serotonin syndrome. Sympathetic hyperactivity may also be an important manifestation of limbic encephalitis. Less commonly, autonomic hyperactivity also involves the parasympathetic system and manifests primarily with bradyarrhythmia or even syncope.

Focal Disorders

Focal disorders affecting the cerebral cortex, diencephalon, or brainstem may manifest with severe consequences of sympathetic activation. Typical examples are ischemic strokes affecting the insular cortex or focal temporal lobe seizures, which may produce cardiac arrhythmias, myocardial injury, and increased risk of sudden death. Other manifestations of temporal lobe seizures include paroxysmal hypertension resembling a pheochromocytoma, ictal piloerection, ictal sweating, facial flushing, or pallor. In rare cases, temporal lobe seizures may also manifest with excessive vagal activity leading to ictal bradycardia and asystole. Sympathetic hyperactivity may also occur as a consequence of brainstem lesions, particularly those involving the medulla.

Limbic Encephalitis and Disorders Associated with Sleep Dysregulation

Sympathetic hyperactivity may be a major manifestation of limbic encephalitis associated with autoantibodies against voltage-gated K^+ channel complexes, including leucine-rich glioma-inhibited 1 (LGI1) and contactin-associated protein 2 (CASPR2). In these disorders, the common coexistence of hyponatremia reflects involvement of the hypothalamus. N-methyl-D-aspartate receptor (NMDAR) encephalitis typically manifests with autonomic hyperactivity following initial stages characterized by memory impairment, seizures, psychosis, and movement disorders. Sympathetic hyperactivity may also accompany disorders of sleep–wake regulation and be associated with confusional state, fluctuating delirium, and excessive or abnormal motor activity, including include delirium tremens, fatal insomnia, and IgLON5 disease.

Autonomic Dysreflexia and Other Causes of Fluctuating Sympathetic Activity

Spinal cord lesions above the T5 level interrupt the descending modulatory pathways that incorporate the segmental spinal autonomic reflexes into specific patterns of response according to the stimulus. This results in autonomic dysreflexia, which is characterized by episodes of unpatterned, massive sympathoexcitation in response to segmental visceral or somatic inputs below the level of the lesion.[70] The most typical example of peripheral nerve disorder associated with autonomic hyperactivity is Guillain-Barré syndrome, where marked variations of blood pressure and heart rate may reflect impaired baroreflex modulation of sympathetic cardiovascular output due to demyelination of baroreceptor afferents. Afferent baroreceptor failure characterized by severe fluctuations of blood pressure may also occur as a sequela of previous neck surgery or radiation affecting the carotid baroreceptors, or in some hereditary disorders such as hereditary sensory and autonomic neuropathy type III (familial dysautonomia).[71]

Central Autonomic Dysregulation, Cardiac Morbidity, and Risk of Sudden Death

Reduced heart rate variability and decreased baroreceptor sensitivity are relevant markers of cardiovascular risk, including predisposition toward ventricular arrhythmias in patients with primary cardiac disease.[72,73] In general, reduced heart rate variability primarily reflects decreased cardiovagal modulation, but sometimes it is associated with indices of increased sympathetic activity, as occurs in patients with ischemic stroke, epilepsy, multiple sclerosis, and Parkinson disease. Sympathetic hyperactivity triggers both supraventricular and ventricular tachycardia; vagal hyperactivity leads to bradyarrhythmias, including atrioventricular block. Imbalance between sympathetic and vagal control of the heart can trigger or predispose to cardiac arrhythmia and risk of sudden death.[74] For example, both excessive sympathetic and cardiovagal activity may predispose to atrial fibrillation. Sympathetic activation prolongs the plateau of the cardiac action potential; in this setting inability to activate repolarizing K^+ currents due to drug effects or hereditary channelopathies may lead to QT prolongation, which predisposes to polymorphic ventricular tachycardia (torsades de pointes) and ventricular fibrillation.[74] Acute neurologic insults leading to sympathetic hyperactivity may trigger reversible myocardial injury known as Takotsubo cardiomyopathy or apical ballooning syndrome.[75] Seizures and cardiac arrhythmias may be the coincident features of channelopathies and may constitute an important trigger of sudden unexpected death in epilepsy (SUDEP). Impaired control of breathing has also been linked to SUDEP.[76] Ictal apnea occurs when seizure activity spreads into the amygdala; amygdala stimulation during the intraoperative mapping elicited apnea, implicating this structure in the conscious control of breathing.[77]

KEY POINTS

- Central control of homeostasis and adaptation to internal or external challenges requires the integrated activity of the hypothalamus, amygdala, insula, and anterior cingulate cortex (ACC).
- The hypothalamus receives and integrates interoceptive, humoral, and emotional signals and functions as a pattern generator for coordinated autonomic and endocrine responses to restore the internal milieu and adapt to challenges to survival.
- The preoptic area has a major role in thermoregulation, electrolyte balance, and sleep induction.
- The paraventricular nucleus (PVH), dorsomedial nucleus (DMH), lateral hypothalamic area (LHA), and other hypothalamic regions participate in integrative circuits controlling responses to stress.
- The posterior lateral hypothalamus, including the orexin (ORX)/hypocretin neurons has a critical role in control of arousal and motivated behaviors.
- The PVH has a critical role in integrated responses to internal stressors.
- DMH triggers sympathetically mediated responses to external stressors such as social stressors and cold exposure.
- The ORX neurons activate cardiovascular and respiratory responses associated with behavioral arousal, reward and motivated behavior, and stress.
- The responses to stress vary according both to the type of stressor and the subject's perception and ability to cope, and are orchestrated by different PAG cell columns.
- There are close reciprocal interactions between the autonomic and the immune systems at multiple levels, including the gut, the CNS, and lymphoid organs.
- The PVH via its projections to the C1 area of the RVLM promotes sympathetic output to lymphoid organs eliciting anti-inflammatory responses.
- The regulation of core temperature involves feedback and feedforward mechanisms integrated at the preoptic area and mediated by sympathetic outputs to the skin.
- Warm-sensitive neurons in the medial preoptic area (MPO) area respond to increases in core temperature, inhibit cold-sensitive neurons, and initiate skin vasodilation and sweating.
- Neurons in the median preoptic area (MnPO) receive inputs from warm and cold receptors and interact with other hypothalamic thermoregulatory groups.
- The DMH contains neurons that initiate thermoregulatory responses to cold via projections to the rostral portion of the raphe pallidus.
- The febrile response is triggered by cytokines that activate endothelial cells to produce prostaglandin E2, which inhibits the warm-sensitive neurons of the MPO.
- The critical areas involved in osmoregulation and fluid homeostasis are located in the SFO, OVLT, and MnPO.
- Increases in plasma osmolality and decreases in plasma volume trigger thirst, secretion of AVP (antidiuretic hormone, ADH), and increased sympathetic activity.
- The arcuate nucleus (ARC, infundibular nucleus) contains different subpopulations olf neurons that exert opposite effects on food intake in response to leptin.
- The antagonistic effects between orexinergic and anorexinergic neurons in the ARC reflect their opposite effects on neurons in the PVH, which elicit homeostatic satiety and reduce total food consumption via projections to the lateral parabrachial nucleus.
- The LHA contains GABAergic neurons that promote reward-related feeding by indirectly increasing the activity of dopaminergic VTA neurons.
- The termination of a meal is triggered by gut signals that activate vagal afferents terminating in the NTS, which project to the lateral PB leading to activation of the centromedial nucleus of the amygdala (CeM).

- Endocannabinoids acting via CB1 receptors in the VTA, hypothalamus, gut, and liver promote accumulation of energy stores.
- The amygdala provides automatic tagging of positive or negative valence to environmental challenges and triggers automatic survival responses via the hypothalamus and brainstem.
- Interoception strongly influences emotion, cognition, and motivation.
- Central autonomic commands from the anterior insula and ACC may be sent as predictive signals about the expected sensory consequences resulting from activation of the target organs.
- The mismatch between feedforward commands and feedback signals generates an error prediction signal that influences cognitive and emotional processing.
- Autonomic hyperactivity is typically characterized by excessive sympathetic activation.
- The most common causes of sympathetic hyperactivity are head trauma, hypoxic brain injury, subarachnoid hemorrhage, autonomic dysreflexia, Guillain-Barré syndrome, and iatrogenic disorders.
- Sympathetic hyperactivity may be an important manifestation of limbic encephalitis associated with NMDA receptor, LGI1, or CASPSR2 autoantibodies.
- Some cardiac arrhythmias secondary to neurologic disorders may be life-threatening.
- Acute neurologic insults leading to sympathetic hyperactivity may trigger reversible myocardial injury known as Takotsubo cardiomyopathy.
- Cardiac arrhythmias may be an important ictal event in temporal, medial frontal, or insular seizures.
- Seizures and cardiac arrhythmias may be the coincident features of channelopathies and may constitute an important trigger of sudden unexpected death in epilepsy (SUDEP).
- Ictal apnea may occur when seizure activity spreads into the amygdala.

REFERENCES

1. Saper CB, Lowell BB. The hypothalamus. Curr Biol 2014;24:R1111–1116.
2. LeDoux J. The amygdala. Curr Biol 2007;17:R868–874.
3. Shoemaker JK, Goswami R. Forebrain neurocircuitry associated with human reflex cardiovascular control. Front Physiol 2015;6:240.
4. Craig AD. Interoception: the sense of the physiological condition of the body. Curr Opin Neurobiol 2003;13:500–505.
5. Vogt BA, Vogt L, Farber NB, Bush G. Architecture and neurocytology of monkey cingulate gyrus. J Comp Neurol 2005;485:218–239.
6. Kreibig SD. Autonomic nervous system activity in emotion: a review. Biol Psychol 2010;84:394–421.
7. Rolls ET. Limbic systems for emotion and for memory, but no single limbic system. Cortex 2015;62:119–157.
8. Siso S, Jeffrey M, Gonzalez L. Sensory circumventricular organs in health and disease. Acta Neuropathol 2010;120:689–705.
9. Langlet F. Tanycyte gene expression dynamics in the regulation of energy homeostasis. Front Endocrinol (Lausanne) 2019;10:286.
10. Dampney RA. Central neural control of the cardiovascular system: current perspectives. Adv Physiol Educ 2016;40:283–296.
11. McEwen BS. Physiology and neurobiology of stress and adaptation: central role of the brain. Physiol Rev 2007;87:873–904.
12. Ulrich-Lai YM, Herman JP. Neural regulation of endocrine and autonomic stress responses. Nat Rev 2009;10:397–409.
13. Grimaldi D, Silvani A, Benarroch EE, Cortelli P. Orexin/hypocretin system and autonomic control: new insights and clinical correlations. Neurology 2014;82:271–278.
14. Nattie E, Li A. Respiration and autonomic regulation and orexin. Prog Brain Res 2012;198:25–46.
15. Bandler R, Keay KA, Floyd N, Price J. Central circuits mediating patterned autonomic activity during active vs. passive emotional coping. Brain Res Bull 2000;53:95–104.
16. Benarroch EE. Autonomic nervous system and neuroimmune interactions: New insights and clinical implications. Neurology 2019;92:377–385.
17. Johnson JD, Barnard DF, Kulp AC, Mehta DM. Neuroendocrine regulation of brain cytokines after psychological stress. J Endocr Soc 2019;3:1302–1320.
18. Tan CL, Knight ZA. Regulation of body temperature by the nervous system. Neuron 2018;98:31–48.
19. Madden CJ, Morrison SF. Central nervous system circuits that control body temperature. Neurosci Lett 2019;696:225–232.
20. Morrison SF. Efferent neural pathways for the control of brown adipose tissue thermogenesis and shivering. Handb Clin Neurol 2018;156:281–303.
21. Zimmerman CA, Leib DE, Knight ZA. Neural circuits underlying thirst and fluid homeostasis. Nat Rev Neurosci 2017;18:459–469.
22. Andermann ML, Lowell BB. Toward a wiring diagram understanding of appetite control. Neuron 2017;95:757–778.
23. Tups A, Benzler J, Sergi D, Ladyman SR, Williams LM. Central regulation of glucose homeostasis. Compr Physiol 2017;7:741–764.
24. Stuber GD, Wise RA. Lateral hypothalamic circuits for feeding and reward. Nat Neurosci 2016;19:198–205.
25. Piazza PV, Cota D, Marsicano G. The CB1 receptor as the cornerstone of exostasis. Neuron 2017;93:1252–1274.
26. Critchley HD. Neural mechanisms of autonomic, affective, and cognitive integration. J Comp Neurol 2005;493:154–166.
27. Cechetto DF, Shoemaker JK. Functional neuroanatomy of autonomic regulation. Neuroimage 2009;47:795–803.
28. Beissner F, Meissner K, Bar KJ, Napadow V. The autonomic brain: an activation likelihood estimation meta-analysis for central processing of autonomic function. J Neurosci 2013;33:10503–10511.
29. Shoemaker JK, Norton KN, Baker J, Luchyshyn T. Forebrain organization for autonomic cardiovascular control. Auton Neurosci 2015;188:5–9.

30. Macefield VG, Henderson LA. "Real-time" imaging of cortical and subcortical sites of cardiovascular control: concurrent recordings of sympathetic nerve activity and fMRI in awake subjects. J Neurophysiol 2016;116:1199–1207.
31. Macey PM, Ogren JA, Kumar R, Harper RM. Functional imaging of autonomic regulation: methods and key findings. Front Neurosci 2015;9:513.
32. Sklerov M, Dayan E, Browner N. Functional neuroimaging of the central autonomic network: recent developments and clinical implications. Clin Auton Res 2019;29:555–566.
33. Kimmerly DS. A review of human neuroimaging investigations involved with central autonomic regulation of baroreflex-mediated cardiovascular control. Auton Neurosci 2017;207:10–21.
34. Critchley HD, Nagai Y, Gray MA, Mathias CJ. Dissecting axes of autonomic control in humans: Insights from neuroimaging. Auton Neurosci 2011;161:34–42.
35. LeDoux J. Rethinking the emotional brain. Neuron 2012;73:653–676.The amygdala. Curr Biol 2007;17:R868–874.
36. Gold PW. The organization of the stress system and its dysregulation in depressive illness. Mol Psychiatry 2015;20:32–47.
37. Pace-Schott EF, Amole MC, Aue T, et al. Physiological feelings. Neurosci Biobehav Rev 2019;103:267–304.
38. Damasio A, Carvalho GB. The nature of feelings: evolutionary and neurobiological origins. Nat Rev Neurosci 2013;14:143–152.
39. Craig AD. Significance of the insula for the evolution of human awareness of feelings from the body. Ann N Y Acad Sci 2011;1225:72–82.
40. Critchley HD, Harrison NA. Visceral influences on brain and behavior. Neuron 2013;77:624–638.
41. Berridge KC, Kringelbach ML. Pleasure systems in the brain. Neuron 2015;86:646–664.
42. Schulz SM. Neural correlates of heart-focused interoception: a functional magnetic resonance imaging meta-analysis. Philos Trans R Soc Lond B Biol Sci 2016;371(1708):20160018.
43. Makovac E, Garfinkel S, Bassi A, et al. Fear processing is differentially affected by lateralized stimulation of carotid baroreceptors. Cortex 2018;99:200–212.
44. Adolfi F, Couto B, Richter F, et al. Convergence of interoception, emotion, and social cognition: a twofold fMRI meta-analysis and lesion approach. Cortex 2017;88:124–142.
45. Cechetto DF. Cortical control of the autonomic nervous system. Exp Physiol 2014;99:326–331.
46. James C, Macefield VG, Henderson LA. Real-time imaging of cortical and subcortical control of muscle sympathetic nerve activity in awake human subjects. Neuroimage 2013;70:59–65.
47. Oppenheimer S, Cechetto D. The insular cortex and the regulation of cardiac function. Compr Physiol 2016;6:1081–1133.
48. Al-Khazraji BK, Shoemaker JK. The human cortical autonomic network and volitional exercise in health and disease. Appl Physiol Nutr Metab 2018;43:1122–1130.
49. Seeley WW. The salience network: a neural system for perceiving and responding to homeostatic demands. J Neurosci 2019;39:9878–9882.
50. Allman JM, Tetreault NA, Hakeem AY, Park S. The von Economo neurons in apes and humans. Am J Hum Biol 2011;23:5–21.
51. Caruana F, Gerbella M, Avanzini P, et al. Motor and emotional behaviours elicited by electrical stimulation of the human cingulate cortex. Brain 2018;141:3035–3051.
52. Guo CC, Sturm VE, Zhou J, et al. Dominant hemisphere lateralization of cortical parasympathetic control as revealed by frontotemporal dementia. Proc Natl Acad Sci U S A 2016;113:E2430–2439.
53. Lacuey N, Hampson JP, Theeranaew W, et al. Cortical structures associated with human blood pressure control. JAMA Neurol 2018;75:194–202.
54. Lane RD, Weidenbacher H, Smith R, Fort C, Thayer JF, Allen JJ. Subgenual anterior cingulate cortex activity covariation with cardiac vagal control is altered in depression. J Affect Disord 2013;150:565–570.
55. Dosenbach NU, Visscher KM, Palmer ED, et al. A core system for the implementation of task sets. Neuron 2006;50:799–812.
56. Taylor KS, Kucyi A, Millar PJ, et al. Association between resting-state brain functional connectivity and muscle sympathetic burst incidence. J Neurophysiol 2016;115:662–673.
57. Barrett LF, Simmons WK. Interoceptive predictions in the brain. Nat Rev Neurosci 2015;16:419–429.
58. Seth AK, Friston KJ. Active interoceptive inference and the emotional brain. Philos Trans R Soc Lond B Biol Sci 2016;371.
59. Evrard HC. The organization of the primate insular cortex. Front Neuroanat 2019;13:43.
60. Watanabe M, Furusho K, Takahashi T, Tamaoka A. Galactorrhea in a patient with aquaporin-4 antibody-positive neuromyelitis optica spectrum disorder: a case report and review of the literature. Neurologist 2015;20:101–103.
61. Pu S, Long Y, Yang N, et al. Syndrome of inappropriate antidiuretic hormone secretion in patients with aquaporin-4 antibody. J Neurol 2015;262:101–107.
62. Dauvilliers Y, Bauer J, Rigau V, et al. Hypothalamic immunopathology in anti-Ma-associated diencephalitis with narcolepsy-cataplexy. JAMA Neurol 2013;70:1305–1310.
63. Benarroch EE. Thermoregulation: recent concepts and remaining questions. Neurology 2007;69:1293–1297.
64. May A, Burstein R. Hypothalamic regulation of headache and migraine. Cephalalgia 2019;39:1710–1719.
65. Schulte LH, Allers A, May A. Hypothalamus as a mediator of chronic migraine: evidence from high-resolution fMRI. Neurology 2017;88:2011–2016.
66. Mravec B, Horvathova L, Cernackova A. Hypothalamic inflammation at a crossroad of somatic diseases. Cell Mol Neurobiol 2019;39:11–29.
67. Cai D, Khor S. "Hypothalamic microinflammation" paradigm in aging and metabolic diseases. Cell Metab 2019;30:19–35.
68. McEwen BS, Morrison JH. The brain on stress: vulnerability and plasticity of the prefrontal cortex over the life course. Neuron 2013;79:16–29.
69. McEwen BS. Allostasis and the epigenetics of brain and body health over the life course: the brain on stress. JAMA Psychiatry 2017;74:551–552.
70. Shouman K, Benarroch EE. Segmental spinal sympathetic machinery: implications for autonomic dysreflexia. Neurology 2019;93:339–345.
71. Kaufmann H, Norcliffe-Kaufmann L, Palma JA. Baroreflex dysfunction. N Engl J Med 2020;382:163–178.

72. Kleiger RE, Stein PK, Bigger JT, Jr. Heart rate variability: measurement and clinical utility. Ann Noninvasive Electrocardiol 2005;10:88–101.
73. Lahiri MK, Kannankeril PJ, Goldberger JJ. Assessment of autonomic function in cardiovascular disease: physiological basis and prognostic implications. J Am Coll Cardiol 2008;51:1725–1733.
74. Franciosi S, Perry FKG, Roston TM, Armstrong KR, Claydon VE, Sanatani S. The role of the autonomic nervous system in arrhythmias and sudden cardiac death. Auton Neurosci 2017;205:1–11.
75. Yoshimura S, Toyoda K, Ohara T, et al. Takotsubo cardiomyopathy in acute ischemic stroke. Ann Neurol 2008;64:547–554.
76. Ryvlin P, Nashef L, Lhatoo SD, et al. Incidence and mechanisms of cardiorespiratory arrests in epilepsy monitoring units (MORTEMUS): a retrospective study. Lancet Neurol 2013;12:966–977.
77. Nobis WP, Schuele S, Templer JW, et al. Amygdala-stimulation-induced apnea is attention and nasal-breathing dependent. Ann Neurol 2018;83:460–471.

Section VI

Cortical Networks and Cognitive Domains

39 Emotion and Social Cognition

OVERVIEW

Emotion constitutes both a psychological and physical reaction that is critical for survival and control of behavior. Emotional processing involves several brain areas, including the amygdala, insular cortex, orbitofrontal cortex (OFC), and cingulate cortex, and their connections with subcortical areas (Figure 39.1). Emotions are experienced as strong feelings that vary according to their valence (pleasant or unpleasant) and intensity and produce physiological changes that prepare the body for immediate action. External or internal stimuli are automatically tagged with either positive or negative valence by the amygdala, leading to coordinated activation of survival, arousal, and reward and motivation circuits[1,2,3] (Figure 39.2). The activation of survival autonomic circuits occurs independently of the conscious experience of emotions but elicits responses that indirectly affect emotional consciousness.[4] Conscious emotional experience is closely bound to changes in bodily sensations (interoception) created by the patterned neural responses to behaviorally relevant stimuli.[5–8] The insular cortex has a major role in such conscious interoceptive awareness.[7] The OFC receives inputs from the amygdala and the insular cortex and represents the reward value of stimuli and outcomes of actions.[9,10] The amygdala, insula, and OFC are connected to the cingulate cortex, which since the initial description of Broca has been viewed as a critical component of the so-called limbic system.[11] However, the concept of a unique limbic system is an oversimplification.[1,12–14] The cingulate cortex has three major subdivisions that together with their connections form six limbic "subsystems."[13] The anterior cingulate cortex (ACC) is involved in emotional processing (anterior emotional subsystem); the midcingulate cortex (MCC) in response selection and feedback-guided decision-making (middle sensorimotor subsystem), and the posterior cingulate cortex (PCC) and retrosplenial cortex in visuospatial orientation and assessment of the self-relevance of objects and events (posterior cognitive map subsystem).[13,14] The anterior emotional subsystem has robust interactions with the amygdala, the middle subsystem with neocortical sensorimotor cortices, and the posterior subsystem with the posterior parietal cortex. The hippocampus contributes to memory in each subsystem. Thus, emotions reciprocally interact with cognition to determine the mental state, which is the combination of all feelings, thoughts, memories, and intentions that are present at a given moment.[15] Emotions determine the value of incentives for goal-seeking behaviors, influence motivation and memory processing, and provide a basis for social cognition.[16] Disorders affecting these functions manifest with profound alterations in decision-making, social cognition, and behavior, as occur in behavioral variant frontotemporal dementia (bvFTD), in focal lesions, or psychiatric disease.[17,18] The aims of this chapter are to review: (1) the connections and mechanisms by which the amygdala participates in emotion social behavior; (2) the contribution of the insular cortex, OFC, and cingulate cortex to the processing of emotions for allocation of value, decision-making, and motivation; and (3) the brain circuits controlling social behavior.

AMYGDALA AND EMOTIONAL RESPONSE

The amygdala is a critical component of the emotion system. It provides automatic tagging of positive or negative valence of environmental stimuli and their intensity and therefore encodes their relevance. Either directly or after Pavlovian conditioning, the amygdala triggers automatic survival responses, contributes to representation of value for reward (incentive)-based behavior and decision-making, modulates episodic memory, and contributes to social cognition.[4]

Intrinsic Circuit

As discussed in chapter 25, the amygdala is a nuclear complex subdivided into a basolateral nuclear group, a centromedial group, an intercalate mass, and the olfactory

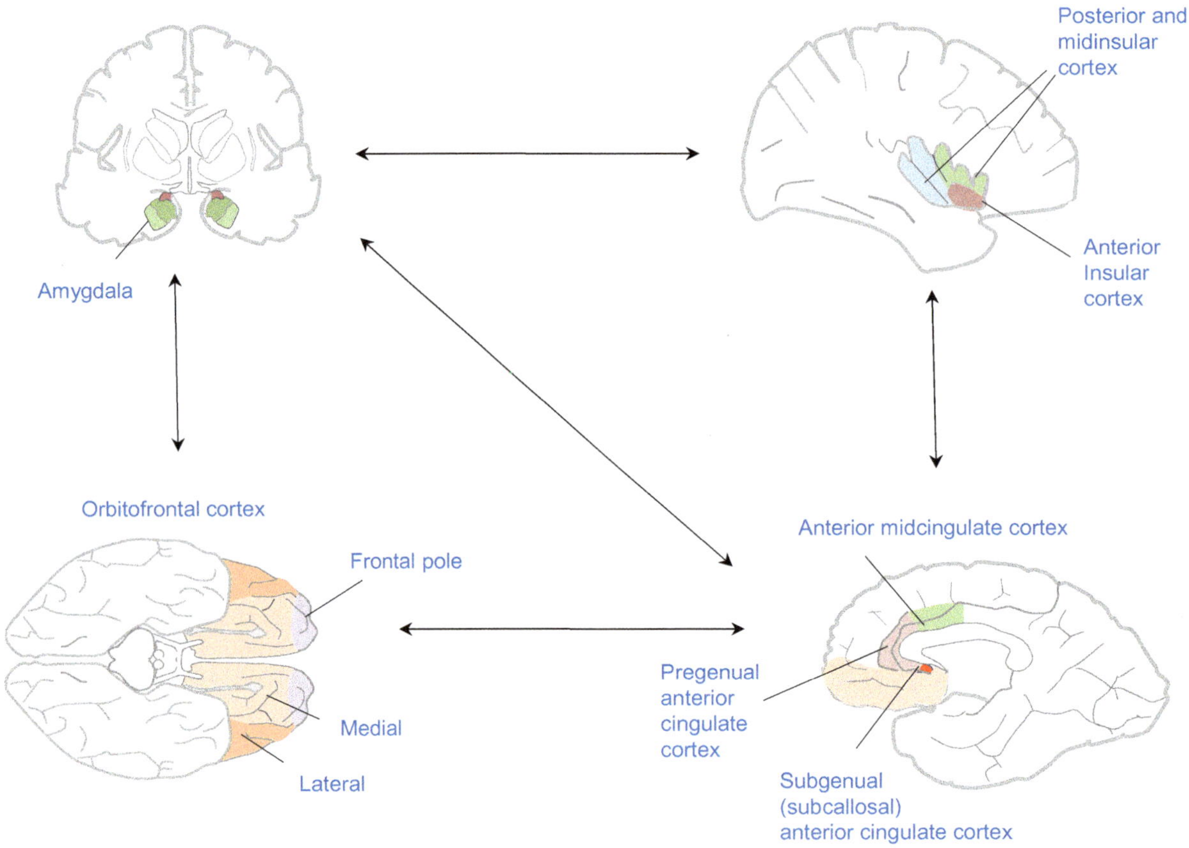

FIGURE 39.1 Core areas for emotional processing
The core components of the emotion system constitute the classical "anterior" limbic system. This circuit includes the amygdala, insular cortex, orbitofrontal cortex (OFC), anterior cingulate cortex (ACC), and midcingulate cingulate cortex (MCC), which are reciprocally interconnected.

amygdala. Information processing within the amygdala involves serial excitatory connections controlled by local GABAergic circuits. The lateral nucleus of the amygdala receives both highly processed visual, auditory, somatosensory, and visceral information from cortical association areas of the ventral stream encoding object feature information ("what" pathway), particularly the anterior temporal cortex, and less elaborated sensory inputs, such as pain, directly via the thalamus. The convergence of cortical and subcortical inputs on single neurons of the lateral nucleus provides the basis for associative (Pavlovian) learning in the amygdala. The lateral nucleus sends excitatory projections to the basal nucleus, which consists of separate subdivisions that target the centromedial nucleus (CeM) and also sends projections to cortical and subcortical areas (Figure 39.3). Local GABAergic neurons control processing at all levels of the intrinsic circuit of the amygdala, including probability of associative conditioned learning in the lateral nucleus, and the influence of the basal nuclei on the CeM. These GABAergic interconnections thus strongly control encoding, learning, retrieval, and extinction of emotional memories.[19,20]

Extrinsic Connections

Via its multiple outputs and interactions, the amygdala has a major role in all aspects of emotional processing (Figure 39.3). It sends extensive reciprocal projections to cortical sensory association areas, which provides survival relevance to specific sensory stimuli and contributes to modulation of sensory processing. Connections of the amygdala with the OFC, either directly or via the mediodorsal nucleus of the thalamus, provide signals that contribute to stimulus value-based coding. Interactions with the ACC and anterior MCC contribute both to learning and extinction of conditioned responses, trigger emotional awareness, and influence decision-making and motivation. There are strong interactions between the amygdala and the hippocampus, which are important for encoding of both emotional and episodic memories. Projections of the basal nucleus of the amygdala to the basal forebrain promote attentional modulation of cortical function, whereas projections to the NAc contribute to reward processing and motivated behavior. Projections from the amygdala to cholinergic and monoaminergic groups of the hypothalamus and brainstem contribute to modulation of the global

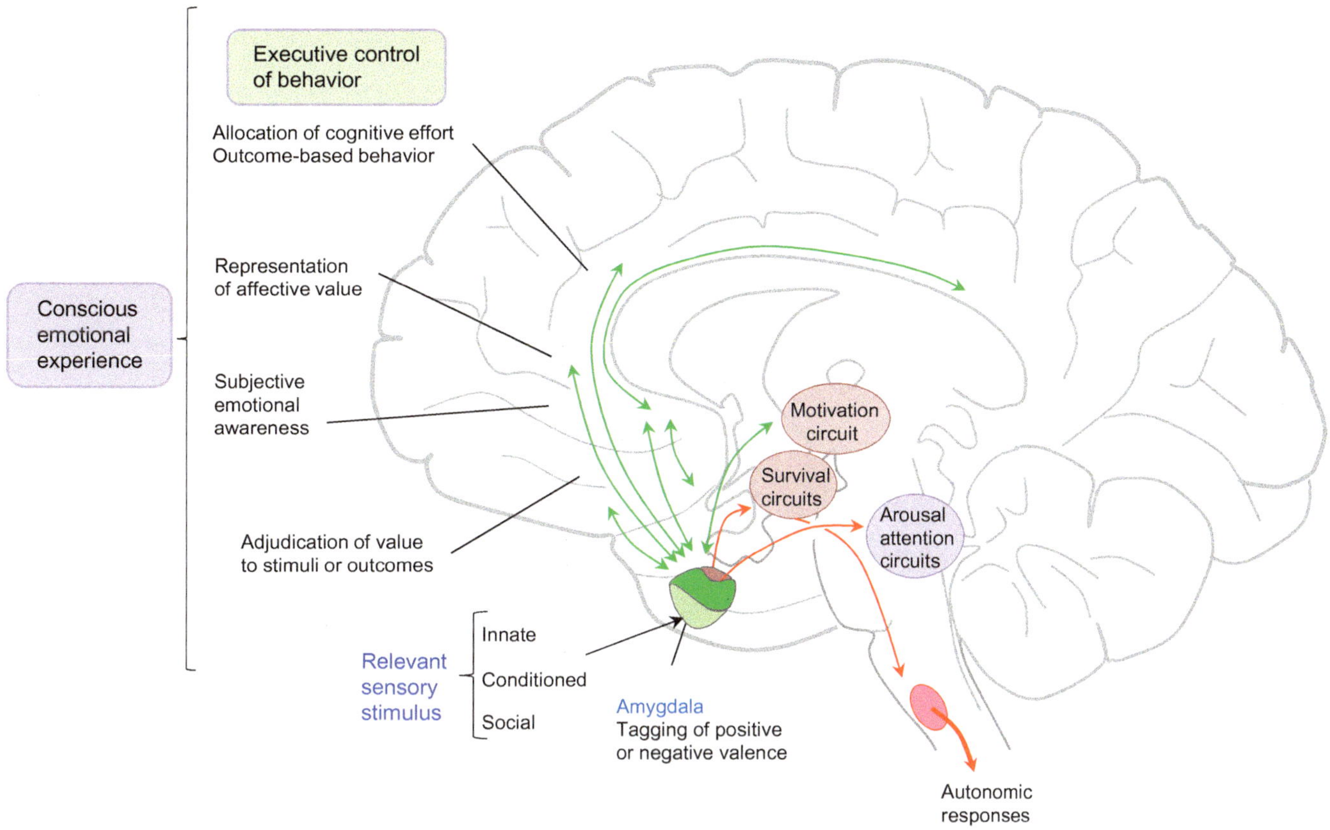

FIGURE 39.2 The multiple aspects of emotion
External or internal stimuli are automatically tagged with either positive or negative valence by the amygdala, leading to coordinated activation of survival, arousal, and reward and motivation circuits. The activation of survival circuits occurs independently of the conscious experience of emotions but elicits responses that indirectly affect emotional consciousness. Emotions reciprocally interact with cognition to determine the mental state and determine the value of incentives for goal-seeking behaviors, influence motivation and memory processing, and provide a basis for social cognition.

behavioral state, including arousal, attention, and sensory processing. The CeM is anatomically and functionally interconnected with the bed nucleus of the stria terminalis, forming a functional complex known as extended central amygdala.[21] Outputs from the extended central amygdala to the hypothalamus and brainstem trigger automatic survival responses. Important targets include the dorsomedial, ventromedial, and lateral hypothalamic areas, midline and posterior nuclei of the thalamus, periaqueductal gray (PAG), nucleus of the solitary tract, and pontomedullary reticular formation. These areas have a critical role in autonomic and motor responses to stress, including sympathetic activation, changes in respiration, vocalization, startle, and freezing.[2] The amygdala may also be activated by appetitive stimuli such as the taste of food, these projections also promote survival responses such as food ingestion.[4]

Conditioned Learning

Some stimuli referred to as primary reinforcers, such as pain and the taste of food, trigger innate and species-specific survival responses. In contrast, biologically neutral stimuli such as a sound or a visual stimulus can acquire behavioral relevance when they occur in conjunction with biologically significant aversive or appetitive stimuli. This constitutes Pavlovian conditioning or associative learning. For example, a neutral or conditioned stimulus (CS) such as a sound acquires a threat status after presented in conjunction with an aversive unconditioned stimulus (US) such as a painful electric shock.[2] Once the association is formed, the CS alone can trigger the innate survival response, such as freezing or startle, and associated autonomic and endocrine activation. The intrinsic circuits in the amygdala are critical for acquisition, consolidation, retrieval, and extinction of associative emotional memories. Associative learning in the amygdala involves synaptic plasticity in these excitatory and inhibitory circuits, resulting in recruitment of subsets of neurons (referred to as "engrams") in the lateral and basal nuclei during learning and their reactivation during memory retrieval, as discussed in chapter 25.[19,20]

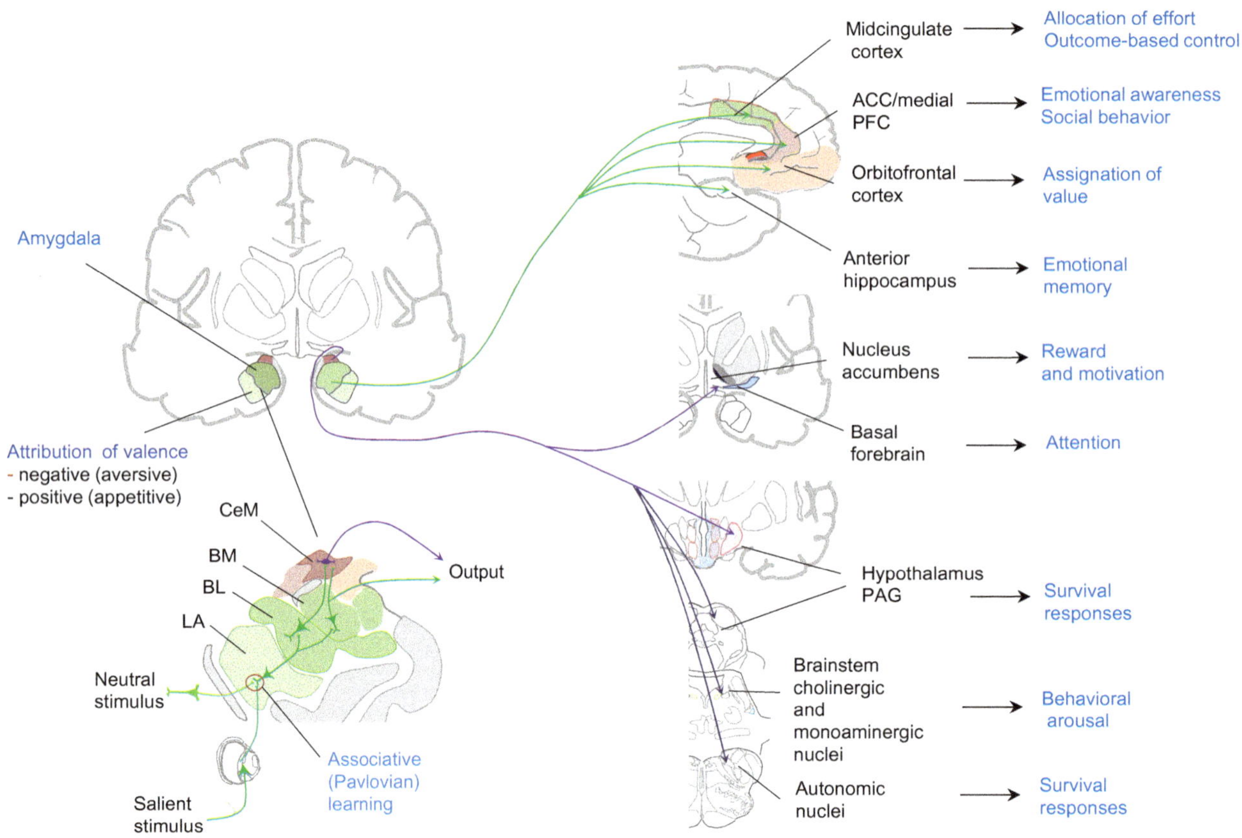

FIGURE 39.3 Intrinsic circuitry and connections of the amygdala

Information processing within the amygdala involves serial excitatory connections controlled by local GABAergic circuits. The convergence of cortical and subcortical inputs on single neurons of the lateral nucleus (LA) provides the basis for associative (Pavlovian) learning. The LA sends excitatory projections to the basal nucleus, which consists of basolateral (BL) and basomedial (BM) subdivisions that target the central nucleus and project to cortical and subcortical areas. The centromedial nucleus (CeM) provides the output of the amygdala to the hypothalamus and brainstem. Connections of the amygdala with the orbitofrontal cortex provide signals that contribute to value-based coding for decision-making. The strong interactions with the hippocampus are important for encoding of both emotional and episodic memories. Projections of the basal nucleus to the basal forebrain promote attentional modulation of cortical function, whereas those to the nucleus accumbens contribute to reward processing and motivated behavior. Projections to cholinergic and monoaminergic groups of the hypothalamus and brainstem contribute to modulation of arousal, attention, and sensory processing. Outputs from the CeM to the hypothalamus and brainstem trigger both innate and conditioned autonomic, endocrine, and motor survival responses.

Dissociation Between Amygdala Activation and Experience of Fear

Fear is an emotional conscious experience that occurs in the presence or perception of a threat to the well-being or survival of the individual. The amygdala is not the substrate for the feeling of fear; however, the physiological responses resulting from activation of the amygdala ("threat" responses) help create a state that enters conscious awareness as a feeling of fear.[22] Functional neuroimaging shows that there is activation of the human amygdala during fear-conditioning paradigms. However, these studies also show a poor correlation between the conscious feeling of fear and anxiety and the behavioral and physiological responses controlled by the survival circuits. For example, exposure to subliminal visual stimuli signaling a threat activate the amygdala and elicit body responses despite the participant's lack of awareness of the visual stimulus or experience of fear. Activation of the amygdala and innate survival responses also occurs in patients with blindsight who are unable to consciously detect threatening visual stimuli.[23]

This may involve direct connections from the pulvinar to the amygdala.[24] In contrast, damage of the amygdala interferes with bodily responses to threats but does not interfere with the conscious experience of emotions, including fear.

Frontal Cortex Regulation of Fear Learning and Extinction

Fear conditioning and extinction involve an interactive network that includes not only the amygdala but also areas of the prefrontal cortex (PFC), ACC, MCC, and anterior hippocampus.[19,25–27] Fear extinction is the gradual elimination of the fear reaction upon repeated exposure of the originally neutral stimulus without presenting the aversive stimulus. Fear extinction is an active learning process that leads to the formation of a new inhibitory memory that competes with the initial fear memory. Therefore, extinction is not permanent but rather context dependent and decays with time. The differential engagement of fear-extinction and fear-learning circuits in the amygdala involves a rapid switch in of different intrinsic inhibitory circuits, particularly within the basal and the central nuclei. Different subsets neurons of the basal nucleus of the amygdala send projections either to the MCC, which is engaged in fear conditioning, or to the ventromedial PFC including the ACC, which promotes extinction of fear memory. Activation of the PFC and MCC during threat situations is associated with the conscious appraisal of threat. The PFC can bidirectionally modulate the expression of previously learned fear (defense) response.[28] The PFC contributes to the initial learning of threat conditioning where there is a delay between the presentation of the CS and the US (a paradigm referred to as "trace" conditioning).[29] Neurons in the dorsolateral PFC involved in working memory may provide a bridging signal between the CS and US where a cue predicts the occurrence of an aversive stimulus that will occur several seconds later. Contextual control of fear extinction allows the appropriate expression of fear responses in a new, but not in a safe context, and requires an input from the hippocampus to both the amygdala and the PFC. Numerous fMRI studies show increased PFC activity and concomitant reduced amygdala activity during cognitive regulation of emotion during stressful situations. These studies also show that individual differences in a person's ability to control fear may be linked to differential activation of the ventromedial PFC. There is activation of the ventromedial PFC and inhibition of the MCC during extinction training; the opposite occurs during extinction recall.

Amygdala Involvement in Emotional and Episodic Memory

Studies using intracranial electroencephalography revealed that the amygdala is involved in selective aspects of memory formation and retrieval and affective processing in humans.[3] The amygdala coordinates the enhancement in consolidation and recall of emotionally salient information via connections with the perirhinal cortex and hippocampus. The human amygdala participates in semantic encoding and recognition of specific objects and individuals independently of context or visuospatial attributes, and discriminates between familiar and novel stimuli. The amygdala also responds differentially to social affective facial cues, increasing firing to relevant novel stimuli and showing habituation to familiar affective stimuli.[3]

Projections from the basal nucleus of the amygdala to the hippocampal formation provide emotional relevance to a particular event, promoting its consolidation in episodic memory.[30] Emotional enhancement of memory consolidation has social implications, as patients with amygdala lesions have difficulties learning traits of others such as likability and trustworthiness. Reciprocally, projections from the hippocampus provide contextual information to the amygdala about the emotional event.

Amygdala Responses to Facial Expression

Facial expression is a fundamental cue for social communication in humans. The fusiform gyrus (fusiform face area) processes information on static features of faces that allow personal identity; the superior temporal gyrus and superior temporal sulcus process information about changeable configurations of the face, such as facial expression, mouth, and eye movements. Both areas send inputs to the amygdala. Multiple fMRI studies show that the amygdala is particularly responsive to facial expressions, particularly fearful facial expression.[31] Deep electrode recordings in neurosurgical patients showed that the amygdala specifically encodes the subjective judgment of emotional faces, driven predominantly by judgments about the eye region of the face stimuli.[32] These responses do not require an intact primary visual cortex. A study in a patient with cortical blindness showed activation of the right amygdala in response to faces with their gaze directed toward but not away from the viewer.[33] The amygdala may also respond to the emotional expression of faces in the context of visual extinction and spatial neglect.[34] However, amygdala processing of highly arousing visual threats requires conscious awareness.[35]

Role of the Amygdala in Adjudication of Value and Framing Effect

Conditioning in the amygdala occurs for both aversive and rewarding stimuli. The amygdala contains intermingled populations of neurons that encode the positive or negative valence and intensity of emotions. For example, some neurons show stronger responses to neutral visual stimuli associated with aversive stimuli (negative value–coding neurons) whereas other neurons show stronger responses to neutral visual stimuli associated with reward (positive value–coding neurons). Functional neuroimaging studies indicate that in humans there is activation of the amygdala in response to both aversive and appetitive stimuli. For example, during a gambling task, there is a correlation between amygdala activation and the strength of the so-called framing effect.[36] Framing effect refers to the susceptibility of behavioral choices according to how the options are presented. This effect is associated with amygdala activity, suggesting a key role for an emotional system in mediating decision biases.[36] In contrast, activity of the orbital and medial PFC prefrontal reduces susceptibility to the framing effect.[36] The amygdala sends robust projections to the thalamic reticular nucleus, which via its inhibitory influence on thalamic relay nuclei functions as a hub of the attentional system that gates thalamocortical signaling.[37] The amygdala–thalamic reticular nucleus circuit can mediate selective attention guided by emotion by enabling focused top-down and flexible bottom-up allocation of attention.[37] This inhibitory selection mechanism can mediate a powerful affective framing effect that may lead to biased decision-making in highly charged emotional situations.[37] In contrast, social framing effects are based on decision-making regarding other people and are associated with activation in the right temporoparietal junction (TPJ) and its functional connectivity with the medial PFC.[38]

INSULAR CORTEX: INTERFACE BETWEEN BODILY FEELING AND EMOTIONAL AWARENESS

The insula has a major role in representations of sensory input from peripheral organs, known as interoception, and forms part of large-scale networks controlling attention and social behavior[39] (Figure 39.4).

Insular Cortex and Interoception

Interoception is a fundamental aspect of emotion and has relevance in many other phenomena, including decision-making and social behavior. As mentioned in previous chapters, the insula has a crucial role in multimodal integration of interoceptive signals such as pain, thermal, and visceral sensation, with proprioceptive, auditory, vestibular, and visual signals and provides one link between interoception, awareness of the body, and emotion.[7,8,40] Functional neuroimaging show insular activation when participants are made aware of their thirst, heartbeat, and

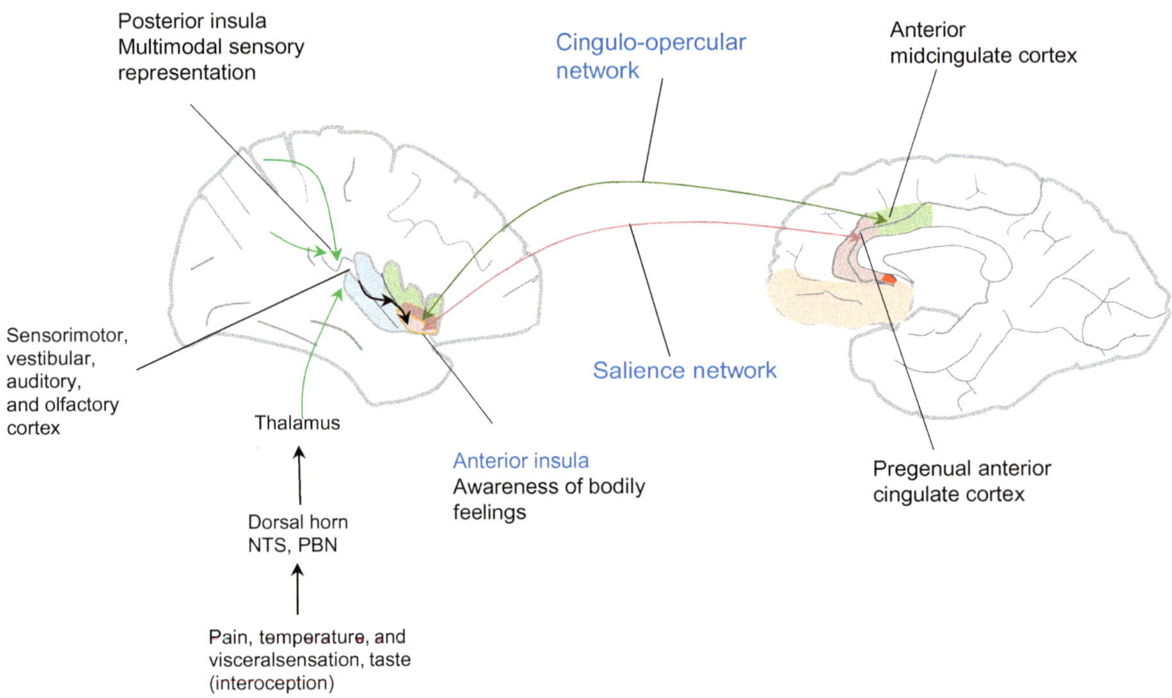

FIGURE 39.4 Information processing in the insula and insula-based networks
The insula has a crucial role in multimodal integration of interoceptive signals such as pain, thermal, and visceral sensation, with proprioceptive, auditory, vestibular, and visual signals and provides one link between interoception, awareness of the body, and emotion. Interoceptive inputs reach the insula via the thalamus, which receives inputs from the dorsal horn, nucleus of the solitary tract (NTS), and parabrachial nucleus (PB). The posterior insula is the primary interoceptive cortex and projects via the midinsula to the anterior insula, which integrates interoceptive signals with emotional and cognitive processing and is involved in conscious experience of bodily sensation. The ventral anterior insula and the pregenual anterior cingulate cortex are hubs of the "salience" network that participates in the awareness of bodily sensations and is also activated during social cognition tasks, including those involving empathy. The dorsal anterior insula and the anterior midcingulate cortex (also referred to as dorsal or supracallosal ACC) are components of the cingulo-opercular control network involved in task set maintenance.

visceral sensations.[40–42] The posterior insula is the primary interoceptive cortex and projects via the midinsula to the anterior insula, which integrates interoceptive signals with emotional and cognitive processing and is involved in conscious experience of bodily sensation.[5–8]

Functional Networks Involving the Insular Cortex

The insular cortex participates in different functional networks with other brain regions involved in emotional processing. Human studies focused on architectonic organization and postmortem MRI,[43] probabilistic tractography,[44] and resting-state fMRI[45] showed that both the insular and cingulate cortex form part of functionally distinct networks that are activated in response to events in the environment that are behaviorally relevant (salient) to the current goals and needs. The ventral anterior insula (frontoinsular cortex) and the pregenual ACC are hubs of the so-called salience network that participates in the awareness of bodily sensations and is also activated during social cognition tasks, including those involving empathy.[46,47] Both the ventral anterior insula and the pregenual ACC contain large layer 5 von Economo neurons, which project to brainstem autonomic areas and are vulnerable to neurodegeneration.[48] The dorsal anterior insula and the anterior MCC (also referred to as dorsal or supracallosal ACC) are components of the cingulo-opercular control network involved in task set maintenance.[49] One recent meta-analysis of fMRI date showed convergence of areas linked to interoception, emotional regulation, and social cognition in the right anterior insula, OFC, inferior frontal gyrus, and amygdala as well as in midtemporal areas and basal ganglia.[50]

ORBITOFRONTAL CORTEX: ASSIGNATION OF VALUE, REVERSAL LEARNING, AND DECISION-MAKING

The OFC has a major role in assignation of value to the available options for decision-making based on comparison between the values of these options.[8,10] The OFC represents the reward value of sensory stimuli such as taste, smells, touch, or facial expressions that are known as primary reinforcers, and conveys this information to other prefrontal areas for decision-making. Value-based behavior involves interactions of the OFC with the amygdala, ACC, and the MCC, both directly and via the mediodorsal nucleus of the thalamus. The amygdala provides value signals to the OFC, which in turns influences coding in the amygdala. Whereas the amygdala may be biased toward encoding both valence and intensity of emotions, the OFC encodes a broader range of variables participating in cognitive regulation of emotions and behavior.[51]

Connectivity and Multimodal Representations

The OFC includes several subregions with distinct connectivity and function[10,52] (Figure 39.5). The medial OFC receives inputs from all sensory modalities and is at the end stage of processing of the ventral stream encoding modality-specific feature ("what") information. Visual inputs are conveyed by the inferior temporal cortex (containing representations of objects and faces), the superior temporal sulcus (containing representations of facial expressions), and temporal pole. The OFC receives taste information from the insular cortex (primary taste cortex), olfactory information from the piriform cortex (primary olfactory cortex), and somatosensory information from the primary and secondary somatosensory cortex and insula.[53] The OFC also receives inputs from the mediodorsal nucleus of the thalamus relaying afferents from the olfactory cortex, amygdala, and inferior temporal cortex. The OFC is also strongly interconnected with the perirhinal cortex, which has a critical role in familiarity-based recognition of stimuli. Together with the amygdala, the OFC constitutes a second tier of processing for representation of affective value of stimuli. There are many intrinsic connections within the OFC, which enables many of its neurons to respond to multiple sensory modalities. For example, the OFC contains a major representation of taste, which is a primary reinforcer and thus, like the amygdala, functions in stimulus-reinforcer association learning between previously neutral stimuli (such as the sight of a food) and primary reinforcers (such as its taste). There are separate representations and responses of individual OFC neurons to different stimuli.[10] For example, different taste stimuli elicit a robust activation of individual OFC neurons; some of them also respond to the combinations of different tastes, combinations of taste and smell (flavor), combinations of taste and texture or temperature of what is in the mouth, or combinations of taste and the sight of food. Primary rewards such as the taste of food are represented in posterior portions of the OFC, whereas more complex or abstract reinforcers such as money gains or losses are represented more anteriorly.

Assignation of Value of Stimuli and Outcomes According to Contingency

A fundament role of the OFC is to guide decision-making by determining what stimulus is rewarding and what stimulus is not, according to the contingencies. For example, the taste or smell of a particular food elicits activation of OFC neurons in the setting of hunger, but the same neurons gradually reduce their response and eventually stop responding after satiety is reached and the food is no longer rewarding. In reward-devaluation paradigms, subjects learn two stimuli that predict two different reward types before one of these outcomes is devalued due to an aversive outcome. In normal conditions, this change in value in one stimulus immediately leads to the selection of the alternative stimulus. Many types of reward and adverse outcome(punishment) are differentially represented in the OFC. Functional neuroimaging in humans show that medial OFC (areas 13 and 11) is activated by taste, smell, and oral texture of foods and that this activation is linearly correlated with the subjective

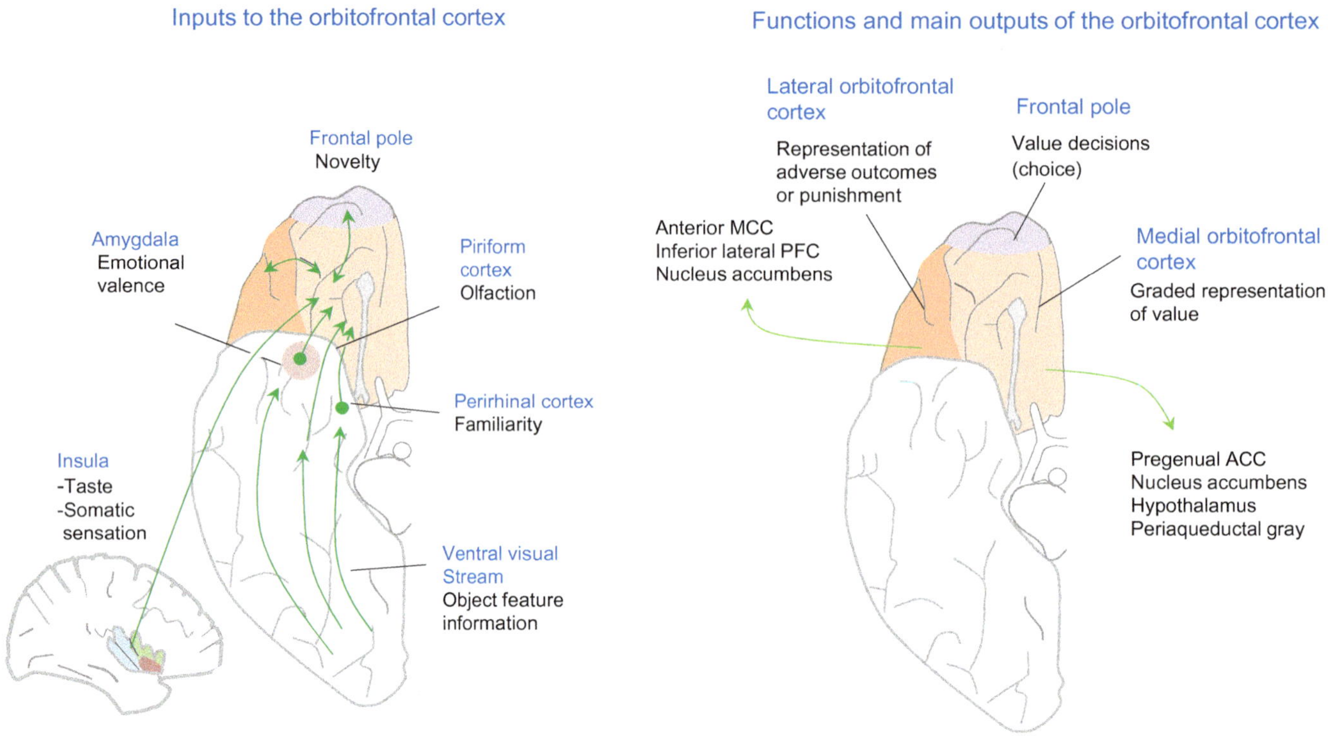

FIGURE 39.5 Connectivity and functional segregation in the orbitofrontal cortex
The orbitofrontal cortex (OFC) includes several subregions with distinct connectivity. The medial OFC receives inputs from all sensory modalities and is at the end stage of processing of the ventral stream encoding modality-specific feature ("what") information. Visual inputs are conveyed by the inferior temporal cortex, superior temporal sulcus, and temporal pole. Taste and somatosensory inputs are provided by the insular cortex and olfactory information by the piriform cortex. The OFC also receives inputs from the mediodorsal nucleus of the thalamus. The OFC is also strongly interconnected with the perirhinal cortex, which has a critical role in familiarity-based recognition of stimuli. Activation of the medial OFC (areas 13 and 11) is linearly correlated with the subjective sense of pleasantness and positive rewards. In contrast, the lateral OIFC signals punishments. The most anterior of the medial OFC (fronto polar cortex, area 10) is involved in binary decisions about values.

sense of pleasantness and positive rewards, such as pleasant odors or earning money. The medial OFC is connected with the pregenual ACC, which is also activated by emotionally pleasant experience.

Reversal Learning

In addition to neurons that encode the expected reward value of stimuli, the OFC contains error neurons that detect nonreward, and neurons that respond, for example, when an expected reward is not obtained. These neurons are termed "negative reward-prediction error neurons." These neurons are located in the lateral OFC (areas 47/12) and are activated by aversive outcomes. The lateral OFC is connected to the ventrolateral PFC and anterior MCC, which are involved in outcome-based action control.[10] The negative reward-prediction error neurons of the OFC may be more suitable to encode negative reward-prediction errors than midbrain neurons, as these OFC neurons encode both the expected reward and the learned reinforcer.[10] The OFC has projections to the ventral striatum, which in turn projects in part via the lateral habenula to midbrain dopamine neurons. The error-encoding neurons of the OFC may have a major role in the mechanism of stimulus-outcome reversal learning. In reversal learning studies, one stimulus is paired with a reward and the other is not. When learning has been acquired, the rewarding stimulus switches, so that the reward is now delivered after the previous unrewarded stimulus. In normal conditions, this leads to a reversal of choice.

Facial Recognition and Social Behavior

Like the amygdala, the OFC contains neurons that respond to facial expression, but in humans the OFC overshadows the amygdala in emotional learning for social behavior.[10,54–56] Faces convey information that is important in social reinforcement in at least two ways that could be implemented by the OFC. Facial expression may represent reinforcement as well as the current reinforcement value based on stimulus-reinforcement association to a particular individual. The role of the OFC on reversal learning also applies during a face discrimination reversal task. In the task, the faces of two different individuals are shown, and when the correct face is selected, the expression turns into a smile whereas turns to angry if the wrong face is selected. After a period of correct performance, the contingencies reverse, and the other face must be selected to obtain a smile expression as a reinforcer. Activation of the lateral OFC occurred specifically in relation to the reversal, that is, when a formerly correct face was chosen, but an angry face expression was obtained.

Influence of Cognition on Encoding of Affective Value

Top-down attentional and cognitive modulation by the dorsolateral PFC can bias affective representations in the OFC, providing a mechanism for cognition to influence emotion.[10] For example, the medial OFC is more strongly activated when a stimulus a "framed" by cognitive labels (suggestions) of an expected pleasant experience. For example for an identical taste stimulus, paying attention to pleasantness activated the medial OFC/pregenual ACC whereas paying attention to intensity, which reflected the physical properties of the stimulus, activated the insular taste cortex. Similarly some OFC neurons respond to novel but not familiar visual stimuli. Associations between previously neutral stimuli such as a visual stimulus with primary reinforcers such as taste are both formed and rapidly reversed in the OFC, which may thus have important role functions in emotions produced by these secondary (learned) reinforces such as the sight of food. These learned (instrumental) reinforcers specify the goals for action and produce emotions.

Attribution of Value and Decision-Making

Whereas neuronal activity in the OFC is related to the reward value of sensory stimuli and changes when reward contingencies change, it is not related to the actions that are being performed. The value of stimuli in the OFC is represented on a continuous scale, with a gradual change in OFC neuronal responses to taste, olfactory, and visual rewarding stimuli that correlates with the subjective pleasantness ratings. This indicates that the OFC may contribute to decision-making by representing on a continuous scale the value of each reward. Different subsets of neurons respond to each different particular reward, which is essential to represent each reward separately. When a choice is made between stimuli with different reward values, the choice made depends on the probability with which each reward will be obtained. Activation of the OFC is related not only to the expected value while the decision was being made but also to the reward magnitude. Activations in the ventromedial PFC may continuously track the subjective utility of available rewards. The representation of reward magnitude, expected reward, and subjective utility of a reward provided by the OFC and ventromedial PFC are important inputs to the decision-making process. When making a decision between two rewards, or whether to work for a reward that has an associated cost, it is important that the exact value of each reward be represented and enters the decision-making process. However, when a decision is reached, is necessary to make a binary choice between one of the two options; the high firing of some neurons may represent one decision (i.e., choice), and the high firing of other neurons represents a different choice. The anterior portion of the medial OFC is connected to the medial PFC (frontopolar area 10), which constitutes a third level of processing involved in making binary choices and decisions regarding stimulus.[10]

CINGULATE CORTEX: INTERACTIVE HUBS FOR AFFECT, COGNITION, AND SELF-REFERENTIAL PROCESSES

The cingulate cortex has a critical role in transferring information from one region of the brain to others and its main function is to promote different behaviors by selecting the relevant network for their implementation.[57] Structural, circuitry, and functional neuroimaging studies indicate that the three subdivisions of the cingulate cortex, ACC, MCC, and PCC, are hubs of three major limbic subsystems each involved in unique aspects of emotional and cognitive processing and form parts of distinct large-scale networks[13,14,57-60] (Figure 39.6).

Anterior Cingulate Cortex: "Anterior Emotional Subsystem"

The ACC has strong connections with the amygdala, insula, and OFC and is primarily involved in emotional processing. The ACC includes a subgenual (subcallosal) and a pregenual regions. The subgenual ACC includes several area 25, subgenual area 24, and ventral portion of area 33—and is primarily activated by negatively valenced episodic memories. For example, activation of subgenual area 24 occurs in association with sadness; that on subgenual area 33 with fear processing of painful stimuli.[61] Functional neuroimaging showed excessive activation of the subgenual (area 25) and adjacent PFC cortex in patients with severe depression, which has provided the rationale for targeting this area with deep brain stimulation (DBS) for treatment of refractory cases. Recordings of single unit activity in the subcallosal cortex in such patients showed that upon viewing emotionally evocative images, the majority of subcallosal neurons selectively responded to negatively valenced emotional content.[62] Area 25 is heavily connected to the CeM, lateral hypothalamus, PAG, and parabrachial nucleus and thus has a strong influence on the autonomic nervous system. Stimulation of the subgenual ACC elicits cardiovagal activation resulting in bradycardia, and sympathetic inhibition, reducing blood pressure.

In contrast to the subgenual ACC, the pregenual ACC is activated by positively affective (pleasant) reward values such as pleasant touch, pleasant temperature, taste, odors, and monetary rewards, and its activation correlates with the subjective state of pleasure. The activation of the pregenual ACC area 32 and adjacent medial PFC reflects emotional awareness. This activation depends on inputs from

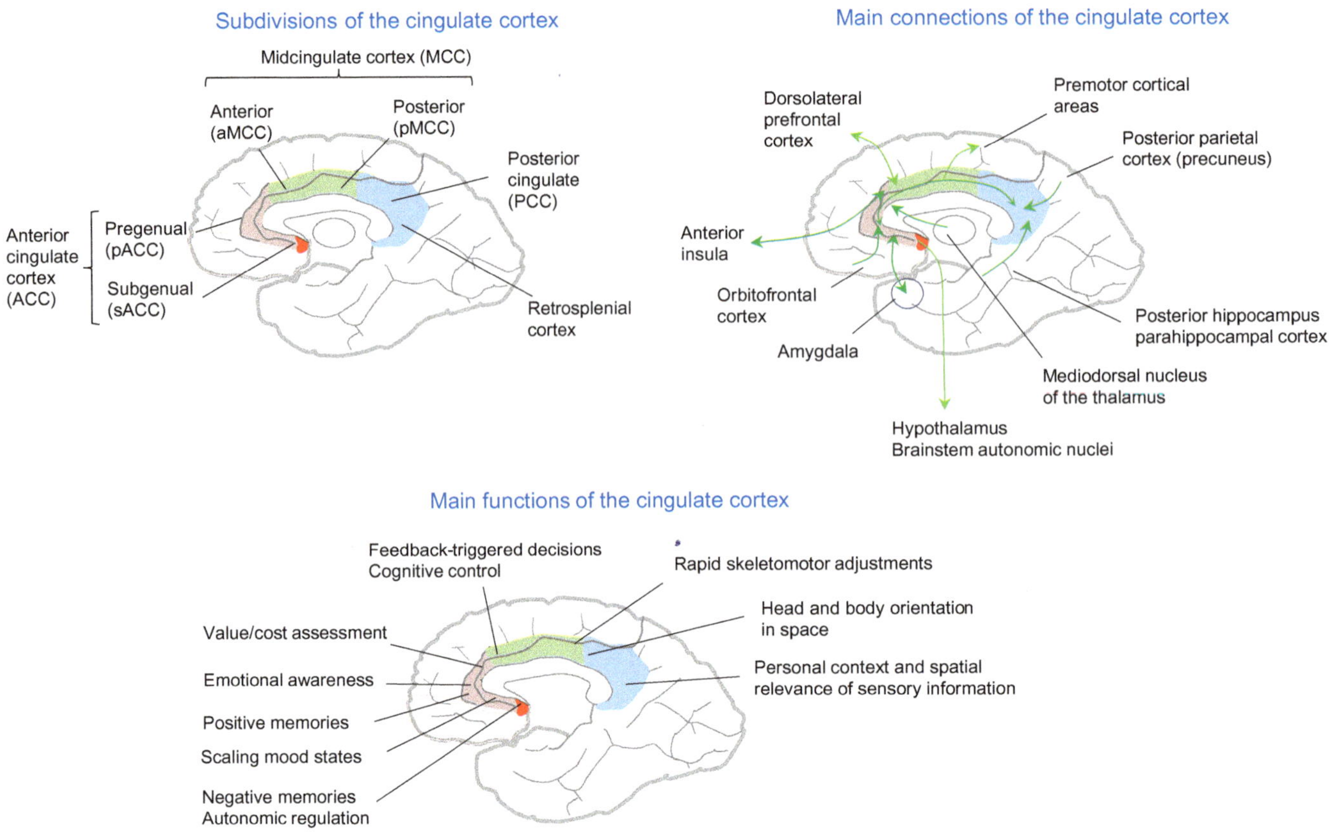

FIGURE 39.6 Main connections and functions of the cingulate cortex
The different subdivisions of the cingulate cortex participate in unique aspects of emotional and cognitive processing and form parts of distinct large-scale networks. The anterior cingulate cortex (ACC) has strong connections with the amygdala, insula, and OFC; is primarily involved in emotional processing; and includes subgenual (subcallosal) and pregenual regions. The midcingulate cortex (MCC) is divided into an anterior MCC involved in cognitive tasks and posterior MCC in skeletomotor orientation. The posterior MCC is involved in rapid cognitive and skeletomotor adjustment. The responses are mediated by neurons in the caudal cingulate motor area. The posterior cingulate cortex (PCC) is a core component of the default mode network, which also includes the ventral medial PFC, cortex, retrosplenial cortex, posterior inferior parietal lobule, lateral temporal cortex, parahippocampal cortex, and hippocampal formation.

the medial OFC, which also processes such pleasant stimuli and outcomes.[10,14] The continuous scaling of value is critical for selecting action outcome in order to select a specific goal during decision-making. A critical feature of decision-making mediated by pregenual ACC area 24 is assessment of the cost of actions. The pregenual ACC is also consistently coactivated with the ventral anterior insula as a hub of the "salience network" that is activated by homeostatically relevant stimuli that control behavior.[46] Some studies showed that the pregenual ACC is also activated during noxious stimulation (particularly visceral pain) and may thus be involved in pain control mechanisms.[63] There is also some evidence that the pregenual ACC may also have an important role in emotional regulation by dampening activity of the amygdala.[64] Stimulation of the pregenual ACC during preoperative evaluation of patients with intractable epilepsy produced anxiety, visceral sensations, and autonomic responses associated with sympathoexcitation.[65]

Midcingulate Cortex: "Middle Sensorimotor Subsystem" for Feedback-Based Action Control

The MCC enables reward outcome information from the OFC and ACC to be associated with action information from the PCC and with output directed to premotor cortical areas. The MCC is divided into an anterior MCC involved in cognitive tasks and posterior MCC in skeletomotor orientation.[59] The pregenual ACC and ventral PCC, which are engaged in emotion, are reciprocally connected and bypass MCC. The MCC is the last stage for action and feedback monitoring given its extensive dorsal projections to sensorimotor cortices. The major role of the dorsal anterior MCC is feedback-mediated decision-making for reward/approach and fear/avoidance decisions. The anterior MCC is activated by emotion-generating stimuli, fear, and reward and contains intermingled nociceptive and reward-coding neurons. Via its connections with the lateral OFC, the anterior MCC is activated by reward prediction errors or punishers[10] and may respond to such adverse outcomes by directing behavioral adaptation when circumstances are changing or when it is necessary to suppress habitual actions and consider an alternative course of action. Thus, at the anterior MCC goal and feedback information are used to modulate activity in brain regions that direct attention and produce motor responses.[66] The anterior MCC, together with the dorsal anterior insula is a component of a cingulo-opercular network (also referred to as "dorsal salience"–control network) involved in task set maintenance.[49] Via its connections with both the ACC and the frontoparietal attention network that includes the dorsolateral PFC, the anterior MCC is engaged in diverse processes including attention, executive function, and allocation of effort during cognitive tasks by monitoring outcomes. The anterior MCC receives strong dopaminergic inputs from the ventral tegmental area and is an important component of the circuits regulating action selection, motivation, and effort. Via its connections to the rostral cingulate motor region, the anterior MCC is involved in action-selection based on action–reward associations.[67] Stimulation of the anterior MCC in presurgical patients with intractable epilepsy elicits complex motor behaviors with an "actotopic" ventral-to-dorsal organization, including whole-body behaviors directed to the extrapersonal space, hand actions in the peripersonal space, and body-directed actions respectively.[65] The posterior MCC is involved in rapid cognitive and skeletomotor adjustments that do not reflect internal emotional assessment of sensory stimuli. For example, in response to a painful stimulus, it is activated before the conscious experience of pain. The responses are mediated by neurons in the caudal cingulate motor area and occur at much shorter latencies that those in the rostral cingulate motor area, suggesting their role in rapid orienting responses and consistent with earlier premotor activity in the posterior than in the anterior MCC.[59]

Posterior Cingulate Cortex: "Posterior Cognitive Map Subsystem"

The PCC is a core component of the default mode network, which also includes the ventral medial PFC, retrosplenial cortex, posterior inferior parietal lobule, lateral temporal cortex, parahippocampal cortex, and hippocampal formation.[68] This network has an important role in integrating autobiographic memory, self-monitoring, and social cognitive functions and becomes active during processes such as episodic memory retrieval, self-referential processes and imagining one's future. The PCC functions as a flexible hub that strongly interacts with other regions, both within the default mode network and within other functional networks. The ventral PCC is engaged in assessment of context spatial relevance and personal relevance of sensory information. Once the personal relevance is coded in the ventral PCC it becomes available to the subgenual ACC via direct connection via the cingulum bundle for combining actions in the anterior MCC. Personal relevance is also encoded in pregenual ACC area 24, where there is attribution of personal relevance to rewards. The dorsal PCC encodes eye, head, and body orientation in space, reflecting its strong input from the dorsal visual stream via the posterior parietal cortex. The dorsal PCC has heavy connections with the posterior MCC, is activated by familiar objects and places, and is involved in rapid visuospatial orientation, before the occurrence of conscious cognitive processing. It has also been proposed that the dorsal PCC and adjacent retrosplenial cortex promote the speed of spatial target detection to coordinate spatial attention.

Based on circuitry and functional studies, it has been proposed that there are six stages by which sensory information has access to the cingulate cortex to evoke skeletomotor and autonomic responses.[13] Sensory information related to objects and events in their context have access to the ventral PCC/retrosplenial cortex when it is personally relevant. Valenced memories depend on reciprocal interactions between the ACC and the ventral PCC. The dorsal PCC drives to orientation of the eyes, head, and body to personally relevant stimuli via the caudal cingulate motor area for attention and intentions along with the anterior MCC. The rostral cingulate motor area and anterior MCC evaluate rewarded and punished outcomes and adjust movement sequences based on feedback to accomplish the intended movements in the appropriate context. The coordinated outputs of both the cingulate premotor areas and subgenual ACC drive the relevant motor and autonomic responses.

SOCIAL COGNITION

Most areas involved in emotion are also involved in social behavior.[69,70] Social behavior comprises social communication, self-understanding, understanding others, and affiliation and attachment. "Emotional intelligence" is the set of emotional abilities that predict success in the real world and includes emotional awareness (recognizing emotional states in oneself), emotion recognition (recognition of emotional states of others, empathy, understanding how emotions shape one's behavior and the behavior of others, emotional memory, and regulation of emotion and associated behaviors.[71] Lesion studies indicate that the core regions involved in these processes are the amygdala, anterior insula, ACC, and ventromedial PFC.[71] Functional MRI studies in in humans indicate that these regions are part of several networks.[70]

Perception of Social Signals

Most studies on social signals have focused on the visual modality. Social visual signals include information about the face, such as facial expression and direction of gaze, and about the body, such as posture and movements. The fusiform face area processes information on static features that allow identification of faces; the superior temporal gyrus and superior temporal sulcus process information about facial expression. Recognition of biological movements, such as locomotion and motor actions, are also important cues for social communication.[72] The superior temporal sulcus contains neurons that respond selectively to full body or hand movements. Recognition of biological motions may involve processing by both the dorsal and ventral visual streams. Neurons of the dorsal visual pathway process perception of action; neurons of the ventral pathway selectively respond to human body configurations, so that biological movements might be recognized by analyzing sequences of body shapes that correspond to "snapshots" of the movement.[72]

The Amygdala as a Hub for Social Cognition Networks

The amygdala is a hub for several networks involved in emotionally driven social perception, affiliation, aversion, and decision-making[73] (Table 39.1, Figure 39.7). The ventral sector of the amygdala, including the lateral and basolateral nuclei and their connections with the lateral OFC and ventrolateral temporal cortex, is part of a social perception network involved in detecting, decoding, and interpreting social signals in the context of current goals and past experiences. These areas are coactivated during tasks of social recognition, such as face identity and facial and body expression. The medial sector of the amygdala and its connections with the ventromedial PFC, ACC, dorsomedial temporal pole and medial temporal lobe, ventromedial hypothalamus, and ventromedial striatum form a social affiliation network that responds to positive social stimuli, such as pictures of loved ones and positive social feedback that elicits empathy, altruistic behavior, and social cooperation. In contrast, the rostrodorsal portion of the amygdala, including the CeM and its functional connections with the MCC and anterior insula, forms a social-aversion network that responds to untrustworthy-appearing faces, negative social feedback, physical and second-hand pain, and pain of social rejection.

Cortical Networks for Social Cognition

In addition to these amygdala-centered networks, there are three cortically based social networks. They include the empathy network, the "mentalizing" network, and the mirror motor network (Figure 39.8). Affective empathy is the ability to share the emotional state of another person and is critical to drive prosocial behavior aimed at helping others. The anterior insula and the ACC/MCC boundary are the core components of the empathy network.[47,74] Signals from the anterior insula related to body states, such as the heart rate, are sent to this region of the cingulate cortex to initiate the selection of responses to emotional events. The ventromedial PFC, including the ventral OFC and the ACC, may also contribute to emotional awareness in the setting of processing of reward value for decision-making. "Mentalizing," or "theory of mind"' refers to the ability to infer, understand, and think about the mental states of the self and other people in terms of their beliefs and desires, particularly in social contexts. Cognitive theory of mind may be assessed, for example, by having participants observe or read stories about others' behavior and then asked to make judgments about their underlying motivations. Affective theory of mind allows understanding how emotions shape our own behavior and the behavior of others. Functional MRI show that the core components of this mentalizing network include the temporoparietal junction, superior temporal sulcus, dorsal and medial PFC, pregenual ACC, and dorsal PCC and adjacent precuneus. Several components of this network overlap with the default mode network and with networks involved in episodic and prospective memory.[75] The mirror motor system is involved

TABLE 39.1 *Amygdala-Based Social Networks*

Network	Social Perception	Social Affiliation	Social Aversion
Sector of the amygdala	Ventrolateral	Medial	Rostrodorsal (including the CeM)
Cortical connections	Orbitofrontal cortex Ventral and lateral temporal cortex	Anterior cingulate cortex Medial prefrontal cortex Medial temporal pole	Midcingulate cortex Anterior insula
Stimuli that elicit network activation	Socially salient facial expressions	Appetitive stimuli Positive social feedback	Negative social feedback Pain of social rejection
Effects of network impairment	Lack of awareness of other's emotional and social behavior	Social and emotional detachment Reduced empathy	Lack of social apprehension Lack of recognition of unworthiness or unfairness

CeM, centromedial nucleus

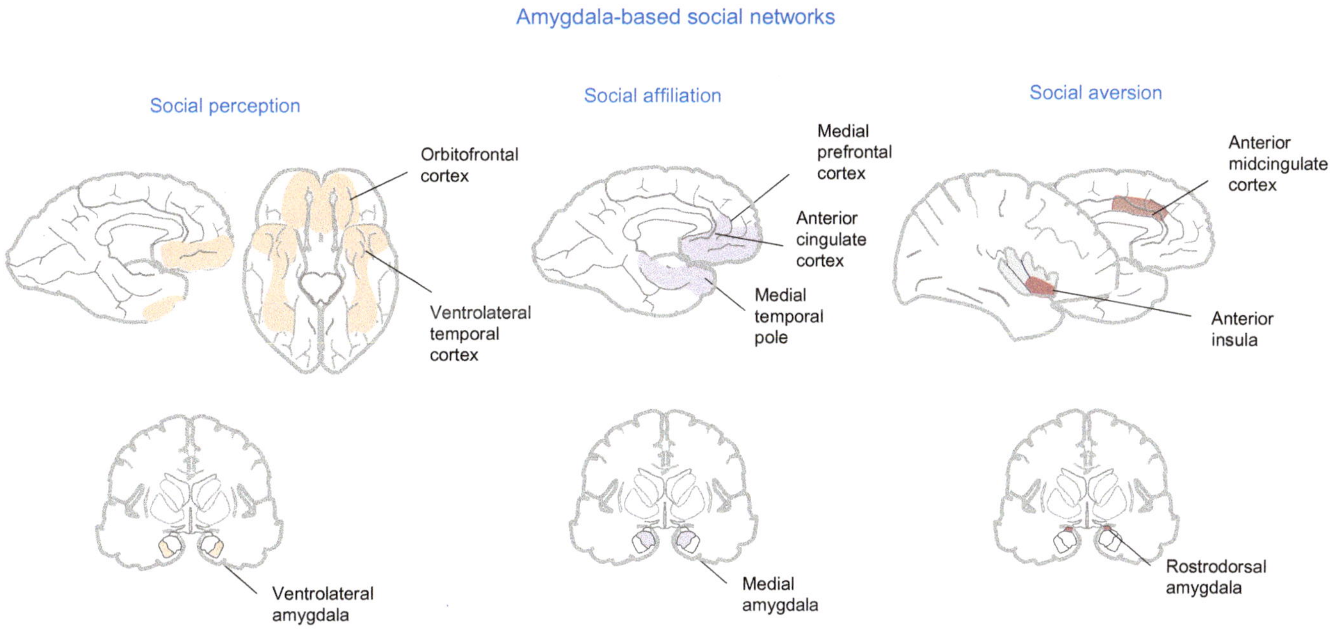

FIGURE 39.7 Social hubs involving the amygdala

The amygdala is a hub for several networks involved in emotionally driven social perception, affiliation, aversion, and decision-making. The ventral sector of the amygdala, including the lateral and basolateral nuclei and their connections with the lateral orbitofrontal cortex and ventrolateral temporal cortex, is part of a social perception network. The medial sector has connections with the ventromedial prefrontal cortex, anterior cingulate cortex, dorsomedial temporal pole and medial temporal lobe, ventromedial hypothalamus, and ventromedial striatum to form a social affiliation network. The rostrodorsal portion of the amygdala, including the centromedial nucleus and its functional connections with the MCC and anterior insula forms a social-aversion network.

in recognition, processing, and understanding actions by observation and inferring of goals of others.[76–78] This basic action-observation circuit includes the ventral premotor cortex and adjacent inferior lateral prefrontal cortex, inferior parietal lobule, and superior temporal sulcus. Neurons in the superior temporal sulcus respond to observed action and encode action regardless of whether the observed action is part of the observer's motor repertoire. In contrast, mirror neurons in the inferior parietal and ventral premotor cortex only respond to observation of actions that are a part of the motor repertoire of the observer. This results in a direct recognition of the observed action based on its similarity with an executed action.[72] In humans, mirror neurons were also recorded in the medial motor areas (supplementary motor area) and hippocampus. The discharge of mirror neurons is influenced by the value of the object on which the action is performed and thus the value of the observed action.

CLINICAL CORRELATIONS

Lesions affecting the amygdala, OFC, ventromedial PFC, anterior/midcingulate cortex, and insula, either in isolation or in various combinations, produce a wide range of disturbances in emotional recognition, decision-making, and social behavior. However, the pattern of activation of these regions in experimental human functional MRI studies does not always predict the clinical manifestations of their involvement by focal lesions.[17]

Frontotemporal Dementia

Current consensus diagnostic criteria for behavioral variant frontotemporal dementia (bvFTD) propose six core features: apathy, disinhibition, loss of empathy, change in eating behavior, stereotypical behavior, and executive dysfunction. The presence of three of the six features is sufficient to meet diagnosis of either possible, probable, or definite bvFTD, depending on the level of additional biological evidence, such as neuroimaging changes, genetic abnormality, or postmortem examination supporting the diagnosis.[79] This disorder is clinically quite heterogeneous. Some manifestations include Diogenes syndrome (i.e., extreme self-neglect and excessive collecting with clutter), late-onset gambling disorder, antisocial behaviors, and violations of the law (including theft and hit and run). Such behaviors may also be observed in about 20% of patients with semantic variant primary progressive aphasia affecting the anterolateral temporal lobe. In bvFTD, disturbances of various facets of social cognition such as emotion recognition, theory of mind, and empathy reflect impaired activity in amygdala-linked social networks.[73] Involvement of the social perception network results in impairment of perception of facial expressions and

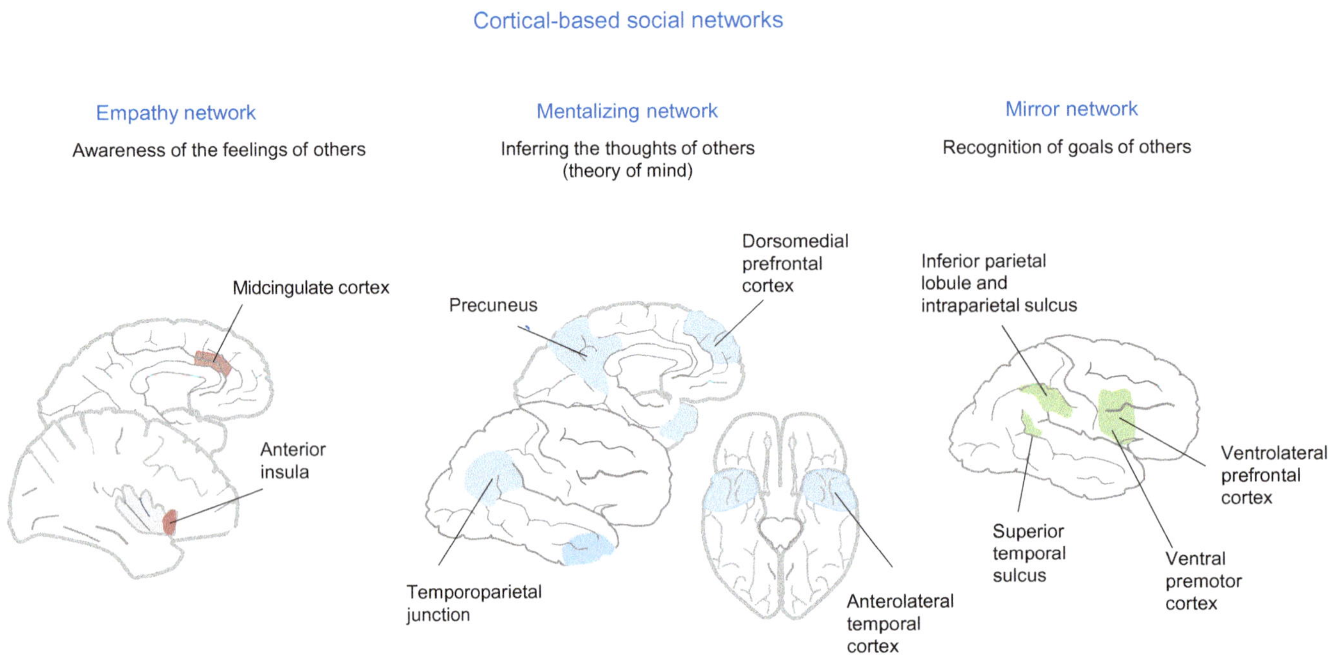

FIGURE 39.8 Cortical networks for emotion
The anterior insula and the boundary region between the anterior cingulate (ACC) and midcingulate (MCC) cortex are the core components of an empathy network that participates in affective empathy, which is the ability to share the emotional state of another person. The components of the "mentalizing" or "theory of mind"' network include the ventromedial and dorsomedial prefrontal cortex, precuneus, and bilateral temporoparietal junction. The mirror network involved in processing and understanding actions and inferring intentions of others includes the ventral premotor cortex and adjacent inferior lateral prefrontal cortex, inferior parietal lobule, and superior temporal sulcus.

lack of awareness or understanding of the social and emotional behavior of others. Impaired activity of the social affiliation network results in social and emotional detachment and indifference and unresponsiveness to feelings, needs, or desires of other people. Impaired activity of the social aversion network leads to lack of social apprehension, so patients are less cautious around strangers, and tend to seek social rewards or make prosocial decisions. Repetitive behaviors are also common in bvFTD and include hoarding, collecting of items, stereotypies of speech, and repetitive actions, which can be simple (e.g., foot tapping) or more complex (e.g., continual trips to the bathroom). These behaviors appear to be driven by impulsive mechanisms rather than as a strategy to ease anxiety, and are therefore, distinct from the repetitive behaviors observed in obsessive-compulsive disorder. In bvFTD, such behaviors can be triggered by environmental stimuli and may represent a complex manifestation of environmental dependency syndrome, resulting from involvement of the orbitomedial PFC. In addition to disinhibition and stereotypical behaviors, apathy affects ~90% of patients early on and essentially all patients at some point of the disease. Similarly to patients with OFC lesions, patients with bvFTD affecting the OFC, amygdala, or both also have severe impairment in value-based decision-making, particularly under ambiguous or risky conditions. These alterations in behavior indicate a functional link between disorders affecting anterior temporal and prefrontal function and thus the interaction among behavioral and executive dysfunction in bvFTD. The von Economo neurons in the frontoinsular and ACC are affected early in bvFTD.[80] Of note, these neurons selectively express the bombesin peptides neuromedin B and gastrin-releasing peptide, which signal satiety; this led to the proposal that loss of von Economo neurons may contribute to disturbances of the control of appetite in these patients.[48]

There are three main molecular groups of frontotemporal lobar degeneration (FTLD) identified so far, which all share a mechanism of abnormal protein accumulation. Most common are FTLD-TDP cases, which show abnormal deposition of the TAR DNA-binding protein 43 (TDP-43) and accounts for ~50% of all cases of FTD. TDP-43 inclusion are subdivided in five subtypes (A–E), each with a distinctive morphological appearance depending on the cellular distribution of TDP-43 and the appearance of the inclusions. The second group (FTLD-TAU) includes cases with increased accumulation of hyperphosphorylated tau protein, and constitutes ~40% of cases. FTLD-TAU is further subdivided depending on the type of abnormally deposited tau, either three-repeat or four-repeat microtubule-binding domains. The classical three-repeat tauopathy is Pick disease, which is associated with intraneuronal tau-positive Pick bodies. Four-repeat tauopathies include corticobasal degeneration (with tau-positive ballooned achromatic neurons and astrocytic plaques), progressive supranuclear palsy (with tau accumulation forming neurofibrillary tangles, neuropil threads, tufted astrocytes, and oligodendroglial coiled bodies), globular glial tau inclusions, and argyrophilic grain disease (punctate staining of tau, pronounced in the medial temporal lobe). The third group (FTLD-FET), which accounts for 5%–10% of cases, comprises cases that show abnormal deposition of the FET (FUS, EWS, TAF15) protein family, proteins involved in RNA transcription. About 10% of cases diagnosed with FTD are explained by single gene abnormalities with autosomal dominant transmission. Three genes account for ~80% of all familial cases: *C9ORF72*, *GRN* (progranulin), and *MAPT* (microtubule-associated protein tau).

Focal Amygdala Lesions

Removal of large portions of the anterior temporal lobes, including the amygdala, in monkeys produces the Klüver-Bucy syndrome, which is characterized by oral exploration of objects; placidity with loss of normal fear and anger responses; and changes in eating behavior. In humans, some of the these manifestations may occur in disorders affecting the amygdala and anterior temporal lobe, including bvFTD, limbic encephalitis, temporal lobe epilepsy, and mucopolysaccharidosis type III. For example, visual agnosia is an important manifestation of progressive visual agnosia syndrome associated with neurodegenerative anterior temporal lobe disease. Changes in food preferences, table manners, and other related oral behaviors can occur early in bvFTD and constitute one of the six core clinical features of the disease. In contrast, excessive oral exploration and hyperorality are important and potentially life-threatening manifestations that occur only in advanced stages. Lipoid proteinosis (Urbach-Wiethe disease), an autosomal recessive disorder caused by mutations in the *ECM1* (extracellular matrix protein 1) gene producing bilateral calcifications of the basolateral amygdala, manifests with cognitive impairment and temporal lobe epilepsy. These patients have specific deficits in recognizing the facial expression of fear, and to lesser extent other emotions; these deficits vary in different patients. Lack of recognition of fearful faces does not occur in all cases.[81] However, these patients may be hypervigilant while viewing emotional facial expressions, particularly fearful expression, due to increased activation of the central and medial nuclei. Some patients have impaired judgment of all emotions in facial expressions regardless of the positive or negative connotations. Patients may have absence of fear even upon exposure to fear-provoking stimuli, and show both lack of avoidance and instead exploratory approach, described as an overwhelming sense of curiosity. The involvement of the amygdala in mesial temporal lobe epilepsy and hippocampal sclerosis may explain some of the clinical features of these seizures, including sensation of fear, memories with strong emotional content, olfactory hallucinations, and autonomic manifestations. Connections between the amygdala CeM and brainstem respiratory and autonomic networks may elicit respiratory depression and cardiac arrhythmias contributing to sudden unexpected death in epilepsy.[82]

Ventromedial and Cingulate Lesions

Focal lesions including the medial OFC and ventromedial PFC may result in profound abnormalities in emotion recognition and social behavior. They include lack of affect, poorly modulated emotional responses, and lack of inhibition of socially inappropriate behavior. These patients fail to use emotions to guide decisions; have impaired recognition of emotions based on facial expression and prosodic cues; and exhibit deficits in cognitive empathy and inability to use social cues to guide behavior. The effects of OFC lesions may be related in part to a failure to rapidly update the reinforcement associations of stimuli when the contingencies are changed. Patients with OFC lesions may have difficulties decoding face and voice expression (which are social reinforcers), in reversing stimulus-reward associations and in emotional behavior. The importance of the OFC in emotion in humans is emphasized by a comparison with the effects of bilateral amygdala damage. Whereas amygdala lesions produce deficits in face decision-making and reduced autonomic responses to conditioning, they may not produce major changes in emotion that are apparent in everyday behavior. The manifestation of OFC lesions are mimicked by those of borderline personality disorder, including impulsivity, affective instability, emotionality, and low extroversion.

Insular Lesions

Consistent with fMRI studies indicating a role of the insula in bodily feeling and self-awareness, large lesions affecting the anterior insula may be associated with alexithymia, a subclinical condition defined as impaired emotional awareness.[83] High-resolution magnetic resonance spectroscopy studies also show that alexithymia reflects a glutamate/GABA imbalance in the pregenual ACC.[84] In humans, lesions involving the dorsal portion of the right insula have been associated with an alteration of the sense of body ownership that is necessary for self-agency.[85] However, the function of the insula as the sole substrate of self-awareness has been challenged by cases in which patients were able to experience everyday emotions and feelings and retain self-awareness despite almost complete or complete bilateral destruction of the insula.[14,86] Despite the role of the posterior insula as a cortical station for pain pathways, unilateral lesions in this region and adjacent parietal operculum can produce pain hypersensitivity or, in the worst cases, debilitating central neuropathic pain syndrome, referred to as operculo-insular pain.[87] Patients with insular lesions may still recognize their own pain, but may be unable to recognize pain in someone else, which is consistent with the role of the anterior insula in empathy for pain.

Psychiatric Disorders

A large number of fMRI studies showed involvement of the amygdala in psychiatric disorders. Anxious but otherwise normal individuals show increased amygdala activity in response not only to threat-related stimuli such as fearful faces but also to nonthreat-related stimuli. In general, increased activity of the amygdala is associated with reduced activity of the ventromedial prefrontal cortex, and functional connectivity between these two structures is a common finding in patients with anxiety disorders, including social anxiety disorder and posttraumatic stress disorder. Early fMRI studies showed that the subgenual ACC and its interconnected areas are activated during sad events, suggesting its role in processing negative emotional information. The OFC and cingulate cortex have been implicated in depression.[88] There is hypermetabolism in the subgenual (subcallosal) ACC in patients with major depression. The subcallosal cortex and underlying white matter ACC (including the subgenual cingulate cortex) is a potential target for DBS for treatment of severe cases.[89,90]

Early fMRI studies also showed that the pregenual ACC is activated by pleasant and happy events, whereas hypoactivity of this region is related to the presence of anhedonia in patients with severe depression.[91] It has been suggested that these manifestations result from overactivity of the lateral OFC, which contains neurons that respond to nonreward and may enter a state maintained by high firing rate due to strong recurrent excitatory synaptic connections thereby maintaining a memory of the nonreward.[10] According to this proposal, enhanced firing of the lateral OFC involved in the nonreward/punishment system triggers negative cognitive states held on-line in other cortical systems, such as the dorsolateral PFC attentional control and language areas. These areas, in turn would have top-down effects on the orbitofrontal nonreward system that help to bias it in a negative direction and thus to increase its sensitivity to nonreward and maintain its overactivity.[10] In contrast, the medial OFC reward-related areas would be underactive in depression.[10]

KEY POINTS

- The core components of the emotion system include the amygdala, insular cortex, orbitofrontal cortex (OFC), and cingulate cortex.
- The amygdala automatically tags external or internal stimuli with either positive or negative valence and triggers coordinated activation of survival, arousal, and reward and motivation circuits.
- The activation of survival circuits occurs independently of the conscious experience of emotions but elicits responses that indirectly affect emotional consciousness.
- Biologically neutral stimuli can acquire behavioral relevance when they occur in conjunction with biologically significant aversive or appetitive stimuli; this constitutes Pavlovian conditioning or associative learning.
- The amygdala-centered defensive survival circuits are separate from the conscious experience of fear.
- Fear extinction is the gradual elimination of the fear reaction upon repeated exposure of the originally neutral stimulus without presenting the aversive stimulus.
- Fear extinction is an active learning process that leads to the formation of a new inhibitory memory that competes with the initial fear memory.
- Contextual control of fear extinction requires interactions of the amygdala with the hippocampus and prefrontal cortex (PFC).
- Numerous fMRI studies show increased PFC and concomitant reduced amygdala activity during successful cognitive regulation of emotion.
- The amygdala coordinates the enhancement in consolidation and recall of emotionally salient information.
- The amygdala responds differentially to social affective facial cues, increasing firing to relevant novel stimuli and showing habituation to familiar affective stimuli.
- The insula provides one link between interoception, awareness of the body, and emotion.
- The medial OFC represents reward value with subjective pleasantness linearly related to its activity and with devaluation reducing its response.
- The lateral OFC detects and represents nonreward as a difference between the expected value and the outcome value or punishment, both of which can be used to change actions.
- The more anterior parts of the OFC, including the medial frontopolar cortex are involved in binary choice (decision-making) between stimuli with different value.
- The cingulate cortex has three major subdivisions that together with their connections, form six limbic subsystems.
- The anterior cingulate cortex (ACC) is involved in emotional processing.
- The midcingulate cortex (MCC) is involved in response selection and feedback-guided decision-making.
- The posterior cingulate cortex (PCC)/is involved in visuospatial orientation and assessment of the self-relevance of objects and events.
- The amygdala functions as a hub for social cognition network, with different portions involved in emotionally driven social perception, affiliation, aversion, and decision-making.

- The ventral anterior insula and the ACC/MCC boundary are the core components of the empathy network.
- The medial PFC and other components of the default mode network are involved in inferring the mental states of the self and other people, which is known as "theory of mind."
- Recognition, processing, and understanding inferring of goals of others involves the mirror motor network.
- Behavioral variant frontotemporal dementia (bvFTD) is characterized by apathy, disinhibition, loss of empathy, change in eating behavior, stereotypical behavior, and executive dysfunction.
- Focal lesions including the medial OFC and ventromedial PFC may result in profound abnormalities in emotion recognition and social behavior.
- Depression is associated with hyperactivity of the lateral OFC and subgenual (subcallosal) ACC and reduced activity in the medial OFC and pregenual ACC.
- Large lesions affecting the anterior insula may be associated with alexithymia, a subclinical condition defined as impaired emotional awareness.
- Patients with insular lesions may still recognize their own pain, but may be unable to recognize pain in someone else.

REFERENCES

1. Rolls ET. Limbic systems for emotion and for memory, but no single limbic system. Cortex 2015;62:119–157.
2. LeDoux J. The amygdala. Curr Biol 2007;17:R868–874.
3. Murray RJ, Brosch T, Sander D. The functional profile of the human amygdala in affective processing: Insights from intracranial recordings. Cortex 2014;6:10–33.
4. LeDoux J. Rethinking the emotional brain. Neuron 2012;73:653–676.
5. Pace-Schott EF, Amole MC, Aue T, et al. Physiological feelings. Neurosci Biobehav Rev 2019;103:267–304.
6. Damasio A, Carvalho GB. The nature of feelings: evolutionary and neurobiological origins. Nat Rev Neurosci 2013;14:143–152.
7. Craig AD. Significance of the insula for the evolution of human awareness of feelings from the body. Ann N Y Acad Sci 2011;1225:72–82.
8. Critchley HD, Harrison NA. Visceral influences on brain and behavior. Neuron 2013;77:624–638.
9. Padoa-Schioppa C, Conen KE. Orbitofrontal cortex: a neural circuit for economic decisions. Neuron 2017;96:736–754.
10. Rolls ET. The orbitofrontal cortex and emotion in health and disease, including depression. Neuropsychologia 2019;128:14–43.
11. Pessoa L, Hof PR. From Paul Broca's great limbic lobe to the limbic system. J Comp Neurol 2015;523:2495–2500.
12. Kötter R, Stephan KE. Useless or helpful? The "limbic system" concept. Rev Neurosci 1997;8:139–145.
13. Vogt BA. Cingulate cortex in the three limbic subsystems. Handb Clin Neurol 2019;166:39–51.
14. Rolls ET. The cingulate cortex and limbic systems for action, emotion, and memory. Handb Clin Neurol 2019;166:23–37.
15. Salzman CD, Fusi S. Emotion, cognition, and mental state representation in amygdala and prefrontal cortex. Annu Rev Neurosci 2010;33:173–202.
16. Berridge KC, Kringelbach ML. Neuroscience of affect: brain mechanisms of pleasure and displeasure. Curr Opin Neurobiol 2013;23:294–303.
17. Feinstein JS. Lesion studies of human emotion and feeling. Curr Opin Neurobiol 2013;23:304–309.
18. Szczepanski SM, Knight RT. Insights into human behavior from lesions to the prefrontal cortex. Neuron 2014;83:1002–1018.
19. Duvarci S, Pare D. Amygdala microcircuits controlling learned fear. Neuron 2014;82:966–980.
20. Bocchio M, Nabavi S, Capogna M. Synaptic plasticity, engrams, and network oscillations in amygdala circuits for storage and retrieval of emotional memories. Neuron 2017;94:731–743.
21. Heimer L, de Olmos J, Alheid GF, Zaborszky L. "Perestroika" in the basal forebrain: opening the border between neurology and psychiatry. Prog Brain Res 1991;87:109–165.
22. LeDoux JE. The slippery slope of fear. Trends Cogn Sci 2013;17:155–156.
23. Striemer CL, Whitwell RL, Goodale MA. Affective blindsight in the absence of input from face processing regions in occipital-temporal cortex. Neuropsychologia 2019;128:50–57.
24. Bertini C, Pietrelli M, Braghittoni D, Ladavas E. Pulvinar lesions disrupt fear-related implicit visual processing in hemianopic patients. Front Psychol 2018;9:2329.
25. Kim JJ, Jung MW. Neural circuits and mechanisms involved in Pavlovian fear conditioning: a critical review. Neurosci Biobehav Rev 2006;30:188–202.
26. Myers KM, Davis M. Mechanisms of fear extinction. Mol Psychiatry 2007;12:120–150.
27. Ciocchi S, Herry C, Grenier F, et al. Encoding of conditioned fear in central amygdala inhibitory circuits. Nature 2010;468:277–282.
28. Gilmartin MR, Balderston NL, Helmstetter FJ. Prefrontal cortical regulation of fear learning. Trends Neurosci 2014;37:455–464.
29. Knight DC, Cheng DT, Smith CN, Stein EA, Helmstetter FJ. Neural substrates mediating human delay and trace fear conditioning. J Neurosci 2004;24:218–228.
30. Girardeau G, Inema I, Buzsaki G. Reactivations of emotional memory in the hippocampus-amygdala system. Nat Neurosci 2017;20:1634–1642.
31. Fusar-Poli P, Placentino A, Carletti F, et al. Functional atlas of emotional faces processing: a voxel-based meta-analysis of 105 functional magnetic resonance imaging studies. J Psychiatry Neurosci 2009;34:418–432.
32. Wang S, Tudusciuc O, Mamelak AN, Ross IB, Adolphs R, Rutishauser U. Neurons in the human amygdala selective for perceived emotion. Proc Natl Acad Sci USA 2014;111:E3110–3119.

33. Burra N, Hervais-Adelman A, Kerzel D, Tamietto M, de Gelder B, Pegna AJ. Amygdala activation for eye contact despite complete cortical blindness. J Neurosci 2013;33:10483–10489.
34. Vuilleumier P, Armony JL, Clarke K, Husain M, Driver J, Dolan RJ. Neural response to emotional faces with and without awareness: event-related fMRI in a parietal patient with visual extinction and spatial neglect. Neuropsychologia 2002;40:2156–2166.
35. Hoffmann M, Lipka J, Mothes-Lasch M, Miltner WH, Straube T. Awareness modulates responses of the amygdala and the visual cortex to highly arousing visual threat. Neuroimage 2012;62:1439–1444.
36. De Martino B, Kumaran D, Seymour B, Dolan RJ. Frames, biases, and rational decision-making in the human brain. Science 2006;313:684–687.
37. John YJ, Zikopoulos B, Bullock D, Barbas H. The emotional gatekeeper: a computational model of attentional selection and suppression through the pathway from the amygdala to the inhibitory thalamic reticular nucleus. PLoS Comput Biol 2016;12:e1004722.
38. Liu J, Gu R, Liao C, et al. The neural mechanism of the social framing effect: evidence from fMRI and tDCS studies. J Neurosci 2020;40:3646–3656.
39. Nieuwenhuys R. The insular cortex: a review. Prog Brain Res 2012;195:123–163.
40. Craig AD. How do you feel—now? The anterior insula and human awareness. Nat Rev Neurosci 2009;10:59–70.
41. Cechetto DF. Central representation of visceral function. Fed Proc 1987;46:17–23.
42. Schulz SM. Neural correlates of heart-focused interoception: a functional magnetic resonance imaging meta-analysis. Philos Trans R Soc Lond B Biol Sci 2016;371.
43. Morel A, Gallay MN, Baechler A, Wyss M, Gallay DS. The human insula: architectonic organization and postmortem MRI registration. Neuroscience 2013;236:117–135.
44. Cerliani L, Thomas RM, Jbabdi S, et al. Probabilistic tractography recovers a rostrocaudal trajectory of connectivity variability in the human insular cortex. Hum Brain Mapp 2012;33:2005–2034.
45. Cauda F, D'Agata F, Sacco K, Duca S, Geminiani G, Vercelli A. Functional connectivity of the insula in the resting brain. Neuroimage 2011;55:8–23.
46. Seeley WW. The salience network: a neural system for perceiving and responding to homeostatic demands. J Neurosci 2019;39:9878–9882.
47. Engen HG, Singer T. Empathy circuits. Curr Opin Neurobiol 2013;23:275–282.
48. Allman JM, Tetreault NA, Hakeem AY, Park S. The von Economo neurons in apes and humans. Am J Hum Biol 2011;23:5–21.
49. Marek S, Dosenbach NUF. Control networks of the frontal lobes. Handb Clin Neurol 2019;163:333–347.
50. Adolfi F, Couto B, Richter F, et al. Convergence of interoception, emotion, and social cognition: a twofold fMRI meta-analysis and lesion approach. Cortex 2017;88:124–142.
51. Salzman CD, Fusi S. Emotion, cognition, and mental state representation in amygdala and prefrontal cortex. Annu Rev Neurosci 2010;33:173–202.
52. Heather Hsu CC, Rolls ET, Huang CC, et al. Connections of the human orbitofrontal cortex and inferior frontal gyrus. Cereb Cortex 2020;30:5830–5843.
53. Rolls ET. Taste and smell processing in the brain. Handb Clin Neurol 2019;164:97–118.
54. Willis ML, Palermo R, McGrillen K, Miller L. The nature of facial expression recognition deficits following orbitofrontal cortex damage. Neuropsychology 2014;28:613–623.
55. Jonker FA, Jonker C, Scheltens P, Scherder E. The role of the orbitofrontal cortex in cognition and behavior. Rev Neurosci 2015;26:1–11.
56. Willis ML, Murphy JM, Ridley NJ, Vercammen A. Anodal tDCS targeting the right orbitofrontal cortex enhances facial expression recognition. Soc Cogn Affect Neurosci 2015;10:1677–11683.
57. Touroutoglou A, Dickerson BC. Cingulate-centered large-scale networks: normal functions, aging, and neurodegenerative disease. Handb Clin Neurol 2019;166:113–127.
58. Vogt BA. Submodalities of emotion in the context of cingulate subregions. Cortex 2014;59:197–202.
59. Vogt BA. Midcingulate cortex: structure, connections, homologies, functions and diseases. J Chem Neuroanat 2016;74:28–46.
60. Yu C, Zhou Y, Liu Y, et al. Functional segregation of the human cingulate cortex is confirmed by functional connectivity based neuroanatomical parcellation. Neuroimage 2011;54:2571–2581.
61. Palomero-Gallagher N, Eickhoff SB, Hoffstaedter F, et al. Functional organization of human subgenual cortical areas: relationship between architectonical segregation and connectional heterogeneity. Neuroimage 2015;115:177–190.
62. Laxton AW, Neimat JS, Davis KD, et al. Neuronal coding of implicit emotion categories in the subcallosal cortex in patients with depression. Biol Psychiatry 2013;74:714–719.
63. Vogt BA. Pain and emotion interactions in subregions of the cingulate gyrus. Nat Rev Neurosci 2005;6:533–544.
64. Etkin A, Buchel C, Gross JJ. The neural bases of emotion regulation. Nat Rev Neurosci 2015;16:693–700.
65. Caruana F, Gerbella M, Avanzini P, et al. Motor and emotional behaviours elicited by electrical stimulation of the human cingulate cortex. Brain 2018;141:3035–3051.
66. Sheth SA, Mian MK, Patel SR, et al. Human dorsal anterior cingulate cortex neurons mediate ongoing behavioural adaptation. Nature 2012;488:218–221.
67. Shackman AJ, Salomons TV, Slagter HA, Fox AS, Winter JJ, Davidson RJ. The integration of negative affect, pain and cognitive control in the cingulate cortex. Nat Rev Neurosci 2011;12:154–167.
68. Raichle ME. The brain's default mode network. Annu Rev Neurosci 2015;38:433–447.
69. Adolphs R. Conceptual challenges and directions for social neuroscience. Neuron 2010;65:752–767.
70. Stanley DA, Adolphs R. Toward a neural basis for social behavior. Neuron 2013;80:816–826.
71. Hogeveen J, Salvi C, Grafman J. "Emotional intelligence": lessons from lesions. Trends Neurosci 2016;39:694–705.
72. Giese MA, Poggio T. Neural mechanisms for the recognition of biological movements. Nat Rev Neurosci 2003;4:179–192.
73. Bickart KC, Dickerson BC, Barrett LF. The amygdala as a hub in brain networks that support social life. Neuropsychologia 2014;63:235–248.
74. de Vignemont F, Singer T. The empathic brain: how, when and why? Trends Cogn Sci 2006;10:435–441.

75. Singer T. The neuronal basis and ontogeny of empathy and mind reading: review of literature and implications for future research. Neurosci Biobehav Rev 2006;30:855–863.
76. Rizzolatti G, Fabbri-Destro M. The mirror system and its role in social cognition. Curr Opin Neurobiol 2008;18:179–184.
77. Spunt RP, Lieberman MD. Dissociating modality-specific and supramodal neural systems for action understanding. J Neurosci 2012;32:3575–3583.
78. Giese MA, Rizzolatti G. Neural and computational mechanisms of action processing: interaction between visual and motor representations. Neuron 2015;88:167–180.
79. Rascovsky K, Hodges JR, Knopman D, et al. Sensitivity of revised diagnostic criteria for the behavioural variant of frontotemporal dementia. Brain 2011;134:2456–2477.
80. Seeley WW, Carlin DA, Allman JM, et al. Early frontotemporal dementia targets neurons unique to apes and humans. Ann Neurol 2006;60:660–667.
81. Becker B, Mihov Y, Scheele D, et al. Fear processing and social networking in the absence of a functional amygdala. Biol Psychiatry 2012;72:70–77.
82. Nobis WP, Schuele S, Templer JW, et al. Amygdala-stimulation-induced apnea is attention and nasal-breathing dependent. Ann Neurol 2018;83:460–471.
83. Jones CL, Ward J, Critchley HD. The neuropsychological impact of insular cortex lesions. J Neurol Neurosurg Psychiatry 2010;81:611–618.
84. Kuhnel A, Widmann A, Colic L, et al. Impaired cognitive self-awareness mediates the association between alexithymia and excitation/inhibition balance in the pgACC. Psychol Med 2020;50:1727–1735.
85. Karnath HO, Baier B. Right insula for our sense of limb ownership and self-awareness of actions. Brain Struct Funct 2010;214:411–417.
86. Damasio A, Damasio H, Tranel D. Persistence of feelings and sentience after bilateral damage of the insula. Cereb Cortex 2013;23:833–846.
87. Garcia-Larrea L, Perchet C, Creac'h C, et al. Operculo-insular pain (parasylvian pain): a distinct central pain syndrome. Brain 2010;133:2528–2539.
88. Akil H, Gordon J, Hen R, et al. Treatment resistant depression: a multi-scale, systems biology approach. Neurosci Biobehav Rev 2018;84:272–288.
89. Dunlop BW, Rajendra JK, Craighead WE, et al. Functional connectivity of the subcallosal cingulate cortex and differential outcomes to treatment with cognitive-behavioral therapy or antidepressant medication for major depressive disorder. Am J Psychiatry 2017;174:533–545.
90. Holtzheimer PE, Husain MM, Lisanby SH, et al. Subcallosal cingulate deep brain stimulation for treatment-resistant depression: a multisite, randomised, sham-controlled trial. Lancet Psychiatry 2017;4:839–849.
91. Walter M, Henning A, Grimm S, et al. The relationship between aberrant neuronal activation in the pregenual anterior cingulate, altered glutamatergic metabolism, and anhedonia in major depression. Arch Gen Psychiatry 2009;66:478–486.

40 Episodic Memory

OVERVIEW

Memory includes a variety of specific processes that allow storage and retrieval of information over variable time periods. These multiple forms of memory have distinct anatomical substrates and are differentially affected by disease. The hippocampus and surrounding areas form a medial temporal system that has a crucial role in episodic memory.[1–3] Episodic memory is the ability to learn, store, and retrieve information about unique personal experiences and events that occur in daily life. This information is channeled to the hippocampus via the entorhinal cortex, which conveys segregated inputs from the perirhinal and the parahippocampal cortex about the elements of an event. Inputs from the perirhinal cortex convey object feature information required for object recognition by familiarity. Inputs from the parahippocampal cortex convey visuospatial information that provides a frame of reference about the context where the events occur. The hippocampal circuits thus provide a spatial and temporal framework for relating experiences, creating a "cognitive map" based on these individual autobiographic events.[4,5] By integrating a reference frame based on landmarks of the environment, the medial temporal system is also critical for navigation. Information processed in the hippocampus is conveyed back to the neocortex for consolidation of episodic memories. The prefrontal cortex (PFC), via its reciprocal interactions with the hippocampus, exerts an executive control on memory encoding and retrieval. The medial temporal system interacts with core areas of the default mode network involved in processing of inner thoughts, including reflecting on past and predicting or simulating future personal events. Functional magnetic resonance (fMRI) in normal subjects[4] and intracranial recordings in patients undergoing epilepsy surgery,[6] have confirmed results from hallmark studies in rodents elucidating the role of different components of the medial temporal lobe system These circuits are affected by aging, Alzheimer disease (AD), and other disorders causing episodic memory disturbances. The aims of this chapter are to review: (1) the features of the hippocampal circuits and their connections that provide the basis for encoding, storage, and retrieval of episodic memory; (2) the role of the medial temporal connections in spatial navigation; (3) the organization and functions of the default mode network; and (4) examples of disorders associated with amnesia.

HIPPOCAMPUS AS THE CORE AREA FOR EPISODIC MEMORY

Episodic memory relates to specific personal events, including information about their content and their context. The hippocampus is essential for spatial representation of the environment and for the ability to remember specific events.[4] The hippocampus is therefore a nodal component in operations such as context-dependent representations of autobiographic memories, mental exploration, and use of recalled information for navigation and decision-making.[7]

Extrinsic Connectivity and Functionally Segregated Input

Neocortical association areas send projections to the perirhinal and parahippocampal cortex. These areas project to the entorhinal cortex, which channels this information to the hippocampus. Cortical inputs to the entorhinal-hippocampal system are functionally segregated[8,9] (Figure 40.1). The perirhinal cortex targets the lateral entorhinal cortex and conveys information from the ventral stream of

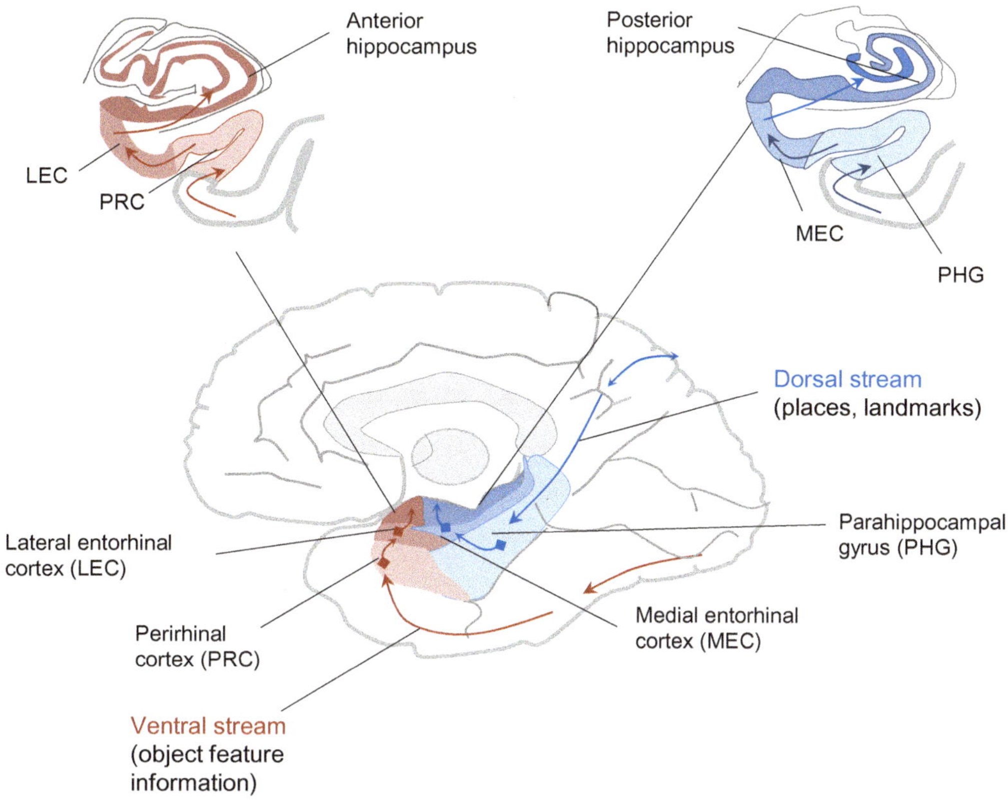

FIGURE 40.1 Sources of extrinsic input to the hippocampal formation
The neocortical inputs to the hippocampus are channeled by the entorhinal cortex. The lateral entorhinal cortex receives inputs from the perirhinal cortex, which conveys sensory information from the ventral pathway provided by the anterolateral temporal cortex and involved in object recognition ("what"/content pathway). This perirhinal-lateral entorhinal input primarily targets the anterior hippocampus and is critical for object recognition based on familiarity. The medial entorhinal cortex receives inputs from the parahippocampal cortex, which conveys spatial information from the posterior parietal cortex ("where"/context pathway). This parahippocampal–medial entorhinal pathway primarily targets the posterior hippocampus and encodes highly specific locations and time signals that allow both spatiotemporal organization of the event memories and navigation.

sensory processing involved in object recognition ("what"/content pathway). This perirhinal–lateral entorhinal input originates in the anterolateral temporal cortex, primarily targets the anterior hippocampus, and is critical for object recognition based on familiarity. In contrast, the parahippocampal cortex projects to the medial entorhinal cortex and conveys information from the dorsal stream involved in spatial processing ("where"/context pathway). This parahippocampal–medial entorhinal pathway originates in the posterior parietal cortex, primarily targets the posterior hippocampus, and encodes highly specific locations and time signals that allow both spatiotemporal organization of the event memories and navigation.[10] Thus, the hippocampal circuits participate in two large-scale networks that support different types of memory.[11]

Intrinsic Hippocampal Circuit

The hippocampus contains several subfields or subdivisions, dentate gyrus, CA3, CA2, CA1, and subiculum (Figure 40.2). These fields are connected by largely unidirectional excitatory pathways. Inputs from the lateral and medial entorhinal cortex converge in the dentate gyrus and CA3, but they remain segregated in different regions of CA1 and subiculum.[8] The intrinsic circuit of the hippocampus is reviewed in more detail in chapter 25 and only few aspects will be emphasized here.

Granule cells of the dentate gyrus provide excitatory inputs via mossy fibers to pyramidal cells of the CA3 or CA2. Pyramidal CA3 (or CA2) neurons are interconnected via recurrent collaterals and provide excitatory inputs to CA1 via the Schaffer collaterals. Pyramidal CA1 neurons project to the subiculum. This intrinsic hippocampal circuit is driven by two separate excitatory pathways from the entorhinal cortex. One pathway involves neurons of layer 2 of the entorhinal cortex, which project via the perforant pathway to the dentate gyrus; granule cells of the dentate gyrus provide mossy fiber input to CA3 (or CA2), which then projects to CA1. The second pathway involves a direct projection from layer 3 of the entorhinal cortex to CA1 and the subiculum. The CA1 neurons integrate novel

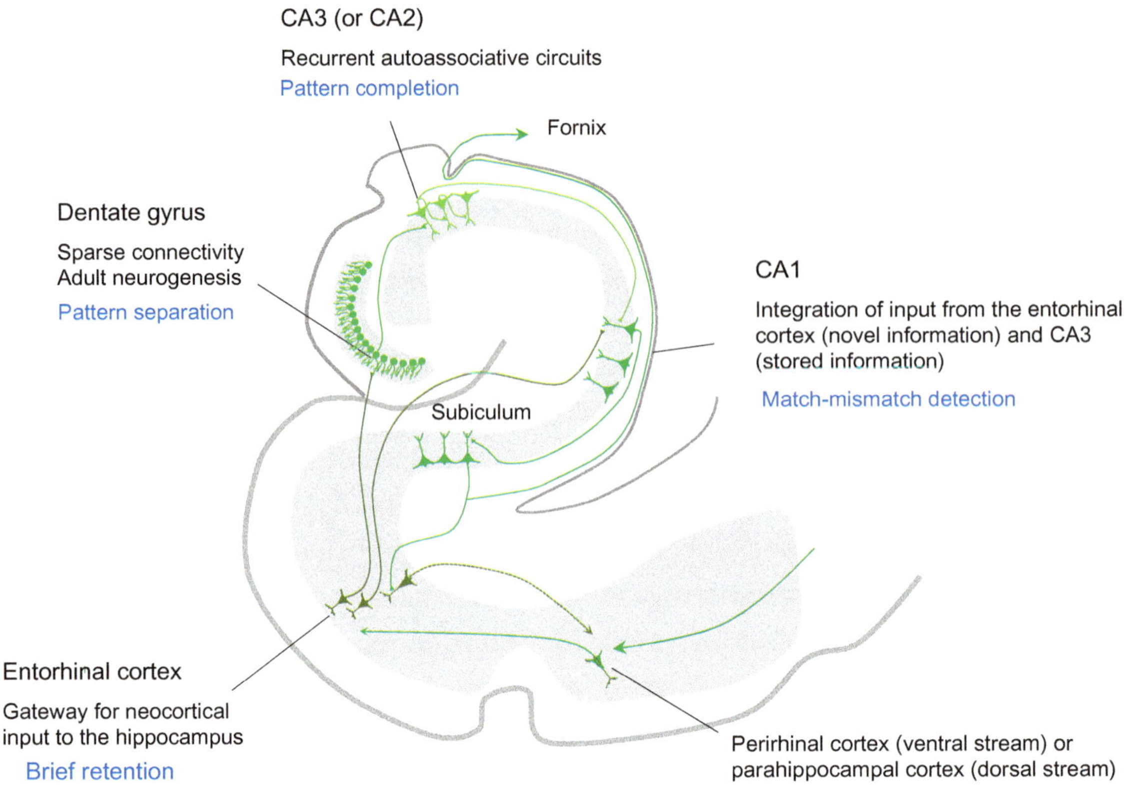

FIGURE 40.2 Intrinsic circuit and functional segregation in the hippocampus
Neocortical association areas send projections to the parahippocampal region, including the perirhinal and parahippocampal cortices. These areas project to the entorhinal cortex, which channels this information to the hippocampus. The hippocampus contains several subfields or subdivisions:, dentate gyrus, CA3, CA2, CA1, and subiculum. Granule cells of the dentate gyrus provide excitatory inputs via mossy fibers to pyramidal cells of the CA3 or CA2 region; CA3 and CA2 neurons are interconnected via recurrent collaterals and provide excitatory inputs to CA1 via the Schaffer collaterals; and CA1 provides outputs to the subiculum. The entorhinal cortex projects to the intrinsic hippocampal circuit via two separate excitatory pathways that participate in different processing of information. One consists of a projection via the perforant pathway to the dentate gyrus and CA3 (or CA2) and finally to CA1. A second pathway involves a direct projection from the entorhinal to CA1 and the subiculum. The dentate gyrus is involved in a pattern separation, which enables processing of similar experiences as distinct memories, even though the general context may be the same. Pattern completion involves CA3 and depends on autoassociative connections that functionally couple coactive CA3 pyramidal cells at the time of encoding. CA1 pyramidal neurons receive direct inputs from both the entorhinal cortex and CA3. Thus, CA1 neurons integrate novel information originating from the entorhinal cortex with stored information provided by CA3.

information originating from the entorhinal cortex with stored information provided by CA3 (or CA2) and are sensitive to mismatches between new and old information.

Functional Segregation Within the Intrinsic Hippocampal Circuit

Formation of new memories simultaneously involves two different processes, referred to as pattern separation and pattern completion. A balance between these two processes allows keeping similar episodes separate while retrieving previous memories based on environmental cues or contexts.[12,13] The ability to distinguish among similar experiences is a key feature of episodic memory. Through pattern separation, day-to-day overlapping experiences (for example parking a car in the same parking lot every day) are recalled as specific memories (for example, parking in today's parking spot as opposed to yesterday's parking spot). The dentate gyrus is selectively involved in pattern separation (Figure 40.2).[13–15] Granule cells of the dentate gyrus have unique anatomical, functional, and cellular features, such as the dependence of their survival on circulating corticosteroids. These cells receive sparse and divergent input from the entorhinal cortex and send strong but sparse projections to CA3; this minimizes overlap between CA3 neurons encoding successive memory traces, thus preventing interference among similar, but distinct memories.[12] Adult neurogenesis in the subgranular zone of the dentate gyrus also provides a substrate for pattern separation.[15–18] Neurons born in the subgranular zone differentiate into excitatory granule cells and are more likely than mature dentate granule neurons to undergo activation and use-dependent plasticity triggered by new information.[16] Whereas mature dentate granule cell populations may encode the more familial features, adult-born dentate granule cells may be particularly important for encoding novel events.[16]

Granule cell activity may be required during initial encoding and early intrahippocampal consolidation of a memory but can be dispensable for its recall. Granule cells may also be required for short-term memory retention and consolidation and for specificity during memory retrieval; these cells can enhance precision of recall by affecting processing at the perforant pathway-CA3-CA1 loop. A tentative circuit mechanism for the discrimination of memory contents, such as similar spatial contexts or individual episodes in the same environment, involves highly excitable adult-born ganglion cells that preferentially contact feedforward inhibitory CA3 interneurons; plasticity at these synapses is critical for discriminative contextual learning. This mossy fiber-recruited feedforward inhibition may suppress activation of CA3 cells that would otherwise be recruited by overlapping perforant pathway input in similar contexts or during repeated encounters of the same environment. This could spare unique sets of context- and episode-specific CA3 pyramidal cells to represent the distinctive elements of each memory. However, in addition to similar-content discrimination, the DG appears to support integrative memory operations, such as the binding of objects and events to spatial contexts and integrating new experiences into existing frameworks.[15] Such granule cells might support integrative or binding functions by recruiting overlapping CA3 ensembles to create links between shared elements of distinct memories.

In contrast to pattern separation, pattern completion is the tendency to lump together similar or related experiences or events. This provides a mechanism for retrieval of memory representations and allows the recall of a complete representation in the presence of a partial or degraded input. Pattern completion involves CA3 (Figure 40.2). The CA3 field is characterized by autoassociative connections that functionally couple co-active CA3 pyramidal cells at the time of encoding. Activation of a sufficient subset of CA3 neurons would propagate to all members of the cell ensemble leading to complete reconstitution of the learned episode.[12,19]

CA1 pyramidal neurons have a major role in distinguishing between novel and familial events by integrating inputs from the entorhinal cortex and CA3. Inputs from the entorhinal cortex terminate in the distal dendrites and signal new information to CA1 cells, whereas CA3 Schaffer collateral inputs terminate in the ascending dendrite of CA1 and signal information stored in the autoassociative CA3 network. The CA1 computes inputs from both sources and may be able between encoding and retrieval modes based on comparison of novel versus already stored information, therefore acting as a match/mismatch detector.[20,21] The shift of hippocampal operation between storage and a retrieval state is in part controlled by acetylcholine and generation of the theta rhythm. During wakefulness, acetylcholine is released from the medial septum in response to novel signals and promotes encoding on new information in CA1 while preventing recurrent connectivity in CA3. During slow-wave sleep, the decreased levels of acetylcholine allow the recurrent activity in CA3 to be transferred to CA1 during sharp wave-ripples, promoting memory consolidation, as discussed in chapter 25.

The intrinsic circuits of the hippocampus receive two major diencephalic inputs that target separate, nonoverlapping, regions and promote information processing in these circuits. The supramammillary nucleus of the posterior hypothalamus is a major component of the ascending brainstem system generating the theta rhythm and sends projections to the dentate gyrus; these projections amplify signals from the entorhinal cortex to the dental gyrus. The nucleus reuniens of the midline thalamus routes information between the hippocampus and medial PFC and projects to CA1 and to the subiculum; these inputs amplify signals from CA3 and entorhinal cortex to CA1.

Hippocampal Outputs

Information processed in the hippocampus is fed back from CA1 and subiculum to layers 5 and 6 of the entorhinal cortex, which project back to the perirhinal and parahippocampal cortex and from there to back to the neocortex. These feedback projections largely respect the topographic organization of the inputs the hippocampus. Outputs to subcortical targets are channeled via the fornix and originate in CA1, subiculum, presubiculum, and parasubiculum. Some projections of the fornix target the septal area, but most primarily target the anterior nucleus of the thalamus, either via direct projections or a relay in the mammillary nuclei (Figure 40.3). The anterior nuclear complex of the thalamus includes three subdivisions, anteromedial, anteroventral, and anterodorsal, which are involved in different functional circuits. The anteromedial nucleus has reciprocal connections with the orbitofrontal, anterior cingulate, and medial prefrontal cortex (PFC) and participates emotional processing. The anteroventral subnucleus receives inputs from the subicular cortex, both directly and via the medial mammillary nucleus and mediates interactions with the retrosplenial cortex, conveying theta rhythm activity important for episodic memory. The anterodorsal nucleus is interconnected with the lateral mammillary nucleus, postsubiculum, and retrosplenial cortex and is involved in spatial navigation. Other hippocampal outputs target the amygdala, nucleus accumbens, and hypothalamus. These inputs originate primarily from the anterior hippocampus.

Extrinsic Hippocampal Connectivity in the Setting of the "Three Limbic Subsystems" Frame

As discussed in the previous chapter, current evidence indicates that the classical "limbic system" is not a unique

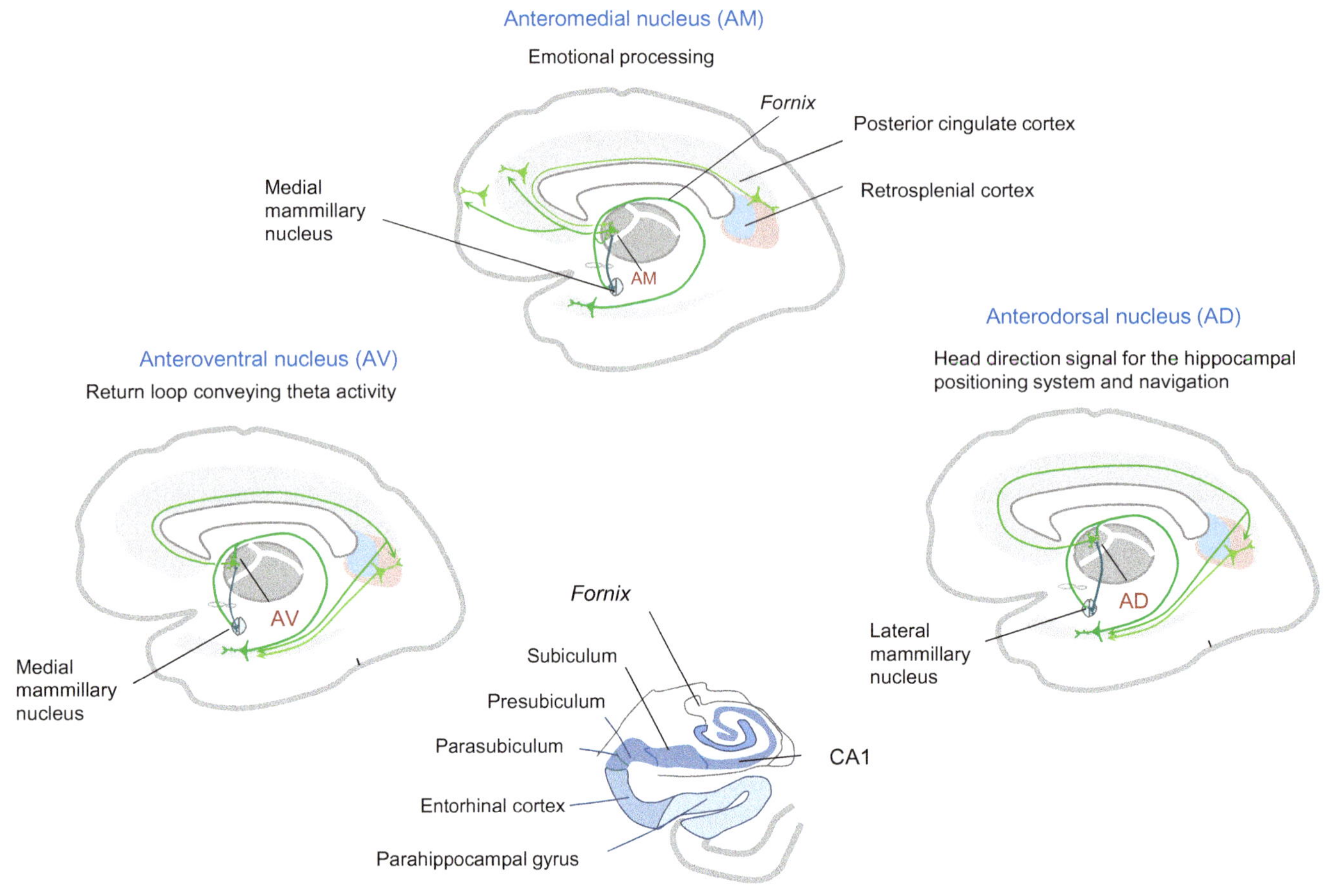

FIGURE 40.3 Hippocampal projections via the anterior nucleus of the thalamus
Outputs to subcortical targets are channeled via the fornix and originate in CA1, subiculum, presubiculum, and parasubiculum. Some outputs via the fornix target the septal area, but the primary target is the anterior nucleus of the thalamus, via either direct projections or a relay in the mammillary nuclei. The anterior nuclear complex includes three subdivisions: anteromedial, anteroventral, and anterodorsal. The anteromedial nucleus has reciprocal connections with the orbitofrontal, anterior cingulate, and medial prefrontal cortex and participates emotional processing. The anteroventral subnucleus receives inputs from the subicular cortex, both directly and via the medial mammillary nucleus, and mediates interactions with the retrosplenial cortex by conveying theta-rhythm activity important for episodic memory. The anterodorsal nucleus is interconnected with the lateral mammillary nucleus, postsubiculum, and retrosplenial cortex and is involved in spatial navigation.

system but rather includes at least three different subsystems, each with different representations along the cingulate cortex and associated areas and with distinct but interacting functions.[22] Consistent with this concept, based on anatomical organization and functional connectivity (as assessed in functional fMRI studies) the anterior, middle, and posterior hippocampus participate in different limbic subsystems.[22] The anterior hippocampus has interconnections with components of the anterior or "emotional" limbic subsystem, including the amygdala, orbitofrontal cortex (OFC), and anterior cingulate cortex (ACC), which process information from the ventral stream (including the perirhinal cortex). This subsystem is involved in reward valuation, and reward-related decision-making. In this system, value representations in the OFC are transmitted to the ACC and anterior midcingulate cortex (MCC) for action-outcome learning. The anterior hippocampus is a likely part of this circuitry, given its heavy interactions with the amygdala and OFC and may have a role in approach-avoidance conflict processing.[22] Emotion can enter the hippocampal memory system from the OFC and can be recalled to the OFC during memory retrieval. However, the emotional and hippocampal networks can operate independently of each other, except when an emotional state may be part of an episodic memory. There is also evidence suggesting functional connectivity between the midhippocampus and the anterior MCC, which is involved in error detection. The right midhippocampus responds to the novelty of spatial and nonspatial relationships. A similar finding has been reported for the MCC for novel lists of words Thus, both the midhippocampus and anterior MCC may have a role in novelty/mismatch detection. The posterior hippocampus has strong connectivity with multiple cortical regions, including the posterior cingulate cortex (PCC), retrosplenial cortex, precuneus, ACC, and MCC as well as ventromedial PFC, middle frontal gyrus, and visual association cortex. This hippocampal system receives information from neocortical areas about spatial location and objects, and can rapidly associate this information to engage in feedback mechanisms. The system can later recall the whole of this information in the CA3 sector from any component and convey the information to neocortical areas by a feedback recall process. The hippocampus may use temporal information to retrieve specific prior experiences, particularly when a representation shares common elements with a similar prior experience. The posterior hippocampus may have the major role of linking events comprising an episodic memory together in a sequential manner across time, which is the defining characteristic of episodic memory. The functional connectivity of the posterior hippocampus suggests that it may have a role in decision-making by predicting the possibilities of what might come next, allowing the OFC and striatum to evaluate the expected choice options to make the correct action at a choice point.[22]

CONSOLIDATION AND RETRIEVAL OF EPISODIC MEMORY

Memory Consolidation

Newly encoded spatial memories are typically fragile and thus require an additional maintenance process of consolidation by which they are stabilized over time.[23] At the network level, one mechanism of consolidation is the offline reactivation of firing patterns of neuronal ensembles that occurred during previous learning. The autoassociative connections of CA3 allow the spontaneous replay of memories even in the absence of the external stimuli. These replay events may help strengthen a given representation in the hippocampus and coordinate the reactivation of multiple neocortical networks to consolidate new long-term memory traces.[24] Reactivation of ensemble activity primarily occurs during episodes of sharp wave-ripple activity during non–rapid eye movement (NREM) sleep and coordinates hippocampal-to-neocortical transfer. This reactivation correlates with reduced acetylcholine levels during this sleep stage.[25,26] Reward-triggered dopamine release in the hippocampus may also promote memory consolidation by strengthening the functional connectivity between the hippocampus and neocortical regions during active encoding.

There are several hypotheses regarding the role of the hippocampus in long-term memory consolidation.[23] The classical view is that episodic memory is initially dependent on medial temporal lobe structures, primarily the hippocampus, but through reactivation over time it becomes more dependent on the neocortex. In humans, activation of the hippocampus during accurate memory retrieval is maximal for the most recent and autobiographic events and declines over the course of approximately nine years, which is parallel to the course of retrograde amnesia. In contrast, activation of widespread cortical association areas gradually increases for more remote memories, particularly semantic memories (facts, names). After consolidation, long-term memories are believed to be represented in interconnected neocortical networks. The medial PFC may have a role in consolidation, as it participates together with the hippocampus in off-line replay of learning-related activity.[27] Newly acquired memories are overlaid with preexisting semantic information, so that common elements become independent of the hippocampus. However new memories are incorporated to a "schema" that contains both semantic knowledge and episodic details. As hippocampal neurons encode both distinct experiences and their common overlapping features (semantic transformation), the hippocampus may have a critical role in linking and reorganizing separate and disparate experiences so that pre-existing semantic networks become hippocampus-dependent.[23]

Role of the Prefrontal Cortex in Memory Consolidation and Retrieval

The PFC contributes to episodic memory by top-down control of memory processing.[28] The medial PFC may have a role in directing neocortical learning during the shift from medial temporal lobe to neocortical representations during memory consolidation. The main functions of the medial PFC would be to detect the congruency of new information with existing information in the neocortex.[29] The activity and functional coupling between the medial PFC and the medial temporal cortex during encoding, offline replay, and retrieval is a function of the congruency of novel information with that previously stored in neocortical networks.[29] Whereas the medial temporal system is required for episodic memory coding of new information, the medial PFC may be able encode information that is congruent with previous semantic knowledge via its interactions with other neocortical areas, independently of the hippocampus.

During retrieval, the PFC may exert a strategic top-down control that allows retrieval of context-appropriate memories while suppressing competing context-inappropriate memories.[30] Electrocorticography studies in patients undergoing epilepsy monitoring showed that successful memory retrieval is associated with increased global network connectivity, reflected by oscillatory phase synchronization among the medial PFC, medial temporal lobe, and parietal cortex.

The PFC and the hippocampus are strongly connected via direct and indirect pathways (Figure 40.4). They include a direct projection from CA1 of the anterior hippocampus and proximal subiculum to the PFC; a bidirectional connection between the medial PFC and the perirhinal and lateral entorhinal cortex; and bidirectional connections via the thalamic nucleus reuniens.[30–32] There is strong oscillatory synchrony at theta frequency between the medial

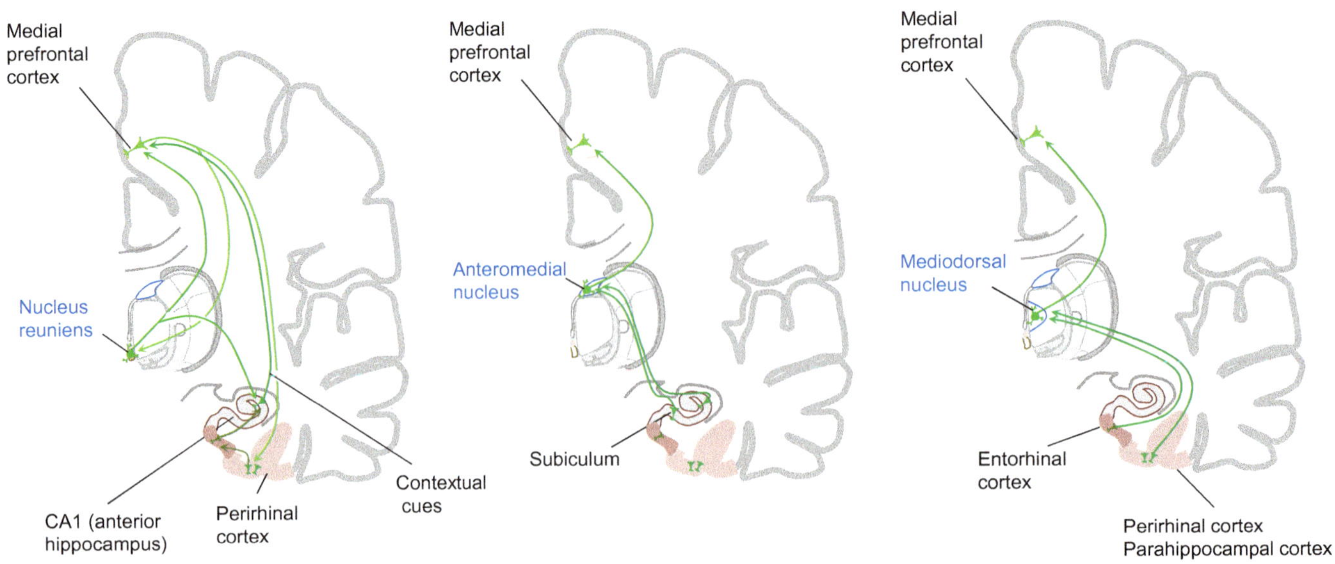

FIGURE 40.4 Medial temporal–prefrontal interactions
Whereas the hippocampus is critical for establishing the relationships between the events and their context, which compose memories for specific experiences, the prefrontal cortex (PFC) contributes to episodic memory by top-down control of memory processing and retrieval. The PFC and the hippocampus are strongly connected via direct and indirect pathways. They include a direct projection from CA1 of the anterior hippocampus to the PFC; a bidirectional connection between the medial PFC and the perirhinal and lateral entorhinal cortices; and bidirectional connections via the thalamic nucleus reuniens. A second pathway is via the anteromedial subdivision of the anterior nucleus of the thalamus, which receives inputs from CA1 and subiculum and also promotes theta synchronization between the hippocampus and the medial PFC. The parahippocampal, perirhinal, and entorhinal cortex project via the mediodorsal nucleus of the thalamus to the PFC. In this system, beta-band synchronization between the medial temporal lobe and the PFC may promote recognition memory and cue-based recollection.

PFC and hippocampus during memory encoding and retrieval.[33,34] Slow gamma oscillations in the medial PFC are strongly linked to attentional processing and flexible rule switching, and are coupled to hippocampal theta oscillations. Hippocampal theta may send contextual cues to the medial PFC during contextual learning. During retrieval, prefrontal theta precedes hippocampal theta.[28] The PFC may provide a top-down control over the retrieval of specific memories by suppressing context-inappropriate representations in the perirhinal and lateral entorhinal cortex[30] and may also suppress irrelevant memories via projections to inhibitory neurons in the hippocampus.[35,36] The nucleus reuniens would coordinate these interactions, resynchronizing and reversing the direction of information flow between these two cortical areas. A second pathway for interactions between the hippocampus and the medial PFC is via the anteromedial subdivision of the anterior nucleus of the thalamus, which receives inputs from CA1 and subiculum and also promotes theta synchronization between the hippocampus and the medial PFC. A third pathway for interaction between the medial temporal memory system and the PFC is provided by projections of the parahippocampal, perirhinal, and entorhinal cortex to the mediodorsal nucleus of the thalamus, which projects to the PFC. In this system, beta-band synchronization between the medial temporal lobe and the PFC may promote recognition memory and cue-based recollection.

SPATIAL NAVIGATION AND TEMPORAL ORGANIZATION OF EPISODIC MEMORIES

Navigation is a fundamental behavior that involves multiple cognitive functions and processes.[37,38] The hippocampus has a critical role in navigation by providing a representation of space.[39] An influential view is that space may represent a frame to organize all experiences within episodic memories, what is referred to as a "cognitive map."[5] Thus, temporally organized activity of hippocampal neurons helps organize these memories both in space and time.[4]

Reference Frames for Spatial Navigation

Spatial navigation is based on both dynamic body-based self-motion cues and static environmental cues.[37] Self-motion information derives from two main sources. The first is the combination of vestibular input, motor efference copy, and proprioceptive feedback, which are first integrated at the level of the brainstem to yield estimates of linear and angular movement and velocity; the second originates from visual perception and signals optic flow.

Both types of information are further processed in areas of the parietal and superior temporal cortex and provide an integrated percept of self-motion. Environmental cues comprise static objects (landmarks) and boundaries that can be used to determine the position and orientation of a subject relative to the environment. These cues predominantly derive from visual information and involve structures of the posterior parietal cortex.

Self-motion and environment cues provide representation of space in three references frames: egocentric, allocentric, and inertial or idiothetic. The egocentric reference frame involves the representation of locations encoded in relation to the navigator's body part axis; the allocentric reference frame is based on the spatial relationship among external features or landmarks of the environment independently of the position and movement of the navigator. The inertial or idiothetic frame is the relative location and orientation based on direction and distance moved from an arbitrary reference point and is referred to as "path integration." For path integration, subjects use self-motion cues such as vestibular information and optic flow to keep track of their own location relative to a starting point. In human fMRI studies, the hippocampus is activated when people use a strategy based on cognitive maps during virtual navigation, including the use of shortcuts for planning of efficient novel routes. In contrast, learning habitual routes depends on the striatum, including the caudate nucleus.[38]

Hippocampal Navigation System

Whereas the egocentric space reference frame is represented in the parietal cortex and associated regions, the allocentric (scene representation) and idiothetic (path integration) frames are represented in the hippocampus and associated regions.[40,41] Space representation in the hippocampus may represent a frame to organize all experiences within episodic memories, what is referred to as a "cognitive map."[5] Temporally organized activity of hippocampal neurons helps organize these memories in both space and time.[4] As initially shown in landmark studies of O'Keefe et al. in rodents, the CA3 and CA1 regions contain *place cells* that selectively fire when the animal is in a specific location of space.[5] This led to the proposal that space provides for a an internal cognitive map for integration of the multimodal features of a given experience or episode.[5] The hippocampal system also uses a path integration reference frame for spatial coding and navigation. The entorhinal cortex and subiculum contain different types of cells that encode self-motion and environment cues. These include *grid cells*, *border cells*, *head direction cells*, and *speed cells*.[39,42] Grid cells in the medial entorhinal cortex are part of an intrinsic path-integration system and provide direct input to place cells in CA1. Border cells fire exclusively along geometric borders of the environment (such as along walls or edges of a platform) and relate the firing of place and grid cells to these fixed features of the environment. Head-direction cells signal the orientation of the subject's head in the horizontal plane and integrate direction and velocity signals into a coherent two-dimensional space. Head-direction cells are present in a network that includes the inferior vestibular nucleus, dorsal tegmental nucleus, lateral mammillary bodies, anterodorsal nucleus of the thalamus, retrosplenial cortex, parasubiculum, and entorhinal cortex.[43]

Functional MRI studies during imagined navigation tasks show that the human hippocampus supports map-like spatial codes[44] and also shows grid-like codes in the entorhinal cortex.[45] These representations have been confirmed by intracranial recordings on presurgical epilepsy patients.[46,47] These studies also show a network that is selectively activated in during virtual navigation, imagined navigation, spatial memory recall, or viewing navigationally relevant stimuli. This network includes the parahippocampal cortex (parahippocampal place area), retrosplenial cortex, and medial parietal cortex (precuneus). These areas respond strongly to passive viewing of scenes (such as buildings, landscapes, and rooms) and participate in processing of navigation-relevant stimuli. The retrosplenial and medial parietal region may be involved in processing and storage of long-term spatial knowledge.[38] The navigation network also includes areas of the PFC that respond primarily to active navigation in relationship to route planning. The hippocampal and entorhinal spatial codes can be used together with frontal lobe mechanisms to plan routes during navigation.[38]

Hippocampus and Encoding of Time

In addition to its representation of space, the hippocampus also represents the temporal organization of memories. Time has a central role in episodic memory. A central process for retrieval of an experience is the ability to remember the order of events that composed the episode. The perception of elapsed time (called interval timing) involves a widespread brain system. Internal timing may involve the interaction of multiple oscillatory patterns in the prefrontal and parietal areas that are activated at different times and integrated in the striatum. In human fMRI studies, the temporoparietal junction is activated when persons are trained to judge the temporal order of stimuli. Mental self-projection both to earlier times in life and to specific locations in space also engages the inferior parietal cortex as a component of different networks. The subnetworks for spatial and temporal processing are connected via medial temporal areas as hubs for spatiotemporal integration. The parahippocampal and the medial entorhinal cortex support memory not only for spatial but also for temporal contexts. Medial entorhinal cortex grid cells, which have highly specific spatial firing patterns during field exploration also fire at sequential moments and signal both elapsed time and distance. Thus, the same cells in the parahippocampal and medial entorhinal cortex that code locations in space also code moments in a temporally structured experience. The hippocampus also contains cells that encode the temporal sequence of events. Spatial and temporal coding in the hippocampus may be segregated or combined across the different subdivisions but appear to be integrated in CA1, which contains not only place cells but also "time cells."[4] Functional MRI studies in humans also show that the hippocampus is activated in relationship to retrieval of temporal order and accuracy of sequence detail.[6]

THE TWO CORTICAL SYSTEMS FOR MEMORY-GUIDED BEHAVIOR

Via its cortical connections, the hippocampus participates in two large-scale networks that support different types of memory: an anterior temporal system and a posteromedial system.[11]

Anterior Temporal System and Familiarity-Based Recognition Memory

The anterior temporal system is primarily involved in recognition memory underlying the sense of familiarity. This system is centered in the perirhinal cortex.[48] The perirhinal cortex is interconnected with the hippocampus via the lateral entorhinal cortex, with the ventrolateral anterior temporal cortex involved in object feature processing and with the lateral orbitofrontal cortex involved in value-based representation (Figure 40.5). These neocortical connections allow the perirhinal cortex to access both highly processed object feature and object value (emotional) information. Neurons in the perirhinal cortex encode the experience-dependent features of objects acquired through learning the associations between these different features and their behavioral context. As the final station of the ventral visual stream, the perirhinal cortex relates the structure with other memorized features of objects. Simultaneously, via its widespread backward projections to the anterior temporal cortex, the perirhinal cortex initiates the signaling between cortical areas required to retrieve associations between attributes of visual objects, thus constituting a hub of the network for semantic memory.[48]

The perirhinal cortex may integrate unique object features across multiple spatial dimensions or sensory modalities and discriminate between objects that have high feature overlap. In addition to its major role in recognition memory based on familiarity, the perirhinal cortex has a role in learning associations about and between words and objects and may also support learning of the affective relevance of objects and participate in emotional processing and social cognition. The human perirhinal cortex is engaged during the encoding and recognition of visual objects, particularly faces. Changes in functional connectivity between the perirhinal cortex and the fusiform face area predicts individual differences in subsequent recognition of faces.[49] High-resolution functional MRI studies in monkeys shows that processing in the perirhinal cortex involves a laminar module whereby the representations in the supragranular layers 2/3 preferentially encode the cue stimulus whereas the representations of the to-be-recalled targets are localized in the infragranular layers, first in layer 5 and then in layer 6. The key memory retrieval process occurs in layer 5/6 of the perirhinal cortex, which primarily targets the upper layers 2/3 of the lateral entorhinal cortex. Backward perirhinal projections targeting the orbitofrontal cortex participate in learning and reversal learning of reward-stimulus association. Perirhinal projections also relay the indirect bidirectional PFC-hippocampal pathway that allows the use of current behavioral context to retrieve relevant memories. Backward perirhinal projections to the temporal lobe contribute to the retrieval of explicit memory traces consolidated in multiple domain-specific and cross-modal cortical areas within semantic memory networks; these traces are then integrated in the anterior temporal lobe. The perirhinal cortex may serve as hub that links episodic memory with semantic memory through a consolidation process whereas the temporopolar cortex may be involved in abstract representations to support the use of well-consolidated semantic knowledge.[48] Overall, the anterior temporal system could facilitate the use of past experiences to infer features about objects and construct knowledge about people.[11]

Posterior Medial System: Contextual Memory, Scene Perception, and Spatial Navigation

The posterior medial system is involved in contextual memory, scene representation, and visual navigation. This system is centered in the parahippocampal cortex, which is connected with the hippocampus via the medial entorhinal cortex and is reciprocally interconnected with the retrosplenial cortex (Figure 40.6). The parahippocampal and retrosplenial areas receive visual inputs from the dorsal stream and are interconnected via the cingulum bundle with the posterior cingulate cortex (PCC), medial parietal cortex (precuneus), medial PFC, and ventrolateral parietal cortex (angular gyrus). These strongly interconnected areas are core components of the default mode network. The posteromedial network plays a role in the processing of contextual information for self-initiated retrieval of episodic memory.[50] This system is particularly active when individuals mentally construct future-oriented, self-relevant scenarios. Both the parahippocampal and retrosplenial cortex area are also involved in spatial memory and navigation and are strongly activated by viewing images of scenes or objects that serve as landmarks for navigation. Whereas the parahippocampal cortex represents information about spatial contexts (scenes), the retrosplenial cortex integrates scene information to allow orientation within the spatial context.

At the late stages of processing, spatial information becomes integrated into the ventral object processing pathway for vision and memory.[51] The direct interactions with the different sectors of the hippocampal formation could help refine information processing within the anterior

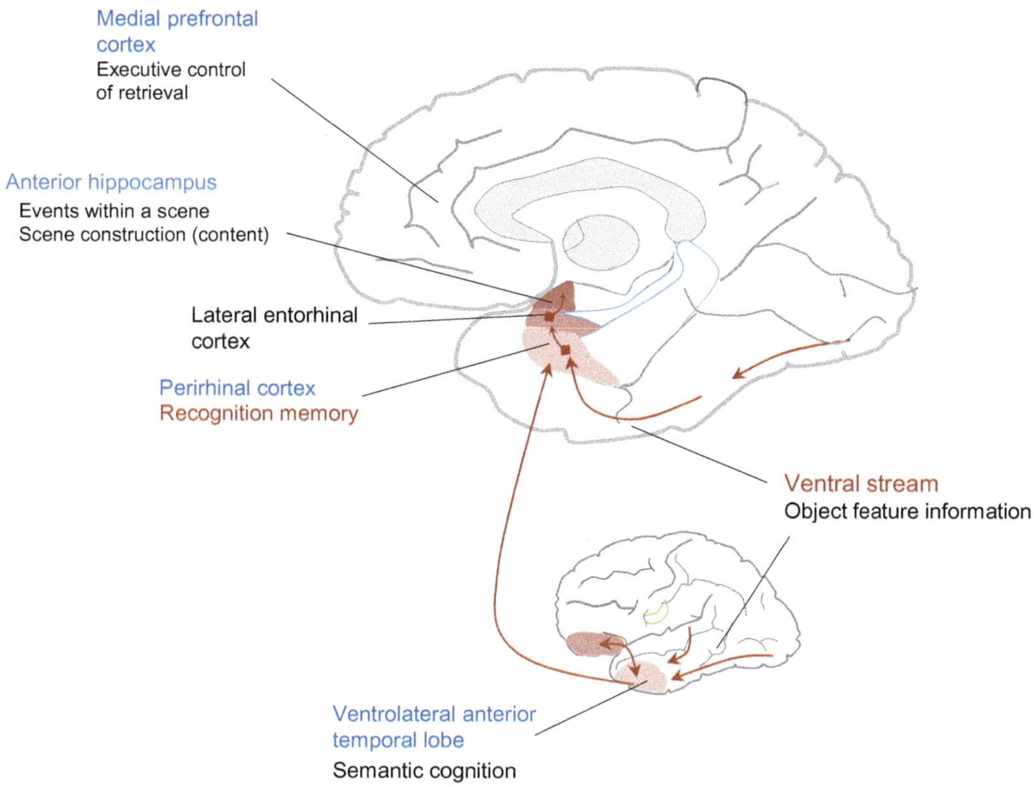

FIGURE 40.5 Anterior temporal system for recognition memory
The anterior temporal system is primarily involved in recognition memory, or sense of familiarity. This system is centered in the perirhinal cortex, which is interconnected with the hippocampus via the lateral entorhinal cortex, with the ventrolateral anterior temporal involved in semantic processing, and with the lateral orbitofrontal cortex. These connections allow access both highly processed object feature and object value information.

temporal and the posteromedial systems. The hippocampal formation may also increase the ability to link the representations of entities in the perirhinal cortex and representations of context in the parahippocampal-retrosplenial system, via convergent inputs of the lateral and the medial entorhinal cortex in the dentate gyrus and CA3.[11]

DEFAULT MODE NETWORK

The brain's default network consists of multiple areas located in large distributed zones of the association cortex, which are active during several forms of internal mentation and suppressed when attention is focused on the external world.[52–55] The default network is involved in representation of self-relevant information, construction of mental scenes based on episodic memory, imagining the future, and inferring the mental state of self and others ("mentalizing" or theory of mind").[52–55] This network may also be critical for the organization and expression of preplanned, reflexive behaviors that are unconstrained by the social and physical environment. Recent evidence indicates that the default network comprises multiple juxtaposed, functionally interconnected individual networks. Different classes of tasks activate distinct juxtaposed regions. The detailed organization of these networks is revealed when intrinsic functional connectivity is studied fully within a single individual.[55]

The default network is composed of multiple widely distributed clusters of areas extending from the frontal pole (areas 9, 10 and, possibly, 11) through the anterior cingulate (areas 24 and 32), the posterior midline including the retrosplenial cortex and the precuneus just ventral to the medial posterior parietal cortex, as well as extensive regions of the temporal association cortex dorsolateral prefrontal cortex.[55] On the basis of meta-analysis of fMRI studies, the default networks have been subdivided into core regions and two separate subsystems, a medial temporal subsystem and a dorsal medial subsystem, each functionally linked with core areas[52–54] (Figure 40.7). Whereas this concept is an oversimplification, it helps to emphasize the putative role of the main components of the distributed networks within the brain default network.

Core Areas and Representation of Self-Relevant Information

The core areas of the default network are activated in most tasks involving self-thought processing and include

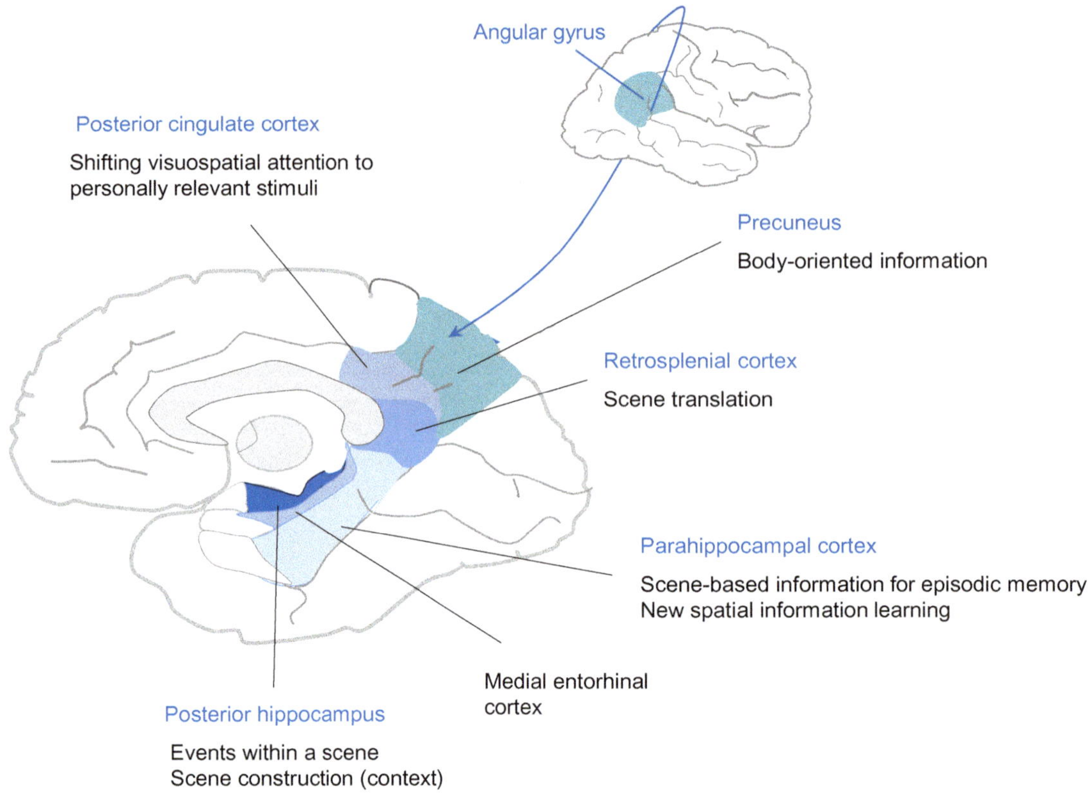

FIGURE 40.6 Posterior medial systems for contextual memory and spatial navigation
The posterior medial system is critically involved in contextual memory, scene representation, and visual navigation. This system is centered in the parahippocampal cortex, which is connected with the hippocampus via the medial entorhinal cortex and is reciprocally interconnected with the retrosplenial cortex. The parahippocampal and retrosplenial areas receive visual inputs from the dorsal stream and are interconnected via the cingulum bundle with the posterior cingulate cortex (PCC), medial parietal cortex (precuneus), medial prefrontal cortex (PFC), and ventrolateral parietal cortex (angular gyrus). This network plays a role in the processing of contextual information for self-initiated retrieval of episodic memory. The posteromedial network also encompasses the head-direction signaling network, and both the parahippocampal and retrosplenial cortex area also involved in spatial memory and navigation. Whereas the parahippocampal cortex represents information about spatial contexts (scenes), the retrosplenial cortex integrates scene information to allow orientation within the spatial context.

the anterior medial PFC, PCC and adjacent precuneus, and angular gyrus. These areas represent personally relevant information and are activated when individuals reference information to themselves, retrieve personal knowledge, recall autobiographical memories, consider their future goals or mental states, and simulate personal future events or social interactions. The anterior medial PFC integrates salient external or internal information with personal affective experience, its perceived value, and prior conceptual or episodic knowledge. The PCC and adjacent precuneus support attention to behaviorally relevant sources of information drawn from memory, perception, or both. The PCC includes a ventral region that is activated during tasks involving self-referential processing, autobiographical memory, spatial navigation, future thinking, and mentalizing; and a dorsal region that is activated in tasks linked to awareness and monitoring of behaviorally relevant environmental stimuli. The angular gyrus has widespread connectivity with other posterior parietal areas involved in perception, attention, spatial cognition, and action; with areas of the anterior lateral temporal cortex involved in storage of semantic knowledge and conceptual processing; and with other default network regions. Via these connections, the angular gyrus may function as a crossmodal hub, allowing the access of internal and external sources of information to conceptual representations of events or items in their spatial and temporal context.

Medial Temporal Subsystem: Construction of Mental Scenes and Imagining the Future

The medial temporal subsystem of the default mode network comprises the retrosplenial and parahippocampal cortex, hippocampus, and the posterior inferior parietal lobe, including the angular gyrus. This subsystem is

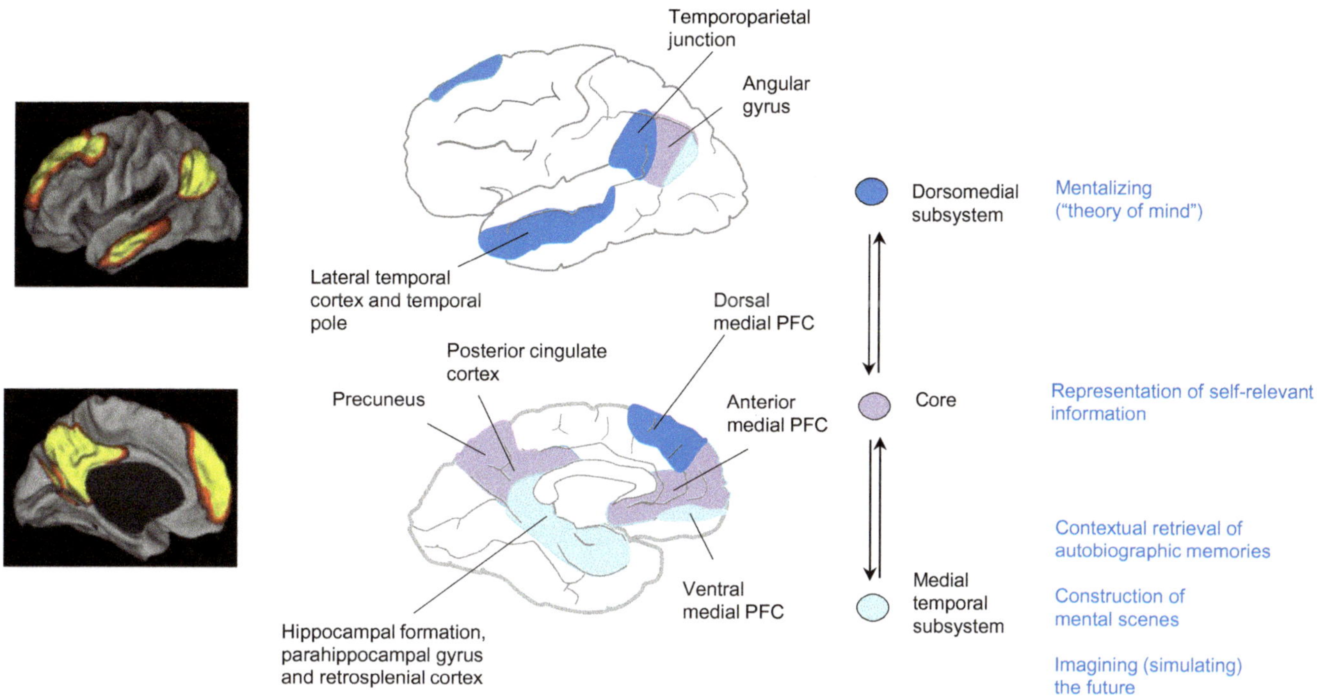

FIGURE 40.7 Default mode network

The default network is involved in representation of self-relevant information, construction of mental scenes based on episodic memory, imagining the future, and inferring the mental state of self and others. The default network has been subdivided into core regions and two separate subsystems, a medial temporal subsystem and a dorsal medial subsystem, each functionally linked with core areas. The core areas are activated in most tasks involving self-thought processing and personally relevant information and include the anterior medial prefrontal cortex (PFC), posterior cingulate cortex and adjacent precuneus, and angular gyrus. The medial temporal subsystem comprises the retrosplenial and parahippocampal cortex, hippocampus, and posterior inferior parietal lobe (including the angular gyrus). This subsystem is activated during tasks involving past and future autobiographical thought, episodic memory, and contextual retrieval and allows an individual to construct coherent mental scenes, reflecting about the past and imagining (simulating) the future. The dorsal medial subsystem of the default network comprises the dorsomedial PFC, temporoparietal junction, lateral temporal cortex, and temporal pole. This subsystem is activated during social cognition tasks and during story comprehension and semantic and conceptual processing, and has a major role in mentalizing, or "theory of mind," which is the process of inferring or reflecting on the mental states of one's self and others. (Functional MRI courtesy of Dr. David T. Jones).

activated during tasks involving past and future autobiographical thought, episodic memory, and contextual retrieval and thus allows the individual to construct coherent mental scenes, reflecting about the past and imagining (simulating) the future. The medial temporal subsystem also interacts with the ventromedial PFC. The ventromedial PFC receives information from both the external world and the body via the orbitofrontal cortex, has connections with the amygdala and ventral striatum, and is thus involved in emotional processing and motivated behaviors. Via its connections with the ventromedial PFC, the default network may function as a link among the individual's personality (including mood control), social behavior, and motivational drive. Imaging studies show that the emotional state, including the anxiety level while performing a task, has a direct effect on the activity of the ventromedial PFC, thus reflecting a dynamic balance between focused attention and a subject's baseline emotional default state.

Dorsal Medial Subsystem: Inferring the Mental State of Self and Others

The dorsal medial subsystem of the default network comprises the dorsomedial PFC, temporoparietal junction, lateral temporal cortex, and temporal pole. This subsystem is activated during social cognition tasks, story comprehension, and semantic and conceptual processing. Key structures within the dorsal medial subsystem, including the dorsomedial PFC and temporoparietal junction, have a major role in mentalizing, or "theory of mind," which is the process of inferring or reflecting on the mental states of one's self and others. The right temporoparietal junction is activated when individuals are asked to reflect on the beliefs of other people. The dorsal medial subsystem also includes regions along the left superior temporal sulcus, which facilitates the retrieval of stored semantic and conceptual, including social, knowledge.

The Default Network at the Apex of the Gradient of Cortical Organization

Emerging evidence indicates that the default network include distributed, parallel nodes comprising many spatially separate heteromodal cortical association areas. The default network is currently viewed as the most distant transmodal association network respect to its relative position in the cortical mantle. Its components occupy the higher-order association cortex that matures late in development, and displays high spatial variability from one person to the next. According to the cortical gradient of microarchitecture and connectivity, the association networks linked to external sensory attention lie closest to the primary sensory areas and are succeeded by the multiple higher-order networks, one after the other; in terms of spatial progression outward from the primary sensory cortex the default network is at the apex of this gradient.[56] Human intracranial recordings of high-frequency signals reflecting population-spiking activity from many thousands of neurons confirm fMRI findings showing suppression of the default network during active externally directed tasks.[57] For example recordings from the posterior cingulate and the medial PFC showed substantially suppression of signals soon after initiation of an externally oriented task. Direct neuronal recordings in humans also show increased high-frequency broadband signals in the posterior cingulate when individuals are engaged in autobiographical memory tasks. The activity of the default mode network may be regulated by thalamic inputs gated by the thalamic reticular nucleus, by cholinergic inputs from the basal forebrain to the prefrontal cortex, and by other subcortical influences.[55]

EFFECTS OF AGING AND NEURODEGENERATION ON NAVIGATION AND EPISODIC MEMORY

Age-Related Navigation Deficits

An important feature of cognitive aging is impaired spatial navigation.[35] The hippocampus, parahippocampal region, and retrosplenial cortex show reduced or absent activation during virtual navigation tasks in older as compared to younger adults. Older adults have difficulties in path integration tasks. Hyperactivity of the CA3 autoassociative network may affect spatial navigation by erroneous retrieval of the same scene map for multiple different space representations, or by the inappropriate generation of distinct place representations for familial environments. There is also impairment in spatial working memory when revisiting a location that was memorized relative to external landmarks; this inability reflects impaired function of the medial PFC.

Amnestic-Type Mild Cognitive Impairment and Alzheimer Disease

Episodic memory decline occurs with increasing age and is a major symptom in amnestic type mild cognitive impairment (MCI) and amnestic dementia due to AD pathology. Alzheimer disease is characterized by accumulation of both amyloid β (Aβ) in the form of plaques and hyperphosphorylated tau in the form of neurofibrillary tangles. The tauopathy that underlies AD typically begins in medial temporal structures before involving the lateral temporal and parietal isocortical areas.[58] Patients with amnestic MCI and amnestic dementia due to AD have several episodic memory deficits. They include impaired storage and recall of new information, where objects are better remembered than words; inability to discriminate between old and new information, leading to increase in false memories and confabulation; and prominent impairment in prospective memory. These patients also have difficulty with pattern separation.[59,60] A key feature in aging, amnestic type MCI, and amnestic dementia due to AD is difficulty discriminating among highly similar items or episodes, reflecting impaired pattern separation. The inability to detect a novelty signal when stimuli are similar but not identical leads, for example, to falsely classifying novel scenes as familiar ones. The substrate for this decline is a shift in hippocampal network dynamics away from pattern separation in the dentate gyrus toward excessive pattern completion in CA3. This reflects excessive activity of the CA3 circuits, which is linked to changes in the perforant pathway and disinhibition in the dentate gyrus and CA3 resulting from loss of GABAergic inhibitory tone.[61] Changes in excitation/inhibition balance may lead to strengthening of CA3 recurrent collaterals, biasing the network toward reactivation of previous experiences at the expense of learning new information. Impaired cholinergic modulation also reduces the influence of novel information arriving via the direct entorhinal cortex-CA1 pathway and favors the reactivation of stored cognitive maps due to increased CA3 influence on CA1.[62] High resolution fMRI studies in patients with amnestic MCI performing an object discrimination task showed hyperactive dentate gyrus/CA3 and hypoactive signals in the entorhinal cortex during task. This may reflect impaired processing in the lateral entorhinal cortex-perirhinal cortex pathway, which is one of the earliest sites of tau pathology both in aging and in AD. Whereas tau pathology in the lateral entorhinal cortex may contribute to CA3 hyperactivity, eventually there is reduction in hippocampal activity in patients with AD. The cognitive disorder in typical AD involves multiple domains—not only declarative memory but also visuospatial, executive, and language functions. The early neuropathology of AD, as reflected by metabolic mapping, tau PET imaging, and neuropathology, affects not only the medial temporal lobe but also the temporoparietal cortex, precuneus, PCC, and retrosplenial cortices, which are core components of the default mode network. With disease progression, patients with AD exhibit impairments in self-reflective, social, and executive aspects of self-generated thought. The functional integrity of the default mode network also diminishes to a lesser extent with normal aging.

Other Neurodegenerative Disorders

Hippocampal sclerosis is a disorder associated with accumulation of TAR-DNA binding protein of 43 kD (TDP-43) resulting in neuronal loss and gliosis preferentially affecting the CA1 region and subiculum, and is a relatively common finding in patients older than 80 years of age with dementia. Asymmetric hippocampal with ipsilateral mammillary atrophy and relative preservation of metabolism in the lateral temporal lobe may help distinguish hippocampal sclerosis from AD.[63] The clinical amnestic syndrome associated with hippocampal sclerosis differs from that of the clinical syndrome of AD by a pure involvement of episodic memory and long evolution in the former, and the involvement of nonmemory domains in the latter.[64]

Primary age-related tauopathy is a neuropathological diagnosis characterized by tau neurofibrillary tangles in the absence of amyloid plaque pathology. In this disorder high tau pathology burden is associated with more rapid decline on tasks involving episodic and semantic memory along with tests of processing speed and attention.[65] However, compared with patients with AD, individuals with primary age-related tauopathy have slower rates of decline on measures of memory, language, and visuospatial performance.[66]

Whereas AD affects the core components and the medial temporal subsystem of the default mode network, this network is also affected in behavioral variant frontotemporal dementia (FTD) and the semantic variant of primary progressive aphasia (PPA), previously known as semantic dementia. These disorders are characterized by reduced activation or connectivity in the default network resulting in impairment of self-generated cognition. Behavioral variant FTD affects the anterior medial PFC dorsal medial subsystem as well as the salience network, with degeneration extending from dorsal to ventral prefrontal regions and into the lateral temporal cortex. This results in the alterations in personality, social functioning, self-reflection, and emotional processing. Semantic variant PPA is associated with degeneration of the lateral temporal lobes extending into medial temporal lobe structures. It typically presents with impairments in semantic knowledge, language, emotion processing, construction of future scenarios (possibly due to the deterioration of conceptual knowledge), and impaired episodic future thinking.

FOCAL DISORDERS AFFECTING THE EPISODIC MEMORY SYSTEM

Focal disorders typically affecting the hippocampus, either in isolation or in association with other portions of the medial temporal lobe memory system, include hypoxic-ischemic injury, herpes simplex encephalitis, autoimmune limbic encephalitis, and ischemic stroke affecting the posterior cerebral artery territory.

Damage of diencephalic structures connected with the hippocampal formation, including the mammillary bodies, anterior and dorsomedial nuclei of the thalamus, and fornix, may also produce a profound amnestic syndrome, as occurs in Wernicke-Korsakoff syndrome. Lesions of the mammillary bodies or fornix impair learning of new episodic information with relative sparing of recognition memory based on familiarity. Many disorders affecting episodic memory may be associated with confabulation. Confabulation is defined as a false memory that the patient believes is true and often involves a statement about an autobiographical event that the patient has never experienced. Confabulation typically occurs with PFC lesions. Prefrontal cortex dysfunction impairs executive control (monitoring) of retrieval that is superimposed on the memory deficit. Patients with PFC lesions are particularly impaired when target information must be remembered under distracting or interfering conditions or when they have to distinguish the source or context of the information learned.

Some focal lesion may produce localizing abnormalities. Damage of the anterior temporal lobe involving the perirhinal and adjacent temporopolar cortex (particularly on the left hemisphere) produces substantial deficits in recognition memory. These deficits may occur despite sparing of the hippocampus and preserved ability to recollect the context associated with specific items. Patients with damage of the right parahippocampal cortex are often unable to recognize familiar buildings or rooms; this is referred to topographical disorientation or landmark agnosia. Lesions of the retrosplenial cortex spare scene perception but impair the ability to use landmarks for orientation; this is referred to as topographical amnesia. These patients are unable to orient themselves within real or imagined landmarks and thus can neither navigate nor describe routes between familiar locations. Lesions affecting the angular gyrus lead to egocentric disorientation; a form of topographic disorientation characterized by difficulties in navigation and impaired memories for landmarks.

TRANSIENT EPILEPTIC AND TRANSIENT GLOBAL AMNESIA

Patients with mesial temporal lobe epilepsy have material-specific memory deficits; with verbal memory impairment lateralized to the dominant hemisphere and visual or visuospatial memory impairment localized to the nondominant hemisphere. Transient epileptic amnesia is a form of anterograde and/or retrograde amnesia that occurs in brief (30–60 min), typically recurrent episodes that commonly occur upon awakening, often in middle-aged or elderly patients with epilepsy. Transient epileptic amnesia is associated with accelerated long-term forgetting and remote memory impairment. Accelerated long-term forgetting is characterized by normal initial learning and recall of information over minutes to hours, followed by an unusually rapid loss of information over days to weeks.[67] Remote memory impairment is the relatively prominent impairment of remote autobiographic or semantic memory compared to recent memory. Transient global amnesia is the acute onset of anterograde and temporally graded amnesia with otherwise normal neuropsychiatric function.[68] It usually lasts less than 24 hours (4–10 hours) and resolves completely except for complete amnesia of the episode. Several pathophysiological mechanisms have been suggested, including transient spreading depression in the setting of migraine. Current evidence indicates that the major mechanism may be venous stasis affecting the medial temporal lobe triggered by Valsalva-type maneuver in the setting of jugular venous insufficiency.

PSYCHIATRIC DISORDERS

Depression is associated with abnormalities in episodic memory. Persons with depression in the absence of neurodegenerative or cerebrovascular diseases typically complain of impaired memory, but on objective testing perform only slightly below the normal range, in contrast to persons with neurodegenerative causes of memory dysfunction, who tend to score very poorly on objective testing once they become symptomatic. Findings in depression include impaired recollection, better memory for negative material but worse memory for positive material, and "overgeneral" memory retrieval. Stress-induced inhibition of adult hippocampal neurogenesis in the dentate gyrus may impair pattern separation during memory encoding of neutral material, leading to impaired recollection of episodic memories. Experimental and postmortem human studies show that hippocampal neurogenesis is suppressed in depression. Antidepressant treatment with selective serotonin reuptake inhibitors, electroconvulsive therapy, and aerobic exercise all promote neurogenesis in the dentate gyrus. In addition, patients with depression have particularly impaired recollection for affectively positive, as opposed to negative autobiographic information. Stress-induced inhibition of midbrain dopaminergic neurons may disrupt encoding and consolidation of rewarding memories, resulting in a selective deficit of retrieval of positive memories. Stress-induced sensitization of the amygdala may lead to exaggerated emotional responses to negative materials, contributing to biased retrieval of autobiographic memory toward negative material.

DYSFUNCTION OF THE DEFAULT MODE NETWORK IN PSYCHIATRIC DISORDERS

Some psychiatric disorders are associated with hyperfunction within the default mode network.[53] This results in excessive forms of self-generated thought, affecting its content, as occurs in mood disorders. Impairment in content regulation often manifests as polarized forms of internal thinking where most thoughts pertain to similar content and there is difficulty in flexibly shifting between different types of self-generated thought. Excessive focus on negatively valenced or past-related thoughts occur in depression, while excessive focus on overly confident, positive, and grandiose thoughts occurs in manic states. Excessively focal or specific thoughts occur in autism spectrum disorders. Thoughts characterized by an exaggerated concern about likelihood of personal harm are associated with many anxiety disorders, including phobias and obsessive-compulsive disorder. The polarized thought content in these psychiatric disorders could reflect trade-offs between hyper- and hypoactivity or connectivity among default network subsystems, or with default mode and other large-scale brain systems. For example, major depressive disorder and bipolar disorder are associated with enhanced activity and connectivity of the default network with key regions of the limbic and/or salience networks.

KEY POINTS

- Memory includes a variety of processes that allow storage and retrieval of information over variable time periods.
- The hippocampus and surrounding areas of the medial temporal lobe have a crucial role in episodic memory.
- Inputs from the perirhinal cortex channeled via the lateral entorhinal cortex to the anterior hippocampus convey object feature information required for object recognition based on familiarity.
- Inputs from the parahippocampal cortex channeled via the medial entorhinal cortex to the posterior hippocampus convey visuospatial and contextual information for visual navigation and episodic memory.
- Information processed in the hippocampus is conveyed back to the neocortex both via cortico-cortical connections and via the thalamus for consolidation of episodic memories.
- Pattern separation is the ability to distinguish among similar experiences for them to be encoded

and recalled as specific memories and involves the dentate gyrus.

- Pattern completion is the tendency to lump together similar or related experiences or events; it provides a fundamental mechanism for retrieval and involves the autoassociative connections in CA3.
- CA1 pyramidal neurons have a major role in distinguishing between novel and familiar events by integrating inputs from the entorhinal cortex (novel information) and CA3 (stored information).
- Information processed in the hippocampus is fed back via the entorhinal cortex to the perirhinal and parahippocampal cortex and then back to the neocortex.
- Long-term memories are represented in interconnected neocortical networks, where newly acquired memories are overlaid with preexisting semantic information.
- The prefrontal cortex (PFC) may exert a strategic top-down control that allows retrieval of context-appropriate memories while suppressing competing context inappropriate memories.[30]
- The hippocampus has a critical role in navigation by providing a representation of space which may represent a frame to organize all experiences within episodic memories, what is referred to as a "cognitive map."
- The perception of elapsed time (called interval timing) involves the interaction of multiple oscillatory patterns in the prefrontal and parietal areas as well as the hippocampus.
- The hippocampus participates in two large-scale networks: an anterior temporal system and a posteromedial system.
- The anterior temporal system is primarily involved in recognition memory and is centered in the perirhinal cortex.
- The posteromedial system is involved in contextual memory, scene representation, and visual navigation and is centered in the parahippocampal cortex.
- The default network is involved in representation of self-relevant information, construction of mental scenes based on episodic memory, imagining the future, and inferring the mental state of self and others ("mentalizing" or "theory of mind").
- Episodic memory decline is a major symptom in amnestic type mild cognitive impairment (MCI) and amnestic dementias due to Alzheimer disease (AD) pathology.
- The tauopathy that underlies AD typically begins in medial temporal structures before involving temporal and parietal isocortical areas.
- One substrate for memory decline in AD is a shift in hippocampal network dynamics away from pattern separation in the dentate gyrus toward excessive pattern completion in CA3.
- An important feature of cognitive aging is impaired spatial navigation.
- Hippocampal sclerosis is a disorder associated with accumulation of TAR-DNA-binding protein of 43 kD (TDP-43) in the CA1 region and subiculum.
- Asymmetric hippocampal with ipsilateral mammillary atrophy and relative preservation of metabolism in the lateral temporal lobe may help distinguish hippocampal sclerosis from AD.
- Whereas AD affects the core components and the medial temporal subsystem of the default mode network, this network is also affected in behavioral variant frontotemporal dementia (FTD) and the semantic variant of primary progressive aphasia (PPA).
- Focal disorders typically affecting the hippocampus, either in isolation or in association with other portions of the medial temporal lobe memory system, include hypoxic-ischemic injury, herpes simplex encephalitis, autoimmune limbic encephalitis, and ischemic stroke affecting the posterior cerebral artery territory.
- Damage of the anterior temporal lobe involving the perirhinal and adjacent temporopolar cortex, particularly on the left hemisphere, produces deficits in recognition memory.
- Patients with damage of the right parahippocampal cortex are unable to recognize familiar landmarks, which is referred to as topographical disorientation or landmark agnosia.
- Patients with lesions affecting the retrosplenial cortex are unable to use landmarks to orient themselves; this is referred to as topographical amnesia.
- Damage of diencephalic structures connected with the hippocampal formation, including the mammillary bodies, anterior and dorsomedial nuclei of the thalamus, and fornix, may also produce a profound amnestic syndrome, as occurs in Wernicke-Korsakoff syndrome.
- Patients with mesial temporal lobe epilepsy have lateralized material-specific memory deficits.
- Transient epileptic amnesia is a form of anterograde and/or retrograde amnesia that occurs in brief recurrent episodes that commonly occur upon awakening, and are associated with accelerated long-term forgetting and remote memory impairment.
- Transient global amnesia is the acute onset of anterograde and temporally graded amnesia that may be in some cases due to venous stasis affecting the medial temporal lobe.
- Depression is associated with abnormalities in episodic memory.

REFERENCES

1. Milner B, Squire LR, Kandel ER. Cognitive neuroscience and the study of memory. Neuron 1998;20:445–468.
2. Squire LR, Stark CE, Clark RE. The medial temporal lobe. Annu Rev Neurosci 2004;27:279–306.
3. Dickerson BC, Eichenbaum H. The episodic memory system: neurocircuitry and disorders. Neuropsychopharmacology 2010;35:86–104.
4. Eichenbaum H. On the integration of space, time, and memory. Neuron 2017;95:1007–1018.
5. O'Keefe J. Place units in the hippocampus of the freely moving rat. Exp Neurol 1976;51:78–109.
6. Johnson EL, Knight RT. Intracranial recordings and human memory. Curr Opin Neurobiol 2015;31:18–25.
7. Lisman J, Buzsaki G, Eichenbaum H, Nadel L, Ranganath C, Redish AD. Viewpoints: how the hippocampus contributes to memory, navigation and cognition. Nat Neurosci 2017;20:1434–1447.
8. van Strien NM, Cappaert NL, Witter MP. The anatomy of memory: an interactive overview of the parahippocampal-hippocampal network. Nat Rev Neurosci 2009;10:272–282.
9. Strange BA, Witter MP, Lein ES, Moser EI. Functional organization of the hippocampal longitudinal axis. Nat Rev Neurosci 2014;15:655–669.
10. Small SA, Schobel SA, Buxton RB, Witter MP, Barnes CA. A pathophysiological framework of hippocampal dysfunction in ageing and disease. Nat Rev Neurosci 2011;12:585–601.
11. Ranganath C, Ritchey M. Two cortical systems for memory-guided behaviour. Nat Rev Neurosci 2012;13:713–726.
12. Marr D. Simple memory: a theory for archicortex. Philos Trans R Soc Lond B Biol Sci 1971;262:23–81.
13. Leal SL, Yassa MA. Integrating new findings and examining clinical applications of pattern separation. Nat Neurosci 2018;21:163–173.
14. Bakker A, Kirwan CB, Miller M, Stark CE. Pattern separation in the human hippocampal CA3 and dentate gyrus. Science 2008;319:1640–1642.
15. Hainmueller T, Bartos M. Dentate gyrus circuits for encoding, retrieval and discrimination of episodic memories. Nat Rev Neurosci 2020;21:153–168.
16. Aimone JB, Deng W, Gage FH. Resolving new memories: a critical look at the dentate gyrus, adult neurogenesis, and pattern separation. Neuron 2011;70:589–596.
17. Piatti VC, Ewell LA, Leutgeb JK. Neurogenesis in the dentate gyrus: carrying the message or dictating the tone. Front Neurosci 2013;7:50.
18. Spalding KL, Bergmann O, Alkass K, et al. Dynamics of hippocampal neurogenesis in adult humans. Cell 2013;153:1219–1227.
19. McNaughton BL, Barnes CA, Rao G, Baldwin J, Rasmussen M. Long-term enhancement of hippocampal synaptic transmission and the acquisition of spatial information. J Neurosci 1986;6:563–571.
20. Duncan K, Ketz N, Inati SJ, Davachi L. Evidence for area CA1 as a match/mismatch detector: a high-resolution fMRI study of the human hippocampus. Hippocampus 2012;22:389–398.
21. Kumaran D, Maguire EA. Match mismatch processes underlie human hippocampal responses to associative novelty. J Neurosci 2007;27:8517–8524.
22. Vogt BA. Cingulate cortex in the three limbic subsystems. Handb Clin Neurol 2019;166:39–51.
23. McKenzie S, Eichenbaum H. Consolidation and reconsolidation: two lives of memories? Neuron 2011;71:224–233.
24. Wilson MA, McNaughton BL. Reactivation of hippocampal ensemble memories during sleep. Science 1994;265:676–679.
25. Buzsaki G. The hippocampo-neocortical dialogue. Cereb Cortex 1996;6:81–92.
26. Hobson JA, Pace-Schott EF. The cognitive neuroscience of sleep: neuronal systems, consciousness and learning. Nat Rev Neurosci 2002;3:679–693.
27. Frankland PW, Bontempi B. The organization of recent and remote memories. Nat Rev Neurosci 2005;6:119–130.
28. Eichenbaum H. Prefrontal-hippocampal interactions in episodic memory. Nat Rev Neurosci 2017;18:547–558.
29. van Kesteren MT, Ruiter DJ, Fernandez G, Henson RN. How schema and novelty augment memory formation. Trends Neurosci 2012;35:211–219.
30. Keene CS, Bladon J, McKenzie S, Liu CD, O'Keefe J, Eichenbaum H. Complementary functional organization of neuronal activity patterns in the perirhinal, lateral entorhinal, and medial entorhinal cortices. J Neurosci 2016;36:3660–3675.
31. Ketz NA, Jensen O, O'Reilly RC. Thalamic pathways underlying prefrontal cortex-medial temporal lobe oscillatory interactions. Trends Neurosci 2015;38:3–12.
32. Cassel JC, Pereira de Vasconcelos A, Loureiro M, Cholvin T, Dalrymple-Alford JC, Vertes RP. The reuniens and rhomboid nuclei: neuroanatomy, electrophysiological characteristics and behavioral implications. Prog Neurobiol 2013;111:34–52.
33. Benchenane K, Peyrache A, Khamassi M, et al. Coherent theta oscillations and reorganization of spike timing in the hippocampal-prefrontal network upon learning. Neuron 2010;66:921–936.
34. Backus AR, Schoffelen JM, Szebenyi S, Hanslmayr S, Doeller CF. Hippocampal-prefrontal theta oscillations support memory integration. Curr Biol 2016;26:450–457.
35. Anderson MC, Bunce JG, Barbas H. Prefrontal-hippocampal pathways underlying inhibitory control over memory. Neurobiol Learn Mem 2016;134 Pt A:145–161.
36. Schmitz TW, Correia MM, Ferreira CS, Prescot AP, Anderson MC. Hippocampal GABA enables inhibitory control over unwanted thoughts. Nat Commun 2017;8:1311.
37. Lester AW, Moffat SD, Wiener JM, Barnes CA, Wolbers T. The aging navigational system. Neuron 2017;95:1019–1035.
38. Epstein RA, Patai EZ, Julian JB, Spiers HJ. The cognitive map in humans: spatial navigation and beyond. Nat Neurosci 2017;20:1504–1513.
39. Moser EI, Kropff E, Moser MB. Place cells, grid cells, and the brain's spatial representation system. Annu Rev Neurosci 2008;31:69–89.
40. Moser EI, Moser MB, McNaughton BL. Spatial representation in the hippocampal formation: a history. Nat Neurosci 2017;20:1448–1464.
41. Rolls ET, Wirth S. Spatial representations in the primate hippocampus, and their functions in memory and navigation. Prog Neurobiol 2018;171:90–113.
42. Sanders H, Renno-Costa C, Idiart M, Lisman J. Grid cells and place cells: an integrated view of their navigational and memory function. Trends Neurosci 2015;38:763–775.

43. Cullen KE, Taube JS. Our sense of direction: progress, controversies and challenges. Nat Neurosci 2017;20:1465–1473.
44. Morgan LK, Macevoy SP, Aguirre GK, Epstein RA. Distances between real-world locations are represented in the human hippocampus. J Neurosci 2011;31:1238–1245.
45. Horner AJ, Bisby JA, Zotow E, Bush D, Burgess N. Grid-like processing of imagined navigation. Curr Biol 2016;26:842–847.
46. Ekstrom AD, Kahana MJ, Caplan JB, et al. Cellular networks underlying human spatial navigation. Nature 2003;425:184–188.
47. Jacobs J, Weidemann CT, Miller JF, et al. Direct recordings of grid-like neuronal activity in human spatial navigation. Nat Neurosci 2013;16:1188–1190.
48. Miyashita Y. Perirhinal circuits for memory processing. Nat Rev Neurosci 2019;20:577–592.
49. Martin CB, McLean DA, O'Neil EB, Kohler S. Distinct familiarity-based response patterns for faces and buildings in perirhinal and parahippocampal cortex. J Neurosci 2013;33:10915–10923.
50. Vann SD, Aggleton JP, Maguire EA. What does the retrosplenial cortex do? Nat Rev Neurosci 2009;10:792–802.
51. Connor CE, Knierim JJ. Integration of objects and space in perception and memory. Nat Neurosci 2017;20:1493–1503.
52. Raichle ME. The brain's default mode network. Annu Rev Neurosci 2015;38:433–447.
53. Andrews-Hanna JR, Smallwood J, Spreng RN. The default network and self-generated thought: component processes, dynamic control, and clinical relevance. Ann N Y Acad Sci 2014;1316:29–52.
54. Fox KC, Andrews-Hanna JR, Christoff K. The neurobiology of self-generated thought from cells to systems: integrating evidence from lesion studies, human intracranial electrophysiology, neurochemistry, and neuroendocrinology. Neuroscience 2016;335:134–150.
55. Buckner RL, DiNicola LM. The brain's default network: updated anatomy, physiology and evolving insights. Nat Rev Neurosci 2019;20:593–608.
56. Sormaz M, Murphy C, Wang HT, et al. Default mode network can support the level of detail in experience during active task states. Proc Natl Acad Sci U S A 2018;115:9318–9323.
57. Fox KCR, Foster BL, Kucyi A, Daitch AL, Parvizi J. Intracranial electrophysiology of the human default network. Trends Cogn Sci 2018;22:307–324.
58. Braak H, Braak E. Staging of Alzheimer's disease-related neurofibrillary changes. Neurobiol Aging 1995;16:271–278; discussion 278–284.
59. Palmer A, Good M. Hippocampal synaptic activity, pattern separation and episodic-like memory: implications for mouse models of Alzheimer's disease pathology. Biochem Soc Trans 2011;39:902–909.
60. Salmon DP. Neuropsychological features of mild cognitive impairment and preclinical Alzheimer's disease. Curr Top Behav Neurosci 2012;10:187–212.
61. Yassa MA, Mattfeld AT, Stark SM, Stark CE. Age-related memory deficits linked to circuit-specific disruptions in the hippocampus. Proc Natl Acad Sci U S A 2011;108:8873–8878.
62. Hasselmo ME, Bower JM. Acetylcholine and memory. Trends Neurosci 1993;16:218–222.
63. Botha H, Mantyh WG, Murray ME, et al. FDG-PET in tau-negative amnestic dementia resembles that of autopsy-proven hippocampal sclerosis. Brain 2018;141:1201–1217.
64. Jicha GA, Nelson PT. Hippocampal sclerosis, argyrophilic grain disease, and primary age-related tauopathy. Continuum (Minneap Minn) 2019;25:208–233.
65. Jefferson-George KS, Wolk DA, Lee EB, McMillan CT. Cognitive decline associated with pathological burden in primary age-related tauopathy. Alzheimers Dement 2017;13:1048–1053.
66. Bell WR, An Y, Kageyama Y, et al. Neuropathologic, genetic, and longitudinal cognitive profiles in primary age-related tauopathy (PART) and Alzheimer's disease. Alzheimers Dement 2019;15:8–16.
67. Kambaja B, Dupont S. Amnesia, memory disturbances and epilepsy. Geriatr Psychol Neuropsychiatr Vieil 2016;14:415–419.
68. Arena JE, Rabinstein AA. Transient global amnesia. Mayo Clin Proc 2015;90:264–272.

41 Language

OVERVIEW

Language is a cognitive function that involves core areas primarily located in the dominant (usually left) hemisphere and interconnected via several pathways. Whereas most studies have focused on spoken language the same organizational principles apply to written and sign language. Thus the focus of this chapter will be on spoken language. The language network includes both relatively functional specialized brain regions and areas that are components of domain-general cognitive control networks.[1] Processing of spoken language requires a set of cognitive operations that allow the transition from sound to meaning for language comprehension, and from meaning to sound for language production. The core areas involved in these processes are located in the inferior frontal gyrus; superior temporal cortex and inferior parietal lobule; anterior temporal lobe; and posterior middle temporal gyrus (Figure 41.1).[2–4] Different portions of these core areas form separate networks for semantic or syntactic processes and are interconnected by two ventral and two dorsal pathways respectively. Speech production is regulated at multiple hierarchical levels. Whereas vocalizations involve an innate brainstem mechanism, production of meaningful speech involves a widespread network that includes prefrontal, premotor, and motor cortical areas as well as the cerebellum. Semantic knowledge is a fundamental cognitive process for all tasks of everyday life, including language comprehension.[3] The main aims of this chapter are to review: (1) the cognitive operations involved in language comprehension and production, (2) the core areas and connecting pathways involved in these processes, (3) the mechanisms of voice and speech production, (4) the semantic networks providing the basis for language and other cognitive functions.

LANGUAGE

Spoken language comprises distinct linguistic units and rules to combine them. A phoneme is a sound feature that makes the difference between two words; these features and their combination are part of phonology. Lexicon is the store of all word forms, including both their syntactic category (e.g., noun or verb) and their respective meaning associated with their semantic features (e.g., human, female). This lexicon is learned and then stored in long-term memory. Syntax is a set of rules that guides the combination of words into phrases and sentences.

Comprehension of Spoken Language

Comprehension of spoken language is the mapping from sound to meaning. This involves three core components: form (i.e., speech sounds or phonemes, word forms or graphemes), syntactic structure, and meaning (semantic knowledge). These three components also apply to written and sign language. Word recognition is the entrance point for the retrieval of semantic and syntactic information from what is referred to as the mental lexicon. This information is encoded and consolidated in long-term memory, primarily in the inferior parietal and temporal neocortex in the course of language acquisition. Language processing also requires the ability to combine these lexical elements from memory to derive complex meaning; this process has been referred to as unification and involves the areas of the left frontal cortex. Linguistic marking of information structure (emphasis) and nonlinguistic input (e.g., co-speech gestures, visual context) are immediately integrated for processing of language.

Production of Spoken Language

Language production is the mapping of meaning into words. The preverbal message is transformed into a sequence of speech sounds. Studies focused on single word production such as picture naming show that the process from the stage of conceptual preparation to the final articulation takes about 600 milliseconds and is then performed in an incremental fashion allowing the production of 2–4

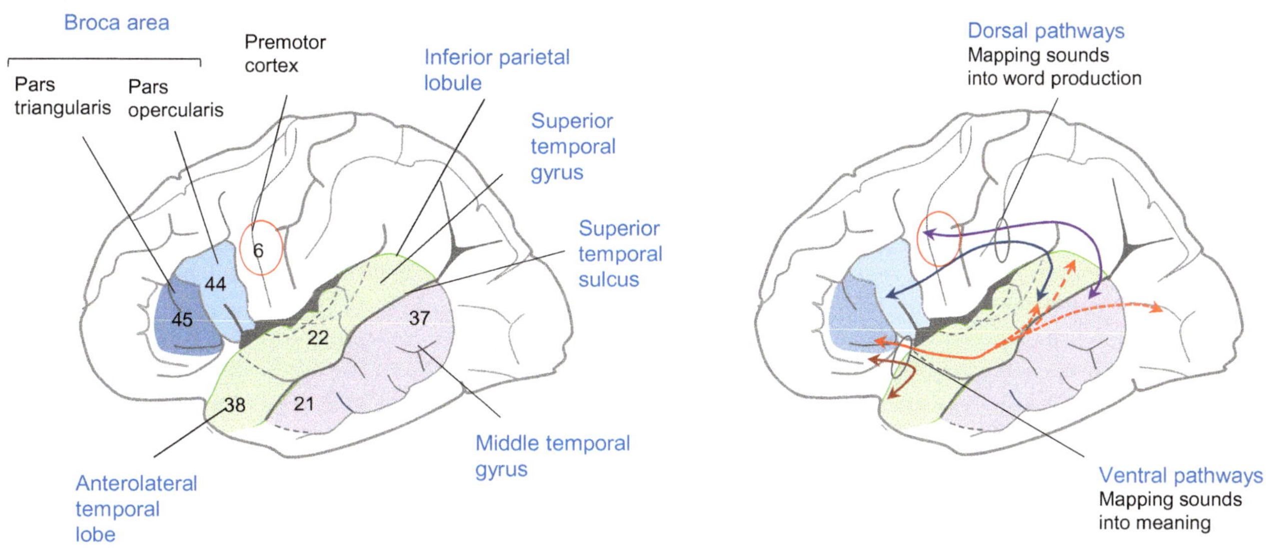

FIGURE 41.1 Core language areas

The core areas for spoken language are located in right-handed and in a substantial proportion of left-handed persons in the inferior frontal gyrus, including Broca area (areas 44/45), posterior superior temporal gyrus, inferior parietal lobule, anterior temporal lobe, and posterior middle temporal gyrus. Similar areas on the right hemisphere also participate in language processing. Different areas in the temporal and parietal cortex store information about word form, word meanings, and syntactic templates and interact with areas in the inferior frontal gyrus, including Broca area and adjacent cortex, which are crucial for unification operations for word production and sentence formation. These areas are interconnected via two dorsal and two ventral pathways.

words per second. Like comprehension, speech production also requires the retrieval of building blocks from memory and their unification at multiple levels. A prominent theory assumes that there is a most basic syntactic operation, called "Merge," that binds two elements, such as "the" and "house" together into a syntactic hierarchy; application of this operation several times leads to the building of sentences.

Core Language Areas

Studies in patients with aphasia lead to the concept that the left perisylvian cortex contains the crucial network for supporting the processing of language. According to the classical Wernicke-Lichtheim-Geschwind model, the key components of the language network are Broca area in the left inferior frontal cortex for speech production, Wernicke area in the left superior temporal cortex and inferior parietal lobule for speech comprehension, and their mutual connections via the arcuate fasciculus for speech repetition. However, functional neuroimaging studies have largely disproved this classical model.[4] Current evidence points instead to the presence of a much more extended network of language processing areas, not only in the left hemisphere, but also in homologous areas in the right hemisphere (Figure 41.1).[5–8] Both Broca and Wernicke areas are functionally heterogeneous. For example, area 44 (pars opercularis) is a distinct portion of Broca region that is coupled to parallel and overlapping large-scale networks and participates in language, cognitive, and motor functions. In addition to Broca and Wernicke areas, the left anterior temporal lobe and the posterior middle temporal gyrus have a major role in language processing. The left anterior temporal lobe is critical for semantic cognition; the posterior medial temporal gyrus appears to be a crucial lexical node due to its heavy connections to both the anterior temporal lobe and other language areas. One alternative model of language processing is the memory, unification, and control model.[9] In this model, different areas in the temporal and parietal cortex store information about word form, word meanings, and syntactic templates that have been laid down in memory during language acquisition and form the building blocks for language comprehension and production. These areas interact with areas in the inferior frontal gyrus, including Broca area and adjacent cortex, which are crucial for unification operations that generate larger structures from the building blocks that are retrieved from memory in temporoparietal regions. These interactions support the three core types of information that are crucial for language—phonological, syntactic, and semantic.

The dorsolateral prefrontal cortex (PFC) and anterior cingulate cortex are involved in executive control of these operations.

Networks for Semantic and Syntax Processing

Lexical-semantic processing is the mapping of words into meaning. This process involves a network that includes areas of the temporoparietal cortex and inferior frontal gyrus. Temporal and parietal regions, particularly the angular gyrus and the supramarginal gyrus, are part of

Wernicke area and may support the storage or representation of lexical–semantic information. The inferior frontal gyrus, including pars triangularis in classical Broca area (area 45) and adjacent pars orbitalis (area 47), is involved in semantic retrieval and manipulation.

Syntax is a set of rules for generation of complex structures such as sentences. The neural substrate for the processing of syntactically complex sentences involves a second large-scale frontotemporal network that includes core regions in the left posterior superior temporal gyrus and sulcus and the pars orbicularis in Broca area (area 44). The left posterior temporal cortex may be important for the retrieval of the syntactic frames that are stored in the lexicon. These individual frames are then connected into a configuration of phrases by recruiting Broca area 44. This area is the site of the low-level syntactic operation of "Merge" that assembles words into hierarchies such as article, noun, or verb. This operation provides for the ability to create structures such as sentences out of single words. For the processing of sentences, Broca area 44 works together with a syntax-related working memory system located in the left inferior frontal sulcus. These two regions are connected by short-range pathways and show functional coupling during the processing of complex syntactic structures. This left inferior frontal network is part of a large-scale network that includes areas in the posterior temporal and parietal lobes and inferior part of the posterior superior temporal sulcus and gyrus, which function as an integrative processor. Both activation of left area 44 and its coupling with the left inferior parietal lobule are reduced in patients with stuttering.[10]

Pathways Within the Language Networks

The core regions in the language network are interconnected by two dorsal and two ventral pathways (Figure 41.2). The two dorsal pathways are involved in mapping sound into production words; the two ventral pathway are involved in mapping of words into meaning. One dorsal pathway supports speech repetition. This process requires the perception of speech, phonological working memory to hold the perceived information, and aspects of speech production such as articulatory planning and execution. The cortical network supporting repetition includes the

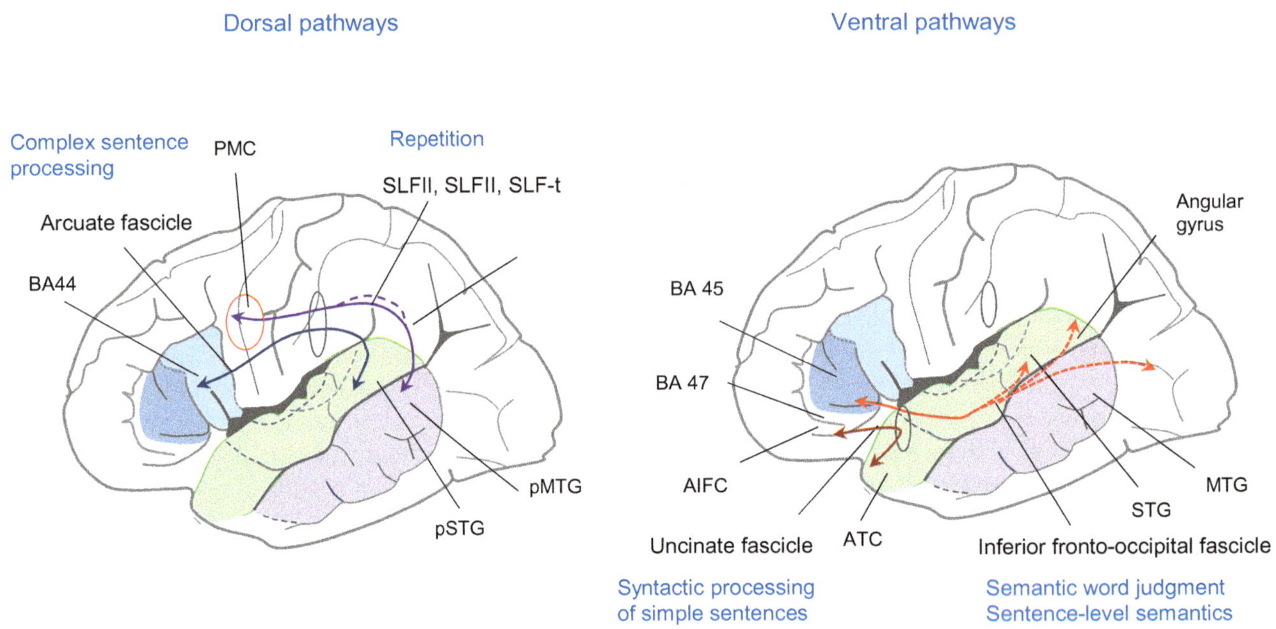

FIGURE 41.2 Pathways within the language network
The core regions in the language network are interconnected by at least two dorsal and two ventral pathways. The two dorsal pathways are involved in mapping sound into production words. One such pathway is via components of the superior longitudinal fascicle (SLF) that indirectly connects the middle temporal gyrus (MTG) to the premotor cortex (PMC) through the inferior parietal cortex; this pathways supports speech repetition. The SLF consists of (SLFI, SLFII, and SLFIII) and a temporoparietal bundle (SLF-tp) that connects the angular gyrus to the temporal cortex. The second dorsal pathway is the arcuate fascicle, which connects the posterior superior temporal gyrus (pSTG) and MTG to Broca area (BA) 44. The two ventral pathways include the uncinate fascicle that connects the anterior temporal cortex (ATC) with anterior inferior frontal cortex (AIFC) and has a role in syntactic processing of simple sentences. The inferior fronto-occipital fascicle connects the posterior temporal, parietal, and occipital cortices with the inferior frontal and dorsolateral prefrontal cortices. After passing through the anterior floor of the external capsule, this fascicle courses medially in the temporal lobe and sends radiations to the middle and superior temporal gyri. These projections participate in semantic processing.

auditory input system in the superior temporal gyrus and planum temporale (supporting phonological discrimination), the inferior parietal cortex (supporting phonological working memory), and the premotor cortex (organizing speech output). The pathway for speech repetition involves different components of the superior longitudinal fascicle (SLF), which indirectly connects the middle temporal gyrus to the premotor cortex through the inferior parietal cortex and includes several components. The SLF II component connects the angular gyrus with the dorsal premotor and prefrontal cortices; the SLF III connects the supramarginal gyrus with ventral prefrontal areas; and the temporoparietal bundle (SLF-tp) connects the angular gyrus to the temporal cortex. The second dorsal pathway is the arcuate fascicle, which is relevant for complex syntactic processing. The arcuate fascicle connects the posterior superior and middle temporal gyrus to Broca area 44 and is strongly lateralized to the left hemisphere. Intraoperative stimulation of the arcuate fascicle leads to phonological and syntactical errors; lesions in this fiber tract impair processing complex syntactic structures.

The two ventral pathways interconnecting core components of the language network participate in processing sounds into meaning. They include the uncinate fascicle and the inferior fronto-occipital fascicle. The uncinate fascicle connects the anterior temporal cortex with the anterior inferior frontal cortex and is involved in syntactic processing of simple sentences. The inferior fronto-occipital fascicle, also known as extreme capsule fiber system, connects the posterior temporal, parietal, and occipital cortices with the inferior frontal and dorsolateral prefrontal cortices. This fascicle also sends radiations to the middle and superior temporal gyri. These projections participate in semantic processing by connecting areas 45 and 47 in the inferior frontal cortex with the areas in the middle and superior temporal gyrus. Areas 45 and 47 support semantic word judgment, categorization, and other aspects of semantic plausibility within sentences; the middle temporal and posterior superior temporal gyrus, together with the angular gyrus, support sentence-level semantics. Intraoperative stimulation of the inferior fronto-occipital fascicle elicited semantic paraphasias.

Interactions Between Core Language Areas

Language processing involves the dynamic interplay between the core areas in the left posterior temporal and parietal areas and left inferior frontal cortical areas. The lexical information of each individual word is rapidly retrieved and unified within the context of a sentence via co-modulation between these anterior and posterior core cortical regions. From the early stages of processing, these core language areas are supported by the attentional network and by context-based predictions. Local connectivity within the posterior temporal cortex and angular gyrus result in activation of neighboring neuronal populations coding for related lexical-semantic information. Feedforward projections from these posterior regions produce selective activation of populations of neurons in the left inferior frontal cortex; these neurons respond with a self-sustaining firing and send efferent feedback signals back to the same temporoparietal regions that were the source of their input. During each word-processing reverberatory cycle, the interaction between the memory component in the temporoparietal region and the unification component in the inferior frontal region leads to strengthening of connections, which maintain lexical information active over time in working memory. There is also a complex interplay between motor and auditory processes during speech production, involving the online comparison of the speech output with an internally generated forward model. Auditory cortical areas are involved in an active comparison between the prediction and the actual sensory input. Subsequently, these areas interact with motor areas to generate a motor response.

Network Activity in Language Areas

The basic linguistic units such as phonemes and words are assumed to be represented by small ensembles of temporarily cooperating neurons. The flexible recombination of feature-selective neurons into different assemblies allows a large number of phoneme combinations to be encoded by a relatively small number of neurons. The generation of transient spatiotemporal patterns of distributed neuronal responses provides for the processing of syntactic sequences and the binding of words into phrases and sentences. The integration of syntactic and semantic information during sentence processing reflects the activation of large numbers of neurons coordinated in different patterns on each occasion. Coherence of small, spatially restricted assemblies involves synchronization of oscillatory activity in the gamma frequency range (30–80 Hz), whereas coherence in large, spatially extended assemblies involves synchronization of oscillations in lower-frequency bands (beta, 15–30 Hz; theta, 4–8 Hz). In tasks with high memory load or requiring extended search of stored information, coherence increases in the theta range within a large-scale network involving inferior frontal and temporoparietal cortex.

Role of the Lateral Prefrontal Cortex in Speech

Auditory information reaches the lateral PFC via a posterodorsal and an anteroventral stream of sensory processing originating from the primary auditory cortex. The posterodorsal stream encodes auditory space (i.e., spatial location of the stimulus). It originates in posterior belt and parabelt regions of the auditory association cortex and projects to the dorsolateral PFC, both directly and via the posterior parietal association cortex. The dorsolateral PFC is engaged in auditory working memory tasks. The anteroventral stream encodes auditory identity (auditory features of an object). It originates in anterior belt and parabelt areas of the auditory association cortex, and projects to the ventrolateral PFC, both directly and via the temporal association cortex in the anterior superior temporal gyrus. The ventrolateral PFC is engaged during selective retrieval of verbal and nonverbal auditory information via its interactions with both the auditory temporal region providing object information and the inferior parietal lobule providing spatial information. Neurons in the ventrolateral PFC respond to human vocalizations and particularly to face-voice combinations, thereby processing and integrating social communication via speech and gestures. These neurons also establish semantic associations, which require interactions between the PFC and the medial temporal lobe. Functional MRI studies show that the ventrolateral PFC is more active in children learning semantic associations compared to proficient adults;[11] in contrast, adults more than children recruit the left intraparietal sulcus].[12]

Central Representation of Writing

Writing is complex process that ranges from visual control to hand control.[13] The posterior part of the left superior frontal sulcus, also known as the "graphemic motor frontal area" (Exner area), and the left superior parietal cortex, including the superior parietal lobule and anterior intraparietal sulcus, are involved in writing. Lesions in these regions are the most common cause of apraxic ("pure") agraphia. Functional neuroimaging studies revealed that these core areas, as well many other areas, are activated not only during writing tasks but also during drawing, naming of pictures, and some oral spelling.[13] These areas include the left ventral premotor area (which may be involved in storage of the motor representation of letters), posterior inferior temporal cortex (visual word form area, which may be involved in the storage or recovery or the visual graphic images of words), and right posterior cerebellum, However, only the graphemic motor area in the superior frontal sulcus showed a writing-specific lateralization to the left hemisphere in right-handed persons, as well as bilateral activity during drawing.[13]

SPEECH

The ability to speak is regulated by complex mechanisms coordinated by high-level cortical signaling, brainstem reflexes, peripheral nerves and muscles controlling the larynx and orofacial movement. Nonlanguage voice production, such as crying, whistling, and sighing use larynx, lips, tongue and jaw movements integrated at the level of the brainstem, In contrast, speech articulation requires the appropriate and control of muscle activity by the cerebral cortex. According to a dual network model, a volitional articulatory motor network originating in the PFC including Broca area cognitively controls a primary vocal motor network located in subcortical areas[14] (Figure 41.3).

Nonverbal Vocalizations

The lowest level of the hierarchical system for voice production includes the medullary reticular formation and phonatory motor and sensory cranial nerve nuclei. The brainstem vocal pattern generator consists of the periaqueductal gray (PAG) and ventrolateral pontine reticular formation. The PAG is an important component of the emotional motor system and receives strong projections from the amygdala, anterior cingulate, insula, and orbitofrontal cortical areas. The PAG provides strong projections to the nucleus retroambiguus, located in the caudal ventrolateral medulla. This nucleus provides inputs to all motoneurons involved in vocalization, including cranial motoneurons innervating soft palate, pharynx, larynx, and spinal motoneurons innervating respiratory muscles necessary for generating vocalization. This level of control is responsible for production of genetically preprogrammed innate vocalizations, including the cry or laugh of an infant. As children develop and become capable of learning and mimicking vocal utterances, innate vocalizations become increasingly more voluntary; for example cry can be produced without an emotional stimulus or suppressed despite the presence of discomfort. This level of vocal control requires input from the dorsal pregenual anterior cingulate cortex to the PAG. The anterior cingulate cortex, together with the lateral hypothalamus, may participate in the uncontrollable laughter that occurs in elastic seizures.[15] However, lesions in other cortical areas connected with the PAG may result in similar manifestations.[16] Lesions affecting either the cingulate cortex or PAG may result in akinetic mutism.[17]

Volitional Articulatory Motor Network

Speech production requires a series of cognitive and motor events. Once phonological planning has begun, fluent speech requires coordination of respiration, phonation, articulation, resonance, and prosody.[18] The voluntary motor articulation network encompasses a widespread network that includes the inferior frontal gyrus (Broca area 44 and 45) ventral premotor cortex (PMv), and the ventrolateral portion of the primary motor cortex (M1, area 4), containing the representation of the larynx and orofacial muscles (Figure 41.3). Functional neuroimaging studies also show recruitment of the supplementary motor area (SMA), presupplementary motor area (preSMA), superior temporal gyrus, inferior parietal lobule, cerebellum, putamen, and thalamus during speech production.[10] The interactions between these areas are bilaterally distributed but interregional connectivity during speaking is stronger in the left than in the right hemisphere.[19,20] A functional MRI study showed that several of these regions also respond to nonarticulation tasks that share features with speech production.[21] The articulation-selective regions only included the left inferior frontal gyrus and left superior temporal cortex. In contrast, the right inferior frontal gyrus, precentral gyrus, SMA, and the cerebellum responded as strongly during the production of nonspeech oral-motor movements and respiration as during articulation. Whereas articulation is a cognitively complex attention-demanding behavior, the articulation-selective regions in the posterior

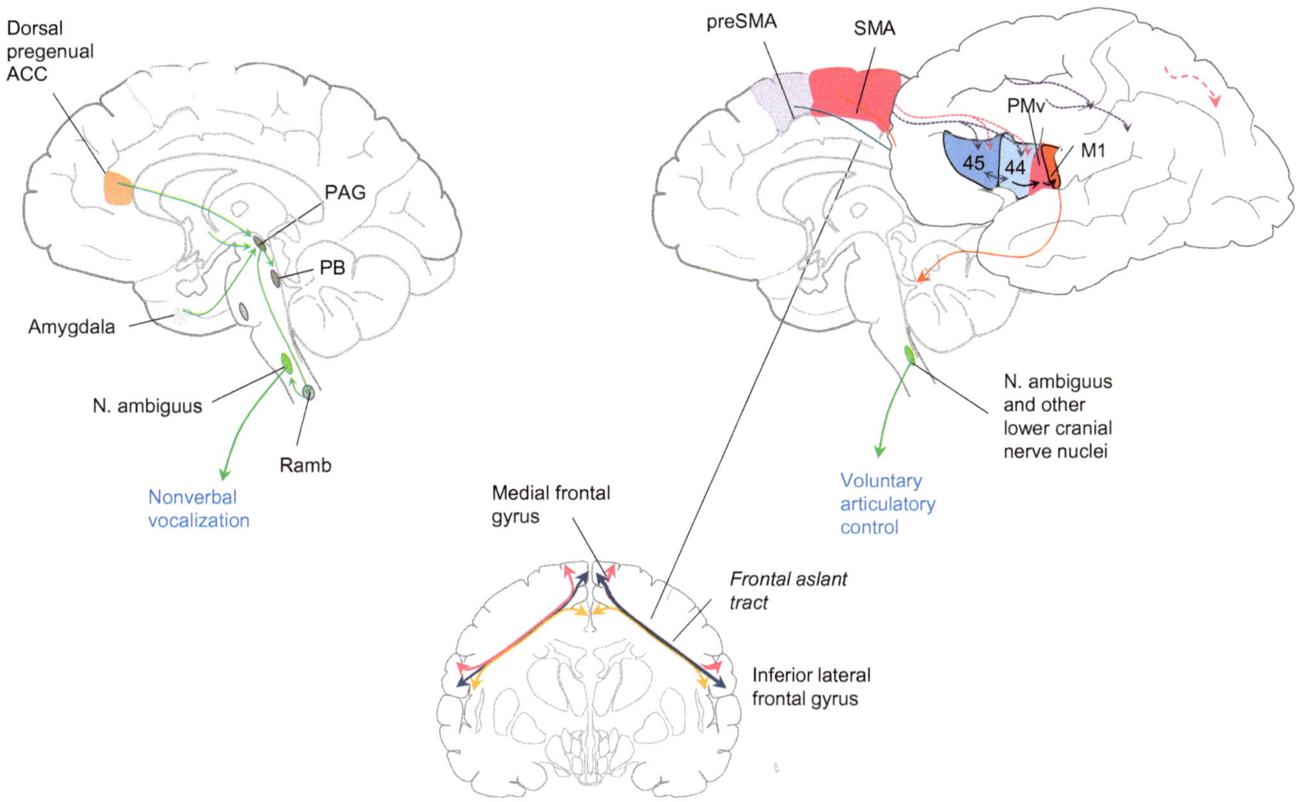

FIGURE 41.3 Control of vocalization and speech

The brainstem vocal pattern generator consists of the periaqueductal gray (PAG), parabrachial nucleus (PB), medullary parvocellular formation (not shown), and nucleus retroambiguus (Ramb), which controls the phonatory motoneurons located in the nucleus ambiguus and other cranial nerve nuclei. Emotional vocal control requires input from the anterior midcingulate cortex to the PAG. Other emotion-related inputs to the PAG originate in the amygdala (Am) and hypothalamus. The voluntary motor articulation network includes the inferior frontal gyrus, including Broca areas 44 and 45, ventral premotor cortex (PMv), and the primary motor cortex (M1) containing the representation of the larynx and orofacial muscles. A direct projection from the laryngeal motor cortex to the nucleus ambiguus enables a direct coordination of complex movements for voluntary vocal control. The supplementary motor area (SMA) and presupplementary motor area (preSMA), as well as the superior temporal gyrus, inferior parietal lobule, cerebellum, putamen, and thalamus (not shown) are components of this network.

left inferior frontal gyrus/frontal operculum and superior temporal gyrus were spatially and functionally distinct from the nearby domain-general frontoparietal network regions involved in attention and executive function.[21]

The ventrolateral PFC is a core region of the volitional articulatory control network. It receives highly processed sensory information of all posterior cortical areas and maintains communicative signals in working memory to guide goal-directed speech output. Broca area 44 contains distinct clusters associated with action processing, sequencing, linguistic working memory, task-switching, and meaning.[22] Broca area coordinates the transformation of information across large-scale cortical networks and formulates an appropriate articulatory code to be implemented by motor cortex.[23] Regarding syntax, Broca area processes start- and endpoints of higher-order motor segments and forms a hierarchical structure of motor plans. In contrast, the PMv and SMA are more involved in in the precise timing of ongoing motor acts and sequences required for articulation.[24] Direct cortical surface recordings in neurosurgical patients showed that during the cued production of words, Broca area becomes silent while motor cortex is activated.[23] Broca area 44 is connected to the anterior PMv, which in turn sends projections to the speech motor cortex. The anterior PMv integrates sensorimotor signals from the posterior parietal cortex with cognitive signals from the ventrolateral PFC, pre-SMA, and anterior midcingulate cortex. The role of the insula in speech control is still poorly understood. The anterior insula is functionally interconnected with Broca area 44, the midinsula with area 4, and the posterior insula with area 22 in the superior temporal gyrus involved in sound processing.[25]

The speech motor cortex in ventral M1 has a dorsal-to-ventral somatotopic representation controlling the movements of the lips, jaw, tongue, and pharynx/larynx along the central sulcus.[19] There is a partially overlapping representation of articulators and two separate representations of the larynx, one ventral to the tongue and a second dorsal to the lips. In addition to a bilateral projection from the motor cortex to orofacial motor nuclei, in humans there is a direct projection from the laryngeal motor cortex to the nucleus ambiguus, which enables fast and direct coordination of complex laryngeal, orofacial, and respiratory movements that facilitate learning and voluntary vocal control.

The volitional articulatory motor network may exert a modulatory control on the nonverbal vocalization network; nonverbal emotional vocalizations may emerge as the voluntary articulatory control vanishes.[26] The lateral frontal cortex may gain control over articulation via disinhibition of articulatory motor activity briefly before the vocal output. For example, experimental studies indicate that vocal tics emerge as a consequence of dysrhythmic alpha coupling between critical nodes in the limbic and motor networks, including the nucleus accumbens, anterior midcingulate cortex, and primary motor cortex.[27]

Role of Medial Frontal Areas in Speech Control

During motor-related cognitive tasks such as action language processing, there is activation of several premotor areas, including not only the ventral and dorsal premotor cortex but also medial frontal motor areas, the SMA, and preSMA. Action sentence processing activates both SMA and preSMA. Whereas the SMA is involved in action language processing related to motor planning and execution, the pre-SMA may be involved in high-order processing such as sequencing, intention of action, or motor inhibition. The frontal aslant tract, so named due to its oblique course in the frontal white matter, is a U-fiber system that connects preSMA, SMA, and anterior cingulate cortex with the posterior inferior frontal gyrus and dorsal anterior insula. Functional neuroimaging, physiological recordings, effects of lesions, and findings in patients with stuttering and primary progressive aphasia indicate that the left frontal aslant tract is strongly associated with speech initiation and verbal fluency. Verbal fluency tasks typically require a participant to produce words beginning with a particular letter (e.g., "f") in phonological fluency tasks, or representing a particular category (e.g., "animals") in semantic or category fluency tasks. Both tasks recruit the left inferior frontal gyrus and the pre-SMA/SMA.

Role of the Right Hemisphere in Language Processing and Speech Control

Whereas the core language regions are lateralized to the dominant (usually left) hemisphere, effects of lesions, Wada test, and split-brain studies suggest that speech perception is bilaterally processed. The nondominant hemisphere appears to be selective for longer-term integration and has a major role in for processing of prosodic features such as emotional tone, which are important facets of everyday communication. The right inferior frontal gyrus may be involved in executive function, specifically inhibitory control. Whereas the left inferior frontal gyrus is involved in speech production, the right inferior frontal gyrus is primarily activated during action inhibition. During speech production tasks, patients who stutter have larger activation of the right inferior frontal gyrus compared to persons who do not stutter, suggesting a hyperactive mechanism to stop speech motor responses in stuttering.[10]

The right inferior frontal gyrus has a role in top-down executive control of motor responses and is recruited during Go/No Go and Stop-Signal experimental paradigms. The right inferior frontal gyrus receives inputs from the preSMA and SMA via the frontal aslant tract and projects to the subthalamic nucleus via the hyperdirect pathway, which triggers action inhibition.

Cerebellum and Speech

The cerebellum regulates the temporal online sequencing and adaptation of basic speech movement patterns into words, phrases, and sentences. Functional MRI studies show substantial activation of fronto-cerebellar network both during the prearticulatory (internal, covert) phase of speech and during overt speech production. This activation is lateralized to the left cerebral cortex and right cerebellum. The cerebellum is actively involved in language and speech production independently of its motor function. The cerebellum participates in language through monitoring and coordinating cortical functions via timing and sequencing mechanisms.[28] Transcranial magnetic stimulation (TMS) using continued theta-burst protocol (inhibitory) over the right posterior lateral cerebellum during a semantic fluency task (groceries or animals) elicited a reduction of ability to switch between subcategories of words in normal subjects.[29] These findings are consistent with the role of the cerebellum in executive control via its interaction with the frontal cortex.

SEMANTIC COGNITION

Semantic knowledge is the transformation of multiple types of sensory information into meaning. This is a fundamental cognitive process that extends beyond language as all tasks of everyday life require knowledge of objects and their action.[3,30] Semantic cognition may depend on two interacting systems, one for object representation and a second for control[3] (Figure 41.4). The semantic object representation system involves the ventrolateral anterior temporal lobes. This system encodes knowledge of objects acquired through learning of high-order associations among widely distributed sources of sensory, affective, motor, and linguistic information. The semantic control network includes the PFC, posterior middle temporal gyrus, intraparietal sulcus, preSMA, and anterior cingulate cortex. This system manipulates the activations within the representational system to

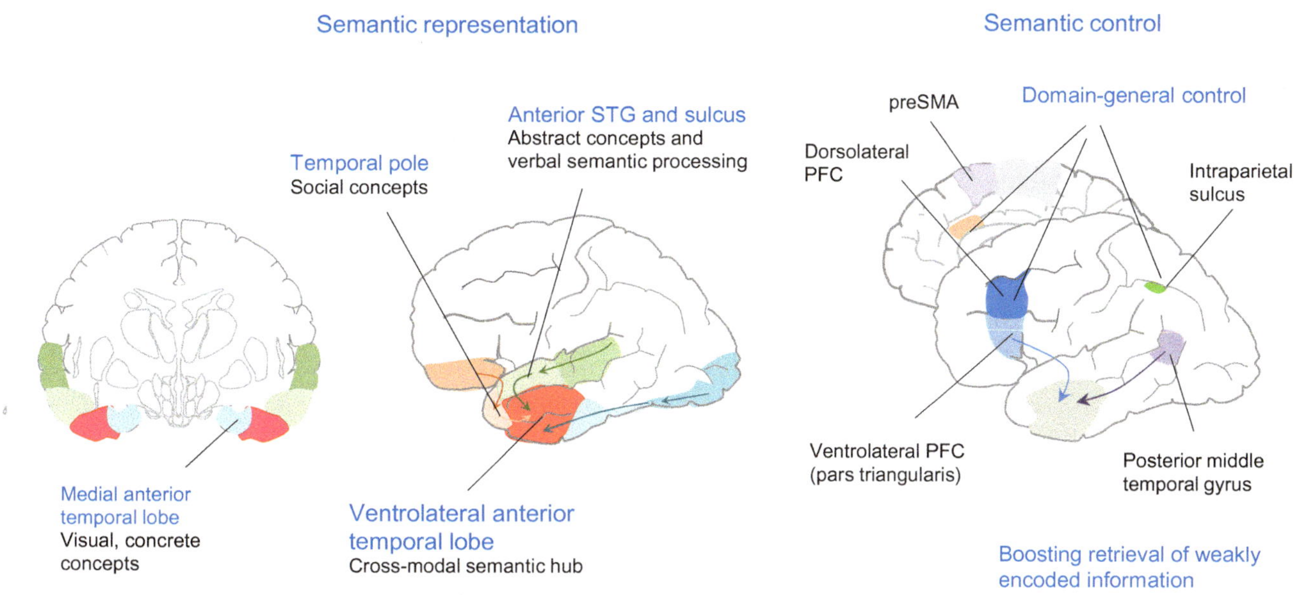

FIGURE 41.4 Areas involved in semantic representation and semantic control
Semantic cognition depends on two interacting systems, one for object representation and a second for control. The object representation system encodes knowledge of objects. Cross-modal interactions among all modality-specific sources of information occur in a transmodal hub located bilaterally in the ventrolateral anterior temporal lobe (ATL). Semantic function varies in a graded manner across subregions in the ATL. The more medial ATL subregions respond more to visual or concrete concepts; the anterior superior temporal gyrus (STG) and sulcus contribute more to abstract concepts and verbal semantic processing; and the temporal pole contributes more to social concepts by virtue of its connectivity to networks that support social cognition and affect. The ventrolateral ATL is equally important for all domains because it connects equally to these areas. The semantic control network includes the prefrontal cortex (PFC), posterior middle temporal gyrus (MTG), intraparietal sulcus (IPS), pre-motor area (preSMA), and cingulate cortex. The ventral PFC and posterior middle temporal gyrus directly connects to the ATL and may boost retrieval of weakly encoded information. The dorsal PFC, preSMA, and anterior cingulate cortex may contribute to more domain-general control.

generate inferences and behaviors required for each specific task context.

Semantic Representation in the Anterior Temporal Lobe

Concepts can be categorized at different levels: superordinate (e.g., animal or tool), basic (e.g., dog or hammer), or specific (e.g., bulldog or reflex hammer).[3] Conceptual representations are constructed from multimodal verbal and nonverbal experiences and promote generalization of knowledge among items and contexts. Cross-modal interactions among all modality-specific sources of information occur in a transmodal hub located bilaterally in the ventrolateral anterior temporal lobe. This area is involved in semantic processing irrespective of input modality (objects, pictures, words, sounds) and conceptual categories. Both the left and the right anterior temporal lobe participate in verbal and nonverbal processing. Functional MRI in healthy individuals, cortical grid-electrode stimulation and electrocorticography in neurosurgical patients, and 18F-fluorodeoxyglucose positron emission tomography in patients with semantic dementia all support the critical role of the ventrolateral anterior temporal lobe as the cross-modal center-point of the hub for naming and comprehension in all sensory modalities. Inhibitory TMS of the lateral anterior temporal lobe produces domain-general semantic slowing, whereas TMS of individual regions projecting to this area produces a category-specific defect. In healthy persons, anterior temporal lobe regions exhibit intrinsic connectivity (as detected by resting-state functional MRI) with modality-specific brain areas. Thus, the ventrolateral anterior temporal has an important role in coordinating the communication among modality-specific areas, thereby encoding semantic similarity among items.[3]

There is also evidence that semantic function varies in a graded manner across subregions in the anterior temporal lobe. The anterior temporal lobe receives projections from several sources that only partially overlap in its different subregions, leading to graded partial differentiations in the gross connectivity across these subregions [3 30]. The connections with the orbitofrontal via the uncinate fasciculus strongly target the temporopolar cortex; prefrontal connections through the extreme capsule and inferior parietal lobule connections via the middle longitudinal fasciculus preferentially terminate in superior anterior temporal lobe regions; and connections from visual areas via the inferior longitudinal fasciculus strongly target the ventral and ventromedial anterior temporal lobe. As a consequence, the temporal pole contributes more to social concepts by virtue of its connectivity to networks that support social cognition and affect; the anterior superior temporal sulcus and superior temporal gyrus contribute more to abstract concepts and verbal semantic processing by virtue of its greater connectivity to language system; and the more medial anterior temporal lobe subregions respond more to visual or concrete concepts.[3] The ventrolateral anterior temporal lobe is equally important for all domains because it connects equally to these areas.

Semantic Control

The distributed semantic control network interacts with the semantic representation network and provides an executive mechanism that constrains how activation propagates through the representation network.[3] The input from the semantic control network is particularly relevant when tasks or contexts require retrieval or infrequent and weakly encoded information; when it is necessary to suppress overlearned responses; or when it is necessary to adjust the responses to contingencies of the task. The semantic control network also supports working memory representations and executive control relevant to the current behavior. In contrast, in well-practiced contexts where the relevant information is robustly encoded, the semantic representation network needs little input from the semantic control network to produce the correct response. Some studies reveal specialization in this control network.[3,31] The ventral PFC and posterior middle temporal gyrus directly connects to the anterior temporal lobe and may boost retrieval of weakly encoded information. The dorsal PFC, preSMA, and anterior cingulate cortex may contribute to more domain-general control. Functional MRI and inhibitory TMS studies show that the PFC has a graded function in semantic control.[31] The ventral PFC and posterior middle temporal gyrus show increased activation during the retrieval of weak semantic associations; the dorsolateral PFC and intraparietal sulcus areas show increased responses to high selection demands; and the intermediate middle-lateral PFC during both types of task. Inhibitory TMS applied to the left inferior frontal region, posterior middle temporal gyrus, or intraparietal sulcus transiently disrupts semantic functioning, particularly in conditions that tax cognitive control. This suggests that both the inferior and superior components of the semantic control network are jointly required for the successful completion of executively demanding semantic tasks.

CLASSICAL APHASIA SYNDROMES DUE TO ISCHEMIC STROKE

In most cases, acute-onset aphasia is caused by left hemisphere strokes due to middle cerebral artery occlusion and affecting core speech areas located around the Sylvian fissure. These classical perisylvian syndromes include Broca aphasia, Wernicke aphasia, conduction aphasia, and global aphasia (Table 41.1). However, despite the unquestionable historical value of the landmark observations from these "fathers" of localization of brain language areas, these terms have several shortcomings.[32] As discussed earlier in this chapter, the classical Broca and Wernicke areas encompass several functional different regions. Furthermore, the description classical "Broca aphasia" and "Wernicke aphasia" were based on cases where there was additional involvement of neighboring areas or white matter tracts. Disorders affecting the watershed areas between the middle cerebral artery and the anterior or posterior cerebellar artery territories or both produce transcortical aphasias. These include transcortical motor aphasia, transcortical sensory aphasia, and transcortical global aphasia (also known as "isolation of speech area"). Other syndromes include pure anomia and optic aphasia. Motor speech impairment mostly reflects damage to components of the dorsal language pathways, whereas impaired speech comprehension is more strongly associated with involvement of the ventral language pathways.[32]

PRIMARY PROGRESSIVE APHASIA

Primary progressive aphasia (PPA) refers to a group of neurodegenerative disorders characterized by early and prominent language impairment in the absence of cognitive, behavioral, or motor symptoms.[33,34] There are three canonical variants of PPA: nonfluent/agrammatic, semantic, and logopenic (Table 41.2). Nonfluent/agrammatic and semantic PPA are considered variants of frontotemporal dementia (FTD) associated with frontotemporal lobar degeneration (FTLD).

Nonfluent/Agrammatic Variant

Nonfluent/agrammatic variant PPA is characterized by inability to comprehend syntactically complex sentences and impaired grammar or syntax (e.g., dropping words, using words out of order, or reversal of terms such as *yes* and *no* or *her* and *him*), with preserved comprehension of single words. This form of PPA is due to involvement of the anterior portion of the language network including Broca area 44 and 45 in the inferior frontal gyrus of the dominant hemisphere. Other areas typically involved are the anterior insula and superior temporal gyrus. About one-third of these patients have a positive family history. Mutations are less frequent than in behavioral variant FTD and include those affecting *MAPT* (microtubule-associated protein tau), *GRN* (progranulin) and *C9ORF72* (chromosome 19 open reading frame 72) genes. Nonfluent/agrammatic variant PPA is neuropathologically heterogeneous and may be associated with 3-repeat tau (Pick disease), 4-repeat tau (progressive supranuclear palsy or corticobasal degeneration), or transactive response DNA-binding protein 43

TABLE 41.1 *Classical Vascular Aphasia Syndromes*

	Broca	Wernicke	Conduction	TCM	TCS	Global	Anomic	Optic
Fluency	Poor	Good	Fair or good	Poor	Good	Poor	Good	Good
Content	Good	Poor	Good	Good	Poor	Poor	Good	Good
Comprehension	Intact for words and simple sentences	Poor	Intact for words and simple sentences	Intact for words and simple sentences	Poor	Poor	Good	Good
Repetition	Poor, nonfluent	Poor, fluent jargon	Good	Good	Poor	Poor	Good	Good
Naming	Worse for verbs	Worse for nouns	Fair or good	Fair or good	Poor	Poor	Worse for nouns	Poor with visual stimuli
Spelling	Poor	Poor	May be spared	May be spared	Poor	Poor	May be spared	Good
Reading	Poor	Poor	May be spared	May be spared	Poor	Poor	May be spared	Poor

TCM, transcortical motor; TCM, transcortical sensory

TABLE 41.2 *Main Features of Primary Progressive Aphasia (PPA) Syndromes*

PPA Variant	Nonfluent/Agrammatic	Fluent/Semantic	Logogenic
Core Features	-Agrammatism in language production -Effortful, halting speech with inconsistent speech sound errors (apraxia of speech)	-Impaired confrontation naming -Impaired single-word comprehension	-Impaired single-word retrieval in spontaneous speech and naming -Impaired repetition of sentences and phrases
Supportive features	-Impaired comprehension of syntactically complex sentences -Spared single-word comprehension -Spared object knowledge	-Impaired object knowledge particularly for low-frequency or low-familiarity items -Surface dyslexia or dysgraphia -Spared repetition -Spared motor speech and grammar	-Phonological errors in spontaneous speech and naming -Spared single-word comprehension and object knowledge -Absence of frank agrammatism
Area involved	Broca area 44 and 45 in left hemisphere Anterior insula Superior temporal gyrus	Anterior temporal lobe bilateral, more on the left side Middle and inferior temporal gyri, fusiform gyri, amygdala	Left Inferior parietal and superior temporal lobe
Genetic mutation;	*MAPT* (tau) *GRN* (progranulin) *C9ORF72*	Rarely genetic	Rarely genetic
Inclusions	Tau TDP-43	TDP-43 type C inclusion in >80% of cases	Alzheimer-type pathology

(TDP-43) inclusions. When apraxia of speech is prominent 4-repeat tau is more likely; with motor neuron disease TDP-43 is more likely. Familiar forms associated with *GRN* or *C9ORF72* mutations are associated with TDP-43 inclusions, whereas MAPT mutations are associated with 3- and/or 4-repeat tau. Patients with PPA may develop abnormal laughter-like vocalizations that increasingly replace speech.[35]

Fluent/Semantic Variant

Semantic variant PPA is characterized by a prominent language deficit at the onset of disease. The most prominent findings are word-retrieval difficulties or difficulty remembering words, particularly nouns. This results in circumlocution (such as *thing to move around* rather than *car*), the use or general category labels (such as *animal* for *cat*), or use of nonspecific fillers (such as *thing* or *place*). Loss of word meaning and impaired naming (anomia) are characteristic. Patients with semantic variant PPA typically exhibit progressive loss of semantic knowledge, which is not modality-specific. In conversation, and on testing, this semantic loss is reflected by marked naming difficulties and reduced use of low-frequency words, in the context of generally preserved insight, at least early in the disease course. Whereas patients with other forms of PPA benefit from verbal cues for naming, patients with semantic variant PPA do not. A supportive feature of semantic variant PPA is the presence of surface dyslexia or surface dysgraphia, which refers to difficulty with irregularly spelled words such as colonel, patch, and debt that do not follow the typical lexical-phonetic rules. Fluent PPA is typically associated with atrophy of the left anterior temporal lobe. Over time, atrophy tends to propagate to the contralateral temporal lobe as well as to the orbitofrontal and posterior brain regions. Often bilateral anterior temporal lobe atrophy may be asymmetric; involvement of the left side is associated with semantic variant PPA, and involvement of the right side with prosopagnosia. Impaired social skills, such as emotion recognition, theory of mind, and empathy, which are typical of behavioral variant FTD can occur in language presentations of FTD. These changes appear to be mediated by a decrease in structural brain integrity in predominantly right-hemispheric regions (orbitofrontal cortex, anterior temporal lobe) and their connecting white matter tracts (e.g., uncinate, superior and inferior longitudinal fasciculi) as well as a decline in functional integrity of the salience network.

Logopenic Variant

Unlike other forms of PPA, logopenic variant PPA is typically associated with Alzheimer disease. Its major manifestations are impaired retrieval of single words, during both spontaneous speech and naming and impaired repetition of sentences or phrases. Associated features include phonological errors during both spontaneous speech and naming, spared word comprehension and object knowledge (unlike semantic PPA), and lack of agrammatism (unlike nonfluent PPA). Logopenic PPA reflects involvement of the left inferior parietal and superior temporal lobes, which contain the representations (memory) of words.

APRAXIA OF SPEECH

Apraxia of speech is a motor speech disorder that reflects impaired capacity to plan and program commands necessary to control movements for normal articulation and phonetic and prosodic speech.[34] This has led to its classification in three types: phonetic (characterized by sound-level errors such as distorted substitutions or additions), prosodic (characterized by slow rate or segmented speech), and mixed. Patients present primarily with inability to articulate words, with preserved ability for writing and typing. Unlike spastic and ataxic dysarthria, apraxia of speech is characterized by trial-and-error articulatory attempts, groping, and distorted substitutions. Primary progressive apraxia of speech results from damage and dysfunction of a widespread distributed cortical and subcortical network involved in planning, production, and monitoring of speech. This includes the motor and premotor cortex and SMA bilaterally, but it is asymmetric in different patients. The anatomical substrate of pure primary progressive apraxia of speech has been thoroughly investigated using positron emission tomography (Figure 41.5). One functional neuroimaging study showed that patients with primary progressive apraxia of speech had reduced connectivity of the SMA with speech and language regions compared to controls.[36] Most patients with primary progressive apraxia of speech do not have genetic mutations associated with FTLD. However, approximately 40% develop a progressive supranuclear palsy/corticobasal syndrome-like disorder approximately 5 years after onset of symptoms. Neuropathologically, the vast majority of cases have an underlying 4-repeat tauopathy most commonly with features of corticobasal degeneration.

Childhood apraxia of speech is a development disorder associated with mutations of multiple genes encoding transcription factors, including *FOXP2* and *SEPT2*.[37]

CEREBELLAR LANGUAGE AND SPEECH DISORDERS

Lesions affecting the cerebellum may manifest with motor and nonmotor disorders of speech. Ataxic dysarthria is the imprecise production of consonants and vowels, irregular articulatory breakdowns, excess and equal stress, and harsh voice quality. It typically occurs with lesions in the superior anterior vermis and paravermis. Patients with apraxic speech disorders, such as developmental apraxia of speech, foreign accent syndrome, neurodegenerative apraxia of speech, and apraxic dysgraphia, have disruption of the cerebro-cerebellar network for processing of oral and written language planning. Cerebellar disease produces

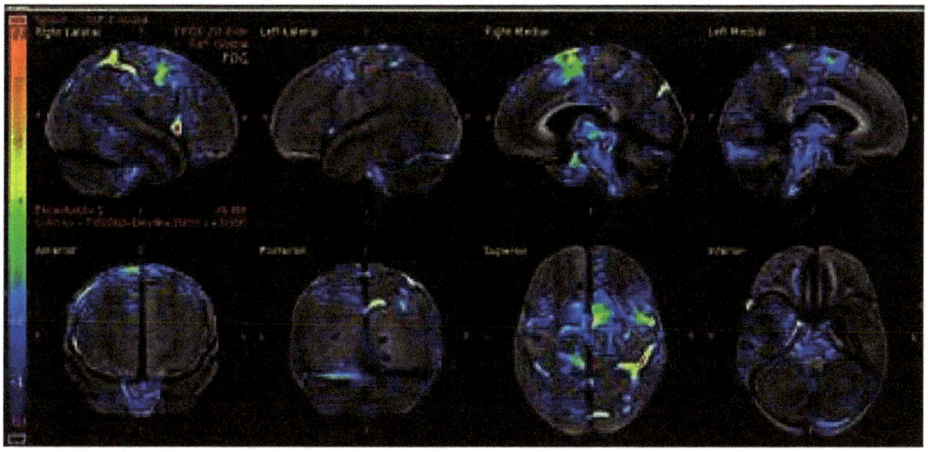

FIGURE 41.5 Involvement of the supplementary motor area in primary progressive apraxia of speech. Fluorodeoxyglucose positron emission tomography (PET) scan in a 72-year-old woman with a 4-year-history of difficulty enunciating words followed by sound level errors and eventually slow speech production. Her examination showed apraxia of speech. The PET scan shows hypometabolism in the supplementary motor area. (Courtesy of Dr. Hugo Botha)

nonmotor linguistic deficits in both children and adults, including reduced phonological fluency, and impaired grammatical and syntactic skills. There are several clinical syndromes that reflect the important role of the cerebellum in high-order cognitive function including language and speech.[28] The cerebellar cognitive affective syndrome consists of a range of cognitive, linguistic, and affective symptoms resulting from cerebellar damage.[38] This syndrome is characterized by executive dysfunction, visuospatial deficits, and language symptoms including agrammatism and anomia, and behavioral affective disturbances such as a blunting of affect or disinhibited behavior. Lesion studies indicate that involvement of the posterior lobe results in cognitive symptoms whereas involvement of the vermis is associated with behavioral affective disturbances. The posterior fossa syndrome may develop following acute cerebellar damage and is characterized by a broad range of linguistic, cognitive, and behavior-affective disturbances. This disorder most often occurs in pediatric patients after surgery for cerebellar neoplasms but is rare in adults. This syndrome may manifest initially with akinetic mutism and may be followed by a profile similar to that of cerebellar cognitive affective syndrome. The cognitive linguistic deficits associated with cerebral lesions have been attributed to cerebello-cerebral diaschisis, which reflects the metabolic impact of a cerebellar lesion on an anatomically and functionally connected area in the contralateral cerebral hemisphere.[28] Other proposed mechanisms include impaired ability of the cerebellum in detecting spatiotemporal patterns of incoming stimuli, resulting in impaired spatial function, language, verbal memory, and sequencing processing; or in the generation of temporarily accurate predictions based on sensory input, which may be important for verbal working memory and predictive articulatory control.

SEMANTIC DEMENTIA

Bilateral damage of the anterior ventral and polar temporal regions results in semantic dementia, which is characterized by impairment of knowledge of objects and concepts across all modalities.[39] Consistent with the role of the ventrolateral anterior temporal lobe as a transmodal hub for all conceptual domains, these patients have semantic impairments for virtually all types of concept, with the exception of simple numerical knowledge. In general, left anterior temporal lobe damage leads to more severe impairment of object recognition and naming (anomia) and right anterior temporal lobe damage to greater inability to recognize objects within categories (associative agnosia), including different faces (prosopagnosia). The likelihood that these patients respond correctly to a given item in a task requiring semantic knowledge depends on several factors including the familiarity of the item (high familiarity leads to better performance) and the specificity of the knowledge that is required by the task (high specificity of unique items leads to worse performance). Neuroimaging shows asymmetrical atrophy and hypometabolism of the anterior temporal pole and anterior fusiform gyrus, usually lateralized to the left hemisphere (Figure 41.6). Functional MRI studies reveal widespread changes in connectivity of the anterior temporal regions. With disease progression, atrophy extends into the contralateral temporal pole and medial prefrontal cortices, which reflects emerging changes in behavior and social cognition. There is also involvement of the middle and inferior temporal gyrus, and amygdala. The most common neuropathological subtype is that of accumulation TDP-43 type C inclusions. The majority of cases are sporadic.[39]

Disorders of semantic control lead to difficulty manipulating and using semantic knowledge but not loss of

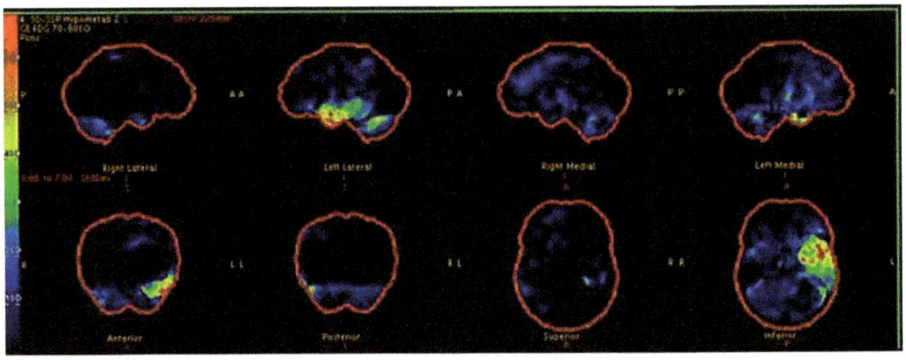

FIGURE 41.6 Hypometabolism in the left anterior temporal lobe in a patient with semantic dementia.

semantic knowledge itself. Impaired semantic control is referred to as "semantic aphasia," which differs in many aspects from semantic dementia.[3,40] Whereas patients with semantic dementia have consistent semantic "store" deficit, patients with semantic aphasia have inconsistent semantic "access" deficits. Patients with semantic aphasia perform poorest on the most demanding tasks and stimuli; they show inconsistent performance across tests; insensitivity to the frequency or familiarity of stimuli; strong influence of the ambiguity or semantic diversity of word meanings; and strong influence of cueing and miscuing on performance.[40] They have associative semantic errors in naming, such as saying "milk" in response to a picture of a cow. The cueing and miscueing effects distinguish patients with semantic aphasia from those with semantic dementia. For example, given a picture of a tiger, both groups of patients fail to name it; but with presentation of the phonological cue "t" patients with semantic aphasia, but not those with semantic dementia, would often succeed and when presented with the clue "l" they will often produce "lion." All these differences are consistent with the view that whereas semantic dementia reflects impairment within the network for semantic representation, semantic aphasia reflects disordered control of activation within that network.[3,40]

KEY POINTS

- The core language areas are located in the left inferior frontal gyrus corresponding to Broca area (pars opercularis-area 44 and pars triangulars-area 45), left posterior temporal and inferior parietal gyrus (including classical Wernicke area), and the left anterior temporal lobe and posterior middle temporal gyrus.
- Area 44 is coupled to parallel and overlapping large-scale networks and participates in language, cognitive, and motor functions.
- Lexical-semantic processing is the mapping of words into meaning, and involves a network that includes left temporoparietal areas and inferior frontal areas.
- Left temporoparietal areas, including the angular gyrus and the supramarginal gyrus, are involved in the storage or representation of lexical-semantic information.
- The inferior frontal gyrus, including pars triangularis (area 45) in classical Broca area and adjacent pars orbitalis (area 47), is involved in semantic retrieval and manipulation.
- Syntax involves a network that includes the left posterior superior temporal gyrus and sulcus and the pars orbicularis in Broca area (area 44).
- The left posterior temporal cortex may be important for the retrieval of the syntactic frames that are stored in the lexicon.
- Broca area 44 is involved in a "Merge" operation that assembles words into hierarchies, such as noun or verb.
- The core regions in the language network are interconnected by two dorsal pathways for mapping sound into word production and two ventral pathways for mapping sound into meaning.
- The superior longitudinal fascicle supports speech repetition.
- The arcuate fascicle is relevant for complex syntactic processing.
- The uncinate fascicle is involved in syntactic processing of simple sentences.
- The inferior fronto-occipital fascicle (extreme capsule fiber system) supports semantic word judgment.
- The posterior part of the left superior frontal sulcus and the left superior parietal cortex are involved in writing.
- Vocalization involves a network that includes the supragenual anterior cingulate cortex, periaqueductal gray and nucleus retroambiguus.
- The voluntary motor articulation network includes the Broca areas 44 and 45, ventral premotor cortex (PMv), ventrolateral portion of the primary motor cortex, supplementary motor area (SMA), presupplementary motor area (preSMA), superior

temporal gyrus, inferior parietal lobule, cerebellum, putamen, and thalamus.

- The left inferior frontal gyrus and left superior temporal cortex are selectively recruited during speech articulation.
- Broca area 44 coordinates the transformation of information across large-scale cortical networks and formulates an appropriate articulatory code to be implemented by motor cortex.
- The speech motor cortex has a partially overlapping representation of articulators and two separate representations of the larynx.
- In humans the direct projection from the laryngeal motor cortex to the nucleus ambiguus, facilitates rapid voluntary vocal control.
- The frontal aslant tract connecting the posterior inferior frontal gyrus and dorsal anterior insula with the preSMA, SMA, and anterior cingulate cortex may have an important role in executive control of speech.
- The right hemisphere appears to have a role in processing of prosodic features such as emotional tone.
- The cerebellum is actively involved in language and speech production.
- The ventrolateral anterior temporal cortex is critical for semantic processing irrespective of input modality.
- A semantic control network provides an executive mechanism that constrains how activation propagates through the representation network.
- Primary progressive aphasias (PPAs) are neurodegenerative disorders characterized by early and prominent language impairment.
- Nonfluent/agrammatic variant PPA is characterized by both inability to comprehend syntactically complex sentence and impaired grammar or syntax.
- Nonfluent/agrammatic PPA is due to involvement of the anterior portion of the language network including Broca areas 44 and 45 in the dominant hemisphere.
- Semantic or fluent variant PPA is characterized by prominent word-retrieval difficulties or difficult remembering words, loss of word meaning, and impaired naming (anomia).
- Fluent PPA is typically associated with atrophy of the left anterior temporal lobe.
- Logopenic variant PPA manifests with impaired retrieval of single words, and impaired repetition of sentences or phrases due to involvement of the left temporoparietal region.
- Apraxia of speech is a motor speech disorder that results from damage and dysfunction of a widespread distributed cortical and subcortical network involved in planning, production, and monitoring of speech.
- Cerebellar disease produces both motor and nonmotor impairment of speech.
- Semantic dementia is the impaired knowledge of objects and concepts across all modalities and results from bilateral damage of the anterior ventral and polar temporal regions.

REFERENCES

1. Fedorenko E, Thompson-Schill SL. Reworking the language network. Trends Cogn Sci 2014;18:120–126.
2. Fedorenko E, Duncan J, Kanwisher N. Language-selective and domain-general regions lie side by side within Broca's area. Curr Biol 2012;22:2059–2062.
3. Ralph MA, Jefferies E, Patterson K, Rogers TT. The neural and computational bases of semantic cognition. Nat Rev Neurosci 2017;18:42–55.
4. Tremblay P, Dick AS. Broca and Wernicke are dead, or moving past the classic model of language neurobiology. Brain Lang 2016;162:60–71.
5. Chang EF, Raygor KP, Berger MS. Contemporary model of language organization: an overview for neurosurgeons. J Neurosurg 2015;122:250–261.
6. Friederici AD. The brain basis of language processing: from structure to function. Physiol Rev 2011;91:1357–1392.
7. Friederici AD. Evolution of the neural language network. Psychon Bull Rev 2017;24:41–47.
8. Poeppel D. The neuroanatomic and neurophysiological infrastructure for speech and language. Curr Opin Neurobiol 2014;28:142–149.
9. Hagoort P. The core and beyond in the language-ready brain. Neurosci Biobehav Rev 2017;81:194–204.
10. Neef NE, Butfering C, Anwander A, Friederici AD, Paulus W, Sommer M. Left posterior-dorsal area 44 couples with parietal areas to promote speech fluency, while right area 44 activity promotes the stopping of motor responses. Neuroimage 2016;142:628–644.
11. Ansari D, Garcia N, Lucas E, Hamon K, Dhital B. Neural correlates of symbolic number processing in children and adults. Neuroreport 2005;16:1769–1773.
12. Matejko AA, Hutchison JE, Ansari D. Developmental specialization of the left intraparietal sulcus for symbolic ordinal processing. Cortex 2019;114:41–53.
13. Planton S, Longcamp M, Peran P, Demonet JF, Jucla M. How specialized are writing-specific brain regions? An fMRI study of writing, drawing and oral spelling. Cortex 2017;88:66–80.
14. Hage SR, Nieder A. Dual neural network model for the evolution of speech and language. Trends Neurosci 2016;39:813–829.
15. Egea-Lucas I, Martinez-Mondejar E, Piqueres-Vidal CF, Frutos-Alegria MT. [Gelastic seizures as the presenting symptom of infarction of the cingulate gyrus]. Rev Neurol 2015;61:211–214.
16. Tran TP, Truong VT, Wilk M, et al. Different localizations underlying cortical gelastic epilepsy: case series and review of literature. Epilepsy Behav 2014;35:34–41.
17. Nagaratnam N, Nagaratnam K, Ng K, Diu P. Akinetic mutism following stroke. J Clin Neurosci 2004;11:25–30.

18. Kent RD, Duffy JR, Slama A, Kent JF, Clift A. Clinicoanatomic studies in dysarthria: review, critique, and directions for research. J Speech Lang Hear Res 2001;44:535–551.
19. Simonyan K. The laryngeal motor cortex: its organization and connectivity. Curr Opin Neurobiol 2014;28:15–21.
20. Simonyan K, Fuertinger S. Speech networks at rest and in action: interactions between functional brain networks controlling speech production. J Neurophysiol 2015;113:2967–2978.
21. Basilakos A, Smith KG, Fillmore P, Fridriksson J, Fedorenko E. Functional characterization of the human speech articulation network. Cereb Cortex 2018;28:1816–1830.
22. Clos M, Amunts K, Laird AR, Fox PT, Eickhoff SB. Tackling the multifunctional nature of Broca's region meta-analytically: co-activation-based parcellation of area 44. Neuroimage 2013;83:174–188.
23. Flinker A, Korzeniewska A, Shestyuk AY, et al. Redefining the role of Broca's area in speech. Proc Natl Acad Sci U S A 2015;112:2871–2875.
24. Koechlin E, Jubault T. Broca's area and the hierarchical organization of human behavior. Neuron 2006;50:963–974.
25. Battistella G, Kumar V, Simonyan K. Connectivity profiles of the insular network for speech control in healthy individuals and patients with spasmodic dysphonia. Brain Struct Funct 2018;223:2489–2498.
26. Lauterbach EC, Cummings JL, Kuppuswamy PS. Toward a more precise, clinically—informed pathophysiology of pathological laughing and crying. Neurosci Biobehav Rev 2013;37:1893–1916.
27. McCairn KW, Nagai Y, Hori Y, et al. A primary role for nucleus accumbens and related limbic network in vocal tics. Neuron 2016;89:300–307.
28. Marien P, Borgatti R. Language and the cerebellum. Handb Clin Neurol 2018;154:181–202.
29. Arasanz CP, Staines WR, Roy EA, Schweizer TA. The cerebellum and its role in word generation: a cTBS study. Cortex 2012;48:718–724.
30. Martin A. GRAPES—Grounding representations in action, perception, and emotion systems: how object properties and categories are represented in the human brain. Psychon Bull Rev 2016;23:979–990.
31. Hallam GP, Carin Whitney C, Mark Hymers M, et al. Charting the effects of TMS with fMRI: Modulation of cortical recruitment within the distributed network supporting semantic control. Neuropsychologia 2016;93:40–52.
32. Fridriksson J, den Ouden DB, Hillis AE, et al. Anatomy of aphasia revisited. Brain 2018;141:848–862.
33. Mesulam MM. Primary progressive aphasia and the left hemisphere language network. Dement Neurocogn Disord 2016;15:93–102.
34. Botha H, Josephs KA. Primary progressive aphasias and apraxia of speech. Continuum (Minneap Minn) 2019;25:101–127.
35. Rohrer JD, Warren JD, Rossor MN. Abnormal laughter-like vocalisations replacing speech in primary progressive aphasia. J Neurol Sci 2009;284:120–123.
36. Botha H, Utianski RL, Whitwell JL, et al. Disrupted functional connectivity in primary progressive apraxia of speech. Neuroimage Clin 2018;18:617–629.
37. Hildebrand MS, Jackson VE, Scerri TS, et al. Severe childhood speech disorder: gene discovery highlights transcriptional dysregulation. Neurology 2020;94:e2148–e2167.
38. Argyropoulos GPD, van Dun K, Adamaszek M, et al. The cerebellar cognitive affective/Schmahmann syndrome: a task force paper. Cerebellum 2020;19:102–125.
39. Landin-Romero R, Tan R, Hodges JR, Kumfor F. An update on semantic dementia: genetics, imaging, and pathology. Alzheimers Res Ther 2016;8:52.
40. Thompson HE, Almaghyuli A, Noonan KA, Barak O, et al. The contribution of executive control to semantic cognition: Convergent evidence from semantic aphasia and executive dysfunction. J Neuropsychol 2018;12:312–340.

42 Executive Control

OVERVIEW

The ability to rapidly and accurately learn and process new information in response to a changing environment, engage in goal-directed tasks, and switch between behaviors according to the context requires attention, working memory, decision-making, and cognitive control. All these processes engage large-scale networks involving different portions of the frontal cortex and interactions with posterior cortical areas in the parietal and temporal lobes. The frontal lobe consists of multiple cytoarchitectonically distinct areas with specific connections to other brain regions.[1] The lateral prefrontal cortex (PFC), medial PFC, orbitofrontal cortex (OFC), anterior cingulate cortex (ACC), and anterior midcingulate cortex (MCC) are fundamental components of separate yet interactive networks. Meta-analyses of functional neuroimaging studies have provided maps of the functional correlates of behavioral functions in these frontal regions[2,3] (Figure 42.1). For example, lateral frontal areas are part of parietal networks involved in attention and executive functions, somatosensory networks involved in motor planning and programming, and the default mode network involved in inner thought processing. Similarly, medial frontal cortical areas have been subdivided into anterior, middle, and posterior regions according to their participation in networks involved in emotional/social, cognitive, and motor functions, respectively. Thus, different areas of the frontal cortex are core regions of large-scale cognitive networks involved in attention,[4–6] working memory,[7–9] decision-making[10,11] and executive control.[12,13] Attention selects task-relevant information. Working memory maintains the relevant information "on-line" over brief periods of time for processing, manipulation, and transformation to guide behavior. Decision-making selects a particular option among a set of alternatives taking into account their reward value, costs, and personal relevance. Motivation is a process by which incentives invigorate and guide behaviors toward goals. Control signals are required for implementation, maintenance, and updating of behavior based on feedback, particularly when it is necessary to overcome distraction or suppress habitual responses when outcomes deviate from expectations. Appropriate cognitive control requires cognitive effort, which is the ability to allocate cognitive resources to the pursuit of a goal.[14,15] Control mechanisms allow the flexible shift of motivated behaviors between those triggered by relevant external stimuli captured by the attention networks and those driven by internal thoughts of personal relevance processed in the default mode network.[16] Based on microstructure, connectivity, and functions, these networks are located along a gradient of hierarchical cortical organization and are flexibly engaged in different cognitive tasks.[17,18] Dysfunction of these large-scale networks is a cardinal feature of neurodegenerative dementias, particularly behavioral variant frontotemporal dementia (bvFTD) and Alzheimer disease (AD); focal lesions affecting different portions of the frontal lobe;[19] including stroke;[20] and psychiatric disorders. Mapping of cognitive and emotional networks using resting-state fMRI may have potential applications for the mapping of cognition and emotion in neurosurgical patients.[21] The aims of this chapter are to review: (1) the areas and mechanisms involved in selective attention and working memory; (2) mechanisms of decision-making, motivation, and allocation of effort; (3) the areas involved in cognitive control; and (4) examples of disorders affecting these large-scale networks.

ATTENTION

Attention is the selection of task-relevant sensory information at the expense of nonrelevant information.[4] The best-studied form of attention is visual attention, using either visual spatial orienting (spatial location-based attention), or visual search (feature-based attention) paradigms.[22,23] Visual spatial attention may include both the focusing of attention at a selected location and an automatic monitoring of other locations for flexibly gating the reallocation of attentional resources. Attentional processing may be biased by either top-down or bottom-up influences.

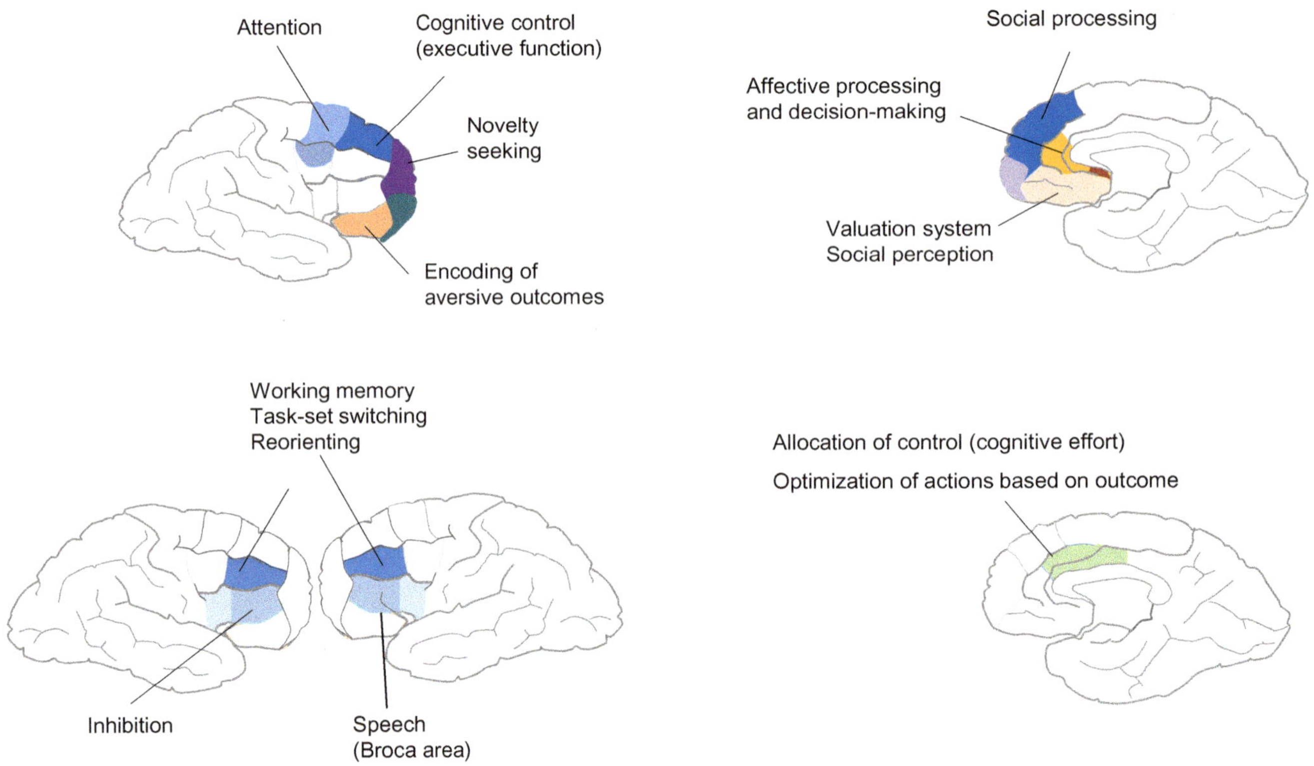

FIGURE 42.1 Overview of functions of the prefrontal cortex
Meta-analyses of functional neuroimaging studies has provided maps of the functional correlates of behavioral functions in the frontal cortex. Areas of the lateral prefrontal cortex (PFC) are subdivided according to their affiliation with other cortical areas and patterns of activation into those that form a part of parietal networks involved in executive functions, the default mode network involved in inner thought processing, and somatosensory networks involved in motor planning and programming). Similarly, medial frontal cortical areas have been subdivided into anterior, middle, and posterior regions according to their participation in networks involved in emotional/social, cognitive, and motor functions (not shown), respectively.

Top-down processing is the goal-oriented voluntary guidance of attention to location, objects, and features of the environment that are relevant to the current behaviors and goals. Bottom-up attention is driven by salient external stimuli. Attention may be reoriented toward objects that are behaviorally relevant because they match current goals, require a completely different course of action, or are signaled as important on the basis of previous experience and long-term memory associations.[4] Reorienting to new objects may also occur reflexively based on their high sensory salience, for example, if they are unexpected based on their features or spatial location. Functional imaging studies show the presence of two separate frontoparietal attention networks, dorsal and ventral, which are defined by their functional connectivity and different roles in attentional processing[4] (Figure 42.2).

Dorsal Attention Network

The dorsal attention network includes the dorsal parietal cortex, particularly intraparietal sulcus and superior parietal lobule; the lateral PFC along the precentral sulcus; and the frontal eye field (FEF).[5,6] This dorsal network is involved in goal-oriented attention. It enables the selection of sensory stimuli based on current internal goals or expectations, sends top-down signals to the sensory cortex to bias processing of appropriate stimulus features and locations, and then links the selected stimuli to appropriate motor responses. The dorsal attention network is activated by the expectation of seeing an object at a particular location or with certain features, by the preparation of a specific response, or by the short-term memory of a visual scene. Via the FEF, this network directs attention and gaze toward sensory stimuli appearing at unexpected locations in the contralateral hemispace. There is both segregation and strong correlation between the activity of the dorsal attention network and that of the visual network (including the primary visual and association visual areas) at rest. During a visual attention task that required dynamic and selective rerouting of visual information, there was a reduced of correlation of the ongoing "idling" activity within the visual network and an increase in the top-down connectivity from the dorsal attention to the visual network.[23]

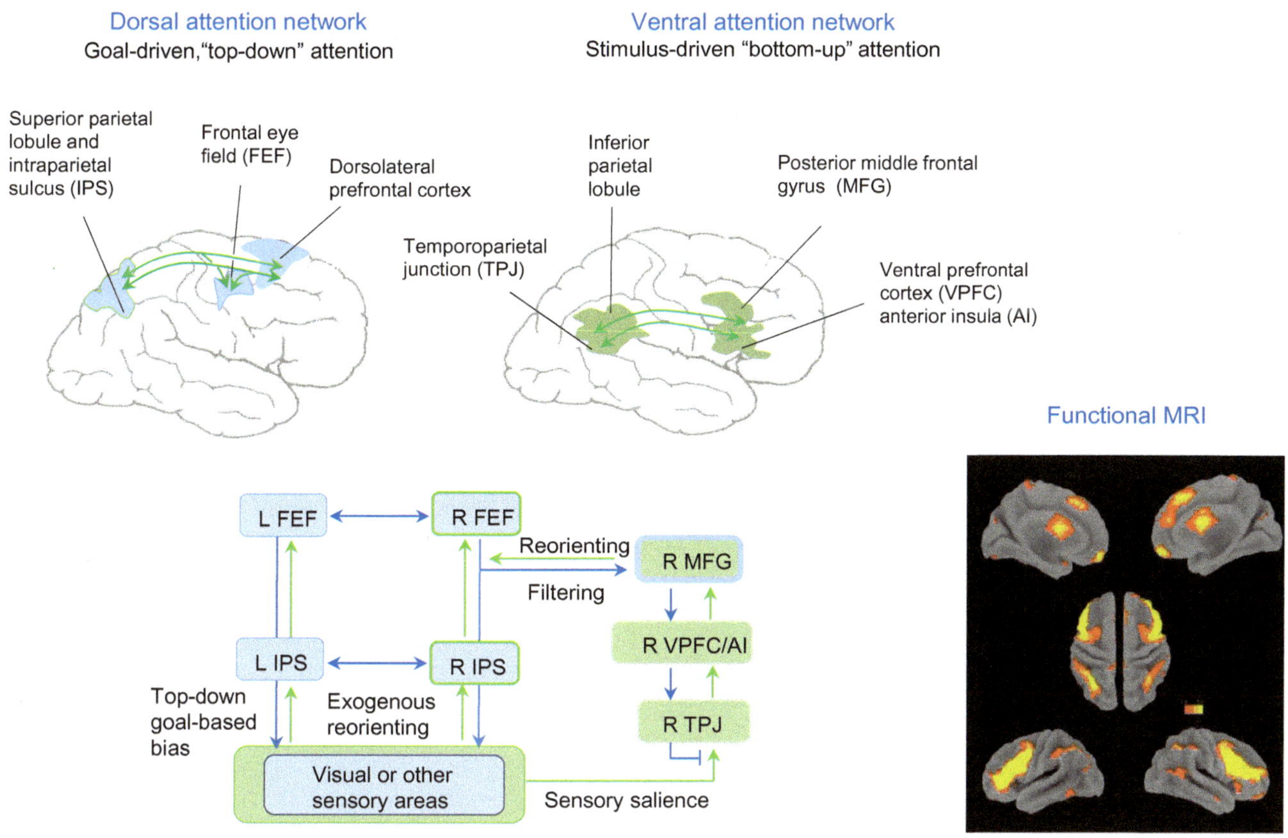

FIGURE 42.2 Attention networks

Functional imaging studies show the presence of two separate frontoparietal attention networks, dorsal and ventral. The dorsal frontoparietal attention network includes the dorsal parietal cortex, particularly intraparietal sulcus (lateral intraparietal area) and superior parietal lobule; the lateral PFC along the precentral sulcus; and the frontal eye field (FEF) and is involved in goal-oriented attention. The ventral frontoparietal network includes the temporoparietal junction and the ventral lateral frontal cortex (parts of middle frontal gyrus, inferior frontal gyrus, frontal operculum, and anterior insula). It is lateralized to the right hemisphere and registers salient events in the environment. The reorienting response is triggered by novel and unexpected stimuli and involves the action of the right hemisphere ventral frontoparietal network that interrupts and resets ongoing activity of the dorsal frontoparietal network. When attention is focused via the dorsal network based on an internal goal (goal-driven), the ventral network is suppressed to prevent reorienting to distracting events. (Functional MRI images courtesy of Dr. David Jones).

Ventral Attention Network

The ventral attention network includes the cortex at the temporoparietal junction, including the posterior superior temporal sulcus, superior temporal gyrus, and ventral part of the supramarginal gyrus, and the ventral lateral frontal cortex, including parts of middle frontal gyrus, inferior frontal gyrus, frontal operculum, and anterior insula. This ventral network is lateralized to the right hemisphere and registers salient events in the environment not only in the visual but also in other sensory modalities and in social situations. A component of this network, the temporoparietal junction-posterior superior temporal sulcus, is highly expanded in humans and contains areas that are engaged not only in attention but also in processing of emotional expression of faces, theory of mind, and memory.[24] The expansion of the temporoparietal junction–posterior superior temporal sulcus has allowed for the elaboration of the cortical areas contained within this region. This has led to the proposal that the temporoparietal junction–posterior superior temporal sulcus is the basis of a third frontoparietal processing stream separate from the classical dorsal ("where") and the ventral ("what" stream); this third stream would underlie the increased social abilities in humans by functioning as a hub that coordinates the activities of multiple brain networks in the exploration of the social scenes typical of the human social experience.[24] The ventral anterior network includes components of both the salience[25] and cingulo-opercular task control[26] networks, including the anterior insula and anterior MCC.[18] There is a rightward asymmetry in white matter connectivity strength between the temporoparietal junction and the insula, which supports the right-sided lateralization in stimulus-driven attention, sensory awareness, interoception, and pain.[27]

Reorienting Response

The reorienting response is triggered by novel and unexpected stimuli.[5] It involves the action of the right hemisphere dominant ventral frontoparietal network that interrupts and resets ongoing activity of the dorsal frontoparietal networks.[5] When attention is focused via the dorsal network based on an internal goal (goal-driven), the ventral network is suppressed to prevent reorienting to distracting events. Upon detection of behaviorally relevant objects or targets, attention is reoriented to the new source of information (stimulus-driven reorienting) as the ventral network interrupts ongoing selection in the dorsal network, which in turn shifts attention toward the novel object of interest. In contrast, the reduced response of the ventral attention network to unimportant objects prevents shifts of attention that could interfere with the performance of a goal-oriented task. This "filtering" response reflects a top-down suppression signal from the dorsal attention network as well as the input from executive control networks acting at the level of the right temporoparietal junction. The right posterior middle frontal gyrus may be a major link between the ventral and dorsal networks.

The different patterns of recruitment of the dorsal and ventral attention networks during goal-oriented behavior and reorienting responses may reflect inputs from the locus coeruleus (LC) noradrenergic system. During focused attention, LC neurons may have a phasic response to target stimuli that shares many similarities with the P300 target-related cortical evoked potential. This response may function as an "interrupt" or "network reset" signal that may allow the flexible configuration of the attention networks once a target is detected. The decrease in tonic LC activity during the transition from an exploratory state to a task-focused state may parallel the deactivation of temporoparietal junction, which would promote engagement on the current task and filtering of distractors.[5,28]

Perceptual Episodes and Attentional Blink

Attention is deployed over an interval that frequently encompasses several stimuli. When numerous stimuli are densely packed in time, attentional selection occurs in brief perceptual episodes. The ability to identify a target is usually hindered if it appears shortly after another target. Two episodes of attentional selection cannot occur very close in time. When two items are presented briefly and in close succession, observers can usually report the first but often fail to report the second. This phenomenon is known as the *attentional blink*.[29–31] A second attentional episode may occur only when the second target follows the first by more than 100 to 250 ms. There are several hypotheses regarding the basis of attentional blink. Evidence indicates that both cognitive control and emotion strongly influence the duration of the perceptual episodes and thus attentional blink.[29–31]

Value-Driven Guidance of Visual Attention

One fundamental component of attention is the attraction of gaze direction toward objects with high reward value.[32] This decision-making process is regulated by the caudate nucleus, which is a component of the oculomotor circuit of the basal ganglia. This circuit is integrated to the dorsal attention network and includes the FEF, substantia nigra pars reticulata (SNr), and superior colliculus. The SNr tonically inhibits saccadic burst neurons of the superior colliculus; in response to a reward signaled by a peak of dopamine, inhibitory inputs from the caudate nucleus to the SNr transiently interrupt the tonic inhibition of the superior colliculus, thus promoting the initiation of a saccadic eye movement toward the high-value objects of attention.[32] A caudate head circuit relays on short-term value memories to trigger eye deviation toward recently valued objects; a caudate tail circuit relays on long-term reward memories to allow the subject's gaze to move automatically to a previously valued object.[32]

Effects of Attention on Sensory Processing and Cortical Oscillations

The dorsolateral PFC and components of the dorsal frontoparietal attention network, including the FEF and lateral intraparietal area, provide modulatory attention-related signals that are fed back to sensory cortex.[33] Neurons in the parietal cortex encode a salience map of the visual scene, encoding which locations in space are of potentially high significance, whereas neurons in frontal cortex carry information about task-relevant stimuli. Visual attention elicits an increase in the high-frequency (gamma, 40–80 Hz) oscillations and decreased the low-frequency (<10 Hz) oscillations in populations of neurons in the visual cortex representing the attended location. There is also synchrony between the frontal and parietal cortex during attentional tasks. There is gamma band synchrony when attention is captured by external stimuli and information from the parietal to the frontal cortex (bottom-up) and beta band synchrony when attention is internally controlled and information flows from the prefrontal to parietal cortex.

Spatial attention to a visual stimulus increases neural responses to the selected stimulus across many levels of processing, including primary and secondary visual areas as well as subcortical regions such as the lateral geniculate nucleus, pulvinar, reticular nucleus of the thalamus, and superior colliculus. Interactions between excitatory pyramidal neurons and inhibitory interneurons are central to the mechanism supporting attention. Interneuron-mediated lateral inhibition suppresses competing stimuli; attention has a much larger impact on the responses of inhibitory interneurons than in pyramidal cells. Activity of inhibitory interneurons also leads to the generation of high-frequency synchronous oscillations within a cortical region. Inter-areal synchronization occurs as these local oscillations synchronize along with the propagation of a bottom-up sensory drive.

A "reverse hierarchy" model of visual attention suggests that selection begins in the prefrontal and parietal cortices, where neurons represent abstract categories, and then filters backward along the cortical hierarchy to "simpler" visual areas. Spatial and feature-based attention interact with one another; attending to a spatial location would select an object at that location. Spatial attention can drive feature-based attention (e.g., attending to a single object in space leads to increases in attention to its properties across the entire cortex); conversely, feature-based attention can drive spatial attention (e.g., the detection of a car in a visual scene drives spatial attention to that location).

Thalamic Mechanisms of Attention

Communication in cortical large-scale networks during attention is mediated not only through cortico-cortical interactions but also through cortico-thalamo-cortical interactions involving the pulvinar and the mediodorsal thalamic nucleus. During spatial selection, interactions via the pulvinar increase synchrony of slow alpha oscillations between two interconnected visual cortical areas. During sustained visuospatial attention, alpha activity in the pulvinar reflects the precise temporal coordination of cortical activity via phasic inhibition of projection neurons in the posterior parietal cortex. Alpha band synchronization driven by posterior parietal cortex to the pulvinar may act to gate or suppress the processing of incoming sensory information at early stages of visual cortex. The major thalamic input to the PFC originates in the mediodorsal nucleus. Projections from this nucleus promote relevant recurrent synaptic interactions in the PFC, which maintains representations of task-rules, for example those required for sensory selection. Via this mechanism, the different subdivisions of the mediodorsal nucleus participate in multiple cognitive processes, including attention, working memory, familiarity-based recognition and retrieval, and emotional processing. The medial (magnocellular) portion of the mediodorsal nucleus is a component of a parahippocampal-prefrontal system involved in familiarity-based recognition and retrieval processing, and also has a central role in emotional processing by interconnecting the amygdala and the posterior orbitofrontal cortex.[34] The lateral (parvocellular) division of the mediodorsal nucleus via its reciprocal connections with the dorsolateral PFC has a major role in working memory; both areas contain neurons that sustain tonic activity during the delay period between the presentation of the cue and the motor output.

The claustrum may also have an important role in attention.[35] This thin, sheet-like structure located between the insular cortex and the putamen is characterized by its reciprocal and topographically organized connections with all neocortical areas including visual, somatosensory, auditory, and motor cortical regions. The claustrum communicates most densely with medial frontal cortical regions and receives prominent inputs from the amygdala, hippocampus, and mediodorsal nucleus of the thalamus. Glutamatergic projections from the claustrum target pyramidal neurons in supra- and infragranular layers but primarily terminate on local inhibitory neurons in layer 4, thereby promoting feedforward inhibition of incoming information in multiple cortical areas.[35] The claustrum may also orchestrate and integrate cortical activity by boosting synchronized cortical oscillations.

WORKING MEMORY

Working memory is the "mental sketchpad" for short-term maintenance of information over brief periods of time (several seconds to minutes) in the absence of sensory input; this process is commonly referred to as "short-term memory." However, in addition working memory allows manipulation and processing of the transiently stored information for guidance of behavior.[7] Both selective attention and cognitive control operations are integral parts of working-memory processing.[7,8,36]

Features of Working Memory

There are several theoretical models of working memory.[37,38] A well-known model is that working memory involves four components, a "phonological loop" for language processing; a "visuospatial sketchpad" for visual processing; an "episodic buffer that allows features to be bound in "chunks," such as shape and color or words in a sentence; and finally a "central executive" involved in focusing of attention, dividing attention along parallel verbal or visual tracks, switching between tracks, and interacting with long-term memory processing.[37] Working memory requires both the storage of sensory information in modality-specific posterior cortical areas during the delay period when the stimulus is no longer present, and recurrent activity in the lateral PFC to focus attention on the relevant stimulus, select information from distractors, and process the held information according to the task. Neurophysiological findings support a separation of prefrontal frontal executive and storage mechanisms in the posterior parietal and temporal cortex. An active maintenance process through reverberating activity provides attentional top-down signals to regions involved in perceptual and long-term memory representations related to the current content of working memory. Both sustained attention and the rehearsal process are crucial for maintaining the information in working memory. This process is potentially vulnerable to distraction and interference by task-irrelevant information. Working-memory capacity is limited; most estimates of the average capacity among healthy young adults suggest that it has a capacity limit of approximately three or four simple items. Capacity increases if the items can be grouped into meaningful units, or "chunks," which can exploit preexisting information about concepts already stored in long-term memory. Working-memory changes across the lifespan and can be modified by training. Recent models assume that short-term retention of information in working memory requires the allocation of attention to internal representations in long-term memory. When a subject is presented with symbolic information to be remembered (e.g., a list of names or a telephone number), the long-term memory representations of this information are accessed and subsequently maintained via attentional mechanism in an elevated state of activation until this information is no longer needed to achieve a goal.

Brain Areas and Connections Involved in Working Memory

Working memory results from the dynamic interaction of a large number of brain regions (Figure 42.3). The specific regions involved depend on a number of factors, including the type of material to be remembered, the task, and the stage of the dynamic interplay of processing components.[7,8] The current view of the mechanisms underlying working memory is based on persistent activity in a recurrent network with fixed connectivity via reverberant excitatory circuits in areas 9/46 of the lateral PFC. The strong lateral inhibition between memory representations causes a winner-take-all dynamics that typically leaves only the winning representation active. The strength of dorsolateral PFC activity varies with the state of arousal: working-memory abilities are greatly impaired during fatigue or stress.[39] Maintenance of working memory results from the interactions between selective attentional processing of sensory information and long-term memory representations. These interactions involve reentrant loops between frontal and posterior cortical areas encoding perceptual information, as well as subcortical structures such as the basal ganglia and the cerebellum. The same brain regions dedicated to sensory processing store sensory information during delay periods during performance of working-memory tasks. Therefore, there is not a single but rather multiple working-memory network interactions.[8] For example,

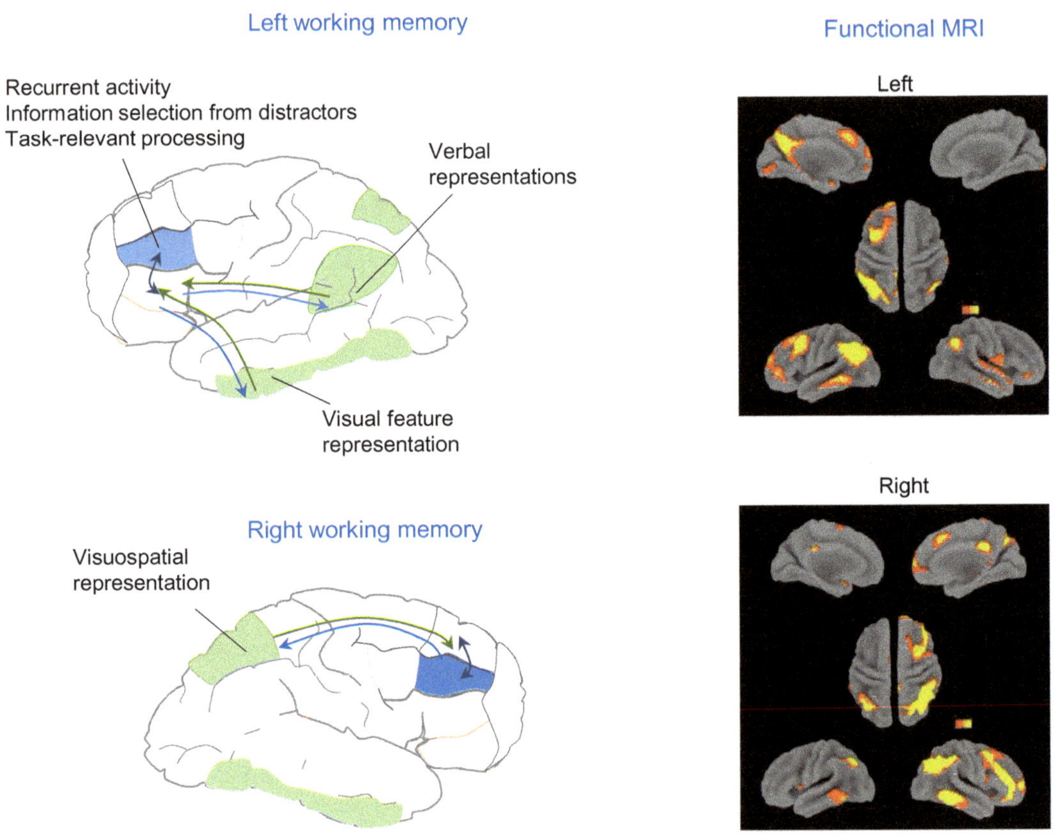

FIGURE 42.3 Areas involved in working memory

Working memory results from the dynamic interaction of a large number of brain regions. Maintenance of working memory involves reentrant loops between frontal and posterior cortical areas encoding perceptual information. Spatial working-memory tasks commonly activate parietal cortex bilaterally predominantly on the right hemisphere; stimulus categories, such as faces and houses, activate category-specific regions of the ventral visual cortex; and the left inferior parietal superior temporal and ventral prefrontal regions are activated during verbal working memory. The lateral prefrontal cortex is critical for information maintenance and manipulation during all working-memory tasks (Functional MRI images courtesy of Dr. David Jones).

spatial working-memory tasks commonly activate parietal cortex bilaterally predominantly on the right hemisphere. Different stimulus categories, such as faces and houses, activate category-specific regions of the ventral visual cortex. The left inferior parietal superior temporal and ventral prefrontal regions are activated during verbal working memory. The lateral PFC is critical for information maintenance during all working-memory tasks.[9] Meta-analyses have demonstrated that the left, particularly ventrolateral, PFC is more involved in verbal working-memory tasks, whereas the right, particularly dorsolateral, PFC is more involved in spatial working-memory tasks. There is substantial overlap between the neural mechanisms supporting working memory and those involved in attention and cognitive control. Together with the lateral PFC, the superior parietal cortex has also been associated with executive aspects of working memory. Both the cerebellum and the striatum are also commonly activated in working-memory tasks. Neuroimaging studies have shown that activity of the medial temporal lobe may be needed for working-memory tasks that require binding and relational processing associated with stored memories.[8]

Processing Hierarchy in the Lateral Frontal Cortex

As discussed previously, a key feature of human cortical organization is the spatial arrangement of areas along a global gradient between sensory motor and transmodal regions.[17] Functional MRI studies show that there is a functional gradient along the anterior-to-posterior axis of the lateral frontal cortex, representing a processing hierarchy according to the task involved. Simple response tasks activate the lateral premotor cortex (area 6), feature-based tasks activate area 8; dimension-based tasks activate the inferior frontal sulcus (areas 45 and 9/46); and task contexts activate the frontopolar cortex (area 10). Thus, the frontopolar regions are preferentially activated in relationship to the abstraction level of goals and task rules, whereas activity toward posterior portions of the lateral frontal cortex becomes progressively more specific to certain situational contexts. This hierarchical organization indicates that the frontopolar cortex influences information processing in posterior regions via widespread back projections down to area 6 at the lowest level. The frontopolar cortex is at the highest of cognitive processing and may have a major role functions such as novelty seeking, multitasking, and prospective thinking. Multitasking requires the ability to hold goals in mind while performing or processing secondary subgoals ("cognitive branching"), ability to remember to carry out an intended act in the future while engaging in another task, and effectively managing time while switching tasks. Prospection, imagining the future, or "metacognition," requires reality monitoring, introspection, self-judgment, and analogical reasoning and involves interactions with components of the default network, which constitutes the final transmodal region along the gradient of cortical organization.[17]

DECISION-MAKING, MOTIVATION, AND ALLOCATION OF EFFORT

Decision-making is the selection of a particular option among a set of alternatives that are expected to produce different outcomes. This requires assignation of value to the available options and comparison of values and outcomes, and depends on both past experience and current motivational state. Motivation invigorates and guides behaviors toward goals.[40] The successful pursuing of a goal requires cognitive control, especially when it is necessary to overcome distraction or strong habitual responses or when outcomes deviate from expectations. Appropriate cognitive control requires cognitive effort, which allocates cognitive resources, such as working memory, to the pursuit of a goal. These functions reflect the coordinated interaction among multiple cortical areas including the OFC, ventromedial PFC, ACC, and MCC and their interactions with the amygdala, ventral striatum (particularly the nucleus accumbens, NAc), and midbrain dopaminergic system (Figure 42.4).[10,14,15,40–44]

Orbitofrontal Cortex: Decisions Based on Outcomes

As discussed in chapter 39, the OFC has a major role in assignation of value to available options and decision-making based on comparison of values.[10,42] The OFC processes sensory stimuli from all modalities to compute their subjective value and reward expectations, in order to estimate the expected outcome that can affect behavioral choices. Some neurons of the medial OFC encode the attributes of potential choices or rewards to be expected, whereas others encode the value of potential outcomes of these choices. Neuroimaging and neuropsychological studies show that activity of the human medial OFC is related with the learning, memory, and monitoring of the reward value of stimuli, including their hedonic quality.[41] Pleasant stimuli or positive rewards activate the medial OFC, which is connected to the pregenual ACC. Activation of these areas correlates linearly with the subjective emotional experience of affective stimuli. Unpleasant stimuli or punishers activate the lateral PFC, which is connected to the anterior MCC. The most anterior portion of the medial OFC, corresponding to the medial frontopolar area 10, is involved in the final binary decision about which among available stimuli is chosen to guide behavior. The classical tests of OFC function are reward devaluation paradigms and stimulus-outcome reversal learning. In reward devaluation tasks, subjects learn two stimuli that predict two different rewards. Then one of these stimuli is devalued due to an aversive outcome. In normal conditions, this change in value in one stimulus immediately leads to the selection of the alternative stimulus. In reversal learning studies, one stimulus is paired with a reward and other is not. When learning has been acquired, the rewarding stimulus switches, so that the reward is now delivered after the previous unrewarded stimulus. In normal conditions, this leads to a reversal of choice.[42]

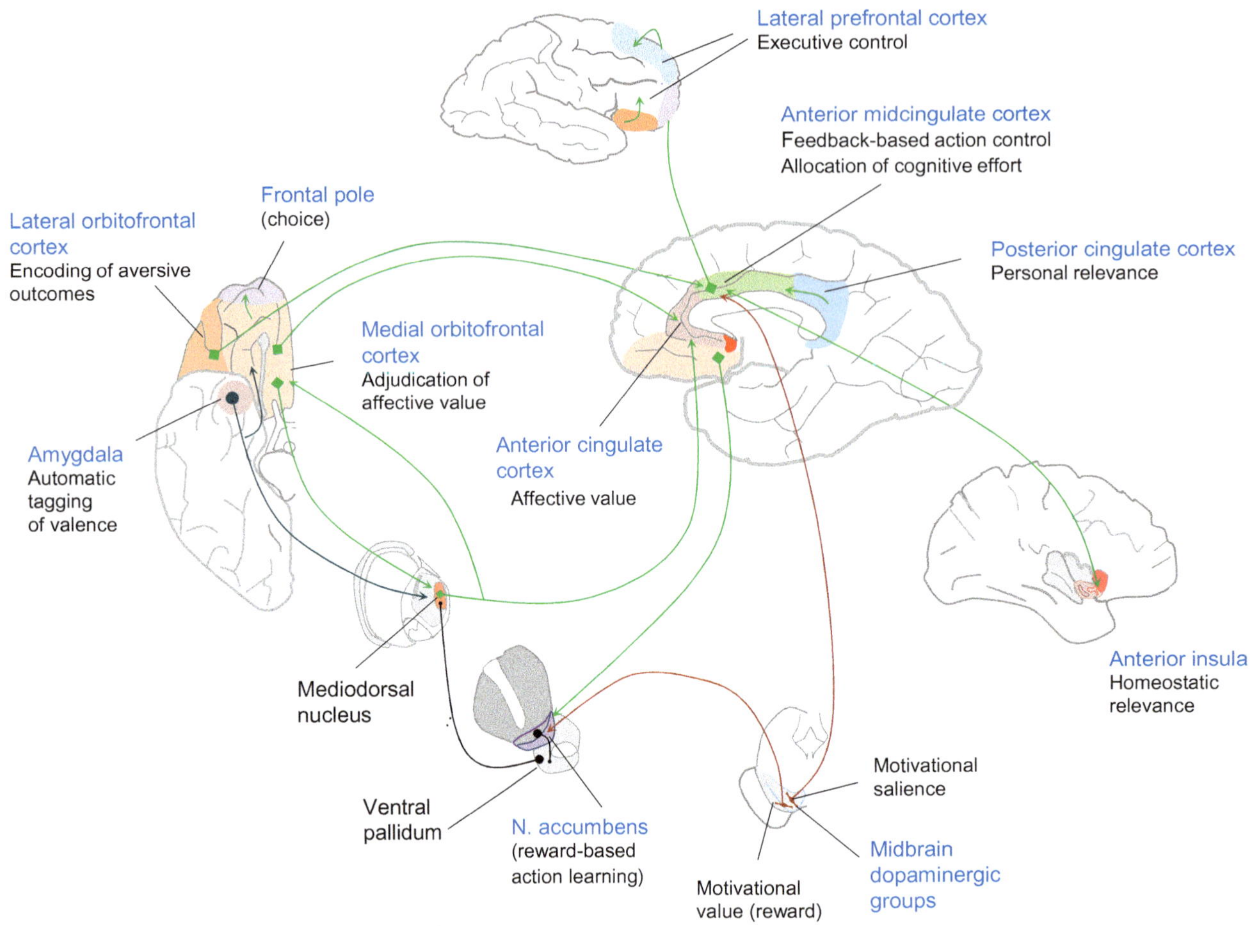

FIGURE 42.4 Areas involved in decision-making and motivation
Assignation of value to stimuli and outcomes, decision-making, cognitive control when it is necessary to overcome distraction, cognitive effort, and motivation reflect the coordinated interaction among multiple cortical and subcortical areas, including the orbitofrontal cortex, ventromedial prefrontal cortex, anterior cingulate cortex, ventral striatum (particularly the nucleus accumbens), and midbrain dopamine neurons.

Cingulate Cortex and Subsystems for Control of Reward-Based and Outcome-Based Behavior

As also discussed in chapter 39, the cingulate cortex harbors at least three subsystems controlling behavior.[43,44] The ACC has an emotional function and includes a subgenual (subcallosal) region primarily activated by negatively valenced stimuli and memories and a pregenual region activated by positively affective (pleasant) reward values with activation that correlates with the subjective state of pleasure. The activation of the pregenual ACC area reflects emotional awareness. The continuous scaling of value in the medial OFC and pregenual ACC is critical for selecting action outcomes in order to select a specific goal during decision-making. The pregenual ACC is also involved in assessment of the cost of actions. The ventral PCC is engaged in assessment of personal relevance of sensory information.[45] Once the personal relevance is coded in the ventral PCC it becomes available to the subgenual ACC. Personal relevance is also encoded in pregenual ACC area 24, where there is attribution of personal relevance to rewards. The MCC enables reward outcome information from the OFC and ACC to be associated with personally relevant space and action information from the PCC to guide motor behavior. The anterior MCC is involved in cognitive motor control and intentional movement generation, which are linked to its major function in feedback-based action responsiveness to error and reward.[43,44]

Subcortical Components of Motivation: Ventral Striatum and Midbrain Dopaminergic System

The key subcortical components of the motivation system are the ventral striatum, particularly the NAc, and the midbrain dopaminergic neurons.[15] The ventral striatum receives partially overlapping inputs from the OFC, medial PFC, and MCC. The caudal ventromedial PFC projects primarily to the NAc; the OFC and insula to the medial caudate and rostral ventral putamen; and the MCC to the head of the caudate.[46] As mentioned in previous chapters, the

NAc consists of a core region and a shell region; the NAc core shares features with other components of the striatum whereas the NAc shell constitutes an interface between the basal ganglia and the emotional limbic subcircuits based on its interaction with the amygdala, hypothalamus, periaqueductal gray, and brainstem autonomic regions. Diffusion tractography shows that the lateral-rostral region of the NAc (putative core) is preferentially connected to other components of the basal ganglia, the frontal pole, OFC, and thalamus; the medial-caudal region of the NAc (putative shell) to the amygdala; and both divisions are connected to the ACC, insula, and hippocampus.[47]

Projections from the NAc target the ventral pallidum and substantia nigra pars reticulata, which in turn project to the ventral anterior and dorsomedial nuclei of the thalamus; these thalamic nuclei project back to the OFC, ACC, and MCC thus closing the so-called limbic circuit of the basal ganglia. The ventral pallidum and substantia nigra pars reticulata also project to the STN, superior colliculus, and pedunculopontine tegmental nucleus.[48,49] Core-based circuits may function in action selection, whereas shell-based circuits participate in encoding the reward value and reinforcing effects of rewards.[48,50] Both the ventral striatum and the MCC receive strong dopaminergic inputs from the ventral tegmental area and substantia nigra pars compacta.[51] The NAc shell primarily receives inputs from midbrain dopaminergic neurons that encode the reward value of stimuli. The dopamine peaks in the striatum promote the selection of the rewarding action.[52] Dopaminergic inputs to the NAc thus promote behavioral activation, approach behavior, exertion of effort, and sustained engagement in tasks.[52–54] In contrast, areas of the PFC, including the anterior MCC, receive dopaminergic inputs from midbrain neurons that encode the motivational salience of stimuli and increase their activity both in response to a positive or a negative outcome. These signals are important to allocate cognitive effort. Whereas the dopamine peaks are important signals for rewards, the reduced firing of dopaminergic neurons may not be the major signal encoding reward-prediction errors or punishers.[10] The lateral OFC (areas 47/12) contains error neurons that detect nonreward and respond when an expected reward is not obtained or when an action leads to an aversive outcome. These OFC negative reward prediction error neurons may be more suitable to encode negative reward-prediction errors than midbrain dopaminergic neurons, as OFC neurons encode both the expected reward and learned reinforcer (stimulus-reward association).[10] The lateral OFC projects to the anterior MCC and ventrolateral PFC, which are involved in outcome-based action control.[10] The OFC also sends inputs to the ventral striatum, which via the globus pallidus projects to the lateral habenula. The lateral habenula responds to negative outcomes and controls the activity of midbrain dopamine neurons. Thus, the error-encoding neurons of the OFC may have a major role in the mechanism of stimulus-outcome reversal learning, by which a previously rewarding stimulus is no longer chosen when it no longer produces an expected favorable outcome or results in punishment.[42]

Anterior Midcingulate Cortex Use of Outcome Information for Cognitive Control of Effort

The anterior MCC has a major role in feedback-mediated decision-making for reward/approach and fear/avoidance decisions, by providing an interface among reward, decision-making, action selection, motivation, and effort allocation.[55] The anterior MCC is primarily engaged in tasks that demand cognitive control to pursue a goal, especially when it is necessary to overcome distraction or strong habitual automatic responses.[56,57] The behavioral relevance of incentives, determined both by the expected size of the reward and the effort cost (demands) to obtaining it, drives the allocation of working-memory resources to accomplish a goal. The anterior MCC monitors action-outcome associations to determine benefits and costs and allocate cognitive effort, then recruits the lateral PFC to implement control.[58] The MCC may monitor both the increased costs and incremental progress and then convey the balance between these variables to the midbrain dopaminergic neurons. Whereas tonic dopamine levels in the lateral PFC promote stability of mental representations, phasic dopamine signals render these circuits into a labile state that allows flexible adaptation of working-memory representations. This phasic dopamine release may also encode a reward-minus-effort signal that promotes the allocation of effort by the anterior MCC. In the ventral striatum, dopamine would first select the action sequences for goal-directed behavior and then invigorate action as the goal is reached.[54] The anterior MCC monitors the outcome of a choice, which is critical for behavioral adjustments.[59] Human studies show activation of the anterior MCC when subjects receive negative feedback following inappropriate behaviors. In experimental animals, neurons in the anterior MCC are activated together with those in the lateral habenula in response to adverse outcomes such as reward omission.[59] Inputs from the lateral habenula indirectly inhibit the activity of dopaminergic neurons encoding stimulus value and projecting to the NAc shell, while directly promoting activity of dopaminergic neurons encoding stimulus valence and projecting to the anterior MCC. As the anterior MCC reciprocally projects to the lateral habenula, these two structures can communicate with each other and cooperate to monitor a negative outcome. Whereas the lateral habenula quickly detects the negative outcome of an ongoing action, the anterior MCC stores information about negative past experiences and signals the appropriate behavioral adjustment during the next choice trial.[59]

COGNITIVE CONTROL NETWORKS

Normal cognitive function depends on tonic alertness, selective attention, and adaptive control of behavior. Tonic alertness is a mentally effortful, self-initiated preparedness to process information and to respond. Selective attention enhances processing of task-relevant sensory inputs. Adaptive cognitive control is required for initiation and maintenance of behavior after a cue, behavioral adaptation in response to errors, and moment-to-moment capacity to shift between mental processes in response to contextual changes (set-shifting or cognitive flexibility). Cognitive control involves three distributed networks, a frontoparietal network, a cingulo-opercular network and the salience network[12,13,60] (Figure 42.5). Each has a unique function in cognitive control, separate from that of downstream processing or attention networks. These control networks are apparent by two years of age and throughout childhood and adolescence and then become integrated with other brain networks supporting maturation of inhibitory control.[61]

Frontoparietal Network

The frontoparietal network comprises bilaterally the dorsolateral PFC, frontopolar PFC, posterior inferior

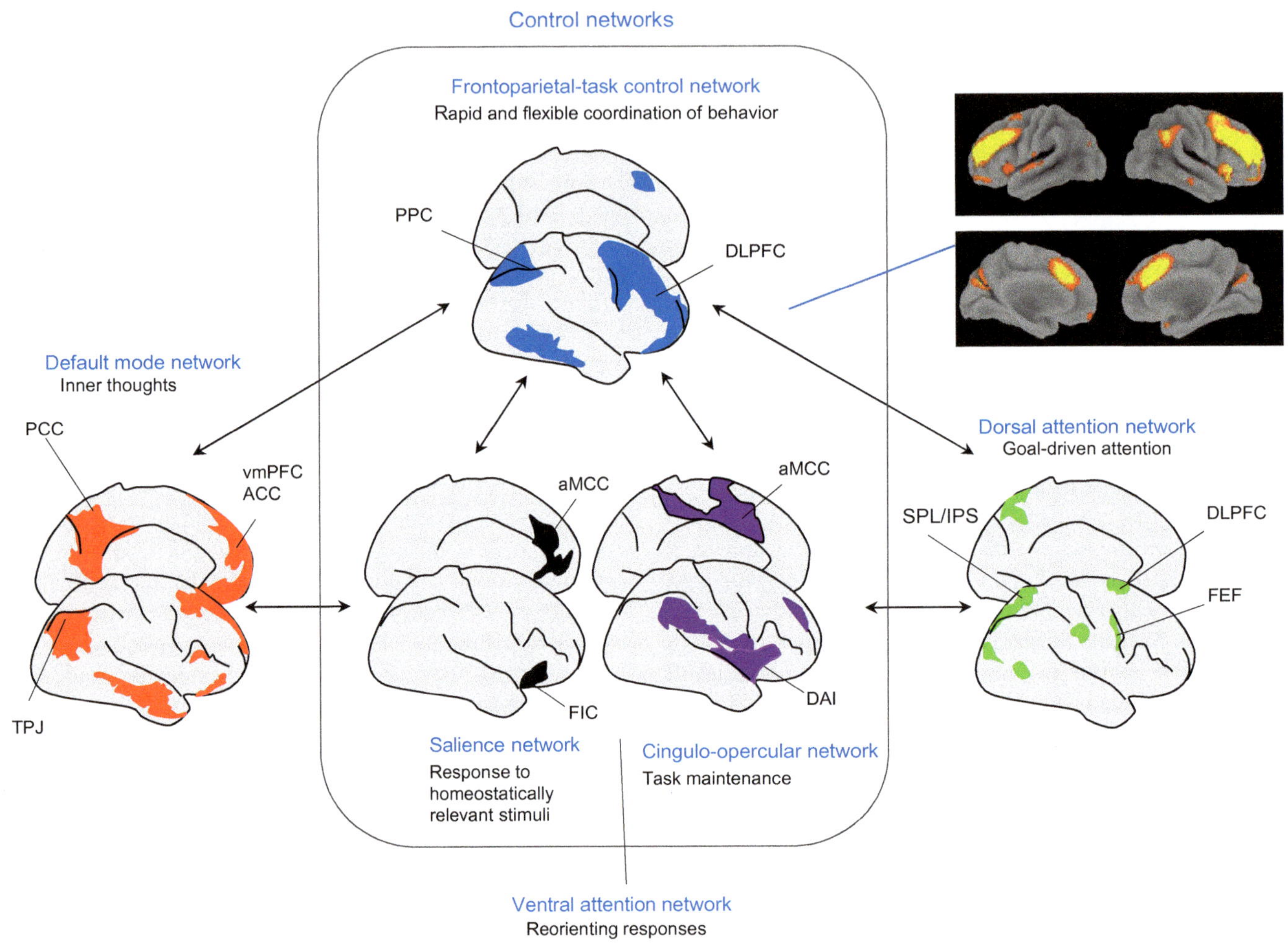

FIGURE 42.5 Executive control networks and interactions with other networks

Cognitive control involves two distributed networks, a cingulo-opercular network and the frontoparietal network. The cingulo-opercular network comprises bilaterally the anterior midcingulate cortex (MCC) and anterior insula/frontal operculum; (AI) interconnected areas include the dorsal anterior prefrontal cortex (PFC) and anterior inferior parietal lobe (supramarginal gyrus). A central function of this network is the maintenance of tonic alertness or vigilance and the stable maintenance of task control and task goals. Components of this network have also been referred to as the "salience" network, which detects behaviorally significant stimuli in the external environment. Large von Economo projection neurons, which are selectively found in anterior insula (AI), anterior MCC, and dorsolateral PFC, may have a major role in these processes. The frontoparietal network comprises bilaterally the dorsolateral PFC (DLPFC), frontopolar cortex, posterior parietal cortex (PPC), posterior inferior parietal lobe, paracingulate gyrus, and portions of the MCC and shares. The cingulo-opercular and the salience networks have their hubs in anterior insular cortex (AI) and anterior MCC. ACC, anterior insular cortex; DAI, dorsal anterior insula; FEF, frontal eye field; FIC, frontoinsular cortex; IPS, intraparietal sulcus; MPFC, medial prefrontal cortex; PCC, posterior cingulate cortex; SPL, superior parietal lobule (Functional MRI courtesy of Dr. David T. Jones).

parietal lobe, paracingulate gyrus, and portions of the MCC. Precision mapping has revealed that the functional topography of this network is variable among normal individuals.[62] The frontoparietal control network is critical for the rapid, accurate, and flexible coordination of goal-driven behavior. It supports rapid and adaptive aspects of cognitive control such as exogenously triggered initiation of control, adjusting control after errors, and moment-to-moment control during repeated rapid task-switching. The frontoparietal network is a flexible hub that shares a high degree of functional connectivity to many brain networks. Regions within the frontoparietal network flexibility adapt the strength of their functional connectivity to a diverse set of networks to accommodate changing task demands. The frontoparietal network is in close anatomic proximity to the dorsal attention network and may combine brain regions that initiate attentional control in response to cues with regions that process performance feedback on a trial-by-trial basis to adjust control settings. However, the frontoparietal control network is not only involved in externally directed tasks but also regulates self-generated mnemonic, social, and emotional information. The frontoparietal control and default networks can cooperate to perform particular mental operations, such as problem-solving tasks involving mental simulations and imagining the steps necessary to attain a personal goal. This emphasizes the concept that the default network processes transmodal information that is not tied to a specific form of informational content, and may act as a hub that integrates representational information across the cortex. The frontoparietal network has a major role in implementing and flexibly modulating control to meet task demands. It demonstrates transient signals resulting from the realization for the need to instantiate control and adaptive control (i.e., performance-related feedback). The strength of functional integration of the frontoparietal network and the rest of the brain is crucial for supporting superior cognitive functioning.[63] Greater connectivity between the frontoparietal and default mode networks during resting state was correlated with higher intelligence scores.[64]

Cingulo-Opercular Network

The cingulo-opercular network comprises bilaterally the anterior MCC and dorsal anterior insula and frontal operculum; interconnected areas include the dorsal anterior PFC and anterior inferior parietal lobe (supramarginal gyrus). A major function of this network is the stable maintenance of task control and task goals.[26] This network may also have a role in maintenance of tonic alertness or vigilance.[13]

Salience Network

Salience is defined as objects, ideas, or events that are very important or noticeable and thus attract attention. Salience is not only relevant for attention but also refers to contexts such as personal relevance of stimuli or events that are meaningful or emotionally provocative. Thus, the concept of salience provides a broad construct that is relevant to the domains of pain, error detection, and attention. The salience network responds to homeostatically relevant stimuli and outcomes.[25] This network has its hubs at the transition between the pregenual ACC and anterior MCC and at the ventral anterior insular (frontoinsular) cortex. These areas contain von Economo neurons that project to the brainstem. The salience network also includes the temporal pole, mediodorsal nucleus of the thalamus, extended amygdala, and midbrain dopaminergic areas. Ascending inputs conveying information about the body are integrated in the frontoinsular cortex. A resting-state functional connectivity study demonstrated strong connections between the anterior insula and the ACC/MCC.

The salience network functions by enabling communication of cortical areas with subcortical regions to integrate interoceptive and visceromotor signals that can be used to guide behavior and has a key role in dynamically switching between external and internal modes of attention.[25,65] Mapping of gradients in connectivity patterns throughout the cortex shows that the salience network is situated between unimodal regions and the frontoparietal control network.[18]

Anterior Midcingulate Cortex as a Nexus for Control

The anterior MCC comprises functionally diverse, flexible network nodes that are involved multiple regulatory behaviors. There is an organizing gradient along the anterior and midcingulate cortex.[18] As in the case of the insular cortex,[66] there may be a continuous gradual gradient of functional connectivity along the ventral-anterior to dorsal posterior axis along the dorsal cingulate cortex, including the ACC and MCC.[18] The anterior MCC is activated during several tasks requiring cognitive control, including novelty detection, error monitoring, and task switching. It participates in several large-scale functional brain networks, including the ventral attention network that corresponds to both the salience and cingulo-opercular task control networks.

There is an overlapping activation of the anterior MCC by pain, negative affect, and cognitive control. This indicates that this region functions as a domain-general hub where emotionally salient inputs are linked to motor centers for expression of affect and execution of goal-directed behavior.[56] The anterior MCC may use information about punishment to control aversively motivated actions. The anterior MCC may serve as a link between higher-level cognitive representations of the ACC and medial PFC and motor output.[18] The function of the anterior MCC in the salience network may be to allow rapid access to the motor system to facilitate appropriate behavioral responses to salient inputs from the environment.

The anterior MCC also signals the expected value of control.[57] One of the functions of the anterior MCC may be to monitor whether the current behavior is serving the demands of the task. Control signals from the anterior

MCC may determine how much cognitive effort should be allocated to the task, taking into account both the benefits and costs of such effort.[57] Signals that indicate the need to respecify the intensity of control include response conflict, delays or errors, negative feedback, and aversive outcomes. The classical example of a task demanding executive control is the Stroop task. In this task, participants are shown a color word and asked to name the color of the font in which it is displayed. When the two dimensions disagree (e.g., "GREEN" written in red text), there is an interference effect, and the subjects have to make a cognitive effort to overcome the automatic tendency to name the word. Control can be integrated across many past experiences in order to appropriate guide the next choice. Human neuroimaging studies show anterior MCC activation in a wide variety of tasks that involve selecting between actions; it is most active when persons explore options not expected to generate immediate reward, or when their decision moves away from long-term expectations based on repetition of the same action.[56–68]

Default Mode Network and Internally Directed Reorienting

The default mode network is involved in internally directed processing, such as introspection, self-referential thoughts, or projecting oneself into a situation.[16] One core component of this network is the PCC, which encodes personal relevance together with the ACC and provides input to the MCC. The activity of the default mode network, which provides a self-centered predictive model of the world, is anticorrelated with that of the dorsal attention network, which detects novel features of the environment.[69] The default mode network is strongly deactivated during a wide range of demanding cognitive tasks that require attention to external stimuli. Engagement of the dorsal attention network in visuospatial processing is associated with suppression of the default network. In contrast, occurrence of self-generated thought reduces the processing of sensory information, a phenomenon that has been termed *perceptual decoupling*. This anticorrelation supports competitive relationships between an internal focus of attention during self-generated thought and attention to concurrent environmental stimuli. This dynamic balance emerges in early childhood and decreases with advancing age.

The salience network, which is a component of the ventral attention network, is involved in the reorienting mechanisms required for shifting from self-thought processes in the default network to activity in the dorsal attention network in order to deal with relevant stimuli or events in the environment. One of the nodal components of the salience network, the right anterior insula, may have an important role in suppressing the default network and reallocating attentional resources to salient events. Because of its functional segregation from both the dorsal attention and default networks the ventral attention (salience) network may be able to flexibly interact either with the dorsal attention network during externally directed behavior or with the default network during an internally directed behavior. The frontoparietal control network is anatomically interposed between the default and dorsal attention networks and may have a potentially important modulatory role in the activation or suppression of either of these other two networks based on switching goal states.

The default network is transmodal area that, on the basis of its connectivity, is located at the final end of a gradient that starts in areas involved in primary sensory/motor functions.[17] The role of the default network in cognition might reflect its position at one extreme of the hierarchy of the gradient of cortical organization, allowing it to process transmodal information that is unrelated to immediate sensory input. Thus, the default mode network is not tied to a specific form of informational content, and may thus act as a hub that integrates representational information across the cortex. Because of its location equidistant to all sensory and motor systems, the default network integrates multiple sensory modalities and systems, including those involved in episodic and semantic memory, reward-guided decision-making, social cognition, and goal-directed working memory. Thus the default mode network permits cognitive processing that is independent of the here and now. Whereas both the ventral attention and default systems may deactivate during goal-oriented behavior, their deactivations depend on different factors. Filtering of the ventral attention network is necessary to protect the system from involuntarily reorienting to environmental stimuli during goal-oriented behavior or when resources are allocated to self-referential processing. Studies using individual-specific precision resting-state functional connectivity showed that several default mode subnetworks exhibited topographical similarity across subjects whereas others represented separate streams by which the default network couples with other canonical large-scale networks, including language and control networks.[70]

"Multiple Demand" Cortical Areas and Subcortical Network Integration

A recent study revealed a core of 10 widely distributed "multiple-demand" parcels per hemisphere that are activated during many tasks and are functionally interconnected.[71] These areas are located along the lateral frontal surface, above the anterior insula, the dorsal part of the lateral frontal surface, dorsomedial frontal surface, within and surrounding the intraparietal sulcus, dorsomedial parietal cortex, and posterior temporal cortex. A study using precision functional mapping-individual-specific analysis revealed distinct subcortical zones of network specificity and multinetwork integration.[72] This study showed that the caudate nucleus is an integration zone for convergence of the default mode and multiple control networks; the ventral intermedius nucleus of the thalamus is a convergence motor integration zone of the cingulo-opercular control and somatomotor networks; and the pulvinar is a convergence integration zone between the dorsal attention and visual networks.[72]

Network Oscillations and Cognitive Control

Cognitive control involves the long-distance integration of activity of local neuronal ensembles, reflected by coupled cortical oscillations. Via cross-frequency phase–amplitude coupling, slower-frequency oscillations coordinate gamma activity over long distances. Alpha oscillations mediate both feedback and feedforward processing and are associated with reduced neural excitability. Thalamocortical interactions primarily via the pulvinar, as well as cortico-cortical interactions may be pivotal in originating cortical alpha oscillations that translate control signals from prefrontal and parietal regions into modulation in other cortical areas. One model proposes that the cingulo-opercular network provides top-down modulation via widespread enhancement of alpha oscillations, leading to a global inhibition of neural activity; this would correspond to an intrinsically maintained tonic alertness and nonspecific disengagement from task-irrelevant brain processing.[73] In contrast, activity of the dorsal attention network initiates a focal reduction of alpha oscillations in task-relevant sensory areas. The frontoparietal control network would participate in exchange of currently relevant information across remote areas by controlling and stabilizing the phase-lag of alpha oscillations between distant neural populations. Theta band activity is also broadly distributed across the brain and reflects active operations during high-level cognitive processes such as memory encoding and retrieval, working memory retention, novelty detection, and top-down control.[74] Frontal midline theta activity originating primarily in the MCC and the pre-supplementary motor area may convey the need of control. This activity manifests as components of the event-related potential detected on surface electrode recordings and reflects control processes elicited by novel information, conflicting stimulus-response requirements, realization of errors, and punishing feedback.

CLINICAL CORRELATIONS

Attention Network Damage and Spatial Neglect

Spatial neglect is characterized by a bias to attend and respond to objects on the contralesional hemispace. Visuospatial neglect most frequently occurs with lesions at the right temporoparietal junction and superior temporal cortex, and less frequently with damage of the frontal lobe, ACC, superior parietal lobule, or thalamus, particularly the pulvinar. Neglect can also result from white matter lesions that affect structural connections between nodes of the attention network. Functional MRI studies indicate that the spatial bias of neglect reflects a physiological imbalance between left and right dorsal parietal cortex caused by structural and physiological abnormalities in the ventral attention network. Left-side neglect is associated with relative hyperactivation of left parietal cortex and impaired functional connectivity within the damaged ventral network involving the right middle frontal gyrus and its white matter connections to the dorsal parietal cortex. Impaired interactions between the ventral and dorsal attention networks may produce an imbalance in parietal spatial maps that result in a tonic attentional bias toward the ipsilesional field. This would be consistent with the "interhemispheric competition" model, in which each hemisphere directs attention toward the contralateral visual field. In the intact brain the two hemispheric processors would be balanced through mutual reciprocal inhibition possibly via callosal connections, or through cortico-subcortical interactions. Functional brain-imaging studies have shown several asymmetries in the strengths of attentional biasing signals across the nodes of the dorsal attention network, which can theoretically account for the observed right hemispheric dominance. Studies in patients suffering from hemineglect following a stroke in the right superior temporal cortex showed reduced activity in the right relative to the left dorsal parietal attention network, even though these brain regions were structurally intact. This results in an imbalance of attentional biasing signals generated by each hemisphere and, thus in the ability to control contralateral hemispace.

Effects of Orbitofrontal Lesions

Focal lesions in the frontal lobe produce cognitive and behavioral alteration that reflect its multiple function as a hub of several distributed cortical networks.[19] The profound effects of lesions of the OFC are typified by the classical case of Phineas Gage, who underwent profound behavioral and personality changes following damage of the left orbitofrontal cortex and its connections from a penetrating head injury.[75,76] Patients with orbitofrontal damage have profound deficits in decision-making. They have impaired inhibition of inappropriate responses leading to impulsivity and risk-taking behavior. These patients make maladaptive decisions and continue to respond to stimuli that are no longer rewarding, even after acknowledging the changes in contingencies. These deficits reflect the importance of the OFC for learning and relearning associations of choices with reward or punishment outcomes, and for updating behavior based on these associations. Lesions affecting the medial orbital and ventromedial prefrontal cortex are also associated with abnormalities in affective and social behavior. Focal lesions including the medial OFC and ventromedial PFC may result in profound abnormalities in emotion recognition and social behavior, as discussed in chapter 39. For example, these patients have poorly modulated emotional responses and fail to use emotions or social cues to guide decisions. Patients with OFC also have impairment in attention, particularly to emotional stimuli, and impairment in temporal context memory, that often result in confabulation.

Several studies indicate abnormalities in the OFC activity and volume in both obsessive-compulsive disorders and drug addiction. These disorders have several features in common, including tight coupling of particular actions to particular external cues, leading to the urge to carry out that action or difficulty suppressing it despite cognitive awareness of probability of an aversive outcome. These cues create a state of anxiety until the habitual behavior is executed. Compulsions therefore constitute an irresistible urge to act, to prevent or reduce anxiety and stress despite a negative outcome. In general, the OFC is hyperactive both at rest and during some tasks compared to that in control persons.

Effects of Medial Prefrontal Lesions

Damage of the dorsomedial PFC, including the anterior MCC, has been associated with inability to detect error, difficulty resolving stimulus conflict, inattention, abulia, and akinetic mutism. Impaired MCC function produces global slowing and increased response variability on tasks requiring cognitive control. However, MCC damage does not impair performance in the Stroop and the Go-NoGo tasks, which measure conflict and error detection and activate the MCC in fMRI studies. This indicates that the anterior MCC depends on the lateral PFC to monitor several types of response conflict. Consistent with the role of the MCC in associating actions with value and updating goal-directed actions based on previous reinforcement, patients with MCC damage are less likely than normal individuals to repeat an action that led to a reward in previous trial. Lesions affecting the MCC also produce lack of motivation, manifested with abulia or, in severe cases, akinetic mutism. This reduction in spontaneous, self-initiated behaviors and spontaneous responses may result from damage of the posterior midcingulate cortex and or its connections with premotor areas. Lesions affecting midline prefrontal areas including the anterior MCC result in inability to maintain a task set with preserved ability to switch tasks. In contrast, lesions in lateral PFC produce deficits in the ability to switch tasks but spare the ability to maintain a task set.

Dysexecutive Syndrome in Neurodegenerative Dementias

Lesions affecting the lateral PFC produce severe deficits in cognitive control and executive functions. Manifestations include difficulty performing working-memory tasks, increased distractibility, impaired retrieval, perseveration, and inability to perform sequential actions. Lesions restricted to the frontopolar cortex may not alter performance in neuropsychological testing but may result in disorganized behavior in situations encountered in everyday life, impaired multitasking, inability to switch between cognitive contexts, impaired estimation of time, and deficits in creativity and original thinking.[19]

Impaired cognitive control and dysexecutive syndrome is a typical feature of behavioral variant frontotemporal dementia (bvFTD) and Alzheimer disease (AD). These disorders are characterized by altered functional connectivity within large-scale networks. Patients with bvFTD have abnormal functional connectivity within the salience, default mode, executive, attention/working memory, and dorsal attentional networks.[77] Whereas behavioral variant FTD is the prototypical neurodegenerative disorder associated with impaired executive function, early involvement of working memory networks may manifest with prominent dysexecutive syndrome in AD. A recent review on 55 participants with AD showed that this disorder may frequently manifest with progressive impairment of executive function such as working memory, cognitive flexibility, and cognitive inhibitory control.[78] In these patients there was hypometabolism of frontal and parietal regions that overlap with working memory network, with relative sparing of the medial temporal lobes (unlike amnestic-type AD), occipital lobe (unlike posterior cortical atrophy variant AD), and left temporal region (unlike language variant AD) (Figure 24.6).[78]

Behavioral Manifestations of Parkinson Disease

Patients with Parkinson disease (PD) have behavioral manifestations that reflect impaired dopaminergic modulation of prefrontal and striatal circuits involved in motivation and decision-making. Dopamine has complex effects on both the PFC and the striatum, via different receptor subtypes. In the lateral PFC, the effects of dopamine exhibit an inverted U curve so that either too little or too much dopamine has deleterious effects on attention and other functions, including cognitive control.[39] Thus, both dopaminergic deficits due to loss of midbrain neurons and excessive dopaminergic replacement therapy may adversely affect behavior. In PD, manifestations such as anxiety, depression, and apathy have been defined as a "hypodopaminergic syndrome," whereas both impulse control disorders and dopamine dysregulation syndrome associated with dopaminergic therapy have been defined as a "hyperdopaminergic syndrome."[79] Depression and apathy often coexist in PD patients, but may occur separately. Both apathy and depression may respond to dopaminergic therapy in a proportion of PD patients. Neuroimaging studies using dopamine transporter (DAT) single photon emission computer tomography (SPECT) showed greater reduction in dopaminergic innervation of the caudate nucleus in de novo untreated PD patients with apathy or depression than in patients without these symptoms.[80,81] Involvement of the caudate, which is part of a frontostriatal circuit for executive control and goal-oriented behavior could explain the cognitive difficulties that accompany depression and apathy.[81]

In one study in patients with early PD, $^{(18)}$F-DOPA uptake in the bilateral ACC and middle frontal gyrus correlated with executive function and verbal fluency, indicating a role of the mesocortical dopaminergic pathways in cognitive dysfunction in early PD.[82]

Impulse control disorders associated with dopaminergic agonist therapy share epidemiological and phenomenological overlap with substance abuse disorders.[79] Chronic administration of dopaminergic agonists may

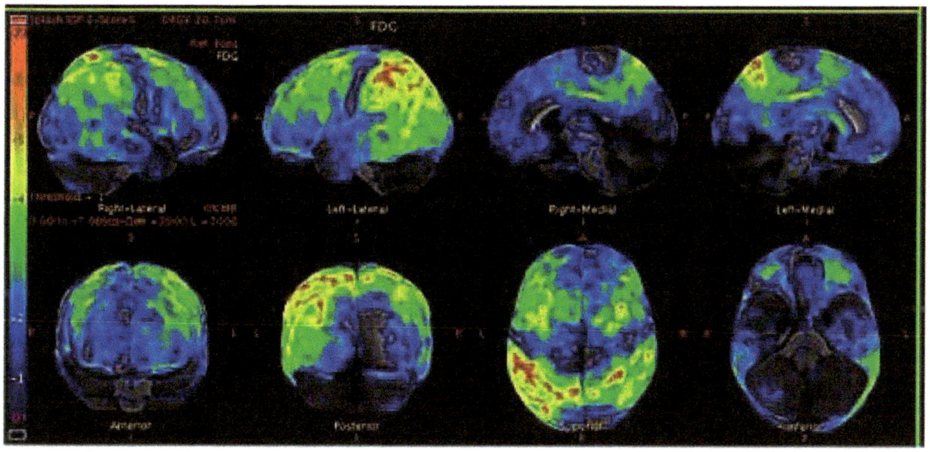

FIGURE 42.6 Involvement of executive control network in Alzheimer disease
18[Fluroro]deoxy glucose positron emission tomography of a 51-year-old patient with Alzheimer disease who presented with difficulty with attention, action, sequencing, and mental calculations, followed by word-finding difficulties. There is hypometabolism in parietal and frontal cortical regions of the dorsal attention and working-memory networks. (Courtesy of Dr. Hugo Botha).

elicit downregulation of D2/D3 inhibitory autoreceptors, enhancing firing of dopaminergic neurons of the ventral tegmental area. The NAc expresses high levels of D3Rs, which mediate the reinforcing effects of dopamine released from ventral tegmental area afferents. Patients with dopamine dysregulation syndrome have enhanced levodopa-induced dopamine release in the ventral striatum; and patients with impulse control disorders have enhanced striatal dopamine release in response to reward-related visual cues or during a gambling task. Pramipexole has a higher affinity for the D3R subtype than other dopamine receptor agonists and elicits upregulation of these receptors in the striatum; upregulation of D3R binding relates to gambling severity and other impulse control disorders in PD.

Impulsivity in Parkinson's disease may be mediated by faulty evaluation of rewards or the failure to inhibit inappropriate choices. A systematic review and meta-analysis of morphometric and functional studies in PD patients with impulse control disorders consistently showed increased activity in the ventral striatum and OFC and decreased activity in the ACC.[83]

A high-resolution diffusion MRI study on reward evaluation and response inhibition networks using high resolution tractography in patients with PD performing a task of gambling in a virtual casino showed that different components of impulsivity were associated with distinct variations of structural connectivity.[84] Risk taking (larger bet sizes) was associated with greater connectivity of the reward evaluation network involving the ventral striatum and ventromedial PFC bilaterally; in contrast, increased exploration of alternative slot machines in the virtual casino was associated with weaker connectivity of the response inhibition network particularly between the right preSMA and STN.[84]

KEY POINTS

- Attention, working memory, decision-making, and cognitive control engage large-scale cortical networks.
- Mapping of gradients in connectivity patterns throughout the cortex shows that cortical are arranged in a consistent spatial order.
- There is a functional gradient along the anterior-to-posterior axis of the lateral frontal cortex, representing a processing hierarchy according to the task involved.
- The dorsal attention network is involved in goal-oriented attention.
- The ventral attention network registers salient events, resets ongoing activity of the dorsal network during reorienting responses, and is lateralized to the right hemisphere.
- Working memory is the short-term maintenance of information over brief periods of time and processing of the transiently stored information for guidance of behavior.
- Working memory is potentially vulnerable to distraction; its capacity is limited, changes across the lifespan, and can be modified by training.
- Decision-making based on the affective value of stimuli or outcomes involves interactions between the orbitofrontal cortex (OFC) and several portions of the cingulate cortex.
- The OFC has a major role in assignation of value to available options and in decision-making based on comparison of values.
- The anterior cingulate cortex (ACC) is involved in evaluation of stimuli, selection between values, and processing of inner thoughts to guide behavior.

- The midcingulate cortex (MCC) uses feedback information about outcomes for cognitive control of motor output and allocation of effort.
- Frontal cortical areas involved in motivation, decision-making, and cognitive control, and effort allocation project to the ventromedial striatum, including the nucleus accumbens (NAc).
- Dopaminergic inputs to the NAc promote behavioral activation, approach behavior, exertion of effort, and sustained engagement in tasks.
- The anterior MCC monitors action–outcome associations to determine benefits and costs to allocate cognitive effort and recruits the lateral PFC to implement control.
- The anterior MCC and the lateral habenula monitor adverse outcome to modify action selection in part by affecting activity of midbrain dopaminergic neurons.
- Adaptive cognitive control is required for initiation and maintenance of behavior, behavioral adaptation in response to errors, capacity, and flexible responses to contextual changes.
- The frontoparietal control network is critical for the rapid, accurate, and flexible coordination of goal-driven behavior.
- The cinguloopercular network is involved in the stable maintenance of task control and task goals.
- The salience network including the anterior insula and anterior MCC has a key role in dynamically switching between external and internal modes of attention.
- Internally directed processing, such as introspection, self-referential thoughts, or projecting oneself into a situation involve the default network.
- Reorienting triggered by the salience network allow shifting from self-thought processes in the default network to the dorsal attention network to deal with environmental relevant events.
- Visuospatial neglect most frequently occurs with lesions at the right temporoparietal junction and superior temporal cortex.
- Orbitofrontal damage produce deficits in decision-making, impaired inhibition of inappropriate responses, impulsivity and risk-taking behavior, impaired emotion recognition and inappropriate social behavior.
- Lesions affecting of midline prefrontal areas including the anterior MCC have resulted in inability to maintain a task set with preserved ability to switch tasks.
- Lesions affecting the lateral PFC impair working memory, cognitive control, and executive function.
- Behavioral variant frontotemporal dementia is the prototypical neurodegenerative disorder associated with impaired executive function.
- Alzheimer disease may also manifest with early and prominent dysexecutive syndrome.
- Patients with Parkinson disease have behavioral manifestations that reflect impaired dopaminergic modulation of prefrontal and striatal circuits involved in motivation and decision-making.

REFERENCES

1. Barbas H. General cortical and special prefrontal connections: principles from structure to function. Annu Rev Neurosci 2015;38:269–289.
2. de la Vega A, Chang LJ, Banich MT, Wager TD, Yarkoni T. Large-scale meta-analysis of human medial frontal cortex reveals tripartite functional organization. J Neurosci 2016;36:6553–6562.
3. de la Vega A, Yarkoni T, Wager TD, Banich MT. Large-scale meta-analysis suggests low regional modularity in lateral frontal cortex. Cereb Cortex 2018;28:3414–3428.
4. Petersen SE, Posner MI. The attention system of the human brain: 20 years after. Annu Rev Neurosci 2012;35:73–89.
5. Corbetta M, Patel G, Shulman GL. The reorienting system of the human brain: from environment to theory of mind. Neuron 2008;58:306–324.
6. Ptak R. The frontoparietal attention network of the human brain: action, saliency, and a priority map of the environment. Neuroscientist 2012;18:502–515.
7. D'Esposito M, Postle BR. The cognitive neuroscience of working memory. Annu Rev Psychol 2015;66:115–142.
8. Eriksson J, Vogel EK, Lansner A, Bergstrom F, Nyberg L. Neurocognitive architecture of working memory. Neuron 2015;88:33–46.
9. Lara AH, Wallis JD. The role of prefrontal cortex in working memory: a mini review. Front Syst Neurosci 2015;9:173.
10. Rolls ET. The orbitofrontal cortex and emotion in health and disease, including depression. Neuropsychologia 2019;128:14–43.
11. Vogt BA. Midcingulate cortex: structure, connections, homologies, functions and diseases. J Chem Neuroanat 2016;74:28–46.
12. Power JD, Petersen SE. Control-related systems in the human brain. Curr Opin Neurobiol 2013;23:223–228.
13. Marek S, Dosenbach NUF. Control networks of the frontal lobes. Handb Clin Neurol 2019;163:333–347.
14. Lee D. Decision making: from neuroscience to psychiatry. Neuron 2013;78:233–248.
15. Haber SN, Behrens TE. The neural network underlying incentive-based learning: implications for interpreting circuit disruptions in psychiatric disorders. Neuron 2014;83:1019–1039.
16. Raichle ME. The brain's default mode network. Annu Rev Neurosci 2015;38:433–447.
17. Huntenburg JM, Bazin PL, Margulies DS. Large-scale gradients in human cortical organization. Trends Cogn Sci 2018;22:21–31.
18. Margulies DS, Uddin LQ. Network convergence zones in the anterior midcingulate cortex. Handb Clin Neurol 2019;166:103–111.

19. Szczepanski SM, Knight RT. Insights into human behavior from lesions to the prefrontal cortex. Neuron 2014;83:1002–1018.
20. Siegel JS, Ramsey LE, Snyder AZ, et al. Disruptions of network connectivity predict impairment in multiple behavioral domains after stroke. Proc Natl Acad Sci U S A 2016;113:E4367–4376.
21. Catalino MP, Yao S, Green DL, Laws ER, Golby AJ, Tie Y. Mapping cognitive and emotional networks in neurosurgical patients using resting-state functional magnetic resonance imaging. Neurosurg Focus 2020;48:E9.
22. Meehan TP, Bressler SL, Tang W, et al. Top-down cortical interactions in visuospatial attention. Brain Struct Funct 2017;222:3127–3145.
23. Spadone S, Della Penna S, Sestieri C, et al. Dynamic reorganization of human resting-state networks during visuospatial attention. Proc Natl Acad Sci U S A 2015;112:8112–8117.
24. Patel GH, Sestieri C, Corbetta M. The evolution of the temporoparietal junction and posterior superior temporal sulcus. Cortex 2019;118:38–50.
25. Seeley WW. The salience network: a neural system for perceiving and responding to homeostatic demands. J Neurosci 2019;39:9878–9882.
26. Dosenbach NU, Fair DA, Miezin FM, et al. Distinct brain networks for adaptive and stable task control in humans. Proc Natl Acad Sci U S A 2007;104:11073–11078.
27. Kucyi A, Moayedi M, Weissman-Fogel I, Hodaie M, Davis KD. Hemispheric asymmetry in white matter connectivity of the temporoparietal junction with the insula and prefrontal cortex. PLoS One 2012;7:e35589.
28. Aston-Jones G, Waterhouse B. Locus coeruleus: from global projection system to adaptive regulation of behavior. Brain Res 2016;1645:75–78.
29. Dux PE, Marois R. The attentional blink: a review of data and theory. Atten Percept Psychophys 2009;71:1683–1700.
30. Snir G, Yeshurun Y. Perceptual episodes, temporal attention, and the role of cognitive control: lessons from the attentional blink. Prog Brain Res 2017;236:53–73.
31. Goodbourn PT, Martini P, Barnett-Cowan M, Harris IM, Livesey EJ, Holcombe AO. Reconsidering temporal selection in the attentional blink. Psychol Sci 2016;27:1146–1156.
32. Hikosaka O, Kim HF, Yasuda M, Yamamoto S. Basal ganglia circuits for reward value-guided behavior. Annu Rev Neurosci 2014;37:289–306.
33. Buschman TJ, Kastner S. From behavior to neural dynamics: an integrated theory of attention. Neuron 2015;88:127–144.
34. Timbie C, Barbas H. Pathways for emotions: specializations in the amygdalar, mediodorsal thalamic, and posterior orbitofrontal network. J Neurosci 2015;35:11976–11987.
35. Goll Y, Atlan G, Citri A. Attention: the claustrum. Trends Neurosci 2015;38:486–495.
36. Gazzaley A, Nobre AC. Top-down modulation: bridging selective attention and working memory. Trends Cogn Sci 2012;16:129–135.
37. Baddeley A. Working memory: theories, models, and controversies. Annu Rev Psychol 2012;63:1–29.
38. Hitch GJ, Allen RJ, Baddeley AD. Attention and binding in visual working memory: two forms of attention and two kinds of buffer storage. Atten Percept Psychophys 2020;82:280–293.
39. Arnsten AF, Wang MJ, Paspalas CD. Neuromodulation of thought: flexibilities and vulnerabilities in prefrontal cortical network synapses. Neuron 2012;76:223–239.
40. Rolls ET. Limbic systems for emotion and for memory, but no single limbic system. Cortex 2015;62:119–157.
41. Kringelbach ML. The human orbitofrontal cortex: linking reward to hedonic experience. Nat Rev Neurosci 2005;6:691–702.
42. Padoa-Schioppa C, Conen KE. Orbitofrontal cortex: a neural circuit for economic decisions. Neuron 2017;96:736–754.
43. Vogt BA. Cingulate cortex in the three limbic subsystems. Handb Clin Neurol 2019;166:39–51.
44. Rolls ET. The cingulate cortex and limbic systems for emotion, action, and memory. Brain Struct Funct 2019;224:3001–3018.
45. Andrews-Hanna JR, Smallwood J, Spreng RN. The default network and self-generated thought: component processes, dynamic control, and clinical relevance. Ann N Y Acad Sci 2014;1316:29–52.
46. Haber SN. The place of dopamine in the cortico-basal ganglia circuit. Neuroscience 2014;282C:248–257.
47. Baliki MN, Mansour A, Baria AT, et al. Parceling human accumbens into putative core and shell dissociates encoding of values for reward and pain. J Neurosci 2013;33:16383–16393.
48. Salgado S, Kaplitt MG. The nucleus accumbens: a comprehensive review. Stereotact Funct Neurosurg 2015;93:75–93.
49. Root DH, Melendez RI, Zaborszky L, Napier TC. The ventral pallidum: subregion-specific functional anatomy and roles in motivated behaviors. Prog Neurobiol 2015;130:29–70.
50. Humphries MD, Prescott TJ. The ventral basal ganglia, a selection mechanism at the crossroads of space, strategy, and reward. Prog Neurobiol 2010;90:385–417.
51. Haber SN. The place of dopamine in the cortico-basal ganglia circuit. Neuroscience 2014;282:248–257.
52. Schultz W. Updating dopamine reward signals. Curr Opin Neurobiol 2013;23:229–238.
53. Watabe-Uchida M, Eshel N, Uchida N. Neural circuitry of reward prediction error. Annu Rev Neurosci 2017;40:373–394.
54. Westbrook A, Braver TS. Dopamine does double duty in motivating cognitive effort. Neuron 2016;91:708.
55. Mogenson GJ, Jones DL, Yim CY. From motivation to action: functional interface between the limbic system and the motor system. Prog Neurobiol 1980;14:69–97.
56. Herbet G, Lafargue G, Duffau H. The dorsal cingulate cortex as a critical gateway in the network supporting conscious awareness. Brain 2016;139:e23.
57. Shenhav A, Cohen JD, Botvinick MM. Dorsal anterior cingulate cortex and the value of control. Nat Neurosci 2016;19:1286–1291.
58. Kennerley SW, Behrens TE, Wallis JD. Double dissociation of value computations in orbitofrontal and anterior cingulate neurons. Nat Neurosci 2011;14:1581–1589.
59. Kawai T, Yamada H, Sato N, Takada M, Matsumoto M. Roles of the lateral habenula and anterior cingulate cortex in negative outcome monitoring and behavioral adjustment in nonhuman primates. Neuron 2015;88:792–804.
60. Sheffield JM, Repovs G, Harms MP, et al. Fronto-parietal and cingulo-opercular network integrity and cognition in health and schizophrenia. Neuropsychologia 2015;73:82–93.
61. Marek S, Hwang K, Foran W, Hallquist MN, Luna B. The contribution of network organization and integration to the development of cognitive control. PLoS Biol 2015;13:e1002328.

62. Marek S, Dosenbach NUF. The frontoparietal network: function, electrophysiology, and importance of individual precision mapping. Dialogues Clin Neurosci 2018;20:133–140.
63. Ito T, Hearne L, Mill R, Cocuzza C, Cole MW. Discovering the computational relevance of brain network organization. Trends Cogn Sci 2020;24:25–38.
64. Hearne LJ, Mattingley JB, Cocchi L. Functional brain networks related to individual differences in human intelligence at rest. Sci Rep 2016;6:32328.
65. Uddin LQ. Salience processing and insular cortical function and dysfunction. Nat Rev Neurosci 2015;16:55–61.
66. Tian Y, Zalesky A. Characterizing the functional connectivity diversity of the insula cortex: Subregions, diversity curves and behavior. Neuroimage 2018;183:716–733.
67. Sheth SA, Mian MK, Patel SR, et al. Human dorsal anterior cingulate cortex neurons mediate ongoing behavioural adaptation. Nature 2012;488:218–221.
68. Sklar S, Walmer M, Sacre P, et al. Neuronal activity in human anterior cingulate cortex modulates with internal cognitive state during multi-source interference task. Conf Proc IEEE Eng Med Biol Soc 2017;2017:962–965.
69. Sridharan D, Levitin DJ, Menon V. A critical role for the right fronto-insular cortex in switching between central-executive and default-mode networks. Proc Natl Acad Sci U S A 2008;105:12569–12574.
70. Gordon EM, Laumann TO, Marek S, et al. Default-mode network streams for coupling to language and control systems. Proc Natl Acad Sci U S A 2020;117:17308–17319.
71. Assem M, Glasser MF, Van Essen DC, Duncan J. A domain-general cognitive core defined in multimodally parcellated human cortex. Cereb Cortex 2020;30:4361–4380.
72. Greene DJ, Marek S, Gordon EM, et al. Integrative and network-specific connectivity of the basal ganglia and thalamus defined in individuals. Neuron 2020;105:742–758 e746.
73. Sadaghiani S, Kleinschmidt A. Brain networks and alpha-oscillations: structural and functional foundations of cognitive control. Trends Cogn Sci 2016;20:805–817.
74. Cavanagh JF, Frank MJ. Frontal theta as a mechanism for cognitive control. Trends Cogn Sci 2014;18:414–421.
75. Damasio H, Grabowski T, Frank R, Galaburda AM, Damasio AR. The return of Phineas Gage: clues about the brain from the skull of a famous patient. Science 1994;264:1102–1105.
76. Van Horn JD, Irimia A, Torgerson CM, Chambers MC, Kikinis R, Toga AW. Mapping connectivity damage in the case of Phineas Gage. PLoS One 2012;7:e37454.
77. Filippi M, Agosta F, Scola E, et al. Functional network connectivity in the behavioral variant of frontotemporal dementia. Cortex 2013;49:2389–2401.
78. Townley RA, Graff-Radford J, Mantyh WG, et al. Progressive dysexecutive syndrome due to Alzheimer's disease: a description of 55 cases and comparison to other phenotypes. Brain Commun. 2020;2(1):fcaa068. doi:10.1093/braincomms/fcaa068.
79. Voon V, Dalley JW. Parkinson disease: impulsive choice-Parkinson disease and dopaminergic therapy. Nat Rev Neurol 2011;7:541–542.
80. Santangelo G, Vitale C, Picillo M, et al. Apathy and striatal dopamine transporter levels in de-novo, untreated Parkinson's disease patients. Parkinsonism Relat Disord 2015;21:489–493.
81. Vriend C, Raijmakers P, Veltman DJ, et al. Depressive symptoms in Parkinson's disease are related to reduced [123I] FP-CIT binding in the caudate nucleus. J Neurol Neurosurg Psychiatry 2014;85:159–164.
82. Picco A, Morbelli S, Piccardo A, et al. Brain (18)F-DOPA PET and cognition in de novo Parkinson's disease. Eur J Nuc Med & Mol Imaging 2015;42:1062–1070.
83. Santangelo G, Raimo S, Cropano M, et al. Neural bases of impulse control disorders in Parkinson's disease: A systematic review and an ALE meta-analysis. Neurosci Biobehav Rev 2019;107:672–685.
84. Mosley PE, Paliwal S, Robinson K, Coyne T, et al. The structural connectivity of discrete networks underlies impulsivity and gambling in Parkinson's disease. Brain 2019;142:3917–3935.

INDEX

Tables, figures, and boxes are indicated by an italic *t*, *f*, and *b* following the page number.